Clinical Sports Medicine

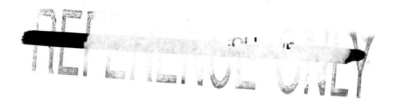

Clinical Sports Medicine

Medical Management and Rehabilitation

Walter R. Frontera MD PhD
Dean and Professor of Physical Medicine and Rehabilitation
University of Puerto Rico School of Medicine
Puerto Rico
Lecturer (and former Professor and Chair)
Department of Physical Medicine and Rehabilitation
Harvard Medical School/Spaulding Rehabilitation Hospital
Boston, MA

Stanley A. Herring MD
Medical Director of Spine Care
Clinical Professor
Departments of Rehabilitation Medicine, Orthopaedics and
Sports Medicine, and Neurological Surgery
University of Washington
Team Physician, Seattle Seahawks
Team Physician, Seattle Mariners
Seattle, WA

Assistant Editor for the CD
Timothy P. Young MD
Department of Physical Medicine and Rehabilitation
Charlotte Institute of Rehabilitation
Charlotte, NC

Lyle J. Micheli MD
O'Donnell Family Professor of Orthopaedic Sports Medicine
Harvard Medical School
Boston, MA

Julie K. Silver MD
Assistant Professor
Department of Physical Medicine and Rehabilitation
Harvard Medical School
Attending Physician
Spaulding Rehabilitation Hospital
Associate in Physiatry
Massachusetts General and
Brigham and Women's Hospital
Boston, MA

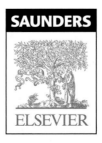

SAUNDERS

ELSEVIER

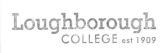

SAUNDERS
ELSEVIER

An affiliate of Elsevier Inc.

ISBN-13: 978 1 4160 2443 9
ISBN-10: 1 4160 2443 3

British Library Cataloguing in Publication Data
A catalogue record for this book is available from the British Library

Library of Congress Cataloging in Publication Data
A catalog record for this book is available from the Library of Congress

Notice

Medical knowledge is constantly changing. Standard safety precautions must be followed, but as new research and clinical experience broaden our knowledge, changes in treatment and drug therapy may become necessary or appropriate. Readers are advised to check the most current product information provided by the manufacturer of each drug to be administered to verify the recommended dose, the method and duration of administration, and contraindications. It is the responsibility of the practitioner, relying on experience and knowledge of the patient, to determine dosages and the best treatment for each individual patient. Neither the Publisher nor the editors or contributors assume any liability for any injury and/or damage to persons or property arising from this publication.

The Publisher

Printed in China
Last digit is the print number: 9 8 7 6 5 4 3 2 1

Working together to grow
libraries in developing countries

www.elsevier.com | www.bookaid.org | www.sabre.org

ELSEVIER BOOK AID International Sabre Foundation

Commissioning Editor: Susan Pioli
Project Development Manager: Cecilia Murphy
Project Manager: Glenys Norquay
Design Manager: Jayne Jones
Illustration Manager: Gillian Murray
Illustrator: Jenni Miller and Cactus
Marketing Manager(s) (UK/USA): Verity Kerkhoff /Matthew Latuchie

Contents

Section 3 • Specific Injuries by Anatomical Location

Preface

Sports medicine is a rapidly evolving interdisciplinary field that has benefited from recent increases in scientific and clinical knowledge in many medical specialties, including physiology, nutrition, primary care, orthopedics, and rehabilitation. This book is unique in that it is a comprehensive sports medicine text that specifically focuses on a rehabilitation approach.

Many sports medicine books limit their content to a specific discipline such as exercise physiology, sports training, or sports injuries. We have taken a different approach and present to the sports medicine practitioner a wide variety of topics in three major areas of the field: basic principles of conditioning and medical care of the athlete, a comprehensive discussion of rehabilitation principles and interventions, and a general (non-surgically oriented) discussion of sports injuries by anatomical area. After reading this book, sports medicine practitioners will understand the scientific basis of sports conditioning and performance, identify the most important medical issues confronting the athlete, recognize the principles of rehabilitation for the injured athlete, and know the most common therapeutic principles of sports injuries in various anatomical areas and sports.

The practice of sports medicine around the world is not uniform and significant variability exists among sports medicine centers and models of care in various countries, even among countries in geographical proximity. We have assembled experts from several continents and countries to reflect this diversity and to make sure that different points of view are represented in the discussion. We, as the editors, would like to thank all of our colleagues around the world for their interest in and contribution to this project. It would be hard to find another discipline or medical specialty with more international flavor than sports medicine. The international nature of sports competition requires that sports medicine practitioners understand the special needs of the traveling athlete in areas such as nutrition, environmental factors, doping control, and many others. These and related topics are discussed in detail in the book.

The practice of sports medicine requires, by definition, a team of professionals with training and expertise in various health-related fields. This book is intended for all medical and non-medical professionals who are members of the sports medicine team, especially the non-surgical medical specialists. The sports medicine practitioner in general and the team physician in particular must have broad knowledge and understanding of a wide variety of scientific and medical issues that could result in deteriorating athletic performance and serious health complications. The relationship of these medical conditions and sports training programs must be recognized and understood. Thus, chapters in Section 1 include principles of conditioning as well as important primary care problems of the athlete and exercise enthusiasts.

The incidence of injuries in many sports has increased with the intensity of the training and competition. Further, the goal of many athletes of all ages after injury is to return to competition as fast as possible. Therefore, rehabilitation has become an important area of research and practice in sports medicine. We recognize these developments in Section 2 of the book with a combination of classical and sports-oriented rehabilitation. Finally, although Section 3 has been dedicated to sports injuries, the book is not a treatise on the surgical management of the injured athlete. However, it may be useful to surgeons who serve as team physicians.

We sincerely hope this book will help the established sports medicine specialist practice excellent sports medicine as well as motivate the beginner to dedicate further study to sports medicine.

Sincerely,
Walter R. Frontera
Stanley A. Herring
Lyle J. Micheli
Julie K. Silver
Timothy P. Young

List of Contributors

Julia Alleyne MD CCFP Dip Sport Med FACSM
Medical Director, Sport C.A.R.E.
Women's College Hospital
Assistant Clinical Professor
Department of Family and Community
Medicine
University of Toronto
Toronto, Ontario

Eduardo Amy MD
Assistant Professor
Sports Injuries Unit
PR Olympic Training Center
University of Puerto Rico
San Juan, Puerto Rico

Joseph F. Audette MA MD
Instructor
Department of Physical Medicine and
Rehabilitation
Harvard Medical School
Boston, MA

Norbert Bachl MD
Professor
Department of Sports and Exercise Physiology
Institute of Sports Science
University of Vienna
Vienna

Allison Bailey MD
Instructor
Department of Physical Medicine and
Rehabilitation
Harvard Medical School
Boston, MA

Ramon Baron MD
Professor
Department of Sports and Exercise Physiology
Institute of Sports Science
University of Vienna
Vienna

Deborah A. Bergfeld MD
Attending Physician
Buffalo Spine and Sports Institute, PC
Buffalo, NY

Joanne Borg-Stein MD
Assistant Professor of Physical Medicine and
Rehabilitation
Harvard Medical School
Medical Director
Spaulding-Wellesley Rehabilitation Center
Wellesley, MA

Andrea Burry MSc MD
Resident
Family Medicine Department
Women's College Hospital
Toronto, Ontario

Robert C. Cantu MA MD FACS FACSM
Chairman, Department of Surgery
Chief, Neurosurgery Service
Emerson Hospital
Concord, MA

Robert V. Cantu MD
Assistant Professor of Orthopaedic Surgery
Department of Orthopaedic Surgery
Dartmouth-Hitchcock Medical Center
Lebanon, NH

**Kal-Ming Chan MBBS MCH(Orth) FRCS(G)
FRCS(E)**
Chair, Professor, and Chief of Service
Department of Orthopaedics and Traumatology
The Chinese University of Hong Kong
Prince of Wales Hospital
Shatin, Hong Kong

David S. Chang MD
Orthopaedic Surgeon
Sports Medicine
Bay Area Sports Orthopaedics
San Francisco, CA

Joseph Jeremy Hsi-Tse Chang MBChB
Resident
Department of Orthopaedics and Traumatology
The Chinese University of Hong Kong
Prince of Wales Hospital
Shatin, Hong Kong

Gian Corrado MD
Clinical Lecturer
Department of Emergency Medicine
University of Michigan
Ann Arbor, MI

José Correa MD
Assistant Professor
Director of Primary Unit
PR Olympic Training Center
University of Puerto Rico
San Juan, Puerto Rico

David M. Crandell MD
Instructor
Department of Physical Medicine &
Rehabilitation
Spaulding Rehabilitation Hospital
Boston, MA

Wayne E. Derman MBChB PhD FACSM
Associate Professor
Sports Science and Sports Medicine
University of Cape Town
Director, Chronic Disease Rehabilitation
Programme
Sports Science Institute of South Africa
Cape Town

Eduardo H. De Rose MD PhD
Professor of Medicine
Porto Alegre

Pierre A. d'Hemecourt MD FACSM
Director
Primary Care Sports Medicine
Children's Hospital Boston
Boston, MA

Sheila A. Dugan MD
Assistant Professor
Department of Physical Medicine &
Rehabilitation
Rush Medical College
Chicago, IL

Brandon E. Earp MD
Instructor
Department of Orthopaedic Surgery
Harvard Medical School
Boston, MA

Emin Ergen MD PhD
Professor of Sports Medicine
Department of Sports Medicine
Ankara University School of Medicine
Ankara

Federica Fagnani BSc
Technician
Sports Medicine Laboratory
Department of Health Sciences
University Institute of Movement Sciences
(IUSM)
Rome

Karl B. Fields MD CAQ
Director
Moses Cone Family Medicine Residency and
Primary Care Sports Medicine Fellowship
Moses Cone Family Medicine
Greensboro, NC

Walter R. Frontera MD PhD
Dean and Professor of Physical Medicine and
Rehabilitation
University of Puerto Rico School of Medicine
Puerto Rico
Lecturer (and former Professor and Chair)
Department of Physical Medicine and
Rehabilitation
Harvard Medical School/Spaulding
Rehabilitation Hospital
Boston, MA

Peter Gerbino MD
Assistant in Orthopedic Surgery
Division of Sports Medicine
Department of Orthopedic Surgery
Children's Hospital Boston
Instructor in Orthopedics
Harvard Medical School
Boston, MA

Arrigo Giombini MD
Medical Doctor
Physiotherapy and Rehabilitation Department
Sports Medicine Unit
University Institute of Movement Sciences
(IUSM)
Rome

Stanley A. Herring MD
Medical Director of Spine Care
Clinical Professor
Departments of Rehabilitation Medicine,
Orthopaedics and Sports Medicine, and
Neurological Surgery
University of Washington
Team Physician, Seattle Seahawks
Team Physician, Seattle Mariners
Seattle, WA

Jeff Hyman BSc MD FRCPC
Assistant Professor of Pediatrics
Children's Clinic
Winnipeg, Manitoba

Robert Kennedy MD
Associate Director
Sports Medicine Department
Saint Joseph's Regional Medical Center
Mishawaka, IN

W. Ben Kibler MD FACSM
Medical Director
Lexington Clinic Sports Medicine Center
Lexington, KY

Mininder S. Kocher MD MPH
Associate Director
Division of Sports Medicine
Children's Hospital Boston
Assistant Professor of Orthopaedic Surgery
Harvard Medical School
Boston, MA

Brian J. Krabak MD MBA
Assistant Professor of Physical Medicine &
Rehabilitation
Assistant Professor of Orthopaedic Surgery

Johns Hopkins Medical Institution
Baltimore, MD

Ted A. Lennard MD
Clinical Assistant Professor
Department of Physical Medicine and
Rehabilitation
University of Arkansas for Medical Sciences
Staff Physician
Springfield Neurological and Spine Institute
Springfield, MO

Bert R. Mandelbaum MD
Orthopaedic Surgeon
Director, Santa Monica Orthopaedic and
Sports Medicine
Orthopaedic Research and Education
Foundation and Fellowship
Santa Monica, CA

Julio A. Martinez-Silvestrini MD
Assistant Clinical Professor, Tufts University
School of Medicine
Staff Physiatrist, Division of Physical Medicine
& Rehabilitation
Baystate Medical Education and Research
Foundation
Springfield, MA

Lyle J. Micheli MD
O'Donnell Family Professor of Orthopaedic
Sports Medicine
Harvard Medical School
Boston, MA

William Micheo MD
Chairman & Professor
Department of Physical Medicine,
Rehabilitation & Sports Medicine
University of Puerto Rico School of Medicine
San Juan, Puerto Rico

Jason H. Nielson MD
Pediatric and Adolescent Sports Medicine
Children's Bone and Spine Surgery
Las Vegas, NV

Attilio Parisi MD
Professor of Nutrition
Sports Medicine Unit
University Institute of Movement Sciences
(IUSM)
Rome

Fabio Pigozzi MD
Professor of Sports Medicine
Head, Sports Medicine Unit
University Institute of Movement Sciences
(IUSM)
Rome

Joel M. Press MD
Medical Director
Spine and Sports Rehabilitation Center
Rehabilitation Institute of Chicago
Chicago, IL

Mark R. Proctor MD
Assistant Professor in Surgery
Department of Neurosurgery
Children's Hospital Boston
Harvard Medical School
Boston, MA

Thomas D. Rizzo Jr MD
Consultant
Department of Physical Medicine &
Rehabilitation
Mayo Clinic
Jacksonville, FL
Assistant Professor of Physical Medicine and
Rehabilitation
Mayo Clinic College of Medicine
Rochester, MN

Roy J. Shephard PhD MD (Lond) DPE
Professor Emeritus of Applied Physiology
University of Toronto
Toronto, Ontario

Julie K. Silver MD
Assistant Professor
Department of Physical Medicine and
Rehabilitation
Harvard Medical School
Attending Physician
Spaulding Rehabilitation Hospital
Associate in Physiatry
Massachusetts General and
Brigham and Women's Hospital
Boston, MA

Stephen M. Simons MD FACSM
Director of Sports Medicine
Saint Joseph's Regional Medical Center
South Bend, IN

Gerhard Smekal MD
Professor
Department of Sports and Exercise Physiology
Institute of Sports Science
University of Vienna
Vienna

Jennifer L. Solomon MD
Clinical Instructor of Physical Medicine and
Rehabilitation
Weill Medical College
Cornell University
New York, NY

Christopher J. Standaert MD
Clinical Assistant Professor
Departments of Rehabilitation Medicine,
Orthopaedics and Sports Medicine, and
Neurological Surgery
University of Washington Medical Center
Seattle, WA

Rachael Tucker MBChB
Research Associate
Division of Sports Medicine
Children's Hospital Boston
Boston, MA

Bülent Ulkar MD PhD
Associate Professor
Department of Sports Medicine
Ankara University School of Medicine
Ankara

Brandee Walte MD
Assistant Professor of Physical Medicine and
Rehabilitation
University of California – Davis Medical Center
Sacramento, CA

Katherine M. Walker MD CAQ
Assistant Director, Sports Medicine Fellowship
Sports Medicine and Injury Center
Cabarrus Family Medicine
Concord, NC

Peter M. Waters MD
Professor of Orthopedic Surgery
Department of Orthopedic Surgery
Harvard Medical School
Boston, MA

Jennifer M. Weiss MD
Assistant Professor of Clinical Orthopaedics
Department of Pediatric Orthopedics
Keck School of Medicine of USC
Children's Hospital Los Angeles
Los Angeles, CA

Anton Wicker MD PhD MS
Head of Department
Physical Medicine and Rehabilitation
Paracelsus University Salzburg
Salzburg

Fiona Chui-Yan Wong MBChB
Resident
Department of Orthopaedics and Traumatology
The Chinese University of Hong Kong
Shatin, Hong Kong

Merrilee Zetaruk MD FRCPC Dip Sport Med
Associate Professor
Department of Pediatrics and Child Health
University of Manitoba
Winnipeg, Manitoba

Jerrad Zimmerman MD
Medical Director of Sports Medicine
Carle Clinic
University of Illinois Team Physician
Urbana, IL

Dedication

We dedicate this book to the sports medicine providers whose knowledge and dedication help to ensure optimal health and performance in the athletes they treat.

General Scientific and Medical Concepts

CHAPTER 1

An Overview of Sports Medicine

Walter R. Frontera

INTRODUCTION

The purpose of this chapter is to present an overview of the scientific and clinical discipline known as sports medicine. In a diverse world like ours, it is not surprising to see that there is no single definition of sports medicine that is accepted by all interested in the field. Clearly, discussions about sports medicine include the positive and negative consequences of acute and chronic exercise and physical activity, sports performance and the health implications of an active lifestyle. Yet, these elements have not been assembled in a statement that is universally accepted.

Different authors and professional groups throughout the world have their own conceptual and practical definitions of sports medicine. This heterogeneity may explain why clinical sports medicine programs around the world vary in the nature and scope of their services. Also, educational and training programs in sports medicine do not have a common curriculum and educational experiences vary from region to region. Sports medicine is sometimes seen as the primary field of interest and sometimes as a sub-specialty within another field, such as cardiology, orthopedics or rehabilitation. It could be argued that sports medicine has been divided into sub-specialties such as the treatment and rehabilitation of sports injuries, the medical care of the athlete, and exercise medicine for public health.

Finally, research in sports medicine covers a wide spectrum of topics and includes an assortment of scientists working in overlapping but distinct areas. Some examples of research topics that can be classified under the umbrella of sports medicine are the genetic determinants of aerobic performance, the molecular mechanism of force production in skeletal muscle, the optimal prescription of exercise for the primary prevention of chronic and degenerative diseases, the surgical technique most appropriate for the reconstruction of the anterior cruciate ligament (ACL) of the knee, and the types of mental training that will enhance performance in specific events such as archery. The wide variety of research questions makes sports medicine an exciting field of study for many. In fact, some researchers whose background is not in sports medicine may use experimental models including exercise to answer questions relevant to other medical specialties. In other words, they use exercise as a technique to study a biological phenomenon unrelated to sports performance.

There is little doubt that a consensus with regards to the definition of sports medicine has not been achieved. Thus, for the purpose of this chapter it may be more relevant and productive to describe sports medicine as it is perceived and practiced around the world and to comment on the various approaches that have resulted from local or regional interests and beliefs. It is not the intention of the author to propose a definition of sports medicine but rather to describe the subject matter. This book is an attempt to assemble the knowledge in the field of sports medicine in a single source, with an emphasis on the medical and rehabilitative aspects.

ORGANIZED SPORTS MEDICINE

Modern sports medicine, as we know it, has been around for decades. During the last 100 years, many countries have established national associations for sports medicine practitioners. For example, the German Society of Sports Medicine was established in 1912 and the French Society of Sports Medicine in 1921. In the Americas, national sports medicine associations were founded in Uruguay in 1941, in the US in 1954 and in Chile in 1955. Several international groups have also been established including the International Federation of Sports Medicine (1928), the Pan American Confederation of Sports Medicine (1976), the European Federation of Sports Medicine Associations (1997) and the Asian Federation of Sports Medicine (1990). The basis for the foundation of these groups, the professional background of their members, and the scientific and clinical emphasis of each vary widely.

One way of illustrating the different views of sports medicine around the world is to examine the institutional organization and affiliation of sports medicine practitioners and clinics. In some countries, sports medicine services and clinics are fully integrated within academic departments in a medical school or in an academic health center; either as an independent department or as a section or division of another department. In these countries, sports medicine is included in the medical school curriculum and there is significant research activity. Physicians in those centers work with sports teams but their primary affiliation is with the academic institution. In other countries, sports medicine services are an integral part of a university faculty of sports science or physical education. Medical doctors are included and actively participate in educational and research programs but the structure is outside of a medical school or academic health center. In yet a third model, in other countries, the main sports medicine service or clinic is part of the National Sports Institute or Sports Ministry, loosely affiliated with an academic institution. In this case, it is the government or the sports federations that provide most of the support needed by the sports medicine service. The sports medicine physician is an employee of the government or sports club and the emphasis is dictated by the immediate health needs of the athletes and not by academic considerations. Finally, there are also large numbers of practitioners who provide services as private doctors, some without formal training but with an interest in sports and the medical needs of the competitive athletes. The latter is an example of sports medicine services offered outside of a system.

KNOWLEDGE BASE

All sports medicine practitioners benefit from the knowledge generated by research in many basic and applied sciences. Some of this knowledge is not unique to the field of sports medicine and serves as the foundation for the practice of many health-related professions and medical specialties. When applied to the physically active individual and/or to the competitive athlete, this knowledge becomes part of the foundation of sports medicine. On the other hand, there is a body of knowledge that has accumulated over the last few decades that is unique to sports medicine. It has emerged from investigations designed to address specific questions related to the limits of human performance, the health benefits of regular physical activity and the healthcare needs of the physically active population. In these investigations, exercise has been the central proposition.

Many scientific disciplines contribute to the knowledge base in sports medicine. *Physiology* and *nutrition* constitute the foundation that successful training programs are built upon. Sports performance cannot be thoroughly understood or enhanced without the sound application of exercise physiology principles and the optimal combination of fluids and nutrition with training loads. In addition, an in-depth understanding of the physiological responses to acute and chronic exercise can guide the development of preventive exercise programs for the general population and the rehabilitation interventions for patients with acute injuries and chronic diseases. Indeed, from the point of view of public health, one of the most important contributions made by sports medicine to society is the generation of new knowledge supporting the hypothesis that an active lifestyle contributes to the primary or secondary prevention of common chronic illnesses such as heart disease, diabetes, osteoporosis and hypertension.

Research on the psychological and biological bases of *human behavior and emotions* provide the framework for the mental preparation needed by the high-performance athlete and for the study of benefits of physical activity and exercise on mental health. The fundamental sciences such as *physics and mathematics* contribute to the understanding of the effects and benefits of therapeutic modalities such as cold and ultrasound used in the rehabilitation of sports-related injuries. *Chemistry and pharmacology* explain the appropriate use and effectiveness of the pharmacological agents in the treatment of pain and inflammation and serve to study the interaction between the metabolic changes associated with physical activity and drug metabolism. Pharmacological principles are equally relevant to the anti-doping efforts and the safe use of exercise training in patients who are taking drugs for therapeutic reasons. Substantial knowledge of the *anatomy and biomechanics* of the musculoskeletal system is essential in the development of proper training and performance techniques for successful sport participation. This knowledge is also fundamental in the development of therapeutic and surgical techniques for the treatment of injuries such as ligamentous tears and muscle-tendon strains.

Clinical research has also contributed significantly to strengthening the science underlying the practice of sports medicine. Research into the optimal training techniques has helped develop recommendations for the elite athlete as well as the general public. Clinical trials of pharmacological, rehabilitative and surgical interventions have contributed enormously to the development of therapeutic protocols for injured athletes. In fact, the results of clinical research in sports medicine have now been used in the development of therapeutic interventions for the non-active individual.

PRACTICAL AND OPERATIONAL DEFINITIONS

The content of study in sports medicine has evolved significantly during the last 50 years. In an editorial for the *Journal of Sports Medicine and Physical Fitness* published in 1977, Professor Giuseppe La Cava, President of the FIMS 1968–1976, described sports medicine as the application of medical knowledge to sport with the aim of preserving the health of the athlete while improving his or her performance. La Cava included sports biotypology, physiopathology, medical evaluation, traumatology, hygiene and therapeutics as the main elements of sports medicine.[1] Absent from this definition is the application of sports medicine to those who are not actively involved in sports.

In 1988, Professor Wildor Hollmann, FIMS president 1986–1994, summarized the main aspects or sports medicine as follows: medical treatment of injuries and illnesses; medical examination before starting a sport to detect any damage that could be worsened by the sport; medical performance investigation to assess the performance capacity of the heart, circulation, respiration, metabolism and the skeletal musculature; performance diagnosis specific to the type of sport; medical advice on lifestyle and nutrition; medical assistance in developing optimal training methods; and scientifically based control of training.[2] This definition is more inclusive and shows the evolution in the knowledge that took place during the 1980s and 1990s.

More recently, many authors have expanded the nature of the clinical activities included in sports medicine. For example, according to Brukner and Khan (1993),[3] clinical sports medicine includes management of medical problems associated with physical activity and exercise; the role of exercise in the treatment and rehabilitation of chronic disease states; performance enhancement through various interventions such as physiological training, and nutritional alterations; prevention, diagnosis, treatment and rehabilitation of sports injuries; special and specific needs of the pediatric, female and older populations of physically active people; healthcare needs of the traveling sports team; and the use and abuse of substances prohibited in sports (doping). This definition expands the frontiers of sports medicine and includes topics that were not previously thought to be within its domain.

Thus, the evolution of the definition shows that sports medicine has become more inclusive of the non-elite athlete and the general public and more interested in topics other than the limits of human performance in competitive sports.

A PERSONAL VIEW

It is clear that sports medicine includes a wide variety of themes and topics and that sports medicine practitioners must be familiar with many basic applied sciences as well as with broadly diverse medical and clinical disciplines.

Sports medicine can be briefly and accurately defined as the study of the *interrelationship between physical activity and health*. In this context, physical activity includes daily and occupational activities, structured exercise training for the non-competitive athlete, and sports participation. This definition considers not only the study of the benefits of physical activity but also the deleterious effects of its absence since it is known that inactivity and deconditioning have negative consequences on human health and performance. Further, the fact that excessive activity, inappropriate training loads and techniques, and movements that test the limits of the musculoskeletal system may lead to injury and disease is also recognized.

Health must be defined (in accordance with the World Health Organization) as a state of physical, psychological and social well-being, not only the absence of disease. Sports medicine is based on the reciprocal relationship between physical activity (in all forms) and health. In other words, in order to achieve health it is not only important but a requirement to participate in regular physical activity, exercise training and/or sports.

This concept applies to the general public as well as to the competitive athlete. Optimal performance is not possible without optimal health. The converse idea is equally important: a state of optimal health can only be achieved by means of appropriate levels of physical activity, exercise, or sport participation. Physical activity, exercise, and sport participation contribute significantly to the prevention of chronic disease and the enhancement of physical and psychological functional

capacity. Thus, it is clear that the sports medicine practitioner must be an advocate for both health for sports and sports for health.

It could be argued that those who benefit from sports medicine services have one thing in common: they are physically active. The practice of sports medicine is not limited by age, gender, or the interest of the practitioner in one organ or system of the human body. Although specialists may develop particular skills and interests in one area, it is the need for a holistic and comprehensive approach that characterizes sports medicine. An interest in the consequences of physical activity, exercise, and sports is the fundamental stimulus of the sports medicine practitioner.

THE SPORTS MEDICINE TEAM

Sports medicine is one of those professional disciplines in which the team approach is synonymous with the standard of care. The team is interdisciplinary in nature and the leader or coordinator of the team's efforts is a physician. The medical leader of the team can be a sports medicine specialist, an orthopedic surgeon, a physiatrist (specialist in physical medicine and rehabilitation), a specialist in internal medicine, a pediatrician, or a physician with experience working with physically active people and athletes. Frequently, the athlete/patient interacts with any or all members of the healthcare team. Members of the sports medicine team may include, but are not limited to, athletic trainers, physiotherapists, nutritionist/dieticians, dentists and psychologists. The interdisciplinary nature of the sports medicine approach is not limited to the competitive athlete and is also applicable to the care of physically active individuals.

In addition to the athlete/patient, other persons may be active participants in the delivery of healthcare services. In the case of a competitive athlete, the coach or manager should be included in important discussions and decisions made about the ability of the athlete to train or compete with the team. The planning of sports medical services as well as the implementation of many medical clinical interventions require, with the consent of the patient/athlete, the active participation of the coach, e.g. the treatment of a sports injury may require a reduction in the training load. Compliance with this recommendation is enhanced if the coach understands the rationale for the action. Further, the managers or administrators of sports teams or delegations should be aware of the nature of the health problem because their decisions directly affect the ability of the healthcare team to maintain the health status and enhance the performance of the athlete.

SPORTS MEDICINE IN DIFFERENT COUNTRIES

In some countries such as Brazil, Cuba, Mexico, Italy, Germany, Spain and Uruguay, sports medicine is a recognized medical specialty. Formal postgraduate training has been instituted in various medical schools and universities, and sports medicine is recognized by the national medical society as a distinct field of interest within medicine. Education in sports medicine in these countries emphasizes the medical and physiological control of the athlete as well as the many other non-orthopedic aspects of sports medicine. In other countries, such as Canada, Switzerland and the US, sports medicine is not recognized as a specialty and training is available in the form of fellowships for physicians who have completed a primary medical specialty (for example, orthopedic surgery, physical medicine and rehabilitation, internal medicine, emergency medicine, or family medicine). However, the scope of some of these fellowships is at times limited to a particular area of sports medicine such as the diagnosis and treatment of sports-related injuries. In many other countries, where neither a residency nor a fellowship is available, physicians complete their professional training and acquire knowledge and expertise in sports medicine by participating in courses, attending seminars and working with physically active people and competitive athletes.

THINGS THAT MAKE SPORTS MEDICINE SPECIAL

An interesting challenge in the practice of sports medicine is the nature of the patient and the interrelationship between the disease and the environment. The underlying mechanism of injury or medical problem must be fully understood because the patient/athlete's objective is to return to the activity that caused the problem. Avoiding the activity associated with the injury or medical problem, except in life-threatening situations, is not an option; the sports medicine team must do everything possible to correct the fundamental problem to avoid re-injury or chronic disease. Although rest and even immobilization might be needed, it is almost never accepted without complaint. This is one reason why rehabilitation is needed to enhance the performance of the athlete, not only in daily activities but most importantly in the sports activities to which the patient/athlete will return.

A BROADENING SCOPE

It is important to highlight the fact that the current international perspective of sports medicine is no longer limited to the elite athlete. Sports medicine has evolved from both the philosophical and clinical perspectives. The application of the sports medicine principles to the general population has become as important (some say more important) as the use of sports medicine knowledge to maintain health and enhance performance in competitive athletes. Furthermore, the use of exercise and physical activity in the prevention, treatment and rehabilitation of some chronic diseases is now considered as effective as more traditional interventions such as the use of pharmacological agents. The importance of exercise and physical activity should be obvious if we consider that in many countries, chronic diseases are the most frequent causes of morbidity and mortality, the prevalence of disability resulting from such diseases is on the rise, and the aging population will experience functional loss and disability.

REFERENCES

1   La Cava G. What is sports medicine: Definition and tasks. J Sports Med Phys Fitness 1977; 17:1-3.
2   Hollmann W. The definition and scope of sports medicine. In: Dirix A, Knuttgen HG, Tittel K, eds. The Olympic book of sports medicine. Oxford: Blackwell Scientific; 1988:xi-xii.
3   Brukner P, Khan K. Clinical sports medicine. New York: McGraw Hill; 1993:3-7.

CHAPTER 2

Principles of Exercise Physiology and Conditioning

Norbert Bachl, Ramon Baron and Gerhard Smekal

METABOLISM DURING EXERCISE

Box 2.1: Key Points

Metabolism during exercise

The human organism can rely on three basic energy sources:

- ATP-PCr system ('high energy phosphates'): primarily for high intensive ('all-out') activities lasting for seconds (3–7 s).
- Glycolysis: anaerobic energy provision from carbohydrates; primarily intensive ('all-out') activities lasting 40 s to 3 min.
- Oxidative system: Oxidation from carbohydrates, fats and proteins; primarily at rest and during lower (more fat oxidation) or higher (more carbohydrates oxidation), intensive endurance events.

The principles of exercise physiology are based on an understanding of the production and use of energy in biological systems. In every cell, the hydrolysis of adenosine triphosphate (ATP) is the immediate energy source for almost all energy-requiring processes.

$$ATP + H_2O \rightarrow ADP + Pi + energy$$

As the store of ATP in the cells is limited, ATP must therefore be continuously replenished. This occurs through aerobic and anaerobic processes in a way that energy rich substances (carbohydrates, fat, proteins and phosphocreatine) are transformed into compounds like H_2O, CO_2, lactate and creatine, by sequences of different chemical reactions. During these processes, part of the change in free energy is used for the resynthesis of ATP. This ATP-ADP-ATP cycle (ADP, adenosine diphosphate) can be considered as the basic mechanism of energy metabolism in all cells and constitutes an intermediate between energy consumption and utilization processes.[1]

Because of the large variation in energy turnover, the skeletal muscle is a unique tissue. The transition from rest to exercise requires an increase in the energy demand and therefore the rate of ATP utilization can increase more than 150 times. This would lead to the utilization of all the ATP stored in the muscles in about 2 to 3 s. However, to guarantee cellular homeostasis and keep the muscular filaments contracting, it is important to maintain a constant muscle ATP concentration, meaning that the rate of ATP regeneration must equal the rate of ATP utilization. This requires different supplying systems of fuel and oxygen as well as the control of the energetic processes involving both feed-forward and feedback mechanisms.[1]

Anaerobic processes of ATP generation

During muscle contraction, ATP is the direct connecting link between fibre shortening (or lengthening), force development and metabolism. In this process, the ATP turnover in muscle is most significantly determined by the quantity of calcium released from the transverse tubular system. The most important regulatory enzymes responsible for energy release from ATP are ATPase like actomyosin-ATPase, Na^+/K^+-ATPase and sarcoplasmatic reticulum Ca^{2+}-ATPase which, in turn, are activated by calcium. The maximum quantity of ATP that can be hydrolyzed during a single contraction depends on the myosin isoenzyme pattern and, therefore, on the type of muscle fibre. In addition, muscles contain phosphocreatine (PCr), which is another high-energy phosphate compound and stored in muscle tissue at a concentration three times that of ATP. Because of the small quantity of ATP available in the cell, the breakdown to ADP immediately stimulates the breakdown of PCr to provide energy for ATP resynthesis. This reaction is catalyzed by the enzyme creatine kinase (CK):

$$ADP + PCr + H^+ \rightleftharpoons ATP + creatine$$

In other words, a fall in the ATP concentration is buffered by PCr, and therefore the ATP concentration in the muscle remains nearly constant at a high level during physical exercise. Even under extreme physical strain leading to exhaustion, the ATP concentration rarely falls below 50% of the baseline value.[2] The 'high energy phosphate' system, however, is limited by the fact that the quantity of releasable phosphate for the energy-production from the high-energy phosphates (PCr and

ATP) during high intensive work is drastically reduced. During short-term intensive physical exercise followed by longer phases of regeneration, or during low-intensity physical loads, high-energy phosphates are mainly re-phosphorylated by the oxidative pathway. The capacity for resynthesis depends on the oxidative capacity of the respective system.[3] In contrast, at highly intensive physical loads of longer duration, the PCr concentration drops rapidly and drastically. In this case, the resynthesis occurs through the anaerobic energy provision from carbohydrates, which leads to the production of lactic acid, a process named anaerobic glycolysis, because this process does not require oxygen.

Glycolysis from glycogen:

$$3\ ADP + 3\ Pi + glycosyl\ unit \rightarrow 3\ ATP + 2\ lactate + 2H^+$$

An increase in pyruvate, $NADH/NAD^+$ ratio or H^+ are metabolic changes that will promote lactate formation. Oxygen deficiency, increased recruitment of fast twitch fibers and low aerobic conditions in the exercising muscle are conditions for this metabolic imbalance. $NADH + H^+$ can be re-oxidized only by the reduction of pyruvate, catalyzed by lactate dehydrogenase (LDH). Lactic acid is produced in this process. The process of $NADH - H^+$ re-oxidation through pyruvate is a very uneconomical interference because only three moles of ATP are obtained from the degradation per mole glycosyl unit, whereas 36 moles/38 moles of ATP can be formed during complete oxidation.[4]

Glycogen phosphorylase plays a key role in anaerobic glycolysis. It breaks down the muscle glycogen and is regulated by Ca^{2+} released from the transverse tubular system through the enzyme phosphorylase-kinase. Generally, the reduced Ca^{2+} release from the tubular system during cumulative fatigue is an indication of the importance of Ca^{2+} in muscle fatigue. Also the enzyme phosphofructokinase, which catalyzes the transformation of fructose 6-phosphate to fructose 1.6-diphosphate in the cytoplasm of the muscle cell, appears to play a decisive role in anaerobic glycolysis in the sense that it is inhibited by the sinking pH value due to the lactic acid production and thus limiting the anaerobic glycolysis. In fact, H^+ ion concentrations influence glycolysis and the PCr concentration during physical exercise.[3,5] A high H^+ concentration reduces the PCr level through the enzyme creatine kinase. Furthermore, local acidosis in the working muscles appears to further reduce the formation of cross-bridges between the myosin heads and the actin molecules of muscle fibers. In this context, it should be mentioned that a metabolic acidosis is not an absolute prerequisite for muscle fatigue because patients with a congenital glycogen phosphorylase deficiency (McArdle's disease) are prone to early fatigue despite the fact that they have no lactate acidosis.[6]

During high intensive exercise, lactic acid can be accumulated for two reasons. As a result of the extremely high glycolysis rate which occurs under intensive physical strain, pyruvate is formed in such large quantities that it cannot be utilized by the mitochondria. In addition, the reduced $NADH + H^+$ occurring in the cytoplasm of muscle cells during glycolysis cannot be re-oxidized at a sufficient rate by the mitochondrial membrane. When very intensive exercise continues to persist,

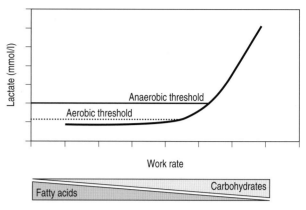

Figure 2.1 Model of the lactate performance curve and the energy supply during increasing work load.

which requires continued anaerobic energy production, the buffer capacity of the organism is exceeded and lactic acid accumulates. Based on these theoretical considerations, the concentration of lactic acid in muscle and blood serves as a reference point for the interaction of the aerobic–anaerobic metabolism under physical strain. Therefore, lactate can be used as one of the most important parameters to determine endurance performance and also to optimize the training processes (Fig. 2.1).

This can be recognized by plotting the blood lactate concentrations *versus* VO_2 ($l \times min^{-1}$; $ml \times kg \times min^{-1}$) during an exercise test with increasing work loads. During the first minutes or even first load steps, the blood lactate concentration as an indirect measure of the lactic acid produced in the exercising muscles remains stable because the energy demand, meaning the ATP-resynthesis rate is met by oxidation of fats and carbohydrates. Although at the beginning of the exercise or when increasing the workload step by step, lactate will be produced in the working muscles because of the delay of the cardio-respiratory supplying reactions, lactate will be metabolized within the muscles and will not be carried to other compartments like blood, a process which is called 'cell to cell shuttle'. From a certain point, when the exercise intensity is higher, fast twitch muscle fibers which have a lower oxidative potential and therefore produce more lactate have to be activated and therefore lactate in the exercising muscles is formed and the blood lactate concentration will increase. This point, which is called the aerobic threshold or first lactate turn point is the beginning of a so-called 'mixed aerobic-anaerobic metabolism'. With increasing intensity a second deflection point can be observed, when more lactate in the exercising muscle will be produced than can be buffered or even removed. From this point called the anaerobic threshold or respiratory compensation threshold, or the second lactate turn point, lactate production increases rapidly, will be accumulated and finally leads to the end of the exercise. If one contrasts the so called 'lactate-performance-curve' of an untrained person, a marathon runner and a 400-m runner, the differences in the interaction of the aerobic–anaerobic metabolism can easily be seen. The untrained person shows a very rapid

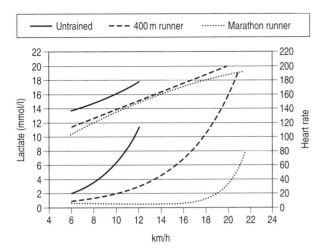

Figure 2.2 Lactate-performance curves and heart rate performance curves of three different trained individuals.

increase and accumulation of the blood lactate concentration from the resting value. In contrast, in the endurance-trained marathon runner, the lactate level remains low with increasing workloads, which is the result of the aerobic adaptations by the endurance training. That means that both – the first and the second lactate turn points – occur at a higher percentage of the athlete's maximal aerobic power. On the other hand, the production rate of lactic acid and resistance against lactate accumulation is decreased. In contrast, the 400-m runner shows an earlier increase of the lactate production because of the specific metabolic adaptations resulting from anaerobic training. Furthermore, the increase of the blood lactate concentration over the anaerobic threshold (second lactate turn point) is longer and more flat, showing that the muscle cells can tolerate the acidification resulting from increasing lactate accumulation better as a consequence of the anaerobic training (Fig. 2.2).[7]

Aerobic processes of ATP generation
In contrast to the anaerobic energy system which provides energy at a high liberation rate but with limited supply, muscles need a continuous supply of energy at rest and during long duration but low intensive activities. This is provided by the oxidative (aerobic) system which has a lower energy liberation rate but a tremendous energy yielding capacity. Aerobic production of ATP occurs in the mitochondria and involves the interaction of the citric acid cycle (Krebs Cycle) and the electron transport chain. Oxygen serves as the final hydrogen acceptor at the end of the electron transport chain. The term maximal aerobic power (VO_2max, VO_2peak) reflects the amount of ATP which can be produced aerobically and therefore the rate at which oxygen can be transported by the cardiorespiratory system to the active muscles. From resting metabolism (3.5 ml/kg per min) the aerobic power production can be increased up to peak values of 35–38 ml/kg per min and 42–45 ml/kg per min in untrained women and men, respectively. Values of 72–76 ml/kg per min and 85–90 ml/kg per min

have been reported in endurance-trained female and male athletes, respectively.

Oxidation of carbohydrate
The first step in the oxidation of carbohydrates is the anaerobic breakdown of muscle glycogen and blood glucose to pyruvate. In the presence of oxygen, pyruvate – the end product of glycolysis – is converted into acetyl-coenzyme A (acetyl-CoA), which enters the Krebs Cycle (citric-acid cycle). The Krebs Cycle is a complex series of chemical reactions that breaks down these substrates into carbon dioxide and hydrogen and forming two ATPs. In addition, six molecules of reduced nicotinamide-adenine-dinucleotide (NADH) and two molecules of reduced flavin-adenine-dinucleotide (FADH 2) are also produced from the glucose molecule, which carry the hydrogen atoms into the electron transport chain where they are used to re-phosphorylate ADP to ATP (oxidative phosphorylation). The complete oxidation of one glucose molecule in skeletal muscle results in a net yield of about 36 or 38 ATPs depending on which shuttle system is used to transport NADH to the mitochondria (Fig. 2.3).[8]

Oxidation of fat
Fat can only be metabolized in the presence of oxygen. The triglycerides are stored in fat cells and within the skeletal muscles and serve as a major energy source for fat oxidation.

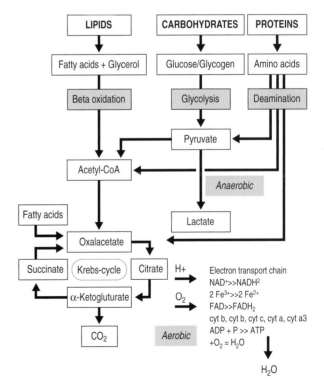

Figure 2.3 'Flow sheet' for energy yielding processes from lipids, carbohydrates and proteins. (Redrawn from Smekal 2004.[8])

For this to happen, the triglycerides are broken down by lipases to their basic units of one molecule of glycerol and three molecules of free fatty acids (lipolysis). After having entered the mitochondria, the free fatty acids undergo a series of reactions in which they are converted to acetyl-coenzyme A, a process called beta-oxidation. From this point, the fat metabolism then follows the same pathway as the carbohydrate metabolism when acetyl coenzyme A enters the Krebs Cycle and the electron transport chain. While the ATP-amount produced varies depending on the oxidation of different fatty acids, the complete oxidation of one (18-carbon) triglyceride molecule results in a total energy yield of about 460 ATPs. Although triglyceride oxidation provides more energy production per gram than carbohydrates, the oxidation of fat requires more oxygen, meaning that fat mostly is oxidized at rest or during moderate exercise when oxygen delivery is not limited by the oxygen transport system. At rest, e.g. the ratio of ATP-production is up to 70% of fat and 30% from carbohydrates, whereas during high intensity exercise, the majority of energy or even the total energy comes from carbohydrates.

Oxidation of proteins

Oxidation of proteins is also utilized to obtain energy at rest as well as during physical exercise.[9] Several amino acids (especially leucine, isoleucine, alanine and valine) contribute to the production of energy. The access to amino acids increases in proportion to the load intensity of any physical activity, but the proportion of energy provided by amino acids during physical exercise appears to be limited to about 10%. However, of practical significance is the fact that amino acids are oxidized in greater quantities when the caloric supply is insufficient and also in the presence of a carbohydrate deficiency. This leads to catabolic states (degradation of functional proteins) and loss of nitrogen. The degradation of functional proteins is problematic because muscles are affected by this phenomenon, which obviously has a detrimental effect on performance capacity.[10]

Power and capacity of energy yielding processes

An important approach to a better understanding of energy demand and energy supply during physical activity and sports is the question as to which substrates are utilized for the production of energy at specific intensities. An important factor in the selection of the substrate is the rate at which energy can be released from the respective substrate, i.e. the maximum achievable release of energy per time unit. Therefore, the maximal intensity of the exercise is limited by the (combined) maximal power of the energetic processes.

The 'high energy phosphates-system' provides the highest rate of energy liberation, but its capacity is limited to only 3–7 s and therefore needs to be replenished constantly providing other processes for ATP resynthesis on a lower energy liberation rate, the glycolytic (anaerobic) and the oxidative combustion of fuels.

Table 2.1 Power and Capacity of Energy Yielding Processes in Human Muscle

	Power (mol ATP/min)	Capacity (mol/ATP)
Pcr	2.5	0.37
Lactate	1.9	0.94
CHOox	1.1	59
FFAox	0.6	Not limited

Pcr, phosphocreatine; CHOox, carbohydrate oxidation; FFAox, free fatty acid oxidation. For details, see Henriksson and Sahlin 2002.[1]

The glycolytic pathway can provide energy rapidly because of the high concentration of glycolytic enzymes and the speed of the chemical reactions involved. However, glycolysis cannot supply as much energy per second as the ATP-PC system. At high intensity exercise, the highest energy liberation from glycolysis occurs during the first 10–15s because acidification of muscle fibers reduces the breakdown-rate of glucose and glycogen. This impairs glycolytic enzyme function and decreases the fiber's calcium binding capacity and thus muscle contraction. This causes an increase of the muscle lactate up to more than 25–30 mmol/kg wt, and later one of blood lactate up to 18–25 mmol/l (Table 2.1).[1]

The muscle cells capacity for anaerobic glycolysis during maximal physical activity is for a period of approximately 1–3 min (shorter or longer depending on the intensity). Activities such as the 200-m free-style swim, 400-m sprint and strength-training activities with short rest periods between sets (e.g. 30 s) rely primarily on glycolysis for energy liberation. Anaerobic systems also contribute to energy production at the beginning of less intense exercise, when oxygen uptake kinetics lag behind the total energy demand placed on the system.

Stored carbohydrates supply the body with a rapidly available form of energy with 1 g of carbohydrate yielding approximately 4.1 kcal (17.1 kJ) of energy. Under resting conditions, muscle and liver take up glucose and convert it into a storage form of carbohydrate, called glycogen, which is, when needed as an energy source, broken down into glucose and can be metabolized to generate ATP anaerobically and aerobically.

The carbohydrate stores of the human organism are limited. They are composed of the circulating glucose in blood, and carbohydrates which are stored in the form of glycogen in the muscle and liver. The quantity of carbohydrates which can be stored in the form of glycogen in the skeletal muscles depends on a number of factors (e.g. nutrition, the state of training, muscle mass, the composition of muscle fibers and several other factors). Therefore, published data about the quantity of stored glycogen in the entire musculature vary between 1000 and 1900 kcal or even slightly more in trained athletes after carbohydrate loading. Taking into consideration that the muscles needed for physical exercise (e.g. the marathon run or biking) only constitute a part of the entire muscle mass, the carbohydrate reserves of the working musculature must obviously be regarded as an important limiting factor during physical strain of long duration and/or high

Table 2.2 Body Stores for Fuels and Energy[a]

	Grams		kcal	
	Untrained	Trained	Untrained	Trained
Carbohydrates				
Liver glycogen	~80	~120	~328	~492
Muscle glycogen	~250	~400	~1025	~1640
Glucose in body fluids	~15	~18	~62	~74
Total	~345	~538	~1415	~2206
Fats				
Subcutaneous	8000	6000	74 000	55 880
Intramuscular	50	300	465	2790
Total	8050	6300	74 465	58 670
Amino acids	100	110	410	451
Proteins	6000	7000	–	–

[a] Estimates based on body size of 70 kg and 12% body fat (male).

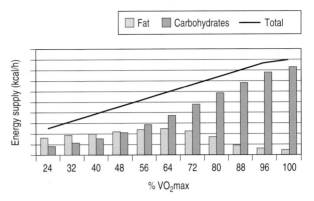

Figure 2.4 Total energy supply and relation of fat and carbohydrates during incremental workload. (Estimated from data by Achten and Jeukendrup 2003.[12])

intensity. The liver also has a storage pool of about 60–80 to a maximum 120 g of glycogen, corresponding to an energy reserve of about 240 to a maximum of 490 kcal.[8] It is important to mention that hepatic glycogen has another important function: it maintains the supply of blood sugar to the brain, which is also important during exercise of high intensity or long duration (Table 2.2).

Carbohydrates are used preferentially as energy fuel at the beginning of exercise and during high intensive loads requiring more than 70% of the maximum oxygen uptake. Compared with the anaerobic energy breakdown, the rate of energy liberation with the oxidation of carbohydrates is about one half and its capacity depends on the amount of glycogen stored in the muscles and in the liver. Without any substitution of carbohydrates during a long duration exercise, carbohydrate capacity allows endurance exercise for about 60–90 (120) min depending on the involved muscular system and the intensity of the physical activity.

Because muscle glycogen stores are limited and can become depleted during longer lasting vigorous exercise, an adequate diet especially for endurance exercise must contain a reasonable amount of carbohydrates, which enhance glycogen synthesis and also glycogen stores in muscles and liver.[11]

Fats are stored well in the organism but oxidized rather slowly. In order to utilize fat from fat deposits as a source of energy, they must be mobilized and transported to the muscle cell in the blood in the form of free fatty acids, bound to albumin. However, fats are also present within the muscle in the form of fat cells between muscle cells, and in the form of droplets inside muscle cells. At low intensities, a large portion of the energy is provided by fat metabolism – mainly by the free fatty acids in plasma. If the intensity of physical activity is increased further, intramuscular fats and carbohydrates are utilized in greater measure to fulfill the energy requirements. Fat oxidation does not increase at higher load intensities, but it is rather markedly reduced. A large body of data shows that the limitation is particularly within the mitochondria. This is also evidenced by the fact that the oxidation of intramuscular fats seems to occur in an incomplete fashion. The most likely theory

at the present time points to a blockade of the transport of long-chain fatty acids through the inner mitochondrial membrane when the rate of glycolysis is high (high intensity load). However, it is evident that in the presence of a markedly increased oxidative capacity of mitochondria, which is found in persons who have undergone endurance training, larger quantities of metabolites resulting from beta-oxidation can be oxidized. In other words, at the same load intensity, less metabolites are formed during glycolysis – which, in turn, has a positive effect on fat oxidation (Fig. 2.4).[12]

As discussed earlier, even in persons with a very good endurance performance, the energy flow rate from fat is limited. If one assumes that the energy requirements for various sports increase with the load intensity, carbohydrates must be utilized to an increasing extent to provide the required energy, because energy flow rates from carbohydrates markedly exceed those that could possibly result from fat.[13,14] An increased carbohydrate utilization reduces the glycogen stores in muscles and liver, which are, as mentioned earlier, limited. Therefore when discussing carbohydrates and fat depots, it is important to mention that dietetic measures can increase the carbohydrate reserves in muscle a few days prior to the actual physical activity.[15] Carbohydrates should also be ingested a few hours before the physical activity in order to optimize and restore the carbohydrate reserves in the muscle and liver.[11] A major reason for this is the fact that the energy production from exogenously supplied carbohydrates during physical strain, even when supplied at optimum concentrations, is relatively low.[16] Therefore the body's fats constitute by far the largest energy depot in the human organism and ensure a constant resynthesis of high-energy phosphates. Fat is also the most efficient depot substrate in the organism because 1 g of fat contains more than double the quantity of energy compared with the other two substrate groups (carbohydrates and proteins). One gram of fat contains 9.3 kcal. In contrast, carbohydrates and proteins contain only 4.1 kcal/g. In other words, a man weighing 80 kg, with a body fat content of 15% has 12 kg of fat in his body and a total energy store of about 110 000 kcal. This is supplemented by the quantity of fatty compounds stored within the muscle (as described earlier). In practice, this means that a normally nourished individual is equipped with a large energy depot which he/she can utilize if necessary. The problem, however, is that because of the limited energy flow per time unit during intensive physical strain, this large depot can be accessed only to a limited (slow) extent. Thus, in intensive physical activity or training, one again is dependent on carbohydrates.

CONDITIONING

In sports, training is defined as the preparation of sportsmen for the highest levels of performance. Sports training is the physical, technical, intellectual, psychological and moral preparation of an athlete by means of physical exercise, i.e. by applying workloads.[17]

Training involves an organized sequence of exercises that stimulates improvements, or adaptations, in anatomy and physiology. These adaptations require adherence to carefully designed training programs with attention focused on factors such as frequency, intensity, type of training, time or duration (FITT) and rest intervals.

The development of effective training programs requires an understanding of fundamental training principles, specific types of training and individual goals. Optimizing training requires knowledge of such principles as specificity, overload, progression, recovery, diminishing returns, supercompensation, reversibility, tapering, periodization, de-training and overtraining. Therefore, principles of training include all methodologies and mechanisms of manipulating training variables which enhance physical performance and have to be applied to the training process of elite athletes as well as untrained persons and patients in the rehabilitation.

IMPORTANT PRINCIPLES OF TRAINING

Box 2.2: Key Points

- Specificity
- Overload
- Progression
- Supercompensation
- Reversibility principle and detraining
- Tapering
- Periodization

Specificity

Specificity implies that the body's acute and chronic responses and adaptations to exercise training are metabolically and biomechanically specific to the type of exercise performed and the muscle groups involved. Thus, the specificity principle has implications for anatomy, neuromuscular recruitment, motor skill patterns, cardiorespiratory function and muscle energy metabolism. Different activities, depending on their duration and intensities require the activation of specific energy sys-

tems. In many cases, all three energy-transfer systems – the ATP-CP system, the glycolytic system and the aerobic system – operate at different times during exercise. Activities of short duration lasting about 6 s rely mainly on the breakdown of the 'high energy phosphates-system'. Therefore, athletes such as sprinters or weightlifters, have to improve primarily the capacity of this energy-transfer system. When a muscle performs endurance exercise such as cycling or running lasting 1 h, the activities rely heavily on the aerobic system and the athletes have to improve the capacity of the aerobic system. Therefore, when designing a training program, it is important to know the specific metabolic profile of a sport or activity and to consider the relative contributions of the aerobic and anaerobic energy pathways to sports performance.

In the context of the specificity principle, the principle of individual differences plays an additional important role.

The principle of individual differences
This principle refers to the concept that individuals respond differently to the same training stimulus.

The variability of the training response may be influenced by such factors as pre-training status, fitness level, genetic predisposition and gender.[18] For example, athletes who are less conditioned make greater gains than those who begin the training program at a higher level of fitness. After several months of training, sedentary adults may improve their aerobic fitness by more than 50%, whereas conditioned athletes may improve by only 3% over the same period of time. At the end however, the athlete has a higher level of fitness.

Therefore, even though they have the same goals they may not reach them by the same means.[19] Because we cannot expect, that all people will response to exercise in the same manner, a proper training program should be modified to take individual differences into account.

Overload principle
The principle of overload is based on the need to train the body at a level beyond that at which it normally performs. Therefore, overload should be a training stimulus, sufficient for chronic adaptations to occur. The amount of overload necessary to elicit a training response depends on the training state of the individual. An untrained individual needs very little overload stimulus to improve his performance. In contrast, to maximize muscular strength in athletes, the muscle needs to be stimulated with a resistance of relatively high intensity.

Exercise *frequency*, *duration* and *intensity* are the variables most often manipulated to provide overload to the systems of the body with specific consideration given to the *mode* of exercise.[16]

As an example, for endurance exercise a minimal overload training stimulus is attained at exercise intensity corresponding to 50% VO_{2max}, 70% of maximum heart rate, or 60% of the heart rate reserve.

Plateaux in performance improvement
With regard to the experience that some individuals appear more 'trainable' than others or even reach a plateau in their

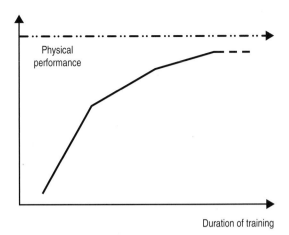

Figure 2.5 Theoretical training curve and ceiling effect.

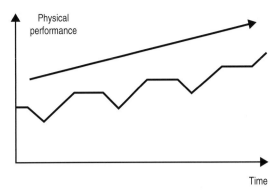

Figure 2.6 Load increments according to the overload principle.

performance improvement the principle of diminishing returns states that performance gains are related to the level of training experience of the individual. Untrained people will experience large gains in performance after a relatively short period of time. In contrast, athletes who have trained for several years will make small performance gains over a long period of time.

At the onset of a training program, rapid gains are made. As training duration continues, the rate of plateau appears to be reached. This plateau may be considered a genetic ceiling (Fig. 2.5).[18]

Progression

As an athlete adapts to a training stimulus, the exercise load (i.e. intensity, duration and/or frequency) must be increased so that improvements will continue. The training program can be progressed by, for example, increasing the load lifted, training frequency, quality and quantity of drills, or exercise stimulus. However, too great an overload may overstress the physiological systems and increase the risk of sports-related overuse injuries and exercise burnout. The training concept that provides an adequate overload stimulus without overstressing the body is optimal.

From the initiation stage to the elite performance stage, workload in training must increase gradually according to each athlete's physiological and psychological abilities. Physiologically, training gradually increases the body's functional efficiency, increasing its work performance (Fig. 2.6).[20]

Supercompensation

The amount of recovery required after a training session is directly related to the magnitude and duration of the exercise stress.

Stimulus-fatigue-recovery-adaptation (SFRA): Conceptually, an appropriate stimulus will result in some level of fatigue, recovery and adaptation such that performance can be eventually improved. This phenomenon is called supercompensation (Fig. 2.7).[21]

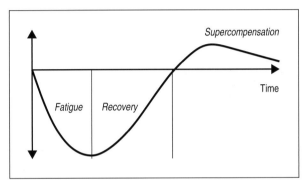

Figure 2.7 Stimulus-fatigue-recovery-adaptation. (Based on Yakovlev 1967.[21])

This concept is not limited to a single exercise response but may be observed over a longer period producing training adaptations.[22] There are a number of observations that support this concept. For example: Verkoshansky[23,24] noted that a unidirectional concentrated load of strength or strength-endurance training for several weeks could result in a diminished speed–strength (power) capability among track and field athletes. Upon returning to normal training, increased performance can often be observed, sometimes beyond baseline values. Verkoshansky[23,24] suggested that these results may be explained by the SFRA concept. Similar results have been observed among junior weightlifters after a planned high volume over-reaching phase; these results among weightlifters appear to be at least partially linked to alterations in anabolic/catabolic hormones.[25,26]

Reversibility principle and detraining

Adaptations to regular physical activities begin to return to pre-training values when the training stimulus is removed. An extreme example of reversibility and detraining occurs during bed rest.[27] Under this condition, VO_2max decreased by 27% in 21 days. A decrease in VO_2max has also been shown for prolonged periods where no training has occurred. Decrements in VO_2max resulting from training cessation initially result from reductions in plasma volume[28] and then from marked reductions in muscle mitochondrial enzyme activity.[29–31] In contrast, no reduction in glycolytic enzyme activities has been shown during detraining. The metabolic causes of decreased performance during strength or power-related training are minimal. This means that training induced gains in strength and muscle power seem to diminish at a slower pace compared with gains in aerobic endurance.

Detraining/retraining

It is evident that both low–moderate and highly-trained individuals who are detrained have a more rapid rate of gains after a return to training. Previous training does not alter the rate of training improvements from aerobic exercise after a period of 2–7 weeks of detraining.

The slogan 'If you don't use it, you lose it' is the main tenet of reversibility. After time off caused by injury, all athletes know that they cannot pick up exactly where they left off. Unfortunately, the body seems to lose muscle much more quickly than it is gained. A general proportion is 3:1. Missing 1 week of training requires 3 weeks to return to the same level.

Regularity and recovery

Performance enhancement requires a balance between overload and recovery. Too much overload and/or too little rest may result in over-reaching and over-training and therefore reduced physical performance. This causes a state of physical, chemical and mental imbalance (Fig. 2.8).[32]

Therefore, recovery is one of the most important principles of training, because during the recovery sessions, the adaptations to training take place. Recovery sessions may not necessarily mean complete rest. Periods of training with lower intensity will guarantee an adaptation without increasing stress. These periods are excellent opportunities for training on technique and tactics.

Tedium

Contemporary training requires many hours of work from the athlete. The volume and intensity of training are continuously increasing, and exercises are repeated numerous times.

Under these conditions, boredom and monotony can become obstacles to motivation and improvement.[33]

The sessions should be different and enjoyable. When boredom sets in, it is very difficult to motivate people to improve their fitness.

Tapering

Tapering is defined as: 'a progressive nonlinear reduction of the training load during a variable period of time, in an attempt to reduce the physiological and psychological stress of daily training and optimize sports performance'.[34]

Peak performance requires maximal physiological stress tolerance. After periods of intensive training, the athlete's exercise tolerance and performance capacity may start to decrease.

Coaches may therefore reduce the training volume and intensity after a 'hard training period' before the next training cycle or major competition. This practice is referred to as tapering. Costill *et al.*[35] showed, that the taper does not decrease conditioning, but actually can increase muscle power, improve psychological states and improve performance. Therefore, athletes should not fear to reduce their training volume for several days in a long-term training program and before an athletic competition.

The length of a tapering period and the training programs depends on the specific sport, the purpose of the taper, the specific period in a training year and individual needs.

Designing a training program

Based on the knowledge of the model of supercompensation, an effective sports training program must include an exercise prescription specifically developed for the individual athlete. This requires manipulation of the four primary program design variables (Table 2.3).[36]

The optimal way to develop an adequate training program is to have the factors related to the sports performance evaluated and use that information to generate a training program specific to the athlete.

Training frequency Training frequency refers to the number of training sessions conducted per day or per week. The frequency of training sessions will depend on an interaction of exercise intensity and duration, the training status of the athlete and the specific sport season.

Recovery from individual training sessions is essential if the athlete is to derive maximum benefit from the subsequent training session. Whereas an Olympic athlete has to train twice a day, it is enough for recreational sportsmen and women to train three times a week.

Training intensity Important for training adaptations in the body is the interaction of training intensity and duration. Generally, the higher the exercise intensity, the shorter the exercise duration. All biological adaptations are specific to the intensity, or effort expended during a training session.

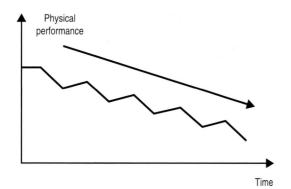

Figure 2.8   If the recovery is too short, the performance trend is negative. (Based on Kipke 1985.[32])

Table 2.3   Training Program Design Variables (FITT)

F	Frequency of training
I	Intensity of training
T	Type of exercise mode
T	Time of exercise duration

Based on Potteiger 2000.[33]

Sprinting requires a high percentage of high intensity training; marathon, triathlon or 24 h running need more training sessions of long duration and low intensity.

Exercise mode: type The exercise mode refers to the specific physical activity performed by the athlete: cycling, rowing, playing basketball, etc. To improve performance, the athlete should select activities that mimic the movement pattern employed in competition as closely as possible.

Exercise duration: time Exercise duration refers to the length of time the training session is conducted. The duration of a training session is often influenced by the exercise intensity: the longer the exercise duration, the lower the exercise intensity (*see* Training intensity).

Periodization

Because fatigue is a natural consequence of training (especially with high volume-loads) – and adaptations are primarily manifested during subsequent unloading periods – fatigue management is exceptionally important in producing an adequate program.

To promote long-term training and performance improvements, the coaches should include variations in training variables organized in planned periods or cycles within an overall program.[37] This program-design strategy is called periodization.

The concept of periodization was proposed in the 1960s by Russian physiologist Matveyev.[38]

Macrocycle
The largest division typically constitutes an entire training year but may also be a period of many months up to 4 years (for Olympic athletes).

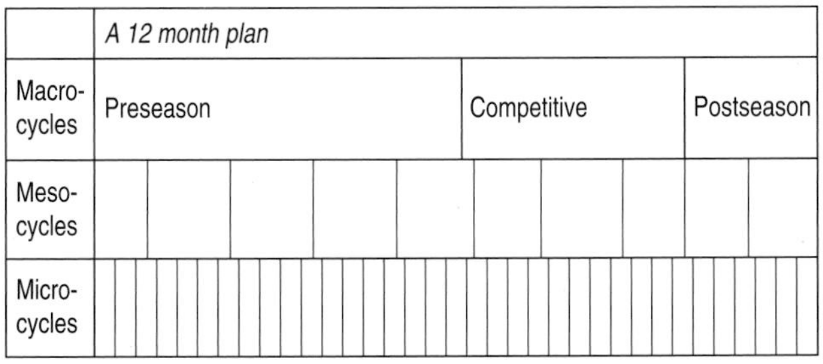

Typically, the training year is divided into phases that include the off-season, pre-season, in-season, and post-season (Fig. 2.9).

Preparatory/pre-season The priority of pre-season training is to maintain a base of cardiorespiratory fitness. Initially, the training program should be composed of long-duration and low-intensity workouts.

Periodic increases in exercise intensity occur when an athlete has adapted to the training stimulus and requires additional overload for continued improvements.

During the preseason, the athlete should focus on increasing training intensity, maintaining or reducing training duration and incorporating all types of training into the program. Workload and type of training (e.g. endurance, strength, flexibility, speed) vary according to each athletes physiological abilities. The strengths and weakness of the individual athlete should determine the amount and frequency of each type of training (*see* Tapering).

Competitive The in-season training program needs to be designed to include competition or race days in the training schedule. Low-intensity and short-duration training days should precede schedule competitions so the athlete is fully recovered and rested.

Transition/Post-season During the active rest period, the main focus should be on recovering from the previous competition season. Low-training duration and intensity are typical for this active rest phase, but enough overall exercise or activity should be performed to maintain a sufficient level of cardiorespiratory fitness, muscular strength and lean body mass (Fig. 2.10, Table 2.4).[38,39]

	A 12 month plan			
Macro-cycles	Preseason		Competitive	Postseason
Meso-cycles				
Micro-cycles				

Figure 2.9 A schematic illustration of the division of the annual training plan into macrocycles, mesocycles and microcycles.

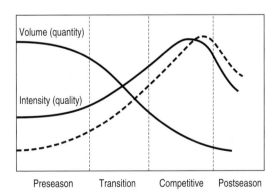

Figure 2.10 Matveyev's model of periodization (1965). (Redrawn from Matveyev 1965.[38])

Table 2.4   Model of Periodization, Sample for Macrocycle, Weight Training

Macrocycle	General Conditioning	Strength	Power	Maintenance	Active Recovery
Sets	3–4	3–4	2–3	1–2	1
Reps	7–10	5–9	3–5	6–10	10–12
Intensity	Low-moderate	High	High	Moderate	Low
Volume	High	Moderate	Low	Moderate	Moderate

Based on Rhea *et al.* 2002.[36]

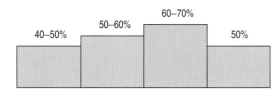

Figure 2.11 Percent increase of training load for a 4-week cycle.

Mesocycle

This divides the macrocycle into two or more periods, each lasting several weeks to several months; the number depends on the goals of the athlete and the number of competitions.

Figure 2.11 illustrates a hypothetical load increment over 4 weeks. The training load increases from step to step by approximately 10%, except in the regeneration week, when it decreases by 20%. The load per step refers to the training program for 1 day, which the athlete must repeat two or three times, depending on the number of training sessions per week (Fig. 2.12).[33]

Microcycle

Each mesocycle is divided into two or more microcycles that are typically 1-week long but could last for up to 4 weeks, depending on the program.

A microcycle is a weekly training program. It is probably the most important planning tool. Throughout the annual plan, the nature and dynamics of microcycles change according to the phase of training, the training objectives, and the physiological and psychological demands.[33]

FUNDAMENTALS OF FITNESS TRAINING

Box 2.3: Key Points

- Training works by altering homeostasis.
- Adaptations occur during recovery.
- Optimization of training and recovery govern progression in a conditioning program.
- Principles of training represent an evidence-based understanding of how training works.
- Optimization of performance trend line by exercising at the optimal training:
  - intensity
  - duration
  - frequency
  - type of training.

Although there is consensus on the importance of the relation between physical activity and health and well-being, the specific dose of physical activity necessary for good health remains unclear.[40] How much, what type, how often, what intensity and how long the physical activity dose should be and how this dose should be quantified and disseminated has led to the promulgation of numerous different public health and clinical recommendations.[41]

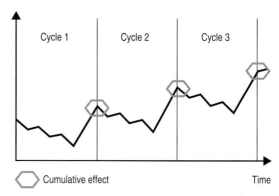

Figure 2.12 Cumulative effect of multiple training sessions.

The Centers for Disease Control and Prevention and American College of Sports Medicine (CDC/ACSM) developed guidelines for moderate and vigorous activity based on an accumulation of epidemiological research over the past several decades.[42,43] The recommended level of moderate activity (MACT) is at least 30 min of moderate-intensity physical activity each day.[43]

For individual training, the President's Council on Physical Fitness and Sports[44] published 'Fitness Fundamentals – Guidelines for Personal Exercise Program', including basics for fitness training:

'Each workout should begin with a warm-up and end with a cool-down. As a general rule, the workouts have to be spread throughout the week and consecutive days of hard exercise should be avoided.

In general, the amount of activity necessary for the average healthy person to maintain a minimum level of overall fitness is as follows:

WARM-UP: 5–10 minutes of exercise such as walking, slow jogging, knee lifts, arm circles or trunk rotations.

MUSCULAR STRENGTH: a minimum of two 20-minute sessions per week that include exercises for all the major muscle groups. Lifting weights is the most effective way to increase strength.

MUSCULAR ENDURANCE: at least three 30-minute sessions each week that include exercises such as pushups, situps, pullups, and weight training for all the major muscle groups.

CARDIO-RESPIRATORY ENDURANCE: at least five 30-minute bouts of continuous aerobic (activity requiring oxygen) rhythmic exercise each week, e.g. walking, jogging, swimming, cycling, rowing, cross-country skiing.

FLEXIBILITY: 10–12 minutes of daily stretching exercises performed slowly, without a bouncing motion. This can be included after a warm-up or during a cool-down.

COOL-DOWN: a minimum of 5–10 minutes of slow walking, low-level exercise, combined with stretching'.

STRUCTURAL AND FUNCTIONAL ADAPTATION OF CARDIOVASCULAR SYSTEM, RESPIRATORY SYSTEM AND SKELETAL MUSCLE TO TRAINING

The cardiovascular system

Long-term regular training causes favorable hemodynamic changes which are associated with structural and functional adaptations. These adaptations are generally described as 'athlete's heart'. From the hemodynamic point of view, sports might be divided into different types (although these types never appear in an 'isolated' form: (1) Endurance sports such as long-distance running, cross-country skiing, in which cardiac output is increased during exercise. (2) Strength sports, such as weightlifting and wrestling are associated with pressure load by a more pronounced increase of blood pressure and only slight increase in cardiac output caused by an enhanced heart frequency. (3) Sports with different combinations, for example rowing, canoeing and cycling. Over a long time, it has been accepted that endurance sports are characterized by a ventricular cavity enlargement, whereas strength sports lead to an increase in wall thickness.

Sports with a high endurance component

Several previous studies[45–48] reject the hypothesis that only left ventricular diameters increase as a result of dynamic endurance training. Data from these investigations show that in dynamic sports, such as long-distance running, athletes had not only larger left ventricular diameters and left ventricular mass but also significantly higher left ventricular wall thickness compared with controls.[48] Scharhag et al.[48] documented not only an increase in left ventricular inner diameter but also significant higher posterior wall thickness and interventricular septal thickness. In a meta-analysis, Fagard[45] compared the echocardiographic parameters of runners and strength athletes with those of control groups, where all groups were matched for age and body surface area. They showed increased left ventricular end-diastolic diameters, increased left ventricular end-systolic wall thickness and increased relative left ventricular wall thickness (synonym: 'hypertrophic index' = ratio between left ventricular wall thickness plus interventricular septal thickness and left ventricular internal diameter) for both, runners and strength athletes versus the control group. The runners showed a larger increase in left ventricular end-diastolic diameter and in left ventricular end-systolic wall thickness. Only the relative left ventricular wall thickness of runners was lower than that of strength athletes. The data of enhanced left ventricular end-diastolic diameters of endurance athletes in comparison with strength athletes has been confirmed by another meta-analysis.[46] In contrast to the results of Fagard, the left ventricular wall thickness was higher in strength athletes. But in this investigation, anthropometric data were not considered so that it cannot be excluded that body size might have influenced these results. Heart enlargement (increase in diameter and wall thickness) in endurance athletes seem to have two main explanations: (1) training regimes of endurance athletes are not exclusively 'dynamic' because in endurance sports, training schedules often include elements of strength training; (2) in 'dynamic' sports, load on the heart is not exclusively that of volume, since blood pressure also increases in endurance events although to a lesser extent than during strength events.

Previous studies using echocardiographic techniques often refer to the left ventricle because echocardiographic measures of the right ventricle are topographically complicated by the lung. Using the technique of magnetic resonance imaging (MRI), it has been shown[48] that regular and extensive endurance training results in similar changes in left ventricular and right ventricular mass, volume and function. Therefore, it can be concluded that regular and extensive endurance train-

ing results in a balanced enlarged heart with similar changes in both ventricles. Similar to muscle cells of peripheral muscles the above described structural changes of the heart are accompanied by ultrastructural and metabolic cellular adaptations resulting in an increased 'aerobic capacity' of heart muscle cells.[49]

Many studies investigating ventricular systolic function are based on the extent and velocity of fiber shortening, ventricular ejection fraction and the velocity of circumferential shortening. In concluding data from literature there is evidence that the ventricular emptying time is somewhat faster in endurance-trained individuals in comparison with untrained.[50,51] But the systolic function during dynamic exercise is usually similar in the group of endurance athletes and untrained controls.[45,46,48] The high stroke volumes observed in endurance-trained athletes are predominantly caused by higher end-diastolic volumes. In this context, it should be mentioned, that during incremental exercise, untrained individuals show a 'plateau' of stroke volume at submaximal heart rates. This phenomenon has been explained by an inadequate filling of ventricles when diastolic periods get shorter at higher heart rates. Comparing trained and untrained individuals, it has been demonstrated,[50] that at high heart rates and work rates not only the ventricular emptying but also the ventricular filling of trained subjects were significant faster in the trained group. Furthermore, these changes in hemodynamic function were much more pronounced during the filling phase than during the emptying phase.[50] The enhanced left ventricular diastolic function of athletes is also documented by measures of transmitral flow velocity, showing enhanced early diastolic ventricular filling (increase of 'passive mitral blood' flow).[46,52,53] These changes are accompanied by progressively increasing stroke volumes with increasing exercise intensity and heart rates.[50] Therefore, the high stroke volumes corresponding to high end-diastolic volumes observed in athletes during dynamic exercise are not only caused by structural but also by functional changes.

Structural and functional adaptations result in changes in the physiological behavior of a trained heart when compared with an untrained one: higher maximal performance, higher cardiac output and a lower heart frequency at rest and at sub-maximal loads. Cardiac output at sub-maximal loads is similar between trained and untrained subjects. But long-term endurance training decreases sub-maximal exercise heart rate by reducing sympathetic and increasing parasympathetic activity in trained subjects.[54] Therefore at sub-maximal loads, cardiac output of trained athletes is reached by higher stroke volumes and lower heart rate.

These structural and functional changes are accompanied by adaptations of the central nervous system, adaptations of the coronary vascular system and adaptations of peripheral vessels (e.g. the common femoral artery).

Sports with high strength component

Resistance exercise is associated with very high arterial pressure. This condition supported the 'old' theory of a 'concentric hypertrophy' caused by 'static exercise' with an increase in wall thickness without any increase in ventricular diameters. But this theory is not tenable considering current literature.[45,46,55] It has been demonstrated that in strength athletes not only the left ventricular wall thickness was increased (in comparison with controls), but also the left ventricular diameter. A study presented by Fagard[45] compared runners and strength athletes with that of controls, where all data were adjusted to age and body surface. It was shown that the percentage of increase in left ventricular wall thickness compared with controls was even lower in strength athletes than that of runners and much lower than that of cyclists. In the study of Pluim et al.[46] the posterior wall thickness of strength athletes was only slightly higher than that of endurance athletes and equal with that of athletes performing 'combined sports' but as mentioned above in this case, the anthropometric data were not considered.

However, this kind of adaptation caused by resistance exercise is reasonable considering that (1) heart rate and cardiac output do not remain unchanged during strength training; (2) pressure overload is limited by relatively short duration of resistance training when compared with endurance training and (3) training regimes and sports activities of strength athletes are often not only static but also dynamic. It should also be mentioned that echocardiographic data of elite strength athletes (e.g. weightlifters, shot putters) have to be considered with caution due to the potential influence of anabolic steroids. This assumption is confirmed by data including anabolic-free weightlifters, anabolic-free bodybuilders and bodybuilders using anabolic steroids.[56] Comparing these athletes, the authors found a significant increase in the hypertrophic index in doped bodybuilders when compared with bodybuilders and weightlifters not practicing doping.

Sports with different combinations of endurance and strength

This category of sports (e.g. rowing, canoeing, cycling, judo) involve elements of both dynamic and static exercise. Therefore, on one hand, mean arterial blood pressure is often increased over 200 mmHg for longer periods. On the other hand, this pressure load is also combined with an extreme volume load. This basic pre-requisite may explain why the largest increases in left ventricular internal dimension, left ventricular mass and left ventricular wall thickness are found in cyclists and rowers.[45,46,55] Fagard[45] documented the highest increase in left ventricular wall thickness, relative left ventricular wall thickness and left ventricular mass in cyclists when compared with runners, strength athletes and controls all adjusted in age and body size. In their meta-analysis, Pluim et al.[46] found the highest mean values for left ventricular left ventricular internal dimension, left ventricular dimensions and left ventricular muscle mass in athletes with combined load profiles compared to runners and strength athletes. Pelliccia et al.[55] measured left ventricular dimensions in 947 elite, male, highly-trained athletes who participated in a wide variety of sports. Only in 16 of the 947 athletes was an end-diastolic wall thicknesses identified 13 mm (normally a borderline for the diagnosis of hypertrophic cardiomyopathy). Fifteen of them were rowers or canoeists and one was a cyclist. It should not be forgotten that dimensions are also influenced by anthropometric dimensions. However, there is evidence that the propensity for developing an athlete's heart is partly genetically determined. Already in the 21st century, longitudinal training studies on identical twins have supported this theory. There is also indication that the ACE-gene (angiotensin-I-converting enzyme) – and probably others – has an effect to heart hypertrophy caused by training. It has been shown that individuals with the DD genotype of ACE-gene show a significantly increased left ventricular mass in response to physical training.[57]

The respiratory system

It is commonly accepted that during exercise, the structural capacity of the 'untrained' lung concerning large diffusion surface area, short alveolar-capillary diffusion distance, substantial ventilatory capacity exceeds the demand of pulmonary O_2 and CO_2 transport in healthy humans at sea level. Certainly the lung adapts to regular training with an increase in maximal voluntary ventilation.[58] These functional adaptations caused by endurance training are accompanied by improvement of oxidative capacity of inspiratory muscles and can be (in part) attributed to a higher mitochondrial enzyme activity of inspiratory muscles. Training also reduces the cross-sectional area of inspiratory muscles – a structural change that reduces the distance for diffusion of gases, metabolites and substrates. It is clear however, that lung diffusion surface, airways and respiratory muscles do not adapt to the same extent as other links in the oxygen transport and utilization system. Therefore, the suggestion of an 'overbuilt' lung has to be re-assessed in the light of high aerobic capacities of extremely endurance-trained individuals. Two main causes have been described, which may contribute in limiting the aerobic capacity via respiratory system during very hard or maximal exercise: the fatigue of diaphragm,[59] and the so-called 'exercise induced arterial hypoxemia' (EIAH).[59] Concerning the fatigue of the diaphragm it has been suggested that this effect is caused by a competitive relationship between working skeletal muscles and respiratory muscles for limited cardiac output, thus redistributing cardiac output to working limb muscles and depriving the diaphragm of adequate blood flow.[59] However, it has been shown that alveolar ventilation is not compromised despite diaphragm fatigue[59] – presumably because accessory respiratory muscles are recruited.[59] EIAH is a phenomenon of arterial O_2 desaturation of 3–15% below resting levels during very heavy and maximal exercise. It has been reported most frequently in fit young individuals (sedentary individuals do not experience EIAH). Until now, the causal mechanism, which favor the development of EIAH is uncertain.

With regard to the respiratory system, it can be stated that: (1) the lung adapts to regular training but to a lesser extent than other systems linked to oxygen transport and utilization system and (2) the contribution of the respiratory system to the limitations of aerobic capacity is (if even present) probably very small. The cause for limitation of aerobic capacity is probably in other systems such as cardiac output, peripheral vessels, such as the common femoral artery, limb blood flow and mitochondrial function and structure of working muscle cells.

The skeletal muscle
Adaptation to endurance training

Endurance training performed on a regular basis induces extensive alterations in the metabolic characteristics of exercising skeletal muscles. These adaptations are accompanied by pronounced changes in energy delivery and utilization. After long-lasting endurance training, exercise at a given intensity results in an enhanced fat oxidation.[60–63] At given exercise loads, muscle glycogen depletion is also prevented after training due to a shift from anaerobic utilization of carbohydrates to an enhanced carbohydrate oxidation and due to an increase in fat oxidation.[62,63]

From the late 1960s, a wealth of data on exercise induced ultrastructural changes in skeletal muscle has become available. Since that time it has been frequently demonstrated that endurance training increases both size and number of mitochondria.[64] This increase in mitochondrial surface area observed in trained skeletal muscle seems to stand for an increased capacity to exchange substrates, oxygen, and carbon dioxide between mitochondrion and cytoplasm.[64] Training adaptations of the mitochondrial system have been shown to include increases in mitochondrial enzyme activities.[63] The observation that a training-induced increase in mitochondrial enzyme activity was accompanied by an increase in oxidative capacity during exercise[61,63] as well as the finding of a coincidental increase of mitochondrial ATP production rates and mitochondrial enzyme activity following longer periods of endurance training,[65] support the theory that the mitochondrial enzymes are decisively involved in the shift from carbohydrates to fatty acids during sub-maximal exercise observed in trained skeletal muscle. This assumption is also indirectly supported by the observation that oxidative Type I fibers contain considerably higher mitochondrial activity of oxidative enzymes than Type II fibers.

There is also common agreement in the literature about the importance of mitochondrial ultrastructural and metabolic adaptations for a training-induced increase in fat utilization of skeletal muscle during prolonged sub-maximal exercise. Recent investigations conducted in isolated mitochondria of skeletal muscle support this theory by clearly demonstrating an increase in mitochondrial ATP production rates, mitochondrial fat oxidation rates and increased muscle oxidative power as a result of training.[65,66] However, these findings support a model of a greater 'pull' by the mitochondria[60] of endurance-trained skeletal muscle compared with their untrained counterparts.

The findings of a substrate flux to the mitochondrion (caused by an increased mitochondrial surface area) and of an oxidative utilization rate (caused by an increased activity of mitochondrial oxidative enzymes in mitochondria) in skeletal muscle are in agreement with the observation of larger intramuscular fat stores of endurance-trained muscle cells.[67] Intramuscular triglycerides (IMTG) which are mainly stored in the form of lipid droplets in the cytoplasm of muscle cells are supposed to contribute to the energy supply of exercising muscles. Because these intramyocellular droplets are located close to muscle mitochondria,[68] the transit time of fatty acids hydrolyzed from droplets to the outer mitochondrial membrane is very short and therefore these fatty acids seem to be readily available for oxidation during exercise. Utilizing ^{1}H nuclear magnetic resonance spectroscopy it has been shown that the IMTG content of working muscles decreases after prolonged sub-maximal exercise.[69] This observation is in agreement with findings showing that higher IMTG content is found in Type-I muscle fibers

than in Type II fibers.[70] However, the higher relative contact surface area between the intracellular lipid droplets and the outer mitochondrial membrane of the trained skeletal muscle has also been interpreted as an adaptive mechanism of trained skeletal muscle to increase fatty acids turnover.

It is important to be aware that oxidative processes are dependent on the microvascular supply of skeletal muscle. Based on available data it has been hypothesized that capillary surface per muscle fiber expressed as capillary to fiber ratio is linked with the mitochondrial volume.[71] These differences in oxygen (and substrate) supply to skeletal muscle seem to be matched by differences in the amount of mitochondrial structure.[71] However, there is clear evidence indicating that capillarization of human and animal skeletal muscle increases as a result of training, prolonging the transit time of red blood cells that pass through the capillaries into the mitochondrion of muscle cells.

Adaptation to strength training

It is also generally accepted that strength training is beneficial to improve athletic performance, enhance general health and fitness and rehabilitate after injury. Resistance training results in adaptations of many physiological systems such as the muscle, the endocrine system and the neuronal control. These adaptations contribute to changes of muscular strength, power, local muscular endurance, speed, balance, coordination, jumping ability, flexibility and the corresponding measures of motor performance.[72,73] However, these adaptations depend on the muscle actions used (mode of exercise, intensity, volume, number of sets and rest periods between sets). This summary is focused on strength, power, muscle hypertrophy and muscular endurance.

Training to maximize muscular strength for sports performance is normally carried out with 100% of one repetition maximum (1 RM) down to 80% 1 RM, whereas a variety of loads within this range seems to be most conductive.[73] Regularly performing this kind of training alters human fiber type profile. The main adaptation to training near maximal loads is a conversion of IIB fibers to IIA.[72,74] This finding is in agreement with the observation of increased IIa myosin heavy chain isoforms (MHC) and decreasing IIb MHC.[75]

Concerning hypertrophy, it has been shown that bodybuilders are different with respect to percentage of cross-sectional area (CSA) fiber type when compared with weightlifters. While weightlifters show a preferential hypertrophy of type II fibers, the bodybuilders obviously succeed in increasing size of both, type I and type II fibers.[72,74] This difference seems to be caused by extremely high loads (= 90% 1 RM) routinely used by weightlifters during training, while bodybuilders spend considerable more time using loads = 80% 1 RM with a higher number of repetitions. However, based on data in literature, there is some evidence that there may be a 'threshold' for optimal growth of muscles at about 80% 1 RM.[72] Furthermore, proceeding from the assumption of a 'hypertrophy threshold' of 80% 1 RM it is also evident, that higher volumes (higher amount of repetitions) can be reached at 80% 1 RM when compared with 100% 1 RM. Additionally, there is also some evidence that hypertrophic response is not optimal when using only sets of 100% 1RM.[76]

Concerning structural adaptations caused by high load/low repetition resistance training, the following observations have been made: (1) Elite weightlifters show a similar number of capillaries per muscle fiber when compared with untrained subjects. However, there is a decrease in capillaries per unit muscle area due to an increase in muscle fiber size.[77,78] In contrast to weightlifters, bodybuilders often show a slight increase in capillaries per muscle fiber with a similar number of capillaries per unit muscle area in comparison with untrained persons.[78,79] (2) Mitochondrial density has been found similar or even slightly decreased[80,81] as result of high load resistance training. (3) High load resistance training does not enhance the activity of enzymes associated with aerobic energy production.[82] Weightlifters normally show similar or even slightly decreased activities of 'aerobic' enzymes than untrained persons. However, higher activities of citrate synthetase and 3-hydroxyacyl-CoA dehydrogenase (HAD) has been demonstrated in bodybuilders when compared with weightlifters.[78] These differences between weightlifters and bodybuilders seem to be caused by differences in training regimes with regard to higher number of repetitions in body building. (4) Concerning the high energy phosphate metabolism, some[83,84] investigators found an improvement of fast ATP restoration caused by higher activities of several enzymes like ATPase, creatine kinase or myokinase as a result of high load resistance training. These changes seem to contribute to the higher contractility, power and speed observed as a result of high load resistance training. (5) Evaluating the effects of high load resistance training to anaerobic glycolytic metabolism data presented in literature are inconsistent. Several investigations demonstrate that 'anaerobic' enzymes like phosphofructokinase or lactate dehydrogenase are unaffected by high load resistance training.[81,84,85] These findings are contrasted by other data showing a slightly higher activity of 'anaerobic' enzymes like lactate dehydrogenase in strength-trained athletes than untrained subjects.[83]

Local muscular endurance can be trained with a special regime of resistance training. This kind of training consists of low to moderate intense training with high repetitions and short recovery between the sets. This kind of training is designed to increase muscular endurance capacity of specific muscle groups with all its structural and functional adaptations such as mitochondrial and capillary density, fiber type transition and buffering capacity.

REFERENCES

1   Henriksson J, Sahlin K. Metabolism during exercise – energy expenditure and hormonal changes. In: Kjaer M, Krogsgaard M, Magnusson P, et al., eds. Textbook of sports medicine: Basic science and clinical aspects of sports injury and physical activity. Oxford: Blackwell Science; 2002:30–48.

2   Meyer RA, Brown TR, Krilowicz BL, Kushmerick MJ. Phosphagen and intracellular pH changes during contraction of creatine-depleted rat muscle. Am J Physiol 1986; 250:264–274.

3   Sahlin K. Control of energetic processes in contracting human skeletal muscle. Biochem Soc Trans 1991; 19:353–358.

4   Blei ML, Conley KE, Kishmerick MJ. Separate measures of ATP utilization and recovery in oral or i.v. glucose intake. Eur J Appl Physiol 1993; 59:327–333.

5   Sahlin K, Söderlund K, Tonkonogi M, Hirakoba K. Phosphocreatine content in single fibers of human muscle after sustained submaximal exercise. Am J Physiol 1997; 273:172–178.

6   Sahlin K, Jorfeldt L, Henriksson KG, et al. Tricarboxylic acid cycle intermediates during incremental exercise in healthy subjects and in patients with McArdle's disease. Clin Sci (Colchester) 1995; 88:687–693.

7   Bachl N, Faigenbaum A. Principles of exercise physiology. In: Micheli L, Smith A, Bachl N, Rolf C, Chan KM, eds. FIMS Team Physician Manual. Sim Sha Tsui, China: Lippincott, Williams & Wilkins; 2001:50–75.

8   Smekal G. Substratutilisation (muskulärer Energiestoffwechsel). In: Pokan R, Förster H, Hofmann P, et al., eds. Kompendium der Sportmedizin. Wien: Springer; 2004:83–101.

9   Carraro F, Naldini A, Weber JM, Wolfe RR. Alanine kinetics in humans during low-intensity exercise. Med Sci Sports Exerc 1994; 263:48–53.

10 Brouns F, Saris WH, Stroecken J, et al. Eating, drinking cycling. A control Tour de France simulation study. Part 1. Int J Sports Med 1989; 10:32–40.

11 Coyle EF. Timing and method of increased carbohydrate intake to cope with heavy training, competition and recovery. J Sports Sci Spec 1991; 9:29–51.

12 Achten J, Jeukendrup AE. Maximal fat oxidation during exercise in trained men. Int J Sports Med 2003; 24:603–608.

13 Romijn JA, Coyle EF, Sidossis LS, et al. Regulation of endogenous fat and carbohydrate metabolism in relation to exercise intensity and duration. Am J Physiol 1993; 265:380–391.

14 Romijn JA, Coyle EF, Sidossis LS, et al. Substrate metabolism during different exercise intensities in endurance-trained women. J Appl Physiol 2000; 88:1707–1714.

15 Hultman E, Sjöholm H. Substrate availability. In: Knuttgen HG, Vogel JM, Poortmans JR, eds. Biochemistry of exercise. Champaign, IL: Human Kinetics 1983:63–75.

16 Wagenmakers AJ. Muscle amino acid metabolism at rest and during exercise: role in human physiology and metabolism. Exerc Sport Sci Rev 1998; 26:287–314.

17 Harre D. Principles of sports training. Introduction to the theory and methods of training. Berlin: Sportverlag; 1982.

18 Hoffman J. Physical aspects of sports training and performance. Champaign, IL: Human Kinetics; 2002.

19 Cross N. Individualization of training programmes. In: Cross N, Lyle J, eds. The Coaching process: principles and practice for sport. Oxford: Butterworth-Heinemann; 1999:174–191.

20 Bompa T. Periodization training for sports. Champaign, IL: Human Kinetics; 1999.

21 Yakovlev NN. Sports biochemistry. Leipzig: Deutsche Hochschule für Körperkultur (German Institute for Physical Culture); 1967.

22 Rowbottom DG. Periodization of training. In: Garret WE, Kirkendall DT, eds. Exercise and sports science. Baltimore: Williams & Wilkins; 2000:499–512.

23 Verkhoshansky YV. Fundamentals of special strength-training in sport. Moscow: Fizkultura i Spovt; 1977.

24 Verkhoshansky YV. Programming and organization of training [translated by A. Charniga, Jr.]. Moscow: Fizkultura i Spovt, Livonia Sportivny Press; 1985.

25 Fry AC, Kraemer WJ, Stone MH, et al. Relationships between serum testosterone, cortisol and weightlifting performance. J Strength Cond Res 2000; 14:338–343.

26 Stone MH, Fry AC. Increased training volume in strength/power athletes. In: Kreider RB, Fry AC, O'Toole ML, eds. Overtraining in sport. Champaign, IL: Human Kinetics; 1997:87–106.

27 Saltin B, Blomqvist G, Mitchell JH, Johnson RL Jr, Wildenthal K, Chapman CB. Response to exercise after bed rest and after training. Circulation 1968; 38:1–78.

28 Coyle EF, Hemmert MK, Coggan AR. Effects of detraining on cardiovascular responses to exercise: Role of blood volume. J Appl Physiol 1986; 60:1857–1864.

29 Chi MY. Effects of detraining on enzymes of energy metabolism in individual human muscle fibers. Am J Physiol 1983; 244:276–287.

30 Costill DL, Fink WJ, Hargreaves M, King DS, Thomas R, Fielding R. Metabolic characteristics of skeletal muscle during detraining from competitive swimming. Med Sci Sports Exerc 1985; 17:339–343.

31 Coyle EF, Martin WH 3rd, Sinacore DR, Joyner MJ, Hagberg JM, Holloszy JO. Time course of loss of adaptations after stopping prolonged intense endurance training. J Appl Physiol 1984; 57:95–99.

32 Kipke L. The importance of recovery after training and competitive efforts. N Z J Sports Med 1985; 13:120–128.

33 Bompa T. Total training for young champions. Champaign, IL: Human Kinetics; 2000.

34 Mujika I. Optimizing performance without falling into detraining. Etienne: IAT, Med.&Biomech; 2002.

35 Costill DL, King DS, Thomas R, Hargreaves M. Effects of reduced training on muscular power of swimmers. Phys Sports Med 1985; 13:94–101.

36 Potteiger J. Aerobic endurance exercise training. In: Baechle T, Earle R, eds. Essentials of strength training and conditioning. Champaign, IL: Human Kinetics; 2000:495–508.

37 Wathen D, Baechle T, Earle R. Training variation: Periodization. In: Baechle T, Earle R, eds. Essentials of strength training and conditioning. National Strength and Conditioning Association. Champaign, IL: Human Kinetics; 2000:513–526.

38 Matveyev L. Die periodisierung des sportlichen trainings. [Translated from Russian]. Moscow: Fiskultura I sport; 1965.

39 Rhea MR, Ball SD, Phillips WT, Burkett LN. A comparison of linear and daily undulating periodized programs with equated volume and intensity for strength. J Strength Cond Res 2002; 16:250–255.

40 Kesaniemi YK, Danforth E Jr, Jensen MD, Kopelman PG, Lefebvre P, Reeder BA. Dose-response issues concerning physical activity and health: an evidence-based symposium. Med Sci Sports Exerc 2001; 33:351–358.

41 Blair S, LaMonte MJ, Nichaman MZ. The evolution of physical activity recommendations: how much is enough? Am J Clin Nutr 2004; 79 (Suppl):913–920.

42 American College of Sports Medicine Position Stand. The recommended quantity and quality of exercise for developing and maintaining cardiorespiratory and muscular fitness, and flexibility in healthy adults. Med Sci Sports Exerc 1998; 30:975–991.

43 Pate RR, Pratt M, Blair SN, et al. Physical activity and public health: a recommendation from the Centers for Disease Control and Prevention and the American College of Sports Medicine. JAMA 1995; 273:402–407.

44 President's Council on Physical Fitness and Sports. Fitness fundamentals – Guidelines for personal exercise programs. Online. Available: http://fitness.gov/fitness.pdf 19 July 2003.

45 Fagard RH. Athlete's heart: a meta-analysis of the echocardiographic experience. Int J Sports Med 1996; 17:140–144.

46 Pluim BM, Zwinderman AH, van der Laarse A, van der Wall EE. The athlete's heart. A meta-analysis of cardiac structure and function. Circulation 2000; 101:336–344.

47 Spirito P, Pelliccia A, Proschan MA, et al. Morphology of the 'athlete's heart' assessed by echocardiography in 947 elite athletes representing 27 sports. Am J Cardiol 1994; 74:802–806.

48 Scharhag J, Schneider G, Urhausen A, Rochette V, Kramann B, Kindermann W. Athlete's heart: right and left ventricular mass and function in male endurance athletes and untrained individuals determined by magnetic resonance imaging. J Am Coll Cardiol 2002; 20:1856–1863.

49 Moore RL. Cellular adaptations of the heart muscle to exercise training. Ann Med 1998; 30:46–53.

50 Gledhill N, Cox D, Jamnik R. Endurance athletes' stroke volume does not plateau: major advantage is diastolic function. Med Sci Sports Exerc 1994; 26:1116–1221.

51 Ferguson S, Gledhill N, Jamnik VK, Wiebe C, Payne N. Cardiac performance in endurance-trained and moderately active young women. Med Sci Sports Exerc 2001; 33:1114–1119.

52 Di Bello V, Santoro G, Talarico L, et al. Left ventricular function during exercise in athletes and in sedentary men. Med Sci Sports Exerc 1996; 28:190–196.

53 Stork T, Mockel M, Muller R, Eichstadt H, Hochrein H. Left ventricular filling behaviour in ultra endurance and amateur athletes: a stress Doppler-echo study. Int J Sports Med 1992; 13:600–604.

54 Carter JB, Banister EW, Blaber AP. Effect of endurance exercise on autonomic control of heart rate. Sports Med 2003; 33:33–46.

55 Pelliccia A, Maron BJ, Spataro A, Proschan MA, Spirito P. The upper limit of physiologic cardiac hypertrophy in highly trained elite athletes. N Engl J Med 1991; 324:295–301.

56 Urhausen A, Kindermann W. Sports-specific adaptations and differentiation of the athlete's heart. Sports Med 1999; 28:237–244.

57 Fatini C, Guazzelli R, Manetti P, et al. RAS genes influence exercise-induced left ventricular hypertrophy: an elite athletes study. Med Sci Sports Exerc 2000; 32:1868–1872.

58 O'Kroy JA, Coast JR. Effects of flow and resistive training on respiratory muscle endurance and strength. Respiration 1993; 60:279–283.

59 Dempsey JA, Sheel AW, Haverkamp HC, Babcock MA, Harms CA. Pulmonary system limitations. Can J Appl Physiol 2003; 28 (Suppl):2–4.

60 Coggan AR, Raguso CA, Gastaldelli A, Sidossis LS, Yeckel CW. Fat metabolism during high-intensity exercise in endurance-trained and untrained men. Metabolism 2000; 49:122–128.

61 Hurley BF, Nemeth PM, Martin WH 3rd, Hagberg JM, Dalsky GP, Holloszy JO. Muscle triglyceride utilization during exercise: effect of training. J Appl Physiol 1986; 60:562–567.

62 Martin WH 3rd, Dalsky GP, Hurley BF, et al. Effect of endurance training on plasma free fatty acid turnover and oxidation during exercise. Am J Physiol 1993; 265:708–714.

63 Phillips SM, Green HJ, Tarnopolsky MA, Heigenhauser GF, Hill RE, Grant SM. Effects of training duration on substrate turnover and oxidation during exercise. J Appl Physiol 1996; 81:2182–2191.

64 Hoppeler H, Howald H, Conley K, Lindstedt SL, Claassen H, Vock P, Weibel ER. Endurance training in humans: aerobic capacity and structure of skeletal muscle. J Appl Physiol 1985; 59:320–327.

65 Starritt EC, Angus D, Hargreaves M. Effect of short-term training on mitochondrial ATP production rate in human skeletal muscle. J Appl Physiol 1999; 86:450–454.

66 Tonkonogi M, Walsh B, Svensson M, Sahlin K. Mitochondrial function and antioxidative defence in human muscle: effects of endurance training and oxidative stress. J Physiol 2000; 15:379–388.

67 Howald H, Boesch C, Kreis R, Matter S, Billeter R, Essen-Gustavsson B, Hoppeler H. Content of intramyocellular lipids derived by electron microscopy, biochemical assays, and (1)H-MR spectroscopy. J Appl Physiol 2002; 92:2264–2272.

68 Vock R, Weibel ER, Hoppeler H, Ordway G, Weber JM, Taylor CR. Design of the oxygen and substrate pathways. V. Structural basis of vascular substrate supply to muscle cells. J Exp Biol 1996; 199:1675–1688.

69 Brechtel K, Niess AM, Machann J, et al. Utilisation of intramyocellular lipids (IMCLs) during exercise as assessed by proton magnetic resonance spectroscopy (1H-MRS). Horm Metab Res 2001; 33:63–66.

70 Hwang JH, Pan JW, Heydari S, Hetherington HP, Stein DT. Regional differences in intramyocellular lipids in humans observed by in vivo 1H-MR spectroscopic imaging. J Appl Physiol 2001; 90:1267–1274.

71 Hoppeler H, Weibel ER. Structural and functional limits for oxygen supply to muscle. Acta Physiol Scand 2000; 168:445–456.

72 Fry AC. The role of resistance exercise intensity on muscle fibre adaptations. Sports Med 2004; 34:663–679.

73 Kraemer WJ, Adams K, Cafarelli E, et al. American College of Sports Medicine. American College of Sports Medicine position stand. Progression models in resistance training for healthy adults. Med Sci Sports Exerc 2002; 34:364–380.

74 Campos GE, Luecke TJ, Wendeln HK, et al. Muscular adaptations in response to three different resistance-training regimens: specificity of repetition maximum training zones. Eur J Appl Physiol 2002; 88:50–60.

75 Hikida RS, Staron RS, Hagerman FC, Walsh S, Kaiser E, Shell S, Hervey S. Effects of high-intensity resistance training on untrained older men. II. Muscle fiber characteristics and nucleo-cytoplasmic relationships. J Gerontol A Biol Sci Med Sci 2000; 55:347–354.

76 Hakkinen K, Pakarinen A. Acute hormonal responses to two different fatiguing heavy-resistance protocols in male athletes. J Appl Physiol 1993; 74:882–887.

77 Kadi F, Eriksson A, Holmner S, Butler-Browne GS, Thornell LE. Cellular adaptation of the trapezius muscle in strength-trained athletes. Histochem Cell Biol 1999; 111:189–195.

78 Tesch PA, Alkner BA. Acute and chronic muscle metabolic adaptations to strength training. In: Komi PV, ed. Strength and power in sport. Oxford: Blackwell Science; 2003:265–280.

79 Schantz PG, Kallman M. NADH shuttle enzymes and cytochrome b5 reductase in human skeletal muscle: effect of strength training. J Appl Physiol 1989; 67:123–127.

80 Chilibeck PD, Syrotuik DG, Bell GJ. The effect of strength training on estimates of mitochondrial density and distribution throughout muscle fibers. Eur J Appl Physiol Occup Physiol 1999; 80:604–609.

81 Wang N, Hikida RS, Staron RS, Simoneau JA. Muscle fiber types of women after resistance training – quantitative ultrastructure and enzyme activity. Pflugers Arch 1993; 424:494–502.

82 Green H, Goreham C, Ouyang J, Ball-Burnett M, Ranney D. Regulation of fiber size, oxidative potential, and capillarization in human muscle by resistance exercise. Am J Physiol 1999; 276:591–596.

83 Tesch PA, Thorsson A, Essen-Gustavsson B. Enzyme activities of FT and ST muscle fibers in heavy-resistance trained athletes. J Appl Physiol 1989; 67:83–87.

84 Komi PV, Karlsson J, Tesch PA, Suorninen H, Heikkinen E. Effects of heavy resistance and explosive-type strength training methods on mechanical, functional and metabolic aspects of performance. In: Komi PV, ed. Exercise and sport biology: International series on sports sciences. Vol. 12. Champaign, IL: Human Kinetics; 1982:90–102.

85 Bishop D, Jenkins DG, Mackinnon LT, McEniery M, Carey MF. The effects of strength training on endurance performance and muscle characteristics. Med Sci Sports Exerc 1999; 31:886–891.

CHAPTER 3

The Role of Diet and Nutritional Supplements

Fabio Pigozzi, Arrigo Giombini, Federica Fagnani and Attilio Parisi

INTRODUCTION

In modern sports, nutritional strategies may have their biggest influence on performance by supporting intensive sports activity and thus promoting adaptations to training that will lead to enhanced performance.

Box 3.1: Key Points

1 Carbohydrate supplementation during exercise is an effective means of improving performance in endurance sports. This can be accomplished without significantly modifying an athlete's normal training protocol or diet.

2 An adequate protein intake can help an individual who is active in aerobic or resistance training to reach his/her potential by preserving muscle tissue and possibly enhancing recovery after strenuous exercise.

3 For the athlete with very high levels of energy expenditure during training, the exercise intensity will inevitably be reduced to a level where fatty acids provide a large part of the energy supply and become an important dietary component.

4 Of special significance in the metabolic mixture are the micronutrients, the small quantities of vitamins and minerals that play highly specific roles in facilitating energy transfer and tissue synthesis. These nutrients can be obtained by consuming well-balanced meals.

5 Minerals function primarily in metabolism where they serve as important parts of enzymes. Sweat loss during exercise usually does not increase the minerals requirements above recommended values.

6 The use of supplements and ergogenic aids represents a controversial area of sports medicine worldwide. The clinician has to be well informed in the more popular supplements and drugs reputed to be ergogenic in order to distinguish fact from fiction.

The foods that an athlete chooses can make the difference between success and failure. A correct food choice will not make a champion out of the athlete who is not talented or motivated but a scanty or inadequate diet can prevent the talented athlete from making it to the top. The goals for adequate nutrition for athletes should include: maintaining energy supply to the working muscles, supporting tissue adaptation, growth and repair, and promoting immune function.

In competition, all important and worthy goals must be met, but the requirements and the strategies adopted will greatly vary depending on the nature of the event.

The purpose for the nutritionist involved in competitive sport is to identify first the nutritional goals of the athlete and then to translate them into dietary strategies, taking into account the individual needs. This general consideration is applied to all sports, but the strategies utilized may be very different because of the different demands of training and competition.

Any form of sport activity will increase the rate of energy expenditure, and for this reason, energy intake must be increased accordingly; also considering that the energy demands of sportsmen and women in training vary depending primarily on body mass and training load.

MACRONUTRIENTS

Role of carbohydrates

Relative to fat or protein, the carbohydrate stores of the body are quite limited: 300–500 g of glycogen are stored in skeletal muscle; 60–100 g are stored in the liver and an additional 15–20 g of glucose is stored in blood and extracellular space.[1] The rate of blood glucose and muscle glycogen use is dependent on both the intensity and duration of exercise. It is also influenced by the availability of other fuel sources, mainly plasma free fatty acids. If carbohydrate stores were the only fuel source available during exercise, they would provide only enough energy to complete a 32 km run.[1]

When the exercise intensity increases linearly, muscle glycogen use increases exponentially. Saltin and Gollnick[2] found that the rate of muscle glycogen use was 0.7, 1.4, and 3.4 mmol/kg per min at exercise intensity of 50%, 75% and 100% of VO_2max, respectively.[2] However, the rate of glycogenolysis is also dependent on the muscle glycogen concentration, the greater the initial muscle glycogen concentration, the faster the rate of glycogenolysis.

Similar to the situation with muscle glycogen utilization, a linear increase in exercise intensity results in an exponential increase in muscle glucose uptake.[3] Björkman and Wahren reported that after 40 min of exercise at an intensity of 25% and 75% VO_2max, leg glucose uptake was 0.4 mmol/min and 1.8 mmol/min, respectively.[1]

This increase in muscle glucose uptake seems to partially offset the decrease in glycogenolysis that accompanies a decrease in the muscle glycogen concentration.[4]

Recovery of the muscle and liver glycogen stores after exercise is a rather slow process, and complete recovery may not be achieved until 24–48 h after the end of an exercise bout. The rate of glycogen resynthesis after exercise is determined largely by the amount of carbohydrates supplied in the diet. The amount of carbohydrates consumed is of far greater importance for this process than the type of carbohydrates.

Carbohydrate loading is a practice used to maximize glycogen storage before competition. This can be accomplished without significantly modifying an athlete's normal training protocol or diet. Sherman and collaborators have recommended that the muscle glycogen stores first be depleted with a hard exercise bout, 7 days before competition.[3] This is followed by a normal 6-day training taper. During the first 3 days of the taper, a mixed diet composed of 45–50% carbohydrate is consumed. During the last 3 days of the taper, the carbohydrate content of the diet should be increased to 70%. A high-carbohydrate meal may also be consumed 4 h before competition, providing an additional supply of carbohydrate without substantially altering the normal exercise hormonal and metabolic milieu.[5] Supplements taken less than 4 h before competition could result in hypoglycemia and an increased reliance on muscle glycogen; however, if supplementation is continued throughout exercise, this should not present a problem as long as the supplement is readily digestible.

Carbohydrate supplementation during exercise is an effective means of improving endurance performance. The major objective of supplementation during exercise is to prevent hypoglycemia. Some authors recommend the consumption of 30–60 g of carbohydrate per hour. The means by which this is provided depend on the type, intensity, duration of the exercise, and the environmental condition under which the exercise is performed. For hot, humid conditions in which dehydration is a concern, liquid supplements composed of 5–6% carbohydrate every 15–20 min is optimal. Dehydration becomes a definite risk during cold weather exercise because colder air contains less moisture than air at warmer temperature and cold stress stimulates the body to increase urine production causing a considerable body fluid loss; for this reason, liquid supplements are suggested during prolonged exercise in cold weather.

For the rapid restoration of muscle glycogen, some authors recommend that 1.0–1.5 g carbohydrate/kg body weight be consumed immediately after exercise. Continuation of supplementation every 2 h, or smaller amounts taken more frequently, will maintain a maximal rate of storage 6 h after exercise.

Supplements composed of glucose or glucose polymers are more effective than fructose for the restoration of muscle glycogen; however, the addition of some fructose to the supplement is recommended because fructose is more effective than glucose in the restoration of liver glycogen. The addition of protein to the supplement may also be of benefit because it increases the pancreatic insulin response and rate of muscle glycogen synthesis.

We think, in conclusion, that there is enough evidence to support the theory that adequate carbohydrate intake is important for the restoration of muscle glycogen stores, and that other dietary strategies related to the timing of intake, type of carbohydrate source or addition of other nutrients may either directly enhance the rate of glycogen-storage recovery or improve the practical achievement of carbohydrate intake targets.

Role of proteins

Humans need dietary protein to provide the essential amino acids that our body cannot synthesize but that are needed in the production of important proteins in the body. Therefore, all humans need to consume a certain proportion of nine essential amino acids including histidine, isoleucine, leucine, lysine, methionine, phenylalanine, threonine, tryptophan and valine. Our total nitrogen need is in excess of that required for the essential amino acids and the body can use this additional nitrogen to synthesize non-essential amino acids needed for protein synthesis.

Most athletes consume more than enough protein in their daily diets. Van Erp-Baart et al. found that protein intake in high-level athletes was highly related to energy intake.[6] Thus, athletes in high-energy-expenditure sports and male athletes were the highest consumers of protein. The highest protein intakes were found in male cyclists in the Tour de France, at approximately 3 g/kg per day (Fig. 3.1). Male bodybuilders consumed approximately 2.5 g/kg per day, whereas female bodybuilders reported diets with approximately 2.0 g/kg per day. Female hockey, volleyball and handball players had the lowest average protein intake, at about 1.0–1.2 g/kg per day. Thus, all of the athletic groups as a whole were consuming a quantity of protein greater than the US recommended dietary allowance (RDA), but some individuals, particularly the low-energy consumers, may have consumed less than this recommended level.

Both muscle protein synthesis and degradation are increased as a result of resistance exercise, with more of an increase in synthesis resulting in net increase of body protein. Scientific evidence shows that protein intake in the range of 1.2–1.8 g/kg per day is optimal for maintaining body protein and allowing maximal muscle protein synthesis.[7] Novice athletes starting a resistance-training program should use the upper end of this range. Long-term consumption of protein at higher levels than this range has not been shown to have any benefit. Preliminary research suggests that consumption of carbohydrate with protein mixtures after resistance exercise may enhance protein increase and metabolic recovery.

Resistance exercise is required to stimulate muscle protein synthesis and in the end, muscle hypertrophy. Thus, underweight patients who ask whether protein supplements would help them gain weight should be advised to begin resistance

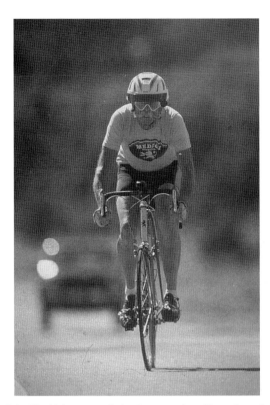

Figure 3.1 The highest protein intakes were found in male cyclists in the tour the France. (From Van Erp-Baart et al. 1989,[6] with permission.)

training in addition to increasing their energy intake. Additional dietary energy, required for protein synthesis to occur, is probably the most important dietary change they can make because they are likely consuming enough protein in their typical diets.

Although the majority of individuals already consume the recommended amount of protein in their daily diets, there are high-risk groups for low protein intake such as women, people who are dieting for weight loss and elderly individuals. A safe minimal competitive body weight should be established for female gymnasts, many of whom use disordered eating behaviors to achieve weight loss. For female gymnasts, the minimal body weight should contain no less than 12–14% body fat. They can decrease the intake of calories by reducing dietary lipid, protein and carbohydrate, but should not totally eliminate any one of these three, consuming at least 1500 cal/day to prevent vitamin and mineral deficiencies.

The low energy intake associated with these groups is more likely to result in a low protein intake. Any individuals thought to be at risk should be asked to keep a food record for 3 days and receive counseling concerning low-fat sources of protein, such as lean meats, low-fat or non-fat dairy products, fish and legumes.

A common question could be whether there is any risk in consuming a high protein diet. A high protein diet is known to be detrimental in individuals with kidney and liver disease. It has been suggested that a chronically high protein diet con-

tributes to the development of kidney disorders. Although there is little experimental evidence to support this concern, it would be advisable to limit protein intake to less than 2 g/kg. Protein intake greater than 2 g/kg has not been shown to be beneficial and may have negative effects on overall dietary quality, excluding high carbohydrate and other nutrient dense foods from the diet.

It is the authors' opinion that an adequate protein intake, in the range of 1.2–1.8 g/kg, can help an individual who is active in aerobic or resistance training to reach his potential by preserving muscle tissue and possibly enhancing recovery after strenuous exercise.

Protein catabolism during exercise becomes pronounced when carbohydrate reserves deplete. The amino-acid alanine plays a key role in providing carbohydrate fuel during prolonged exercise via gluconeogenesis. During strenuous exercise of long duration, the alanine-glucose cycle accounts for up to 10–15% of the total amount of energy expenditure.

Role of fats

If carbohydrates are not available or available only in a limited amount, the intensity of the exercise must be reduced to a level where the greater part of the energy requirement can be met by fat oxidation.[8]

For the athlete with very high levels of energy expenditure in training, the exercise intensity will inevitably be reduced to a level where fatty acid oxidation will make a substantial contribution to energy supply and fat will provide an important energy source in the diet. Marathon and triathlon are examples of sports that depend on fat oxidation (Fig. 3.2).

Plasma triacylglycerols (TGs), free fatty acids (FFAs) and muscle triacylglycerols (TG) are oxidizable lipid fuel sources for skeletal muscle metabolism during prolonged exercise. Plasma FFAs are a major fuel oxidized by skeletal muscle, and their rate of use by muscle depends on several factors, including their plasma concentration, transport from plasma to the mitochondria, and intracellular metabolism. Mobilization of FFAs from adipose tissue is the first step in FFA metabolism, and it depends on the rate of adipose tissue lipolysis. Adipose tissue lipolysis increases with exercise duration and intensity up to approximately 60–65% of VO_2max.[8]

Evidence suggests that FFAs are transported from plasma to the mitochondria by FFA carrier proteins that include the plasma membrane and cytosolic plasma membrane fatty acid-binding protein ($FABP_{PM}$) and cytoplasmic fatty acid-binding protein ($FABP_c$). Plasma FFA use can also be regulated at the mitochondrial transport step by changes in the activity of carnitine palmitoyltransferase (CPT-1).[9,10]

Although results from biopsy and tracer studies indicate that muscle TG contribute to skeletal muscle oxidative metabolism during exercise, their exact contribution is difficult to ascertain in quantitative terms.[11]

Dietary strategies can modulate substrate use during exercise and can potentially affect exercise performance. High carbohydrate availability before exercise is associated with an increase in blood glucose and plasma insulin concentrations which can, in the end, decrease the rate of adipose tissue

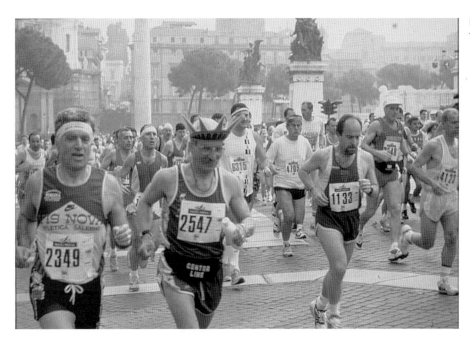

Figure 3.2 Marathon is an example of sport that depends on fat oxidation.

lipolysis and the availability of plasma FFAs. Increased glucose flux has also been shown to decrease lipid oxidation by directly inhibiting the transport of FFAs across the mitochondrial membranes. High lipid availability can be altered by short-term or long-term exposure to high-fat diets. The value of feeding a high-fat diet in preparation for competition is still a matter of considerable debate. There is evidence both for and against the hypothesis that training on a high-fat diet a few weeks before competition can improve performance by promoting fat utilization and sparing glycogen stores. It is likely that differences in diet composition exercise models, and in the training status of athletes, make comparisons between studies very difficult.

MICRONUTRIENTS

Vitamins

Of special significance in the metabolic mixture are the micronutrients, the small quantity of vitamins and minerals that play highly specific roles in facilitating energy transfer and tissue synthesis. For example, the body requires, each year, only about 350 g (12 oz) of vitamins from the 820 kg (1820 lb) of food consumed by the average adult.[5]

Some 13 different vitamins have been isolated, analyzed, classified and synthesized, and have established recommended dietary allowance (RDA) levels. Vitamins are classified as either fat-soluble or water-soluble. The fat-soluble vitamins are vitamins A, D, E and K; the water-soluble vitamins are vitamin C and the B-complex vitamins (based on their common source distribution and common functional relationships): pyridoxine (B_6), thiamine (B_1), riboflavin (B_2), niacin (nicotinic acid), pantothenic acid, biotin, folic acid (folacin or folate, its active form in the body) and cobalamin (B_{12}).

Fat-soluble vitamins

Because fat-soluble vitamins dissolve and store in the body's fatty tissues, they need not be ingested daily. In fact, years may elapse before symptoms of a fat-soluble vitamin insufficiency become evident. The liver stores vitamins A and D, whereas vitamin E is distributed throughout the body's fatty tissues. Vitamin K is stored only in small amounts, mainly in the liver. Dietary lipid provides the source of fat-soluble vitamins; these vitamins, transported as part of lipoproteins in the lymph, travel to the liver for dispersion to various body tissues.

Fat-soluble vitamins should not be consumed in excess without medical supervision. There is no evidence that daily supplementation above the recommended level of fat-soluble vitamins can be beneficial for sports performance. However, a daily moderate to large excess of vitamin A and D can produce serious toxic effects. For example, an excess of vitamin A in adults can cause nausea, headache, drowsiness, loss of hair, diarrhea and loss of calcium from bones; kidney damage can result from an excess of vitamin D.

Water-soluble vitamins

The water-soluble vitamins act largely as coenzymes, with small molecules combining with a larger protein compound (apoenzyme) to form an active enzyme that accelerates the interconversion of chemical compounds. Coenzymes participate directly in chemical reactions; when the reaction runs its course, coenzymes remain intact and participate in additional reactions. Water-soluble vitamins, similar to their fat-soluble counterparts, consist of carbon, hydrogen and oxygen atoms. They also contain nitrogen and metal ions including iron, molybdenum, copper, sulphur and cobalt.

Because of their solubility in water, water-soluble vitamins disperse in the body fluids without being stored to any appreciable extent. Sweating, even during strenuous physical activity, produces negligible losses of water-soluble vitamins.

An excess intake of water-soluble vitamins becomes voided in the urine. Water-soluble vitamins probably exert their influence for 8–14 h after ingestion, then their effectiveness begins to decrease. For maximum benefit, for example, vitamin C supplements should be consumed at least every 12 h.

Although vitamins contain no useful energy for the body, they do serve as essential links and regulators in metabolic reactions that release energy production from food. Vitamins also control the processes of tissue synthesis and aid in protecting the integrity of the cells' plasma membrane.

The vitamin needs of athletes do not exceed those of sedentary counterparts. Well-balanced meals provide an adequate quantity of all vitamins, regardless of age and physical activity level. Indeed, individuals who expend considerable energy exercising do not need to consume special foods or supplements that increase the vitamin content above recommended levels. In addition, at high levels of daily physical activity, food intake is generally increased in order to sustain the added energy requirements of exercise. Additional food through a variety of nutritious meals proportionately increases vitamins intake. Different athletic groups receive relatively low intakes of vitamins B_1 and B_6.[12–14] Adequate intake of these two vitamins occurs if the daily diet contains fresh fruit, grains and uncooked or steamed vegetables. Individuals on meatless diets should consume a small amount of milk, milk products, or eggs because vitamin B_{12} exists only in foods of animal origin.

Antioxidants role of specific vitamins

Although regular physical activity is known to have many beneficial effects, it results in an increased production of radicals and other forms of reactive oxygen species (ROS).[15–18] In fact, evidence exists to implicate ROS as an underlying cause in exercise-induced disturbances in muscle homeostasis (e.g. redox status), which could result in muscle fatigue or injury.[19,20,21]

Muscle cells contain complex cellular defense mechanisms to minimize the risk for oxidative injury. Two major classes of endogenous protective mechanisms work together to reduce the harmful effects of oxidants in the cell: enzymatic and non-enzymatic antioxidants. Key antioxidant enzymes include superoxide dismutase, glutathione peroxidase and catalase. These enzymes are responsible for removing superoxide radicals, hydrogen peroxide or organic hydroperoxides and hydrogen peroxide, respectively. Important non-enzymatic antioxidants include vitamins E and C, beta-carotene, GSH, uric acid, ubiquinone and bilirubin. Vitamin E, beta-carotene and ubiquinone are located in the lipid regions of the cell, whereas uric acid, GSH and bilirubin are in water compartments of the cell.

To date, limited reports have examined the effects of antioxidant supplementation on muscular performance in humans. Furthermore, many of these studies suffer experimental design weaknesses, and most studies have investigated the effects of a single antioxidant rather than investigating the combined effects of both lipid-soluble and water soluble antioxidants. So far, the most widely studied antioxidant vitamin is vitamin E,

whereas few studies have examined the effects of other antioxidants on human performance.[22]

Although several studies have indicated that supplementation with vitamin E and vitamin C[23] decreases exercise-induced oxidative stress in humans, little evidence shows that antioxidant supplementation can improve human performance.

One well-designed study has reported an improvement in human performance following supplementation with antioxidants. In this study, Reid *et al.* administered 150 mg of N-acetylcysteine to human subjects and measured muscular fatigue during low-frequency electrical stimulation. Results revealed an improvement in muscular endurance following treatment with this antioxidant.[24]

To date, limited evidence shows that dietary supplementation with antioxidants improves human exercise performance. However, because of the paucity of research on this topic, many additional studies are required before a firm conclusion can be reached about the effects of antioxidant treatment on human exercise performance. Future studies should examine the potential synergistic effects of several different antioxidants on human performance.

Nutrition and immune function

A fundamental characteristic of the immune system is that it involves multiple functionally different cell types which permit a large variety of defense mechanisms.

A heavy schedule of training and competition can lead to immune impairment in athletes, which is associated with an increased susceptibility to infections, particularly upper respiratory tract infections (URTI).[25] This exercise-induced immune dysfunction seems to be mostly due to the immunosuppressive actions of stress hormones such as adrenaline and cortisol. Nutritional deficiencies can also impair immune function and there is a vast body of evidence that many infections are increased in prevalence by specific nutritional deficiencies.[25]

Dietary immunostimulants

β-Carotene (pro-vitamin A) acts both as an antioxidant and an immunostimulant, increasing the number of T-helper cells in healthy humans and stimulating natural killer cell activity when added *in vitro* to human lymphatic cultures.[26] Furthermore, elderly men who had been taking β-carotene supplements (50 mg on alternate days) for 10–12 years were reported to have significantly higher natural killer cell activity than elderly men on placebo.[26] However, supplementing runners with β-carotene was not found to have a significant effect on the incidence of URTI after a 90-km ultramarathon.[27]

Several herbal preparations are reputed to have immunostimulatory effects, and consumption of products containing *Echinacea purpurea* is widespread among athletes. However, few controlled studies have examined the effects of dietary immunostimulants on exercise-induced changes in immune function. In one recent double-blind, placebo-controlled study, the effect of a daily oral pre-treatment for 28 days with pressed juice of *E. purpurea* was investigated in 42 triathletes before and after a sprint triathlon. A sub-group was also treated with magnesium as a reference for supplementation with a micronutrient important for optimal muscular function. The most important finding was that during the 28-days pre-treatment period, none of the athletes in the *Echinacea* group felt ill, compared with three individuals in the magnesium group and four in the placebo group.[28] Pre-treatment with *Echinacea* appeared to reduce the release of soluble IL-2 receptor before and after the race and increased the exercise-induced rise in IL-6.

Probiotics are food supplements that contain 'friendly' gut bacteria. There is now a reasonable body of evidence that regular consumption of probiotics can modify the population of the gut microflora and influence immune function.[25] Some studies have shown that probiotic intake can improve rates of recovery from rotavirus diarrhea, increase resistance to enteric pathogens and promote anti-tumor activity. Furthermore, there is some evidence that probiotics may be effective in alleviating some allergic and respiratory disorders in young children. However, to date, there are no published studies of the effectiveness or safety of probiotic use in athletes.

Minerals

Approximately 4% of the body's mass (about 2 kg for a 50-kg woman), consist of a group of 22 mostly metallic elements, collectively called minerals.

Minerals serve as constituents of enzymes, hormones and vitamins, and exist in combination with other chemicals (e.g. calcium phosphate in bone, iron in the heme of hemoglobin) or exist singularly (free calcium in body fluids).

Minerals, essential to life, are classified into major (seven minerals required in amounts of more than 100 mg daily) or minor or trace minerals (14 minerals required in amounts of less than 100 mg daily).

Mineral supplements, like vitamins, generally confer little benefit in terms of sports performance because these minerals are readily available in our food and water. Some supplementation may be necessary, however, in geographic regions where the soil or water supply lacks a particular mineral.

While vitamins activate chemical processes without becoming part of the by-products of the reactions they catalyze, minerals often become incorporated within the structures and existing chemical in the body.

Minerals provide structure in forming bones and teeth, activate numerous reactions that release energy during carbohydrate, fat and protein metabolism. In addition, minerals are essential for synthesizing biologic nutrients, such as glycogen from glucose, triglycerides from fatty acids, and glycerol and proteins from amino acids. The fine balance between catabolism and anabolism would be disrupted without the essential minerals. Minerals also form important components of hormones.

Iron

Iron deficiency is one of the most prevalent nutrient deficiencies observed in female athletes.[29] This high incidence of iron deficiency is usually attributed to several factors. First, female athletes often have poor iron intake, which is usually attributed to a diet poor in foods high in heme iron, such as meat, fish and poultry. These diets have a low caloric content restricting energy intake. If energy intake is restricted, total daily iron intake will be lower unless a supplement is added to the diet. Second, many female athletes follow vegetarian diets, which provide no heme iron. Therefore, the bioavailability of the iron consumed is reduced. Finally, female athletes may have increased iron losses through menstrual blood and iron lost in sweat, feces and urine.

Examination of the dietary iron intake of female athletes who do not take iron supplements shows large variations in iron intake, depending on when the data were collected. Studies published in the late 1980s and early 1990s typically reported the dietary iron intakes of female athletes to be less than the RDA of 15 mg/d[28]; however, recent studies report higher iron intakes in female athletes from the diet only.[30]

The increased prevalence of fortified foods in the typical US diet and the diets of athletes has increased the intake of many micronutrients, including iron; however, this increased intake of iron did not reduce the prevalence of iron deficiency in these athletes. The diagnosis of asiderotic anemia results from the hemachrome which shows the presence of microcythemia (with small red blood cells), with decrease in the values of sideremia and ferritin, while transferrin is normal or increased. Altered values in the long run can lead to a decrease in the hemoglobin. Reports of the incidence of poor iron status in active women are variable and often depend on the sport and the type of athlete examined. When ferritin concentrations are used as the assessment criteria (either <12 or <20 μg/l are typically used), 15–60% of female athletes are reported to have low iron stores.[29] This number is somewhat higher than the incidence of iron deficiency seen in the non-athletic US adolescent and adult female population (20–30%).[29] Because of the high incidence of iron deficiency in active women, assessment of iron status, including dietary iron intake, should be routinely performed in female athletes. Care should also be taken to determine whether changes in iron status reflect alterations in iron stores and are not artificially caused by the changes in plasma volume that occur with training.

Recommended dietary allowances for iron are for adult male 10 mg/day and for adult female in fertile age, 20 mg/day. Supplements should not be used indiscriminately because excessive iron can accumulate to toxic levels and contribute significantly to ailments like diabetes, liver disease and joint damage.

Electrolytes and fluid

The recommended daily dietary allowances for sodium, potassium and magnesium are approximately 1100–3100 mg, 1900–5600 mg and 350 mg, respectively. These values are based on the average human and do not consider the potentially substantial losses that accrue in active individuals, particularly those involved in endurance training.

Sweat, although hypotonic, does contain small amounts of sodium, chloride, potassium and lesser quantities of other substances.[31,32] Sweat sodium concentration generally ranges from 10–70 mEq/l but is generally 10–30 mEq/l in physically active, heat-acclimated individuals. As sweating rates increase, the salt content of sweat increases. Heat acclimatization increases sodium and chloride reabsorption and secretion of a more hypotonic sweat.[33] Dietary factors also influence the amount of salt in sweat. For example, during periods of low dietary sodium intake, aldosterone secretion acts to increase renal and sweat gland sodium reabsorption to preserve body sodium content. The result is secretion of sweat with lower than usual amounts of sodium.

The maintenance of salt balance is important for minimizing risk for heat-related injuries. Physical activity increases salt losses. In hot climates, it can produce sodium deficits in excess of 8 g/day.[33] Salt balance is also important for restoring water balance because sustained rehydration can only be achieved by replacing the electrolytes lost daily in sweat and urine.[34,35] However, salt supplementation has not been shown to improve exercise performance or exercise-heat tolerance.[33]

Nevertheless, in hot weather conditions, if prolonged exercise is planned, some dietary salt supplementation may be required to sustain sodium balance. In general, the added caloric intake associated with exercises provides the necessary sodium, so no additional salt beyond what is in food is necessary.

Magnesium deficiencies caused by sweating seem unlikely. The concentration of magnesium in sweat is low, ranging from 0.02–0.3 mmol/l and 0.8–5 mmol/l. The average daily intake of magnesium is 10–15 mmol.[30,35] Studies examining muscle magnesium concentration during repeated days of heavy sweating (daily sweat losses of >3 l) found no change in muscle magnesium over time.[36]

Potassium is lost in sweat at a rate of approximately 0.3–15.0 mEq/l. The rate of loss does not change with prolonged sweating or heat acclimation. Costill reported that plasma and muscle potassium were well maintained during 4 days of heavy sweating (3 l/day) even on a low-potassium (25 mmol/day) diet.[36] With the exception of the first few days of heat exposure or during periods of long-duration physical activity in hot climates, dietary electrolyte supplementation seems unnecessary. Generally, a normal dietary intake provides sufficient electrolytes to maintain electrolyte balance. Under such conditions, salting food to taste or drinking electrolyte beverages may be indicated to sustain daily water-salt balance.

The American College of Sports Medicine recommends that individuals consume 400–600 ml of water 2 hours before exercise, independent of body weight.[37] This volume adequately offsets any deficit accumulated in the earlier hours and provides sufficient time for renal mechanisms to regulate total-body water and osmolality. Drinking water is sufficient. However, consumption of a commercial sports drink provides carbohydrate which also optimizes muscle and liver glycogen stores before exercise. If possible, an additional 200–300 ml is recommended during the final minutes before beginning competition so that exercise is started with water entering the circulation during the initial minutes of exercise. As such, fluid losses are offset at the onset of water loss, rather than after a deficit has occurred.

Exercise performance can be compromised by a body water deficit, particularly when exercise is performed in hot climates. It is recommended that individuals begin exercise when adequately hydrated. As mentioned above, this can be facilitated by drinking 400–600 ml of fluids 2 h before beginning exercise, but mainly by drinking sufficiently during exercise to prevent dehydration from exceeding 2% body weight. A practical recommendation is to drink small amounts of fluid (150–300 ml) every 15–20 min of exercise, varying the volume depending on sweating rate.

During exercise lasting less than 90 min, water only is sufficient for fluid replacement. During prolonged exercise longer than 90 min, commercially available carbohydrate electrolyte beverages should be considered to provide an exogenous carbohydrate source to sustain carbohydrate oxidation and endurance performance. Electrolyte supplementation is generally not necessary during exercise because dietary intake is adequate to offset electrolytes lost in sweat and urine; however, during initial days of hot weather training or when meals are not calorically adequate, supplemental salt intake may be indicated to maintain sodium balance.

SUPPLEMENTS AND ERGOGENIC AIDS

Products that claim to be performance enhancing are popular with recreational and elite athletes. Some of these products are classified as drugs, others as supplements.

None of the supplements and ergogenic aids described are included in the 2005 World Anti-doping Agency (WADA) prohibited list. Only caffeine has been placed on the 2005 Monitoring Program. WADA, in consultation with other signatories and Governments, has established a monitoring program regarding substances which are not on the prohibited list, but which WADA wishes to monitor in order to detect patterns of misuse in sport.

Often, performance-enhancing products are purchased based on popular magazine advertisements or peer or coach recommendations rather than professional medical advice.[38] Furthermore, some products are popular and marketed as ergogenic, despite a lack of objective evidence to support claims of an ergogenic effect (Table 3.1).[39] In the US for example, ergogenic claims of supplements can be made without control by the Food and Drug Administration (FDA), since the controversial passage of the Dietary Supplement Health and Education Act in 1994.[40] We will describe some of these products and the scientific studies that have tested their efficacy in enhancing exercise or sports performance.

Creatine
Creatine supplementation is the most popular nutritional supplement today. According to the *Nutrition Business Journal*, sales in the year 2000 were estimated at more than US$300m in the US only; a 3-fold increase since 1997.

Table 3.1 List of Supplements and their Effectiveness

Supplement	Proposed Action	Effectiveness
Creatine	Increase the rate of CP resynthesis; improvement of capability to maintain repetitive burst of intense exercise with little recovery time	Scientific evidence
β-Hydroxy-β-methylbutyrate	Increase strength and lean body mass preventing muscle breakdown	No scientific evidence in trained individuals
Proteins and amino acids	Development further of muscle hypertrophy and strength	No scientific evidence
Pyruvate	Ergogenic effect, glucose oxidation, lipid breakdown	Potential effect at high dose; need of further investigations
Caffeine	Ergogenic effect in endurance activity	Scientific evidence
Carnitine	Increase fat acid oxidation, glycogen sparing effect	No scientific effect
Bicarbonate and other buffers	Reduction of metabolic acidosis in high intensity work (exercise lasting from about 30 s to a few minutes)	Some scientific evidence but collateral effects

Creatine was discovered by Chevreul in 1832 but the first reported use of creatine by elite athletes did not occur until the 1992 Summer Olympic Games in Barcelona by British track and field athletes. During the last 10 years, the use of creatine has become popular, particularly in anaerobic sporting events.

Several prevalence studies among college athletes report a utilization rate of 41–48% among men.

Creatine is a naturally occurring compound made from the amino acids glycine, arginine, and methionine. Primarily synthesized in the liver, pancreas and kidney, 95% of the creatine is stored in skeletal muscle. These stores are broken down at a relatively constant rate of 2 g/dl into creatinine, which is excreted by the kidney. Exogenous sources of creatine include fresh fish and meat. Daily turnover is approximately 2 g creatine concentrations in skeletal muscle average 125 mmol/kg of dry muscle, with a higher capacity for storage in type II muscle fibers. In its phosphorylated form, creatine contributes to the rapid resynthesis of adenosine triphosphate during short-duration maximal bouts of anaerobic exercise. This mechanism forms the basis for creatine supplementation. Most research studies on creatine supplementation examining exercise performance involved doses of 20–30 g/day for 5–7 days.

In 1992, Harris and collaborators[41] showed that oral creatine supplementation resulted in a significant increase in the total creatine content of the quadriceps femoris muscle, in some subjects reaching as high as 50%. Further studies by Balsom and colleagues have shown that creatine supplementation may delay or decrease anaerobic glycolysis during brief maximal exercise.[42] These effects may enhance anaerobic training, leading to strength and performance gains in these athletes.

Exercise performance in humans taking creatine supplements has been studied extensively.[43,44] Typical designs of these studies have been longitudinal, prospective, randomized and placebo controlled. A relatively small group of athletes was included in most studies. Athletes were evaluated with a sport-specific test before and then after several weeks (in most studies) of creatine supplementation.

In weightlifters, the number of repetitions at a specified percentage of the single-repetition maximum, increases approximately 20–30% after a short-term creatine supplementation period (Fig. 3.3).

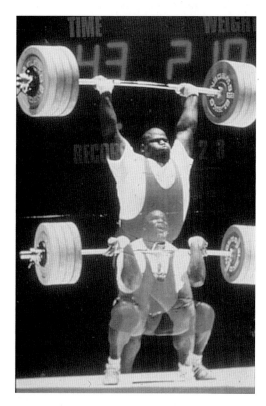

Figure 3.3 Short-term creatine supplementation increases 20–30% the number of repetitions at a specified percentage of single maximum-repetition in weightlifters.

In cyclists, most studies have shown that creatine supplementation is effective in maintaining muscular force and power output. In swimming, performance has been measured with repeated short sprints of maximal intensity. Results have been mixed, with some studies showing a significant reduction in sprint times, whereas others have found the opposite and concluded that creatine supplementation is not effective in swimmers (Fig. 3.4). Differences in these studies may be attributed to different outcome measures, the complex mechanism of the swimming stroke, or different supplementation regimens.[45]

In track and field sprinters, several studies have shown an improvement in mean sprint times in the range of 1–2%, whereas the authors of two other studies concluded that creatine had no effect on single sprint times (Fig. 3.5).[46]

In terms of body composition changes, creatine supplementation appears to increase body weight and lean body mass by approximately 1–2 kg during a short-term supplementation cycle.

In several studies, creatine has been shown to be ineffective. These include supplementation in older athletes (60–87 years of age) and in aerobic sports, although the latter study[45] did find an approximate 18% benefit in the final 'kick' phase of an aerobic event.

In summary, these studies suggest that creatine can be an effective ergogenic supplement when used for simple, short-duration, maximal-effort anaerobic events.

Since the introduction of creatine in the early 1990s, there have been a number of isolated case reports of renal side-effects associated with its use. Although creatine is commonly thought to lead to dehydration, to date, there has been no study that has demonstrated negative side-effects with the use of creatine in athletes. It should be cautioned, however, that the studies that have been done are mostly of short duration and in healthy individuals. We do not know the long-term effects of this supplement, nor do we have sufficient data on the possible effects on other creatine-containing tissues such as

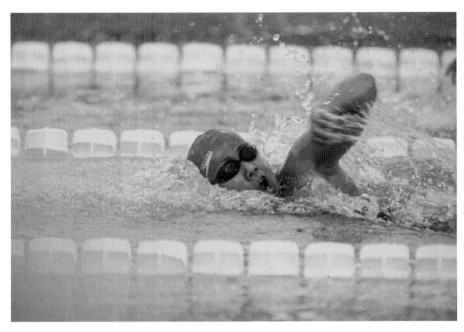

Figure 3.4 Creatine supplementation is not effective in swimmers.

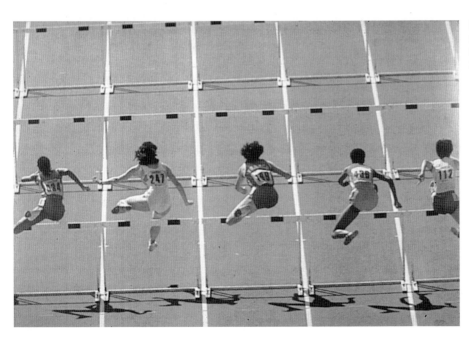

Figure 3.5 Improvement in mean sprint times was found in track and field sprinters after creatine supplementation. (From Bosco et al. 1997,[46] with permission.)

the brain, cardiac muscle, or testes. In addition, several authors caution that long-term administration of creatine will likely lead to the downregulation of the creatine carrier protein and, thus, an increased resistance to the compound.

The exact maintenance dose required to retain muscle creatine stores for various populations is not known; however, a daily dose of approximately 0.03 g/kg should be adequate to replace the normal breakdown of creatine and maintain elevated creatine stores.[47]

Several types and forms of creatine are available. The most common type of creatine examined in scientific studies is creatine monohydrate. Whether other types of creatine, such as creatine citrate and creatine phosphate, have ergogenic effects is unknown. Initially, creatine was available only in either powder or capsules; now it is available in several forms (e.g. gel, candy and gum) and is also an ingredient in many liquid protein and carbohydrate supplements. The efficacy of some of these other forms (e.g. gums of creatine) in delivering the required doses remains to be demonstrated. Doses may vary depending on the serving size of the particular product. Thus, care should be taken when consuming creatine-containing products to ensure their purity and that the appropriate and intended dose only is consumed.

Many unanswered questions in fact remain concerning creatine supplementation, including strategies to maximize creatine accumulation in muscle; doses needed to load muscle (should be much lower than the 20–25 g/day used thus far, for example, 3–5 g/day); doses required to maintain elevated creatine stores in muscle; aspects related to the matrix of delivery, timing of intake, it is not clear in fact, how long before the beginning of training session the creatine has to be assumed, individual variability in creatine accumulation and factors regulating the creatine receptor on muscle and transport in tissues.

Thus, although it appears that short-term supplementation with creatine is safe; many concerns have been raised that the effects of long-term use of large doses of creatine are unknown, and that its use may represent a risk for health. Concerns seem to focus primarily on the possible effects on renal function, in particular in individuals with impaired renal capacity. Studies on the response to long-term creatine use are in progress at this time, but results are not yet available. However, there have been no reports of adverse effects in any of the studies published in the literature, or in any athletes taking creatine supplements.

β-Hydroxy-β-methylbutyrate

β-hydroxy-β-methylbutyrate (HMB) is a metabolite of the essential amino acid leucine. It is promoted as a supplement to increase strength and lean body mass, not because it is truly anabolic, but by preventing muscle breakdown.

HMB is metabolized to hydroxymethylglutaryl coenzyme A, which has been hypothesized to be the rate-limiting enzyme when cholesterol synthesis is in demand.[48] Because cholesterol synthesis is needed in membrane repair, it is thought that HMB supplementation can decrease muscle damage and enhance the process of recovery. Despite the popularity and heavy marketing of this product, it has yet to be proven effective, and studies on the ergogenic effect of HMB have been controversial.[49]

Knitter et al. studied 13 untrained individuals supplemented with 3 g/day of HMB for 6 weeks, and found that the HMB group had a lower increase in creatine phosphokinase and lactate dehydrogenase after a 20 km run, supporting the hypothesis that HMB may prevent muscle damage. However, the study does not concern performance, and does not support, or refute, the cholesterol synthesis theory.[50]

In a study funded by two sports supplement companies, Gallagher and colleagues studied untrained college men during 8 weeks of resistance training, supplementing one experimental group (n = 12) with 3 g/day of HMB, the other group (n = 11) with 6 g/day HMB.[51] The results were mixed and therefore difficult to draw conclusions from. One repetition maximum strength did not improve in either group. The 3 g/day group did show a greater increase in peak isometric torque than placebo, but interestingly, also greater than the 6 g/day group. No differences were observed in body fat among the three groups, but the 3 g/day group showed a greater increase in fat-free mass than placebo. Strangely, the 6 g/day group did not show a greater increase in fat free mass than placebo. The authors conclude that HMB appears to increase peak isometric and isokinetic torque values, and increase fat free mass. Such a conclusion seems not to be warranted as the two experimental groups varied in their results.

In another study on untrained individuals, Jowko et al. studied 3 g/day HMB supplementation with resistance training in nine men, and found beneficial results in six of seven strength tests compared with placebo, but not significant changes in body fat or lean body mass.[52]

The results of HMB on trained individuals are less promising. A recent study by Slater and colleagues found that HMB supplementation for 6 weeks did not affect strength or body composition in trained men. It is thought that this may be due to the training-induced suppression of protein breakdown.[53]

On a positive note, Gallagher and colleagues found that HMB did not adversely affect lipid profiles, hepatic enzyme levels or renal function in their study participants.[54] The safety of HMB was further addressed by Nissen and colleagues at Iowa State University and no untoward effects were seen, although the longest study was only 8 weeks' duration.[55]

HMB, is probably safe when taken for 8 weeks or less and may have a role as an ergogenic aid in untrained individuals. However, the data on trained individuals are far less convincing. Further research, not only on performance but also on the cholesterol synthesis hypothesis, would be of value in understanding the role of HMB in exercise and muscle breakdown.

Proteins and amino acids

Arguably, proteins and amino acids are the most heavily marketed category of sports supplements. Despite the known role of amino acids and protein synthesis in the development of muscle hypertrophy and strength, the need for additional supplementation over and above the amount provided in the diet, is highly questionable. It is generally accepted that athletes have a greater daily protein requirement than sedentary people. The recommended daily allowance is 0.8 g/kg per day for adults, but ranges from 1.2–1.8 g/kg per day for athletes, with the higher range being reserved for strength athletes.[56]

Despite the acceptance of the additional protein needs of athletes, most athletes eat well enough to obtain the required amount of protein in their diet, and there is little evidence to support the additional consumption of protein or amino acids for enhancing sports performance.[57] Williams and collaborators studied seven untrained individuals supplemented with a glucose/amino product for 10 weeks. They utilized a clever design, whereby alternate legs within the same individuals were trained on successive days, so each individual in a training group served as his or her own control. The study design minimized the inter-individual variability inherent in other small sample size studies. The investigators found no strength benefits of the supplementation.[58] In another study, Jentjens and colleagues found that the addition of protein and amino acids to a carbohydrate diet did not enhance post-exercise muscle glycogen synthesis.[59] A widely cited, double-blind, crossover study by Lemon and colleagues in 1992 found that supplemental protein intake did not increase muscle mass or strength in novice bodybuilders.[60]

The branched chain amino acids (BCAAs) are leucine, isoleucine and valine. Theoretically, these amino acids decrease protein-induced degradation, which can lead to a greater fat-free mass.[57] The data on BCAAs as an ergogenic aid are not convincing. For example, Davis and collaborators studied the effects of BCAA administration with sports drink in individuals who performed intermittent, high-intensity running, with no beneficial effect noted.[61] Some studies have suggested that BCAAs may reduce exercise-induced muscle damage based on creatine phosphokinase and lactate dehydrogenase levels, but did not evaluate performance.[62] BCAAs, while representing an essential component of diet, are not ergogenic even when taken in large quantities as a dietary supplement. In this regard, Wagenmakers asserts that BCAAs may be ergolytic (detrimental to performance) due to a negative effect on aerobic oxygenation.[63]

In fact, excessive acceleration of the metabolism of BCAA drains 2-oxoglutarate in the primary aminotransferase reaction and thus reduces flux in the citric acid cycle and impedes aerobic oxidation of glucose and fatty acids.

While protein and amino acids are essential components of the regular diet, studies on supplemental protein are not convincing. Individuals wishing to take amino acid or protein supplements should be told that a proper diet is sufficient, and that dietary protein provides 20 essential and nonessential amino acids, including those that are marketed as 'ergogenic', such as leucine, isoleucine, lysine, alanine and glutamine.

Pyruvate

Pyruvate is a carboxylic acid produced by the metabolism of glucose. In 1990, Stanko and colleagues published two studies that involved upper and lower limb endurance capacity in individuals who consumed pyruvate.[64] The results of these studies caught the eye of the supplement industry and pyruvate was aggressively marketed by companies as being performance enhancing for endurance events. The unproven mechanism was that pyruvate enhances glucose oxidation.

The analysis of these studies, however, shows that both involved untrained individuals and a very small sample size

(8–10 individuals), and neither study used pyruvate alone. The upper limb study[64] utilized dihydroxyacetone and a pre-event high carbohydrate diet. The dose of pyruvate utilized (25 g) was also much higher than that marketed by supplement companies, which is usually 5 g. High doses can cause gastric distress, which also raises doubts about the feasibility of conducting true double-blind trials. Furthermore, pyruvate is usually marketed alone. The pyruvate/dihydroxyacetone combination product is commonly known as DHAP.

Morrison and colleagues[65] did a recent study that incorporated a randomized double-blind crossover design ($n = 7$), and found that 7 g of pyruvate for 7 days did not improve cycling performance time (approximately 90 min cycling). Equally important, blood pyruvate levels did not even increase, despite the supplementation. In a separate study by Morrison, included in the same paper,[65] nine recreationally active individuals ingested 7, 15, and 25 g of pyruvate, but again no effect was found on blood pyruvate, glucose or lipid metabolism. This is of particular interest because pyruvate is also marketed as a weight-loss and cholesterol-lowering agent; neither effect has been proven.[66] Unlike the studies by Stanko and colleagues, those by Morrison involved trained individuals, and most sports medicine specialists will find them more clinically relevant.

The studies by Stanko et al.[64] may reveal some potential of high dose pyruvate/dihydroxyacetone in untrained individuals, but the dose necessary cast significant doubt on the feasibility of this regimen, particularly in trained athletes.

Caffeine

Caffeine is an adenosine-receptor antagonist and a stimulant of the dimethyl-xanthine class. The mechanism for the ergogenic effect of caffeine remains somewhat inconclusive in humans, although rat studies clearly show that caffeine inhibits adenosine receptors,[67] and such receptors are located throughout the human body. A theory that has been put forward is the stimulation of adrenaline secretion, resulting in the mobilization of free-fatty acids an important fuel for muscle. This increase in fat utilization decreases carbohydrate utilization, thus delaying glycogen depletion.[68] Recent studies have failed to support this theory.[69]

The evidence supporting caffeine's ergogenic potential is strong, particularly during aerobic activity.[70] In a double-blind, crossover study, Kovacs and colleagues studied 15 well-trained male triathletes and cyclists in a 1-h cycling time trial at 75% maximal exercise capacity.[70] Three different dosages of caffeine were consumed: 154 mg (2.1 mg/kg), 230 mg (3.2 mg/kg) and 328 mg (4.5 mg/kg). Even when consumed in the lowest dosage, there was improvement in time trial performance. Interestingly, the highest dosage was no more efficacious than the middle dosage, indicating a possible saturation effect of caffeine as an ergogenic aid. Urinary concentrations of caffeine were also measured, and did not reach levels higher than 2.5 µg/ml. This is below the disqualification limits imposed by the International Olympic Committee (IOC) and WADA (12 µg/ml; until the year 2003). Caffeine is not on the WADA 2005 prohibited list, but is placed in a monitoring program established by WADA regarding substances which are not on the prohibited list, but which WADA wishes to monitor in order to detect patterns of misuse in sport.

In a double-blind, crossover study involving physical activity of short duration, Bruce and collaborators found enhancement of the 2000-m rowing performance after caffeine consumption of either 6 or 9 mg/kg.[71] The improvement in time averaged 1%, with a 3% improvement in power output when comparing both caffeine groups to placebo. One strength of Bruce's study is that all eight study participants were well trained.

Even for sprint activity, caffeine has shown ergogenic potential in a single cycling or swimming sprint.[72]

The doses of caffeine used in studies range from 2–9 mg/kg (about 250–700 mg caffeine), taken 1 h or less prior to the event. Clearly, an ergogenic effect of caffeine in aerobic activity is demonstrated in doses that would not reach the disqualifying levels which have been imposed in the past by the IOC and WADA, as it takes approximately 9 mg/kg consumed to achieve a urinary concentration of 12 μg/ml.[70]

Negative effects of caffeine are minimal; however, those on the central nervous system include anxiety and dependency. Although coffee is not considered the ideal method of consumption of caffeine (tablets are the usual recommendation), it should be emphasized that coffee tablets can vary greatly in their caffeine content. The content of caffeine in common foods and drinks is summarized by Harland.[73]

Carnitine

Fatty acid uptake into the cell and translocation across the mitochondrial membrane are key steps in fat oxidation. Carnitine combines with fatty acetyl-coenzyme A (acyl-CoA) in the cytoplasm and allows fatty acid to enter the mitochondrion. The first step is catalyzed by carnitine palmitoyl transferase 1 (CPT1) and trans-membrane transport is facilitated by acyl carnitine transferase. Within the mitochondrion, the action of carnitine palmitoyl transferase 2 (CPT2) regenerates free carnitine and the fatty acyl-CoA is released for entry into the β-oxidation pathway.

Within the mitochondrion, carnitine also functions to regulate the acetyl-CoA concentration and the concentration of free CoA. Free CoA is involved in the pyruvate oxidation and thus plays a key role in the integration of fat and carbohydrate metabolism. It has been proposed that an increased availability of carnitine within the mitochondrion might allow the cell to maintain a higher free CoA concentration, with a stimulatory effect on oxidative metabolism.

Because of the key role of carnitine in the oxidation of both fat and carbohydrates, it has been proposed that carnitine supplementation may improve exercise performance. On this basis, carnitine is widely sold in sports shops as a supplement for endurance athletes. It is also sold as a weight loss product with claims of increased fat oxidation. Carnitine is present in the diet in red meat and dairy products, so it might be thought that individuals who follow a vegetarian diet might be at increased risk of deficiency, but carnitine can also be synthesized from lysine and methionine in the liver and kidney. Studies on the effects of exercise and diet on muscle carnitine concentrations in humans (muscle accounts for about 98% of the total body carnitine con-

tent) have only been carried out relatively recently, and there have been few attempts to measure the effects of supplementation on muscle carnitine levels. Barnett and colleagues[74] and Vukovic and colleagues[75] reported that short-term supplementation with carnitine (4–6 g/day for 7–14 days) had no effect on muscle carnitine concentrations or on the metabolic response to exercise. Even when fatty acid mobilization was stimulated by high fat meals or heparin, there was no effect of carnitine supplementation on fat oxidation.

In contrast to these negative findings, some published reports suggest that carnitine supplementation can increase the contribution of fatty acids to oxidative metabolism and thus promote the use of body fat stores and spare glycogen stores. In a comprehensive review of the literature, Spriet[76] identified eight studies that examined the effects of supplementation on the metabolic response to endurance exercise, and found that three of these studies reported an increase rate of fat oxidation. There is more recent evidence to support this, with one study showing an increased oxidation of 13C-labelled palmitate after 10 days of carnitine supplementation.[77] This finding is not however, evidence that weight loss and a reduction in body fat content will result from carnitine supplementation.

Bicarbonate and other buffers

Anaerobic glycolysis allows higher rates of ATP resynthesis than can be achieved by aerobic metabolism, but the capacity of the system is limited and fatigue follows rapidly. The metabolic acidosis that accompanies glycolysis can inhibit key glycolytic enzymes, interfering with Ca^{2+} transport and binding, and directly with the actin–myosin interaction. Induction of a metabolic alkalosis by ingestion of $NAHCO_3$ before exercise can increase both the muscle buffering capacity and the rate of efflux of H^+ from the active muscles, potentially delaying the attainment of a critically low intracellular pH.[78]

Improvements in performance are typically seen in exercise lasting from about 30 s to a few minutes, but several studies have failed to find positive effects, even when they have used exercise of this duration. Effective doses have been large, typically about 0.3 g/kg body mass. There are, of course, potential problems associated with the use of such large doses of bicarbonate. Vomiting and diarrhea are symptoms that are frequently reported as a result of ingestion of even relatively small doses of bicarbonate. One study[79] has investigated the potential of sodium citrate as an exogenous buffer, because sodium citrate might be associated with less gastrointestinal discomfort than sodium bicarbonate.

Sodium citrate does not buffer directly like sodium bicarbonate: the dissociation constant for citrate/citric acid lies well outside the body's pH range, but the consumption of protons during its oxidation effectively generates bicarbonate. McNaughton[79] found that ingestion of sodium citrate had a positive effect on work output, without adverse gastrointestinal symptoms but it failed to have a significant effect on performance in other studies. This a good example of a physiological benefit that does not translate into an enhanced sports performance. For this reason, the true effect remains unclear.

Ingestion of other substances could produce an indirect buffering effect similar to that of sodium citrate. One of these substances is sodium lactate, which would also consume protons when it is metabolized. Using lactate as a buffer may seem counter-intuitive to those who believe that lactic acid causes fatigue but it must be remembered that intracellular acidity causes fatigue, not the accumulation of lactate ions.

Brooks[80] found that lactate can serve as an energy source for exercising muscles. In the study of Fahey and collaborators,[81] the ingestion of 80% poly-lactate and 20% sodium lactate as a 7% solution in water increased blood pH and bicarbonate compared with ingestion of a glucose polymer drink.

CONCLUSION

For today's athletes, the availability of specific food nutrients is of great importance, as physical activity places significant demands on energy expenditure and frequent injuries increase the need for tissue repair and synthesis. For this reason, athletes should establish their nutritional goals and should also be able to translate them into a dietary strategy that will meet these goals.

The use of dietary supplements is widespread in sport, even though most supplements used are probably ineffective.

Although a few supplements have ergogenic potential, their applicability is limited to certain types of exercise and individual variability is a significant factor.

Therefore, it is necessary especially for those who are responsible for athletic teams, to become educated about these products and updated with information about new supplements as they emerge. It is important that athletes understand that supplement use can have a role when food intake is restricted, or as a short-term remedy where a deficiency syndrome has been clearly demonstrated. In addition, there is very little effort on the side of the manufacturers to investigate the potential side-effects of these supplements. Therefore, every athlete that decides to take these products must proceed with extreme caution, above all because the risk of a positive drugs test resulting from the use of sports supplements contaminated with prohibited substances is real.

REFERENCES

1 Björkman O, Wahren J. Glucose homeostatis during and after exercise. In: Horton ES, Terjung RL, eds. Exercise, nutrition, and energy metabolism. New York: MacMillan Library Reference; 1998:100–108.

2 Saltin B, Gollnick PD. Fuel for muscular exercise: Role of carbohydrate. In: Horton ES, Terjung RL, eds. Exercise, nutrition and energy metabolism. New York: MacMillan Library Reference; 1988:45–71.

3 Sherman WM, Costill DL, Fink WJ, et al. Effect of exercise-diet manipulation on muscle glycogen and its subsequent utilization during performance. Int J Sport Med 1981; 2:114–118.

4 Ivy JL, Kuo CH. Regulation of GLUT4 protein and glycogen synthase during muscle glycogen synthesis after exercise. Acta Physiol Scand 1998; 162:295–304.

5 Montain SJ, Hopper MK, Coggan AR, et al. Exercise metabolism intervals after a meal. J Appl Physiol 1991; 70:882–889.

6 Van Erp-Baart AMJ, Saris WHM, Binkhorst RA, et al. Nationwide survey on nutritional habits in elite athletes: Part I. Energy, carbohydrate, protein, and fat intake. Int J Sports Med 1989; 10:3–10.

7 Rankin JW. Nutritional aspects of exercise: Role of protein in exercise. Clin Sports Med Philadelphia 1999; 18:499–511.

8 Coyle EF, Jeukendrup AE, Wagenmakers AJM, et al. Fatty acid oxidation is directly regulated by carbohydrate metabolism during exercise. Am J Physiol 1997; 273:E268.

9 Turcotte LP, Kiens B, Richter EA. Saturation kinetics of palmitate uptake in perfused skeletal muscle. FEBS Letts 1991; 279:327–329.

10 Turcotte LP, Richter EA, Kiens B. Increased plasma FFA uptake and oxidation during prolonged exercise in trained vs. untrained humans. Am J Physiol 1992; 262:791–799.

11 Turcotte LP. Fatty acid binding proteins and muscle lipid metabolism. In: Hargreaves M, Thompson M, eds. Biochemistry of exercise. Champaign, IL: Human Kinetics; 1999:201–215.

12 Van Der Beek EJ. Vitamin supplementation and physical exercise performance. Sports Sci 1991; 9:77–90.

13 Rokitzki L, Sagredos AN, Reub F, et al. Assessment of vitamin B_6 status of strength and speedpower athletes. J Am Coll Nutr 1994; 13:87–91.

14 Haymes EM. Vitamin and mineral supplementation to athletes. Int J Sport Nutr 1991; 1:146–169.

15 Borzone G, Zhao B, Merola AJ, et al. Detection of free radicals by electron spin resonance in rat diaphragm after resistive loading. J Appl Physiol 1994; 77:812–818.

16 Davies K, Quintanilla A, Brooks G, et al. Free radicals and tissue damage produced by exercise. Biochem Biophys Res Commun 1982; 107:1198–1205.

17 Gutteridge JM, Halliwell B. Iron toxicity and oxygen radicals. Baillières Clin Haematol 1989; 2:195–256.

18 O'Neill CA, Stebbins CL, Bonigut S, et al. Production of hydroxyl radicals in contracting skeletal muscle of cats. J Appl Physiol 1996; 81:1197–1206.

19 Reid M, Haack K, Franchek K, et al. Reactive oxygen in skeletal muscle: I. Intracellular oxidant kinetics and fatigue in vitro. J Appl Physiol 1992; 73:1797–1804.

20 Ji LL, Stratman F, Lardy H. Antioxidant enzyme systems in rat liver and skeletal muscle. Arch Biochem Biophys 1988; 263:150–160.

21 Nashawati E, Dimarco A, Supinski G. Effects produced by infusion of a free radical-generating solution into the diaphragm. Am Rev Respir Dis 1993; 147:60–65.

22 Rokitzki L, Logemann E, Sagredos AN, et al. Lipid peroxidation and antioxidant vitamins under extreme endurance stress. Acta Physiol Scand 1994; 151:149–158.

23 Alessio HM, Goldfarb AH. Lipid peroxidation and scavenger enzymes during exercise: Adaptive response to training. J Appl Physiol 1988; 64:1333–1336.

24 Reid MB, Stokic DS, Koch SM, et al. N-acetylcysteine inhibits muscle fatigue in humans. J Clin Invest 1994; 94:2468–2474.

25 Calder PC, Field CJ, Gill HS. Nutrition and Immune Function. Wallingford: CABI Publishing; 2000.

26 Santos MS, Meydani SN, Leka L, et al. Natural killer cell activity in elderly men is enhanced by beta-carotene supplementation. Am J Clin Nutr 1996; 64:772–777.

27 Peters EM, Campbell A, Pawley L. Vitamin A fails to increase resistance to upper respiratory infection in distance runners. South Afr J Sports Med 1992; 7:3–7.

28 Berg A, Northoff H, Konig D. Influence of Echinacin (E31) treatment on the exercise-induced immune response in athletes. J Sports Sci 1998; 17:26–27.

29 Clarkson PM, Haymes EM. Trace mineral requirements for athletes. Int J Sport Nutr 1994; 4:104–119.

30 Beals KA, Manore MM. Nutritional status of female athletes with subclinical eating disorders. J Am Diet Assoc 1998; 98:19–39.

31 Vellar OD, Askevold A. Studies on sweat losses of nutrients: III. Calcium, magnesium and chloride content of whole body cell-free sweat in healthy unacclimatized men under controlled environmental conditions. Scand J Clin Lab Invest 1968; 22:65–71.

32 Verde T, Shephard RJ, Corey P, et al. Sweat composition in exercise and in heat. J Appl Physiol 1982; 53:1540–1545.

33 Allan JR, Wilson CG. Influence of acclimatization on sweat sodium concentration. J Appl Physiol 1971; 30:708–712.

34 Pitts GC, Johnson RE, Consolazio FC. Work in the heat as effected by intake of water, salt and glucose. Am J Physiol 1944; 142:253–259.

35 Noakes TD. Fluid replacement during exercise. In: Holloszy J, ed. Exercise and sport science reviews, Vol 21. Baltimore: Williams & Wilkins; 1993:297–330.

36 Costill DL. Sweating: Its composition and effects on body fluids. Ann NY Acad Sci 1984; 301:160–174.

37 American College of Sports Medicine. Position stand on exercise and fluid replacement. Med Sci Sports Exerc 1996; 28:i–vii.

38 Abbott A. What price the Olympic ideal? Nature 2000; 407:124–127.

39 Sheppard HL, Raichada SM, Kouri KM, et al. Use of creatine and other supplements by members of civilian and military health clubs: a cross-sectional survey. Int J Sport Nutr Exerc Metab 2000; 10:245–259.

40 Dietary Supplements Health and Education Act of 1994. Public law 103–417. 21USC 3419 r (6). United States of America 103rd Congress; 1994.

41 Harris RC, Söderlund K, Hultman E. Elevation of creatine in resting and exercised muscle of normal subjects by creatine supplementation. Clin Sci 1992; 83:367–374.

42   Balsom PD, Ekblom B, Söderlund K, et al. Creatine supplementation and dynamic high-intensity intermittent exercise. Scand J Med Sci Sports 1993; 3:143-149.

43   Earnest CP, Snell PG, Rodriguez R, et al. The effect of creatine monohydrate ingestion on aerobic power indices, muscular strength and body composition. Acta Physiol Scand 1995; 153:207-209.

44   Cooke WH, Barnes WS. The influence of recovery duration on high-intensity exercise performance after oral creatine supplementation. Can J Appl Physiol 1997; 22:454-467.

45   Engelhardt M, Neumann G, Berbalk A, et al. Creatine supplementation in endurance sports. Med Sci Sports Exerc 1998; 30:1123-1129.

46   Bosco C, Tihanyi J, Pucspk J, et al. Effect of oral creatine supplementation on jumping and running performance. Int J Sport Med 1997; 18:369-372.

47   Green AL, Hultman E, MacDonald IA, et al. Carbohydrate ingestion augments skeletal muscle creatine accumulation during creatine supplementation in humans. Am J Physiol 1996; 271:821-826.

48   Nissen SL, Abumrad NN. Nutritional role of the leucine metabolite β-hydroxy-β-methylbutyrate (HMB). Nutr Biochem 1997; 8:300-311.

49   Slater GJ, Jenkins, D. β-hydroxy-β-methylbutyrate (HMB) supplementation and the promotion of muscle growth and strength. Sport Med 2000; 30:105-116.

50   Knitter AE, Panton L, Rathmacher JA, et al. Effects of beta-hydroxy-beta-rnethylbutyrate on muscle damage after a prolonged run. J Appl Physiol 2000; 89:1340-1344.

51   Gallagher PM, Carrithers JA, Godard MP, et al. Beta-hydroxy-beta-methylbutyrate ingestion, Part I: effects on strength and fat free mass. Med Sci Sports Exerc 2000; 32:2109-2115.

52   Jowko E, Ostaszewski P, Jank M, et al. Creatine and beta-hydroxy-beta-methylbutyrate (HMB) additively increase lean body mass and muscle strength during a weight-training program. Nutrition 2001; 17:558-566.

53   Slater G, Jenkins D, Logan P, et al. Beta-hydroxy-beta-methylbutyrate (HMB) supplementation does not affect changes in strength or body composition during resistance training in trained men. Int J Sport Nutr Exerc Metab 2001; 11:384-396.

54   Gallagher PM, Carrithers JA, Godard MP, et al. Beta-hydroxy-beta-methylbutyrate ingestion. Part II: Effects on hematology, hepatic and renal function. Med Sci Sports Exerc 2000; 32:2116-2119.

55   Nissen S, Sharp RL, Panton L, et al. Beta-hydroxy-beta-methylbutyrate (HMB) supplementation in humans is safe and may decrease cardiovascular risk factors. J Nutr 2000; 130:1937-1945.

56   Lemon PW. Beyond the zone: protein needs of active individuals. J Am Coll Nutr 2000; 19:513S-521S.

57   Williams MH. Facts and fallacies of purported ergogenic amino acid supplements. Clin Sports Med 1999; 18:633-649.

58   Williams AG, Dord M Van den, Sharma A, et al. Is glucose/amino acid supplementation after exercise an aid to strength training? Br J Sports Med 2001; 35:109-113.

59   Jentjens RL, Loon LJ Van, Mann CH, et al. Addition of protein and amino acids to carbohydrates does not enhance post exercise muscle glycogen synthesis. J Appl Physiol 2001; 91:839-846.

60   Lemon PW, Tarnopolsky MA, MacDougall JD, et al. Protein requirements and muscle mass/strength changes during intensive training in novice bodybuilders. J Appl Physiol 1992; 73:767-775.

61   Davis JM, Welsh RS, Volve KL De, et al. Effects of branched-chain amino acids and carbohydrate on fatigue during intermittent, high-intensity running. Int J Sports Med 1999; 20:309-314.

62   Coombes JS, McNaughton LR. Effects of branched-chain amino acid supplementation on serum creatine kinase and lactate dehydrogenase after prolonged exercise. J Sports Med Phys Fitness 2000; 40:240-246.

63   Wagenmakers AJ. Amino acid supplements to improve athletic performance. Curr Opin Clin Nutr Metab Care 1999; 2:539-544.

64   Stanko RT, Robertson RJ, Galbreath RW, et al. Enhanced leg exercise endurance with a high-carbohydrate diet and dihydroxyacetone and pyruvate. J Appl Physiol 1990; 69:1651-1165.

65   Morrison MA, Spriet LL, Dyck DJ. Pyruvate ingestion for 7 days does not improve aerobic performance in well-trained individuals. J Appl Physiol 2000; 89:549-556.

66   Sukala WR. Pyruvate: beyond the marketing hype. Int J Sport Nutr 1998; 8:241-249.

67   Fredholm BB, Battig K, Holmen J, et al. Actions of caffeine in the brain with special reference to factors that contribute to its widespread use. Pharmacol Rev Mar 1999; 51:83-133.

68   Graham TE. Caffeine and exercise: metabolism, endurance and performance. Sports Med 2001; 31:785-807.

69   Greer F, Friars D, Graham TE. Comparison of caffeine and theophylline ingestion: exercise metabolism and endurance. J Appl Physiol 2000; 89:1837-1844.

70   Kovacs EM, Stegen JHCH, Brouns F. Effect of caffeinated drinks on substrate metabolism, caffeine excretion and performance. J Appl Physiol 1998; 85:709-715.

71   Bruce CR, Anderson ME, Fraser SF, et al. Enhancement of 2000m rowing performance after caffeine ingestion. Med Sci Sports Exerc 2000; 32:1958-1963.

72   Collomp K, Ahmaidi S, Chatard JC, et al. Benefits of caffeine ingestion on sprint performance in trained and untrained swimmers. Eur J Appl Physiol Occup Physiol 1992; 64:377-380.

73   Harland BE. Caffeine and nutrition. Nutrition 2000; 16:522-526.

74   Barnett C, Costill DL, Vukovic D, et al. Effect of L-carnitine supplementation on muscle and blood carnitine content and lactate accumulation during high-intensity sprint cycling. Int J Sport Nutr 1994; 4:280-288.

75   Vukovic MD, Costill DL, Fink WJ. Carnitine supplementation: effect on muscle carnitine and glycogen content during exercise. Med Sci Sports Exerc 1994; 26:1122-1129.

76   Spriet LL, Gibala MJ. Nutritional strategies to influence adaptations to training. J Sports Sci 2004; 22:127-141.

77   Muller DM, Seim H, Kiess W, et al. Effects of oral L-carnitine supplementation on in vivo long-chain fatty acid oxidation in healthy adults. Metabolism 2002; 51:1389-1391.

78   McNaughton LR. Bicarbonate and citrate. In: Maughan RJ, ed. Nutrition in sport. Oxford: Blackwell Science; 2000:393-403.

79   McNaughton L. Sodium citrate and anaerobic performance: implications of dosage. Eur J Appl Physiol 1990; 61:392-397.

80   Brooks GA. The lactate shuttle during exercise and recovery. Med Sci Sports Exerc 1986; 18:360-368.

81   Fahey TD, Larsden JD, Brooks GA, et al. The effect of ingesting polylactate or glucose polymer drinks during prolonged exercise. Int J Sport Nutr 1991; 1:249-256.

CHAPTER 4

Doping and Sports

Eduardo H. De Rose

HISTORICAL ASPECTS

Antiquity

The use of doping is as old as humanity. It is curious that Csaky[1] mentions that doping started in Paradise, when Eve gave the apple to Adam, to make him as strong as God. The first document related to the use of doping agents is a painting of the Chinese Emperor, Shen Nung, from 2737 BC, showing him with leaves of 'MaHuang' (Ephedra). The Emperor is considered to be the Father of Chinese Medicine and is believed to have introduced the art of acupuncture.[2]

In the ancient Olympic Games, at the end of the third century BC, according to Galen and other authors of the time, athletes believed that drinking herbal teas and eating mushrooms could increase their performance during the competitions.[3] Another interesting form of doping of this time was to prepare a powder with the oil, dust and sweat adhering to the skin of the athlete after the competition. This mix was removed in the dressing room with the 'strigil', a metallic instrument with the shape of an 'L' as show in Figure 4.1. The athlete sold it to other participants, who believed that by drinking the mix, they would have the same physical capabilities of the champion, a myth that was not accepted by Judge Conrado Durantez, a Spanish historian of the Ancient Olympia.[4]

In the South-American sub-continent, stimulants ranging from harmless tea and coffee, up to strychnine and cocaine, were used to increase performance. Spanish writers report a use from the Incas of chewing coca leaves, to help cover the distance between Cuzco and Quito, in Ecuador.[5] In 1886, the first fatality caused by doping was reported, when a cyclist named Linton died after an overdose of stimulants in a race between Bordeaux and Paris.[6]

Origin of the word

La Cava[7] ascertained that the origin of the term doping is controversial, but seems to have derived from a South-African dialect, and for the Boers was an infusion used in the religious festivities – the 'doop'.

Burstin[8] shows that during the construction of the channel, in Amsterdam, the workers used the term 'doopen', when they want to increase their capacity of work. In 1886, the first fatality caused by doping was reported and in 1889, the term 'doping' is referred to in an English dictionary in the generic sense of a drug used to stimulate horses, and from the hippodromes to the stadiums, it is defined today as any substance or method used to increase the performance, which can be detrimental to the health of the athlete or the ethics of the Game.

DOPING IN THE FIRST OLYMPIC GAMES (1886–1932)

The first fatal case of doping documented in the literature was a French cyclist, in a race near Paris in 1886. The Modern Olympic Games were inaugurated by Baron Pierre De Coubertin in Athens, 1896.[9] The philosophy of the Baron considered competing more important than winning and, as a consequence, the incidence of doping was very low, restricted to limited contamination in cycling, track and field events. The mix most used to increase performance was a cocktail of cocaine, ephedrine and strychnine. The cyclist used at this time, besides the mentioned cocktail, an elixir made with coca leaves and wine, produced by a Corsican chemist, Angelo Mariani.

In 1928, during the Second Winter Games in Saint Moritz, Switzerland, sport physicians from many countries came together to create the International Federation of Sports Medicine (FIMS) to preserve the Olympic athletes and to provide a forum to discuss their problems.[10] The first International Federation (IF) to ban the use of doping agents in its sport was the track and field International Association of Athletics Federation (IAAF) in 1928.

In Germany, Hausschild developed Pervitin in 1934, and, in England, Methedrine was synthesized. (Both of these were used for night flights, long marches and other feats of endurance during the Second World War. Amphetamine was produced for the first time in 1938, being used as stimulant during the period of the war.[6])

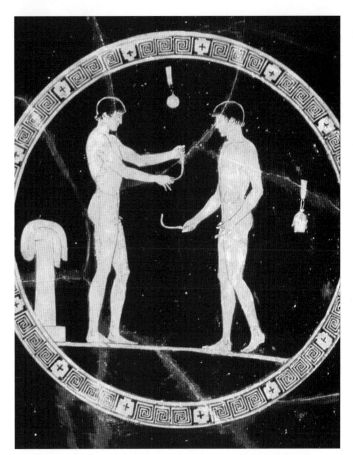

Figure 4.1   Greek ancient athletes using the 'strigil' after a competition. (*Source:* Olympia Museum.)

THE OLYMPIC GAMES (1936–1964)

During the years 1936 to 1964, six Olympic Games were held (excluding the period of the Second World War). The important aspect of this cycle was the use of the Olympic Games in Berlin as a political instrument, to promote the Arian race and political systems of Germany. Together with these political aspects, the commercialization of the Games also began in 1936. This changed the ideal of Coubertin, and winning was now more important than competing.

The substances most used after the Second World War were amphetamines and anabolic steroids. (Anabolic steroids were used during the post-war time, when the Americans discovered the concentration camps and believed that these male hormone steroids could recuperate the prisoners' muscular system.[4])

In 1954, Soviet athletes started to use anabolic steroids to increase muscular mass and, consequently, power. This was followed soon after by weightlifters and bodybuilders and then reached the athletes of all track and field events, and then the other sports.

At the Olympic Games in Rome (1960), a cyclist (Jensen) from Scandinavia died because of an overdose of Isopropylamine and Amphetamine, taken with strong coffee.

Because of that, Lord Porrit was appointed to create a Medical Commission in the International Olympic Committee (IOC), and in the Olympic Games of Tokyo, doping controls

were performed on the cyclists during some competitions, but due to some difficulties, the control could not be totally implemented.[11]

The fight against doping in Europe

Anti-doping measures were initiated by Austria in 1962. In 1965, the Council of Europe defined doping in Strasbourg, and Belgium, France and Greece adopted an anti-doping legislation. The International Federations of cycling (UCI) and football (FIFA) started their doping control programs in 1966.[12]

The International Olympic Committee (IOC) in 1962, in Moscow, passed a resolution against doping. After Lord Porrit resigned to be appointed member of honor of the International Olympic Committee, Prince Alexander De Merode was appointed to control the use of doping agents in the Games, and named in 1967 a Medical Commission that, under his chairmanship, held the first meeting on 27 September of the same year at Lausanne (Switzerland) and started medical controls in the Olympic Games of 1968 (Fig. 4.2).[12]

THE OLYMPIC GAMES (1968–1980)

The newly created Medical Commission, established by the IOC in 1967 for the Winter Games of Grenoble and the Olympiad of Mexico City, both held in 1968, was formed under the leadership of Prince De Merode, a member of the IOC from Belgium.

The Prince invited, among others, some experts to be members: Professor Giuseppe La Cava, the President of the International Federation of Sports Medicine; Professor Ludwig Prokop, from Austria; Professor Arnold Becket, from London and chairman of an anti-doping laboratory; Dr Albert Dirix, Vice President from the Belgium Olympic Committee and Dr Eduardo Hay, Medical Director of the Olympic Games of Mexico City.[12] They published the first list of banned pharmacological classes with the substances given in Box 4.1.

Italy and Uruguay adopted an anti-doping legislation in 1971. The first control of anabolic steroids was done in London in 1974 by Professor Raymond Brooks. In 1975, just before the Olympic Games of Montreal, anabolic steroids were added to this list (Box 4.2).

For the Olympic Games of Montreal in 1976, the same list was maintained but two beta-2 agonists were permitted: salbutamol and terbutaline, as long as the IOC-MC was previously informed of their use. This marks the origin of the Therapeutic Use Exemption (TUE). During this period, doping was founded in all Olympic Games, except the Games of Moscow (1980). The lists of cases can be seen in Table 4.1.

Anabolic steroids were controlled for the first time in Montreal (1976). This is considered an important cornerstone of the IOC Medical Commission, because this substance had been widely used by athletes since 1950.

THE OLYMPIC GAMES (1984–2004)

In 1984, the Council of Europe adopted the European Anti-doping Charter for Sports. At the Olympic Games in Los

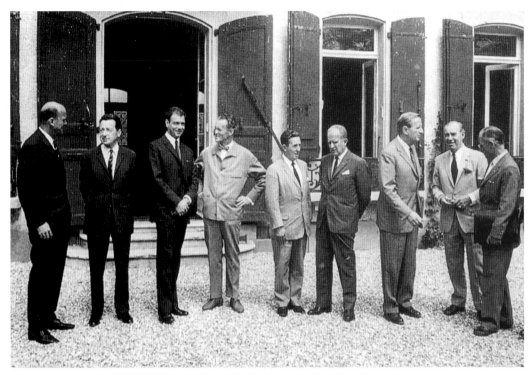

Figure 4.2 The first meeting of the Medical Commission at 'Vila Mon Repos', in Lausanne, chair by Prince Alexander De Merode. (*Source*: Archives of the International Olympics Committee.)

Box 4.1: 1968 IOC List of Doping Substances

1 Psychomotor stimulant drugs
2 Sympathomimetic amines
3 Miscellaneous central nervous system stimulants
4 Narcotic analgesics.

Box 4.2: 1975 IOC List of Doping Substances

1 Psychomotor stimulant drugs
2 Sympathomimetic amines
3 Miscellaneous central nervous system stimulants
4 Narcotic analgesics
5 Anabolic steroids.

Table 4.1 Positive Cases in the Olympic Games from 1968 to 1980

City	Samples	+ Stimulant	+ Anabolic
Mexico City	667	1	0
Munich	2079	7	0
Montreal	1896	3	8
Moscow	1645	0	0

Angeles, there were 11 positive cases (these can be viewed in Table 4.2).

It is interesting to note that the case of Ephedrine (Japan) was caused by a tea of herbal products (Ginseng) and the case of Nandrolone (Finland) was in an athlete that denied the use and which caused great concern at the time. Later it was proved that the athlete had a blood transfusion before the Games and the substance was in reality transmitted by the blood and used months before.

False medical certificates of hypertension were used to justify utilization of beta-blockers in shooting. Blood transfusions were used in cycling and manipulation of the urine was performed in weightlifting. For this reason, the IOC Medical

Table 4.2 Positive Controls in the Los Angeles Olympic Games (1984)

n	Sport	Substance	Country
01	Volleyball	Ephedrine	Japan
02	Weightlifting	Nandrolone	Lebanon
03	Weightlifting	Nandrolone	Algeria
04	Wrestling	Methenolone	Switzerland
05	Volleyball	Testosterone	Japan
06	Athletics	Nandrolone	Greece
07	Athletics	Nandrolone	Finland
08	Weightlifting	Nandrolone	Austria
09	Weightlifting	Nandrolone	Switzerland
10	Weightlifting	Nandrolone	Greece
11	Athletics	Nandrolone	Iceland

Commission modified the list of banned pharmacological classes in 1987, including beta-blockers and diuretics. Restricted substances and forbidden methods were also included, to prevent the use of local anesthetics and corticosteroids, as well as blood transfusions and manipulation of the urine.

A system of escorts was also created to accompany the athlete after their selection, to avoid a physical manipulation of the urine. Probenecid was detected for the first time by Professor Donike, in the Pan-American Games of Caracas, Venezuela, and was included in the list of manipulation of the urine. According to the new list, if the pH is not between 5.0 and 7.0, and the density is lower then 1.005, the sample would be considered not valid and a new one requested, although both samples are sent to the accredited laboratory for analysis (Box 4.3).

In Seoul, Korea, in the Olympics of 1988, many cases were detected and, among them, Ben Johnson, who was one of the most well-known athletes of his time, having a great impact in the media all over the world. Table 4.3 shows the positive doping cases of Seoul.

In Seoul and Calgary, since there was evidence of the use of erythropoietin (EPO) and growth hormone, the IOC Medical Commission included in the list of banned pharmacological classes, the peptide hormones, and marijuana was included in the list of restricted substances. The class of anabolic steroids was changed to androgenic anabolic steroids, since many athletes used anabolic steroids and then stopped before the Games to avoid detection. Out-of-competition doping control started after this Olympic Games (Box 4.4).

In Barcelona, Spain, only five cases were detected, two of them being Clembuterol. The other cases were caused by Strychnine, Norephedrine and Mesocarb. The countries and the modalities may be found in Table 4.4. After the Games, a new change in the list of banned pharmacological classes and methods. The concept of 'related substances' was changed to include not only chemical structure but also pharmacological action. For this reason, a new class of anabolic agents was established, including the anabolic androgenic steroids and also the beta-2-agonists.

The pharmacological class of beta-blockers was removed from the banned area and changed to the restricted area, but

Table 4.3 Positive Doping Cases in the Seoul Olympic Games (1988)

n	Sport	Substance	Country
01	Pentathlon	Caffeine	Australia
02	Weightlifting	Furosemide	Bulgaria
03	Weightlifting	Pemoline	Spain
04	Weightlifting	Furosemide	Bulgaria
05	Weightlifting	Stanozolol	Hungary
06	Athletics	Stanozolol	Canada
07	Weightlifting	Stanozolol	Hungary
08	Weightlifting	Furosemide	Afghanistan
09	Judo	Furosemide	England

Box 4.4: 1992 IOC Doping Classes, Methods and Restrictions

1 Doping classes:
  A Stimulants
  B Narcotics
  C Androgenic anabolic steroids
  D Beta-blockers
  E Diuretics
  F Peptide hormones and analogues:
    i Chorionic gonadotrophin (hCG)
    ii Corticotrophin (ACTH)
    iii Growth hormone (hGH)
    iv Erythropoietin (EPO).
2 Doping methods:
  A Blood doping
  B Pharmacological, chemical and physical manipulation.
3 Classes of drugs subjected to certain restrictions:
  A Alcohol
  B Marijuana
  C Local anesthetics
  D Corticosteroids.

Box 4.3: 1987 IOC List of Doping Classes and Methods

1 Doping classes:
  A Stimulants
  B Narcotics
  C Anabolic steroids
  D Beta-blockers
  E Diuretics.
2 Doping methods:
  A Blood doping
  B Pharmacological, chemical and physical manipulation.
3 Classes of drugs subjected to certain restriction:
  A Alcohol
  B Local anesthetics
  C Corticosteroids.

Table 4.4 Positive Doping Cases in the Barcelona Olympic Games (1992)

n	Sport	Substance	Country
01	Volleyball	Strychnine	China
02	Marathon	Norephedrine	Russia
03	Athletics	Clembuterol	USA
04	Athletics	Clembuterol	USA
05	Athletics	Mesocarb	Lithuania

was banned in some sports, like shooting, archery, pentathlon, equestrian, diving and sailing. The most important decision after this Game was to include the possibility of blood sampling to permit a better determination of use of hormones, in conjunction with the urine sampling (Box 4.5).

Box 4.5: 1993 IOC Doping Classes, Methods and Restrictions

1 Doping classes:
   A Stimulants
   B Narcotics
   C Anabolic agent:
      i Anabolic steroids
      ii Beta-2 agonists
   D Diuretics
   E Peptide hormones and analogues:
      i Chorionic gonadotrophin (hCG)
      ii Corticotrophin (ACTH)
      iii Growth hormone (hGH)
      iv Erythropoietin (EPO).
2 Doping methods:
   C Blood doping
   D Pharmacological, chemical and physical manipulation.
3 Classes of drugs subjected to certain restrictions:
   A Alcohol
   B Marijuana
   C Local anesthetics
   D Corticosteroids
   E Beta-blockers.

Box 4.6: 1998 IOC Prohibited Classes of Substances and Prohibited Methods

1 Prohibited classes of substances:
   A Stimulants (bromantan was included here)
   B Narcotics
   C Anabolic agents:
      i Anabolic androgenic steroids
      ii Beta-2 agonists
   D Diuretics
   E Peptide and glycoprotein hormones and analogues:
      i Chorionic gonadotrophin (hGH)
      ii Corticotrophin (ACTH)
      iii Growth hormone (hGH)
      iv Erythropoietin (EPO).
2 Prohibited methods:
   A Blood doping;
   B Pharmacological, chemical and physical manipulation.
3 Classes of drugs subject to certain restrictions:
   A Alcohol
   B Marijuana
   C Local anesthetics
   D Corticosteroids
   E Beta-blockers.

The Olympic Games of Atlanta, USA in 1996 were the Games celebrating 100 years of the Olympic Movement, and there were only two cases of anabolic steroids detected, in track and field events. However, 10 athletes from Russia and Bulgaria were considered positive because of Bromantan, a new stimulant amphetamine drug that had been produced for the Russian Army. These athletes, penalized by the IOC Medical Commission, were later reinstated by the Tribunal Arbitral of Sports (TAS) and were not considered doping cases. After these Games and before the Winter Games of Nagano, Bromantan was added to the list (Box 4.6).

For the Sydney Olympic Games, in Australia, the IOC-MC established the following list of banned substances and methods, including three peptide hormones and one prohibited method, and changed the term marijuana to cannabis (Box 4.7). In the Sydney Olympic Games, blood was collected in the aerobic sports and there were for the first time, controls after the opening of the Olympic Village, and before the start of the Games, tests in blood and urine were made.

That was also the last time the IOC-Medical Commission made the list of forbidden substances and methods. This was directed in the last Olympics by chairman Prince De Merode (Fig. 4.3) who judged all the positive cases. (He died 3 years later from cancer). In the Winter Games of Salt Lake City and the Olympiad of Athens, the list was made by the newly formatted World Anti-doping Agency (WADA) and the chairman of the Medical Commission was Professor Arne Ljungqvist, an IOC Member from Sweden and Chairman of the Medical Commission of IAAF. The World Anti-doping Agency produced a report on the doping controls in the Games

Box 4.7: 2000 IOC Prohibited Classes of Substances and Prohibited Methods

1 Prohibited classes of substances:
   A Stimulants
   B Narcotics
   C Anabolic agents:
      i Anabolic androgenic steroids
      ii Beta-2 agonists
   D Diuretics;
   E Peptide hormones, mimetics and analogues:
      i Chorionic gonadotrophins (hCG) (only in males)
      ii Pituitary and synthetic gonadotrophins (LH) (only in males)
      iii Corticotrophins
      iv Growth hormone (hGH)
      v Insulin-like growth factor (IGF-1)
      vi Erythropoietin (EPO)
      vii Insulin
2 Prohibited methods:
   A Blood doping
   B Administering artificial oxygen carriers or plasma expanders
   C Pharmacological, chemical and physical manipulation.
3 Classes of prohibited substances in certain circumstances:
   A Alcohol
   B Cannabinoids
   C Local anesthetics
   D Glucocorticosteroids
   E Beta-blockers.

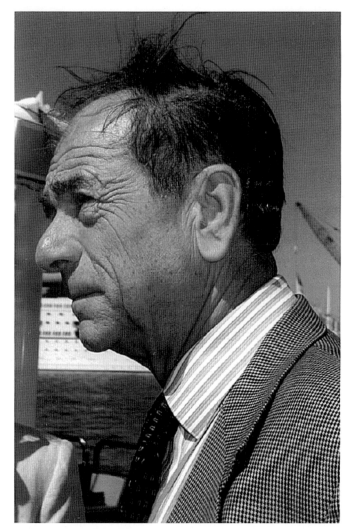

Figure 4.3 Prince Alexander De Merode in 2000, acting in the Sydney Olympic Games.

conduct in-competition doping controls, not only in Greece but in all countries, in the athletes participating in the Games. The high number of the positive controls in weightlifting is not the result of a random distribution, like in the other sports. Weightlifting has an out-of-competition control in all the athletes participating 1 week before the Games.

A total of 2800 controls were conducted by the IOC Medical Commission. In the period before the Games, 11 positives were found, mainly in weightlifting. Table 4.6 shows the results found during this time.

After the Games, the report showed 14 positive results (Table 4.7), from which three were refusals of the athletes to perform doping control after the competition. The refusals, according to an anonymous letter to the IAAF, were motivated by the desire to avoid the detection of the use of certain devices (Fig. 4.4). A balloon, with manipulated and clean urine, is inserted in the anus of the athlete before the competition, and the yellow catheter remains undetectable under the perineum and the penis. During the collection of urine in the doping room, the athlete contracts the gluteus and the elevator of the anus, eliminating the fake urine. Figure 4.5 shows one

(www.wada-ama.org) and stated that, with the exception of minor problems, 2052 samples were analyzed and reported, and nine were detected as positive (Table 4.5). The IOC stipulated an 'Olympic Period', including a period before the Games and after the opening of the Olympic Village, from 30 July to 29 August 2004, and decided that it would be possible to

Table 4.6 Positives Out-of-Competition Doping Controls in the Athens Olympic Games (2004)

n	Sport	Country	Substance
1	Box	Kenya	Stimulant
2	Track and field	Greece	No show
3	Track and field	Greece	No show
4	Track and field	Uzbekistan	Anabolic agent
5	Weightlifting	Kurdistan	Anabolic steroids
6	Weightlifting	Russia	Anabolic steroids
7	Weightlifting	Morocco	Anabolic steroids
8	Weightlifting	Moldavia	Anabolic steroids
9	Weightlifting	Hungry	Anabolic steroids
10	Weightlifting	India	Anabolic steroids
11	Weightlifting	Turkey	Anabolic steroids

Table 4.5 Positive Controls in the Sydney Olympic Games (2000)

Country	Sport	Substance
Bulgaria	Weightlifting	Furosemide
Bulgaria	Weightlifting	Furosemide
Bulgaria	Weightlifting	Furosemide
Latvia	Rowing	Nandrolone
Rumania	Gymnastics	Ephedrine
Armenia	Weightlifting	Stanozolol
Germany	Wrestling	Nandrolone
Mongolia	Weightlifting	Furosemide
Norway	Rowing	Nandrolone

Table 4.7 Positive Doping Controls in-Competition in the Olympic Games (2004)

n	Sport	Country	Substance
1	Weightlifting	Myanmar	Anabolic steroids
2	Weightlifting	India	Diuretic
3	Weightlifting	Greece	Anabolic steroids
4	Track and field	Russia	Anabolic steroids
5	Track and field	Hungary	Refusal
6	Track and field	Belarus	Anabolic agent
7	Rowing	Ukraine	Stimulant
8	Weightlifting	Hungary	Refusal
9	Track and field	Russia	Anabolic steroids
10	Weightlifting	Hungary	Anabolic steroids
11	Wrestling	Puerto Rico	Anabolic steroids
12	Weightlifting	Venezuela	Anabolic steroids
13	Track and field	Hungary	Refusal

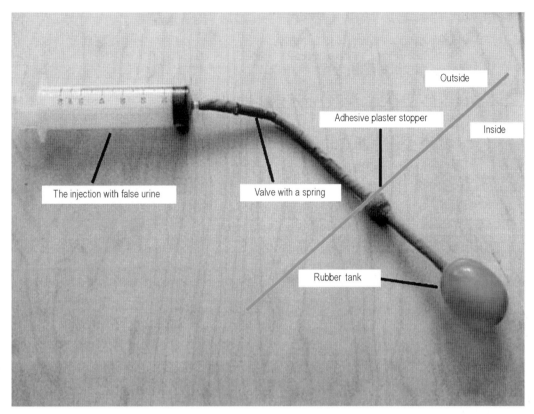

Figure 4.4   Device probably used by the athletes in the Athens Games. (Courtesy of International Association of Athletics Federations.)

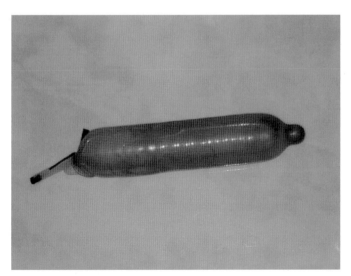

Figure 4.5   Device detected by the author in a World Championship.

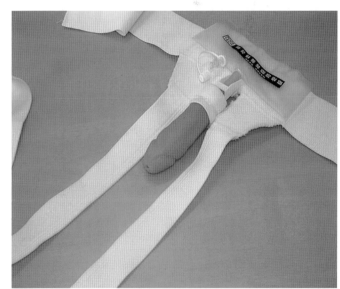

Figure 4.6   Device found on the internet by WADA experts. (Courtesy of World Anti-doping Agency.)

type of simple device; a male preservative full of 'clean urine' found inside the trunk of the athlete during a world championship, to deliver the fake urine for doping control. Figure 4.6 shows another type of device, found by WADA, on the internet, also used to provide fake urine in the collections of the urine sample for doping control. This device is very

sophisticated and has a system to maintain the urine at body temperature.

In the Athens Olympic Games, for the first time, human growth hormone was researched in the blood in 380 athletes, even though the method had only a small window of detection. All positive cases were judged by the Disciplinary Commission

Table 4.8 Positive Doping Controls in the Games from 1984 to 2004

Year	City	Total number	E-stimulants	Anabolic	Others
1984	Los Angeles	1887	1	11	0
1988	Seoul	1998	2	3	4
1992	Barcelona	1842	3	2	2
1996	Atlanta	1795	0	2	0
2000	Sydney	2052	1	3	4
2004	Athens	2800	2	7	5

of the IOC, formed by three members, with the final approval of the Executive Committee, being then informed to the press, without passing through the Medical Commission that only supervised randomly the operation of doping control and the medical care of the athletes in the Games (Table 4.8).

THE CREATION OF THE WORLD ANTI-DOPING AGENCY (WADA)

The idea of the creation of an international agency to regulate doping controls started during the Tour de France, in the year of 1998. During this competition, the controllers of the Government of France, which has a very strict national law on doping, faced problems in relation to the International Federation concerned.

Because of that, and the repercussion in the press of Europe, the president of the IOC called an International Congress on Doping in Lausanne, Switzerland. The conclusion of this congress, that had the presence of most of the Ministers of Sport from Europe, was the decision to create an international body that would substitute the IOC in the control of the fight against doping in a harmonized way, with half of the position of the Foundation being formed by the Governments of all continents and half of the Foundation being formed by the Olympic Movement.

The Agency started the activities in Lausanne, but later it was moved to Montreal, Canada, to avoid misinterpretation by the close proximity of the IOC. The Agency understood that the risk of being considered as a department of the IOC would be great.

The World Anti-doping Code was established in an International Congress held in Copenhagen in 2003 and was enforced in January 2004, with a complete list of banned substances and methods.[13] The Agency has today commissions working in the areas of Medicine and Science, Education and Ethics and has two important programs: the Independent Observer Program, that certifies World and Regional competitions, and the Outreaching Program, directed to athletes in major competitions.

ACTUAL DEFINITION OF DOPING

The first definition of doping, when the control in anti-doping started, was only relevant to an artificial increasing of the performance of an athlete, using drugs or forbidden methods.

The actual definition of doping, in accordance with the World Anti-doping Code enforced in Copenhagen refers to: the use of substances or methods able to artificially increment the performance of the athletes; the fact that these substances will be harmful to the health of the athletes; and that it is against the spirit of the Game.[13]

Doping is contrary to the principles of the Olympics, of Sports, and of Medical Ethics, even Sports Medicine Ethics. It is as forbidden to use doping, as it is to recommend, propose, authorize, relevate or facilitate the use of any substance or method included in this definition.

The permanent progress of Pharmacology, Sports Medicine and Sciences of Performance gives new forms of artificially incrementing performance and makes necessary a strong legislation, dynamic, actual and flexible.

EXISTING DOPING CONTROLS

Doping control may be made today in urine or in blood or both together. Basically, according to the World Anti-doping Code,[13] there are two types of anti-doping control to be done in the urine.

Controls in-competition (IC)
The 'in-competition' doping controls are done immediately after the end of a sports activity.

Controls out-of-competition (OOC)
The 'out-of-competition' control can be made at any moment: in the training, in the accommodation of the athlete, or even immediately before or after a competition.

Substances
The substances controlled in both kinds of tests are not the same. According to the Code, the 'in-competition' test includes all the banned classes of drugs and methods, but the 'out-of-competition' test is more selective, including only anabolic agents, beta-2 agonists, agents with anti-estrogenic activity, masking agents, and all the banned methods. Stimulants, narcotics, or cannabis are not analyzed in this type of control.

Other kinds of control
During a 'Game Period': this comprises control 'in-competiton' during all of the period, from the opening to the closing of the Athletic Village, and the 'health controls' done just before competitions, in events such as cycling, ski-ing and skating, to control the levels of the blood in the competitors. In this last case, it is possible to take an athlete from a specific competition.

List of substances and methods banned by the World Anti-doping Agency (WADA)
The prohibited list of WADA is revised every year by the List Committee, and after approval of the Executive Committee, is placed on the web at the beginning of October, for the information of all those in the Olympic Movement, countries, National Anti-doping Agencies, athletes and others. The list is adopted by

WADA each consecutive year and used in all areas, giving for the first time, real harmonization over the sport and political world.

The prohibited list for 2006 is published by WADA in English and French, and if there is some conflict between both idioms, English should prevail. The list opens with a sentence that states that 'the use of any drug should be limited to medical justified indications' and begins by mentioning substances prohibited at all times (Box 4.8).[14]

This list identifies substances that are susceptible to unintentional anti-doping rules violations because of their general availability in medicinal products. A doping violation involving such substances may result in a reduced sanction provided that

---

Box 4.8: Prohibited Substances and Methods

Substances and methods prohibited at all times

Prohibited substances

S1 Anabolic agents:
   1 Anabolic androgenic steroids (AAS)
      a Exogenous AAS
      b Endogenous AAS
   2 Other anabolic agents.
S2 Hormones and related substances:
   1 Erythropoietin (EPO)
   2 Growth hormone (hGH), insulin-like growth factor (IGF-1) and mechano-growth factors (MGFs)
   3 Gonadotrophins (LH, hCG)
   4 Insulin
   5 Corticotrophins.
S3 Beta-2 agonists
S4 Agents with anti-estrogenic activity:
   1 Aromatase inhibitors including, but not limited to, anastrozole, letrozole, aminogluthemide, exemestane, formestane, testolactone
   2 Selective estrogen receptor modulators (SERMs) including, but not limited to, raloxifene, tamoxifen, toremifene
   3 Other anti-estrogenic substances, including, clomiphene, cyclofenil, fulvestrant.
S5 Diuretics and other masking agents.

Prohibited methods

M1 Enhancement of oxygen transfer:
   a doping, including the use of autologous, homologous or heterologous blood or red blood cell products of any origin, other than for medical treatment
   b Artificially enhancing the uptake, transport or delivery of oxygen, including but not limited to perfluorochemicals, efaproxiral (RS13) and modified hemoglobin products
   c Gene doping.
M2 Chemical and physical manipulation
M3 Gene doping

Substances and methods prohibited in-competition

Prohibited substances

S6 Stimulants
S7 Narcotics
S8 Cannabinoids
S9 Glucocorticosteroids

Substances prohibited in particular sports

P1 Alcohol
   Ethanol is prohibited in-competition only, and the doping violation threshold may be decided by each IF concerned. Detection will be conducted by analysis of breath and/or blood.
P2 Beta-blockers
   Beta-blockers are prohibited, unless otherwise specified, only in-competition.

Specified substances are listed below:

- All inhaled beta-2 agonists, except clenbuterol
- Probenecid
- Cathine, cropropamide, crotetamide, ephedrine, etamivan, famprofazone, hepataminol, isometheptene, levmethamfetamine, meclofenoxate, p-methylamphetamine, metylephedrine, niketamide, norephedrine, octapamine, ortetamine, oxilofrine, phenpromethanine, propylhexedrine, selegiline, sibutramine
- Cannabinoids
- All glucocorticosteroids
- Alcohol
- All beta-blockers.

---

the athlete can establish that the use of the substance was not intended to enhance performance.

THERAPEUTIC USE EXEMPTION (TUE) OF RESTRICTED AND BANNED SUBSTANCES

There follows a summary of the International Standard for Therapeutic Use Exemption, published as an element of the World Anti-doping Code of WADA on 1 January, 2005. The Code, in its Article 44, allows the athlete, through their physicians, to apply for the Therapeutic Use Exemption (TUE). The use of the TUE is to make it possible, for therapeutic reasons, to prescribe an athlete a restricted or forbidden substance. This information should be kept confidential by the Medical Committees of the International Sports Federation (IF) who are responsible for granting it. It is always important to mention that a TUE should be submitted and approved at least 21 days before the competition. A TUE is not for the sport-life of an athlete and should have a period of validity. After expiration, it can be requested again by the athlete.

The World Anti-doping Agency may reverse the grant or denial of a TUE and, in the latter instance, the decision of WADA can be appealed against via the Council Arbitral of Sports (CAS) in Lausanne, Switzerland. To clear the athlete for a TUE, the Committee should verify if the athlete had a significant impairment of health if the medication is suspended during an event. The medication used however, should not produce an additional enhancement of performance and no alternative medication should exist.

The athlete should provide written consent for the transmission of all information related to the case, to the members of the Medical Commission that will judge the case and, if necessary, a third opinion may be requested. In this case, the identity of the athlete should be withheld. All members of the

TUE Tribunals should sign a confidentiality agreement and keep all information reserved. The Commission that judges the TUE should have at least three members and all must have experience in the treatments of athletes.

In terms of language, a TUE may be translated to another idiom, but English and French should remain mandatory. The name of the athlete and the sport should be very clear, and the athlete must list any previous request. The applicant must include a comprehensive medical history of the pathology, laboratory investigations or imaging studies that are relevant to the case. Information should be given on medication used, as well as the dose, frequency, route and duration of the administration. The decision of the Commission should be available 30 days after the receipt of information. If WADA should revise or change a decision, another 30 days is needed.

Some substances included in the List of Prohibited Substances are frequently used to treat medical conditions often found in the athletic population. In this case, a full application is not necessary, and an abbreviated process can be established. The medication that can justify the use of an abbreviated process are the permitted beta-2 agonists (formoterol, salbutamol, salmeterol and terbutaline), used by inhalation only, and glucocorticosteroids, used by non-systemic routes. The abbreviated process will only be considered for retroactive approval in emergency treatment in an acute situation, or due to exceptional circumstances, especially if time and opportunity did not permit submission of the application.

The TUE are granted by the International Federation concerned and the National Anti-doping Organization (NADO) should be informed of the athlete, with a copy to WADA. The clearinghouse for all types of TUEs should be the World Anti-doping Agency and strict confidentiality of the medical information should be guaranteed. The proper request forms for abbreviated and full TUE should be go to the NADO of the athlete, or copied from the WADA website (www.wada-ama.org).

The use of supplements and herbal products

The great majority of the products called supplements, in the pharmacological market, which include among others, vitamins, minerals and amino acids, are not controlled in terms of contents by many of the world governments. A study made by the Schanzer in the accredited laboratory of Cologne,[15] sponsored by the IOC, showed clearly that some of these products do not contain what they claim according to the labels, but also do contain pro-hormones, nandrolone and testosterone, all of which may cause a positive doping result.

Because of this, athletes should only use traditional products previously tested, to avoid the problem of a contamination that, even unintentionally, may not avoid a sanction.

Some products with a base in herbal products, like MaHuang or Ginseng, may contain banned substances or be contaminated by them. In some countries of the world, particularly in South America, athletes should avoid drinking tea of cocaine, which can be present in the urine as metabolic of this drug.[16]

As it is not possible to assure the quality of this type of product, and also considering the fact that the use of supplements is not scientifically related in the literature to increase performance, the athlete should exert common sense in their use.

The WADA statistics of doping use

In 2004, at the request in a meeting of the Foundation Board, WADA published (see www.wada-ama.org) an overview of results reported by the 31 accredited laboratories in the world related to the previous year. In 2005, this analysis was again repeated. Since the last statistic was done by the IOC in 2000, before transfer of the laboratory to the control of WADA, this is the most recent study made.[17] Some interesting information has been found from the statistics of 2004. First, is the relation expressed in Table 4.9 from Olympic and non-Olympic Sport.

Of course, it is not possible to speak of a 'normal' result in doping control, but if around 1.5% of positive results were found, according to a so-called epidemiology of doping, this is inside the average found in the last 35 years. Table 4.9 shows that the adverse analytical finding rate in non-Olympic sports is greater then the Olympic Sports, the average found in the year 2004 being 1.72%. An adverse finding is a result that shows only evidence of the use of a forbidden method, not the use itself.

Figure 4.7 shows that the most common substances are the anabolic steroids (36.0%), followed by the glucocorticosteroids (16.6%), cannabinoids (15.7%), stimulants (11.6%), the beta-2 agonists (11.5%) and the masking agents (4.8%).

Table 4.9   Relation Between Olympic and Non-Olympic Sports

Type of Sport	Sample A	Adverse Finding	Adverse Finding (%)
Olympic	128 591	2145	1.67
Non-Olympic	40 596	764	1.88
Total	169 187	2909	1.72

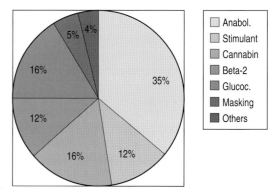

Figure 4.7 Distribution of substances identified in each drug class. Anabol., anabolic steroids; Cannabin., cannabinoids; Beta-2, beta-2 agonists; Glucoc., glucocorticosteroids. (Courtesy of World Anti-doping Agency.)

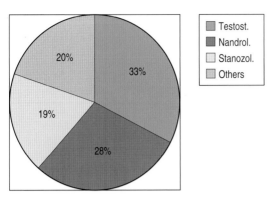

Figure 4.8 Breakdown of the drug class of anabolic steroids. Testost., testosterone; Nandrol., nandrolone; Stanzol., stanozolol. (Modified from World Anti-doping Agency.)

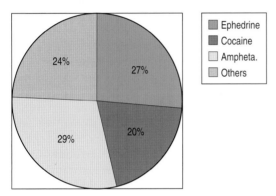

Figure 4.9 Breakdown of the drug class of stimulants. Ampheta., amphetamines. (Modified from World Anti-doping Agency.)

In the breakdown of the anabolic steroids, it is seen that the first substance to be identified is testosterone (32.9%), followed by nandrolone (28.5%) and stanozolol (19.0%). Figure 4.8 shows the breakdown of the drug class of anabolic steroids.

In the breakdown of the drug class of stimulants, it is seen that the results expressed in Figure 4.9, show that amphetamine is the most found substance (29.3%), followed by ephedrine (26.7%) and cocaine metabolites (19.3%). It is interesting to note that cocaine is not used as a performance enhancing drug, but as a social drug, although it is detected in the doping control.

Table 4.10 shows the Olympic sports that presented a greater number of adverse findings in this year. Cycling is the

Table 4.10 Sport with Higher Number of Adverse Analytical Finding

Sport	Total	Adverse A	Adverse (%)
Cycling	13 199	607	4.60
Boxing	2205	70	3.17
Weightlifting	5234	158	3.02
Baseball	8736	250	2.86
Ice hockey	2359	54	2,29

main sport, but it is surprising that boxing, weightlifting, baseball and ice hockey follow.

It is important to mention that adverse analytical findings of the laboratories are not equal to positive cases. All the TUE must be excluded and the possibility of defense for the athlete provided.

THE RIGHTS AND RESPONSIBILITIES OF THE ATHLETES

According to the material provided by WADA,[18] this area may be divided into two major points: Rights of the Athletes and Responsibilities of the Athletes.

Rights of the athletes

The rights of the athletes are as follows:
- Check the credentials of the Doping Control Officer (DCO) to any type of control
- Be notified by writing of a selection process
- Be informed about the consequences of a refusal to cooperate
- Be informed about the correct sequence of the control
- With the consent of the DCO, always accompanied by an escort, the athlete can:
  a Receive a prize
  b Do a warm down
  c Receive medical attention
  d Attend a press conference
  e Elect not to stay in the doping station, if there are other competitions in the day
  f Select the equipment that will be used
  g Be observed in the passing of the urine by someone of the same gender
  h Receive a signed copy of all the documents.

Responsibility of the athletes

The responsibilities of the athletes are:
- To know the norms of the World Anti-doping Agency (WADA), National Organization of Doping Control (NADO), the National Olympic Committee (NOC), the International and National Federation of Sports
- To inform your personal physician and your pharmacologist that you are an athlete and are submitted to doping controls
- To consult your NADO, NOC or IF with anticipation if you will need to use any medical treatment that is related to a banned drug in your sport, to receive a special consent by a TUE
- To keep an actual list of all the medications, supplements, and herbal products that you are using to declare in the event of a doping control
- To be careful in the ingestion of supplements or herbal products if they may contain banned substances
- To bring always an identification with photo with you, to show it to a DCO in the case of a doping control
- In a competition or out of competition, in the case of a doping control, to remain all the time under the sight of his escort or DCO until the conclusion of his control

- To hydrate with previously sealed non-alcoholic beverages
- To be prepared to begin a doping control process as soon as notified and be in the doping control collection room until is sample is closed
- Assure that all your documentation is correctly made and to receive your copy.

THE INTERNATIONAL CONVENTION AGAINST DOPING IN SPORT

It is important to understand that the World Anti-doping Agency is an entity based in private rights, which bring together the Olympic Movement and Governments. WADA often encounters difficulties in collecting fees from Governments, because often the countries cannot transfer funds to an entity of public rights. To solve this problem, the General Conference of UNESCO approved a Convention against Doping in Sport.

The Resolution is the strongest decision from UNESCO and countries are expected to cooperate to adopt the legislation and to adapt their state laws to the convention. The draft was prepared by experts and will be signed by each Minister of Sports that agrees with it.

This Convention defines the Accredited Doping Laboratories, the Anti-doping Organizations, the anti-doping rules violation, the terms athlete, code, competition and doping control, as well as the criteria of no advance notice, out-of-competition, in-competition, prohibited list and the therapeutic use exemption. The Convention of UNESCO, in other words, adopts the World Anti-doping Code and makes it an instrument of public right, making it possible for Governments to accept it and adapt the national legislation to reach a total harmonization, which is expected to happen by the Turin Winter Games in 2006.

GENE DOPING – FUTURE TECHNOLOGY

The future of doping is considered by WADA to be gene doping. It is already mentioned in the list of banned substances and the gene manipulation is defined by the Agency as 'the non-therapeutic use of cells, genes, genetic elements, or modulation of the gene expression, having the capacity to enhance athletic performance'.

Since the discovery of the human genoma, which permits us to better treat many diseases, it is evident that it could be used to try to increase the athlete's performance.[19] The concerns of the Agency are also expressed by its chairman Richard Pound in a recent publication, 'gene doping may represent a new frontier in athletic performance enhancement, but we are working hard to ensure that these emerging medical techniques are not used to create super athletes'.[20]

If one considers athletes on the whole, genetic potential was one of the most important factors of performance, because until now it could not be altered. Today, these characteristics are studied by kinanthropometry, but it will soon be possible to create a genetic screening at an early age, comparing the human genoma with the genetic potential in each sport, which will allow the selection and training of the athlete, according to their inherent abilities.[21]

The use of viral factors to deliver a gene to the athlete is effective and expensive. However, if compared with non-viral factors, they have a higher toxicity and can produce an immune reaction which may sometimes cause rejection. The non-viral factors are only effective locally, and in consequence have a less general effect. They are easily prepared and have a low risk of contamination.[22]

Today, we consider that theoretically, gene doping may increase in patients and also in athletes in the production of red cells through erythropoietin, the muscle hypertrophy in muscle disease or in healthy subjects using the IGF-1, the mechano-growth factor (MGF) and myostatin, and also the production of new vessels, which would be useful not only for patients with cardiovascular diseases but also as a method to increase oxygen transfer in athletes.[23]

Today, gene doping still holds a question over its head. Can it be stopped, or can the cells multiply themselves causing diseases and death? May the immunological risk be uncontrolled and complicated by the response of the body? Can the cell mutations be transferred to following generations? The medical, ethical and legal implications should be evaluated by the physicians and scientists that are dealing with such techniques.[24-26]

The Medical and Science Committee of the World Anti-doping Agency established a Gene Doping Panel in 2005, chaired by Professor Theodore Friedman, a pediatrician who is the director of the gene therapy program at the University of San Diego, USA. He believes that this technology is evolving rapidly, as the science involved is relatively simple and can be performed by well-trained people in thousands of laboratories all over the world. Many scientists believe that by the Olympics of Beijing, it will be possible to have some degree of gene doping.

Will it be possible to detect gene doping? In the opinion of many scientists, the answer is yes. Going back to the history of doping, the same question often arose then and the answer was always yes. Anabolics were detected, including testosterone. Masking agencies and hormones were also detected, as well as manipulation of the anabolic steroids. If enough is invested in research, and WADA is supporting at least five projects now, it is inevitable that we will have the necessary detection when this kind of doping reaches our athletes.

REFERENCES

1 Csaky TZ. Doping. J Sport Med Phys Fitness 1972; 2:117–123.
2 Loriga V. Il doping. Roma: CONI; 1988.
3 Mottram DR. Drugs in sport. Champaign: Human Kinetics; 1988.
4 De Rose EH, Nobrega ACL. O Doping na Atividade Esportiva. In: Lasmar N, Lasmar R, eds. Medicina do esporte. Rio de Janeiro: Editora Revinter; 2002.
5 Montanaro M. I problema del doping. In: Venerando A., ed. Medicina dello sport. Roma: Universo; 1974.
6 Gasbarrone E, Leonelli F. Il doping. In: Silvy S, ed. Manuale di medicina dello sport. Roma: Editrice Universo; 1992.
7 La Cava G. Manuale pratico di medicina sportiva. Torino: Minerva; 1973.
8 Burstin S. Cinq ans de contróle médical antidopage au millieu sportif. Med Sport 1972; 4:204–208.
9 Muller N. Pierre de Coubertin: textes choisis (II). Zurich: Weidmann; 1986.
10 De Rose EH. A Medicina do Esporte através dos tempos. In: Oliveira MAB. Nobrega ACL, ed. Tópicos especiais em medicina do esporte. São Paulo: Editora Atheneu; 2003.
11 Dirix A. Doping – Theorie et pratique. Br J Sports Med 1972; 1(2):250–258.
12 Dirix A. Medical guide. 2nd edn. Lausanne: International Olympic Committee; 1992.
13 WADA. The World Anti-doping Code (version 3.0). Montreal: WADA; 2003.
14 WADA. The prohibited list. Montreal: WADA, Science and Medical Committee; 2005.
15 Schanzer W. Analysis of non-hormonal nutritional supplements for anabolic-androgenic Steroids – An International Study. Cologne: DSHS; 2002.
16 Feder MG, Cardoso JN, De Rose EH. Informações sobre o uso de medicamentos no esporte, 2ª. edição. Rio de Janeiro: COB; 2000.
17 WADA. Report of the accredited laboratories. Montreal: WADA; 2005.
18 WADA. Athlete's guide to the doping control program. Montreal: WADA; 2003.
19 Friedman T, Koss J. Gene transfer and athletes: an impending problem. Molec Ther 2001; 3:819–820.
20 Pound R. Taking the lead. Play True 2005; 1(1)
21 Wolfarth B, Rivera MA. Oppert, IM, et al. A polymorphism in the α-adrenoceptor gene and endurance status. Med Sci Sport Exerc 2000; 32:1709–1712.
22 Machida SM, Booth FW. Insulin-growth factor 1 and muscle growth: implications for satellite cell proliferation. Proc Nutr Soc 2004; 63:337–340.
23 Fischetto G. New trends in gene doping. New Stud Athletics 2005; 20:41–49.
24 Svensson E, Black HB, Dugger DLJ, et al. Long term erythropoietin expression in rodent and non human primates following intramuscular injection of a replication defective adenoviral vector. Hum Gene Ther 1997; 8:1797–1806.
25 Tenenbaum L, Lethonen E, Monaham PE. Evaluation of risks related to the use of adeno-associated virus based vectors. Curr Gene Ther 2003; 3:545–564.
26 Zhou S, Murphy JE, Escobedo JA, Dwarki VJ. Adeno-associated virus-mediated delivery of erythropoietin leads to sustained elevation of hematocrit in non human primates. Gene Ther 1998; 5:665–670.

CHAPTER 5

Traveling with Sports Teams

Brian J. Krabak and Brandee Waite

INTRODUCTION

One of the most rewarding and challenging jobs of the sports medicine practitioner is traveling with a team. On the surface, there is excitement about jetting off to fabulous venues and traveling as a key member of the team. Just below the surface are numerous responsibilities and duties that fall squarely on the shoulders of the team physician.

It is true that in some high profile sporting events, the physicians travel on chartered or private flights, have luxury accommodations and are on the sidelines for fantastic moments in sports. Only a small percentage of elite and professional sports offer this type of experience. The vast majority of sports team travel is conducted with budget restrictions that require travel of only essential team staff, with each person assuming additional responsibilities. The hours can be long and often require evenings and weekends away from family, as well as weekdays away from customary medical practice. In addition, international travel can raise safety issues depending upon the area of travel.

Most sports medicine practitioners truly enjoy their work and therefore accept the difficulties of travel in exchange for the rewards of working with the team. They enjoy having patient-athletes who are dedicated to maximizing their health and fitness. They often spend their leisure time following or playing some of the sports they cover. For the practitioner who accepts the challenges and responsibilities of diligent preparation, coordination, communication and follow through, traveling with the team is a labor of love.

PREPARATION

Preparation for traveling with a team begins long before the bags and team are loaded onto the bus or plane. The duties surrounding team medical care can change with each trip. It is imperative that preparations for each excursion are tailored to the specific needs of each trip and the nature of the sports competition. Information on team members, travel supplies, venue accommodations, and potential difficulties should be researched in advance.

Box 5.1: Key Points

- Be prepared.
- Know the background of all athletes and staff.
- Educate the athletes and staff regarding potential medical issues specific to traveling and the region of competition.
- Have the appropriate medical supplies with you or resources to obtain medical supplies as needed.

Assessing team fitness

In preparation for travel, the medical practitioner should be aware of which team members are traveling and any medical or health issues they have. A pre-participation or pre-season physical will alert the treating physician to any potential medical issues. Pertinent information that can be helpful while traveling includes a need for certain types of medications and prior treatment of a variety of medical conditions. Early detection of a specific diagnosis or concern will allow time for the physician to work-up and treat the issue. In addition, documentation of the initial physical examination will detect any abnormalities or asymmetries (i.e. asymmetric pupil sizes or ligament excursion) that might incorrectly be diagnosed as a new injury. If possible, a brief medical record highlighting the pertinent medical issues or physical examination findings should be carried while traveling to avoid any confusion.

Being familiar with the athletes and their previous or current injuries allows for anticipation of potential needs while on the road. Some athletes may need medical evaluations prior to the departure date to assure that they are physically able to travel and compete. In addition to caring for athletes, the traveling practitioner may also be responsible for the medical care of the coaches, athletic trainers, or officials traveling with the team. If this is the case, take the time to request a past medical history from each of those traveling. If faced with an emergent situation, it will be well worth it to know if 'Coach Smith' had a myocardial infarction 6 months ago or 'Official Jones' is on warfarin for atrial fibrillation.

Medical staff training

In addition to knowing the staff regarding potential healthcare issues, it is important to know who will be assisting in the medical care of the athletes. There may be other physicians providing specialty care, nurses, chiropractors, athletic trainers, physical therapists or massage therapists. The head physician or trainer usually requires that all medical support staff have current basic CPR training (BLS – basic life support). The need for advanced training (ACLS – advanced cardiac life support) may or may not be necessary, depending upon the athlete's medical conditions and support facilities available to the physician. Basic first aid training may also be required. The head practitioner should know the skill level of the supporting medical team, require appropriate certifications and designate duties accordingly. In many instances, there is only one person on the medical team. In that situation, he or she must be willing to assume additional roles within their level of training and have a plan for obtaining additional help if an urgent or emergent situation arises.

For large scale competition, such as World Championships or Olympic Games, a variety of healthcare providers will be needed to provide adequate care. The exact number and type of individuals needed will vary depending upon the number of athletes, length of competition and equipment needs. Each team will have a head physician who should be trained in all aspects of sports medicine. The head physician can be from a variety of professions (physiatry, orthopedics, family medicine), but should be competent in treating all aspects of sports medicine. They should be able to take care of primary care issues such as asthma, allergies, rashes and infections, and musculoskeletal injuries including fractures, muscle strains and ligament injuries. Some teams travel with a mixture of physicians with one focusing on the primary care issues (family medicine) and the other on musculoskeletal injuries (physiatry or orthopedics).

The rest of the sports medicine team will vary depending upon the team needs. It is helpful to have at least one physical therapist or athletic trainer to assist with preventative warm-up programs or modalities, stretching and massage to treat injuries. A massage therapist is often utilized to assist with muscle soreness or soft tissue injuries. Some teams utilize a chiropractor to assist with any injuries requiring manipulation. Further personnel that could be considered, but are less likely, include, e.g. a nutritionist or psychologist, depending upon the team's needs.

Destination information

In order to make appropriate plans for emergent situations, it is necessary to research the destination prior to departure. There are a number of things one should know about the travel sites in order to assure a successful trip. When competing internationally, there may be immunizations required for travel in the countries. In some tropical regions, travelers are required to take prophylactic antimalarial pills or use insect repellants during their stay. Other concerns include Dengue fever and rabies. Most major hospitals will have a Travel Medicine Clinic as a resource for information and immunizations. Other resources include The Center for Disease Control and Prevention (www.cdc.gov/travel), which keeps a wealth of information on traveling throughout the world. Required

Table 5.1 Common Travel Vaccinations

Vaccination	Time of Protection
Hepatitis A vaccine	Lifelong
Hepatitis B vaccine	Lifelong
Influenza (flu) vaccine	1 year
Meningococcal vaccine	3 years
MMR vaccine	Lifelong
Polio vaccine	Lifelong after one time booster
Tb skin test (PPD)	Test yearly to assess for Tb
Tetanus-diphtheria, toxoid absorbed Td	10 years
Typhoid Vivotif vaccine-oral TY21a	5 years
Varicella (chickenpox) vaccine	Lifelong
Yellow fever vaccine	10 years

immunizations will depend upon the region and changes with time. Table 5.1 lists some of the common vaccines and length of protection.

It is imperative that the team understands the local climate and environmental conditions for competition. Multiple factors including temperature, humidity, altitude and pollutants will affect athlete performance (see Common travel illnesses). Transitioning from a hot to cold temperature will affect the body's homeostatic regulatory system. Athletes might train indoors, but need to compete outdoors in hotter or colder temperatures. Inappropriate acclimatization may lead to hyper- or hypothermia. A marked change in humidity will affect the body's ability to perspire which may lead to hyperthermia. Athletes training at sea level, but competing at higher altitudes will need to acclimatize to the new altitude level. The effects of altitude are almost immediate, including shortness of breath, headache, dizziness, nausea and fatigue. Unfortunately, it may take several weeks to adapt to the new altitude level. Finally, regulation of air pollutants will vary from country to country. Excessive pollutants may exacerbate pulmonary conditions including exercise-induced asthma that will compromise athlete performance.

Diet can be another regional concern. Access to clean drinking water is of utmost importance in promoting appropriate hydration status for the athletes and preventing traveler's diarrhea. Traveler's diarrhea is mainly due to bacteria in the water or food due to poor sanitation, poor packaging or improper handling of food in restaurants or markets. Unfortunately, it is unclear as to which athlete is more likely to be susceptible to such an illness. Though a variety of anecdotes, including eating spicy food, has been reported to prevent traveler's diarrhea, the best prevention is to avoid local drinking water. In some countries, local tap water or food washed in local water should be avoided and water should be boiled or bottled with an unbroken seal before use. Ice cubes should be avoided. Arrangements may need to be made for an adequate bottled water supply.

A variety of treatment options are available to purify water for drinking. Boiling of water for at least 1 min (at sea level) or 3 min (elevation >2000 m) will kill most bacteria and parasites. Chemical disinfection including the use of iodine and a neutralizer to make the water more palatable can be effective for a variety of pathogens, but will not kill *Cryptosporidium*. Finally, water filtration systems are available, but vary in regard to the process for which they filter out any pathogens. Reverse-osmosis filters or pore sizes less than 1 μm are designed to filter out such pathogens as *Giardia* or *Cryptosporidium*.

Cultural and regional differences in foods and meals may also be an issue. The team should be aware if the regional diet is similar or comparable with their usual food. If exotic foods are unpalatable or nutritionally deficient, the athletes' energy and performance may be negatively affected. Dairy products are not always pasteurized, including milk, butter, cheese and ice cream. Raw vegetables are easily contaminated during preparation and uncooked vegetables should be avoided. Fresh fruit should be avoided unless washed and peeled by the athlete. Street vendor food should be avoided as it has been associated with an increased risk of illness. Cooked food should be eaten immediately, as food allowed to sit around for hours will develop bacterial growth over time. It is wise to plan ahead for any potential nutritional issues specific to the region of travel.

Prior knowledge of the lodging arrangements at the destination is also important. Accommodations can vary from country to country and will depend upon the event. Lodging with loud noises, excess light or rooms that allow smoking could be quite disruptive to the athletes' rest. Depending upon the venue, accommodation may be a tent, local dormitories, hotels or villages specific for the athletic staff. Ascertain if there are private rooms or if sharing is expected. Be aware of the possibility of the room being used as a treatment room as well.

In addition to accommodation details, the team physician should be aware of the medical treatment facilities at the event venue and in the local area. The team usually has its own medical bag with supplies (detailed in the next section). It helps to know if the venue has private treatment rooms or partitions. It is possible that healthcare may be expected for the opposing team, spectators, or venue employees. Find out if the event is scheduled to have paramedics standing by. If desired, local EMT providers can usually send a unit to be on standby if there is a need and it is requested in advance. Find out whether or not an ambulance is on-site, find out where the nearest hospital is, what emergency services are provided there and how patients can be transported in an emergency. For events in the wilderness, it is necessary to assess emergency evacuation routes including use of all-terrain vehicles or helicopter support, in cases where an athlete is severely injured and has limited access.

Finally, a physician traveling internationally should understand the team's health insurance and malpractice coverage. Every athlete and staff member should have health insurance coverage in case of an emergency. Many insurance plans will reimburse any expenses incurred during travel up to a certain amount. Supplemental health insurance may be helpful, especially if someone needs emergent evacuation from a particular site. Malpractice coverage will vary as well. Some institutions provide malpractice coverage throughout the world. Other plans may offer coverage restricted to the US. However, sometimes the supporting athletic organization will obtain supplemental malpractice coverage. You should check with the malpractice coverage organization to understand the full extent of coverage.

Supplies for emergencies

Preparation of supplies for emergencies during travel should also be established before a trip. The medical bag should be checked and fully stocked. The contents of the medical bag vary somewhat by team and event.[1,2] Table 5.2 provides an example of standard supplies. However, the exact contents will depend upon the teams' needs. Determine if the medical staff or athletic trainers will be responsible for checking, stocking and transporting the bag during travel and at the event. The bag should be precisely organized so that items are clearly labeled, easy to find and always kept in the same location within the case or bag (Fig. 5.1).

In addition to planning what should be in the medical bag, the team physician should also know what should *not* be in the bag. For international travel, the physician should be aware of the local laws to avoid bringing illegal medications into a specific country. In Japan, it is illegal to bring stimulants such as pseudoephedrine or codeine into the country. While in the Middle East, a variety of narcotics may lead to an arrest. All prescription medication should be carried in its original bottle. In addition, a letter from a physician stating the nature and use of the medication is quite helpful. The United States Department of State website can provide a wealth of information regarding any potentially illegal substances while traveling to a specific country (http://travel.state.gov/travel).

It is imperative that the physician be aware of which substances are banned by any governing bodies of the team's sport. Some websites with current guidelines include the World Anti-doping Agency (www.wada-ama.org), United States Olympic Committee (www.usoc.org), the International Association of Athletes Federation (www.iaaf.org/antidoping/downloads), or the National Collegiate Athletic Association (www.ncaa.org). The physician should periodically check the appropriate organization's website, as substances and medications will change over time.

Team communication

It is up to the head medical practitioner to assure that the rest of the team members are informed about medical and health travel issues. For local trips, this is not much of an issue. Long distance and international travel however, may present additional health challenges. Depending on the destination, issues of proper hydration, environmental and climatic conditions, and sanitation may warrant team education prior to travel. Personal safety reminders and education may be needed. Athletes should also be reminded about the potential risks of sexual activity and counseled to use judgment and protection. Cultural differences may necessitate education about appropriate public behavior and attire to avoid embarrassing, difficult, or dangerous public interactions.

Physician checklist

There is much to be scheduled, checked, and planned prior to traveling with the team. Having a standard check list (Table 5.3) of tasks denoting a timeline (count-down to departure) can be very helpful. The successful team practitioner plans ahead and prepares for a trip in a timely manner to avoid last minute

Table 5.2 Team Physician Medical Supplies: Bag Contents

I Airway management	Hibiclens or hydrogen peroxide
Bag valve mask	Sterile water
Forceps	Tefla pads
Laryngoscope	Duoderm
Straight and curved laryngoscope blades	Bioclusives
Extra batteries	Kling gauze
Extra bulbs	Bandaids
ET tubes (sizes 6–9)	Topical antibiotic packets
Oral airways (sizes 5.5–12)	Benzoin
60 cc syringe	Steri-strips
10 cc syringe	Tape
No. 11 blade	Skin glue
Cricothyroidotomy kit	VI Medications (depends upon region)
No. 14 intercath	Injectable
II I.V. kit	Marcaine
Tourniquet	Lidocaine with/without epi
Alcohol pads	Morphine
Angiocaths 14G, 21G, 18G	Epi pen
Butterfly 19G, 21G, 23G	Phenergan
Gauze	Ketorolac (Toradol)
Tape	Celestone
I.V. tubing sets	Oral
I.V. fluid (LR, D51/2NS, NS)	Acetaminophen (Tylenol)
III Eye kit	Ibuprofen or naproxen
Eye shield	Ciprofloxacin
Oval eye pads	Norfloxacin
Cotton tipped applicator	Azithromycin
Eye solution	Benadryl
Tape	Tylenol with codeine
Fluorescein drops	Albuterol inhaler
Tobramycin drops	Loperamide
Proparacaine drops	Phenergan
Cobalt blue light	Methylprednisolone
Mirror	Pepto-Bismol
Pen light	VII Physician diagnostic kit
IV Suture and injection kit	Tongue depressors
Syringes (3 cc, 5 cc, 10 cc)	Cotton-tipped applicator
Marcaine	Latex and vinyl gloves
Lidocaine	Pen light
Needles (16G, 18G, 22G, 25G)	Oto/ophthalmoscope
Alcohol pads	Stethoscope
Betadine swabs	Sphygmomanometer
Needle holder, scissors, pick-ups	Reflex hammer
Suture (3-0, 4-0, 5-0, 6-0)	Urine dip sticks
Antibiotic ointment	Thermometers
Gauze	VIII Miscellaneous
Bandaids	Cervical collar
Tape	Pens
Benzoin	Injury assessment forms
Steri-strips	Prescription pad
Sterile gloves	Sharps container
V Wound care	Biohazard bag
Betadine swabs	
Alcohol pads	

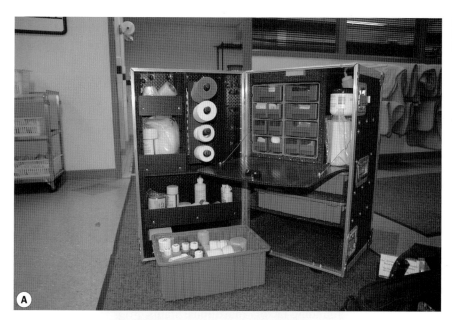

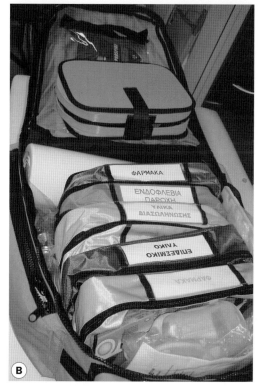

Figure 5.1 (A) Medical cabinet for storage of supplies. (B) Medical backpack with organization of supplies into pouches.

problems. Some general topics to include on this list are checking on the venue, accommodations, required health precautions, emergency numbers/contacts, team education issues and the medical bag. In addition to a medical checklist, having a personal check list can help you to be fully prepared not only for the medical care duties, but also for the personal and fun aspects of the trip.

TRAVEL

Traveling with a team for sporting competition can be both exciting and stressful. Questions related to air or road travel

are often directed to the medical personnel. Psychological and emotional issues related to travel and competitive stress affect team members and staff. Sports-related injuries, incidental

Box 5.2: Key Points

- Traveling can have a physical and emotional impact on athletes and their performance.
- Jet lag may impede performance and should be treated pro-actively as appropriate.
- Maintain proper nutrition including hydration.

Table 5.3   Physician Travel Preparation Checklist

Weeks prior to departure
  Review location logistics
  ☑ Venue medical facilities
  ☑ Accommodations
  ☑ Visas/Passports as appropriate
  ☑ Local hospitals/local contacts
  ☑ Secure any special medications
  ☑ Local weather patterns (temperature, humidity, sun exposure) assessing
     time needed for acclimatization
  Team health concerns
  ☑ Team immunizations
  ☑ Regional health concerns
  ☑ Emergency contact info
Days prior to department
  Team health concerns
  ☑ Review medical supplies and secure items
  ☑ Review any medical precautions with athletes and staff
  ☑ Encourage hydration during travel
  Personal concerns
  ☑ Review personal medical supplies
  ☑ Review personal travel gear
  ☑ Passport

injuries and travel-related illnesses need to be dealt with in a timely fashion. In addition to the preparation discussed in the previous section, successful management of these issues requires knowledge and readiness to act.

Transportation-specific issues

Different methods of travel share some common potential problems that can be simply avoided. More common problems include jet lag, dehydration and muscle cramping from immobility.

Jet lag is a term used to describe a host of symptoms an individual feels after rapidly traversing several time zones. It is believed to occur when a person's internal circadian rhythms and body clock are dyssynchronous with the environment after traveling across time zones.[3] Symptom intensity increases the greater the disparity in time change between home and destination. Symptoms include general malaise, fatigue, insomnia, headaches and gastrointestinal upset. Approximately 0.5–1 day per time zone crossed is needed to reset circadian rhythms to local time, and is generally slower following eastward compared with westward travel.[4] Exposure to the light/dark cycle at the destination is believed to be the major factor in resetting the circadian rhythms.

Treatment options vary based on the individual's preference but include altered sleeping times while traveling, prescribed medications and supplements. The use of medications includes short-acting zolpidem or melatonin. However, long-acting medications, such as diphenhydramine, should be avoided as they might lead to sedation of the athlete and a 'hangover feeling'. There is some evidence that oral melatonin combined with appropriate light/dark entrainment and timely physical exercise can decrease the time it takes to re-entrain to the local time zone.[5,6]

Various studies have attempted to assess the impact of time zone changes on athletic performance.[7–9] A study of athletic performance following travel through multiple time zones has shown some athletes to have mood alterations, and decreased aerobic power, aerobic capacity and dynamic strength.[8] However, another study showed mixed results for measures of muscle strength and muscular endurance.[9] More studies are needed to support or refute the extent to which traveling through time zones affects athletic performance.[7]

Several studies have suggested existence of a 'peak time' for athletic performance related to the internal clock/circadian rhythms. Peak athletic performance has been hypothesized to occur in synchrony with peak circadian body temperatures from approximately 1800 to 2000 hours. It is also purported that the trough temperature (and athletic performance) occurs in the early morning, approximately 0400 to 0600 hours. The studies did not control for all of the multiple potential confounding factors (nutritional status, prior rest, environment and body temperature, among others) and thus cannot be considered conclusive.[4] Studies examining the effect of time zone changes on performance in the National Football League and the National Basketball Association suggest that west coast teams traveling east display a winning advantage for night games, where east coast teams traveling west display a disadvantage.[10–12] The studies propose that a possible factor is that the west coast teams are competing in sync with the circadian peak for athletic performance. Further studies are needed to be conclusive. However, the implication is that athletes do show some competitive advantage when competing in sync with circadian athletic peaks. This may be helpful information if a team has any choice of what time of day to compete when on the road.

Hydration is another factor that affects performance and cramping. Long road trips in warm weather or flights with re-circulated air can certainly lead to mild to moderate dehydration if travelers do not adequately replace water loss by drinking water or sports drinks *en route*. Alcohol intake only contributes to dehydration, especially on flights and should be strongly discouraged. In addition to proper hydration, team members should be reminded to eat at appropriate times during travel. Meals or *per diem* food funds should be provided to the athletes for car or bus trips. Airlines may provide a meal service, but this is becoming less available. Team staff should be prepared to keep the team properly fed or the athletes should be reminded to bring their own food.

Finally, with prolonged transportation by bus, car, or airplane, athletes should be reminded to change position every hour or so to avoid a potential deep venous thrombosis and minimize cramping from immobility in the seated position. Prevention strategies include stopping every few hours at a rest stop (car or bus) or walking in the aisle (bus or airplane).

Common travel illnesses
Traveler's diarrhea

The most common pathogens for traveler's diarrhea include bacteria, viruses and parasites. The primary bacterial strains include *Escherichia coli* and *Shigella*, while viruses or parasites might include *Giardia* or *Entameba*. Symptoms will typically include watery diarrhea, nausea, vomiting, abdominal cramps and low-grade fever. Other rare symptoms include bright red blood in the diarrhea and dehydration with resultant fatigue. Fortunately, the symptoms are often mild and self-limiting. Symptoms will resolve in 1–4 days without antibiotics, but can be shortened to 12–24 h, with antibiotics.[13]

Though diarrhea, nausea and vomiting are self-limited, they can be distressing and negatively affect an athlete's performance. Aggressive hydration with oral rehydration fluids including electrolyte supplement should be instituted and are essential to recovery. Athletes experiencing symptoms for more than 2–3 days or exhibiting signs including orthostasis, tachycardia or disorientation should receive intravenous fluid. Antimicrobial medications (Table 5.4) taken at the onset of the diarrhea will shorten the duration of the symptoms. Ciprofloxacin is typically used, though for more severe cases doxycycline or norfloxacin may be used. Combining loperamide, used to decrease the number of diarrheal stools, with ciprofloxacin, may shorten the recovery time. For very mild cases, bismuth subsalicylate will help with the symptoms but must be taken up to four times a day. Finally, preventive measures include avoidance of tap water, ice cubes and salads or fruit washed in local water.

Upper respiratory tract infections

Upper respiratory tract infections are often quite common. Often, athletes will present with a cough, shortness of breath and decreased performance. Associated symptoms might include wheezing, fever or chills. They may be acquired with a change in the environment with an exposure to various strains of viruses. Often, the symptoms are self limiting and treated symptomatically. However, many standard medications are banned by the governing bodies of most athletic competitions, so care is needed when choosing treatments. Antihistamines, throat lozenges and nasal sprays can be helpful. Antiviral agents are not recommended. In the case of possible bacterial infection, antibiotics may be initiated. If there is concern about cross-infection with other athletes, the infected athlete should be isolated until their symptoms have improved.

Heat-related illnesses

Traveling to different regions or countries may include a significant change in temperature from the departure city. Athletes competing in areas significantly warmer and more humid than their home have the potential to experience heat-related illnesses as heat dissipation is altered. Risk factors include lack of acclimatization, dehydration, fatigue, alcohol and caffeine use, peer pressure and overmotivation.[14] A 10-year study of American high school and college athletes revealed that 10% of deaths were caused by exertional heatstroke.[15] Prevention includes proper hydration and acclimation to the environment.

The clinical spectrum of heat-related illnesses ranges from mild heat cramps to heatstroke. The key to successful management is prevention and early recognition of the symptoms. Heat cramps refers to brief, intermittent cramping of large muscles after physical exertion. The symptoms can become quite painful causing the athlete to stop competition. Prevention includes proper hydration and perhaps, increased dietary salts.[16] Although the etiology is unclear, treatment will include rest in a cool environment and rehydration with an electrolyte solution. For severe cramps, intravenous fluids may be warranted and diazepam may help to relax the muscle.[16]

Athletes presenting with heat exhaustion will typically experience fatigue and decreased athletic performance. They may note associated headaches, dizziness, nausea and irritability. Similar to heat cramps, treatment will include cessation of the athletic activity and rest in a cool environment. A variety of cooling measures have been described including the use of ice packs or ice water immersion for temperatures greater than 40°C.[17] Oral hydration with an electrolyte solution should be attempted first prior to the initiation of intravenous fluids. Intravenous fluids should be initiated if the athlete has severe vomiting and becomes hemodynamically unstable.

Heatstroke is a medical emergency and requires quick treatment to prevent death. It typically occurs with high core body temperatures of 41°C, which leads to thermal injury of tissues. However, symptoms may be experienced with lower core body temperatures. Symptoms include mental status changes (coma, convulsions and confusion) and cessation of sweating in addition to severe hyperthermia. Treatment includes immediate aggressive cooling measures (ice water submersion), intravenous fluids and emergent transport to a hospital (Table 5.5).[16]

Table 5.4 Common Medications for Traveling

Antibiotic	Prophylactic Dose	Treatment Dose
Azithromycin		1000 mg once or 500 mg daily for 3 days
Ciprofloxacin	500 mg	500 mg once or twice a day for trip
Doxycycline	100 mg	200 mg the first day and then 100 mg twice a day for 3 days
Norfloxacin		400 mg twice a day for 3 days
Sulfamethoxazole + Trimethoprim	1DS tab	2DS tabs once or 1DS daily for 3 days
Medication		
Bismuth subsalicylate	2 tabs after each meal and at night	2 tabs every 2–4 h as needed
Loperamide		4 mg once, then 2 mg after each loose stool, max 16 mg per day

Table 5.5 Heat-Related Illnesses

Type	Temperature	Symptoms/Signs	Plan of Care
Heat cramps	36–38 ˚C	*Symptoms*: brief intermittent muscle cramping *Signs*: palpable muscle spasm	*Treatment*: Rest, stretching, oral hydration ± salts *Consider*: i.v. fluids and Valium for severe cases
Heat syncope	36–38 ˚C	*Symptoms*: syncope *Signs*: transient loss of consciousness	*Treatment*: Rest, lie athlete supine with feet raises
Heat exhaustion	37–40 ˚C	*Symptoms*: fatigue, headache, dizziness, nausea, irritability and mild disorientation *Signs*: hypotension, tachycardia, confusion	*Monitor*: ABCs, monitor temperature and vital signs *Treatment*: rest, cool environment, oral or i.v. fluids
Heatstroke	>40 ˚C	*Symptoms*: fatigue, nausea, profound mental status changes, visual disturbances, vomiting *Signs*: hypotension, arrhythmias, possible loss of sweating, hyperventilation, confusion or coma	*Monitor*: ABCs, monitor temperature and vital signs, *Treatment*: rest, cool urgently (ice baths/water immersion, i.v. fluids *Transport to emergency facility*

ABCs, airway, breathing, circulation; i.v., intravenous.

Cold-related illnesses

Similar to heat-related illnesses, athletes competing in areas significantly colder than their home have the potential to experience cold-related illnesses. Fortunately, the majority of the time, the symptoms are mild in nature and can be managed easily. Contributing factors include poor acclimatization, improper clothing, the time of exposure to cold temperatures, concurrent use of medications, dehydration, sleep deprivation and fatigue. Symptoms will include chills, nausea, fatigue and dizziness. With hypothermia (temperature less that 35 ˚C), athletes may experience tachypnea, altered consciousness and incoordination.[18]

Treatment of mild hypothermia requires immediate removal of the athlete from the cold environment. Removal of any wet clothing and slow passive re-warming with blankets is important. Hydration is essential and warm, sweet drinks should be considered if the athlete can take fluids orally. Caffeinated drinks should be avoided. For more severe hypothermia or associated frostbite, the athlete should be transported to a hospital for further care.

Altitude

Acute mountain sickness (AMS) occurs when acclimatization to altitude lags significantly behind the ascent and is basically manifestation of hypoxia. The severity will depend upon multiple factors, including the altitude attained, rate of ascent, length of altitude exposure and level of exertion.[19] AMS encompasses a spectrum of illness from mild to severe (including high altitude cerebral edema, or HACE). The diagnosis of early AMS is a throbbing, bitemporal or occipital headache, typically worse at night and upon awakening. The headache is usually associated with one or more of the following: gastrointestinal upset, fatigue, weakness, dizziness, light-headedness, confusion or insomnia. Dyspnea on exertion is common for AMS, but dyspnea at rest would suggest high altitude pulmonary edema (HAPE). Physical examination is quite varied depending upon the severity of the symptoms, but pulmonary rales and lack of increase urine output is not uncommon.[20] In more severe HACE, the athlete will wish to be left alone, have difficulty performing activities of daily living and eventually may slip into a coma.

Treatment is based on early diagnosis and continued monitoring of systems. Symptoms will usually improve within 24–48 h, but worsening symptoms require a descent to lower altitude. Indications for immediate descent include pulmonary edema and neurologic changes. For mild AMS, the treatment consists of halting the ascent, rest, oral hydration and analgesics (acetaminophen, aspirin or ibuprofen) are helpful. Use of acetazolamide (125–250 mg twice a day orally) can speed acclimatization.[21] Studies suggest that prophylactic acetazolamide 125–250 mg taken orally twice daily started 24 h prior to ascent is effective in decreasing symptoms of AMS.[22]

Skin rashes

Dermatologic disorders are relatively common depending upon the sport. The most common disorders are due to infectious or inflammatory conditions. The following discussion is meant as an overview and specific details should be obtained from more focused articles.

Infectious causes may be fungal, viral, bacterial or parasitic sources.[23] Fungal (tinea), viral (herpes simplex) and bacteria (streptococci or staphylococci impetigo) infections are quite common, especially in wrestlers, football and basketball players. Infections may occur in areas of macerated skin from sweating, including the groin or feet. Environmental factors include competition in hot and humid climates, improper cleaning, prolonged equipment use without cleaning and close skin to skin contact. Prevention is extremely important, including educating athletes about the avoidance of towel or equipment sharing, proper hygiene, use of sandals in the shower and pharmacologic medication, as appropriate. Treatment options will depend upon the source of the infection but include the use of topical or oral antifungal medication (i.e. fluconazole), oral antiviral medications (i.e. famciclovir) and antibacterial medications (i.e. dicloxacillin or cephalexin), as appropriate. Athletes may need to wait 5–7 days or until any lesions are scabbed and dry before returning to competition.

Common inflammatory conditions include contact dermatitis and urticaria. Contact dermatitis may be allergic or from contact with an irritating agent. Athletes may experience allergic reactions from equipment, medications or environmental exposures (plants or chemicals on the field). Athletes especially sensitive to latex, rubber products or adhesives should take special care to avoid such products. Outdoor competitions including exposure to new plants or poison ivy should be limited as much as possible. Treatment includes the use of topical corticosteroids and the avoidance of any offending products.[24] Urticaria (or hives) may occur in both hot and cold climates. The erythematous plaques often resolve over 24 h and in response to the use of antihistamines. Corticosteroid medications are typically ineffective.

Sexually transmitted diseases (STDs)

For some athletes, traveling to a new location is an exciting time to experience new things. Unfortunately, athletes may exhibit some high-risk behaviors that could lead to subsequent medical issues. Unsupervised athletes may partake in excessive drug and alcohol use or high risk sexual behavior. High school and college aged athletes are at increased risk for such behavior leading to morbidity or mortality. College athletes appear to consume more alcohol compared with their non-athletic peers.[25] In addition, college athletes exhibit greater risky sexual behavior, including more sexual partners and less condom use, resulting in a greater number of diseases compared with their non-athletic peers.[25]

Unfortunately, substance abuse may lead to unprotected sexual activity and subsequent sexually transmitted diseases. Common diseases include chlamydia, gonorrhea, syphilis or HIV. Prevention is the key to avoiding such illnesses. The team physician should speak to all athletes about substance abuse and sexual activity prior to traveling. All athletes should be counseled about the potential risks and encouraged not to have random sexual encounters. They should be advised to use condoms during any sexual activities to prevent disease and pregnancy. During the recent Olympic Games, the Athlete Village Central Medical Clinic supplied athletes with condoms in the hope of preventing STDs. Treatment for sexually transmitted diseases will depend upon the source of infection. Common medications include azithromycin (chlamydia), acyclovir (herpes), penicillin (syphilis) or newer medications for HIV.

RETURNING HOME

Arriving home does not quite signify the end of travel responsibility for the physician. Several issues should be resolved prior to the end of the trip. Any athlete or team member who needs follow-up care should be scheduled for an evaluation prior to their final dismissal. Speaking with the coaches, trainers and/or athletes will alert the physician to any lingering issues or questions. A member of the medical staff should assess which supplies have been used and all medical supplies should be re-stocked. Finally, the members of the team should provide input into what worked well for the team and identify any protocol that should be revised to ensure future success.

CONCLUSION

The responsibilities of the team physician are vast and the schedule can be demanding. For the practitioner who chooses the role of traveling team physician, the difficulties and sacrifices are offset by the gratification of working with motivated athlete-patients. Providing medical care in the competitive sports venue is a competitive market itself among sports medicine physicians. Demonstration of effective planning, appropriate knowledge of pertinent issues, and the ability to maintain rapport with the team and staff will make you a sought-after team care provider.

REFERENCES

1 Brukner P, Khan K, eds. Medical care of the sporting team. In: Clinical sports medicine. New York: McGraw-Hill; 1993:654-657.
2 Buettner CM. The team physician's bag. Clin Sports Med 1998; 17:365-373.
3 O'Connor P, Morgan W. Athletic performance following rapid traversal of multiple time zones. Sports Med 1990; 10:20-30.
4 Youngstedt SD, O'Connor PJ. The influence of air travel on athletic performance. Sports Med 1999; 28(3):197-207.
5 Atkinson G, Drust B, Reilly T, et al. The relevance of melatonin to sports medicine and science. Sports Med 2003; 33:809-831.
6 Cardinali D, Bortman G, Liotta G, et al. A multifactorial approach employing melatonin to accelerate resynchronization of sleep-wake cycle after a 12 time-zone westerly transmeridian flight in elite soccer athletes. J Pineal Res 2002; 32:41-46.
7 Atkinson G, Reilly T. Circadian variation in sports performance. Sports Med 1996; 21:292-312.
8 Hill DW, Hill CM, Fields KL, et al. Effects of jet lag on factors related to sports performance. Can J Appl Physiol 1993; 18:91-103.
9 Wright JE, Vogel JA, Sampson JB, et al. Effects of travel across time zones (jet-lag) on exercise capacity and performance. Aviat Space Environ Med 1983; 54:132-137.
10 Jehue R, Street D, Huizenga R. Effect of time zone and game time changes on team performance: national football league. Med Sci Sports Exerc 1993; 25:127-130.
11 Smith R, Guilleminault C, Efron B. Circadian rhythms and enhanced athletic performance in the national football league. Sleep 1997; 20:362-365.
12 Steenland K, Deddens J. Effect of travel and rest on performance of professional basketball players. Sleep 1997; 20:366-369.
13 Brukner P, Khan K. Traveling with a team. In: Bruckner P, Khan K, eds. Clinical sports medicine. New York: McGraw-Hill; 1993:658-665.
14 Epstein Y, Moran DS, Shapiro Y, et al. Exertional heat stroke: a case series. Med Sci Sports Exerc 1999; 31:224.
15 Camp SP Van, Bloor CM, Mueller FO, et al. Nontraumatic sports death in high school and college athletes. Med Sci Sports Exerc 1995; 27:641-647.
16 Eichner ER. Treatment of suspected heat illness. Int J Sports Med 1998; 19:150-153.
17 Gaffin SL, Garnder J, Finn S. Current cooling method for exertional heatstroke. Ann Intern Med 2000; 132:678.
18 Danzl DF. Accidental hypothermia. In: Auerbach P, ed. Wilderness medicine. St Louis, MO: Mosby; 2001:135-177.
19 Roach RC, Maes D, Sandoval D, et al. Exercise exacerbates acute mountain sickness at simulated high altitude. J Appl Physiol 2000; 88:581-585.
20 Hackett PH, Roach RC. High-altitude medicine. In: Auerbach P, ed. Wilderness medicine. St Louis, MO: Mosby; 2001:2-43.
21 Grissom CK, Roach RC, Sarnquist FH, et al. Acetazolamide in the treatment of acute mountain sickness: Clinical efficacy and effect on gas exchange. Ann Intern Med 1992; 116:461-465.
22 Carlsten C, Swenson ER, Ruoss S. A dose-response study of acetazolamide for acute mountain sickness prophylaxis in vacationing tourists at 12,000 feet (3630m). High Alt Med Biol 2004; 5:33-39.
23 Adams BB. Dermatologic disorders of the athlete. Sports Med 2002; 32:309-321.
24 Fischer AA. Sports-related cutaneous reactions: Part II: allergic contact dermatitis to sports equipment. Cutis 1999; 63:202-204.
25 Nattiv A. Puffer J, Green G. Lifestyle and health risks of college athletes: a multi-center study. Clin J Sports Med 1997; 7:262-272.

CHAPTER 6

General Medical Problems of the Athlete

Julia Alleyne and Andrea Burry

ANEMIA

Box 6.1: Key Points

- Athletes with low hemoglobin may have a high plasma volume causing a dilutional effect and treatment is not necessary.
- Check for true anemia through diet recall, detailed gastrointestinal and geni and blood analysis as it may reduce athletic performance.
- Iron supplementation, dietary modifications and monitoring.

Overview and incidence

Anemia, or low hemoglobin, is an important consideration in sport, as iron deficiency may adversely affect athletic performance. Anemia is generally defined as a hemoglobin concentration under 14 g/dl in a man or under 12 g/dl in a woman. Anemia is classically divided into three categories; microcytic, normocytic and macrocytic, based on the size of the RBC or the MCV. All of these categories of anemia are caused by specific conditions (Table 6.1).

There are some important considerations to take into account when interpreting a low Hb value in athletes. Athletes often have a lower Hb concentration than the general sedentary public and therefore, what is an 'abnormal' laboratory value may actually be 'normal' for the athletic population. Also, routine laboratory blood testing does not take into account the RBC mass. If the plasma blood volume is higher (as it may be in athletes) the Hb may be diluted and read as 'low', when in fact the red cell mass is normal.[1]

The three most common causes of anemia in athletes are iron-deficiency anemia, sports anemia or pseudoanemia and footstrike hemolysis.

Iron deficiency anemia is a true anemia commonly found in athletes, especially females. Iron is incorporated into the formation of hemoglobin and is important in sports performance because of its role in oxygen transport. Inadequate iron intake, absorption or excessive loss limits the amount of iron available for this and other intracellular processes.[2]

Iron deficiency anemia is common in non-athletic populations and is likely the most common nutritional deficiency in the western world. The issue of whether iron deficiency is more common in athletes has always been a point of controversy. Large studies have shown that iron deficiency occurs in about 20% of menstruating women and 1–6% of postmenopausal women and men.[3] Some studies have shown a higher prevalence of iron deficiency in female athletes than the general population, while others have failed to show a difference when compared with proper controls.[4,5] This suggests that exercise itself is not a risk factor for the condition, but athletes may be more prone to developing it.

Pseudoanemia, although not a true anemia, is the most common anemia in endurance athletes. As mentioned in earlier, endurance athletes tend to have lower Hb levels than the general population despite a normal red cell mass. This is due to an expansion of plasma volume and a subsequent dilutional effect. This 'sports anemia' due to dilution of RBCs is referred to as pseudoanemia and is an adaptation of exercise and does not seem to inhibit athletic performance. It is not a pathologic condition and it normalizes with training cessation in 3–5 days. The Hb level in a well-conditioned athlete may be 1–1.5 g/dl lower than the laboratory quoted 'normal'. The physician looking after athletes must be able to recognize this as a pseudoanemia and exclude iron deficiency anemia. There is no treatment for pseudoanemia other than recognizing it as distinct from other pathological anemias.

Table 6.1 Categories of Anemia

Microcytic (MCV <75 fL)	Normocytic (MCV 75–95 fL)	Macrocytic (MCV >95 fL)
Iron deficiency	Chronic disease	Folate deficiency
Thalassemia minor	Hemolysis	B_{12} deficiency
Lead poisoning	Rapid bleeding	Hypothyroidism
Sideroblastic anemia	Malignancy	Liver disease
		Malignancy
		Drugs

Modified from Fields 1997.[2] MCV, mean corpuscular volume (red blood cell size).

Footstrike hemolysis refers to the bursting of RBCs in the circulation, from the impact of footfalls.[1] Rowing and swimming also have been shown to have similar intravascular hemolysis and hence, such destruction of RBCs may be due to exertion as opposed to the footstrike itself.[6] This hemolysis is usually mild and rarely if ever drains iron stores and causes anemia. Diagnosis can be made when one has the combination of an elevated red cell volume, reticulocytosis and a low serum haptoglobin. Treatment revolves around lessening the foot impact, i.e. wearing well-cushioned shoes, attaining and maintaining an ideal weight and running on soft surfaces. It is unknown at this point how to treat hemolysis from non-impact sports, however, since it is so mild, treatment is rarely required.

Relation to sport

The underlying development of iron deficiency anemia is either due to blood loss or poor iron intake through diet. Other sources have been suggested but do not appear to contribute to a clinically apparent anemia. Iron loss in sweat accounts for a very minimal amount. Similar studies (Fields 1997) have been done investigating iron loss from urine, the GI tract or from footstrike hemolysis; none of these appear to deplete iron stores in sufficient amounts to cause anemia.[2] The main culprit then seems to be dietary in nature. Athletes, especially women, involved in sports such as long-distance running, ice skaters and gymnasts, through restrictive diets, consume too little iron to meet their daily needs. Vegetarian athletes are particularly at risk because the iron in vegetables and grains is not as readily absorbed as that in red meat.

Signs and symptoms

Athletes with iron deficiency anemia may be asymptomatic, while others may experience muscle weakness, palpitations or shortness of breath. They usually seek medical attention because of fatigue or decreased performance.[2] A complete history should be taken to rule out significant GI or GU sources, although this is uncommon in a younger population, it may be significant in older athletes.

Investigations

Laboratory investigations should include a complete blood count, serum ferritin and total iron binding capacity.[3] Findings of iron deficiency anemia will include microcytic, hypochromic RBCs, a serum ferritin less than 10 µg/l and a low iron saturation. Once diagnosis is made, the etiology of the deficiency must be established. Again, one must be astute to the fact that athletes may present with 'non-athletic' causes of anemia, so GI or GU related causes must be ruled out.

Management

Treatment of iron deficiency anemia requires iron supplementation such as ferrous sulfate or gluconate in doses of 600 mg two to three times daily. Maintenance dosing is 600 mg once daily. Absorption is best when taken between meals and with orange juice as ascorbic acid improves iron absorption. Iron rich foods, such as lean red meats should be incorporated into the diet. With dietary changes and iron supplementation, the athletes' Hb should return to normal within a couple of months, and relief of symptoms may occur within days to weeks. Most recommend therapy for 6–12 months to fully replenish iron stores and some may require lifelong therapy especially if the cause of the deficiency is diet related.[3]

Summary

Iron deficiency is a common problem with special significance for athletes due to the demands of their physical lifestyle. The cause appears to be primarily dietary in nature, however, other more serious causes must be taken into account. The diagnosis can be made quite easily with relatively non-invasive means and treatment in the form of a supplement can improve symptoms within weeks.

ASTHMA

Box 6.2: Key Points

- Exercise-induced asthma (EIA) is a common condition that affects athletes but may be underdiagnosed by 30%, due to its inconsistent presentation.
- It is often triggered by dry, cold conditions.
- History and physical exam may not reveal abnormalities; often a trial of pharmacotherapy and/or formal challenge testing is required.
- The most effective treatment for exercise-induced asthma is a short-acting beta-agonist given within 15 min of exercise.
- When properly treated, exercise-induced asthma does not hinder athletic performance or one's ability to perform in intense competition.

Overview and incidence

Asthma is one of the most common chronic illnesses of young people, affecting between 5 and 15% of the North American population. Asthma is characterized by reversible airway obstruction caused by bronchial smooth muscle spasm, inflammation of the endobronchiole tree or both.[7] Asthma has a significant impact on lifestyle; accounting for missed work or school days and limiting physical activities.

Exercise-induced asthma (EIA) or exercise-induced bronchospasm (EIB) is a type of asthma that is characterized by a transient increase in airway resistance following intense physical exercise. It can be present with chronic asthma, but, most often is a separate disease. The signs and symptoms of EIA are similar, but not identical to those of chronic asthma and many athletes often go undiagnosed as a result. There are special diagnostic tests available to aid in diagnosis and a number of new therapies available to treat EIA. With proper diagnosis and treatment, athletes with EIA should be able to participate in any level of sports competition.

While chronic asthma is primarily caused by inflammation due to a hyper-responsiveness of the airways to inhaled stimulants, the mechanism of EIA is not totally understood. There are two current theories (Storms 2003); the hyperosmolarity theory and the airway re-warming theory.[8] The hyperosmolarity theory assumes that during exercise, water is lost from the airway surface leading to a hypertonic and hyperosmolar condition in the airway cell. This causes the release of inflammatory mediators like histamine, prostaglandins and leukotrienes that eventually lead to bronchoconstriction. The airway re-warming theory states that during exercise, hyperventilation causes cooling of the surface airway cells. Subsequently, following exercise, the 're-warming' causes dilatation of small bronchiolar vessels around the airway, leading to airway lining hyperemia, fluid exudation into the submucosa of the airway wall from the blood vessel, mediator release and subsequent bronchoconstriction.

EIA affects up to 35% of athletes and up to 90% of chronic asthmatics.[9] There have been numerous studies showing a high prevalence of EIA in recreational and elite athletes. Vacek (1997) showed that the incidence of EIA in Canadian high school athletes was 13.2% as determined by a 15% decrease in peak expiratory flow rate on a Free Running Asthma Screening Test (FRAST).[10] Interestingly, almost 30% of these cases were new diagnoses; indicating that symptoms often go unnoticed by the athlete. Kukafka et al. (1998) showed similar results in American high school athletes by the same challenge test and criteria.[9] The prevalence of EIA in elite athletes is similarly high (Table 6.2). In the 1996 summer Olympic Games, 16.7% of the American athletes had a diagnosis of asthma.[11] The events with the highest prevalence were cycling and mountain biking; none of the weightlifters or divers had a diagnosis of EIA and this may be related to the endurance component of the sport or the re-breathing that occurs with prolonged endurance. A similar study by the same authors showed that 22.4% of the athletes on the US team at the 1998 Winter Games had a previous diagnosis of asthma or used asthma medications or both.[12] Nordic, cross-country and short-track skiing had the highest prevalence of EIA by previous diagnosis or current medication use at 60.7% in contrast with only one (2.8%) of the 36 athletes who participated in bobsled, biathlon, luge, and ski jumping. The incidence was 24% in athletes who participated in alpine, long-track, figure skating, snowboarding and curling. This data is beneficial as it is one of the first studies to chronicle the winter sports, however, there was no actual clinical challenge testing done in the field of play.

Taken together, these data suggest that asthma is quite common in athletes and is more prevalent than in the general population. Athletes whose sport is performed in cold weather or dry environments have a much higher incidence of EIA compared with those whose sport is performed in warm/humid conditions.

Relationship to sport

Even though the prevalence of EIA in the elite athletic population is significantly greater than that of the general population, it does not appear to hinder performance. Several well-known elite and successful athletes have EIA. In the 1984 Olympics, 67 out of 597 US athletes had EIA and they accounted for 41 medals.[7] Among the individuals with EIA who performed at the 1998 Winter Games, one team gold medal, one individual silver and one individual bronze medal were won.[13] When properly treated, EIA does not hinder athletic performance and intense competition.

Signs and symptoms of EIA

EIA is associated with airway obstruction and a decrease in forced expiratory volume at 1s (FEV1).[8] Symptoms of EIA are varied and usually begin several minutes after the start of vigorous exercise and peaks after 5–10 min and can persist for 60–90 min before ending spontaneously.[14] Some athletes complain of respiratory problems: coughing, wheezing, shortness of breath and/or chest pain during of after exercise, while others may complain of fatigue, stomach/intestinal aches and/or headaches (Table 6.3).[8,15] The wide variety of symptoms makes diagnosis difficult as athletes may attribute their symptoms to their own lack of conditioning and not seek medical attention.[8] It is important that everyone involved with the athletic population be astutely aware of the typical and atypical symptoms of EIA so that effective treatment can be sought.

A thorough history and physical exam is the first step towards making a diagnosis of EIA, although in many cases it will not reveal any abnormalities. Pertinent questions to ask concern: a history of increased symptoms with triggers such as pollen or animal dander, cold air exposure and with certain sports known to have a higher incidence of EIA such as skating and cross-country skiing; a family history of asthma and personal history of allergic rhinitis or sinusitis also increase the likelihood of EIA. A full physical exam should be done with special attention paid to an ear, nose, throat and respiratory exam to assess any signs of nasal allergies, sinusitis, otitis or wheezing. Most patients with EIA will have a normal respiratory examination in the physician's office.[8]

In someone with a normal physical exam, but in whom EIA is suspected by history, spirometry should be performed in the office. This can be normal in an athlete with EIA when done at

Table 6.2 Incidence of EIA among Elite Athletes

Sport	(%)
Cross-country skiers	50
Ice hockey players	35
Speed skaters	43
Figure skaters	35
Cross-country runners	14

Adapted from Storms 2003.[8] EIA, exercise-induced asthma.

Table 6.3 Symptoms of EIA

Typical	Atypical
Cough: during/after exercise	Stomach cramps
Wheezing	Headache
Shortness of breath: during/after exercise	Feeling 'out of shape'

Adapted from Storms 2003.[8] EIA, exercise induced asthma.

rest. If suspicion for EIA is still sufficiently high but there are no objective physical findings, a trial of pharmacotherapy could be initiated. If the response is less than expected, then formal PFTs or challenge testing would be appropriate next steps.[14]

Investigations

Challenge testing is important for four reasons: (1) to confirm a diagnosis of EIA, (2) to screen athletes who participate in EIA prone sports, (3) for epidemiologic studies to evaluate prevalence of EIA and (4) for proof of EIA in competitive athletes to allow them to take anti-asthmatic medications.[8] As of June 2001, the IOC requires clinical proof of EIA for all competitions since the number of athletes notifying the IOC of their need to take beta-agonists has increased over the past few years. In addition to written notification, the athlete must submit a detailed report of symptoms, medical records pertaining to their diagnosis of asthma and either a positive bronchodilator test, positive exercise challenge test in lab or field, or a positive methacholine challenge test.

There are several tests one can perform to prove or disprove a diagnosis of asthma. The eucapnic voluntary hyperventilation (EVH) challenge has been used to assess EIA in athletes.[15] It has also been recommended by the IOC for testing Olympic athletes. It involves breathing at a pre-determined rate, 60–85% of maximal ventilation rate (MVV). The respiration rate for the challenge is estimated by assuming MVV to be 35 times FEV1. EVH challenge is administered between pre and post-spirometry using a dry-air mixture of 4.5% CO_2 to ensure eucapnia while protecting against a hyperventilation-induced hypocapnia. Any decrease in FEV1 is assumed to be positive for EIA.

A field exercise challenge test *versus* a laboratory exercise challenge test can be beneficial diagnostically, as it is conducted in conditions representing the sport-specific temperature environment and the competition venue conditions.

The methacholine inhalation challenge has been used to classify the severity of a patient's asthma, however, most agree that that it is not specific to the bronchoconstriction associated with exercise.[15]

Management

Non-pharmacologic

The first advice to give an athlete with a recent diagnosis of EIA is to advise about others types of exercise that are less likely to produce symptoms. For those already competing in an asthma-prone sport, this is not practical, but, for a recreational athlete, may be quite feasible.[8] Also, an adequate warm-up, at least 10 min prior to exercise has been shown to reduce the severity of EIA. One could also try covering the mouth and nose with a scarf or balaclava during cold weather.[14]

Pharmacologic

The most effective treatment for EIA is a short-acting beta-agonist within 15 min of exercise.[8] If this is not adequate then Cromolyn (or other mast cell stabilizer) can be added to the beta-agonist. Cromolyn is an anti-inflammatory agent that works with the beta-agonist to inhibit the early bronchospastic phase of EIA by inhibiting mast cell mediator release.

Inhaled corticosteroids have been shown to be useful in EIA and are safe and effective when used in the recommended dosage. Another class of inhalers that may be worth trying are the anticholinergics.

If the pre-exercise therapy is not effective, then daily anti-asthmatic therapy should be added on top of the pre-exercise therapy. These daily medications can be used alone or in combination and include inhaled corticosteroids, leukotriene receptor antagonists, long-acting beta-agonists and theophyllines. Athletes with chronic persistent asthma can also be treated with the same daily controller medications in addition to the pre-exercise therapy medications.

Although there is no evidence to confirm that inhaled beta-2 agonists enhance performance in doses required to treat EIA, a documented history of asthma as identified by the IOC Medical Commission is required for these medications to be allowed in competition.

Information on banned/approved substances can be found on the WADA website (www.wada-ama.org). These lists are subject to change and these sites should be contacted regularly to ensure that there will not be any problems during the competition.

Conclusion

EIA is a common and treatable condition. One first should confirm the athlete does have EIA and not chronic asthma, as the treatments are slightly different and the risk of permanent lung damage from untreated chronic asthma is significant. In making the diagnosis, a through history and physical exam including forced FEV1 should be performed. A trial of inhaled β-agonist with/without anti-inflammatory agents can be tried if the diagnosis is unclear. If there is no improvement, formal pulmonary function testing should be performed to rule out any underlying lung pathology.

DIABETES

Box 6.3: Key Points

- Divide meal planning into the pre-competition, competition and post-competition phases.

- Monitor consistently for disease complications.

- Some athletes may be restricted from participation if they have signs of vascular insufficiency or unstable glucose levels.

Diabetes mellitus is a metabolic condition that affects the pancreas leading to abnormally high blood glucose levels due to deficiency in insulin production. This breaks down carbohydrates into glucose which requires insulin to be transported for cellular activity. When the insulin is impaired, the glucose levels rise in the circulating plasma and this can be harmful to exposed tissues in the eyes, nerves, renal tissue and cardiac system. There are three types of diabetes: Type I (formerly known as insulin-dependent diabetes), Type II (formerly known as non-insulin dependent diabetes) and gestational diabetes, occurring during pregnancy. Treatment revolves around nutrition, exercise and medication.

Competition nutrition

There are a growing number of athletes with diabetes as sport and physical activity has become linked with health and treatment. There are no actual studies at this time identifying the overall incidence but the participation in sport of athletes with diabetes is not uncommon. Athletes with diabetes must be attuned to their blood glucose levels and their diet requirements during training and competitions. This becomes easier with the experience that the athlete has with the diabetes control.

Eating before training and competition

Diabetic athletes should consume a carbohydrate based meal 3–6 h before exercise with a small snack closer to the event if needed. The recommended pre-event carbohydrate intake is 1g/kg body weight within the hour before exercise (toast with jam or juice) and up to 4g/kg body weight within 3–4 h before exercise (pancakes, bread or fruit). Additional carbohydrate intake about 20 min before an event may also be required by some; crackers, muffins, yogurt are good choices.[16] Type I diabetics should also ensure that their blood glucose is between 4 and 8 mmol/l. Exercising with high blood sugar will disrupt normal metabolic control and result in poor performance.

Eating during training/competition

Everyone needs carbohydrate (CHO) during exercise events that last longer than 60–90 min. Ingesting CHO during prolonged activity can improve performance by maintaining blood glucose later in exercise. Non-diabetic athletes have been shown to maintain blood glucose levels and perform better when given 1g/kg of CHO at 20 min of exercise and 0.25 g/kg every 20 min thereafter, compared with athletes not given CHO.[17] Diabetic athletes are more at risk of rapid hypoglycemia and as such, CHO feedings during exercise are extremely important. A minimum of 30–60 g of CHO (in solid or liquid form) should be consumed hourly, preferably at 15–30 min intervals. Appropriate adjustments of insulin doses are also needed to allow hepatic glycogenolysis to continue, therefore reducing the risk of hypoglycemia.[17]

Eating post-training/competition

Nutrition in the post-competition phase should be viewed as replenishment for energy used and then preparation for the next competitive session.

Replenishment should be gradual with monitored glucose levels and should include moderate levels of neutral fluids like water, tea and milk.

It is advised that two small meals be consumed within the first 2.5h post-competition. Meals servings should include 1–2 CHO serving, 1 protein serving and 1 dairy or vegetable serving.

Blood glucose should be done at 15 min post-competition and again at 30 min post the second meal.

Complications of diabetes in sport

There are several complications of exercise in the diabetic athlete, of which the diabetic as well as training personnel and other team members should be aware. These are mainly hypoglycemia, ketoacidosis as well as the complications of the diabetes itself that may be aggravated by exercise and sport.

Hypoglycemia

Hypoglycemia is a fear of most diabetic athletes. The symptoms of hypoglycemia are similar to symptoms experienced during vigorous exercise; sweating, headache and tremulousness and are often difficult to distinguish. Uncorrected hypoglycemia can lead to confusion, loss of consciousness and even convulsions. The diabetic athlete should always carry some form of easily digestible carbohydrate (glucose tablets or glucose-electrolyte solution) and should take it at the first signs of hypoglycemia.[18] Prevention of hypoglycemia requires rigorous blood sugar testing before, during and after exercise so that diet and insulin dosing can be adjusted accordingly. Most diabetics will require 15–30g of glucose per half hour of training.

Diabetic ketoacidosis

Exercise is contraindicated in diabetics with poor glucose control or medical instability, as it can lead to ketoacidosis in poorly-controlled diabetics and in those who commence exercise with an insulin deficiency. Exercise increases glucose levels through the release of counter-regulatory hormones. Therefore, athletes should be well-controlled prior to commencing a vigorous exercise program.

Well-known complications of diabetes include autonomic and peripheral neuropathy, retinopathy and nephropathy. Autonomic neuropathy is a potential problem during exercise because of the impaired sympathetic and parasympathetic activity which can cause abnormal heart rate and blood pressure responses. Athletes with autonomic neuropathy are at high risk for sudden death and myocardial infarction during exercise. Therefore, high intensity activity should be avoided, swimming and stationary bicycling would be better activity choices.

Peripheral neuropathy also causes a problem with sports that may be traumatic to the feet, like running. Non-weight bearing alternatives are suggested. Proper footwear should be worn at all times and feet should be inspected on a regular basis.

Diabetics with evidence of retinopathy should avoid sports that increase blood pressure, in fact, systolic blood pressure should not be elevated greater than 170 mmHg.[16] Weightlifting and other sports that cause significant increases in blood pressure can cause retinal hemorrhage and should be avoided. Activities such as swimming, cycling and walking would be more appropriate for these individuals.

Contraindications to participation

The benefits of exercise in both Type I and Type II diabetics have been firmly established. These mainly relate to better glycemic control, improvement of cardiovascular fitness as well as social and psychological well-being. However, an exercise program is not without risk in a diabetic patient and as such, there are a few absolute contraindications to participation in competitive exercise and/or sports. Even if a diabetic individual is unable to participate in competitive sports, some degree of exercise is possible. The physician should consult the Clinical Practice Recommendations published by the ADA for advice.[18]

Poor blood glucose control

New diabetes or those who are poorly controlled should not begin an exercise program or participate in a sport until they achieve metabolic control (Berg 2001). Exercising with lack of insulin in the blood can cause hyperglycemia and ketosis during exercise. Hypoglycemia is also a consequence of exercise and may occur during or after exercise. It can be related to too much insulin, too little food, too much exercise or a combination of factors. It can take some time before an athlete is comfortable with adjusted meals and insulin so that they avoid blood sugar extremes. Only when good control is demonstrated by target HbA1c and blood glucose monitoring, should competitive training be introduced.

Poor cardiac reserve

Diabetic patients are at significantly higher risk than the general population for cardiovascular disease and silent ischemia. An exercise ECG and/or other tests of circulation and exercise capacity should be administered to patients 40 years of age and older and those who have had diabetes for 25 years or more.[19] The results of these tests should aid the decision making process about whether or not competitive exercise is safe.

Peripheral vascular disease (PVD)

This may be an area of concern in athletes involved with sport that causes foot/lower extremity trauma.

Patients with vascular insufficiency or sensory neuropathy may incur injury to their feet without their knowledge. Diabetics with PVD have a slower rate of healing and an increased risk of infection. Certain sports are more traumatic to the foot and should be avoided, these include running, basketball, martial arts and diving.[19] Diabetic athletes should inspect their feet daily for wounds or callus development.

Retinopathy

Strenuous activities such as contact sports, jumping, scuba diving and weight training are not recommended for patients with retinopathy because of the risk of hemorrhage.[19] Limits may also need to be set on activity in other sports in diabetics with proliferative retinopathy.

DERMATOLOGY

Box 6.4: Key Points

- Athletes such as wrestlers are more prone to infectious skin conditions due to the increased perspiration with skin contact among competitors causing a higher incidence of infections.

- Many athletic organizations have specific criteria regarding participation in competition and dermatological infection. Most require proof of treatment for at least 2 days prior to the event and require complete coverage of infected lesions.

Participation in physical exercise can be associated with a variety of skin problems from infections, mechanical trauma and environmental exposure. The diagnosis of specific skin conditions can be both interesting and challenging for the primary care sports medicine physician and requires some familiarity with common skin conditions associated with athletics. Some problems may require a referral to a dermatologist, but most can be successfully treated by a primary care physician who is educated in common athletic skin conditions.

Bacterial infections

Impetigo

Impetigo is a bacterial infection caused by staphylococcus or β-hemolytic streptococcus. It begins as an erythema, but can rapidly develop into blisters and honey-colored crusted lesions.[20] It most commonly occurs on the face; however, it is very contagious and can spread rapidly to any part of the body.

Diagnosis: Impetigo is diagnosed on its classical clinical appearance (Fig. 6.1). Athletes involved in skin contact sports such as wrestling and rugby are at highest risk of developing impetigo.

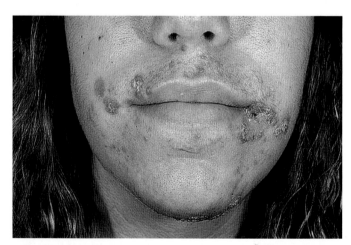

Figure 6.1   Impetigo occurs most often on the face. (Reproduced from Bacterial Infections. In: Skin Disease: Diagnosis and Treatment. Habif TP (ed). Philadelphia: Mosby Inc 2005, pp. 137; with permission of Elsevier, copyright 2005.)

Treatment: Oral and topical antibiotics are used to treat impetigo. Most frequently used are erythromycin, cloxacillin or first generation cephalosporins. Topical treatment works best when one uses warm water soaks to remove crusts before applying mupirocin four times a day for 7–10 days.[20]

Prevention: Impetigo is contagious and as such, many athletic organizations have restrictions for athletic participation. Most require an athlete to have 3 or more days of antibiotics and be free of new lesions for 2 days prior to competition. All lesions must be covered during practice or competition.

Folliculitis

Folliculitis is an infection of the hair follicles usually caused by staphylococcus aureus or can be caused by pseudomonas when it is contracted in whirlpools and hot tubs.

Diagnosis: Inflammatory changes usually occur at the base of the hair follicle and can occur clinically as macules, papules or pustules.[20] Areas usually affected are the skin under protective gear, i.e. shoulder pads and in particularly sweaty areas like the trunk and under arms. Deeper infections can occur and can lead to abscess formation (furuncle and carbuncles).

Treatment: Most cases do well with anti-bacterial soaps, benzoyl peroxide, topical mupirocin as well as oral tetracycline or erythromycin. Severe cases that have developed into furuncles require drainage of the abscess.

Prevention: As with impetigo, most organizations require athletes with folliculitis to have at least 3 days of antibiotics and be without new lesions for at least 2 days prior to competition.

Hot tub folliculitis Hot tub folliculitis is caused by *Pseudomonas aeruginosa*, which is commonly found in hot tubs and whirlpools. The submerged part of the body develops erythematous papules and pustules. The condition is usually self-limiting. Treatment is supportive with antipruritics and/or 5% acetic acid compresses. If the athlete presents with systemic symptoms, one can administer a course of oral ciprofloxacin.[21]

Viral infections
Cutaneous herpes simplex

Herpes simplex viral infection type I (HSV-I) is the most common viral skin infection in athletes. HSV is transmitted by skin–skin contact and is commonly seen in wrestlers and as such is often referred to as *Herpes gladiatorum*.[22] It is spread by contact with the athlete's active lesion or contact with infectious secretions on the mat.

Diagnosis: The diagnosis of HSV is usually clinical. The typical presentation is a prodrome of symptoms including pain, itching and burning in the area of contact before an eruption of multiple vesicles on an erythematous base.[20] Confirmatory tests are also available and include a Tzanck smear of the base of the vesicle or a viral culture of a new lesion.[22]

Treatment: Treatment should begin as soon as the individual is experiencing symptoms. Acyclovir, 400 mg p.o., t.i.d.-p.i.d. for 5–7 days, is usually the treatment of choice however, other anti-viral medications may also be useful.[20] Using oral anti-viral therapy shortens the duration of the disease and significantly reduces viral shedding. Relief from symptoms may be obtained by using NSAIDs, and various creams for the pruritic reaction.

Prevention: HSV is highly contagious; therefore, mats and other equipment must be thoroughly and frequently washed with viricidal solutions. The infected athlete much also be removed from participation for at least 5 days or until the lesions have crusted over. As an extra precautionary measure, even crusted over lesions should be covered.

Verruca vulgaris (plantar warts)

Plantar warts are caused by infection with the human papilloma virus.[20] They are common and extremely annoying to the athlete.

Diagnosis: They are usually diagnosed by their appearance which is a well-circumscribed, firm, slightly elevated lesion.[22] They interrupt normal skin lines and when pared down, they reveal black spots; remnants of thrombosed capillaries (Fig. 6.2).

Prevention: Exposure to the virus in locker rooms and showers is the route of transmission. Therefore, wearing a sandal or an aquatic shoe in these environments should reduce the risk.

Treatment: The best treatment is daily application of a salicylic acid. It is best applied at night after paring the wart. It may take up to 3 months for the wart to completely resolve. More aggressive therapies, such as cryotherapy are also useful; however, this can cause painful ulceration and hence impair mobility.

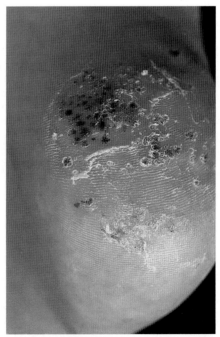

Figure 6.2 Herpes gladiatorum is characterized by grouped vesicles on an erythematous base. (Reprinted from Kirnbauer R, Lenz P , Okun MM. Human Papillomavirus. In: Bolognia JL, Jorizzo JL, Rapini RP (eds). Dermatology. Mosby: Philadelphia 2003, pp. 1222, Fig 79.8; with permission of Elsevier, copyright 2003.)

Fungal infections
Tinea pedis (athlete's foot)
This infection causes an erythematous, scaly eruption on the plantar surface of the foot as well as fissures in the skin between the toes.[20] Occasionally, these areas can become secondarily infected. The most common etiologic agent is the dermatophyte *Trichophyton rubrum*, also *T. mentagrophytes* and *Epidermophyton floccosum*.[20]

Diagnosis: Diagnosis is usually made by classic clinical appearance (Fig. 6.3). The differential includes eczema, contact dermatitis and psoriasis.[20] If unsure, skin scrapings on a KOH will show fungal elements in positive cases, fungal cultures can also be used.

Prevention: Warm, moist conditions support fungal growth. As a result, Tenia pedis is usually from shared surfaces, such as shower or locker room floors. One can avoid infection primarily by wearing shoes or sandals in these areas and by paying attention to proper foot hygiene. Natural fiber socks may also help to prevent infection by whisking the moisture away from the skin.

Treatment: Tinea pedis is best treated with a topical antibiotic cream such as clotrimazole or nystatin 2–3 times a day. In addition, the affected areas should be washed often with soap and water and kept dry during athletic activities with talcum powders.

Tinea Cruris (jock itch)
Tinea cruris is a similar process to tinea pedis and is caused by the same agents. All of the same preventative strategies suggested for tenia pedis will also work here. Poor hygiene may be a factor.

Diagnosis: Similar to tinea pedis, there is a sharply delineated erythematous, scaly rash in the moist folds of the groin and inner thighs sparing the scrotum and penis.[20] The athlete may experience pain and pruritus. The differential includes contact dermatitis, mechanical intertrigo, candida intertrigo and erythrasma.

Treatment: Topical antibiotic creams will work here as in tenia pedis. Topical low-potency steroids may be useful in combination with the anti-fungal creams to lessen pruritus. The area should also be kept dry; this can be accomplished with talcum powder or another drying agent.

Tinea corporis (ringworm)
Tinea corporis is a superficial infection of non-hairy skin (face, trunk, limbs). It occurs as an erythematous scaling ring with raised borders. It is very pruritic and contagious, especially among wrestlers.[20]

Diagnosis: Diagnosis is usually made on clinical appearance and/or by KOH prepared skin scrapings because this is a test a team physician can do in the office (Fig. 6.4).

Treatment: Again topical antibiotic creams work best as with the other tinea infections. Extensive lesions should be treated with griseofulvin, 500 mg orally twice a day. All lesions should be covered with a pas-permeable membrane before a wrestler can compete so that spread is decreased.[20]

Subungual hematoma
Subungual hematoma is often referred to as runner's toe or tennis toe. It is a hemorrhage in the distal nail bed that results from the toe frequently pushing on the toebox of the shoe.[20] These are most common in tennis and football and other such sports that require stopping and turning (Fig. 6.5). Most are painless, however, some may cause pain as pressure builds up in the closed space.[22] Properly fitting footwear can prevent this injury as can keeping toenails trimmed regularly.[23] In painful cases, drainage with a needle through the nail plate can reduce the pressure and the associated tenderness.[23]

Calluses
Calluses are hyperkeratotic lesions that develop on the hands or feet as a result of prolonged friction or pressure. Hand cal-

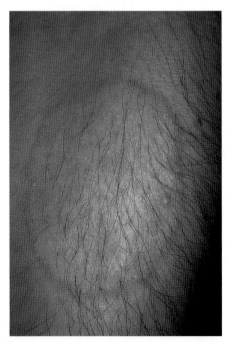

Figure 6.4 Tinea corporis. In classic ringworm, lesions begin as flat scaly spots that develop a raised border which extends out at variable rates in all directions. The advancing scaly border may have raised papules or vesicles. (Reprinted from Sobera JO, Elewski BE. Fungal Diseases. In: Bolognia JL, Jorizzo JL, Rapini RP (eds). Dermatology. Philadelphia: Mosby 2005, pp. 1117, Fig 77.5A, with permission of Elsevier, copyright 2005.)

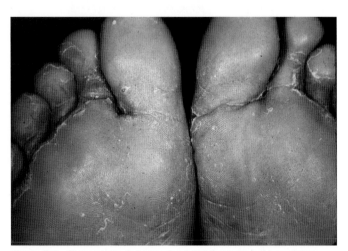

Figure 6.3 Tinea pedis. Infection involving the toes and interdigital spaces. (http://www.doctorfungus.org/ imageban/images/ init_images/381mike.jpg Courtesy of www.doctorfungus.org © 2005).

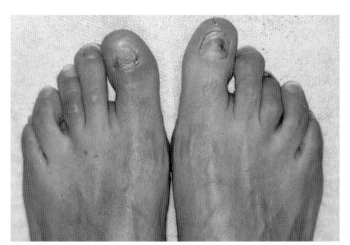

Figure 6.5 Subungual hematoma and nail bed hemorrhages in a squash player. (From Tosti A, Pazzaglia M. Occupational nail disorders. In: Scher RK and Daniel III CR, eds. Nails: diagnosis, therapy, surgery. 3rd edn. New York: Elsevier; 2005: 210; Figs 18–20.)

luses are common in sports such as weightlifting. When calluses are on the feet they are usually over a bony prominence.[20] Treatment is usually not necessary unless they are associated with pain. One can pare down the thickened skin and apply a salicylic acid plaster (40%). Prevention is always best and one should ensure that footwear/equipment is fitting properly. Donut pads can be used over susceptible bony prominences.

Blisters

Blisters are fluid-filled bullae that occur as a result of a disruption of the dermal–epidermal junction due to friction. The areas most affected are the heel and ball of the foot, as well as the plantar surfaces of the great toes.[24] Hands can also be affected in racquet sports and weightlifting. Treatment may be required when the blister is sufficiently large. In these cases, it is best to drain the fluid using a sterile needle and leave the overlying skin intact to act as protection to the underlying, unprotected skin.[23] The drained blister should be covered with an occlusive pressure dressing to facilitate healing. Hydrocolloid or hydrogel dressings such as DuoDERM or Second Skin are helpful if the skin roof is lost.[22] The area should be kept clean and an antibiotic ointment such as a Polysporin may also be applied to prevent infection. The hallmark of blister treatment is prevention. This includes wearing properly fitting shoes and appropriate socks and/or gloves made of synthetic materials that whisk moisture away as well as limiting certain 'at risk' behaviors, i.e. increasing intensity of exercise too quickly, or running in wet shoes.

Sunburn

Training for triathlons, track and field, swimming and several other sports requires prolonged sun exposure and prevention of sunburn is paramount. This can be accomplished in ways similar to that of the general population, i.e. wearing protective clothing and application of sunscreens of at least SPF 15. Agents that contain cinnamates and benzophenones or Parsol 1789 are advisable.[25] Avoiding the sun between the hours of

1000 and 1400 hours is also suggested, but not always possible in training athletes. If sunburn does occur, treatment should include cool compresses and analgesics.

Those that experience excessive sun exposure are also at risk for premature aging of the skin and skin cancers. All athletes with this history and especially those that are fair-skinned or who have had frequent sunburns, should have regular screenings for any ominous skin changes.

GASTROINTESTINAL IRRITATION

Box 6.5: Key Points

- Dietary analysis is a critical factor in the diagnosis and management of gastrointestinal disorders.
- The relationship between anxiety and mood changes with gastrointestinal symptoms should be considered for accurate management.
- Dietary changes should be attempted in practice and trial situations and not as a first attempt in competition.

Overview

Gastrointestinal symptoms in sport are common and usually benign in nature but can certainly have a negative effect on training, performance and optimal preparation. Common symptoms associated with exercise include nausea, heartburn, loss of appetite, abdominal cramps, diarrhea and constipation. The cause of gastrointestinal symptoms may be related to reduced blood flow to the abdominal viscera, acidic changes in the upper tract and changes in the rate of gastric emptying and intestinal motility. Assessment should always include the elimination of pathological disorders such as gastric ulcers, inflammatory bowel disease, tumor and eating disorders.

Incidence

Upper gastrointestinal symptoms such as heartburn, reflux, nausea and even vomiting are more common than lower gastrointestinal symptoms such as diarrhea, constipation, rectal bleeding and abdominal cramping. In patients with established gastric reflux, 20% indicate that exercise is a contributing factor. The incidence of occult bleeding can be high in endurance athletes especially runners and this may be further increased by the frequent use of aspirin and non-steroidal anti-inflammatories (Schwartz). The common abdominal 'stitch' is thought to be related to spasm of the diaphragm or possibly air-trapping in the colon.

Relationship to sport

The impact of exercise on the gastrointestinal system has been inconclusive and indicates that moderate exercise is usually well-tolerated and can benefit patients with inflammatory bowel disease, however high intensity exercise inhibits gastric emptying, interferes with gastrointestinal absorption, and causes many gastrointestinal symptoms, most notably gastrointestinal bleeding.[26]

Gastrointestinal hemorrhage of the stomach is the most frequently reported site in athletes and is most commonly identified in runners. The etiology is unknown but theories include a generalized ischemia to the area, direct trauma from the diaphragm and elevated adrenalin and cortisol levels.

Gastroesophageal reflux (GER) in the athlete, increases with intensity of exercise, is more common with endurance sports, and worse with postprandial exercise.[27]

Common presenting symptoms

Upper gastrointestinal symptoms may be related to gastric reflux and produce symptoms such as heartburn, chest pain and nausea. Gastric emptying rate has been linked to the onset of gastroesophageal reflux (GER) symptoms especially in the initial stages of stomach fullness. Symptoms may be related to gastric hormonal levels, meal size, dietary fibre, acidity and athlete anxiety.

In addition to a dietary intake history, the athlete should be questioned on potential changes in gastric vomiting, stool color and volume and rectal bleeding.

'Runner's Diarrhea' is a term that applies to the urgency to defecate while running and this appears to be related to the intensity of the exercise and potential contributing anxiety. Athletes may have to stop their activity to empty their bowels and their stool may be more watery than usual but usually the color is unaltered. Infective diarrhea may be present when sport is combined with travel however, the diarrhea persists whether the athlete is active or not and is often associated with a stool color change.

A general functional inquiry should include questions related to weight loss, malaise, fever and chills. Medication review should include the use of caffeine, alcohol, tobacco, antibiotics, NSAIDs and sport drinks.

Signs on physical exam

The athlete should always be evaluated for sites of gastrointestinal bleeding and potential bloating and fullness. Hydration status should be evaluated including vital signs, urine color and output and skin turgor. Orthostatic blood pressure can be assessed in the supine position and then after 5 min in the standing position. A decrease in systolic pressure of 20 points or any increase in heart rate of 20 beats can be indicative of dehydration. Abdominal palpation may reveal areas of tenderness, spasm, significant pain or a mass. Auscultation of the abdomen may reveal hyperactive or hypoactive bowel sounds requiring further investigation. Lastly, it is always helpful to palpate the thyroid gland and other key lymphatic glands for enlargement.

Investigations

Investigations should include imaging of the gastrointestinal tract with barium contrast radiography, endoscopy and colonoscopy as indicated. Blood work may identify slow blood loss through reduced iron and ferritin stores. Hemo-occult blood stool testing may be helpful but the sensitivity is low on this test and so clinical history would still dictate further investigations. Stool samples for culture and sensitivity may also be useful to identify agents such as Campylobacter, salmonella or shigella. In addition, screening for absorptive deficiencies such as lactose intolerance is often helpful in long-term management.

Management

Nutritional practices are the foundation of treatment and include avoidance of fat and high protein prior to competition. In certain illness specific conditions, dietary recommendations may include reduction of acid, and an increase of iron or calcium within meal planning. Fluids should be administered in small, frequent doses and may include some carbohydrates. Fibre should be reduced if diarrhea is present.

Medications should be selected and tried in a practice setting to ensure their predicted response during competition. For upper gastrointestinal symptoms, antacids can be used 30 min prior to competition and H2 receptor antagonists such as ranitidine may be required on a daily basis (Table 6.4).

Motility altering drugs are helpful for symptoms related to quick emptying of the gastrointestinal tract. For the upper gastrointestinal symptoms, prokinetic agents may improve the contractility of the esophageal sphincters. The careful use of antidiarrheal agents may be helpful short-term but are not recommended for ongoing long-term use, as they can depress the central nervous system.

In the case of acute distress, hydration is essential to prevent any progression of stomach or bowel ischemia.

There are many causes of diarrhea, most of which are infectious. The most common causative organisms are bacteria, such as *E. coli, salmonella, shigella and Campylobacter*. Parasites or protozoa such as *Giardia lamblia, Entamoeba histolytica, Cyclospora* and *cryptosporidium* occur much less

Table 6.4 Common Medications and Treatment Dosages

Medical Condition	Medication	Treatment Dosage
Diarrhea	Loperamide HC	4 mg initially, then 2 mg following each loose bowel movement to a maximum of 8 mg/day
	Bismuth subsalicylate	Two oral tablets every 1–2 h, with a maximum of 16 tablets per day
Reflux symptoms	Histamine-2 blockers such as Ranitidine	150 mg twice daily
	Esomeprazole magnesium	20–40 mg once daily for maximum of 4 weeks
Nausea and vomiting	Dimenhydrinate	75–150 mg every 8 h to a maximum of 375 mg/day

Table 6.5 Foods and Drugs that can Cause Diarrhea

Foods and Drugs	Ingredient Causing Diarrhea
Apple juice, pear juice, sugar-free gum, mints	Hexitol, sorbitol, mannitol
Apple juice, pear juice, grapes, honey, dates, nuts, figs, soft drinks (especially fruit flavors)	Fructose
Table sugar	Sucrose
Milk, ice cream, yogurt, frozen yogurt, soft cheese, chocolate	Lactose
Antacids containing magnesium	Magnesium
Coffee, tea, cola drinks, some over-the-counter headache remedies	Caffeine
Fat-free potato chips, fat-free ice cream	Olestra

Compiled from: Merck manual of diagnosis and therapy, Section 3. Gastrointestinal disorders, Ch. 27 Diarrhea and constipation. Online. Available: http://www.merck.com/mrkshared/mmanual/tables/27tb1.jsp

frequently. Cholera, a bacteria, is a very rare cause of diarrhea among travelers. Sometimes, diarrhea is not due to infection, but can be attributed to lifestyle choices in alcohol or adjustment to food preparation and spicing (Table 6.5). Diarrhea may be mild with just some cramps and a few loose bowel movements per day, or be much more severe.

The most important aspect of treatment is replenishment of lost fluids. This can be accomplished with flat carbonated drinks, electrolyte mixtures or clear juices. It is important to continue eating but to reduce your food choices to easily digestible carbohydrates such as rice, bread and bananas. Medications may be used for symptomatic relief and antibiotics can be required if fever, pus or additional symptoms occur.

INFECTIONS

Box 6.6: Key Points

- Infection prevention is a key component of performance management including environmental assessment of travel.
- Early detection improves successful outcomes considerably.
- Containment of infectious spread is a priority in games management.

Overview

Infections in sport are a concern to athletes and healthcare professionals alike as they require immediate attention for safe care of the ill athlete and rigorous infection control for the prevention of disease spread to healthy athletes. Athletes are often in close quarters for travel, meals and sleeping and this makes infection control procedures challenging. Many factors have contributed to the rise in athlete infections including the sharing of water bottles, the severity of blood-borne infections like HIV and the increasing international travel. Injuries in sport where blood products are exposed contain potential

threats to the attendees and a cause for concern with Games organizers.

Incidence

Infections such as Hepatitis A, B and C are more common in young people and can be associated with travel and open wound blood exposure. HIV is a worldwide concern and it has affected the sport world with awareness and concern for all athletes. The Epstein–Barr virus causing infectious mononucleosis is very common among young people, contagious and can significantly interfere with an athletes training.

Upper respiratory infections are common and often occur with travel due to airplane air circulation of infections and change in weather conditions. Upper respiratory infections are common infections and include pharyngitis, sinusitis, epiglottitis, laryngotracheitis and the common cold. Viruses play a significant role in the pathogenesis of many of these infections. Bacteria and other organisms also are responsible. Some 80% of upper respiratory infections are caused by viruses and are treated symptomatically for relief. Bacterial infections are usually associated with high fever temperatures and greenish nasal or phlegm discharge. When a viral infection has become prolonged over weeks, bacterial infections are common as a secondary onset.

Relationship to sport

The key factors influencing the management of infections in sport include:
1. Safe athlete participation while infected
2. Infection control for others
3. Safe return to sport after infection.

Common infections in athletes include upper respiratory infections often seen in endurance athletes, skin infections identified in contact sports and water-borne infections particular to water sports.

Common presenting symptoms

The presence of fever, myalgia, tachycardia, fatigue and swollen glands signal that an infection is systemic and greater precautions must be taken to curtail sport participation.

Infectious mononucleosis may display symptoms of fever, sore throat, headache, loss of appetite and nausea. Splenomegaly occurs in about 50% of affected cases and this peaks in about the second or third week of infection.

Signs on physical exam

Assessment should include a complete physical examination including visualization of the ears, nose and throat and palpation of the glandular chains. Vital signs including temperature, heart rate, blood pressure and respiratory rate are key to managing the symptoms.

In hepatitis, identification of jaundice in the conjunctiva, palms and abdomen can assist with the diagnosis. Palpation of the liver and spleen are essential.

In mononucleosis, the patient may have an exudative pharyngitis with swollen cervical lymph nodes and a fever.

Influenza may present with generalized fatigue, muscle weakness and non-specific tenderness of the abdomen.

Investigations

The investigations of an infection should include the identification of the pathogen if possible. This may require a throat swab, stool sample or blood sample for antibody identification. Further blood work may identify the immune status of the athlete and titres can determine the acuteness of the infectious contact in some cases.

Management

Management of infections require a sensible approach to containment. It must be determined whether the athlete is suffering from a single system infection like a localized skin infection or a sinus infection as opposed to a generalized systemic infection such at influenza, mononucleosis or hepatitis. The next question is to determine if the athlete is febrile or afebrile. Generally, an athlete with a localized infection who is afebrile will be able to continue training to 80% of maximum and is safe to enter competition.

On the other hand, if an athlete is systemically ill, then he should refrain from training and competition. Re-integration to sport must be gradual and should resume only after all symptoms have subsided and general energy and appetite have resumed.

SPORT PSYCHIATRY

This is an emerging area of sport management and not identical to sport psychology. Sport psychiatry encompasses the areas of emotional wellness and mood instability that often require intrapersonal counseling, medication and long-term cognitive-behavioral changes.

Common diagnoses include generalized anxiety, depression and mood instability and eating disorders. Schizophrenia, although less common, has an increased incidence of new diagnosis in the youth and young adult age groups which coincides with the average age of competitive athletes. Athletes are not immune to social issues such as substance abuse, legal implications, gambling, financial stress and physical abuse and often may be susceptible due to lifestyle chaos. Athlete screening should include awareness and openness to emotional and social dysfunction.

A reasonable approach for athlete disclosure of emotional problems includes a trusting relationship with an impartial member of the sports medical organization. Disclosure may occur when the athlete is ready or it may occur during crisis. The medical team should include mental health professionals who are on-call for such situations.

Prevention of crisis can be managed with open educational sessions addressing the common problems of athlete mental health and useful strategies for dealing with issues. Medication may be warranted and should first be cleared with competition doping agencies in order to choose the best possible solutions.

REFERENCES

1   Eichner ER. Hematological problems in athletes. Principles and practice of primary care sports medicine. Philadelphia, PA: Lippincott Williams & Wilkins; 2001.
2   Fields KB. The athlete with anemia. Malden, MA: Blackwell Science; 1997.
3   Shaskey DJ, Green GA. Sports haematology. Sports Medicine 2000; 29:27–38.
4   Balaban EP, Cox JV, Snell P, Vaughan RH, Frenkel EP. The frequency of anemia and iron deficiency in the runner. Med Sci Sports Exerc 1989; 21:643–648.
5   Risser WL, Lee EJ, Poindexter HB, et al. Iron deficiency in female athletes: its prevalence and impact on performance. Med Sci Sports Exerc 1988; 20:116–121.
6   Selby GB, Eichner ER. Endurance swimming, intravascular hemolysis, anemia, and iron depletion. New perspective on athlete's anemia. Am J Med 1986; 81:791–794.
7   Orenstein DM. The athlete with asthma or other pulmonary disease. Principles and practice of primary care sports medicine. Philadelphia, PA: Lippincott Williams & Wilkins; 2001.
8   Storms WW. Review of exercise-induced asthma. Med Sci Sports Exerc 2003; 35:1464–1470.
9   Kukafka DS, Lang DM, Porter S. et al. Exercise-induced bronchospasm in high school athletes via a free running test: incidence and epidemiology. Chest 1998; 114:1613–1622.
10 Vacek L. Incidence of exercise-induced asthma in high school population in British Columbia. Allergy Asthma Proc 1997; 18:89–91.
11 Weiler JM, Layton T, Hunt M. Asthma in United States Olympic athletes who participated in the 1996 Summer Games. J Allergy Clin Immunol 1998; 102:722–726.
12 Weiler JM, Ryan EJ. Asthma in United States Olympic athletes who participated in the 1998 Olympic winter games. J Allergy Clin Immunol 2000; 106:267–271.
13 Wilber RL, Rundell KW, Szmedra L, Jenkinson DM, Im, J, Drake SD. Incidence of exercise-induced bronchospasm in Olympic winter sport athletes. Med Sci Sports Exerc 2000; 32:732–737.
14 Sinha T, David AK. Recognition and management of exercise-induced bronchospasm. Am Fam Physician 2003; 67:769–774.
15 Rundell KW, Jenkinson DM. Exercise-induced bronchospasm in the elite athlete. Sports Med 2002; 32:583–600.
16 Brukner P, Khan K. Diabetes and exercise. Clinical sports medicine. 2nd edn. New York: McGraw-Hill; 2003.
17 Franz MJ. Nutrition, physical activity and diabetes. Alexandria, VA: American Diabetes Association; 2002.
18 American Diabetic Association. Standards of medical care in diabetes. Diabet Care 2005; 28:S4–S36.
19 Berg K. The athlete with Type 1 diabetes. Philadelphia, PA: Lippincott Williams & Wilkins; 2001.
20 Lillegard WA, Butcher JD, Fields KB. Dermatologic problems in athletes. Oxford: Blackwell Science; 1997.
21 Freiman A, Barankin B, Elpern DJ. Sports dermatology part 2: swimming and other aquatic sports. Can Med Assoc J 2004; 171:1339–1341.
22 Ramirez AM, Van Durme DJ. Dermatology. In: Birrer RB, Griesemer BA, Cataletto MB, eds. Philadelphia, PA: Lippincott Williams & Wilkins; 2002:
23 Freiman A, Barankin B, Elpern DJ. Sports dermatology part 1: common dermatoses. Can Med Assoc J 2004; 171:851–853.
24 Mellion MB, Sitorius MA, Butcher JD. Medical problems in athletes. Boca Raton: CRC; 1994.
25 Helm TN, Bergfeld WF. Sports dermatology. Philadelphia, PA: Lippincott Williams & Wilkins; 2001.
26 Bi L, Triadafilopoulos G. Exercise and gastrointestinal function and disease: an evidence-based review of risks and benefits. Clin Gastroenterol Hepatol 2003; 1:345–355.
27 Parmelee-Peters K, Moeller JL. Gastroesophageal reflux in athletes. Curr Sports Med Rep 2004; 3:107–111.

CHAPTER 7

Special Considerations in the Pediatric and Adolescent Athlete

David S. Chang, Bert R. Mandelbaum and Jennifer M. Weiss

INTRODUCTION

In the modern age of television and video games, America's youth is experiencing an alarming increase in the prevalence of overweight and obesity (defined as greater than 85th percentile and 95th percentile of body mass index (BMI), respectively). Unfortunately, this phenomenon is not regionalized to the US but rather poses an international problem. Published trends in Australia, Britain, Spain, Canada and the US all demonstrate overwhelming data of overweight and obesity of epidemic proportions. In Australia, from 1985–1997, the prevalence of overweight and obesity combined doubled and that of obesity alone tripled among youths (ages 7–15 years).[1] In a region of Spain, the prevalence of overweight between the years 1985 and 1995 nearly doubled among boys and girls aged 6–7 years.[2] In Canada, the prevalence of boys and girls (ages 7–13 years) classified as overweight was 33% and 26%, respectively.[3] In 2000, data collected from the NHANES (National Health and Nutrition Examination Surveys) demonstrated the prevalence of overweight was 15.5% among adolescents aged 12–19 years, 15.3% among children aged 6–11 years, and 10.4% among children aged 2–5 years.[4] From 1988–1994, the prevalence was 10.5%, 11.3% and 7.2%, respectively. According to data presented by the US Department of Health and Human Services, in the last two decades, overweight among children and teens has doubled. In 2000, one-quarter of US children watched 4 or more hours of television daily. In 2001, only 32% of students in grades 9 through 12 participated in daily school physical education; down from 42% in 1991.

At the other end of the youth activity spectrum is the ever increasing popularity of team athletics, especially soccer and basketball. The multifaceted, positive influence of team sports and routine exercise on young athletes includes physical, psychological and social benefits. However, too much of a good thing can become harmful. More commonly, today's young athlete participates not only in school teams but also in community club teams and tournament teams, thereby creating a 'perpetual season' without adequate rest periods. In addition, many youth athletes participate in multiple sports with overlapping seasons, effectively subjecting their developing bodies to year-round physical stress with no off-season to recuperate. In essence, the American youth have been polarized to those who are inactive and those who are overly active, each with their own significant health risks.

BENEFITS OF SPORTS

The spirit of the Olympic Games is embraced by the phrase '*citius, altius, fortius*', which means 'faster, higher, stronger'. Indeed, this spirit has permeated the arena of American youth athletics with substantial benefits. With routine exercise, children gain fitness, increase strength, reduce body fat, lower cholesterol and triglycerides. Certainly, sports and exercise provide a healthy antidote to the alarming epidemic of child overweight, obesity, and type II diabetes mellitus now observed in the US and internationally.[5–7] Overweight and obesity in children, as in adults, can lead to numerous, significant medical comorbidities such as arterial hypertension, left ventricular hypertrophy, hyperlipidemia, non-alcoholic-steatohepatitis, sleep apnea syndrome, as well as orthopedic, psychological and social problems.

A prospective, randomized trial involving 18 high schools assessed the impact of an educational program (ATHENA – Athletes Targeting Healthy Exercise and Nutrition Alternative) on student-athletes' health and social behavior.[8] A total of 928 students from 40 high school sports teams were enrolled in the study with a mean age of 15.4 years. ATHENA involved 8 weekly 45-min sessions incorporated into a team's usual practice activities. Curriculum content was gender-specific, peer-led and explicitly scripted. Topics included sports nutrition, effective training, negative effects of drug use and other unhealthy behaviors on sports performance, media image of females, and prevention of depression. Athletes randomized to the ATHENA program reported lower use of diet pills and athletic-enhancing substances (amphetamines, anabolic steroids, and sport supplements). They engaged in fewer incidences of high-risk social behaviors such as riding with an alcohol-consuming driver, more seat-belt use and less new sexual activity. The authors concluded that team athletics at the high school level are natural vehicles to promote an educational program to promote healthy lifestyles, deter negative social and athletic behaviors, and minimize other health-harming behaviors. 'Planet Health', another school-based educational program not necessarily catering to student-athletes, focused on decreasing television viewing, decreasing consumption of high-fat foods, increasing fruit and vegetable intake, and increasing moderate and vigorous physical activity. This program reduced the prevalence of obesity among girls in intervention schools compared with controls but no difference was detected among boys.[9]

Team athletics and routine exercise benefit the young athlete psychologically. Vigorous aerobic activity and structured aerobic activity in adolescents and children was found to improve cardiovascular fitness and to increase self-esteem while reducing depression.[10] Naturally, body appearance has a significant impact on self-esteem and self-confidence. A study of university students revealed that for females, BMI was the strongest positive predictor of body dissatisfaction and social physique anxiety.[11] In middle school children, body dissatisfaction was prevalent, especially for females.[12] In addition, body dissatisfaction was negatively related to fitness levels and BMI was positively related to body image measures. The authors suggest that early intervention to decrease body dissatisfaction in this age group is necessary. Indeed, early onset of obesity increases the risk of body dissatisfaction.[13] Additionally, in a cohort of females 7–16 years, a correlation was established between social physique anxiety and a negative body image and risk for developing an eating disorder.[14]

Youth sports and exercise participation can help curtail the negative social consequences associated with overweight and obesity. Overweight women were found to have completed fewer years of school (0.3 years less), to be less likely married (20% less likely), to possess lower household incomes (US$6710 less per year), and to have higher rates of household poverty (10% higher) than non-overweight women, independent of their base-line socioeconomic status and aptitude-test scores.[15] Likewise, overweight men were less likely to be married (11% less likely). In another study, obese girls (compared with normal weight girls) were less sociable, performed less well in school, and reported more emotional problems including suicide attempts.[16] Obese and underweight boys also reported some adverse social and educational issues.

RISKS

Box 7.1: Key Points

- Physical overtraining
- Psychological 'burn out'
- Medical considerations

The modern-day, young athlete is faced with increased training, competition, pressure to succeed, and relatively shorter periods of rest and recovery – all of which contribute to potential disastrous consequences physically, physiologically,

and psychologically. Overtraining and extended seasons with inadequate rest periods lead to overuse injuries that now plague the young athlete. Physiologically, children and adolescents are not fully mature and may have difficulty with heat mal-adaptation and dehydration. Before puberty, body size, body composition, and physiology are similar between girls and boys. Adult women have a larger surface area-to-mass ratio than men and may offer them an advantage in tolerating dry heat.[17] Younger athletes are more prone to heat mal-adaptation due to their immature cardiovascular systems, especially in humid and extremely warm conditions.[18] Symptoms can be avoided or minimized with pre-competition carbohydrate and glycogen loading, adequate hydration (before, during and after the event) and acclimatizing the young athletes to heat.[19]

The young athlete is often at high risk for psychological 'burnout'. The athletes at the greatest risk are those who compete at high intensity year round, such as swimmers, gymnasts, soccer players, and dancers. As the pressure mounts for improved performance and successful outcomes, children may no longer enjoy playing and competing in their respective sports. Injuries and pain may be feigned, preventing the child to continue to fully participate in their sport. Effective and frequent communication among the young athlete, the parents, and the coaching staff is essential to recognize early signs of 'burnout' and to initiate interventional strategies to help the child. Athletic performance is psychologically affected by both intrapersonal (self-motivation, cognitive capacity and coping skills, affective orientation and mental training skills) and interpersonal (social support and the athlete–coach relationship) factors.[20] Finding a balance of these intrapersonal and interpersonal factors is necessary for the young athlete to restore enjoyment in competition.

MEDICAL CONSIDERATIONS

Exercise-induced bronchospasm, exercise-induced bronchoconstriction, and exercise-induced asthma (EIA) are synonymous terms that describe the phenomenon of transient airflow obstruction following physical exertion.[21] The symptoms of EIA include shortness of breath, cough, chest tightness and wheezing. Bronchospasms may occur around 10–15 min after the initiation of exercise, peak at around 8–15 min after the conclusion of exercise, and resolve approximately 60 min later. Exercise-induced asthma (EIA) is largely underdiagnosed in the high school athletic population and affects up to 35% of athletes and 90% of asthmatics.[22-24] Although questionnaires and health histories can readily identify at-risk athletes, the true challenge lies in reliably screening young athletes for EIA. In a 1998 study, 10% of high school American football athletes reported a history of treated asthma, but an additional 9% of the remaining athletes were identified as having EIA via the 'free running test'.[25] The authors concluded that a substantial rate of EIA existed in high school athletes, especially in the urban setting, and that active screening was necessary to identify these young athletes. The free running test proves to be a relatively reliable screening tool for EIA, whereas pre-participation physicals, and self-reporting questionnaires, and peak expiratory flow rates (PEFRs) are less reliable.[26,27] PEFRs conducted in the laboratory setting still remain an important *diagnostic* tool.[21]

Traditional asthma medications are used to suppress EIA. Physical exertion does not produce a prolonged airway reaction as with an allergic response. Short-acting β-agonists are considered the first-line therapy and protect 80–95% of affected individuals. Non-pharmacological therapy can be employed to minimize symptoms. Approximately 40–50% of athletes with EIA experience a refractory period after exercise. Breathing warm, humidified air through the nose and trachea during rest may offer protection from symptoms that last up to 3 h.[28] Certainly, physical fitness and aerobic conditioning can help mitigate symptoms but does not eliminate them.[21]

Sudden death is a rare but tragic occurrence in young athletes with the majority (85%) being attributable to cardiac causes.[29] The prevalence of sudden death in the high school and college athletic population ranges between 1 in 100 000 and 1 in 300 000 resulting in approximately 50 sudden cardiac deaths per year among athletes.[29,30] In a 1996 study by Maron *et al.*, the median age of patient dying of cardiac causes was 17 years, with a range of 12–40 years.[29] Some 90% of the cases were male. White athletes comprised 52% of the cases and black athletes 44%. Basketball and American football accounted for 68% of the sudden death cases. The majority of athletes (90%) succumbed during or immediately after a training session or competition, with 63% of deaths occurring between 1500 and 2100 hours. The most common cause of cardiac sudden death in the pediatric and adolescent athletic population is hypertrophic cardiomyopathy (36%) followed by congenital coronary artery anomalies (13%).[29,31] Hypertrophic cardiomyopathy (HCM) is more prevalent in black athletes (48%) compared with white athletes (26%). Pre-participation medical examinations were found to be of limited value in detecting potential cardiac anomalies, identifying only 3% of affected athletes examined with risk factors. Twelve lead electrocardiogram (ECG) studies can identify patterns left ventricular hypertrophy and inverted T-waves in the inferior and precordial leads that are consistent with the athletic, conditioned heart. If these ECG changes are found in conjunction with left ventricular septal wall hypertrophy of greater than 13 mm, a diagnosis of HCM may be appropriate.[30]

Hypertrophic cardiomyopathy is inherited in an autosomal-dominant pattern with variable expression. The trait results in variable expression of the cardiac sarcomere leading to the disorganized cellular architecture of the left ventricle.[30] Symptoms of HCM may include chest pain, shortness of breath, lightheadedness or syncope. Often, athletes with HCM report no symptoms and the first clinical presentation may be sudden cardiac death. A careful cardiac history during the pre-participation examination may help identify athletes at risk for familial transmission of HCM. Although ECG has been found to be a much more effective screening tool than cardiac history and physical examination in detecting cardiovascular abnormalities, the cost-effectiveness of routine ECG screening of adolescent athletes has not been demonstrated.[30,32]

YOUNG ATHLETE RECOMMENDATIONS

> **Box 7.2: Key Points**
>
> - Initiation of sport
> - Common overuse injuries
> - Stress fractures
> - Injury prevention

For the young athlete, age of initiation to sport and exercise is an important consideration. Introduction to play should be gradual with a systematic progression to the various demands of the particular sport. 'No pain, no gain', the philosophy of the great 1960s American football coach, Vince Lombardi, is no longer applicable in modern youth sports. Overtraining and overplaying without scheduled cyclical rest phases can only lead to injury and burnout. Today, 'less is more' as successful athletes emphasize quality and diversity of training, rather than quantity and duration of training. Children cannot be approached as merely smaller-sized adults. Indeed, young athletes exhibit complex physical, physiological, and psychological differences based on their age and sex. Development of the elite athlete requires a systematic process of selection and progression of increasing levels of focus and competition. Sports, fitness, and exercise are essential for children at all stages for optimal physical, physiological, and psychological development.

Overuse injuries

Not surprisingly, in recent decades, the sports medicine community is witnessing greater numbers of overuse stress injuries in young athletes. Heightened awareness and improved diagnostic means have also contributed to better recognition of these entities. Overuse injuries occur when repetitive, submaximal stress is subjected to normal tissue in the absence of adequate time for healing. In growing children, the problem is compounded when bony growth outstrips soft tissue adaptation, leading to increased propensity for injury. Most commonly, injury patterns are seen at musculoskeletal tissue junctional sites such as bone-ligament, bone-tendon or tendon-muscle. Clinical examples of these common overuse syndromes in youth are Osgood–Schlatter, Sinding–Larsen–Johansson, Sever's apophysitis, and Panner's disease.

Stress fractures

Stress fractures are defined as mechanical failures of bone caused by repetitive mechanical loading beyond the tolerance of bone. In 1885, the Prussian physician Breithaupt first described stress fractures in the feet of marching soldiers. In 1897, these fractures were characterized on roentograms by Stechow. In 1905, the military surgeon Belcher first documented the fatigue fracture of the femoral neck.[33] Even well into the twentieth century, our understanding of stress fractures came largely from the military literature. In 1987, Matheson *et al.*

reported on 320 stress fractures in an athletic population and found that tibial and fibular stress fractures were more commonly associated with younger athletes while femoral and tarsal stress fractures were more commonly associated with older athletes.[34] Similarly, Walker *et al.* reviewed 34 stress fractures in 32 skeletally immature patients and found that the most common site was the tibia (47%), followed by the fibula (21%) and the femur (12%).[35] Nearly all patients healed with conservative treatment and were able to return to normal activity. A review of stress fractures in collegiate athletes at one institution revealed that the tibia (37%) was the most commonly involved bone but that the foot (44%) was the most commonly involved region.[36] Stress injuries were more prevalent among women (1.9%) than men (1.1%), with female distance runners exhibiting the highest incidence (6.4%).[36]

Prevention

'An ounce of prevention is worth a pound of cure'.

Female athletes in the intercollegiate and adult age groups have rates of anterior cruciate ligament (ACL) tears on the order of two to eight times higher than that of male athletes. Due to the recent significant increase in team athletic participation with female athletes at the high school and collegiate ranks, a 9-fold and 5-fold higher incidence of ACL tears compared with male athletes in the same cohort was discovered, respectively.[37–39] A multitude of variables explain this discrepancy including anatomical, environmental, hormonal, and biomechanical risk factors. In 2000, a study was initiated with young female soccer athletes (ages 14–18 years) in Southern California, implementing a neuromuscular training program to determine its efficacy in reducing the incidence of ACL injuries (Table 7.1). That year, 1041 players from 52 teams were trained with the Performance Enhancement injury Prevention (PEP) program developed by the Santa Monica Orthopaedic and Sports Medicine Group.

An additional 1905 players from 95 teams served as the age and skill matched control group. The control group reported 32 ACL tears (1.7 injuries/player/1000 exposures) compared with the PEP group with two ACL tears (0.2 injuries/player/1000 exposures).[40] This resulted in an overall 88% reduction in ACL tears in the PEP group compared with an age and skill-matched control group for the 200 season.[40] In 2001, 844 players from 45 teams were enrolled in the PEP group while 1913 players from 112 teams served as the non-randomized, age and skill-matched control. The control group reported 35 ACL tears (1.8 injuries/player/1000 exposures) compared with the PEP group with four ACL tears (0.47 injuries/player/1000 exposures). This resulted in an overall 74% reduction in ACL tears in the PEP group compared to an age and skill-matched control group for the 2001 season (Fig. 7.1).[40]

Subsequently, a collaborative study between Santa Monica Orthopaedics and Sports Medicine Group and the Center for Disease Control yielded a randomized controlled trail comparing the PEP program to control in NCAA Division I women's soccer teams. A total of 61 teams with 1394 athletes completed the study (561 PEP, 833 control). ACL injuries totaled seven in the PEP group (0.15 injuries/player/1000 exposures) compared

Table 7.1 Prevent Injury and Enhance Performance Program

Exercise	Distance	Repetitions/Time
1. Warm-up		
Jog line to line	50 yd	1
Shuttle run	50 yd	1
Backward running	50 yd	1
2. Stretching		
Calf stretch	NA	2×30 s
Quadriceps stretch	NA	2×30 s
Hamstring stretch	NA	2×30 s
Inner thigh stretch	NA	2×30 s
Hip flexor stretch	NA	2×30 s
3. Strengthening		
Walking lunges	20 yd	2 passes
Russian hamstring	NA	30 s
Single-toe raises	NA	30, bilaterally
4. Plyometrics		
Lateral hops	2- to 6-in cone	30 s
Forward hops	2- to 6-in cone	30 s
Single-legged hops	2- to 6-in cone	30 s
Vertical jumps	NA	30 s
Scissor jumps	NA	30 s
5. Agilities		
Shuttle run	40 yd	1
Diagonal run	40 yd	1
Bounding run	45–50 yd	1

NA, not applicable.

with 19 in the control group (0.28 injuries/player/1000 exposures) ($p = 0.13$). ACL injuries were significantly reduced in practice exposures with no ACL injuries in the PEP group compared with seven ACL injuries in the control group (0.13 injuries/player/1000 exposures) ($p<0.01$). There was no significant difference in ACL injury reduction in game exposures

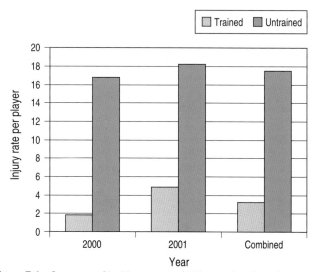

Figure 7.1 Summary of incidence rate of ACL tears by player for years 2000 and 2001.

(PEP 7 *versus* control 12; *p* = 0.66). Non-contact ACL injuries in the control group (ACL tears 10, 0.15 injuries/player/1000 exposures) occurred at over three times the rate than in the PEP group (ACL tears 10, 0.04 injuries/player/1000 exposures) (*p*<0.01). The difference in rates of non-contact ACL injuries between PEP and control groups approached significance in the second half of the season.

Based on these studies, ACL injury incidence has remained consistently lower in the PEP program group compared to the control. This suggests that a pre- and intra-season neuromuscular and proprioceptive training program may have direct benefit in decreasing the number of ACL injuries incurred by female athletes. Continued longitudinal studies and studies with younger female soccer players are currently under way.

Shoulder

Box 7.3: Key Points

- Shoulder dislocations – Basic science
- Traumatic instability
- Atraumatic instability
- Little Leaguer's shoulder

Glenohumeral dislocations and subluxations can occur relatively frequently in adolescent athletes, especially in contact sports such as American football, rugby, and martial arts. The mechanism of injury is typically traumatic – often from a fall on an outstretched arm, collision, or sudden wrenching movement.[41] Atraumatic mechanisms are rare but can occur with innocent maneuvers such as raising the arm or movement during sleep. A bimodal distribution of shoulder dislocations has been described with peaks in the second and sixth decades.[41] Nearly all dislocations involve anterior displacement with only 2% of cases displacing posteriorly.

In the pediatric and adolescent population, traumatic dislocations commonly result in recurrent instability. Reported rates of recurrent dislocations are as high as 100% in the adolescent population.[42] Rowe reported that 70% of patients who have experienced a dislocation can expect a recurrent dislocation within 2 years.[41] In another series, 86% of patients sustained a recurrence within 5 years of the initial injury.[43] Persistent instability with recurrent dislocations led 16 of 32 adolescent patients to undergo a shoulder stabilization procedure.[44] Male patients may demonstrate a higher propensity for recurrence with 71% of recurrences in a small study.[45] Risk of recurrence has been observed to be inversely related to age at the time of injury with recurrence rates of 83–90% of patients younger than 20 years, 60–63% of patients between ages 20 and 40 years, and 10–16% in patients older than 40 years.[45] In a cohort of 11–18 year olds, recurrence rates were higher if the initial dislocation occurred during participation in sports (82%) compared with those whose initial dislocation occurred in a non-sports activity (60%).[44]

Although the glenohumeral joint is considered a ball-and-socket joint, it is more analogous to a golf ball on a golf tee relying on a number of soft-tissue static and dynamic stabilizers to maintain its reduction. Since the bony containment of the humeral head is minimal, stability is dependent on competent static stabilizers (superior glenohumeral ligament, middle glenohumeral ligament, inferior glenohumeral ligament, and labrum) as well as the dynamic stabilizers (rotator cuff, long head of the biceps, latissimus dorsi, and pectoralis major). The dynamic stabilizers work in concert to generate compressive forces at the glenohumeral joint to afford stability throughout a motion arc.[46]

As with other regions of the body, the ligaments and tendons about the shoulder are largely comprised of collagen protein. In newborns, the ratio of type III collagen to type I collagen is much higher than that in adults. Type III collagen is soluble, supple, and elastic. Type I collagen contains disulfide bonds with cross-linked bridges between collagen filaments. Thus, type I collagen is insoluble, relatively tough, and non-elastic. As a child matures, the ratio of type III collagen to type I collagen in the soft tissues decreases. Therefore, in younger patients the soft tissues about the shoulder with higher type III collagen content is more elastic and more prone to dislocations and subsequent recurrences.[46]

Traumatic instability

Glenohumeral joint instability can be classified based on four factors: degree, direction, etiology, and frequency. Degree of instability should be determined as complete disassociation between the humeral head and glenoid (dislocation) or subtotal disassociation without complete dislocation (subluxation). Direction of instability can be described as anterior, posterior, inferior, or multidirectional. Anterior dislocations are the most common accounting for 90% of traumatic cases. Posterior dislocations are much less common, as in the adult population, and are typically secondary to seizures or electrical shock. Inferior dislocations, or luxatio erecta, occurs very rarely and usually results from a hyperabduction injury with extreme trauma.[47,48] Patients with multidirectional shoulder instability experience excessive global (anterior, posterior, inferior) laxity with pain, rather than instability, as the chief complaint.[49] Most patients can address their symptoms with a six-month course of physical therapy. Etiology of instability may be categorized into (1) traumatic and (2) atraumatic. Atraumatic instability can be further sub-divided into (1) voluntary and (2) involuntary. Atraumatic instability occurs only in the presence of multidirectional joint laxity. Frequency of instability can be divided as acute (single, recent episode), chronic (remote episode), or recurrent (multiple episodes).

Traumatic dislocations result from significant injury with an appropriate mechanism and are frequently observed in collision and contact sports. The most common causes of traumatic shoulder dislocations are American football (33%), fall (16%), basketball (13%), wrestling (10%), hockey (6%), baseball/softball (6%), swimming (2%), tennis (2%) and other (12%).[50] Typically, with a fall on an outstretched hand (FOOSH), the glenohumeral joint abducts and externally rotates. The humeral head displaces anteriorly with resulting damage to the anterior capsule and glenohumeral ligaments. The posterior humeral head may become compressed against the anterior glenoid rim, resulting in a Hill–Sachs impaction lesion of the posterior humeral head. A Perthes (described in 1906) or Bankart (described in 1938) lesion of the anterior labrum may result when shear forces avulse the capsule-labral complex off the anterior glenoid.[51,52] Bankart lesions were found to be present in 70% of patients requiring surgery for traumatic instability (Figs 7.2, 7.3).[53]

Patients with traumatic anterior shoulder dislocations present with pain and obvious deformity about the affected shoulder girdle. Inspection reveals a prominent acromion with an associated sulcus below it. The humeral head resides anteriorly in the axillary region. Examination includes a thorough neurologic and vascular assessment, as the axillary nerve is injured in 5–35% of first-time dislocators.[54] Radiographic work-up includes three views: anteroposterior (AP) view, scapular-Y (lateral) view, and axillary view. Often, the axillary view offers the most reliable visualization of the proper positional relationship between the humeral head and

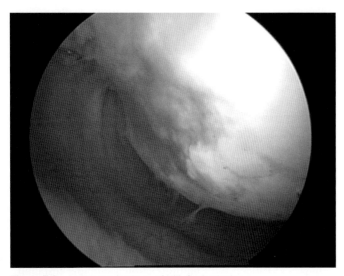

Figure 7.2 Arthroscopic photo of Hill–Sachs lesion.

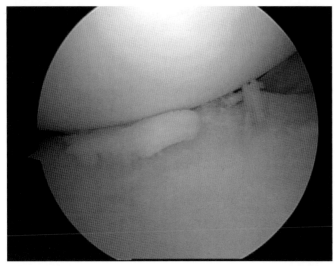

Figure 7.3 Arthroscopic photo of Bankart lesion.

glenoid to assess reduction of the joint. Careful review of the films identifies potential Hill–Sachs lesions and glenoid rim fractures.

Closed reduction can be performed on the field if the athlete can tolerate the pain and muscle spasms are at a minimum. In the emergency room setting, closed reduction can be achieved with gentle maneuvers while the patient is under conscious sedation. A number of reduction maneuvers have been described in various textbooks including the traction-counter-traction technique, the Stimson's maneuver, and the abduction maneuver.[54–56] Post-reduction radiographs include at least the AP and axillary views. A thorough post-reduction examination is conducted to ensure neurologic and vascular integrity in the extremity.

There is controversy regarding extended periods of immobilization and delay in return to sport to minimize recurrent dislocations. The literature presents mixed evidence on the efficacy of prolonged immobilization (4–6 weeks) and delay in return to sport (3–6 months). Compliance in the pediatric and adolescent athletic population is typically low for prolonged immobilization, strict activity modifications and sports limitations, and regimented physical therapy.

Surgical stabilization has provided significant functional improvement in patients with recurrent dislocations. A prospective study comparing non-operative treatment *versus* arthroscopic Bankart repair in West Point cadets after acute, initial glenohumeral dislocations revealed an 80% *versus* 14% incidence of recurrent instability, respectively.[57] Similar subsequent studies confirm the benefit of arthroscopic stabilization over non-operative, rehabilitative treatment.[58,59] In the recent years, arthroscopic stabilization techniques have improved dramatically and their success rates are approaching those of open procedures.[60] Studies analyzing arthroscopic shoulder stabilization in the young population have demonstrated similar successful outcomes. Good and MacGillivray reviewed treatment options for traumatic shoulder dislocations in adolescent athletes and concluded that surgical treatment significantly reduced the incidence of recurrent instability.[61] In specific studies regarding traumatic dislocations in young patients, Bottoni *et al.* (patient age range 18–26 years) and DeBerardino *et al.* (patient age range 17–23 years) reported recurrent instability rates of 11% and 12% following arthroscopic stabilization.[62,63] Specific studies in athletes in the 11–18 year age group still need to be conducted.

Atraumatic instability

In the pediatric and adolescent population, atraumatic instability is the most common type. Proper initial diagnosis of the condition can be difficult as the chief complaint is often pain rather than instability itself. In addition, children and adolescents exhibit a wide spectrum of normal, asymptomatic glenohumeral laxity. In a study of 75 normal adolescents (150 shoulders), signs of shoulder instability were observed in 57% of boys and 48% of girls.[64] A positive posterior drawer sign was most commonly detected in this cohort followed by a positive sulcus sign.

Patients with atraumatic instability all demonstrate multidirectional instability. A distinction must be made between voluntary and involuntary dislocators. Voluntary (habitual) instability is associated with painless subluxation or dislocation of the shoulder. Children with voluntary subluxation of the shoulder possess a favorable prognosis with no risk of early glenohumeral osteoarthritis and should not be treated with surgical stabilization during childhood.[65] The mainstay of treatment for this population is rehabilitation.

Patients with involuntary atraumatic instability also often present with complaints of pain rather than instability. Laxity of the glenohumeral joint capsule may be acquired with repetitive extreme motion about the shoulder, especially with athletes involved in swimming (backstroke and butterfly strokes), gymnastics, baseball, volleyball, and tennis. Congenital etiologies such as Marfan's or Ehlers–Danlos syndrome may account for generalized laxity. Some 80% of atraumatic instability patients treated with a specific regimen of muscle-strengthening exercises obtained good or excellent results as opposed to only 16% in patients with traumatic instability in the same study.[66] An open, inferior capsular shift remains the standard surgical procedure for patients who have failed conservative treatment with exercise alone.[49]

Little Leaguer's shoulder

In 1953, Dotter first described a fracture through the epiphyseal cartilage of the proximal humerus in a 12-year old pitcher as Little Leaguer's shoulder. Little League is a baseball league for youth players ages 5–18 years and encompasses international competition which has culminated into the Little League Baseball World Series that is held in Williamsport, Pennsylvania each year in August. Currently, Little Leaguer's shoulder encompasses the spectrum of pathology from overuse inflammation of the proximal humeral physis to actual fracture of the physis. In short, Little Leaguer's shoulder can be described as a proximal humeral epiphyseal overuse syndrome from any repetitive throwing or serving activity. The specific etiology of this condition is not clear. During the throwing motion, significant rotational stress is experienced by the proximal humeral physis, which is then vulnerable to repetitive use injury. Patients present with pain in the proximal shoulder, especially when throwing hard. The pain presents gradually, with an average duration of symptoms of 7.7 months.[67] Patients present at an average age of 14 years and a majority have played baseball continuously for at least 12 months. Radiographic findings will demonstrate a widened proximal humeral physis with possible associated lateral metaphyseal fragmentation, demineralization, or sclerosis. Rest from throwing for 3 months resulted in resolution of symptoms and return to baseball in 21 of 23 patients (91%).

Elbow

Box 7.4: Key Points

- Little Leaguer's elbow
- Osteochondritis dissecans

The elbow is especially vulnerable to overuse injuries in youth athletes, particularly throwing athletes and gymnasts. The condition Little Leaguer's elbow describes pain with corresponding radiographic changes on the medial aspect of the elbow in preadolescent and adolescent baseball pitchers.[68] Extreme valgus during the acceleration phase of throwing results in simultaneous compressive loads to the lateral elbow and tension forces on the medial elbow.[69,70] With Little Leaguer's elbow, adolescent athletes present with tenderness, swelling, and loss of motion. Radiographs will often demonstrate separation widening and fragmentation of the medial epicondylar apophysis.[68,71] Catchers and pitchers are most prone to this condition and nearly all may demonstrate hypertrophy of the medial epicondyle or medial humeral cortex in the throwing arm.[71] Positive radiographic findings such as separation or fragmentation of the apophysis is only associated with soreness in about half of the boys studied. Flexion contractures of greater than 5° may develop in anywhere from 8–20% of the adolescent throwers, depending on the study.[71]

Lateral compression injuries to the youth elbow manifest largely as Panner's disease or osteochondritis dissecans (OCD) of the capitellum. Much more rare are OCD of the radial head and angular deformity of the radial neck, which may also result from lateral compression forces to the elbow.[72] Panner's disease is an articular osteochondrosis first described in 1927. Early radiographic findings demonstrate fissuring, irregularity, and fragmentation of the capitellum. The process is spontaneous in onset and usually self-limiting. Involvement is typically unilateral and affects predominantly boys in the first decade. Panner's disease has an association with Little League pitchers and youth gymnasts.[70] Patients present with a several weeks history of pain and stiffness in the elbow.

OCD refers to an inflammation of the osteochondral articular surface. Whereas Panner's disease presents largely in children under the age of 10 years, OCD of the capitellum affects adolescents and young adults engaged in throwing or upper extremity weight-bearing activity. Some authors have suggested that Panner's disease and OCD represent two entities in the continuum of disordered endochondral ossification.[73] Symptoms associated with OCD present insidiously in the dominant elbow. Locking and catching sensations may suggest the presence of loose bodies. Physical examination may reveal lateral elbow pain, especially about the capitellum. Range of motion loss will be primarily with extension rather than flexion or rotation. Imaging with plain radiographs and magnetic resonance imaging (MRI) will help confirm the diagnosis. On plain films, a focal area of lucency about the anterior capitellar subchondral bone may be evident. Sclerotic changes may be noted on more chronic cases. Careful attention should be made to identify loose bodies, which are frequently associated with OCD. MRI may demonstrate marrow edema in the capitellar epiphysis prior to obvious changes on plain film. Treatment depends on the stability of the cartilage. Staging systems by Difelice *et al.* emphasize the importance of identifying the stability of the osteochondral fragment.[74] Initial treatment involves rest and bracing for 3–6 weeks followed by return to activity at 3–6 months.[75] Surgery is indicated for refractory cases. Arthroscopic or open techniques may be employed to excise loose bodies, débride lesions, perform abrasion chondroplasty or subchondral drilling. Arthroscopic treatment of adolescent baseball players (average age 13.8 years) was found to provide excellent, early elbow rating scores but did not guarantee return to sport.[76]

Knee

Box 7.5: Key Points

- Anterior cruciate ligament injury
- Discoid meniscus
- Tibial spine fracture
- Tibial tubercle fracture
- Osteochondritis dissecans
- Bipartite patella
- Patello-femoral pain syndrome
- Osgood–Schlatter disease
- Sinding-Larsen-Johansson disease
- Patellar sleeve fracture

The knee in a child is quite different from the knee in an adult. Skeletally immature athletes suffer different knee injuries and overuse syndromes than do adult athletes. Even when the injuries are similar to adult injuries, treatment is often different. It is thus important to understand the skeletally immature knee in terms of its injuries, prognoses and treatments.

ACL

Increased prevalence of ACL tears in skeletally immature athletes has been attributed to increased sports participation, increased awareness, and the technology of magnetic resonance imaging (MRI). Whatever the cause, surgical intervention remains controversial. Most orthopedists who care for skeletally immature athletes agree that surgical intervention should be offered to the child who cannot or will not rest the knee until skeletal maturity. However, patients and families must be counseled regarding the risk of physeal damage, no matter which surgical intervention is offered.[77] Among experts in pediatric orthopedics and sports medicine, surgical methods differ in terms of general technique, graft choice, and fixation methodology.

Surgical technique

When reconstructing the ACL in the immature knee, the surgeon must decide how to address the open physes in the femur and tibia. If the patient is near skeletal maturity, many authors advocate use of standard transphyseal techniques. Patellar tendon autografts are routinely used in the adolescent patient at Tanner stage 3 with closed or nearly-closed physes and little growth left. Although some authors advocate the use of patellar tendon autograft in patients with open physes, more authors recommend the use of hamstring autograft in this peri-adolescent population at Tanner stage 2 with a few centimeters of remaining growth.[78–82] This is supported by animal model

research which shows that soft tissue graft across an open physis inhibits bony bar formation.[83]

Modifications to traditional intraarticular ACL reconstruction may protect the physes of the periadolescent knee. The tibial tunnel angle should be increased such that the drill-hole across the tibial physis is as round as possible, as opposed to oval. If bone is used in the graft, it should be fixed away from the physis.[78] Similarly, graft fixation hardware should be placed away from the physis. Such fixation can be achieved using the Smith and Nephew Endobutton for the femur.

The last group of prepubescent patients are under the age of 12, Tanner stage 1, and have a substantial amount of growth remaining. Especially in this younger patient who is not near skeletal maturity, nonoperative management should be discussed and attempted. If this fails, extraarticular, non-transphyseal ACL reconstruction should be used in this population.

Basic research involving animal models demonstrates that drilling across and tensioning even a soft tissue graft across the wide-open physis causes growth disturbance.[84,85] For this reason, physeal-sparing techniques are used to reconstruct ACLs in knees that are not approaching physeal closure. The transepiphyseal technique spares the growth plate while providing an intraarticular graft.[80] The iliotibial band reconstruction described by Kocher and Micheli offers a combined intra- and extra-articular technique that has promising results with a low incidence of failures.[86]

Partial ACL tears in the skeletally immature knee can often be treated with rehabilitation. Surgery should be considered if physical examination reveals a positive pivot shift or a Lachman grade C or D. Otherwise, 70% of patients with partial ACL tears can avoid surgery with physical therapy alone.[87]

Discoid meniscus

The discoid meniscus is a variant of normal anatomy, almost always found laterally. This lateral meniscal variant is often bilateral. Arthroscopy performed for an unrelated indication may reveal an asymptomatic discoid meniscus. In this scenario, no intervention is recommended. A child with a discoid meniscus usually presents with painless snapping or clicking, sometimes accompanied by intermittent effusion. If the child does not experience pain, no intervention is recommended. However, the family should be counseled that there is a risk of presentation of symptoms later in childhood or even in adulthood.

Watanabe et al. classify discoid menisci according to shape and stability. According to this classification system, a complete discoid meniscus covers the entire lateral tibial plateau. An incomplete discoid meniscus covers more of the lateral plateau than normal. An incomplete, or Wrisburg variant, is the unstable variant.[88] Klingele et al. examined the incidence of peripheral rim instability in discoid menisci.[89] Symptomatic stable discoid menisci are treated by saucerization. Symptomatic unstable discoid menisci are treated by stabilization of the meniscus to the capsular rim. Menisci that are unstable anteriorly are stabilized using inside out suture technique. To avoid damage to the popliteal vessels, safe and sturdy posterior instability can be achieved using all inside newer generation suture devices.

There is often little space in the lateral compartment when a complete discoid meniscus is present. Especially when performing this procedure in a child's knee under the age of 8 years old, the surgeon should consider using a 6 mm arthroscope.

Tibial spine fracture

The mechanism leading to tibial spine fractures is tibial rotation in relation to the femur while the knee is in an extended position. This same mechanism can lead to an ACL tear. It is unclear why stress on an incompletely ossified tibial eminence leads to failure of the eminence before the ligament in some cases. Kocher et al. theorize that notch size is the determining factor.[90] When the tibial spine fractures, it is through the cancellous bone under the subchondral plate.

The McKeever system classifies tibial spine fractures according to the amount of fracture displacement. Type I fractures are nondisplaced. Type II fractures are partially displaced or hinged with angular elevation. Type III fractures are completely displaced with no bony apposition. Zariczny further subcategorizes type III fractures. Type IIIA fractures are displaced but normally aligned. Type IIIB fractures are displaced and angulated.

Physical examination will reveal an effusion along with a positive anterior drawer sign. Lateral radiographs confirm the diagnosis. MRIs should also be performed, as meniscal tears can accompany this fracture. Treatment is based on the amount of fracture displacement. Type I fractures are treated with immobilization with the knee extended. In type II fractures, reduction is attempted by extending the knee. If closed reduction is successful, the knee is immobilized in extension. Repeat imaging is recommended at 1 week to be sure that the fragment does not displace. In Type III fractures and irreducible type II fractures, operative intervention is necessary to reduce and fix the piece. This can be performed arthroscopically or through an open mini-arthrotomy. The menisci should be examined and are often found to block reduction.[91] Fixation technique options include tension band with wire or nonabsorbable suture, or screw fixation. Fixation should not violate the proximal tibial physis.

Long-term results after tibial spine fractures are good. Although many patients are left with relative laxity on Lachman examination, they do not tend to complain of subjective instability.[92] Poor results are correlated with poor reduction of the fracture fragment.[91]

Tibial tubercle fracture

Fracture of the tibial tubercle occurs at a discreet time with regards to physeal closure. The mechanism is similar to that of patellar tendon rupture. The Ogden classification divides tibial tubercle fractures into three types based on fracture pattern. Type I fractures hinge open, with the fracture line extending distally through the tubercle. In Type II fractures, the proximal aspect of the fracture exits parallel to the tubercle physis. Type III fractures are Salter–Harris III fractures, which cross the proximal tibial physis and are intraarticular. Physical examination usually only reveals a knee effusion in type III tibial tubercle fractures. The patient usually cannot perform a straight leg raise if the fragment is displaced.

Treatment of nondisplaced tibial tubercle fractures is long leg casting in extension. Displaced fractures require reduction

and fixation. The authors' preferred method of fixation is with two parallel cancellous screws utilizing washers that do not violate the proximal tibial physis (Fig. 7.4).

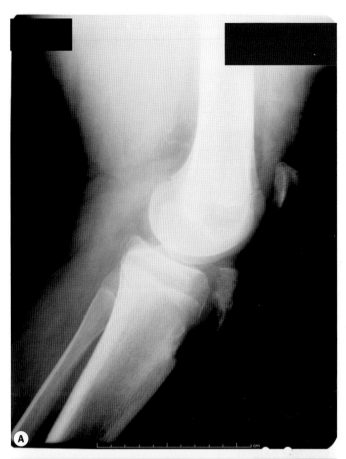

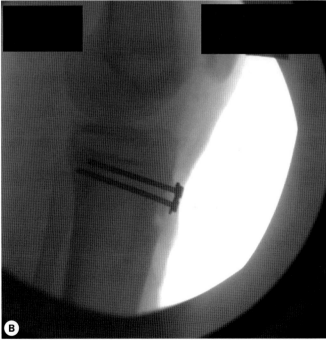

Figures 7.4 (A) Tibia tubercle fracture in a 14 year old with proximal displacement. (B) Open reduction, internal fixation with two cancellous screws and washers.

OCD of the knee

Juvenile osteochondritis desiccans (OCD) of the knee is believed to be an overuse injury. The mechanism is thought to be repetitive impact to the bone. However, some authors believe in genetic or predisposing factors due to the high (20%) bilateral incidence.[93] The most common location for OCD in the skeletally immature knee is the posterior aspect of the medial femoral condyle.

Treatment of juvenile OCD begins with rest, which should last from 6–24 months. Rest can be accompanied by immobilization, especially to improve patient compliance. Indications to operate on juvenile OCD include unstable lesions, failed non-operative management, and near skeletal maturity.

Operative treatment depends on the stage of the lesion. Stable lesions are treated with antegrade or retrograde drilling. Unstable lesions can be fixed using screws or absorbable darts. Fixation should be augmented with bone graft, which can be harvested from the proximal tibia.

Chronic lesions that cannot be fixed are treated according to size and location. Small lesions (less than 1–2 cm) are treated with microfracture. Larger lesions between 2 and 4 cm in size can be treated with osteochondral autograft transfer system (OATS) or mosaicplasty. Lesions that are larger than 4 cm in diameter can be treated with allograft OATS or autologous cartilage implantation (ACI). Recently, ACI outcomes at an average of 47 months were reported on adolescent patients, ages 12–18 years.[94] Some 96% of the patients reported good or excellent results. Similarly, 96% of the patients returned to impact sports with 60% performing at or higher than the pre-injury level. Importantly, all patients with pre-operative symptoms less than 1 year were able to return to preinjury-level athletics, while only 33% with pre-operative symptoms of greater than 1 year were able to do so.

Bipartite patella

The bipartite patella is an unfused (or incompletely fused) secondary ossification center of the superolateral patella. This secondary ossification center usually appears in early adolescence and is usually asymptomatic. When symptoms do occur, there is usually point tenderness over the superolateral patella accompanied by knee effusion. The unfused secondary ossification center is usually visualized on plain radiographs.

Initial treatment consists of rest, anti-inflammatory medications, activity modification and physical therapy focusing on stretching of the quadriceps. Rarely do patients fail this regimen of non-operative treatment. There is controversy regarding the appropriate operative management of the bipartite patella. Fragment excision is described to have good results. Other authors have described fusion of the ossification center to the remainder of the patella via internal fixation. Recently, good results have also been reported with lateral release of the retinacular attachment to the superolateral accessory ossification center. Release of this lateral retinacular attachment is thought to relieve pressure on the accessory patellar ossification center's cartilaginous attachment to the rest of the patella, thus relieving the pain (Fig. 7.5).

Patello-femoral pain syndrome

Patello-femoral pain syndrome is largely due to instability in the pediatric population. This instability ranges from maltracking to

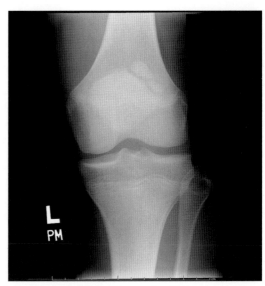

Figure 7.5 Symptomatic bipartite patella with two accessory ossicles superolaterally.

subluxation to frank dislocation. These entities are treated with the same algorithm employed for adult patients. If one is to consider bony surgery for this entity, care must be taken to choose a procedure that does not disturb the tibial tubercle physis. The Galeazzi procedure uses the medial hamstrings to provide medial stabilization to the patella. The Roux–Goldthwaite procedure transfers the lateral aspect of the patellar tendonous insertion medially.

Some anterior knee pain in the skeletally immature patient remains idiopathic in nature. This sort of benign knee pain is a diagnosis of exclusion, once instability and intraarticular pathology have been ruled out. It has been suggested that the patient and family require little more than reassurance, as most patients' pain improves over time without treatment.[95] Consideration should be given to the patient's lower extremity alignment. Patients with genu valgum and pes planus may benefit from arch supports. Physical therapy, focusing on stretching and strengthening of the lower extremities, patellar mobilization, patellar taping, vastus medialis strengthening, and abductor stretching provides relief for many patients. Surgical intervention probably does not play a role for this problem.

Osgood–Schlatter's disease

Osgood–Schlatter's disease is a traction apophysitis, or irritation, caused by the pull of the patellar tendon on the tibial tubercle in a growing child or adolescent.[96–98] First line treatment of Osgood–Schlatter's apophysitis is nonoperative. This consists of rest, icing, anti-inflammatory medication, bracing, orthotics, and even cast immobilization. Physical therapy is also useful, focusing on hamstring and quadriceps stretching.

Surgical treatment has been described for patients who have failed non-operative management of Osgood–Schlatter's disease. Many procedures have been described, including epiphysiodesis (drilling) of the tibial tubercle physis, ossicle excision, and tibial tuberoplasty.[99–101] The authors' preferred operative management for refractory Osgood–Schlatter's disease is ossicle resection accompanied by tibial tuberoplasty.

Sinding–Larsen–Johansson disease

Sinding–Larsen–Johansson disease is a traction apophysitis affecting the distal pole of the patella. It is the patellar distal pole version of Osgood–Schlatter disease – both entities can manifest simultaneously in the same patient.[102] This can also be thought of as patellar tendonitis or jumper's knee in the skeletally immature athlete.

Physical examination reveals tenderness over the distal pole of the patella that is activity related. Treatment is similar to the non-operative management of Osgood–Schlatter disease, consisting of rest, icing, anti-inflammatory medication, bracing and physical therapy. Sinding–Larsen–Johansson disease symptoms rarely last more than 1 year. Non-operative management is effective, and surgical intervention is not necessary.

Patellar sleeve fracture

Patellar sleeve fractures occur through the distal pole of the patella in child. Because the fracture occurs mostly through cartilage, the diagnosis is reliant on physical examination more than radiographs. Point tenderness occurs at the distal pole of the patella and disruption of the extensor mechanism is appreciated by inability of the patient to perform a straight leg raise. MRI can confirm the diagnosis but should not be necessary given the classic physical exam findings.[103]

Treatment of the patellar sleeve fracture consists of open reduction and internal fixation. The distal fragment is often fragmented. The classical recommendation for fixation is with a tension band wire construct.[104] The authors' preferred method of fixation is a tension band construct using nonabsorbable, heavy suture. This negates the need for second surgery to remove the hardware (Fig. 7.6).

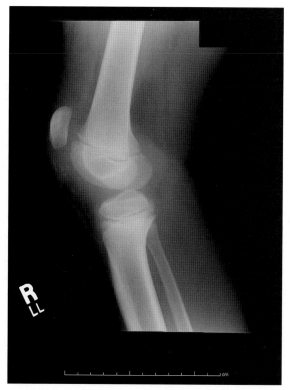

Figure 7.6 This patellar sleeve fracture was initially missed by the emergency room physician.

REFERENCES

1 Booth ML, Chey T, Wake M, Norton K, et al. Change in the prevalence of overweight and obesity among young Australians, 1969-1997. Am J Clin Nutr 2003; 77:29-36.

2 Moreno LA, Sarria A, Fleta J, et al. Trends in body mass index and overweight prevalence among children and adolescents in the region of Aragon (Spain) from 1985-1995. Int J Obes 2000; 24:925-931.

3 Willms JD, Tremblay MS, Katzmarzyk PT. Geographic and demographic variation in the prevalence of overweight Canadian children. Obes Res 2003; 11:668-673.

4 Ogden CL, Flegal KM, Carroll MD, Johnson CL. Prevalence and trends in overweight among U.S. children and adolescents, 1999-2000. J Am Med Assoc 2002; 288:1728-1732.

5 Pontiroli AE. Type 2 diabetes mellitus is becoming the most common type of diabetes in school children. Acta Diabetol 2004; 41:85-90.

6 Deckelbaum RJ, Williams CL. Childhood obesity: the health issue. Obes Res 2001; 9:239S-243S.

7 Wabitsch M, Hauner H, Hertrampf M, et al. Type II diabetes mellitus and impaired glucose regulation in Caucasian children and adolescents with obesity living in Germany. Int J Obes Relat Metab Disord 2004; 28:307-313.

8 Elliot DL, Goldberg L, Moe EL, et al. Preventing substance use and disordered eating: initial outcomes of the ATHENA (athletes targeting healthy exercise and nutrition alternatives) program. Arch Pediatr Adolesc Med 2004; 158:1084-1086.

9 Gortmaker SL, Peterson K, Wiecha J, et al. Reducing obesity via a school-based interdisciplinary intervention among youth. Arch Pediatr Adolesc Med 1999; 153:409-418.

10 Crews DJ, Lochbaum MR, Landers DM. Aerobic physical activity effects on psychological well-being in low-income Hispanic children. Percept Mot Skills 2004; 98:319-324.

11 Hausenblas HA, Fallon EA. Relationship among body image, exercise behavior, and exercise dependence symptoms. Int J Eat Disord 2002; 32:179-185.

12 Hausenblas HA, Symons Downs D, Fleming DS, Connaughton DP. Body image in middle school children. Eat Weight Disord 2002; 7:244-248.

13 Wardle J, Waller J, Fox E. Age of onset and body dissatisfaction in obesity. Addict Behav 2002; 27:561-573.

14 Thompson AM, Chad KE. The relationship of social physique anxiety to risk for developing an eating disorder in young females. J Adolesc Health 2002; 31:183-189.

15 Gortmaker SL, Must A, Perrin JM, et al. Social and economic consequences of overweight in adolescence and young adulthood. N Engl J Med 1993; 329:1008-1012.

16 Falkner NH, Neumark-Sztainer D, Story M, et al. Social, educational, and psychological correlates of weight status in adolescents. Obes Res 2001; 9:32-42.

17 Sanborn CF, Jankowski CM. Physiologic considerations for women in sport. Clin Sports Med 1994; 13:315-327.

18 Drinkwater BL, Horvath SM. Heat tolerance and aging. Med Sci Sports 1979; 11:49-55.

19 Inbar O, Bar-Or O, Dotan R, Gutin B. Conditioning versus exercise in heat as methods for acclimatizing 8- to 10-year-old boys to dry heat. J Appl Physiol 1981; 50:406-411.

20 Iso-Ahola SE. Intrapersonal and interpersonal factors in athletic performance. Scand J Med Sci Sports 1995; 5:191-199.

21 Milgrom H, Taussig LM. Keeping children with exercise-induced asthma active. Pediatrics 1999; 104:e38.

22 Rice SG, Bierman CW, Shapiro GG, et al. Identification of exercise-induced asthma among intercollegiates athletes. Ann Allergy 1985; 55:790-793.

23 McFadden ER, Gilbert IA. Exercise-induced asthma. N Engl J Med 1994; 330:1362-1367.

24 Rupp NT, Guill MF, Brudno DS. Unrecognized exercise-induced bronchospasm in adolescent athletes. Am J Dis Child 1992; 146:941-944.

25 Kukaftka DS, Lang DM, Porter S, et al. Exercise-induced bronchospasm in high school athletes via a free running test. Chest 1998; 114:1613-1622.

26 Hammerman SI, Becker JM, Rogers J. Asthma screening of high school athletes: identifying the undiagnosed and poorly controlled. Ann Allergy Asthma Immunol 2002; 88:380-384.

27 Feinstein RA, LaRussa J, Wang-Dohlman A, et al. Screening adolescent athletes for exercise-induced asthma. Clin J Sport Med 1996; 6:119-123.

28 Godfrey S, Springer C, Bar-Yishay E, et al. Cut-off points defining normal and asthmatic bronchial reactivity to exercise and inhalation challenges in children and young adults. Eur Respir J 1999; 14:659-668.

29 Maron BJ, Gohman TE, Aeppli D. Prevalence of sudden cardiac death during competitive sports activities in Minnesota high school athletes. J Am Coll Cardiol 1998; 32:1881-1884.

30 Basilico FC. Cardiovascular disease in athletes. Am J Sports Med 1999; 27: 108–121.

31 Goble MM. Sudden cardiac death in the young athlete. Indian J Pediatr 1999; 66:1–5.

32 Fuller CM, McNulty CM, Spring DA, et al. Prospective screening of 5,615 high school athletes for risk of sudden cardiac death. Med Sci Sports Exerc 1997; 29: 1131–1138.

33 Shin AY, Gillingham BL. Fatigue fractures of the femoral neck in athletes. J Am Acad Orthop Surg 1997; 5:293–302.

34 Matheson GO, Clement DB, McKenzie DC, et al. Stress fractures in athletes. A study of 320 cases. Am J Sports Med 1987; 15:46–58.

35 Walker RN, Green NE, Spindler KP. Stress fractures in skeletally immature patients. J Ped Ortho 1996; 16:578–584.

36 Arendt E, Agel J, Heikes C, Griffiths H. Stress injuries to bone in college athletes. Am J Sports Med 2003; 31:959–968.

37 National Federation of State High School Associations. High School Participation Survey. Indianapolis, IN: National Federation of State High School Associations; 2002.

38 National Collegiate Athletic Association. NCAA Injury Surveillance System Summary. Indianapolis, IN: National Collegiate Athletic Association; 2002.

39 Myer GD, Ford KR, Hewett TE. Rationale and clinical techniques for anterior cruciate ligament injury prevention among female athletes. J Athl Train 2004; 39:352–364.

40 Mandelbaum BR, Silvers HJ, Watanabe DS, et al. Effectiveness of a neuromuscular and proprioceptive training program in preventing anterior cruciate injuries in female athletes: 2-year follow-up. Am J Sports Med 2005; 33:1003–1010.

41 Rowe CR. Prognosis in dislocations of the shoulder. J Bone Jt Surg 1956; 38A:957–977.

42 Marans HJ, Angel KR, Schemitsch EH, et al. The fate of traumatic anterior dislocation of the shoulder in children. J Bone Jt Surg 1992; 74A:1242–1244.

43 Postacchini F, Gumina S, Cinotti G. Anterior shoulder dislocation in adolescents. J Shoulder Elbow Surg 2000; 9:470–474.

44 Deitch J, Mehlman CT, Foad SL, Obbehat A, Mallory M. Traumatic anterior shoulder dislocation in adolescents. Am J Sports Med 2003; 31:758–763.

45 McLaughlin HL, Cavallaro WU. Primary anterior dislocation of the shoulder. Am J Surg 1950; 80:615–621.

46 Walton J, Paxinos A, Tzannes A, et al. The unstable shoulder in the adolescent athlete. Am J Sports Med 2002; 30:758–767.

47 Freundlich BD. Luxatio erecta. J Trauma 1983; 23:434–436.

48 Yamamoto T, Yoshiya S, Kurosaka M, Nagira K, Nabeshima Y. Luxatio erecta (inferior dislocation of the shoulder): a report of 5 cases and a review of the literature. Am J Orthop 2003; 32:601–603.

49 Schenk TJ, Brems JJ. Multidirectional instability of the shoulder: pathophysiology, diagnosis, and management. J Am Acad Ortho Surg 1998; 6:65–72.

50 Lawton RL, Choudhury S, Mansat P, Cofield RH, Stans AA. Pediatric shoulder instability: presentation, findings, treatment, and outcomes. J Ped Ortho 2002; 22:52–61.

51 Perthes G. Uber operationen bei habitueller schulterluxation. Dtsch Ztschr Chir 1906; 85:199–227.

52 Bankart ASB. The pathology and treatment of recurrent dislocation of the shoulder joint. Br J Surg 1938; 26:23–28.

53 Rowe CR, Zarins B. Recurrent transient subluxation of the shoulder. J Bone Jt Surg 1981; 63A:863–872.

54 Delee J, Drez D, eds. Delee & Drez's Orthopaedic sports medicine: Principles and practice, 2nd edn. Philadelphia, PA: WB Saunders; 2003.

55 Browner B, Jupiter J, Levine A, Trafton P, eds. Skeletal trauma: fractures, dislocations, ligamentous injuries, 2nd edn. Philadelphia. PA: WB Saunders; 2002.

56 Bucholz RW, Heckman JD, eds. Rockwood and Green's fractures in adults, 5th edn. Philadelphia, PA: Lippincott Williams & Wilkins; 2001.

57 Arciero RA, Wheeler JH, Ryan JB, et al. Arthroscopic Bankart repair versus nonoperative treatment for acute, initial anterior shoulder dislocations. Am J Sports Med 1994; 22:589–594.

58 Kirkley A, Griffin S, Richards C, et al. Prospective randomized clinical trial comparing effectiveness of immediate arthroscopic stabilization versus immobilization and rehabilitation in first traumatic anterior dislocations of the shoulder. Arthroscopy 1999; 15:507–514.

59 Boszotta H, Helperstorfer W. Arthroscopic transglenoid suture repair for initial anterior shoulder dislocation. Arthroscopy 2000; 16:462–470.

60 Stein DA, Jazrawi L, Bartolozzi AR. Arthroscopic stabilization of anterior shoulder instability: a review of the literature. Arthroscopy 2002; 18:912–924.

61 Good CR, MacGillivray JD. Traumatic shoulder dislocation in the adolescent athlete: advances in surgical treatment. Curr Opin Pediatr 2005; 17:25–29.

62 Bottoni CR, Wilckens JH, DeBerardino TM, et al. A prospective, randomized evaluation of arthroscopic stabilization versus nonoperative treatment in patients with acute, traumatic, first-time shoulder dislocations.

63 DeBerardino TM, Arciero RA, Taylor DC, Uhorchak JM. Prospective evaluation of arthroscopic stabilization of acute, initial anterior shoulder dislocations in young athletes. Two- to five-year follow-up. Am J Sports Med 2001; 29:586–592.

64 Emery RJ, Mullaji AB. Glenohumeral joint instability in normal adolescents: incidence and significance. J Bone Jt Surg Br 1991; 73:406–408.

65 Huber H, Gerber C. Voluntary subluxation of the shoulder in children. A long-term follow-up study of 36 shoulders. J Bone Jt Surg Br 1994; 76:118–122.

66 Burkhead WZ, Rockwood CA. Treatment of instability of the shoulder with an exercise program. J Bone Jt Surg 1992; 74:890–896.

67 Carson WG, Gasser SI. Little Leaguer's Shoulder: a report of 23 cases. Am J Sports Med 1998; 26:575–580.

68 Brogdon BG, Crow NE. Little leaguer's elbow. Am J Roentgenol Radium Ther Nucl Med 1960; 83:671–675.

69 Adams JE. Injury to the throwing arm: a study of traumatic changes in the elbow joints of boy baseball players. Calif Med 1965; 102:127–132.

70 Kobayashi K, Burton KJ, Rodner C, Smith B, Caputo AE. Lateral compression injuries in the pediatric elbow: Panner's disease and osteochondritis dissecans of the capitellum. J Am Acad Ortho Surg 2004; 12:246–254.

71 Hang DW, Chao CM, Hang YS. A clinical and roentgenographic study of Little League elbow. Am J Sports Med 2004; 32:79–84.

72 Ellman H. Anterior angulation deformity of the radial head. An unusual lesion occurring in juvenile baseball players. J Bone Jt Surg Am 1975; 57:776–778.

73 Ruch DS, Poehling GG. Arthroscopic treatment of Panner's disease. Clin Sports Med 1991; 10:629–636.

74 Difelice GS, Williams RJ 3rd, Cohen MS, Warren RF. The accessory posterior portal for shoulder arthroscopy: Description of technique and cadaveric study. Arthroscopy 2001; 17:888–891.

75 Peterson RK, Savoie FH, Field LD. Osteochondritis dissecans of the elbow. Inst Course Lect 1999; 48:393–398.

76 Byrd JW, Jones KS. Arthroscopic surgery for isolated capitellar osteochondritis dissecans in adolescent baseball players: minimum three-year follow-up. Am J Sports Med 2002; 30:474–478.

77 Kocher MS, Saxon HS, Hovis WD, Hawkins RJ. Management and complications of anterior cruciate ligament injuries in skeletally immature patients: survey of the Herodicus Society and the ACL Study Group. J Pediatr Orthop; 22:452–457.

78 Shelbourne KD, Gray T, Wiley BV. Results of transphyseal anterior cruciate ligament reconstruction using patellar tendon autograft in Tanner stage 3 or 4 adolescents with clearly open growth plates. Am J Sports Med 2004; 32:1218–1222.

79 Edwards PH, Grana WA. Anterior cruciate ligament reconstruction in the immature athlete: long-term results of intra-articular reconstruction. Am J Knee Surg 2001; 14:232–237.

80 Anderson A. Transepiphyseal replacement of the anterior cruciate ligament in skeletally immature patients. A preliminary report. J Bone Jt Surg Am 2003; 85: 1255–1263.

81 Hawkins CA, Rosen JE. ACL injuries in the skeletally immature patient. Bull Hosp Jt Dis 2000; 59:227–231.

82 Matava MJ, Siegel MG. Arthroscopic reconstruction of the ACL with semitendinosus-gracilis autograft in skeletally immature adolescent patients. Am J Knee Surg 1997; 10:60–69.

83 Stadelmaier DM, Arnoczky SP, Dodds J, Ross H. The effect of drilling and soft tissue grafting across open growth plates. A histologic study. Am J Sports Med 1995; 23:431–435.

84 Edwards TB, Greene CC, Baratta RV, Zieske A, Willis RB. The effect of placing a tensioned graft across open growth plates. A gross and histologic analysis. J Bone Jt Surg Am 2001; 83:725–734.

85 Houle JB, Letts M, Yang J. Effects of a tensioned tendon graft in a bone tunnel across the rabbit physis. Clin Orthop 2001; 391:275–281.

86 Kocher MS, Micheli L. Growth plate sparing combined intra-articular and extra-articular anterior cruciate ligament reconstruction with iliotibial band in skeletally immature preadolescent children. Boston: Harvard Medical School.

87 Kocher MS, Micheli LJ, Zurakowski D, Luke A. Partial tears of the anterior cruciate ligament in children and adolescents. Am J Sports Med; 2002:30:697–703.

88 Watanabe M, Takeda S, Ikeuchi A. Atlas of arthroscopy. 3rd edn. Tokyo: Igaku-Shoin; 1979.

89 Klingele KE, Kocher MS, Hresko MT, Gerbino P, Micheli LJ. Discoid lateral meniscus: prevalence of peripheral rim instability. J Pediatr Orthop 2004; 24:79–82.

90 Kocher MS, Mandiga R, Klingele K, Bley L, Micheli LJ. Anterior cruciate ligament injury versus tibial spine fracture in the skeletally immature knee: a comparison of skeletal maturation and notch width index. J Pediatr Orthop 2004; 24:185–188.

91 McLennan JG. The role of arthroscopic surgery in the treatment of fractures of the inter-condylar eminence of the tibia. J Bone Jt Surg Br 1982; 64:477–480.

92 Wiley JJ, Baxter MP. Tibial spine fractures in children. Clin Orthop Relat Res. 1990:54–60.

93 Schenck R, Goodnight J. Osteochondritis Desiccans. J Bone Jt Surg Am 1996; 78:439–456.

94 Mithofer K, Minas T, Peterson L, Yeon H, Micheli LJ. Functional outcome of knee articular cartilage repair in adolescent athletes. Am J Sports Med 2005; 33:1147–1153.

95 Sandow MJ, Goodfellow JW. The natural history of anterior knee pain in adolescents. J Bone Jt Surg Br 1985; 67:36–38.

96 Cohen B, Wilkinson RW. The Osgood-Schlatter lesion. Am J Surg 1958; 95:731.

97 Mital MA, Matza RA, Cohen J. The so-called unresolved Osgood-Schlatter lesion: a concept based on fifteen surgically treated lesions. J Bone Jt Surg 1980; 62:732–739.

98 Osgood R. Lesions of the tibial tubercle occurring during adolescence. Clin Orthop Relat Res 1993; 286:1903.

99 Binazzi R, Felli L, Vaccari V, Borelli P. Surgical treatment of unresolved Osgood-Schlatter Lesion. Clin Orthop Relat Res 1993; 289:202–204.

100   Glynn MK, Regan BF. Surgical treatment of Osgood–Schlatter's disease. J Pediatr
      Orthop 1983; 3:216–219.
101   Flowers MJ, Bhadreshwar DR. Tibial tuberosity excision for symptomatic
      Osgood–Schlatter disease. J Pediatr Orthop 1995; 15:292–297.
102   Medlar R, Lyne E. Sinding–Larsen–Johansson disease. J Bone Jt Surg Am 1978;
      60:1113.
103   Bates D, Hresko M, Jaramillo D. Patellar sleeve fracture: Demonstration with MR imag-
      ing. Radiology 1994; 193:825–827.
104   Tolo V. Skeletal trauma in children. In: Green S, ed. Skeletal trauma. Philadelphia: WB
      Saunders; 1998:443–444.

CHAPTER 8

Special Considerations in the Female Athlete

Joanne Borg-Stein, Sheila A. Dugan and Jennifer L. Solomon

INTRODUCTION

The female athlete distinguishes herself from her male counterpart by possessing unique biomechanical, physiological and psychosocial characteristics that influence sports performance and participation. An appreciation of these gender differences is critically important for the sports medicine clinician.

PARTICIPATION AND HISTORICAL PERSPECTIVE

Women's participation in organized and recreational athletics at all levels is at an all time high and continues to grow. Globally, more young women are participating in soccer, softball, basketball, swimming and track and field events. Mature adults and senior women are participating in gender specific fitness programs and health clubs. Recent gender specific epidemiologic studies have demonstrated the benefit of exercise in women for the prevention of chronic disorders such as cardiovascular disease and osteoporosis.[1,2]

According to the International Olympic Academy, female sports participation has been on the rise ever since the ancient Olympic Games. The representation of female Olympic competitors increased from 10% to 20.6% between 1952 and 1976. The paths of opportunities for females to compete at the international level have never been more promising than in modern times.[3,4]

In the US, at the collegiate level, the NCAA (National Collegiate Athletic Association) keeps records of numbers of participants in all divisions. For the 2000–2001 season, the total number of female participants was 149 115 compared with 206 573 for men. By comparison, during the 1981–1982 season the ratio was 64 390 women compared with 167 055 men. Thus, the rate of participation of women in NCAA athletics has almost tripled in the past 20 years and has outpaced the rate of increase of male athletic participants. Extensive information on NCAA sports participation rates, expenditures, and injuries is available on the website.[5]

At the high school level, participation in sports continues to grow. Growth in female sports outpaces that of male sports. The number of boys participating in 1971 was 3 666 917 and the number of girls 294 015. The most recent survey (1999–2000) of participants found 3 861 749 boys and 2 675 874 girls (www.nfhs.org)

GROWTH AND MATURATION: AGE AND GENDER ASSOCIATED VARIATION IN PERFORMANCE

Box 8.1: Key Points

- Body size, body composition and physiology are basically similar in boys and girls before puberty.
- Female athletes are more flexible than male athletes.
- Female athletes have a less intense adolescent spurt in strength and power.
- In senior adults, gender responses to strength training and detraining are equivalent.

Body size, body composition and physiology are basically similar in boys and girls before puberty. The adolescent growth spurt and puberty mark the period in life when sex differentiation and development begin. Peak height velocity for girls ranges from 10.5 to 13 years and for boys, 12.5 to 15 years. Peak weight velocity and menarche occur approximately 6 months and 1 year, respectively after the height peak. On average, women have a larger surface area-to-mass ratio; lower bone mass; and wider, shallower pelvis compared with men. The implication of these characteristics is that women may have an advantage in the heat, are at more risk for osteoporosis, and may be predisposed to experience knee problems.[6]

Studies comparing motor performances of elite male and female athletes in the same sport suggest that sex differences are not marked, with the exception of greater upper and lower body strength and power in males later in adolescence.[7,8] On the other hand, trends for the agility tests and balance indicate small sex differences in most age groups.[9] In contrast, female athletes are more flexible than male athletes at all ages, and have a less intense adolescent spurt in muscle strength and power.[10]

Comparing the aerobic power of young male and female athletes in the same sport, the differences in maximal oxygen uptake are small in early adolescence, 4–8% between 9 and 13 years, but increase to greater than 22% between 15 and 17 years with studies in elite distance runners. The sex difference is likely related to the larger muscle mass and heart size, and greater hemoglobin concentration in adolescent males, all of which influence the ability to transport and utilize oxygen.[11] Expressing VO$_2$max in relation to body weight somewhat decreases the gap between male and female values. Relative VO$_2$max values for prepubescent girls are 90–95% and for late adolescent girls are roughly 80% of male values.[12]

In senior adults, gender responses to strength training and detraining are equivalent. Studies measuring the response to strength training as measured by muscle volume and improvements in one repetition maximum have demonstrated equivalent gains in older men and women.[13,14] Longitudinal studies of master athletes suggest that age-related losses in maximal oxygen uptake did not differ by gender.[15,16]

THE FEMALE ATHLETE AND PREGNANCY

Box 8.2: Key Points

- The level of fitness and activity before pregnancy is the main determinant of exercise during pregnancy.
- Following an uncomplicated vaginal delivery, exercise may begin as soon as the woman feels ready to exercise.
- Athletes post-partum should incorporate aerobic conditioning, general and sports specific training, as well as pelvic floor and abdominal strengthening to correct pregnancy induced laxity and weakness.

Exercise and pregnancy

Women are being encouraged by their healthcare providers to exercise moderately during pregnancy unless they have any of the contraindications noted in the recommendations of the American College of Obstetrics and Gynecology. The ACOG recommendations include both absolute and relative contraindications to exercise (Tables 8.1–8.3).[17] The level of fitness and activity before pregnancy is the main determinant of exercise participation during pregnancy.

Exercise recommendations have evolved over the last several decades. The data currently available do not support the

Table 8.1   Exercise and Pregnancy: Absolute Contraindications to Aerobic Exercise During Pregnancy

Hemodynamically significant heart disease
Restrictive lung disease
Incompetent cervix/cerclage
Multiple gestation at risk for premature labor
Persistent second- or third-trimester bleeding
Placenta previa after 26 weeks' gestation
Premature labor during current pregnancy
Ruptured membranes
Preeclampsia/pregnancy-induced hypertension

From American College of Obstetrics and Gynecology 2003.[17]

Table 8.2   Exercise and Pregnancy: Relative Contraindications to Aerobic Exercise During Pregnancy

Severe anemia
Unevaluated maternal cardiac arrhythmia
Chronic bronchitis
Poorly controlled type I diabetes
Extreme morbid obesity
Extreme underweight (BMI <12)
History of extremely sedentary lifestyle
Intrauterine growth restriction in current pregnancy
Poorly controlled hypertension
Orthopedic limitations
Poorly controlled seizure disorder
Poorly controlled hyperthyroidism
Heavy smoker

BMI, body mass index. From American College of Obstetrics and Gynecology 2003.[17]

Table 8.3   Exercise and Pregnancy: Warning Signs to Terminate Exercise While Pregnant

Vaginal bleeding
Dyspnea prior to exertion
Dizziness
Headache
Chest pain
Muscle weakness
Calf pain or swelling (need to rule out thrombophlebitis)
Preterm labor
Decreased fetal movement
Amniotic fluid leakage

From American College of Obstetrics and Gynecology 2003.[17]

idea that detailed exercise prescriptions should be viewed as a necessary safety measure for most healthy, physically active pregnant women. Save for a few pregnancy related considerations, the approach should be not different from that used with a non-pregnant individual. For an otherwise healthy woman, the minimal list of precautions include: localized pain, hemorrhage, persistent uterine contractions, physician concern that the pregnancy has complications, and any sudden change in feelings of well-being.[18]

The importance of rest-activity cycles, hydration and nutrition should be stressed and built into an overall training program. The woman should wear loose fitting clothing in ventilated areas, to help prevent persistent elevation in body temperature.[19] More recent studies have not confirmed any increase risk to mother or fetus with moderate aerobic or strength training exercise in women with uncomplicated pregnancy.

Heart rate is a relatively unreliable parameter during pregnancy. Perceived exertion and/or actual oxygen consumption should be used to assess intensity. A two point shift in an individual's level of perceived exertion indicates the need to either decrease or increase the work load. Symptoms of fatigue, localized pain and poor performance indicate the need for action and suggest worn equipment or overtraining in the pregnant as well as the non-pregnant female. If the activity elicits an unusual and/or potentially deleterious physiological response (unusual cardiac activity, pain, hyperthermia, etc.) it should be modified. If the pregnancy is not entirely normal, modifications may be required.[18]

The American College of Gynecology provides general guidelines for exercise during pregnancy.[17] For pregnant women previously active in recreational sports and exercise, the 2003 ACOG guidelines recommend women should continue to be active during pregnancy and 'modify their usual routine as medically indicated'. For competitive athletes engaged in strenuous sports, they note that information is limited and recommend 'close medical supervision'. The guidelines warn against activities with high risk of falling or abdominal trauma. They make specific mention of avoiding scuba diving and being thoughtful about acclimatization for high-altitude exercise.

Following an uncomplicated vaginal delivery, exercise may begin as soon as the woman feels ready to exercise, often within one week. Athletes in training should incorporate aerobic conditioning, general and sports specific strength training, as well as pelvic floor and abdominal strengthening to correct pregnancy induced laxity and weakness.[20]

Musculoskeletal concerns of the pregnant athlete

> ### Box 8.3: Key Points
>
> - Ligamentous laxity, related to the production of the hormones relaxin and estrogen during pregnancy, is associated with connective tissue remodeling and may predispose to pelvic, sacroiliac and low back pain of pregnancy.

Physiologic changes of pregnancy can put the athlete at risk for specific types of injury. Soft-tissue edema of pregnancy and increased fluid retention can predispose to tenosynovial injury or nerve entrapment. Ligamentous laxity, related to the production of the hormones relaxin and estrogen during pregnancy,

is associated with connective tissue remodeling and may predispose to pelvic, sacroiliac and low back pain of pregnancy.[21] Normal weight gain of pregnancy in combination with ligamentous laxity may increase the stress on lower extremity joints. Hyperlordosis of pregnancy in combination with symphysis pubis widening may also contribute to increasing mechanical strain on the low back, sacroiliac, and pelvic regions.[22]

A comprehensive discussion of the peripheral neurologic and musculoskeletal aspects of pregnancy is beyond the scope of this chapter. The reader is referred to published reviews.[19,22] However, the following is an outline of the key regional musculoskeletal causes of pain or injury in athletically active pregnant and post-partum women, with which the sports medicine clinician should be familiar.

- Pubic pain of pregnancy
  - Pubic symphysis inflammation
  - Osteitis pubis: bony resorption and re-ossification about the symphysis pubis
  - Rupture of the symphysis pubis
  - Pelvic dislocation: extremely rare.
- Low back pain of pregnancy
  - Mechanical strain
  - Pelvic ligamentous laxity
  - Sacroiliac pain
  - Vascular compression
  - Spondylolisthesis
  - Discogenic pain and lumbar disc herniation
  - Referred pain from hip pathology
  - Sacral or vertebral stress fracture.
- Peripheral nerve entrapment of pregnancy and the puerperium
  - Median neuropathy at the wrist (carpal tunnel syndrome)
  - Meralgia paresthetica (lateral femoral cutaneous neuropathy)
  - Femoral neuropathy and other intrapartum maternal nerve injuries
  - Lumbosacral plexopathies.
- Upper limb pain of pregnancy
  - De Quervain's tenosynovitis: inflammation of the abductor pollicis longus, and extensor pollicis brevis in the first dorsal compartment of the wrist.
- Lower limb pain of pregnancy
  - Transient osteoporosis of the hip or knee
  - Avascular necrosis of the femoral head
  - Acetabular labral injury
  - Transient laxity and strain of the ACL
  - Medial meniscus tear
  - Patello-femoral stress
  - Stress fracture.

THE FEMALE ATHLETE TRIAD

History

The female athlete triad describes the interrelated findings of inadequate eating, menstrual abnormalities and skeletal demineralization in female athletes that can lead to poor health and injuries, in particular osteoporosis and stress fractures.

Box 8.4: Key Points

- The female athlete triad describes the interrelated findings of inadequate eating, menstrual abnormalities, and skeletal demineralization in female athletes that can lead to poor health and injuries, in particular osteoporosis and stress fractures.

- Identification of disordered eating and prevention of the energy imbalance can prevent the development of hypothalamic mediated menstrual disorders and subsequent bone demineralization.

The term was coined at the 1984 American College of Sports Medicine (ACSM) meeting and by the early 1990s, a Task Force On Women's Issues in Sports Medicine was convened. In 1997, the ACSM published a Position Stand on the Female Athlete Triad.[23] It is currently being updated and continues to be a focus of the Strategic Health Initiative on Women, Sport and Physical Activity of the ACSM.

Inadequate eating

Inadequate eating in female athletes occurs along a continuum from failing to take in sufficient calories for the amount of energy expended to frank eating disorders such as anorexia nervosa and bulimia nervosa. Anorexia nervosa is defined as: body weight 15% below expected; morbid fear of fatness; feeling fat when thin; and amenorrhea.[24] Bulimia nervosa is defined as: binge eating twice per week for at least 3 months; loss of control over eating; purging behavior; and overconcern with body shape.[24] There is a higher incidence of eating disorders in female athletes, with prevalence ranging from 16% to 64% in female athletes surveyed, compared with 5% of females in the population at large.[25–27]

Disordered eating can stem from attempts to control body weight to enhance performance or appearance. Norwegian elite athletes had a higher prevalence of eating disorders when participating in sports emphasizing leanness or specific weight such as gymnastics, figure skating and wrestling.[28] There is sports-specific variation in body fat percentages from pentathletes and runners at the low end to swimmers and skiers at the high end, representing the body's adaptation for performance enhancement.[29] Unfortunately, athletes may supersede this natural adaptation by imposing stringent caloric or nutrient restriction or by excessive training. Some research suggests that exercise itself may suppress the appetite.[30]

Menstrual abnormalities

Menstrual disturbances in female athletes have been recognized and studied over the last two decades. These disturbances range from reduction in the length of the luteal phase and suppression of luteal function in regularly menstruating athletes to frank amenorrhea. Delayed menarche was associated with exercise, in particular the timing and level of training.[31] Higher intensity training at an earlier age was associated with later onset of menses (age 15) in ballet dancers and athletes trained before menarche, compared with sedentary controls (age 13).

Research on energy balance has identified restricted energy availability, rather than stress or lean body composition, as the factor that initiates exercise-induced menstrual disturbances.[32] Low carbohydrate availability in particular may be linked to reproductive disorders. Dietary supplementation to eliminate a difference between dietary energy intake and exercise energy expenditure can prevent or eliminate these menstrual disturbances.

Clinicians and researchers are working on identifying and reliably measuring biomarkers that can be used in the clinic to identify carbohydrate deficiency and fat stores, such as skin fold measurements and urinary ketones. Insulin-like growth factors and intracerebral catecholamines have been identified as important metabolic mediators of energy availability in exercise related menstrual irregularities.[33] Thyroid hormones and leptin levels may provide insight into the catecholestrogenic system.

Skeletal demineralization

The third component of the female athlete triad is bone demineralization, including premature osteoporosis at its worst. Peak bone density may never be achieved if young female athletes have primary amenorrhea and are unable to build bone during formative years. Secondary amenorrhea can cause a decline in bone density similar to that of a postmenopausal woman.[34] Unfortunately, this bone loss may be irreversible.[35] Studies have shown that estrogen supplementation has not increased bone density in amenorrheic athletes.[36] More recent studies, of anorexia nervosa patients, have demonstrated that low dose oral contraceptives given in combination with recombinant human insulin-like growth factor (IGF)-1 increased bone density.[37] However, this combination has not been studied in female athlete triad patients.

Treatment of the female athlete triad

Once female athletes with disordered eating, abnormal menstruation and bone demineralization are identified, appropriate work-up and referrals are required (Fig. 8.1). Dietary modifications may be necessary to provide appropriate nutrients and energy balance. A sports nutritionist can facilitate data collection on energy intake and calorie expenditure and athlete education. For eating disorders, psychological testing and individual and family therapy is necessary. A behavioral modification program can be helpful for aberrant eating habits. Identification of comorbid conditions associated with eating disorders including electrolyte imbalances, cardiac arrhythmias, impaired gastrointestinal motility and anemia, among many other life-threatening disorders, is mandatory for the team physician. Referral for specialty medical care and hospitalization may be required.

The reader is referred to an obstetrics and gynecology text for a complete overview of primary and secondary amenorrhea, oligomenorrhea and delayed menarche.[38] In the sexually active athlete presenting with amenorrhea, pregnancy should be ruled out. The physical exam should include Tanner staging, body fat estimation, and thyroid, breast and pelvic examination. Laboratory testing should include pregnancy, thyroid functioning and hormonal testing. Depending on the individual athlete, additional diagnostic tests including the progestin challenge, endometrial biopsy, magnetic resonance imaging of the pituitary and/or pelvic sonography may be indicated. Optimal management includes the return of natural menses after normalizing energy balance.[34] However, hormone replacement therapy (HRT) may be necessary to resume cyclical menstrual bleeding, with both estrogen and progesterone to avoid the endometrial hyperplasia associated with unopposed estrogen.[39] The management of exercise-induced amenorrhea continues to be speculative with some authors advocating HRT in the setting of stress fracture.[40]

Bone demineralization can present with stress fracture. Dual energy X-ray absorptiometry is the most accurate method of measuring bone mineral density (BMD). The diagnostic work-up and management of stress fractures is addressed in a separate section of this chapter. The World Health Organization (WHO) criterion for the diagnosis of osteoporosis is a BMD greater than 2.5 standard deviations below the youthful mean.[41] Osteopenia is defined as a BMD between 1.0 and 2.5 standard deviations below the youthful mean. While these criteria are used in female athletes of all ages, normative data for BMD of adolescent girls are not available, limiting the ability to adequately define pathological bone loss in this age group. Oral contraceptive pills or HRT should be considered in amenorrheic athletes who are unsuccessful with attempts at non-pharmacological interventions to return normal menses.[39,42] While no studies have been done with female athletes, osteopenic females with eating disorders demonstrated increased bone density with combination phar-

macological therapy including HRT and IGF-1.[37] Recombinant human leptin administered to leptin deficient women with hypothalamic amenorrhea showed improved reproductive, thyroid and growth hormone axes and markers of bone formation.[43]

Prevention through awareness
Identification of disordered eating and prevention of the energy imbalance can prevent the development of hypothalamic mediated menstrual disorders and subsequent bone demineralization. Athletes presenting with stress fractures should be screened for disordered eating and menstrual disorders. The National Collegiate Athletic Association (NCAA), the American College of Sports Medicine (ACSM) and other organizations provide educational materials for athletes, families, coaches and athletic directors. Principles of proper nutrition and nutrients are a mandatory part of preseason training and regularly reinforced in team meetings. Annual medical examinations must include gynecological screening.

EPIDEMIOLOGY OF INJURY

Box 8.5: Key Points

- Generally, there is little difference in the pattern of injury between men and women competing in comparable sports; with the exception of the increased incidence of ACL tears in the female athlete.

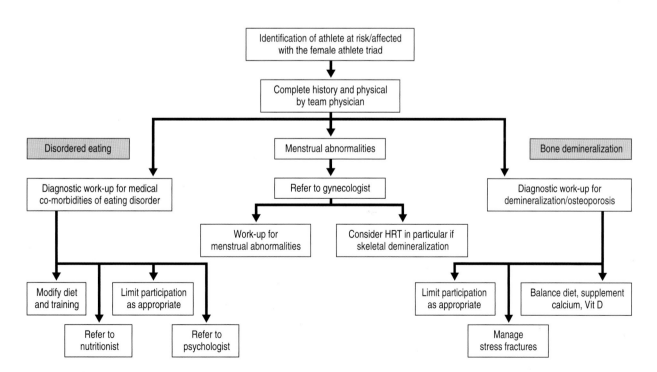

Figure 8.1 Overview of the management of the female athlete triad. HRT, hormone replacement therapy.

Research institutes provide injury rates at the collegiate and high school level. The NCAA injury surveillance system publishes reports that are available for comprehensive review by sport and type of injury (www.ncaa.org). In a recent study of sports injuries from Turkey, there were no differences between 17–28-year-old men and women in percentages of injured athletes. The differences among various sports in the percentage of injured athletes were statistically significant. The most frequently injured body regions were the foot and ankle in basketball, volleyball, soccer and running, but in wrestling, the knee. The findings suggest that injury rates are associated with the sport rather than sex of the player.[44]

In a 2001 study of 3767 NCAA division III 18–22-year-old athletes competing in seven sports, the data suggested very little difference in the pattern of injury between men and women competing in comparable sports. The seven like sports were basketball, cross-country running, soccer, swimming, tennis, track and water polo. The only minor gender differences were seen in swimming and water polo. Female swimmers reported more back/neck, shoulder, hip, knee and foot injuries, and female water polo players reported more shoulder injuries.[45]

Other studies have documented that female athletes sustain more knee injuries than male athletes, specifically ACL sprains. Anterior knee pain is also more common in women athletes than men. The relationship between gender and increased rate of ACL tears has been well documented; however, the relationship between gender and other lower extremity injuries is less clear.[46]

Shoulder and elbow injuries in the female athlete

Box 8.6: Key Points

- Shoulder injuries in female and male athletes occur at similar rates for comparable sports; however, studies have shown that women suffer more serious shoulder injuries in volleyball, more shoulder pain with impingement, and more elbow injuries in amateur golf than men.

- Women have shorter arm length and shorter body length thus requiring more strokes for swimming than men.

- Gender-based anatomic differences about the elbow include greater extension of the female elbow due to differences in the olecranon process.

Shoulder injuries in female and male athletes occur at similar rates for comparable sports.[47] However, studies have shown that women suffer more serious shoulder injuries in volleyball, more shoulder pain with impingement, and more elbow injuries in amateur golf than men.[48–51] Studies demonstrate greater differences in upper body than lower body strength between men and women.[52] Men with larger shoulder girdles may have a higher center of gravity, which can increase one's ability to develop upper extremity strength.[53] These

gender differences in the musculoskeletal system may shed some light on the disparate upper extremity injury rates. Women have shorter arm length and shorter body length thus require more strokes for swimming the same distance. Women historically have poorer conditioning than men. Gender-based anatomic differences about the elbow include greater extension of the female elbow due to differences in the olecranon process.[54] Some authors argue that increased joint laxity, more common in women, may equate to increased injury risk. However, in multiple studies of ligamentous laxity at the knee, there is no direct link between laxity and higher injury rate.[55–57] Women may be at an increased injury risk if training with resistance training equipment designed for the male body.

The most common shoulder injuries seen in athletes include impingement syndrome, rotator cuff tendonitis or tendinopathy, and instability. Swimming, racquet sports and sports requiring throwing are associated with impingement syndromes. In the setting of ongoing pain, maladaptive movement patterns can develop and evaluation of the scapulothoracic joint is included on physical examination. Although uncommon, stress fractures about the shoulder girdle and rib cage should be considered in postmenopausal rowers or younger rowers with exercise induced menstrual irregularity.[58]

The most common elbow injuries include lateral and medial epicondylitis and valgus extension overload. As with other sports injuries, the mechanism of injury relates to sport specific activities. Lateral epicondylitis occurs equally between men and women, however a study of female tennis players over the age of 40 showed an increased risk when participating in more than 2 h of racquet time per week.[59] The reader is directed to the shoulder and arm chapter for further details on the assessment and treatment of sports-related shoulder and elbow injuries. Despite their inequity is upper body strength, men and women experience similar relative strength gains with training.[60] Biceps and rotator cuff strengthening contribute to the stiffness and rigidity of the glenohumeral ligaments, decreasing instability. Restoration of normal movement patterns and strength of the scapular stabilizers avoids recurrent injury. Maintaining full range of motion (ROM), especially of the hip and neck in throwing athletes, allows for appropriate force generation and dissipation. As in all sports injuries, sports specific training precedes return to play.

Low back pain in the female athlete: background

In the general population, low back pain (LBP) is the most common musculoskeletal complaint, affecting as many as 80% of the population at some point in their lives. Athletes are also commonly affected by low back pain. LBP is well documented in various sports including swimming,[61] weightlifting,[62] racquet sports,[63] gymnastics,[61] American football,[64] rowing[65] and triathlons.[66] LBP is a common cause of limited play and practice time.[67] However there is a lack of studies pertaining to female athletes with low back pain. A review of low back pain in high-level rowers over a 10-year period found a 25% incidence in women and 15.2% incidence in men.[68] A prospective

Box 8.7: Key Points

- Male and female athletes are predisposed to the same conditions that result in low back pain.
- Potential causes are numerous and include muscle spasm, muscle strain, discogenic pain, posterior element pain (spondylolysis, spondylolisthesis and facet joint pain) and sacroiliac joint pain.
- Conservative treatment is often successful and includes rest, NSAIDs, heat, and physical therapy that targets the involved muscles and emphasizes stretching and strengthening.
- More studies are needed to examine the specific risk factors in the female athlete.

study of 257 college athletes, both men and women participating in nine varsity sports revealed that 9.3% required treatment for low back pain during the ensuing academic year.[69] In a 3-year study of adolescent athletes, Kujala and colleagues found that athletes participating in ice hockey, soccer, figure skating and gymnastics sustained a significantly higher incidence of disabling low back pain than age-matched controls.[70] The incidence of injury to the pars interarticularis can be as high as 11% in young female gymnasts compared with the norm of 2.3% in non-athletic females.[71]

Few studies have tried to identify risk factors that predispose female athletes to these injuries. However, a study of female soccer players failed to reveal a relationship between low back pain with menstrual cycle or with the use of oral contraceptives.[72] Keene and collaborators also found a higher incidence of overuse and lumbar spine injuries in females compared to males. However, male and female athletes are predisposed to the same conditions that result in low back pain.[73]

The majority of athletes with low back injuries are likely to have benign symptoms.[74] The majority of athletes respond well to conservative non-operative treatment and will return to their sport in an expedited manner. Potential causes are numerous and include muscle spasm, muscle strain, discogenic pain, posterior element pain (spondylolysis, spondylolisthesis and facet joint pain), and sacroiliac joint pain. Saal found that in athletes, posterior element pain accounted for 70% of the injuries involving the low back independent of gender.[75] Discogenic pain is though to account for 25% of low back injuries in male and female athletes.[75] However, it is this author's opinion that discogenic low back pain is underdiagnosed. This section will discuss the history, physical examination, diagnosis and treatment of spondylolysis, spondylolisthesis, facet syndrome, radiculopathy and discogenic pain. These are the common diagnoses seen in female athletes with low back pain.

Spondylolysis/spondylolisthesis/facet syndrome

The incidence of spondylolysis (a defect in the pars interarticularis) in the general population is approximately 6%, most often is asymptomatic, and occurs mostly between the ages of 5 and 10.[76] The athletic population is more prone to this injury and is more likely to be symptomatic.[77] Repetitive flexion/

extension motion causes significant amount of stress on the pars interarticularis and can lead to microfractures and eventually to lysis. Sports including gymnastics, figure skating, and divers are most prone to this injury. The incidence in female gymnasts was found to be four times greater than aged and sex matched controls.[78]

Athletes with spondylolysis/spondylolisthesis (a 'slippage') will typically complain of a dull or aching sensation in lumbar sacral region with or without buttock pain. Spondylolisthesis is the slip of one vertebrae relative to another and spondylosis is defined as a fracture in the pars interarticularis. Radiating symptoms below the knee are rare. Some patients will report the onset of symptoms after extension, arching or twisting whereas other will not recall a history of trauma. Symptoms are typically exacerbated with lumbar extension.

Physical examination Athletes with spondylolysis/spondylolisthesis typically have a hyperlordotic posture with relatively tight hamstrings. One-legged lumbar extension reproduces pain on the ipsilateral side. Palpation of the bony eminences along the middle of the patient's back also known as the spinous processes may reveal a 'step-off' defect. Patients with pain in extension may be more likely to have facet-joint disease or spondylolysis because extension increases the pressure on the posterior elements of the spine. The neurological examination is typically normal; however if radicular signs and symptoms are present it may indicate a high grade spondylolisthesis.

The differential diagnosis of posterior element pain includes lumbar strain/sprain, spondylolysis/spondylolisthesis, facet syndrome, sacroiliac joint dysfunction, and other sources of pain other than the spine. Women with gynecological issues may also experience low back pain that presents with similar signs and symptoms. Low back pain has been shown to be present in up to 10% of patients with endometriosis.[79]

Imaging and diagnostic procedures: Antero-posterior and lateral X-rays may be obtained. If spondylolysis is suspected, an oblique X-ray should be obtained. A defect may be detected in the neck of the 'Scotty dog'; however, defects are commonly missed on X-ray. The lumbar vertebral body will appear as a 'scotty dog' on oblique X-ray images. The pedicle of the vertebra denotes the eye of the dog. The transverse process denotes the nose, superior articular facet the ear, pars interarticularis the neck, and the inferior articular facet the foot. If clinical suspicion is high, a single photon emission computerized tomographic (SPECT) bone scintigraphy can be helpful in identifying stress reactions of the pars not seen on X-rays. A CT scan has also been shown to be a sensitive test in confirming the diagnosis of spondylolysis as well as distinguishing other causes of a positive bone scan or X-ray. Magnetic resonance imaging may also aid in the identification of a pars defect. Lateral X-rays of the spine aid in identifying the presence of spondylolisthesis. This is graded 1 to 4, depending on the degree of displacement or forward slippage of one vertebra in relation to the adjacent inferior vertebra. Grade 1 represents up to 25% displacement; 26–50% is grade 2; 51–75% is grade 3; grade 4 is 76–100%.

Lumbosacral radiculopathy

Lumbosacral radiculopathy is caused by compression or ischemia of a nerve root. The most common cause of lumbosacral radiculopathy is a disc bulge, protrusion, extrusion, or sequestration, accounting for as much as 98% of all cases, with the majority occurring at the L4–5, L5–S1 levels. Other causes of lumbosacral radiculopathy include osteophytes, Z-joint hypertrophy, cyst, tumor, or other causes of neural foraminal stenosis.

Athletes typically complain of numbness, tingling, burning, or electric, radiating pain shooting down the thigh and/or leg in a band-like manner. The distribution of symptoms depends on the level of nerve root involvement. Patients with discs causing the symptoms may complain of exacerbation of symptoms with forward flexion (this position increases pressure on the disc).

Physical examination Gait evaluation may reveal a Trendelenburg gait, which is when a patient cannot maintain the pelvis level while standing on one leg, the contralateral leg hangs lower and the patient is said to have a positive Trendelenburg gait, and may be seen in a patient with an L5 radiculopathy and resulting weakness in the gluteus medius. Sensory, muscle, and reflex testing should be performed and may reveal dysesthesia, weakness, and/or diminished reflex in the involved segment(s) (Table 8.4).

Dural tension signs such as straight leg raise or sitting root test, should be evaluated in a patient with a suspected radiculopathy. These may be performed with the patient in the seated or supine position. When the femoral nerve is implicated as being potentially involved, the patient may be placed in the prone position and the reverse straight leg raise performed.

Imaging and diagnostic procedures: AP and lateral X-rays may be obtained. MRI may also be obtained and is optimal for evaluating the soft tissues that may be involved. It is important to remember that more than a third of all asymptomatic people will have MRI findings of disc abnormalities.[80] However, when the patient's symptoms, straight leg raising test, and MRI findings are correlated, the specificity of the diagnosis of radiculopathy caused by the disc is increased dramatically. Therefore, it is important to treat the patient, not the MRI findings.

Internal disc disruption/discogenic pain

The term internal disc disruption (IDD) was suggested first by Crock in 1970 on the basis of a large group of patients whose disabling back and leg pain became worse following operations for suspected disc prolapse.[81] He defined IDD as a condition marked by alterations in the internal structure and metabolic functions of the intervertebral disc, usually preceded by an episode of spinal trauma.[82]

Typically, athletes present with low back pain in the lumbosacral region. The distribution of referred pain may be anywhere in the lower limb but usually is present more proximally rather than distally. Pain is typically episodic and is worse in the morning. Aggravating factors include prolonged sitting, axial loading, and Valsalva maneuvers. Physical examination is often vague, but typically the neurological examination is normal.

The 'gold standard' to diagnose discogenic low back pain, a provocative discography with post-discogram CT is performed. This is a percutaneous procedure performed under fluoroscopic guidance in which dye is injected into the disc. When the patient's daily pain is provoked at one disc level but not at adjacent levels, the test is considered positive for discogenic pain. After the injection, the patient receives a CT scan in order to evaluate the extravasation, if any, of the dye. In a patient with discogenic pain, the pain originates from the nerve fibers that are located primarily in the outer one third of the annulus fibrosus. Therefore, in patients with discogenic pain, the dye is often seen to extravasate from the nucleus pulposus to the outer third of the annulus fibrosus.

Treatment of athletes with low back pain

The goal is to return the athlete to training and competition, as quickly and safely as possible. Conservative treatment is often successful and includes relative rest, NSAIDs, heat, and physical therapy that targets the involved muscles and emphasizes stretching and strengthening. Lutz *et al.* described a five stage rehabilitation program: stage 1: early protected mobilization; stage 2: spinal stabilization; stage 3: spine safe strengthening

Table 8.4 Lower Extremity Neurological Examination

Root level	T12–L3	L4	L5	S1	S2,S3,S4
Function	Hip flexion (T12-L3) Knee extension (L2-L4) Hip adduction (L2-L4)	Foot inversion/dorsiflexion	Toe extension/hip abduction	Foot eversion/ plantarflexion	Toe clawing. No testing

Myotome	- iliopsoas (T12-L3)
	- quadriceps (femoral n. L2-L4)
	- adductor brevis, longus and
	  magnus (obturator n. L2-L4)
		- tibialis anterior	- extensor digitorum longus
			- extensor hallucis longus
			- gluteus medius
				- peroneus longus and
				  brevis
				- gastroc-soleus
				- gluteus maximus
					- intrinsic foot
					  muscle. No testing

Dermatome	L1-inguinal ligament L2-mid-thigh L3-medial side of knee	Medial leg and medial site of foot (saphenous n. and superficial peroneal n.)	Lateral leg and dorsum of foot (lateral sural cutaneous n. and superficial peroneal n.)	Lateral side of foot (sural n.)	S2-posterior thigh S3,S4-anal area
Reflex	None	Patellar	Tibialis posterior	Achilles	Superficial anal reflex

and conditioning; stage 4: return to sports and stage 5: maintenance.[83] Each athlete is unique and therefore a one-treatment-fits-all protocol is discouraged. These stages are only intended to provide a guideline. It is important to note that an athlete should not return to their sport until he or she is pain free, has obtained full pain free range of motion, and full strength as observed with manual muscle testing.

Treatment of athletes with posterior element pain focuses on promoting abdominal stabilizing with emphasis on forward flexion rather than extension based exercises. A posterior pelvic tilt focuses on strengthening of the abdominal muscles and the stabilization of the lumbar paraspinal muscles. A program which also emphasizes stretching of the hamstrings helps reduce excessive lordosis.

Several studies advocate the use of a thoracolumbar brace in athletes with spondylolysis to limit extension and promote healing of the defect. Iwamoto and Wakano found that 87.5% of athletes who were treated conservatively with activity restriction and antilordotic lumbosacral bracing could return to their original sporting activities in an average of 5.4 months.[84]

Patients with low back pain that is found to be originating from facet-joint disease may be treated with intra-articular injections or radiofrequency neurotomy of the involved nerves. This is a percutaneous procedure performed under fluoroscopic-guidance. The nerves may regenerate and the procedure may need to be repeated periodically if pain returns.

Athletes with radiculopathy may undergo a fluoroscopically-guided epidural steroid and anesthetic injections. The injectate may be delivered via either a caudal, interlaminar, or transforaminal approach. Failure to use fluoroscopic-guidance may result in a relatively high rate of needle misplacement. Percutaneous radiofrequency neurotomy, using fluoroscopic-guidance, is another minimally invasive option for patients with radicular symptoms.

When patients fail to respond to broad conservative measures, surgery should be considered. Progressive neurological symptoms are another indication for surgery.

In summary, both males and females are vulnerable to low back pain. Different athletic events place a diverse tension on the lumbar spine. Early aggressive diagnosis with a comprehensive treatment approach is needed. More studies are needed to examine the specific risk factors in the female athlete.

Pelvis and hip injuries

As in other regions of the body, there are gender differences in the anatomy of the hips and pelvis. The bony pelvis includes three bones, the right and left ilium and the sacrum, forming the right and left sacroiliac joints (SI joints). The hip joint includes the femur articulating with the acetabulum. The female pelvis is broader. Women with broader and shallower pelvises may have greater hip range of motion.[85] The combination of greater femoral neck anteversion and shorter limb length leads to a lower center of gravity for women compared to men.[86] Neuromuscular differences in firing patterns of motor units may arise from these anatomic differences, but have not yet been proven to increase injury risk.[87] The ligaments, fascia and muscles of the pelvic girdle

---

Box 8.8: Key Points

- The female pelvis is broader.
- Women with broader and shallower pelvises may have greater hip range of motion.
- The combination of greater femoral neck anteversion and shorter limb length leads to a lower center of gravity for women compared with men.
- While there have been no specific studies in female athletes, it may be that imbalances in muscle flexibility and strength may predispose female athletes to pelvic girdle and hip pain.

---

support the forced closure (outside forces to withstand load) of the SI joint working in concert with form closure (bony congruency of joint surfaces).[88] Alterations in force closure occur during pregnancy due to increasing abdominal girth, changes in load transfer, and deconditioning in addition to ligamentous laxity due to the hormones relaxin and estrogen. Thus inadequate force closure may be the cause of the increase rate of SI joint pain in pregnant women.[89] While there have been no specific studies in female athletes, it may be that imbalances in muscle flexibility and strength may predispose female athletes to pelvic girdle and hip pain. Form closure is less congruent in women due to the shape of the pelvis and less extensive joint surfaces, which may make women more reliant of muscles and ligaments for stability. The muscular system may be unable to withstand the added forces especially during extensive periods of training or with repetitive unidirectional loading.

Pelvic and hip injuries can be divided into bony and soft tissue causes. Bony causes include osteoarthritis, stress fractures, avulsion injuries, acetabular labral tears, osteitis pubis or avascular necrosis of the head of the femur. Soft tissue conditions include muscle strains, tendonitis, bursitis, and nerve entrapment. Individual chapters on the hip and pelvis will review the evaluation and management of these conditions. A section on stress fractures is included in this chapter, including femoral and pelvic stress fractures. To reiterate, femoral neck stress fractures must be included in the differential of any runner or dancer presenting with hip pain, especially in the setting of menstrual dysfunction, as left untreated the morbidity is substantial. Retrospective survey studies of older women with hip osteoarthritis relate high sports exposure in earlier years with X-ray changes, pain and need for total hip arthroplasty.[90,91] Prospective studies are needed to assess for a dose-response curve to identify harmful levels of exercise.

Pelvic floor dysfunction describes pain or abnormal function of the muscular sling within the bony pelvis. The pelvic floor supports viscera, sphincter function, hip and trunk movement, and sexual function. Dysfunctions are commonly divided into hypertonic versus hypotonic. Hypertonic, or high tone, dysfunctions include pain and excessive muscle tension and can present with associated constipation and dyspareunia (pain with intercourse). Hypotonic, or low tone, dysfunctions can present with incontinence and may be related to collagen changes, previous childbirth or gynecological surgery, or nerve injury. Exercising women presenting with pelvic floor pain may relate it to a previous acute onset or a more insidious pattern; their medical visit often comes about when their athletic performance declines or they are no longer capable of exercising. The myriad tissues that refer pain to the pelvic floor must be considered in the differential diagnosis. This list includes, but is not limited to, the genitourinary or colorectal systems, intraarticular hip pathology (such as acetabular labral tears), lumbosacral radiculopathy, plexopathy or peripheral neuropathy, including the pudendal nerve and its division, or muscles of the abdominal wall or lumbar spine. While evaluation and management of pelvic pain and urinary incontinence is beyond the scope of this chapter, practitioners need to include direct questions of female athletes regarding history of urinary incontinence, at a minimum, to identify women with pelvic floor dysfunction. If left unidentified, it can deter individuals from continued sports participation.

Knee injuries in the female athlete

Box 8.9: Key Points

- Compared with males, females have a greater likelihood of sustaining knee injuries involving the ACL (4.9 greater likelihood), collateral ligament (2.5 greater likelihood) and meniscus (1.9 greater likelihood).

- The reason for the increased incidence of female knee pain and injuries is likely multifactorial with gender differences in neuromuscular responses, hormonal influences, and anatomy.

- An association between the menstrual cycle and ACL injuries has been reported.

- Women tend to demonstrate alterations in strength, relaxation time, and muscular fatigability during the menstrual cycle.

- Hormone levels may play a larger role than we are currently aware especially since they may have a direct impact on hamstrings to quadriceps strength ratios and knee joint mechanics.

Since the passage of Title IX Educational Assistance Act of 1972 in the US, which required institutions that received federal funds to provide equal access to males and females in all curricular and extracurricular activities, women's participation in sports, at both high school and collegiate levels, has considerably increased.[92] This corresponded to an increase in exercise and physical activity for females. Soon after this rapid increase in sports participation, there were subjective reports of excessively high numbers of female athletes sustaining serious knee injuries during jumping and cutting sports. Early studies, in the 1970s, examined a female's physiologic potential in conditioned and non-conditioned states.[93,94] The findings from these initial studies laid the groundwork for the development of biomechanical and biochemical risk factors for sports related female knee injuries. Most female injuries are a result of their participation in the sport rather than their gender.[95] However, anatomical, hormonal and functional differences between males and females must be considered when caring for the female athlete. Most sports medicine research has been conducted on males and as a result, long-term research on female athletes is lacking. The reasons why particular injuries are more common in female athletes are not well understood.

According to the NCAA, more injuries seem to occur during practices than during games in both men and women. Whereas, more knee injuries, including anterior cruciate ligament (ACL), collateral ligament, and meniscal tears occur during games. Compared with males, females have a greater likelihood of sustaining knee injuries involving the ACL, as shown in Box 8.9.[96] In addition, females have an increased incidence of anterior knee pain and patello femoral disorders.[97–99] Females participating in jumping and cutting sports are 4–6 times more likely to sustain a serious knee injury than males participating in the same sports.[100,101] Among serious knee injuries, the incidence of ACL injury is one of the most dramatic differences between female and male athletes. Gray et al. reported the incidence of ACL ruptures in female basketball players to be more than 5 times higher than in male basketball players.[102] Ferretti et al.[103] demonstrated a 4-fold increase of serious knee ligament injuries in female versus male National Championship level volleyball players. Malone et al.[104] reported a 6.2-fold higher incidence of ACL injuries among female basketball players as compared with male basketball players and that the incidence was even higher with non-contact ACL injuries. Serious knee injuries, especially ACL injuries, in female athletes frequently result in the loss of entire athletic seasons and typically require surgical reconstruction and extensive rehabilitation. In the case of university or college athletes, this may result in the loss of scholarship funding and strain academic performance.[105] In the case of Olympic athletes, prolonged departure from training or competing may greatly reduce an Olympian's competitive ability and may result in the loss of selection to compete in Olympic games. ACL injuries is thus a major constituent of knee pain in female athletes and most of the orthopedic research on female athletic knee injuries is centered around the ACL.

Anterior knee pain in female athletes includes patellar subluxation, dislocation, malalignment, and fractures. In addition, other causes of knee pain include: patello-femoral syndrome, osteochondral fractures, pathological plica, cartilaginous and osteochondral loose bodies, osteochondritis dissecans, and skeletally immature-related diseases. Tendinous disruption of the quadriceps and patella will also result in anterior knee pain. Inflammatory conditions, such as bursitis, tendonitis, osteoarthritis, and the various inflammatory arthritides must be considered as potential causes of anterior knee pain. It is important to keep in mind that referred pain from the lumbar spine can contribute to symptoms of anterior knee pain. The reason for the increased incidence of female knee pain and injuries is likely multifactorial with gender differences in neuromuscular responses, hormonal influences and anatomy.

Zelisko et al. have suggested that differences in pelvic structure and lower limb alignment, including Q-angle, may be responsible for the increased incidence of knee injuries in female athletes.[99] However, Gray and colleagues found no association between any anatomical measure, including the Q-angle, and the incidence of ACL injuries.[102] Furthermore, Emerson reported that females have small intercondylar notch widths relative to the size of the ACL.[106] Shelbourne and colleagues argued that a narrow femoral notch leads to a small ACL, which would predispose the female knee to ACL injury.[107] The anatomical theories to explain the disparity of injury rates between men and women remain controversial. The differences in dynamic movement patterns as opposed to static anatomical differences between male and female athletes seem to be more explanatory for the disparity in knee injury rates. Some 80% of ACL injuries occur via a non-contact mechanism, and the majority of these occur at landing from a jump.[108] Females tend to be in a more upright position, with less hip and knee flexion and with more knee valgus angulation when landing from jumps. The more upright position with an externally rotated pronated lower limb may predispose the athlete to knee injury.[109] Reducing the varus and valgus torques, the abduction and adduction moments, at the knee and hip at landing may aid in stabilization of the knee joint and prevent serious knee injury.[110] Hewett and colleagues demonstrated an average reduction of 80% of one bodyweight, in peak landing forces and decreases in abduction or adduction moments at the knee of approximately 50% after applying a plyometric strength and flexibility training program to the female athletes studied.[101]

Strong quadriceps contractions in the setting of a decelerating knee at low knee flexion angles predispose the ACL to injury. This predisposition is further exaggerated in the individual with decreased hamstring contractions. Female athletes tend to contract their quadriceps to a greater degree than their hamstrings as compared with male athletes at landing and in response to anterior tibial translation. Moreover, female athletes show more anterior knee laxity and less knee flexor strength than males.[101,110]

Female athletes primarily contract their quadriceps in response to a force directed anteriorly to the back of the calf. Males on the other hand counter this anterior tibial translation by initially contracting their hamstrings.[57] Hamstrings act to resist forces which strain the ACL, whereas quadriceps contraction at low knee flexion angles (<45°) acts to increase strain on the ACL.[111] Chandy and Grana found a significantly larger number of female than male high school athletes had knee injuries which required surgery. They recommended that conditioning of the quadriceps and hamstrings should be accented during training.[112] As a result, many schools and sports organizations in the US have developed and incorporated jump training programs into their conditioning regimens in jumping sports. These programs emphasize stretching, plyometric exercises, and weightlifting to increase performance and decrease injury risk to jumping athletes[110].

High speed isokinetic strength testing (180°/s) has been conducted to determine hamstrings to quadriceps ratios as well as side to side hamstring strength. Davies postulates that hamstring strength should be 80–100% of quadriceps strength at high speeds and that hamstrings to quadriceps ratios lower than 60% may be correlative to pathology and can predispose

an athlete to ACL injury.[113] Knapik et al. examined hamstring strength and found that dominant leg knee flexor strength 15% or greater than the non-dominant side is indicative of a higher risk of lower limb injury in female collegiate athletes. In addition, a dominant hip extensor which is 15% or more flexible than the non-dominant side has been shown to be predictive of injury.[114]

An association between the menstrual cycle and ACL injuries has been reported. Wojtys and colleagues observed a lower number of ACL injuries occurring during menses or follicular phase of the menstrual cycle.[115] Myklebust and colleagues demonstrated that a significantly greater number of ACL injuries occurred in the premenstrual period or luteal phase.[116] Female hormones, estrogen and progesterone, appear to play an important role in the injury rates in female athletes. The direct effect of these hormones on ligamentous and soft tissue structures has been under investigation. Estrogen receptors have been identified in fibroblasts from the human ACL and the presence of physiological concentrations of estradiol decreases ligamentous strength.[117,118] Samuel et al. has shown relaxin to reduce soft tissue tension.[119] The female neuromuscular system has been known to be directly and indirectly affected by the level of estrogen. Women tend to demonstrate alterations in strength, relaxation time, and muscular fatigability during the menstrual cycle. Sarwar et al. observed an appreciable increase in quadriceps strength, a slowing of relaxation, and an increase in fatigability of the quadriceps during the ovulatory phase, when estrogen reaches peak secretion rates, in women not taking oral contraceptives, but not in women taking oral contraceptives.[120] Hormone levels may play a larger role than we are currently aware especially since they may have a direct impact on hamstrings to quadriceps strength ratios and knee joint mechanics. It is therefore paramount to inquire about the menstrual history and contraceptive use of injured female athletes as well as athletes reporting to training camp. We may be able to lessen the rate of female ACL injuries by adjusting practice, training, and conditioning schedules and regimens in accordance with menstrual cycles and when female athletes would be at a higher risk of injury.

Knee injury prevention falls in line with training and conditioning and includes education. Potentially dangerous maneuvers that should be altered through training to prevent ACL injuries have been identified. Griffin has reported that athletes involved in sports such as volleyball, soccer, and basketball, should land in a more bent-knee position and decelerate before cutting.[121] Implementing these techniques has suggested a decrease in injury rates. Caraffa and colleagues found that athletes who participated in proprioceptive training before their competitive season had a decreased incidence of knee injuries.[122] The study was carried out in which three hundred soccer players during three soccer seasons were instructed to train 20 min per day using different types of wobble-boards with five different phases of increasing difficulty. The first phase consisted of balance training without any balance board; phase 2 involved training on a rectangular balance board; phase 3 of training on a round board; phase 4 of training on a combined round and rectangular board; phase 5 of training on a so-called BAPS (biomechanical ankle platform system) board. Johnson has demonstrated a decrease in knee injuries in

Vermont ski instructors through education and public awareness of the high occurrence and mechanisms of ACL injuries.[123] In this study, the ski instructors were shown videotapes of ACL injuries and were encouraged to create preventive strategies of their own through 'guided discovery'. It is clear that a comprehensive approach to training athletes is crucial in reducing and preventing knee injuries. Combining dynamic, sports-specific, biomechanically correct movements with neuromuscular enhancement techniques and constant and consistent feedback through education and awareness will afford athletes the best arsenal in preventing knee injuries. Hewett and colleagues demonstrated that female athletes who underwent a neuromuscular training program developed greater dynamic knee stability than female athletes who did not participate in training.[124] The conclusion was that participation in this type of training will demonstrate greater dynamic and passive stability as compared with untrained female athletes.

Patello-femoral syndrome (PFS) is a common finding in female athletes with knee pain. Unlike ACL injuries, female athletes are more prone to developing PFS than males secondary to anatomic differences. These include increased pelvic width, increased femoral anteversion, and a resultant increased Q-angle.[125] The diagnosis of PFS can usually be reached from the history alone. PFS had been commonly misdiagnosed as intra-articular pathology, peripatellar tendonitis or bursitis, Osgood–Schlatter disease, chondromalacia patella and osteochondritis dissecans.[126] The increased Q-angle imposes an increased valgus load on the patella thereby creating increased pressure on the patella facets which can lead to cartilage softening and retinacular stress around the patella with ensuing anterior knee pain.[127] Patients with PFS usually report unspecified onset of vague, aching anterior knee pain. In two thirds of the cases, the pain will be bilateral and a family history of similar symptoms may be reported. Pain is classically worse with activity, particularly with deep knee bends, running hills, squats and negotiating stairs. Female athletes are especially prone to PFS as their exercise and training routines commonly employ squats, running hills, and deep knee bends all under increased loading. Female athletes afflicted with PFS should maintain aerobic fitness and sport-specific skills even during the acute phase of treatment provided these activities do not cause or worsen pain. The rehabilitation should include exercises with the knee close to full extension, such as short-arc knee extensions, for the quadriceps particularly strengthening the vastus medialis oblique which is considered to be the key step in the rehabilitation program. The short-arc exercises reduce the joint reaction and compression forces that typically occur with full-arc knee exercises. Once the athlete is able to perform all activities pain free and both limbs are equal in strength, rehabilitation is complete. This treatment paradigm for PFS tends to have good outcomes. Persistent pain despite compliance with an appropriate rehabilitation program should warrant further investigation into the etiology of the athlete's knee pain.

Foot and ankle injuries

Anatomic differences specific to the foot between male and female athletes have not been identified, however, compensatory hyperpronation of the feet has been linked to wider pelvis

---

Box 8.10: Key Points

- Anatomic differences specific to the foot between male and female athletes have not been identified; however, compensatory hyperpronation of the feet has been linked to wider pelvis and increased genu valgus of the female lower limbs.
- Hallus valgus is more common in girls and women.
- There are no gender differences in the most common ankle sprain mechanism (inversion).
- Women are less likely that men to suffer Achilles tendonitis.
- Morton's neuroma is 7–10 times more frequent in women than men.

---

and increased genu valgum of the female lower limbs.[128,129] Hallux valgus, another abnormality linked to abnormal biomechanics, is more common in girls and women.[130,131] Foot and ankle injuries occur at a higher rate than any other lower extremity injury in male and female athletes from adolescence through college age in the US.[95,132,133] Ankle sprain was the most common injury in a study of young elite female basketball players.[134] There are no gender differences in the most common ankle sprain mechanism (inversion), type (lateral), or ligament involved (anterior talofibular > calcaneofibular and posterior talofibular). Women were less likely than men to suffer Achilles tendonitis.[135] Morton's neuroma, on the other hand, is 7–10 times more frequent in women than men.[136] Classical ballet predisposes females to particular foot injuries due to compensating for limited hip turnout. Females had poorer outcomes after fasciotomy for compartment syndrome than their male counterparts in the setting of chronic symptoms.[137]

Gender differences have been noted in metatarsal stress fracture rates in female compared with male soldiers.[138] While it has been proposed that women have smaller and narrower bones that limit absorption and redistribution of ground reaction forces with running, one must always remember to assess nutritional and menstrual status in any female athlete presenting with a stress fracture.[139]

STRESS FRACTURES IN THE FEMALE ATHLETE

Stress fractures are common overuse injuries affecting both male and female athletes, and are seen in a wide variety of sporting activities. Stress fractures occur when the skeleton's reparative capacity cannot keep up with the repetitive load that is being applied. Contributing factors include training errors, underlying bone health and anatomic and biomechanical variations. Stress factors are more commonly reported in female athletes. An athlete with a stress fracture may lose considerable time away from their sport; however, the majority will resolve with non-operative treatment. Uncommonly, these injuries can be more serious and require surgical intervention which may threaten the athlete's profession. It is imperative that health care professionals caring

Box 8.11: Key Points

- Stress fractures are common overuse injuries and are reported more frequently in female than male athletes.
- Clinicians need to have a high index of suspicion for this injury.
- Athletes typically present with pain which is aggravated by activity.
- Imaging is utilized to confirm the diagnosis.
- Conservative treatment is usually successful.
- It is imperative that risk factors for susceptibility to stress fractures be identified and addressed.
- More research is needed to identify the precise risk factors in stress injuries to bone.

for athletes have a high index of suspicion for the diagnosis as well as an understanding of treatment and potential contributing factors.

Epidemiology

Stress fractures were first described in the military population in 1955.[140] With the growth of athletics and awareness stress fractures are now recognized as a frequent injury. The true incidence is not known. Stress fractures have been reported in athletes who partake in many sports including running, gymnasts, dancers, basketball, swimmers, lacrosse and rowers.[141-144] The sport with the greatest reported incidence is running. Bennell et al. reported a 20% incidence of stress fractures in a prospective study of competitive track and field athletes.[142] Others have reported a 13% incidence of stress fractures in a large study of recreational runners.[143]

Numerous studies have concluded that women suffer from stress fractures more frequently than males. The reported relative risk ranges from 1.5 to 12 times greater in females than males.[141,144-146] The majority of this epidemiological data was taken from the military population, and therefore, the difference in the stress fracture rate between women and men in an athletic population may not be as dramatic. There was no significant difference in the incidence of stress fractures between male and female track and field athletes, as reported by Bennell et al. The increased risk of stress fractures in female athletes is closer to 3.5.[144,147,148] However, more studies are needed to accurately access gender as an independent variable.

Most stress fractures are reported in the tibia regardless of gender.[148] Stress fractures involving the pelvis, femur and metatarsals are more commonly reported in women than in men.[141]

Risk factors

A stress fracture occurs when stress applied to the skeleton is greater that its ability to repair itself. The exact pathogenesis of stress fractures is unclear, but most likely involves a multi-faceted relationship between mechanical, hormonal, nutritional, and genetic factors.[149]

The female athlete triad, which involves disordered eating, amenorrhea, and osteoporosis has been implicated as a key risk factor.[150] This topic has been discussed elsewhere in this chapter and will not be further mentioned.

Osteoporosis and reduced bone mineral density (BMD) have been correlated with the development of stress fractures in female athletes. Bennell et al. found that mean BMD was somewhat lower in female athletes with stress fractures than in their contemporaries without stress fractures. However, the difference was not statistically significant.[142] A large scaled controlled study is needed to determine if BMD is an independent risk factor.

Other risk factors include hormonal and nutritional; however, further studies are necessary to clarify the exact relationship. Training errors are the most important predisposing factors in the development of stress fractures in both female and male athletes.

Diagnosis

Early diagnosis of stress fractures allow for prompt treatment and allows athletes to return to their sport in the shortest period of time. It is important to identify fractures that need immediate surgical intervention.

Classically, athletes present with pain associated with a particular activity which has gradually been worsening. Continuing the activity is coupled with progression of symptoms and eventually the pain is persistent and prohibits the athlete from performing. A detailed and history including training patterns, addition of new equipment, and nutritional and menstrual histories should be taken.

Athletes may present with mild swelling at the site of injury, and difficulty with full weight bearing on the affected limb. Point tenderness at the site of fracture is almost always present. Transmission of pain with percussion near the fracture site is also common.[140]

The fulcrum test described by Johnson et al. aids in the diagnosis of femoral shaft stress fractures.[151] The athlete sits on the edge of the examining table and the examiner places her or his arm under the thigh and applies pressure to the dorsum of the knee. The examiner's arm is moved proximal to distal to test the entire femur. A sharp pain indicates the likely possibility of a femoral shaft stress fracture. Decreased range of motion of the hip, and pain with maximum internal rotation, are often present in femoral neck stress fractures. In addition, the heeltap or hop test may be positive in femoral neck or pelvis stress fractures. The examiner should also note the presence of biomechanical or anatomical variations such has leg length discrepancies or foot pronation.

The initial diagnostic image of choice is the plain radiograph even though they often appear normal. Typical findings include periosteal bone reaction, cortical lucency, callus formation, or a fracture line.[152] Some studies report that only 50% of stress fractures will ever be evident on plain radiographs.[140]

The technetium-99 diphosphonate bone scan is nearly 100% sensitive in diagnosing stress fractures.[153] However, bone scans have poor specificity but are improved with the three-phase bone. It is still difficult to locate the precise fracture site in the foot. Magnetic resonance imaging (MRI) is now considered the standard. Magnetic resonance imaging has improved specificity over the bone scan, and is equally sensitive. Shin *et al.* have shown an improved accuracy rate with MR imaging over bone scan in diagnosing femoral neck stress fractures in endurance athletes.[154]

Treatment

The majority of stress fractures can be treated successfully with conservative management. The initial step is to cease the causative activity so that healing can occur. Nonsteroidal anti-inflammatory drugs, ice and elevation are utilized for pain control. Initially, crutches may be helpful if weight bearing on the affected limb is painful. Bracing or casting is only rarely required. Tibial stress fractures may heal more quickly when treated with a pneumatic leg brace.[155]

The majority of stress fractures will heal in 6–12 weeks. Athletes are encouraged to continue with a personalized exercise program incorporating non-weight-bearing activities to maintain flexibility, muscle strength, and cardiovascular fitness. This is an excellent opportunity to identify and correct predisposing factors to prevent athletes from sustaining recurrent fractures. Clement recommends that an athlete be pain-free for 10–14 days prior to resuming sport specific training.[156] Other clinicians recommend a delay in return to sports until healing is evident on radiographs.

The treating physician must also be aware that certain stress fractures, such as those of the femoral neck and tarsal navicular, have a tendency toward displacement and must be managed with aggressive non-weight-bearing and immobilization and surgical fixation should be considered. Treatment of stress fractures that are not responding to conservative treatment should be re-evaluated. The use of an electrical bone stimulator has been advocated to be an effective treatment.[157]

Surgical treatment is rarely needed and is usually limited to those sites at risk for complete or displaced fractures including the tarsal navicular, fifth metatarsal and femoral neck. Non-healing stress fractures of the anterior tibia (associated with the 'dreaded black line' seen on radiographs) often require bone grafting and internal fixation. After an athlete has undergone surgery, the return to pre-injury level is mixed and depends on the location of the fracture.

Once an athlete is cleared to return, conditioning should be individualized, and the development of a structured training program that the athlete agrees to follow has been shown to decrease the incidence of stress fractures.[158] In general, mileage should not be increased more than 10% per week, and total mileage should not exceed 50 miles per week.[159] Cross training should also be encouraged with the incorporation of a strength training program to improve muscle mass which may decrease the risk of stress fractures. Nutritional counseling should also be implemented. Oral contraceptives are commonly used by female athletes, however the evidence on whether stress fractures are reduced are still inconclusive. The treatment of the athlete that demonstrates the female athlete triad is difficult. A multidisciplinary approach that involves the physician, trainer, nutritionist, and psychotherapist is required.

Conclusion

Stress fractures are common overuse injuries and are reported more frequently in female than in male athletes. Clinicians need to have a high index of suspicion for this injury. Athletes typically present with pain which is aggravated by activity. Imaging is utilized to confirm the diagnosis. Conservative treatment is usually successful. It is imperative that risk factors for susceptibility to stress fractures be identified and addressed. More research is needed to conclude the precise risk factors in stress injuries to bone.

REFERENCES

1 Deuster PA. Exercise in the prevention and treatment of chronic disorders. Women's Health Issues 1996; 6:320-321.

2 Manson JE, Greenland P, LaCroix AZ, et al. Walking compared with vigorous exercise for the prevention of cardiovascular events in women. N Engl J Med 2002; 347:716-725.

3 Cahn SK. Coming on strong: Gender and sexuality in twentieth-century women's sport. London: Harvard University Press; 1994.

4 Kluka DA. Women, sport, and leadership: Paths through the Olympic movement. International Council for Health, Physical Education and Recreation 1992; 28(3):4-8.

5 The National Collegiate Athletic Association (NCAA). 2002-2003 Gender-equity report. The National Collegiate Athletic Association; 2005. Online. Available: http://www.ncaa.org Jan 2005.

6 Sanborn CF, Jankowski CM. Physiologic considerations for women in sport. Clin Sports Med 1994; 13:315-327.

7 Geithner CA, O'Brien R, Gabriel JL, Malina RM. Sex differences in the motor performance of elite young athletes. Med Sci Sports Exerc 1999; 31:S170.

8 Bencke J, Damsgaard R, Saekmose A, Jorgensen P, Jorgensen K, Klausen K. Anaerobic power and muscle strength characteristics of 11 years old elite and non-elite boys and girls from gymnastics, team handball, tennis and swimming. Scand J Med Sci Sports 2002; 12:171-178.

9 Klika RJ, Malina RM. Sex differences in motor performance in elite young alpine skiers. Med Sci Sports Exerc 1999; 31:S319.

10 Maline RM. Performance in the context of growth and maturation. In: Ireland ML, Nattiv A, eds. The female athlete. Philadelphia, PA: Saunders; 2002:59.

11 Eisenmann JC, Milina RM. Body size and endurance performance. In: Shephard RJ, ed. Endurance in sport. 2nd edn. Oxford: Blackwell Science; 2000:37.

12 Malina RM, Bouchard C, eds. Aerobic power and capacity during growth. Growth, maturation and physical activity. Champaign, IL: Human Kinetics; 1991:205-217.

13 Lemmer JT, Hurlbut DE, Martel, GF, et al. Age and gender responses to strength training and detraining. Med Sci Sports Exerc 2000; 32:1505-1512.

14 Roth SM, Ivey FM, Martel GF, et al. Muscle size responses to strength training in young and older adult men and women. J Am Geriatr Soc 2001; 49:1428-1433.

15 Wiswell RA, Hawkins SA, Jaque SV, et al. Relationship between physiological loss, performance decrement, and age in master athletes. J Gerontol A Biol Sci Med Sci 2001; 56:618-626.

16 Hawkins SA, Marcell TJ, Victoria JA, Wiswell RA. A longitudinal assessment of change in VO$_2$max and maximal heart rate in master athletes. Med Sci Sports Exerc 2001; 33:1744-1750.

17 American College of Obstetrics and Gynecology (ACOG). Exercise during pregnancy and the postpartum period. Clin J Obstet Gynecol 2003; 46:496-499.

18 Clapp JF. Exercise during pregnancy. In: Bar-Or O, Lamb DR, Clarkson PM, eds. Perspectives in exercise science and sports medicine, Vol. 9: Exercise and the female: A life span approach. Carmel, CA: Cooper Publishing Group; 1996:413-441.

19 Borg-Stein J, Dugan SA, Gruber J. Musculoskeletal aspects of pregnancy. Am J Phys Med Rehabil 2005; 84:180-192.

20 Christian SS, Christian JS, Stamm CA, McGregor JA. Return to activity postpartum. In: Nattiv A, ed. The female athlete. Philadelphia, PA: Saunders; 2002:191–195.

21 Weiss M, Nagelschmidt M, Struck H. Relaxin and collagen metabolism. Horm Metab Res 1979; 11:408–410.

22 Ritchie JR. Orthopedic considerations during pregnancy. Clin Obstet Gynecol 2003; 46:456–466.

23 Otis CL, Drinkwater B, Johnson M, et al. American College of Sports Medicine position stand: the female athlete triad. Med Sci Sports Exerc 1997; 29:I–IX.

24 American Psychiatric Association. Diagnostic and statistical manual of medical disorders: IV. Washington: American Psychiatric Association; 1994:539–550.

25 Rosen LW, McKeag DB, Hough DO, et al. Pathogenic weight-control behavior in female athletes. Phys Sport Med 1986; 14:79–86.

26 Dummer GM, Rosen LW, Heurner WW. Pathogenic weight control behavior of young competitive swimmers. Phys Sport Med 1987; 15:75.

27 Sundgot-Bergen J. Prevalence of eating disorders in elite female athletes. Int J Sports Nutr 1993; 3:29.

28 Sundgot-Bergen J. Risk factors for development of eating disorders in female elite athletes. Med Sci Sports Exerc 1994; 26:414–419.

29 Drinkwater BL. Women and exercise: physiological aspects. Exerc Sports Sci Rev 1984; 12:21–51.

30 Oscai LB. The role of exercise in weight control. Exerc Sports Sci Rev 1973; 1:103–123.

31 DeSouza MJ, Arce JC, Metzger DA. Endocrine basis of exercise-induced amenorrhea. In: Costa DM, Guthrie SR, eds. Women and sports: interdisciplinary perspectives. Champaign: Human Kinetics; 1995:185–210.

32 Loucks AB. Introduction to menstrual disturbances in athletes. Med Sci Sports Exerc 2004; 35:1551–1552.

33 DeCree C. Sex steroid metabolism and menstrual abnormalities in the exercising female: a review. Sports Med 1998; 25:369–406.

34 Drinkwater BL. The female athlete triad. Presented at the 13th annual conference on exercise sciences and sports medicine: Women, exercise and sports. San Juan, Puerto Rico, March 1999.

35 Keen AD, Drinkwater BL. Irreversible bone loss in former amenorrheic athletes. Osteoporos Int 1997; 7:311–315.

36 Hergenroeder AC. Bone mineralization, hypothalamic amenorrhea, and sex steroid therapy in female adolescents and young adults. J Pediatr 1995; 126:683–689.

37 Grinspoon S, Thomas L, Miller K, et al. Effects of recombinant human IGF-1 and oral contraceptive administration on bone density in anorexia nervosa. J Clin Endocrinol Metab 2002; 87:2883–2891.

38 Stenchever MA, Droegemueller W, Herbst AL, et al., eds. Comprehensive gynecology. 4th edn. St Louis, MO: Mosby; 2001:1–1325.

39 Shangold M. Menstruation. In: Shangold M, Mirkin G, eds. Women and exercise: physiology and sports medicine. 2nd edn. Philadelphia, PA: FA Davis; 1988:129–145.

40 Vereeke West R. The female athlete: the triad of disordered eating, amenorrhea, and osteoporosis. Sports Med 1998; 26:63–71.

41 Kanis JA, Melton LJ, Christiansen C, et al. The diagnosis of osteoporosis. J Bone Miner Res 1994; 9:1137–1141.

42 Snow-Harter C. Athletic amenorrhea and bone health. In: Agostini R, ed. Medical and orthopedic issues of active and athletic women. Philadelphia, PA: Hanley & Belfus; 1994:164–168.

43 Welt CK, Chan JL, Bullen J, et al. Recombinant human leptin in women with hypothalamic amenorrhea. N Engl J Med 2004; 351:987–997.

44 Dane S, Can S, Gursoy R, Ezirmik N. Sports injuries: relations to sex, sport, injured body region. Percept Mot Skills 2004; 98:519–524.

45 Sallis RE, Jones K, Sunshine S, Smith G, Simon L. Comparing sports injuries in men and women. Int J Sports Med 2001; 22:420–423.

46 Dugan SA. Sports-related knee injuries in female athletes What gives? Am J Phys Med Rehabil 2005; 84:122–130.

47 Arendt EA. Orthopedic issues for active and athletic women. Clin Sports Med 1994; 13:483–503.

48 Aagaard H, Jorgensen U. Injuries in elite volleyball. Scand J Med Sci Sports 1996; 6:228–232.

49 Kennedy JC, Hawkins R, Christoff WB. Orthopedic manifestations of swimming. Am J Sports Med 1978; 6:309–322.

50 Teitz CC. The upper extremities. The female athlete. American Academy of Orthopedic Surgeons Monograph series (AAOS); 1997.

51 McCarroll JR. The frequency of golf injuries. Clin Sports Med 1996; 15:1–7.

52 Fleck SJ, Kraemer WJ. Designing resistance training programs. 2nd edn. Champaign: Human Kinetics; 1997.

53 Meth S. Gender differences in muscle morphology. In: Swedan N, ed. Women's sports medicine and rehabilitation. Gaithersburg: Aspen; 2001:3–6.

54 Atter MJ. Science of flexibility. 2nd edn. Champaign: Human Kinetics; 1996.

55 Grana WA, Moretz JA. Ligamentous laxity in secondary school athletes. JAMA 1976; 240:1975–1976.

56 Hutchinson MR, Ireland ML. Knee injuries in female athletes. Am J Sports Med 1995; 19:288–302.

57 Huston LJ, Wojtys EM. Neuromuscular performance characteristics in elite female athletes. Am J Sports Med 1996; 24:427–436.

58 Holden DL, Jackson DW. Stress fractures of the rib in female rowers. Am J Sports Med 1985; 13:342–348.

59 Gruchow HW. An epidemiologic study of tennis elbow, incidence, recurrence and effectiveness of prevention strategies. Am J Sports Med 1979; 7:234–238.

60 Ebben WP, Jensen RL. Strength training for women: debunking myths that block opportunity. Phys Sports Med 1998; 26:86–97.

61 Goldstein JD, Berger PE, Windler GE, Jackson DW. Spine injuries in gymnasts and swimmers. An epidemiologic investigation. Am J Sports Med 1991; 19:463–468.

62 Mazur LJ, Yetman RJ, Risser WL. Weight-training injuries. Common injuries and preventative methods. Sports Med 1993; 16:57–63.

63 Chard MD, Lachmann SM. Racquet sports – patterns of injury presenting to a sports injury clinic. Br J Sports Med 1987; 21:150–153.

64 Halpern B, Thompson N, Curl WW, et al. High school football injuries: identifying the risk factors. Am J Sports Med 1988; 16:S113–S117.

65 Reid DA, McNair PJ. Factors contributing to low back pain in rowers. Br J Sports Med 2000; 34:321–322.

66 Manninen JS, Kallinen M. Low back pain and other overuse injuries in a group of Japanese triathletes. Br J Sports Med 1996; 30:134–139.

67 Tall RL, DeVault W. Spinal injury in sport: Epidemiologic considerations. Clin Sports Med 1993; 12:441–448.

68 Hickey GL, Fricker PA, McDonald WA. Injuries to elite rowers over a 10-yr period. Med Sci Sports Exerc 1997; 29:1567–1572.

69 Nadler SF, Wu KD, Galski T, et al. Low back pain in college athletes: A prospective study correlating lower extremity overuse or acquired ligamentous laxity with low back pain. Spine 1998; 23:828–833.

70 Kujala UM, Taimela S, Erkintalo M, et al. Low back pain in adolescent athletes. Med Sci Sports Excer 1996; 28:165–170.

71 Spencer CW III, Jackson DW. Back injuries in the athlete. Clin Sports Med 1983; 2:191–215.

72 Keene JS, Albert MJ, Springer SL, et al. Back injuries in college athletes. J Spinal Disord 1989; 2:190–195.

73 Brukner P, Kahn K. Clinical sports medicine. New York: McGraw-Hill; 1993.

74 Watkins RG. Lumbar disc injury in the athlete. Clin Sports Med 2002; 21:147–165.

75 Saal JA. Rehabilitation of sports-related lumbar spine injuries. Phys Med Rehabil 1987; 4:613–638.

76 Stinson JT. Spondylolysis and spondylolisthesis in the athlete. Clin Sports Med 1993; 12:517–527.

77 Congeni J, McCulloch J, Swanson K. Lumbar spondylolysis. A study of natural progression in athletes. Am J Sports Med 1997; 25:248–253.

78 Jackson DW, Wiltse LL, Dingeman RD, Hayes M. Stress reactions involving the pars interarticularis in young athletes. Am J Sports Med 1981; 9:304–312.

79 Geraci M, Alleva J. Physical examination of the spine and its functional kinetic chain: the low back pain handbook. Philadelphia, PA: Hanley & Belfus; 1997:49–70.

80 Greenberg JO, Schnell RG. Magnetic resonance imaging of the lumbar spine in asymptomatic adults. Cooperative study – American Society of Neuroimaging. J Neuroimaging 1991; 1:2–7.

81 Crock HV. A reappraisal of intervertebral disc lesions. Med J Aust 1970; 1:983–989.

82 Crock HV. Internal disc disruption. A challenge to disc prolapse fifty years on. Spine 1986; 11:650–653.

83 Lutz GE, Vad VB, Wisneski RJ. Segmental instability: Rehabilitation considerations. Sem Spine Surg 1996; 8:332–338.

84 Iwamoto J, Takeda T, Wakano K. Returning athletes with severe low back pain and spondylolysis to original sporting activities with conservative treatment. Scand J Med Sci Sports 2004; 14:346–351.

85 Cyphers M. Flexibility. Personal trainer manual – the resource for fitness instructors. San Diego: Council on Exercise; 1991:275–292.

86 Sady SP, Freedson PS. Body composition and structural compositions of female and male athletes. Clin Sports Med 1984; 3:755–777.

87 Cirullo JV. Lower extremity injuries. In: The athletic female; American Orthopaedic Society for Sports Medicine. Champaign: Human Kinetics; 1993:267–298.

88 Vleeming A, Stoeckart R, Volkers ACW, et al. Relation between form and function on the sacroiliac joints, part 1. Spine 1990; 15:133–135.

89 Prather H. Pelvis and hip injuries in the female athlete. In: Swedan N, ed. Women's sports medicine and rehabilitation. Gaithersburg: Aspen; 2001:35–54.

90 Lane NE, Hochberg MC, Pressman A, et al. Recreational physical activity and the risk of osteoarthritis of the hip in elderly women. J Rheumatol 1999; 26:849–854.

91 Vingard E, Alfredsson L, Malchau H. Osteoarthritis of the hip in women and its relationship to physical loads from sports activities. Am J Sports Med 1998; 26:78–82.

92 Bodnar LM. Historical role of women in sports. Am J Sports Med 1980; 8:54–55.

93 Protzman R. Physiologic performance of women compared to men. Am J Sports Med 1979; 7:191–194.

94 Anderson JL. Women's sports and fitness programs at the US military academy. Phys Sportsmed 1979; 7:72.

95 Clarke K, Buckley W. Women's injuries in collegiate sports. Am J Sports Med 1980; 8:187–191.

96 Injury Surveillance System NCAA. Overland Park, KS: National Collegiate Athletic Association; 1991–1998.

97 Ireland ML, Wall C. Epidemiology and comparison of knee injuries in elite male and female United States basketball athletes [abstract]. Med Sci Sports Exerc 1990; 22:582.

98 Ireland ML. Problems facing the athletic female. In: Pearl AJ, ed. The athletic female. Champaign, IL: 1993.

99   Zelisko JA, Noble HB, Porter M. A comparison of men's and women's professional basketball injuries. Am J Sports Med 1982; 10:297.

100   Arendt E, Dick R. Knee injury patterns among men and women in collegiate basketball and soccer: NCAA data and review of literature. Am J Sports Med 1995; 23:694-701.

101   Hewett TE, Stroupe AL, Nance TA, Noyes FR. Plyometric training in female athletes: decreased impact forces and increased hamstring torques. Am J Sports Med 1996; 24:765-773.

102   Gray J, Taunton JE, McKenzie DC, et al. A survey of injuries to the anterior cruciate ligament of the knee in female basketball players. Int J Sports Med 1985; 6:314-316.

103   Ferretti A, Papandrea P, Conteduca F, Mariani PP. Knee ligament injuries in volleyball players. Am J Sports Med 1992; 20:203-207.

104   Malone TR, Hardaker WT, Garrett WE, Feagin JA, Bassett FH. Relationship of gender to anterior cruciate ligament injuries in intercollegiate basketball players. J South Orthop Assoc 1993; 2:36-39.

105   Freedman KB, Glasgow MT, Glasgow SG, Bernstein J. Anterior cruciate ligament injury and reconstruction among university students. Clin Orthop 1998; 356:208-212.

106   Emerson RJ. Basketball injuries and the anterior cruciate ligament. Clin Sports Med 1993; 12:317-328.

107   Shelbourne K, Davis T, Klootwyk T. The relationship between intercondylar notch width of the femur and the incidence of anterior cruciate ligament tears. Am J Sports Med 1998; 26:402-408.

108   Noyes FR, Mooar PA, Matthews DS, Butler DL. The symptomatic anterior cruciate-deficient knee. Part I: the long-term functional disability in athletically active individuals. J Bone Jt Surg Am 1983; 65:154-162.

109   Ireland ML, Ott SM. Special concerns of the female athlete. Clin Sports Med 2004; 23:281-298.

110   Hewett TE, Lindenfeld TN, Riccobene JV, Noyes FR. The effect of neuromuscular training on the incidence of knee injury in female athletes: a prospective study. Am J Sports Med 1999; 27:699-706.

111   More RC, Karras BT, Neiman R, Fritschy D, Woo SL. Daniel DM. Hamstrings: an anterior cruciate ligament protagonist. An in vitro study. Am J Sports Med 1993; 21:231-237.

112   Chandy TA, Grana WA. Secondary school athletic injury in boys and girls: a three-year comparison. Physician Sports Med 1985; 13:106-111.

113   Davies G. Compendium of isokinetics in clinical usage. 4th ed. La Crosse, WI: S&S Publishers; 1984.

114   Knapik JJ, Bauman CL, Jones BH, Harris JM, Vaughan L. Preseason strength and flexibility imbalances associated with athletic injuries in female collegiate athletes. Am J Sports Med 1991; 19:76-81.

115   Wojtys EM, Huston LJ, Lindenfeld TN, Hewett TE, Greenfield ML. Association between the menstrual cycle and anterior cruciate ligament injuries in female athletes. Am J Sports Med 1998; 26:614-619.

116   Myklebust G, Maehlum S, Holm, Bahr R. A prospective cohort study of anterior cruciate ligament injuries in elite Norwegian team handball. Scand J Med Sci Sports 1998; 8:149-153.

117   Liu SH, al-Shaikh R, Panossian V, et al. Primary immunolocalization of estrogen and progesterone target cells in the human anterior cruciate ligament. J Orthop Res 1996; 14:526-533.

118   Booth FW, Tipton CM. Ligamentous strength measurements in pre-pubescent and pubescent rats. Growth 1970; 34:177-185.

119   Samuel CS, Butkus A, Coghlan JP, Bateman JF. The effect of relaxin on collagen metabolism in the nonpregnant rat pubic symphysis: the influence of estrogen and progesterone in regulating relaxin activity. Endocrinology 1996; 137:3884-3890.

120   Sarwar R, Beltran NB, Rutherford OM. Changes in muscle strength, relaxation rate and fatigability during the human menstrual cycle. J Physiol 1996; 493:267-272.

121   Griffin LY. The Henning program. In: Griffin LY, ed. Prevention of noncontact ACL injuries. Rosemont, IL: American Academy of Orthopedic Surgeons; 2001:93-96.

122   Caraffa A, Cerulli G, Projetti M, Aisa G, Rizzo A. Prevention of anterior cruciate ligament injuries in soccer. A prospective controlled study of proprioceptive training. Knee Surg Sports Traumatol Arthrosc 1996; 4:19-21.

123   Johnson RJ. The ACL injury in female skiers. In: Griffin LY, ed. Prevention of noncontact ACL injuries. Rosemont, IL: American Academy of Orthopedic Surgeons; 2001:107-111.

124   Hewett TE, Myer GD, Ford KR. Prevention of anterior cruciate ligament injuries. Curr Women's Health Rep 2001; 1:218-224.

125   Fulkerson JP, Arendt EA. Anterior knee pain in female athletes. Clin Orthop 2000; 372:69-73.

126   Thomee R, Augustsson J, Karlsson J. Patellofemoral pain syndrome: a review of current issues. Sports Med 1999; 28:245-262.

127   Goldberg B. Chronic anterior knee pain in the adolescent. Pediatr Ann 1991; 20:186-187, 190-193.

128   Haycock CE, Gillette JV. Susceptibility of women athletes to injury: myths vs. reality. JAMA 1976; 236:163-165.

129   Hunter LY. The female athlete. Med Times 1981; 109:48-57.

130   Root ML, Orien WD, Weed JH, et al. Normal and abnormal function of the foot. Los Angeles: Clinical Biomechanics; 1977.

131   Yu G, Landers P, Lu K, et al. Foot and ankle disorders in children. In: Devalentines S, ed. Juvenile and adolescent hallux abductor valgus deformity. Edinburgh: Churchill Livingstone; 1992:369-405.

132   Garrick JG, Requa RK. The epidemiology of foot and ankle injuries in sports. Clin Podiatr Med Surg 1989; 6:629-637.

133   Gross RH. Foot and ankle disorders. Adolesc Med 1998; 9:599-609.

134   Hickey GJ, Fricker PA, McDonald WA. Injuries of young elite female basketball players over a six-year period. Clin J Sports Med 1997; 7:252-256.

135   Soma CA, Mandelbaum BR. Achilles tendon disorders. Clin Sports Med 1994; 13:811-823.

136   Arendt EA, Teitz CC. The lower extremities. In: Teitz CC, ed. The female athlete. Rosemont: American Academy of Orthopedic Surgeons; 1997:45-62.

137   Micheli LJ, Solomon R, Solomon J, et al. Surgical treatment of chronic lower leg compartment syndrome in young female athletes. Am J Sports Med 1999; 27:197-201.

138   Protzman R, Griffis G. Stress fractures in men and women undergoing military training. J Bone Jt Surg 1977; 59:825.

139   Rossum Costa C De, Morris AA, Swedan N. The foot and ankle. In: Swedan N, ed. Women's sports medicine and rehabilitation. Gaithersburg: Aspen Publishers; 2001:90-103.

140   Knapp TP, Garrett WE. Stress fracture: general concepts. Clin Sports Med 1997; 16:339-355.

141   Bennell KL, Brukner PD. Epidemiology and site specificity of stress fractures. Clin Sports Med 1997; 16:179-196.

142   Bennell KL, Malcolm SA, Thomas SA, et al. The incidence and distribution of stress fractures in competitive track and field athletes: a twelve month prospective study. Am J Sports Med 1996; 24:211-217.

143   Brunet ME, Cook SD, Brinker MR, et al. A survey of running injuries in 1505 competitive and recreational runners. J Sports Med Phys Fitness 1990; 30:307-315.

144   Callahan LR. Stress fractures in women. Clin Sports Med 2000; 19:303-314.

145   Burr DB. Bone, exercise, and stress fractures. Excer Sport Sci Rev 1997; 25:171.

146   Hullko A, Overa S. Stress fractures in athletes. Int J Sports Med 1987; 8:221.

147   Nattiv A, Armey TD Jr. Stress injury to bone in the female athlete. Clin Sports Med 1997; 16:197.

148   Matheson GO, Clement DB, McKenzie DC, et al. Stress fractures in athletes. Am J Sports Med 1987; 15:46.

149   Arendt EA. Stress fractures and the female athlete. Clin Orthop 2000; 372:131-138.

150   Yeager K, Agostini R, Nattiv A, et al. The female athlete triad: disordered eating, amenorrhea, osteoporosis. Med Sci Sports Exerc 1993; 25:775-777.

151   Johnson AW, Weiss CB, Wheeler DL. Stress fractures of the femoral shaft in athletes – more common than expected: a new clinical test. Am J Sports Med 1994; 22:248-256.

152   Brukner PD, Bennell KL. Stress fractures in female athletes: diagnosis, management, and rehabilitation. Sports Med 1997; 24:419-429.

153   Montelone GP. Stress fractures in the athlete. Orthop Clin North Am 1995; 26:423-432.

154   Shin AY, Morin WD, Gorman JD, et al. The superiority of magnetic resonance imaging in differentiating the cause of hip pain in endurance athletes. Am J Sports Med 1996; 24:168-176.

155   Swenson EJ, DeHaven KE, Sebastianelli WJ, et al. The effect of a pneumatic leg brace on return to play in athletes with tibial stress fractures. Am J Sports Med 1997; 25:322-328.

156   Clement DB. Tibial stress syndrome in athletes. J Sports Med 1974; 2:81.

157   Reeder MT, Dick BH, Atkins JK, et al. Stress fractures: Current concepts of diagnosis and treatment. Sports Med 1996; 22:198.

158   Jakobsen BW, Kroner K, Schmidt SA, et al. Prevention of injuries in long-distance runners. Knee Surg Sports Traumatol Arthrosc 1994; 2:245-249.

159   James SL. Running injuries of the knee. Instr Course Lect 1998; 47:407-417.

CHAPTER 9

Special Considerations in the Older Athlete

Roy J. Shephard

INTRODUCTION

Aging is associated with a progressive decline in most biological functions, but changes are somewhat less marked in athletic than in sedentary individuals. These changes have implications for physiological and medical evaluation, as well as for competitive performance. Nevertheless, most people can enjoy competition to an advanced age. The sedentary person faces decreases in peak aerobic power, muscle force and endurance, flexibility and balance, with a progressively diminished ability to undertake the activities of daily living. Regular athletic participation is helpful in retarding functional loss. Although continuing sport participation may have little impact on longevity, enhanced function extends the period of independent living, enhancing quality-adjusted life expectancy. The interpretation of physiological and medical data is sometimes difficult in older athletes, as test results often show features that would be regarded as abnormal in a younger person. Nevertheless, a slow but progressive increase in training intensity and duration is a very safe recommendation for most older people, and it should increase rather than decrease the individual's quality-adjusted life expectancy.

In sports where maximal aerobic power and flexibility are of primary importance, competitive performance declines progressively from early adulthood; thus, the first category of Masters swimmers is aged 19–24 years, with additional categories established for every 5 years of age through the 90–94 year age category. In contrast, in sports that demand specific skills and experience, performance may improve through to late middle-age; thus, a Masters category of golf competition is first distinguished for those over 50 years of age. Such categories contrast sharply with the conventional gerontological classification of sedentary people, where distinction is drawn between the young old (those with little overt loss of function, typically aged 65–75 years), the middle old (those who are experiencing some physical limitations when performing daily activities, typically aged 75–85 years) and the very old or frail elderly (typically, those over 85 years of age; a few in this age group remain healthy and very active, but many are by then severely incapacitated or confined to institutions).

Some athletes face substantial physical limitations by the age of 85 years. Others continue sport participation into their 90s, although because of a decreased number of registrants and changing attitudes towards events,[1] the intensity of competition is usually decreased among older individuals.

In this chapter, we will first examine the physiological basis of the functional losses associated with aging, and the potential to slow or even reverse these changes by an appropriate conditioning program. We will then look at the influence of an active lifestyle on longevity, health and quality adjusted life expectancy. Finally, we will discuss the impact of aging upon clinical and physiological evaluation, and the advice that a physician should offer to older individuals who wish to participate in Masters competitions.

Box 9.1: Key Points

How old is old?

Sports demanding endurance and flexibility:

- Age categories start at 19 years

Sports demanding specific skills:

- Age categories start at 50 years

Sedentary adults:

- Young old (65–75 years)
- Middle old (75–85 years)
- Very old (>85 years).

PHYSIOLOGICAL BASIS OF FUNCTIONAL LOSSES IN OLDER INDIVIDUALS

In theory, the best way to determine the extent of functional loss with aging would be to make longitudinal observations over a period of 30–50 years. However, most longitudinal studies cover no more than 5–10 years. In practice, it is difficult to follow a substantial group of adults for a longer time, and longitudinal data thus define the rate of functional loss rather poorly. Some longitudinal observations show a rapid loss of function in athletes, probably because the hours devoted to training decrease as subjects age, whereas other reports show a lesser rate of functional loss than that typical of sedentary people. Those who volunteer for a longitudinal study are usually atypical members of the community, and the initial bias in subject selection is exacerbated by the subsequent 'drop-out' process. Further, involvement in laboratory testing may in itself modify conditioning and other aspects of personal lifestyle, particularly in the sedentary comparison group.

The great majority of reports are thus based on the age-related changes seen in cross-sectional data. Conclusions about the functional loss with age are then impacted by secular changes in training, nutrition and environment that affect performance at any given age. The slopes showing age-related decreases in functional capacity have reasonable validity through to the age of 65 years, but in older age groups, it is important to remember that data are obtained only on those individuals who have remained in sufficient health to agree to continued testing.

Peak oxygen transport

As in younger individuals, performance of endurance sport is determined largely by peak oxygen transport, or peak aerobic power. Some early longitudinal data found a more rapid aging of peak aerobic power in athletes than in sedentary individuals, presumably because the rigor of training decreased as the active individuals became older (Fig. 9.1).[2] Other longitudinal observations on small samples of physically active individuals have seen almost no loss of peak aerobic power over periods of 20 years or more. In such samples, one may presume that the physical condition of the subjects at recruitment was only moderate. A progressive improvement with conditioning thus counteracted the inherent effect of aging.[3,4] In other words, observers were comparing the unfit middle-aged men who entered the study with the same individuals who had become fit 20–30 years later.

Most authors now agree that the peak aerobic power decreases progressively between the ages of 25 and 65 years, both in athletes and in sedentary individuals. Large cross-sectional studies of Masters athletes where older cohorts have maintained training volumes suggest that over the course of adult life, the age-related loss of peak aerobic power averages from 2.8 to 4.2 ml/kg per min per decade, with much of the loss occurring after the age of 50 (Fig. 9.2).[1] This is appreciably less than the 10-year loss of 5–6 ml/kg per min usually seen in sedentary individuals. Such observations agree with findings from a small longitudinal study, in which 15 men were followed for 33 years, beginning at an average age of 45 years. Throughout this period, they trained consistently at 77–84% of the heart rate reserve, 3–4 times per week. Much as in sedentary subjects, peak heart rates decreased by 25 beats/min, but the decrease in peak oxygen transport was only 5.8–6.8% rather than the loss of 10% per decade seen in sedentary individuals.

Box 9.2: Key Points

Physiological demands of independent living

- Peak aerobic power >15 ml/kg per min.
- Sedentary individuals reach this threshold at age 80–85 years.
- Athletic individuals can maintain independence for an additional 10–20 years.

Findings are less well-established for individuals over the age of 65 years, because a high proportion of elderly people are affected by one or more chronic disorders that reduce peak aerobic power. However, recent data suggest that even in the absence of such disease, the loss of peak oxygen intake shows an accelerating decline. The threshold of maximal aerobic

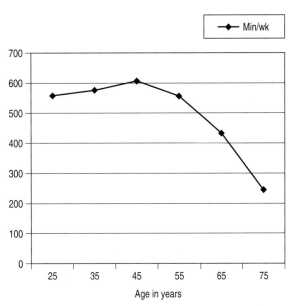

Figure 9.1 The influence of the average age in years upon the average time that male Masters athletes devote to training (min/week). (Data for graph modified from tables in Kavanagh *et al.* 1989.[2])

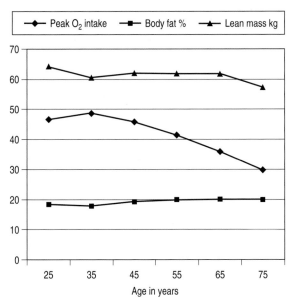

Figure 9.2 The influence of the average age in years upon the functional status of male Masters athletes. Graphs for peak oxygen intake (ml/kg per min), body fat (%) and lean body mass (kg). (Modified from tables in Kavanagh *et al.* 1989.[2])

power needed for independent living (around 15 ml/kg per min) is thus reached at an age of 80–85 years in sedentary people, but 10–20 years later in athletes. In the study of Paterson and associates,[5] no independently living seniors had a peak aerobic power of less than 15 ml/kg per min. Retrospective questioning of another group of seniors established that a physically active lifestyle at an age of 50 years reduced the likelihood of institutionalization as seniors.[6] Equally, a person who is approaching the independence threshold can set back the date of institutionalization by as much as 10–20 years by undergoing a progressive conditioning program.

Cardiovascular changes

Box 9.3: Key Points

Decreases in cardiac function with aging

- Lower peak heart rate
- Decreased ventricular compliance
- Decreased inotropic responses
- Increased after-loading

All contribute to a reduced stroke volume at peak effort.

A part of the age-related decrease in peak oxygen transport reflects the adverse impact of age upon cardiovascular function, including: a decrease in maximal heart rate, from about 195 beats/min at age 25 to around 170 beats/min in sedentary subjects and 160–165 beats/min in athletes at age 65; a decrease in compliance of the heart wall that hampers diastolic filling of the ventricles and thus peak stroke volume; a decrease in the inotropic response of the ventricular muscle to the catecholamines secreted during exercise, thus leading to less complete emptying of the ventricles during systole, further reducing peak stroke volume; and an increase in the after load against which the ventricle must contract (due a combination of more rigid arteries, an increase in systemic blood pressure, and weaker skeletal muscles); the increase of after load reduces the stroke volume yet further.

For these various reasons, most authors accept that as peak effort is approached, the stroke volume is less well sustained in elderly individuals than in their younger peers. One widely cited study[7,8] suggested that the elderly patient could exploit the Frank–Starling relationship, compensating for the decrease in maximal heart rate by an increase of end-diastolic volume and thus of peak stroke volume. However, the individuals studied were not typical of the general population, since they had all agreed to participate in the multi-year Baltimore longitudinal study of aging, and in an attempt to isolate the effects of aging *per se*, ischemic heart disease had been excluded by a combination of ECG and scintigraphy. Many athletes also have little atherosclerosis at an age of 65 years, but a more important criticism of the Baltimore study is that the supposed peak heart rates were relatively low. It thus seems likely that the cardiovascular stress tests were sub-maximal rather than maximal,

and if observations had been pursued to a true peak effort, a decrease rather than an increase in peak stroke volume would have been seen in older subjects.

Other aspects of aging influencing peak oxygen transport

Box 9.4: Key Points

Factors contributing to age-related loss of peak aerobic power

- Cardiorespiratory impairment
- Reduction in weekly training
- Accumulation of body fat.

In many people, an important factor contributing to the decline in peak oxygen intake with age is a lower intensity of weekly training. Many athletes are no longer willing to engage in the long hours of conditioning that they accepted as young adults (Fig. 9.1). Sedentary comparison groups also become progressively more inactive as they age, and if peak oxygen transport is expressed per kilogram of body mass (which is the critical value in most events requiring body displacement), cardiorespiratory losses are compounded by a progressive accumulation of body fat (Fig. 9.2). One large cross-sectional study attributed 50% of the age-related decrease in peak oxygen transport to decreases in habitual physical activity and the accumulation of body fat.[9]

The peak aerobic power of a sedentary individual responds well to an appropriately graded and progressive conditioning program. In percentage terms, gains can be as large (15–20%) as in young adults, although because of low initial readings, the absolute training response decreases with age.[10] The practical contribution of such training to functional capacity is highlighted when the response is compared with the anticipated rate of aging. An increase in peak aerobic power of 5 ml/kg per min is equivalent to a 10-year reduction in biological age.

Muscle strength

Box 9.5: Key Points

Loss of muscle strength with aging

- Begins at age 35–40 years
- Up to 25% loss by 65 years
- Loss of lean tissue
- Selective loss of type II (fast twitch) fibres
- Poorer synchronization of motor units
- Large recovery of strength possible with training – due to both improved coordination of contractions and synthesis of lean tissue.

The peak force of most muscles is well sustained through to the age of 35–40 years; thereafter, there is an accelerating loss of strength, due primarily to a loss of lean tissue, but exacerbated by some reduction in muscle quality.[11] Through to the age of 70 years, lean body mass is better conserved in Masters athletes than in sedentary individuals,[1] but both lean tissue and strength are lost subsequently, even if a vigorous training program is maintained (Fig. 9.2). The probable explanations include an age-related decrease in the secretion of androgens and other growth stimulating factors, a loss of muscle quality and associated myosin dysfunction.

The rate of functional deterioration varies from one muscle group to another. Nevertheless, the typical cumulative effect is a loss of about 25% of young adult strength by the age of 65 years, with an acceleration of this loss during the retirement years.[12] The loss of lean tissue mass is compounded by a decrease in fiber number, with a selective atrophy of the type II (fast-twitch) muscle fibers,[11,13] and a decrease in the synchronization of motor unit firing in older adults.

Training-induced gains in peak muscle force can be quite impressive, particularly in very old individuals who are initially sedentary. Fiatarone and colleagues[14] found a 113% increase of muscle strength in a small group of institutionalized nonagenarians who undertook high intensity resistance exercises. Initially, much of the increase in performance was due to a better coordination of muscle contractions, but as training continued, tomography demonstrated a substantial increase of lean tissue in the exercised muscles. Other investigators found a 29% increase in the cross-sectional area of type IIb fibres in the thigh muscles when elderly individuals undertook 50 weeks of weighted stair climbing; control subjects showed a 22% decrease of fibre area over the same period.[15]

Deterioration in other body systems
Flexibility
The development of cross-bridges between individual filaments of collagen causes a decrease of flexibility with aging. Often, this is exacerbated by the development of osteoarthritis at key joints. A progressive loss of function is readily demonstrated by such simple tests as the 'sit and reach test'.[16] The deterioration of collagen can probably be slowed by regular flexibility exercises. Cross-sectional studies show an association between habitual physical activity and flexibility.[17,18] Further, flexibility has been increased in a number of young-old groups by appropriate training programs.[19–22] Thus, a 2-year program of aerobic, strength and flexibility exercises yielded an 11% increase in flexibility, as assessed by hamstring length.[21] Likewise, a 9% improvement of sit-and-reach score was seen when 57–77-year-old women undertook a 12-week program of stretching, walking and dancing.[20]

The impact of sport participation upon osteoarthritis is controversial. Events such as running seem to have little adverse effect,[23] but the risk of osteoarthritis is increased by participation in a number of contact sports,[24] particularly if injuries have been sustained. A recent report from the

---

Box 9.6: Key Points

Loss of flexibility with aging
- Deterioration of collagen structure
- Osteoarthritis from heavy physical activity, especially if associated injuries.

Framingham longitudinal study found that the seven individuals who had the greatest level of physical activity had a seven fold increase in the risk of osteoarthritic disorders.[25] Decreases in flexibility are not large enough to affect everyday activities until an age of at least 70 years, but they have an adverse effect upon some types of athletic performance from the early twenties.

Once a joint has been damaged, benefit may be obtained from exercise that strengthens the muscles around the affected articulation. Regular physical activity can also be helpful in reducing body mass, and thus the load supported by the injured joint surfaces. When the acute inflammation has passed, regular physical activity is important in maintaining mobility and overall cardiorespiratory function; weight-supported activities (for instance, cycle ergometry or exercises in a heated pool) are best suited to this purpose.[26]

Balance

Box 9.7: Key Points

Age-related deterioration of balance
- Postural hypotension
- Poorer proprioception
- Poorer pressure sensors
- Slower reflexes
- Weaker muscles
- Deterioration of special senses.

A combination of postural hypotension, slower righting reflexes, less powerful muscles and an impairment of proprioceptors, pressure sensors and special senses lead to a progressive deterioration of balancing ability in the elderly. This can be demonstrated objectively as an increase of postural sway when attempting to stand still. If there is substantial loss of function, the affected individual becomes vulnerable to falls, particularly when exercising.[27]

A combination of a faster reaction speed, stronger muscles, enhanced joint proprioception and better control of blood pressure reduces the risk of falls for active seniors.[28] Several reports have suggested that regular muscle strengthening exercises can substantially reduce body sway and enhance balance in older people.[29–31] One report noted that involvement in a simple walking program reduced the likelihood of a fall by 15–20%.[32] Another study found 12 weeks of stretching, walking and dancing[20] improved balance by 12%.

Osteoporosis

A progressive loss of bone calcium and a deterioration of the skeletal organic matrix increase the older athlete's vulnerability to fractures from falls. In extreme old age, fractures can even be caused by sudden muscular contractions. At any given age, bone density is lower in women than in men, and the risk of osteoporosis is correspondingly greater in females than in males.[33]

In general, regular load-bearing physical activity helps to augment peak bone density by the end of the growing years, and subsequently it conserves bone structure in both men and women. Nevertheless, runners who train many hours per week may fail to develop a good bone density, particularly if their intake of calcium and vitamin D is restricted, and their protein intake is insufficient to maintain a positive nitrogen balance; this problem is common among young women who have trained to the point of disturbing menstrual function in sports where a slim body build contributes to competitive success (the female athletic triad).[34] A 5-year follow-up compared typical Masters runners with sedentary controls. Both initially and at the end of the trial, the average bone density was much higher for Masters athletes than for controls.[35] However, both groups showed a substantial decrease of lumbar spinal density over the 5-year interval, and indeed the greatest losses of bone mineral were seen in athletes who curtailed their running schedules over the period of observation.

INFLUENCE OF SPORT PARTICIPATION UPON LONGEVITY, HEALTH AND QUALITY ADJUSTED LIFE EXPECTANCY

Longevity

Substantial subject numbers are needed to calculate survival curves, and practical considerations generally preclude the random assignment of participants to athletic and control groups for such a purpose. The usual approach is thus to make a cross-sectional comparison of survival rates between athletes and sedentary individuals. The effectiveness of regular physical activity in extending lifespan depends on an individual's success in maintaining an active lifestyle, and benefits apparently vary inversely with the age when regular physical activity is begun.

In general, investigators have found that sport participation has a favorable effect upon longevity. However, one divergent study noted that individuals who had played in major sports while at university had no advantage of survival relative to control groups by the time that they reached middle age.[36] There are two probable reasons for this paradoxical finding. Many study participants had been selected for university sports teams in part because they had a muscular body build (a characteristic which in itself has a negative impact on life expectancy). Perhaps more importantly, many of the team members failed to continue their sport involvement as they became older, and indeed by middle age, were more obese than their supposedly sedentary counterparts.[37] A more encouraging report from Finland showed that endurance athletes have a 4–6 year advantage of longevity relative to control subjects, but it is difficult to dissociate this finding from their lean, ecto-

morphic body build and the low prevalence of cigarette smoking which is characteristic of endurance competitors.[38,39]

Multivariate analyses have attempted to adjust mortality rates for confounding variables, but the magnitude of confounding effects is so large that the success of such statistical adjustments remains questionable. For instance, a high socioeconomic status is associated with a physically active lifestyle, and a comparison of the highest and lowest socioeconomic quintiles across Europe and North America shows that the highest quintile has a survival advantage of 6.3 years in men and 2.8 years in women,[40] irrespective of participation in sport. Likewise, abstinence from cigarette smoking can in itself extend life expectancy by an average of 8 years.

A follow-up of 636 men initially aged 45–64 years showed that active members of the cohort had a substantial survival benefit relative to those who were inactive for the first 15 years; after 13.3 years 22% of active men had died, compared with 29% of those who were inactive; however, survival curves converged over the next few years, so that prospects for the two groups were similar between 75 and 80 years of age.[41] The main effect of regular physical activity was to avoid premature death (before the age of 75 years) rather than to prolong the period of frail old age. An active lifestyle thus promotes what Fries has called a 'squaring' of the mortality curve.[42] One cross-sectional study even suggested that after the age of 80 years, vigorous physical activity may increase the mortality rate slightly, although moderate physical activity continues to yield a small benefit relative to sedentary individuals.[43]

Box 9.8: Why do Endurance Athletes have a 4–6 Year Advantage of Life Expectancy?

- Benefit of physical activity
- Ectomorphic body build
- Non-smokers
- High socioeconomic status.

A 19–23-year follow-up of Harvard alumni (Fig. 9.3)[44] suggested that after making statistical adjustments for confounding variables, initiation of a weekly leisure-time energy expenditure of some 8 megajoules (MJ) at the age of 34 years enhanced life expectancy by about 1.5 years.[45] However, if adoption of a physically active lifestyle was deferred to the age of 70 years, the gain in life expectancy was only a few months. The extension of lifespan seemed somewhat greater if the 8 MJ/week was accumulated through sport rather than through lower intensity activities such as walking. One analysis of this data proposed that a threshold intensity of effort of 6 METS was required in order to extend lifespan.[46] However, if a threshold intensity of effort is indeed needed to increase longevity, then it seems likely that this threshold will decrease as a person becomes older.

Health and quality of life

Perhaps the most exciting recent development for those interested in the promotion of healthy aging has been the transition

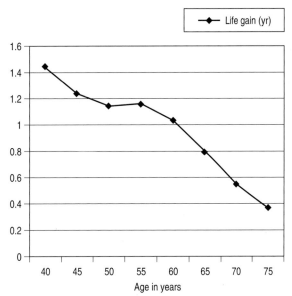

Figure 9.3 Average increase in lifespan (years) associated with beginning an exercise energy expenditure of 8 MJ/week at specified ages. (Graph modified from tabular data of Paffenbarger *et al.* 1990.[44])

from efforts to extend an individual's lifespan to a focus upon quality-adjusted life expectancy. Good arguments can be made for prescribing exercise as a means of reducing overall mortality and disease-specific mortality. However, in many of the frail elderly, the quality of life has become very poor; when assessed by a time-trade-off or a standard gamble,[47,48] values are sometimes no more than 50% of those seen in a young adult.

Regular exercise will do little to reduce some causes of an impaired quality of life, such as defects of vision and hearing. However, the life of an elderly person is often made difficult by general frailty and limitations of mobility; here regular exercise plays an important preventive and therapeutic role, decreasing the likelihood that the individual will become physically dependent. Indeed, an increase in quality-adjusted life expectancy seems one of the most important reasons to encourage athletes to continue regular physical activity into old age.[48] Regular exercise enhances the quality of life not only by countering physical frailty, but also by decreasing the likelihood of acute and chronic disease, augmenting social contacts and improving mood state.

Factors modifying the quality of life

Appropriate amounts of regular physical activity tend to enhance immune function, thus decreasing the likelihood of acute infection. Such regimens decrease the risk of a multiplicity of the chronic diseases where benefit has been established in younger individuals[49] (for example, hypertension, cardiac and peripheral vascular disease, and chronic obstructive lung disease). They also substantially reduce the likelihood of developing obesity, diabetes, osteoporosis, cancer and other chronic medical problems of old age. Regular physical activity enhances appetite and increases the regularity of bowel movements. If the exercise is taken early in the day, sleep is facilitated, and particularly if the exercise is vigorous and prolonged, mood-state may be improved. All of these factors contribute to an improved quality-adjusted life expectancy.[48]

Perhaps most importantly, an active lifestyle increases functional capacity, thus reducing the likelihood of developing dependency at any given age.

Factors modifying functional capacity

> ### Box 9.9: Key Points
>
> **Exercise and quality of life**
> - Functional losses of aging reversed
> - Enhanced immune function reduces acute disease
> - Reduced risk of certain chronic diseases
> - Increased social contacts
> - Enhanced mood state
> - Improved sleep, appetite and bowel function.

Functional capacity of the elderly individual is challenged by decreases in peak aerobic power, muscle strength, flexibility and balance.

Peak aerobic power

A sustained bout of aerobic activity becomes fatiguing if it demands more than 40% of peak oxygen intake, and the progressive, age-related decline of oxygen transport eventually brings most seniors to the point where they lack the oxygen transporting ability needed to undertake the normal activities of daily living independently. Typically, a minimum peak oxygen intake of 15 ml/kg per min is required for independence.[5] When function drops below this minimum, walking up a slight incline, carrying a small bag of groceries from the store, and normal domestic activities become intolerably fatiguing. At any given age, a typical endurance athlete has an advantage of at least 10 ml/kg per min over his or her sedentary peers, and the aerobic threshold for institutionalization is thus delayed for 10–20 years; in the meantime, most physically active individuals have died of some intercurrent disease.

Peak muscle force

The age-related decreases in peak muscle force and power are often important factors causing a loss of independence, particularly in elderly women. Strength becomes inadequate to perform normal activities of daily living, such as carrying household items, opening containers, lifting the body mass from a chair or a toilet seat, and eventually even getting out of bed. Resistance exercises of the type practiced by strength athletes augment muscle strength, improving gait, boosting the preferred speed of walking, and correcting many of these physical limitations.[50]

Flexibility, balance and falls

A progressive decrease in joint flexibility restricts the possible range of activities for most seniors. Difficulty may be encountered when entering a car, or climbing stairs to enter a house or a bus. Eventually, it becomes impossible to climb into a bath, or even to dress without assistance. A person who has problems of balance and is susceptible to falls also faces a very restricted life. As noted above, appropriate training programs enhance flexibility by some 10%, delaying the time when the loss of flexibility has become sufficiently marked to impede the activities of daily living. Regular physical activity also enhances balance and stabilizes blood pressure, thus reducing the likelihood of falls. Further, in the event of tripping over some unperceived obstacle, faster reflexes and stronger muscles enable more rapid righting movements.

Quantitative estimate of impact of an exercise regimen on quality of life

We will now make a tentative estimate of the impact that the regular physical activity of an athlete can have on the quality of life in old age through changes in the risks of acute and chronic infection, enhancement of mood state and decreases in the risk of dependency. It is convenient to assess this in terms of quality-adjusted life years. For instance, if a person survives for 10 years, but the average quality of life over this period is only 80% of optimal, then survival is rated at eight quality-adjusted life years.

Acute infections

Individuals who engage in regular physical activity are, in general, less susceptible to acute infections, because regular physical activity enhances immune function.[51] However, the impact on quality-adjusted life expectancy is likely to be quite small. Commonly, older people sustain two upper respiratory infections per year, each lasting for approximately 15 days. The subjective impact of such an infection has not been formally quantitated; undoubtedly, it varies from one person to another, but for many people it may perhaps cause a 10% reduction in the quality of life.

An optimal dose of physical activity may perhaps boost immune function sufficiently to reduce the risk of infection by 25%, or a total of 7.5 days per year.[1,52] This in turn will enhance the overall quality-adjusted life expectancy by $(7.5/365) \times 0.1$, 0.0021 quality-adjusted life years in any given year, or 0.02 quality-adjusted life-years per decade.

Chronic disease

Robine and Ritchie[40] examined the impact of various chronic diseases upon healthy life expectancy. They estimated the average decrease in this index at 4 years for circulatory disorders, 5 years for locomotor problems and 2 years for respiratory problems (i.e. a total loss of 11 years of healthy life expectancy). If we assume that a functional problem in any one of these body systems reduced the quality of life by an average of 30%, then the cumulative impact of chronic disease would be a loss of 11 (0.3), or 3.3 quality-adjusted life years over middle and old age.

For many of the conditions discussed by Robine and Ritchie, regular physical activity plays both a preventive and a rehabilitative role. Setting the magnitude of the exercise response at a 30% reduction in the prevalence of chronic disease, the gain from maintaining a physically active lifestyle could be a cumulative effect as large as 0.3 (3.3), or 0.99 quality-adjusted life years during middle and old age.

Mood state

A combination of anxiety, depression and other disorders of affect commonly impairs mood-state, particularly in older individuals. If optimal mood is arbitrarily set at 100%, then disorders of mood state seem likely to reduce this by at least 10% (i.e. a reduction in the quality of daily life from 100% to 90%). There is then a cumulative loss of one quality-adjusted life year for each 10 years of survival.

One measure of the favorable impact of physical activity upon mood state[53] is the decrease in the demand for medical consultations and hospital admissions associated with regular exercise. A quasi-experimental study of middle-aged individuals showed that a moderate work-site exercise program decreased the need for such services by 25%.[54] Given the age-related tendency to depression, benefit may be greater in the elderly than in those who are middle-aged. However, on the conservative assumption of a 25% benefit, as seen in the working population, the quality-adjusted life expectancy would increase by 0.25 years for each ten calendar years of survival, or a benefit of one quality-adjusted life year for the period 40–80 years of age.

Dependency

The causes of institutionalization are varied,[55] and many cannot be avoided by maintaining vigorous exercise. In some cases, elderly people experience difficulty in ambulation or transfer. Others complain of frequent falls. There may be a failure to eat or drink adequately, or incontinence. A decrease in manual dexterity, a loss of self-esteem, intellectual deterioration, a sudden stroke or blindness, and the loss of support from significant others are all potential crises that precipitate admission to an institution.

The energetic cost of many physical activities increases slightly with aging. But a more important problem is that peak aerobic power, muscle strength or flexibility deteriorate to the point where the individual can no longer undertake the activities of daily living. The impact upon the individual's quality of life depends on personal coping mechanisms, and the availability of environmental aids. But for many people, there is a progressive transition from partial to total dependency over a period of 10 years (often from 75–85 years of age). We may imagine the quality of life declining gradually from 90% to 50% of its optimal value in this period when dependency develops; there is thus an average loss in life quality of 20% over the decade (a cumulative loss of 2.0 quality-adjusted life years). In many elderly people, total dependency (with a quality of life of perhaps 50% rather than 90% of optimal) continues over a final year of life; this causes a further loss of 0.4 quality-adjusted life years, for a total dependency-related loss of 2.4 quality-adjusted life years.

Regular physical activity is likely to postpone many types of functional deterioration,[56] perhaps by as much as 10–20 years, with the likelihood that the individual will die of some intercurrent condition before dependency develops. But the impact

Table 9.1 Cumulative effects of exercise participation upon quality-adjusted life years (QALY) between 40 and 80 years of age

	QALY
Reduced acute infections	0.08
Reduced chronic infections	0.99
Enhanced mood state	1.00
Reduced dependency	1.20
Total benefit	3.27

of exercise on other causes of dependency such as stroke or blindness is more limited. Thus, the upper limit of benefit is likely to be a 50% reduction in dependency, decreasing the cumulative dependency-related loss from 2.4 to 1.2 quality-adjusted life years in the final 11 years of life (Table 9.1).

Overall impact of an exercise regimen on quality-adjusted life expectancy

During middle age and early old age, exercise will lead to gains in quality-adjusted life years by reducing susceptibility to acute and chronic infections and enhancing mood state, and these benefits are augmented by a decrease in dependency. Summing up the changes postulated above, we may anticipate an overall benefit of (0.08 + 0.99 + 1.00 + 1.20), or about 3.27 quality-adjusted life years during the final four decades of life.

The figure is, as yet, imprecise, and there may be some overlap between the effects that we have attributed to the prevention of chronic disease and the maintenance of functional independence. Nevertheless, the anticipated increase in the quality of life is larger than any gain in calendar life expectancy that can be achieved by initiating an exercise program in middle age or later life (Fig. 9.3). Moreover, most people are more attracted to an enhanced quality of life than to a mere extension of calendar lifespan. Indeed, the average person will explain the reason that they choose to exercise is that it makes them 'feel better'.

METHODS OF EVALUATION AND PRACTICAL ADVICE TO THE OLDER ATHLETE

Given the many benefits that a senior can derive from regular physical activity, it is important that health professionals who interact with senior athletes offer appropriate and effective encouragement to continuation of a physically active lifestyle. If a person is already engaging in regular athletic competition without symptoms, no specific evaluation may be needed. Indeed, the imposition of unnecessary requirements of testing and evaluation may have a negative impact upon sport involvement.

Clinical evaluation and information on physical function may be warranted when judging a person's ability to com-

mence a physically demanding training program such as preparation for a marathon run, but again it is important that appropriate progressive conditioning not be restricted if minor abnormalities are found at clinical or physiological examination. The results of specific physiologic tests are more useful in providing feedback to shape and encourage the conditioning of an athlete, to assess the success of rehabilitation following injury and to regulate the progress of training.

Clinical examination

> **Box 9.10: Key Points**
>
> - Immediate risk of cardiovascular death increases 5-fold *during* vigorous exercise.
> - Danger more than compensated by halving the risk *following* a bout of exercise.
> - Sedentary individual has a greater need of medical examination than an athlete.

Not all older adults require a detailed clinical assessment before athletic events. Admittedly, vigorous exercise increases the risk of a cardiovascular catastrophe by as much as 5-fold while the activity is being performed, and sport-related deaths often attract widespread publicity. However, such risks are more than compensated by a reduced probability of cardiovascular incidents during the remainder of the day.[57,58] It is thus arguable that an older sedentary person is in greater need of a detailed clinical evaluation than a participant in a Masters event. There is no simple test to detect those athletes who are vulnerable to a cardiac catastrophe. The traditional approach to evaluation has included a full clinical examination, followed by a range of laboratory tests including routine blood and urine analysis, and a progressive stress test with electrocardiogram recording and direct or predicted estimation of peak aerobic power.[59-61] Unfortunately, there is little agreement on the interpretation of test results in elderly individuals, and minor abnormalities observed during a standard examination commonly lead to unnecessary exclusions from exercise and sport programs.[62] For example, the findings from a stress electrocardiogram have little practical value when a healthy middle-aged or older adult is contemplating entering a training program. Application of Bayes theorem shows that in such a person, as many as two thirds of apparently positive findings are in fact false positive results. Testing thus creates a great deal of unnecessary fear and iatrogenic illness; indeed, more accurate information might have been obtained by simply tossing a coin.[63] The proportion of false positive results depends on the true prevalence of abnormalities within the test sample. Thus, the prognostic significance of an apparently abnormal electrocardiogram increases with the age of the individual.

Simple approaches to an initial triage of athletes include use of the PAR-Q questionnaire,[64] together with a consideration of standard cardiac risk factors[65] and any family history of premature death. In addition to an adverse family history and

Box 9.11: Key Points

- Exercise stress testing has little value in apparently healthy middle-aged adults because of a high incidence of false positive results.
- False positive results create much unnecessary fear and iatrogenic illness.
- Accuracy of the stress ECG increases as the age of the patient increases, due to greater prevalence of disease.

the presence of overt cardiac risk factors, possible warning signs of an impending cardiac catastrophe identified from retrospective analysis of individual exercise-induced cardiac incidents include a vague period of malaise in the 24 h preceding the episode, a bout of exercise that is unduly heavy or competitive relative to the state of conditioning of the individual, and reluctance to admit tiredness in the face of younger opponents or an exhausting event.[66] These simple warning signs can often be elicited by a coach or paramedical assistant before referral of the athlete to a physician.

Box 9.12: Key Points

Triage of athletes

- PAR-Q questionnaire
- Cardiac risk factors
- Adverse family history
- Malaise in previous 24 h
- Excessive competition relative to current physical condition
- Continuing exercise in face of severe fatigue.

Detailed clinical evaluation is warranted if there is an acute fever, poorly controlled diabetes, severe hypertension, severe asthma, a history of unstable chest pain, unstable congestive heart failure, acute musculoskeletal pain or repeated falling episodes; commonly, such individuals will be excluded from sport until their condition has stabilized.[61] Hernias, cataracts, retinal bleeding and joint injuries are other temporary contraindications to many types of sport.[61] A few more permanent contraindications to sport participation include an inoperable and enlarging aortic aneurysm, a malignant cardiac arrhythmia, severe aortic stenosis, end-stage congestive heart failure, and severe exercise-induced behavioral disturbances.[61]

The biggest role for the sport physician often lies in the prevention and treatment of injuries and overtraining. Activities such as swimming, skiing and cycling may need to be curtailed if there is a history of episodes of unconsciousness (due, for example, to disorders of cardiac rhythm). Age-related deteriorations in vision, hearing and balance may all increase vulnerability to injury. Sports demanding good balance may need to be avoided if there is an intrinsic deterioration in balance, or dizziness is induced by the use of antihypertensive drugs and other forms of medication.

Modern treatment of retinal detachment is such that a diabetic retinopathy is not a contraindication to participation in most types of sport.[67] Because of a deterioration in collagen structure, muscle strains and tears occur more readily than in a young person, and in order to prevent injury, an older competitor should allocate a longer period to gentle stretching and warm-up prior to an exercise bout. If an injury is sustained, it is important to look for specific predisposing and causative factors. A diabetic neuritis may impede the healing of superficial injuries. Both muscle strains and stress fractures may be caused by a too rapid progression of training, and in older athletes where relatively light trauma causes a bone injury, the possibility of osteoporosis should be explored. With the exception of Volpi and associates,[68] most authors have found that the rate of protein synthesis decreases with aging[69,70] and the healing of both bone and muscle injury is thus likely to proceed more slowly in elderly than in younger individuals; however, recovery is helped if a high protein diet is combined with an adequate and suitably adapted reconditioning program.[14]

Box 9.13: Key Points

Signs of overtraining

- Decrease of performance
- Deterioration of mood state
- Increase of resting pulse rate
- Persistent fatigue
- Swelling of the ankles
- Repeated infections
- Impaired immune function.

For any given intensity of training, the risk of overtraining is probably greater in seniors than in younger athletes. However, the main warning signs are much as in a younger individual: a decrease in performance despite continued training, and a depression of mood state.[71] There may also be an increase in the resting pulse rate, persistent fatigue and swelling of the ankles. A decrease in the secretion of mucosal immunoglobulins due to overtraining compounds the age-related decrease in natural killer cell activity;[72] this increases vulnerability to acute infections,[73] and exacerbates the deterioration in performance induced by overtraining. An excess of training is easier to treat if caught in its early stages; the only effective approach is a temporary relaxation of training schedules.

Technical problems of physiological assessment

Given a relatively small number of clients, adequate equipment and sufficient personnel, a detailed physiological assessment is best carried out in an exercise testing laboratory, rather than a physician's office. Potential measurements include peak aerobic power, resting and exercise blood pressure, the resting and exercise electrocardiograms, muscle strength, body fat content, flexibility, balance and reaction speeds.

Box 9.14: Key Points

Potential physiological tests

- Peak aerobic power
- Resting and exercise blood pressures
- Resting and exercise ECGs
- Muscle strength
- Body fat content
- Flexibility
- Balance
- Reaction speeds.

Peak aerobic power

It is best to report oxygen transport data as peak rather than maximal oxygen consumption. Traditional definitions of an oxygen consumption plateau are imprecise in individuals with a low peak oxygen intake, and a fair proportion of seniors fail to reach accepted criteria of a plateau. Peak aerobic power can be estimated by a treadmill or cycle ergometer test, carried to subjective exhaustion under the supervision of a physician. It is best to measure oxygen consumption directly, but if values are predicted from the treadmill stage that is reached (as in the Naughton test), be sure that the subject does not support body weight and thus the rate of working by use of the handrail.

The stress test findings have only limited value in classifying the individual competitor. Because of inter-individual differences in motivation to maximal effort, day-to-day variations in physical condition, the effects of any intercurrent illness and technical errors, about one test in 40 will under-estimate a person's true aerobic power by as much as 10 ml/kg per min, equivalent to a 20-year error in the determination of both functional capacity and biological age.[10] Further, the test results only indicate the person's ability to carry out one form of exercise. Abilities may differ substantially between test modes; for example, a cycle ergometer will give a misleading impression of the capacities of a distance runner.

If submaximal predictions of aerobic power are derived from field test data, such as cycle ergometer power output, a step test, a shuttle run, or a 6 min walk test, errors in the assessment of physical status are even larger (standard deviations from the directly measured value of 20% or more, sometimes with a superimposed systematic error). This underlines the difficulty in using any form of field test to determine the aerobic fitness of an individual, whether the intent is to develop an appropriate training regimen or to predict performance.[10] Possibly, errors may be somewhat smaller if data on a given individual are compared from week-to-week, as a means of monitoring the course of conditioning.

Blood pressure

The resting blood pressure is usually determined in a doctor's office, using a standard clinical sphygmomanometer cuff, although portable battery-operated devices now allow the self-measurement of blood pressure in a person's home. The person who is being evaluated must be thoroughly relaxed; nervousness in a doctor's office can boost recorded pressures

by 10 mmHg, and this is an important argument in favor of home measurements.[74] It is also important to allow adequate preliminary seated rest. Automated devices control technique, but when using a standard cuff, the observer must deflate the cuff slowly, and avoid rounding blood pressure readings to numbers ending with a five or a zero. The systolic reading is indicated by the pressure at which pulsation (the Korotkov sounds) is first heard under the sphygmomanometer cuff, and the diastolic reading corresponds to the fifth phase (the pressure at which the pulsating sounds disappear).

The exercise systolic reading can be measured in similar fashion, but it is difficult to determine the diastolic reading during exercise; diastolic pressures change relatively little, and many investigators have thus made the simplifying assumption that they do not change.

Electrocardiogram

The main points to look for in the resting electrocardiogram are abnormalities of rhythm that could cause temporary loss of consciousness, and any indications of recent or pending myocardial infarction.

The exercise electrocardiogram (ECG) is often quite difficult to interpret in older people, because of baseline abnormalities. If a horizontal or downsloping depression of the ST segment of the ECG in excess of 1 mm (0.1 mV) develops near maximal effort, this implies a statistical increase in the risk of a heart attack, but unfortunately the proportion of false positive responses is high, and ST depression is not in itself justification for prohibiting sport participation.[63] ST segmental depression is more likely to be a true positive finding if the person shows other cardiac risk factors (such as a history of cigarette smoking, a high resting blood pressure, abnormal blood lipids, and a family history of sudden, premature death).

Muscle strength

Muscle strength can be assessed using isotonic, isometric or isokinetic test devices. All such measurements require good cooperation from the participant. The peak muscle force recorded in this fashion depends not only on the active muscle mass, but also on the individual's ability to coordinate the contraction of individual motor units. Less directly, determinations of lean tissue mass (total body mass minus fat mass) can assess overall muscle development, independently of subject cooperation.

Simple field estimates of local muscle strength and endurance include the number of sit-ups and modified push-ups that the individual can perform in one minute. Unfortunately, strength scores are highly specific to the muscle group that has been tested; thus, the force recorded by a hand-grip dynamometer will give little information on a person's ability to perform sports where the leg muscles play a dominant role. Leg strength contributes to the restoration of balance, and is important in the prevention of falls. Grip, shoulder and arm strength are also important to the performance of both specific athletic activities and daily tasks around the home.

Body fat

Most categories of young athlete carry very little body fat, but some older competitors accumulate enough adipose tissue to have a negative impact upon their performance (Fig. 9.2). Body fat is best determined by underwater weighing, but because of dental problems, some older people find difficulty in retaining a mouthpiece while underwater. The amount of superficial fat can be estimated quite simply by applying standard Lange or Harpenden calipers to a double-fold of skin and subcutaneous tissue at selected body sites (for example, the triceps, subscapular and suprailiac skinfolds). Unfortunately, the skinfolds do not examine the amount of intra-abdominal fat (which is important from the viewpoint of cardiovascular risk); however, this can be estimated from measures of abdominal circumference. In elderly people, the skin is thinner than in young adults, and it often has only a loose attachment to underlying tissue. It is thus important to ensure that fat-containing subcutaneous tissue is included in the measured skinfold. Age-specific equations should be used to convert the summated skinfolds to body density and thus to an estimated percentage of body fat; such equations allow for not only the thinner skin of the older person, but also the progressive bone demineralization that reduces the average density of their lean tissues.

Flexibility

Flexibility can be examined in the laboratory, using a goniometer, and a simple field assessment can be made by means of the sit-and-reach test. As with muscle strength, flexibility is specific to the joint that is tested, particularly in older people (where joint mobility is often restricted by local arthritic conditions).

Balance and reaction speed

Balance and reaction speed are critical to the prevention of falls. The overall balance can be assessed from the extent of body sway, as shown by the forces generated when standing on a force plate. A stabilometer provides a simple overall assessment of the time a person can stand astride a balanced beam and keep it from hitting the ground. For field surveys, it is also possible to time the interval a person can remain on one foot with the eyes closed (the 'stork stand' test). Individuals with a poor balance need advising against participation in sports where risk is increased by a deterioration in the sense of balance.

The speed of reaction is commonly assessed from the time needed to make an electrical contact in response to a signal, such as a colored light or a noise. It comprises both the true reaction time (delays in the processing of information by the brain) and the movement time needed to execute a response at a given joint. Because of differences in the length of nerve pathways and the efficiency of various muscle groups, determinations must be made for each of the movements of interest for the sport under consideration.

Exercise prescription and overtraining

The optimal pattern of training for the older individual involves a very gradual progression in the frequency, duration and intensity of training, such that no more than a pleasant tiredness is felt a few hours following a given training session. If the initial duration and intensity are moderate, then conditioning on at least 5 days per week is well tolerated. One popular and successful plan of endurance training has been called

the 'rubber band' technique. Beginning with a 30 min session at a given intensity, duration is progressively increased to 45 min. Assuming that this is well tolerated, the session duration is shortened to 30 min but the intensity is increased; duration is then again increased progressively to 45 min. The regimen normally continues to progress in this fashion until the desired level of training is attained. However, the schedule should be reduced if any incipient signs of overtraining are noted, as discussed above.

In young adults, there is a j-shaped relationship between the volume of training that is undertaken and the immune response. A moderate conditioning program generally enhances immune function, but excessive bouts of acute or chronic exercise have a depressant effect,[51] increasing vulnerability to infections. The same seems true of Masters' athletes. Many competitors report that moderate training enhances their protection against minor infections, but if they exceed a critical weekly running distance (varying with the individual, but typically about 50 km/week), they become more vulnerable to infection.[1] The issue of tailoring training programs to maximize immune function has particular importance in the elderly, since aging in itself is associated with a deterioration in various aspects of immune response, particularly a decrease in natural killer cell function. Auto-immune disease and cancers also become more prevalent in the elderly, and a variety of chronic pathologies predispose to infection.[75] There have been relatively few studies of changes in immune function with exercise in the elderly, but available information points to both prevention and reversal of age-related functional losses by programs of regular, physical activity.[72]

Specific issues for the physician supervising competitive master athletes
Musculoskeletal injuries

Other factors being equal, the older person is at increased risk of musculoskeletal injury. The risk of sport-related injury among those who exercise hard is quite high,[76] although this danger is offset in part by the fact that a strengthening of muscle and bone decreases the likelihood of injury during the activities of ordinary daily life. In the series of master athletes studied by Kavanagh et al.[2] about a half of participants were injured in the course of a year. In some, the injuries were relatively minor, but in about one third of patients, problems were sufficiently severe to interrupt training for a month or more.

Changes in collagen structure and resulting loss of flexibility predispose to strains and tears for any given applied force. Kallinen and Alén[77] found some 38% of the injuries seen in elderly men arose from overuse, predominantly in the upper limbs; sprains and muscle injuries were particularly likely during strength training. Preventive measures include a review of history for previous muscle and joint problems, adequate preliminary warm-up, and careful monitoring for overtraining.

A progressive decrease in both the density and the quality of bone predispose to skeletal injuries. This is compounded by a decrease in the field and acuity of vision (with increased chances of collision in the absence of compensatory increases of neck movement), and a slowing of righting reflexes due to decreases in muscle strength and reaction speed.[78] Methods for the prevention of injury are much as in a younger person, including clearing the playing area of unnecessary obstacles, ensuring a smooth and appropriately textured playing surface, and the wearing of recommended protective equipment.

Special medical problems

As age advances, an increasing proportion of those participating in sport face some form of chronic disease. It is important for participants to carry a good record of any medication, to make sure that participation in sport does not lead to a neglect of necessary treatment, and to evaluate how far vigorous physical activity may modify the absorption and the elimination of any drugs that are being taken. A decrease of blood flow to the viscera is likely to slow the absorption of drugs taken by mouth, but an increased blood flow to muscle accelerates the absorption from intra-muscular injection sites. Renal and hepatic elimination are also likely to be slowed by vigorous exercise.

Many elderly people have problems of balance, and if these are severe, it is important to avoid activities such as cycling and skiing, where balance is at a premium. Others have irregularities of cardiac rhythm which can cause episodes of loss of consciousness, and it is then important to avoid activities where this could prove fatal (for example, swimming or diving without an observant partner).

Type II diabetes mellitus is frequent among the elderly. A careful ophthalmic examination should be undertaken for signs of impending retinal detachment which may be exacerbated by sport-related body impacts. A check should also be made for neurological complications leading to decreased pain sensitivity and proprioception. Bouts of vigorous activity can reduce the need for insulin injections, giving a danger of insulin coma unless medication is decreased appropriately. It is finally important to insist on good skin hygiene, in order to control the risk of boils and other more serious skin conditions in diabetic individuals.

Travel considerations

Age is no longer a barrier to travel, and active older individuals now explore all of the extreme environments of our planet. Air travel is generally well-tolerated, although on long journeys thrombosis may develop in varicose veins, particularly if periodic exercise of the legs is difficult because of a crowded cabin. On long flights, cabin pressure may also drop to the equivalent of 2500 m altitude, imposing a hypoxic stress on individuals with cardio-respiratory limitations. Hot environments are less well tolerated by the elderly,[79] and limiting conditions for summer competition should be adjusted accordingly. The cold conditions of winter sports and Antarctic exploration increase the preloading of the heart. The person who has developed chronic obstructive lung disease also seems to have an increased vulnerability to cold-induced bronchospasm.[80] In the event that cold exposure is increased by some type of catastrophe (such as an injury to a member of the party), the poorer peripheral circulation of the elderly also increases vulnerability to frostbite.

Ski lifts carry many elderly people to high altitudes. Perhaps because most elderly athletes do not exercise as hard as their younger peers, the acute risk of high altitude illness does not seem to increase with age,[81] but those with bouts of myocardial ischaemia at sea level are likely to find that this is exacerbated. Many elderly people continue underwater exploration. Risks in this group include loss of consciousness while underwater, and a sudden bout of hypotension on leaving the water.

For a variety of reasons, older individuals are more vulnerable to many forms of infection,[10] and once infected the disease may have more serious consequences than in a younger individual. It is thus important to ensure that requisite vaccinations are updated prior to travel, and if a physician is traveling with a team, appropriate medications should be carried for any major infections prevalent in the area to be visited.

CONCLUSION

Older individuals show a slower response to athletic training than young adults. Nevertheless, remarkable gains in physical condition can be achieved by a gently progressive exercise regimen, to the point that many aspects of biological age can be reduced by 10–20 years. The risk of sudden death is increased substantially during training and competition, but this is more than offset by a reduced risk of cardiovascular catastrophe during intervals between training. Sport is safe for the majority of older adults, and physicians should not restrict participation unnecessarily. Regular, vigorous physical activity not only gives immediate pleasure, but also improves the quality of life by enhancing mood state, decreasing the risk of chronic diseases and decreasing the likelihood of dependency in the final years of life.

REFERENCES

1   Shephard RJ, Kavanagh T, Mertens DJ. Personal health benefits of Masters athletic competition. Br J Sports Med 1995; 29:35–40.
2   Kavanagh T, Mertens DJ, Matosevic V, et al. Health and aging of Masters athletes. Clin J Sports Med 1989; 1:72–88.
3   Kasch FW, Boyer JL, van Camp SP, et al. Effect of exercise on cardiovascular ageing. Age Ageing 1993; 22:5–10.
4   Kasch FW, Boyer JL, Schmidt PK, et al. Ageing of the cardiovascular system during 33 years of aerobic exercise. Age Ageing 1999; 28:531–536.
5   Paterson DH, Cunningham DA, Koval JJ, et al. Aerobic fitness in a population of independently living men and women aged 55–86 years. Med Sci Sports Exerc 1999; 31:1813–1820.
6   Shephard RJ, Montelpare WJ. Geriatric benefits of exercise as an adult. J Gerontol 1988; 43:86–90.

7   Lakatta EG. Cardiovascular regulatory mechanisms in advanced age. Physiol Rev 1993; 73:413–467.
8   Lakatta EG. Aging and cardiovascular structure and function in healthy sedentary humans. Aging (Milano) 1998; 10:162–164.
9   Jackson AS, Beard EF, Wier LT, et al. Changes in aerobic power of men ages 25–70 yr. Med Sci Sports Exerc 1995; 27:113–120.
10 Shephard RJ. Aging, Physical Activity and Health. Champaign, IL: Human Kinetics; 1997.
11 Aoyaji Y, Shephard RJ. Aging and muscle function. Sports Med 1992; 14:376–396.
12 Fiatarone-Singh MA. Exercise, Nutrition and the Older Woman. Boca Raton, FL: CRC Publishing; 2000.
13 Lexell J. Aging and human muscle: observations from Sweden. Can J Appl Physiol 1993; 18:2–18.

14 Fiatarone M, O'Neill EF, Ryan ND, et al. Exercise training and nutritional supplementation for physical frailty in very elderly people. N Engl J Med 1994; 330:1769–1775.

15 Cress ME, Thomas DP, Johnson J, et al. Effect of training on Vo_2max, thigh strength and muscle morphology in septuagenarian women. Med Sci Sports Exerc 1991; 23:752–758.

16 Fitness Canada. Fitness and lifestyle in Canada. Ottawa, ON: Government of Canada; 1983.

17 Duncan PW, Chandler J, Studenski S, et al. How do physiological components of balance affect mobility in elderly men? Arch Phys Med Rehabil 1993; 74:1343–1349.

18 Voorips LE, Lemmink KA, van Heuvelen MG, et al. The physical condition of elderly women differing in habitual activity. Med Sci Sports Exerc 1993; 25:1152–1157.

19 Brown M, Holloszy JO. Effects of a low intensity exercise program on selected physical performance characteristics of 60- to 71-year olds. Aging 1991; 3:129–139.

20 Hopkins DR, Murrah B, Hoeger WWK, et al. Effect of low impact aerobic dance on the functional fitness of elderly women. Gerontol 1990; 30:189–192.

21 Morey MC, Cowper PA, Feussner JR, et al. Two-year trends in physical performance following supervised exercise among community-dwelling older veterans. J Am Ger Soc 1991; 39:986–992.

22 Rider RA, Daly J. Effects of flexibility training on enhancing spinal mobility in older women. J Sports Med Phys Fitness 1991; 31:213–217.

23 Lane N, Micheli B, Bjorkengren A, et al. The risk of osteoarthritis with running and aging: A 5-year longitudinal study. J Rheumatol 1993; 20:461–468.

24 Vingård E, Alfredson L, Goldie I, et al. Sports and osteoarthrosis of the hip: An epidemiologic study. Am J Sports Med 1993; 21:195–200.

25 McAlindon TE, Wilson PW, Aliabadi P, et al. Level of physical activity and the risk of radiographic and symptomatic knee osteoarthritis in the elderly: the Framingham study. Am J Med 1999; 106:151–157.

26 Minor MA, Hewett JE, Webel RR, et al. Efficacy of physical conditioning exercise in patients with rheumatoid arthritis and osteoarthritis. Arthr Rheum 1989; 32:1396–1405.

27 Overstall PW, Downton JH. Gait, balance and falls. In: Pathy MSJ, ed. Principles and practice of geriatric medicine. Chichester: John Wiley & Sons; 1998.

28 Jaglal SB, Kreger N, Darlington G. Past and recent physical activity and risk of hip fracture. Am J Epidemiol 1993; 138:107–118.

29 Iverson BD, Gossman MR, Shaddea SA, et al. Balance performance, force production and activity levels in non-institutionalized men 60 to 90 years of age. Phys Ther 1990; 70:348–355.

30 Hu M-H, Woollacott MH. Multisensory training of standing balance in older adults. I. Postural stability and one-leg stance balance. J Gerontol 1994; 49:52–61.

31 Judge JO, Lindsey C, Underwood M, et al. Balance improvements in older women: Effects of exercise and training. Phys Ther 1993; 73:254–263.

32 MacRae PG, Feltner ME, Reinsch S. A 1-year exercise program for older women: Effects on falls, injuries, and physical performance. J Aging Phys Activ 1994; 2:127–142.

33 Drinkwater B. Physical activity, fitness and osteoporosis. In: Bouchard C, Shephard RJ, Stephens T, eds. Physical activity, Fitness and Health. Champaign, IL: Human Kinetics; 1994:724–736.

34 Loucks AB. Reproductive changes and the endurance athlete. In: Shephard RJ, Åstrand PO, eds. Endurance in sport. Oxford: Blackwell; 2000:718–730.

35 Michel BA, Lane NE, Björkengren A, et al. Impact of running on lumbar bone density: A 5-year longitudinal study. J Rheumatol 1992; 19:1759–1763.

36 Montoye HJ, Van Huss WD, Olson HW, et al. The longevity and mortality of college athletes. Lansing, MI: Phi Epsilon Kappa Fraternity, Michigan State University; 1957.

37 Yamaji K, Shephard RJ. Longevity and causes of death of athletes: a review of the literature. J Hum Ergol 1977; 6:13–25.

38 Karvonen MJ, Klemola H, Virkajarvi J, et al. Longevity of endurance skiers. Med Sci Sports 1974; 6:49–51.

39 Sarna S, Kaprio J. Life expectancy of former athletes. Sports Med 1994; 17:149–151.

40 Robine JM, Ritchie K. Healthy life expectancy: Evaluation of global indicator of change in population health. BMJ 1991; 302:457–460.

41 Pekkanen J, Marti B, Nissinen A, et al. Reduction of premature mortality by high physical activity: A 20-year follow-up of middle-aged Finnish men. Lancet 1987; i:1473–1477.

42 Fries JF. Aging, natural death and the compression of morbidity. N Engl J Med 1980; 303:130–135.

43 Linsted KD, Tonstad K, Kuzma J. Self-report of physical activity and patterns of mortality in Seventh-Day Adventist men. J Clin Epidemiol 1991; 44:355–364.

44 Paffenbarger R, Hyde RT, Wing AL. Determinants of health and longevity. In: Bouchard C, Shephard RJ, Stephens T, et al., eds. Exercise, fitness and health. Champaign, IL: Human Kinetics; 1990:33–48.

45 Paffenbarger RS, Hyde RT, Wing AL, et al. Some interrelations of physical activity, physiological fitness, health and longevity. In: Bouchard C, Shephard RJ, Stephens T, eds. Physical Activity, Fitness and Health. Champaign, IL: Human Kinetics; 1994:119–133.

46 Paffenbarger RS, Lee I-M. Physical activity and fitness for health and longevity. Res Quart 1996; 67:S11–S28.

47 Guyatt GH, Dego RA, Charlson M, et al. Responsiveness and validity in health status measurement: A clarification. J Clin Epidemiol 1989; 42:403–408.

48 Shephard RJ. Habitual physical activity and the quality of life. Quest 1996; 48:354–365.

49 Bouchard C, Shephard RJ. Physical activity, fitness and health: The model and key concepts. In: Bouchard C, Shephard RJ, Stephens T, eds. Physical activity, fitness and health. Champaign, IL: Human Kinetics; 1994:77–88.

50 Bassey EJ, Fiatarone MA, O'Neill EF, et al. Leg extensor power and functional performance in very old men and women. Clin Sci 1992; 82:321–327.

51 Shephard RJ. Physical activity, training, and the immune response. Carmel, IN: Cooper Publications; 1997.

52 Nieman DC, Berk LS, Simpson-Westerberg K, et al. Effects of long-endurance running on immune system parameters and lymphocyte function in experienced marathoners. Int J Sports Med 1989; 10:317–323.

53 North TC, McCullagh G, Todd IC, et al. Effect of exercise on depression. Ex Sport Sci Rev 1990; 18:379–416.

54 Shephard RJ, Corey P, Renzland P, et al. The influence of an industrial fitness program upon medical care costs. Can J Publ Hlth 1982; 73:259–263.

55 Mathews AM. Contributors to the loss of independence and the promotion of independence among seniors. Ottawa, ON: Community Health Division, Health & Welfare, Canada; 1989.

56 Cress ME, Buchner DM, Questad KA, et al. Exercise: effects on physical functional performance in independent older adults. J Gerontol 1999; 54:242–248.

57 Shephard RJ. Sudden death: A significant hazard of exercise? Br J Sports Med 1974; 8:101–110.

58 Siscovick DS. Risks of exercising: Sudden cardiac death and injuries. In: Bouchard C, Shephard RJ, Stephens T, Sutton JR, McPherson BD, eds. Exercise, fitness and health. Champaign, IL: Human Kinetics; 1990:707–714.

59 Evans WJ. Exercise training guidelines for the elderly. Med Sci Sports Exerc 1999; 31:12–17.

60 Feigenbaum MS, Pollock ML. Prescription of resistance training for health and disease. Med Sci Sports Exerc 1999; 31:38–45.

61 American College of Sports Medicine. Exercise and physical activity for older adults. Med Sci Sports Exerc 1998; 30:992–1008.

62 Shephard RJ. PAR-Q, Canadian Home Fitness Test and exercise screening alternatives. Sports Med 1988; 5:185–195.

63 Shephard RJ. Prognostic value of exercise testing for coronary heart disease. Br J Sports Med 1982; 16:220–229.

64 Thomas S, Reading J, Shephard RJ. Revision of the physical activity readiness questionnaire (PAR-Q). Can J Sport Sci 1992; 17:338–345.

65 American College of Sports Medicine. ACSM's guidelines for exercise testing and prescription. Philadelphia, PA: Lippincott, Williams & Wilkins; 2000.

66 Shephard RJ, Kavanagh T. Predicting the cardiac catastrophe in the post-coronary patient. Can Fam Phys 1978; 24:614–618.

67 Lightman DA, Schachat A. Eye diseases in the elderly. In: LeMura LM, Duvillard SP von, eds. Clinical exercise physiology. Philadelphia: Lippincott, Williams & Wilkins; 2004.

68 Volpi E, Sheffield-Moore M, Rasmussen BB, et al. Basal muscle amino acid kinetics and protein synthesis in healthy young and older men. JAMA 2001; 286: 1206–1212.

69 Welle S, Thornton C, Jozefowicz R, et al. Myofibrillar protein synthesis in young and old men. Am J Physiol 1993; 264:693–698.

70 Toth MJ, Matthews DE, Tracy RP, et al. Age-related difference in skeletal muscle protein synthesis: relation to markers of immune activation. Am J Physiol 2005; :883–891.

71 Verde T, Thomas S, Shephard RJ. Potential changes of heavy training in highly trained distance runners. Br J Sports Med 1992; 26:167–175.

72 Shinkai S, Konishi M, Shephard RJ. Aging and immune response to exercise. Can J Physiol Pharmacol 1998; 76:562–572.

73 Mackinnon LT. Hooper S. Mucosal (secretory) immune system responses to exercise of varying intensity and to overtraining. Int J Sports Med 1994; 15:179–183.

74 Furberg CD, Black DM. The systolic pressure in the elderly pilot program: Methodological issues. Eur Heart J 1988; 9:223–227.

75 Shephard RJ. Exercise, aging, and immune resistance to infections and neoplasms. In: Huber G, ed. Healthy aging. Activity and sports. Werbach-Gamburg, Germany: Health Promotion Publications; 1997:174–180.

76 Kallinen M, Marku A. Aging, physical activity and sports injuries: An overview of common sports injuries in the elderly. Sports Med 1995; 20:41–52.

77 Kallinen M, Alén M. Sports-related injuries in elderly men still active in sports. Br J Sports Med 1994; 28:52–55.

78 Stelmach GE. Physical activity and aging: Sensory and perceptual processing. In: Bouchard C, Shephard RJ, Stephens T, eds. Physical activity, fitness and health. Champaign, IL: Human Kinetics; 1994:504–510.

79 Kenney WL. Body fluid and temperature regulation as a function of age. In: Lamb DR, Gisolfi CV, Nadel E, eds. Exercise in older adults. Carmel, IN: Cooper Publications; 1995:305–351.

80 Killian KJ. Exercise-induced bronchial obstruction. In: Torg J, Shephard RJ, eds. Current Therapy in sports medicine. 3rd edn. Philadelphia, PA: Mosby; 1995:676–678.

81 Balcomb AC, Sutton JR. Advanced age and altitude illness. In: Sutton JR, Brock RM, eds. Sports medicine for the mature athlete. Indianapolis, IN: Benchmark Press; 1986:213–224.

CHAPTER 10

Special Considerations in the Disabled Athlete

David M. Crandell

'This Ability'

Disability sport covers a broad range of sports and sports-related activities for children and adults. It encompasses adapted physical education for children, rehabilitation and recreation for many individuals with acquired and/or congenital physical and cognitive impairments, and for some, elite competition as part of the natural development of sports participation.

Disability sport
- Physical education
- Rehabilitation
- Recreation
- Competition

Although rooted in the context of rehabilitation goals of increased flexibility, strengthening, endurance, balance, coordination, mobility, functional skills, sports participation has its own intrinsic values, especially for individuals with disabilities. Regular physical activity and sports participation has been observed to improve the ability to perform activities of daily living, protect against the development of chronic diseases, decrease anxiety and depression, enhance the feeling of well-being, and improve weight control. Beyond the pure sense of enjoyment that comes along with both individual and team sports participation, the athlete with a disability also gains confidence, a sense of achievement and skills that translate well beyond the competition venue, resulting in improved community integration and employment.

> 'The pleasure of sport is to discover at every moment that you have arrived and you have overcome – that you have achieved your goals, which you thought to be possible only in your dreams'.
> (Béatrice Hess, France: Paralympic Gold Medalist, Swimming)

Through sports, every person, with or without a disability, has the opportunity and ability to reach their potential. Technological improvements coupled with disability legislation like the Americans with Disabilities Act (ADA),[1] the United Nations Standard Rules on the Equalization of Opportunities for Persons with Disabilities[2] and the European

---

Box 10.1: Key Points

- Athletes with disabilities are athletes and the incidence, type, mechanism and treatment of most of sports-related injuries is generally the same as for able-bodied athletes.

- There is a broad spectrum of athletes with physical impairments and as levels of participation increase, it is essential for the sports medicine practitioner to gain an understanding of the special considerations and needs of these athletes.

- More research is needed in the prevention and treatment of sports injuries to athletes with disabilities.

Union Disability Strategy,[3] have led to increased awareness, access and opportunities for individuals with disabilities throughout the world in many domains, including sports and recreation. Sports can be a powerful medium to accentuate the 'ability' and not the impairment, functional loss, or disability (Table 10.1).[4]

Athletes with disabilities are true athletes. Caring for these athletes, in many ways, is comparable with caring for able-bodied athletes. As sports participation has grown overall, there has also been increased interest and involvement by sports medicine practitioners in the study and care for athletes with disabilities. Unfortunately, one of the striking weaknesses in most sports medicine training programs in the US is little contact with athletes with disabilities.[5] There are special considerations related to the physiology and biomechanics of athletes with disabilities that do require additional attention and preparation. This review focuses on elite athletes with physical impairment since they have been the most studied, but much of this information can be applied to recreational or first-time participants as well.

Rehabilitation to recreation to competition

There are approximately 500 million people with a disability around the world, roughly 10% of the world's population.[6]

Table 10.1 World Health Organization Definitions

Health Condition	Impairment	Activity Limitation	Participation Restriction
Spinal injury			
Without intervention	Paralysis	Incapable of running the 1500 m	Unable to be on athletic team
With intervention	Paralysis	Run in racing wheelchair	Team membership

---

Box 10.2: Key Points

- The disability sport movement started with informal games in the 1940s that later developed into national and international competitions.
- The Paralympic Games provide unique opportunities for thousands of elite athletes with a disability.
- Increased sports participation among the disabled has led to improved performance and sporting excellence.

Many participate in sport on a recreational level with far fewer 'raising the bar' to compete on the level of elite sport.

The origins of the disability sport 'movement' started with informal games at veterans' hospitals in the US in the early 1940s. By playing wheelchair basketball in the gymnasium, veterans re-discovered the joy of sports participation after injury. Intra-hospital games led to eventual state and national competitions by the late 1940s. During this time, Sir Ludwig Guttman, a neurosurgeon working on a spinal injuries unit at Stoke Mandeville Hospital near Aylesbury, England, introduced sport as recreation and as part of his rehabilitation program of his patients. Dr Guttmann believed that 'by restoring activity of mind and body, by instilling self-respect, self-discipline, a competitive spirit and comradeship, sport develops mental attitudes that are essential for social reintegration'.[7] On 28 July, 1948 on the opening day of the Olympic Games in London, Dr Guttmann organized an archery competition on the front lawn of the hospital, between 16 wheelchair 'competitors' from the spinal injuries unit and a disabled ex-serviceman's home in London. The Stoke Mandeville Games became an annual event. Four years later, four Dutch paraplegic veterans traveled to compete in the first International Stoke Mandeville Games. Sports such as athletics (track and field), swimming, snooker (billiards), table tennis, basketball and fencing had also been introduced. In the US, in 1957, Ben Lipton, Director of the Bulova Watch School, a popular job-training site for the disabled, orchestrated the first US National Wheelchair Games, in the grounds of the Bulova factory in Queens, New York.

Despite these early successes, physicians were slow to express support for sports for the disabled and some, including Dr Guttmann himself, had concerns about athletes with spinal cord injuries 'over-exerting' themselves. For this reason, there were no wheelchair races beyond 200 m at Stoke Mandeville, until a successful 1500 m wheelchair race was completed at the Pan-American Wheelchair Games in Mexico City, Mexico in 1975. That same year, unofficial registrant ('bandit'), Bob Hall wheeled the Boston Marathon in a time of 2:58 in a slightly modified, standard wheelchair. Two years later, after intensive lobbying efforts, the Wheelchair Division of the Boston Marathon was established. Bob Hall, in a custom-racing wheelchair he designed, became the first wheelchair champion, having shaved 10 min off his initial time.

Paralympics

In the beginning, only athletes competing in wheelchairs (spinal cord injury, post-polio, spina bifida, high-level amputees) participated, but as the disability sport movement grew, other athletes (with visual impairments, cerebral palsy, upper and lower limb amputations or intellectual disabilities) were included (Table 10.2). Elite sport competitions became a natural development and in 1960, the first Paralympic Summer Games took place in Rome, where the Olympic Games had just been held. The word 'Paralympic' is derived from the Greek, 'para' meaning 'parallel' combined with the word 'Olympic'.

The Paralympic Games have grown since the initial competition in Rome, when 400 athletes from 23 nations competed.

Table 10.2 Athens 2004 Summer Paralympics

	Spinal Injury	Amputee	Visually Impaired	Other[a]	Dwarf	Cerebral Palsy
Archery	X	X		X		X
Athletics	X	X	X	X	X	X
Boccia	X					X
Cycling	X	X	X			X
Equestrian	X	X		X		X
Football 5-a-side			X			
Football 7-a-side						X
Goal ball			X			
Judo			X			
Powerlifting	X	X		X		
Sailing	X	X	X	X	X	X
Shooting						
Swimming	X	X	X	X	X	X
Table tennis	X	X		X	X	X
Volleyball sitting	X	X		X		
Wheelchair basketball	X	X		X		X
Wheelchair fencing	X	X				
Wheelchair Rugby	X	X		X		
Wheelchair tennis	X	X		X		

[a]Athletes with multiple sclerosis, muscular dystrophy, Friedreich's ataxia, arthrogryposis, osteogenesis imperfecta, Ehlers–Danlos syndrome.

In the 2004 Athens Summer Games close to 4000 athletes, representing 136 countries, participated. Approximately 1200 women represented their countries and female athletes competed in judo and volleyball for the first time.[8] Founded in 1989, the International Paralympic Committee (IPC) is one of the largest sports organizations in the world and provides unique opportunities for the vast majority of athletes with a disability. Its membership includes over 160 National Paralympic Committees and four International Sport Organizations for the Disabled (Table 10.3). Since the 1988 Summer Games in Seoul, the Paralympics have taken place shortly after the Olympics in the same host city and utilizing the same venues. Following a recent agreement by the International Olympic Committee (IOC) and the IPC, the local organizing committee for the Olympics also stages the Paralympics Games.

A total of 15 of the 19 Paralympic sports are equivalent to Olympic sports. The unique Paralympic Sports are boccia for athletes with cerebral palsy, goalball for the visually impaired, and powerlifting and wheelchair (quad) rugby for wheelchair athletes (see Fig. 10.1 and Table 10.4). The first Paralympic Winter Games were held in Ornskoldvik, Sweden, in 1976, with approximately 140 amputee and visually impaired athletes from nine countries who participated in Alpine and Nordic skiing. At the Salt Lake City 2002 Winter Paralympic Games, 416 athletes, representing 36 nations competed in Alpine and Nordic skiing (including the biathlon) and sledge ice hockey. New sports and disciplines are being developed for future Winter Paralympic Games,[9] with wheelchair curling making its debut as a medal sport in 2006, in Torino, Italy (Table 10.5).

Elite athletes

The disability sports movement has continued to evolve and with it, there has been an increased public awareness and interest by the media (Fig. 10.2). There is now an ESPY Award[10] given

Table 10.3 International Sports Organizations for the Disabled (ISODs)

Cerebral Palsy International Sports and Recreation Association (CP-ISRA)	Netherlands
International Blind Sports Federation (IBSA)	Spain
International Sports Federation for Persons with an Intellectual Disability (INAS-FID)	Sweden
International Wheelchair and Amputee Sports Federation (IWAS)	UK

Table 10.4 Torino 2006 Winter Paralympics

Alpine skiing
Ice (sledge) hockey
Nordic skiing
Wheelchair curling

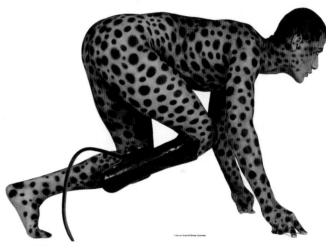

Figure 10.2 Marlon Shirley, USA, World Record Holder 100 m (Courtesy of US Paralympics ©Tim Lanterman).

Figure 10.1 Wheelchair (quad) rugby (©Lieven Coudenys: www.coudenys.be).

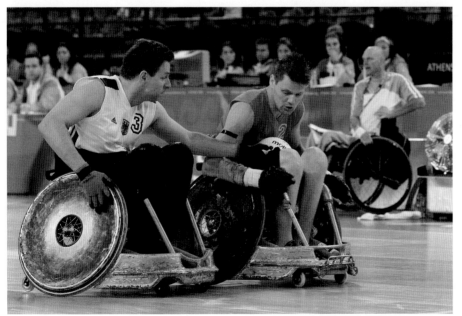

out to the best male and best female disabled Athlete of the Year at the annual award ceremony, along with able-bodied amateur and professional athletes. Athletes with disabilities demonstrate their ability with sport performances that are comparable or exceed those of able-bodied athletes. The record for the Boston Marathon is 1:18:27 by Ernst Van Dyk of South Africa in 2004 (Fig. 10.3). Van Dyk competes in the men's wheelchair division and is the current reigning Boston marathon champion, winning his fifth consecutive race in 2005. By comparison, Cosmas Ndeti of Kenya holds the Men's Open record with a time of 2:07:15 in 1994. Two-time Paralympic gold medalist in the 100 m winner Marlon Shirley of the US has a world record time of 11.08 (just 1.31 s slower than the able-bodied record of 9.77) and he does this on a prosthetic leg and foot. Marla Runyan, a middle distance runner with visual impairment, has qualified for both the US Paralympic and US Olympic teams.

'Disabled' athletes themselves are now defining their own limits. The 'Ironman' triathlon competitions now have triathletes with disabilities regularly competing. Paul Martin of the US broke the Ironman World Record for leg amputees at the 2005 Ironman Couer d'Alene in the record time of 10:09:15 (Fig. 10.4). Martin finished 89th overall in the competition consisting of a 2.5 mile swim, 100 mile cycle and a marathon run. And in a different kind of race, one against the elements, Eric Weihenmayer, a blind mountaineer, ascended to the peak of Mount Everest in 2003.

As progress has been made towards increasing sports participation more broadly, there has also been an effort to increase the level of sporting excellence and performance. The Australian Paralympic Athletics (track and field) team developed an integrated approach[11] to caring for athletes including strength and conditioning, biomechanics, sports psychology, coach education and sports medicine. They were able to improve the physical condition of the athletes, improve technique, improve coaching knowledge, integrate sports medicine and science, identify new talent and ensure the athletes had support to allow sufficient time to train. As a result of this integrated approach, the Australian team went from seventh in the Athletics medal count in Atlanta in 1996 to No. 1 in the Sydney Summer Paralympic Games in 2000. The 'Aussies' fell to No. 2 in Athens behind the new formidable Chinese team, who began utilizing an integrated sports medicine approach.

The US Paralympics, part of the US Olympic Committee (USOC) is working to raise the level of performance of US disabled athletes. They have established new programs such as the Paralympic Academy, which is designed as a national initiative to enhance the health and wellness of children with disabilities in the US. Their goal is to increase participation of children with disabilities in physical education by 30%.[12] US Paralympics is also helping recent combat veterans to return to sports participation with an active military outreach program.

Doping

The prevalence of doping among athletes with disabilities is not known, but there is no reason to believe that the problem is any different from that in able-bodied sports.[13] In order to

Figure 10.3 Ernst Van Dyck, South Africa, wins Boston Marathon, 2004 (Courtesy of Boston Globe and Ernst Van Dyck, with permission).

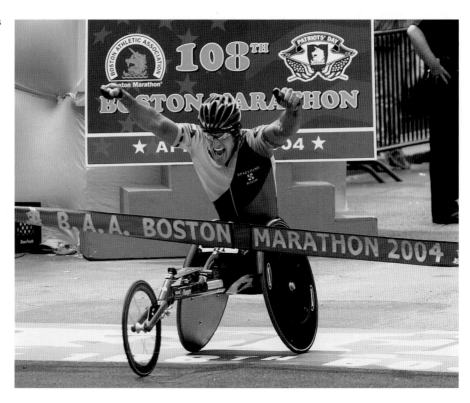

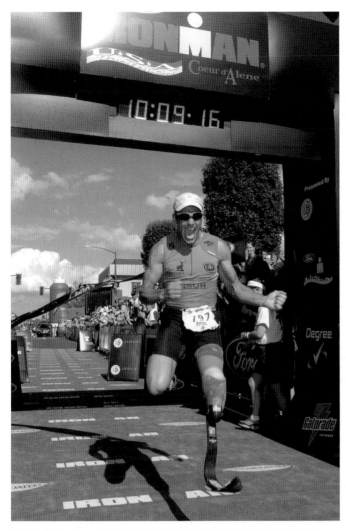

Figure 10.4 Paul Martin, USA, Ironman Triathlete (Courtesy of Paul Martin and Jennifer Reese, Action Sports International, with permission).

decrease the use of drugs, the Doping Disables Project was launched in July 2000 to educate athletes and coaches on specific doping issues for athletes with disabilities. In 2004, the IPC, together with the International Disabled Sports Federations and the National Paralympic Committees, established the IPC Anti-doping Code[14] in conformity with the general principles of the World Anti-doping Code. The IPC also agreed with the World Anti-doping Agency on an out-of-competition testing plan. The rationale for doping control is the same: to protect the athlete from potentially harmful effects some drugs can produce and to ensure fair and ethical competition. Ten anti-doping rule violations were found in Athens in 2004, two were out-of competition violations and eight were in the powerlifting competition.[8] Members of the IPC Medical and Scientific Committee are looking to ensure a strong testing program along with better education for the athletes and coaches. Recognizing that some disabled athletes take prohibited substances (medications) for 'therapeutic' purposes, a Therapeutic Exemption process is used which is sport- and case-specific. The medication must be clinically necessary and

must not offer the athlete an advantage, otherwise, it will be ruled as a doping violation.

CLASSIFICATION

Box 10.3: Key Points

- Various classification systems are used by the disabled sports to equalize competition among the athletes.

A classification system is an integral component to disability sports competitions and allows for equitable competition. It also assures that training and skill are the determining factors, not the level of disability. This is not unlike the able-bodied system, where age, gender or body weight is accepted as a significant factor for equalizing competitive performance. There are various classification schemes that have been based on a medical, disability specific, combined or functional/sports specific models. There is an established minimal degree of impairment for each sport. During recent years, more emphasis has been placed on combining classes and on the scientific validation of the classification systems. An ideal classification system would be complex enough to achieve fairness, yet simple enough to ease understanding and acceptance (Table 10.5).[15]

EPIDEMIOLOGY OF INJURIES

'Athletes with disabilities don't get injured, they just get reclassified'.

(Popular disabled sport adage, author unknown)

Much of the sports injury research for athletes with disabilities has been limited to presenting data from a single event or large competition. Ferrara and colleagues have published studies from injury data from Paralympic competitions dating back to 1976[16,17] that have been helpful in defining the general patterns of injuries and diseases in athletes with disabilities. They found that the number and type of injuries/illnesses were not significantly different from elite athletes without disabilities. Utilizing the athletic injury/report form used by the USOC, Ferrara found that acute illnesses, e.g. upper respiratory infection (URI) were most common followed by muscular strains. Acute injuries were twice as likely as chronic.[15] The authors' own unpublished observations from the 1995 Wheelchair and Amputee National Championships in Boston and the US team injury data from the 1999 Pan-Am Paralympic Games in Mexico City, support these conclusions.[18]

Ferrara's review[16] showed that, among athletes participating in Summer Paralympic events, abrasions, strains, sprains, contusions are the most common injuries. Lower extremity injuries were more common in ambulatory athletes (amputee, cerebral palsy, visually impaired) and upper extremity injuries seem to be more common in athletes who use wheelchairs. The low number of fractures and dislocations observed is attributed

Table 10.5   Classification Systems

Cycling	
Visual impairment	
Men or women	Tandem bike with sighted pilot
Mixed gender	Tandem bike with sighted pilot
Locomotor impairment	
L1	Minor or no lower limb impairment
L2	Disability in one leg, but able to pedal normally w/ or w/o prosthesis
L3	Lower extremity disability, pedal using one leg, w/ or w/o upper limb disability
L4	Severe disability affecting both lower limbs, w/ or w/o upper limb disability
Cerebral Palsy	
Division 4	Athletes with least severe disability (CP Class 8, 7), competing on bicycles
Division 3	Athletes in Division 3 (CP Class 6, 5), competing on tricycles
Division 2	Athletes in Division 2 (CP Class 6, 5), competing on bicycles
Division 1	Athletes with more severe disability (CP Class 4–1) competing on tricycles
Alpine skiing	
Visual impairment	
B1	Totally blind
B2	Partially sighted with little remaining sight
B3	Partially sighted with more remaining sight
Standing	
LW1	Double above-knee amputees
LW2	Outrigger skiers
LW3	Double below-knee amputees
LW4	Skiers with prosthesis
LW6/7	Skiers without poles
LW5/8	Skiers with one pole
LW9/1	Disability of arm and leg (after amputation)
LW9/2	Disability of arm and leg (cerebral palsy)
Sitting	
LW10	Monoskiers – high degree of paraplegia
LW11	Monoskiers – lower degree of paraplegia
LW12/1	Monoskiers – lower degree of paraplegia
LW12/2	Monoskiers – double above knee amputees

to the low number of contact sports. To my knowledge, there are no published reports on catastrophic injuries during competitions including athletes with disabilities.[19]

There is very limited injury data regarding Winter Paralympic events and disabled skiing injuries (Fig. 10.5). Mono-ski technology has improved to allow for safer, independent loading on the ski chairlift reducing a potential source of injury. With increased speeds, helmet use in disabled skiing is standard, as in the able-bodied skiers. Competitions in cycling, equestrian and hockey also require helmets, but other high risk sports, e.g. wheelchair rugby and basketball, do not. More research is required in the area of sports-related concussions in disabled athletes.[20]

AUTONOMIC DYSFUNCTION

Box 10.4: Key Points

- Autonomic dysreflexia (AD) can occur in athletes who have spinal injuries at or above the 6th thoracic neurologic level, usually caused by bladder distention.

- Athletes with AD can present with headache and elevated blood pressure and require early recognition and removal of noxious stimuli.

- If a precipitating cause of AD cannot be determined readily and the athlete remains symptomatic, hospitalization is required to both treat the severe hypertension and determine more occult causes.

Dysreflexia

Spinal cord injury (SCI) not only results in motor and sensory impairment, but autonomic dysfunction that can pose potentially serious problems for SCI athletes. In addition to sparking the disabled sports movement, Guttmann also did outstanding research work with SCI patients, and in 1947, along with Whitteridge, described how distention of viscera had 'set up a response of autonomic mechanisms, which had profound effects on the cardiovascular activity in parts of the body above the level of the spinal lesion'.[21] What they described was autonomic dysreflexia (AD) or hyperreflexia, an acute syndrome manifested by excessive, uncontrolled sympathetic output that can occur in athletes in any sport who have spinal injuries at or above the 6th thoracic neurologic level.[22] An athlete with a high SCI, but with an incomplete lesion, is less likely to develop AD.[23]

AD is caused by a spinal reflex mechanism that remains intact despite the athlete's injury.[22] Noxious stimuli such as bladder or bowel distention or a sports injury (e.g. a thigh contusion) can trigger a generalized sympathetic response resulting in vasoconstriction below the neurologic lesion and a rise in blood pressure (BP). Descending central (brain stem) inhibitory signals, which would typically counteract the rise of BP, are blocked at the level of the SCI and can result in severe hypertension. Normal baroreceptor reflex sensitivity[24] results in increased parasympathetic outflow to the heart. The increased vagal activity results in a reflex bradycardia and peripheral vasodilation above the level of the lesion, but not enough to counter the BP elevation.

The athlete with AD can present with headache, facial flushing, nasal congestion and sweating above the level of the injury. Below the level, the skin may be cool and pale. The main physical finding is an elevation of BP. It is important to remember that the resting BP of an individual with SCI often is low at rest with systolic BP around 90 mmHg. This means that systolic readings of 120–140 mmHg may be considered elevated. The physical signs of AD may be similar in younger disabled athletes, but AD may be more difficult to identify, because they may not be able to articulate their symptoms well.[25]

Any noxious stimulus occurring below the level of the injury can trigger an episode of AD, with bladder distention the most

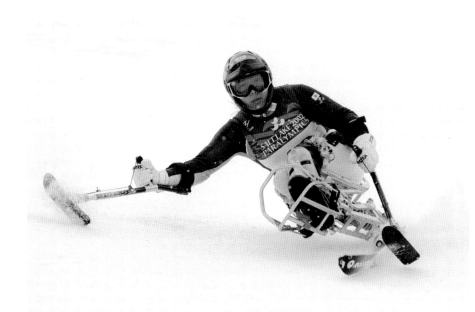

Figure 10.5 Alpine, slalom: 2002 Salt Lake Paralympic Winter Games. Kuniko Obinata (Jap), class LW12/2 (sitski). Won bronze in slalom and giant slalom (©Lieven Coudenys: www.coudenys.be).

common presentation. This can be caused by a blocked catheter or insufficient intermittent catheterization, especially just before competition with long delays in some of the staging areas. The second most common cause is bowel distention caused by fecal impaction. Low-grade dysreflexic symptoms can be seen even with proper bladder and bowel management and the development of mild symptoms can prompt the athlete to tend to their bladder or bowel programs. Other triggers can be pressure sores from prolonged training or frequent competition in racing wheelchairs. Racewear that is too tight may also cause AD as a price for improved aerodynamics.

Treatment for AD involves early recognition and intervention to remove the noxious stimulus and pharmacological treatment may be warranted. Untreated severe hypertension can lead to seizures, cerebral hemorrhage and even death. Antihypertensive agents with rapid onset and short duration are recommended. Nifedipine and nitrates are most commonly used. The rapid and reliable action of immediate release-form Nifedipine makes it a good drug for AD, but its adverse effects in able-bodied persons with cardiac disease may make it not readily available.[26] Topical nitrates are widely available and Captopril has also been shown to been effective in a recent pilot study.[27] Nitrates are contraindicated if the athlete has taken Sildenafil (Viagra) or similar agents (Table 10.6).[28]

If a precipitating cause of AD is not determined and the athlete remains symptomatic, check for less frequent causes. The athlete may need hospitalization for treatment of the hypertension and to determine more occult causes. Because of the loss of sensation, athletes with SCI can have significant pathology with minimal symptoms, e.g. acute abdomen or lower limb fracture.

If AD treatment is successful, BP and heart rate will quickly normalize. The athlete should be monitored for 2 h, checking BP and monitoring symptoms, to make sure AD does not recur. You can utilize this time to educate the athlete on further prevention strategies and explain when to seek medical attention if symptoms do recur.

Boosting

As reported earlier, low-grade dysreflexic symptoms can be seen even with proper bladder/bowel management and quality sports medicine care. During training and competition, some tetraplegic wheelchair racers had noticed that the 'dysreflexic state' actually reduced perceived exertion for pushing and faster speeds were achieved.[29] Athletes have been known to voluntarily induce AD before or during an event in an attempt to enhance their performance by clamping off a urinary catheter to produce bladder distention. This procedure, known as 'boosting' is thought to increase BP and thus cardiac output, giving the athlete a competitive advantage. The IPC considers boosting to be unethical and unsafe and athletes are banned from voluntarily inducing this condition during competition. Enforcement is a practical problem. Since AD occurs spontaneously, you would have to prove that the state was intentionally induced. If an athlete shows signs of dysreflexia in a pre-race warm-up area, he or she may be taken out of the competition by the sports medicine staff or competition officials.

Thermoregulation

Box 10.5: Key Points

- The combination of heat, humidity and exercise can pose potential injury for disabled athletes, especially those with spinal injuries.
- Athletes with disabilities are more susceptible to heat accumulation because of decreased sweating ability and vasodilatory responses.
- Optimizing hydration during pre-exercise, competition and post-exercise can reduce dehydration as a leading risk factor for heat illness.

Table 10.6   SCI Consortium Clinical Practice Guidelines[28]

Autonomic dysreflexia

  1 Recognize the signs and symptoms of autonomic dysreflexia

  2 Check the athlete's blood pressure

  Elevation 20-40 mmHg above baseline, adults; 15-20 mmHg adolescents; 15 mmHg children 'typical' blood pressure 90-110 mmHg[a]

  3 If BP elevated, sit athlete up, which may cause an orthostatic decrease in blood pressure, and proceed to identify cause. If BP not elevated and athlete has signs and symptoms of AD, proceed to identify cause[b]

  4 Loosen any constrictive clothing or devices, e.g. straps or tights

  5 Begin quick survey for instigating 'noxious' stimuli. Start with urinary system as bladder distention is most common cause of AD

Bladder management[c]

  1 If athlete does not have an indwelling catheter in place, catheterize[d]

  2 If athlete has an indwelling catheter, check for kinks and correct placement

  If blocked, gently irrigate with a small amount (10-15 ml) of warm saline, avoid pressing on the bladder

  If does not drain, remove and replace catheter

  If drains and BP remains elevated, suspect another cause, e.g. fecal impaction

Bowel management[e]

  If BP >150 mmHg, consider pharmacologic treatment prior to checking for fecal impaction. If fecal impaction is suspected and the elevated BP is <150 mmHg, check the rectum for stool:

  1 With a gloved hand, insert a lubricated finger in to the rectum and instill 2% lidocaine jelly

  2 Wait 2 min, if possible for sensation to decrease

  3 With a gloved hand, insert a lubricated finger into the rectum and check for the presence of stool and gently remove if possible

  4 If AD becomes worse, stop the manual evacuation, instill more lidocaine jelly and retry

[a]Use correct size cuff.
[b]While identifying and eliminating cause, check BP and HR frequently.
[c]Distention most common cause of AD.
[d]Instill 2% lidocaine jelly (if available) into urethra and wait 2 min if possible. *Note:* catheterization itself can exacerbate AD, use clinical judgment.
[e]Distention second most common cause of AD.

Although both extremes of temperature are problematic for athletes with disabilities, much, if not all the research, has been related to hyperthermia, not hypothermia. Hypothermia is a concern for disabled athletes participating in winter sports, e.g. alpine skiing, nordic skiing, and recreational snowmobiling. The combination of heat, humidity and exercise can be dangerous in athletic populations,[29] especially those with spinal injuries. Limiting environmental exposure and monitoring closely for signs and symptoms of heat illness are important for the sports medicine practitioner.

The capacity of an athlete to regulate their body temperature is related to the amount of heat produced in the muscles and to the ability to dissipate that heat to the environment mostly through the skin.[30] Despite decreased active muscle mass and less relative heat production, some athletes with disabilities are still more susceptible to heat accumulation because of decreased sweating ability and decreased vasodilatory responses. This autonomic dysfunction is due to the loss of autonomic nervous control of sweating and skin blood flow below the level of injury.

Price and Campbell[31,32] have studied the thermoregulatory responses in spinal cord injured athletes. In a comparison of able-bodied (AB) and paraplegic athletes (PA), they found that under experimental conditions, both types of athletes were able to handle the thermal strain and that PA were at no greater thermal risk than AB. They found differing degrees of thermal imbalance between the paraplegics and the tetraplegics (TP) during exercise and during recovery, with more positive heat storage in the TP groups.

When they examined the effects of the level of the spinal cord injury upon the thermoregulatory responses of wheelchair athletes during prolonged exercise (60 min) in warm conditions (32°C, 43% relative humidity), one of the most significant findings was that both trained paraplegics and tetraplegics were able to complete the exercise test. Thus, physical training may protect against heat illness.

Recently, Yaggie et al.[33] also found that the sweat characteristics of trained individuals with tetraplegia may improve with increased physical activity and training due to increased secretory activity of sweat glands above the level of injury. Hagobian et al.[34] have reported on positive results with a new cooling device in tetraplegics. They found that the RTX cooling device, which utilizes negative pressure and focuses on the arteriovenous anastomoses contained beneath the heat exchanging surfaces of the hands and feet, attenuated the rise in body temperature in wheelchair (quad) rugby players with spinal cord lesions above T5 after exercising in the heat.

Athletes with cerebral palsy (CP) may also experience thermoregulation concerns. Maltais[35] has shown that when young athletes with CP exercise for 60 min at 35°C and 50% relative humidity, they store excessive body heat due to increased heat production. Bar-Or recommends that CP athletes should have longer rest periods in the shade and adequate hydration during all training and competitions.[36]

Several blind athletes on the US track and field team have albinism, which is the genetic cause of their visual loss. If they also have the cutaneous form of albinism, they are especially susceptible to sun-related exposure due to the lack of skin pigmentation, which can result in severe heat illness. While competing in the 1994 IPC World Athletics Championships in Berlin in July, a US blind middle distance runner required intravenous resuscitation after each of her 1500-m semifinals and finals events. Optimizing hydration during pre-exercise, competition and post-exercise can reduce dehydration as a major modifiable risk factor leading to heat illness. Proper scheduling of events to certain times of the day (distance events in the early morning or toward evening), providing shelters and proper clothing can also reduce risk (Table 10.7).[37]

Venous pooling

As a result of the diminished or absent venous 'muscle pump' in the legs of athletes with SCI, there is decreased venous

Table 10.7   Guidelines for Preventing Heat-Related Injury[37]

Advance preparation	Advance knowledge of the climatic conditions
	Daily posting of the temperature and humidity can serve as an alert to athletes, medical staffs, team managers and coaches
Acclimatization	This requires a high level of fitness and training with maximum acclimatization to exercise in extreme heat can be achieved in about 2 weeks.
	Simulating hot humid environments can be helpful
Recognition of heat illness symptoms and signs	Important to educate athletes about symptoms of heat stress
	There is considerable variability in heat tolerance
	Heat sensitivity among particular athletes needs to be communicated to all staff
Shade and clothing	Outdoor competition should have adjacent tented or shaded facilities
	There should be ready access to drinking water as well as water for wetting exposed body surfaces
	Exercise clothing should be of light color, loose and made of a breathable material
Hydration	Adequate hydration is fundamental and intake should be monitored
	A systematic schedule of fluid intake before, during and after training and events should be maintained
Sports medicine support	Includes environmental protection and ready access to water
	Adequate response capabilities including i.v. hydration and resuscitation may be necessary
	Ready ambulance transport and pre-arranged hospital preparedness

return to the heart. Some wheelchair athletes use abdominal binders and tight stockings to increase lower body positive pressure to induce a re-distribution of blood flow during exercise. This decreases venous capacitance and facilitates venous return. Still the legs can be a source of swelling and result in AD and infrequently a deep vein thrombosis (DVT). A 43-year-old T4 paraplegic member of the United States National Sledge Hockey Team developed subacute onset of right leg swelling while attending an international tournament in Canada.[38] Several days prior to his 10 h bus trip to the competition, he sustained 'incidental' trauma to his right leg resulting in mild swelling. During the competition, he was strapped into his sledge for several 1-h long matches with occasional collisions with other players. His leg became more swollen and he developed spasms. He was withdrawn from the competition and subsequent Doppler ultrasound was interpreted as possible popliteal DVT. He was placed on low-molecular weight heparin and warfarin for the bus ride home. He continued on warfarin without clinical improvement until a repeat ultrasound revealed a calf hematoma and no DVT. The anticoagulation was stopped and the player received therapeutic ultrasound to help mobilize the hematoma with gradual resolution. Alternate diagnoses for lower extremity swelling need to

be considered in the SCI athlete to optimize treatment and avoid iatrogenic complications.

SENSORY DYSFUNCTION

Box 10.6: Key Points

- The lack of sensation can result in pressure ulceration over bony prominences.
- Sensory dysfunction can make both history taking and the physical examination more challenging in the disabled athlete.

The lack of sensory perception can also be of problematic concern for the sports medicine practitioner working with athletes with disabilities. This can be manifested in the development of pressure ulcers, most commonly over bony prominences like the ischial tuberosities or trochanters in SCI athletes. Most elite athletes complete regular pressure relief by unweighting with their upper limbs or shifting position in their wheelchair. In preparation for an event, athletes may be spending more time in their racing chairs where their cushion and seating support system may be inadequate. Some athletes even prefer not to use a cushion while competing. With a proper cushion, pressure relief for the soft tissues can be provided and sports performance not altered. Recent studies have shown that there may be some sensory 'communication' to body areas below the level of neurological injury even in athletes with complete SCI.[39] This may help cue athletes to do pressure relief more consistently.

Insensate skin may have been a factor in two second-degree burns sustained during showering by athletes with SCI who participated in the 1995 US National Wheelchair and Amputee Championships. Athlete accommodations were at college dormitories and it was unclear whether the shower water temperature settings were too high, or rather the athletes may have spent too long in a poorly accessible shower trying to get clean. Physical therapists and athletic trainers must utilize extra caution with the use of heating or icing modalities and provide frequent monitoring.

Sensory dysfunction can also make taking a history and performing a physical examination more challenging in disabled athletes. With underlying osteopenia, athletes with SCI may sustain long bone fractures, even with minor trauma, and 'classical' signs of fracture may be absent.[40] In a research setting, osteopenia of the distal femur and proximal tibia was shown to be partly reversed by the use of Functional Electrical Stimulation (FES)-assisted training.[41]

Blind track and field athletes compete in seemingly risky events such as the javelin, with apparent safety to fellow competitors, coaches and spectators. It is essential that tournament officials are in complete control of the track and field events to avoid injury from any thrown implement or mishaps from crossing the track at the wrong time to gain access to field event competitions. Appropriate staffing is required to guide athletes with vision impairment to be safe at the competition and off-site venues.

UPPER LIMB SYNDROMES

Shoulder

Shoulder pain is extremely common in individuals with SCI and athletes with disabilities who compete in wheelchairs. Multiple studies have reported shoulder pain prevalence of over 50% in individuals with SCI, with pain more common in tetraplegics and in those with complete injuries.[42–44] Because athletes' shoulders are also needed for basic daily functions such as transfers, shoulder pain and impairment have significant functional significance beyond sports participation.

In a study of athletes with various types of disabilities, Bernardi et al.[45] found that shoulder pain was the most common pain experienced in swimming, athletics and wheelchair basketball. The pain either occurred during the sport (training or competition) or as a consequence of physical exercise. The positive finding was that in 71% of cases, the pain lasted less than a week and only 8.7% experienced pain for more than one month (Tables 10.8, 10.9). Curtis and Black have reported on shoulder pain in women wheelchair basketball players.[46] Wheelchair basketball is characterized by intermittent, high-intensity pushing and maneuvering, as well the overhead activities of shooting, passing and rebounding. This might predispose these athletes to increased risk for impingement. They reported

52% of the players experienced shoulder pain. Of note, the highest intensity pain was reported during household chores, wheelchair propulsion on steep ramps or inclines, lifting overhead or while sleeping. Unfortunately, the study results did not provide significant information about the impact of the shoulder pain on training and game performance.

Finley and Rodgers[47] have recently compared shoulder pain in athletes and non-athletes. In studying 52 manual wheelchair users, they found that 61.5% of the subjects reported shoulder pain. A total of 29% had pain at the time of the study and there was an increased incidence of shoulder pain with time. Some 44% had clinical signs of rotator cuff impingement and 50% had signs of biceps tendonitis. They found anterior instability in 28% of those with a painful shoulder. They found no difference in the incidence of shoulder pain, past or present, between athletes and non-athletes. They concluded that sports participation neither increases nor decreases the risk of shoulder pain in the manual wheelchair user.

Wrist

Athletes with disabilities, especially wheelchair users, may often present with wrist pain. This can be from a musculoskeletal injury or entrapment neuropathy.[48] An athlete with an injury at the C6 level has intact wrist extensor muscles with paralysis of the wrist flexor muscles. Because of this forearm muscle imbalance, body weight loads tend to be borne by the wrist joints during transfers.[49] Athletes with CP are at risk for wrist injuries as a result of falls. In running competitions, athletes with more severe spasticity have a tendency to 'unwind' at the end of a sprint and then 'crash' at, or just after the finish line. 'Falling On an OutStretched Hand' (FOOSH) can result in wrist or more proximal upper limb injury. As an example, a female wheelchair shot-putter with history of healed scaphoid fracture fell on a transfer to her throwing chair and was re-injured. She was withdrawn from the competition due to ongoing wrist symptoms and splinted. Her wheelchair mobility remained problematic and a diagnosis of a new fracture was not made until she returned home and underwent more definitive studies (Table 10.10).

Carpal tunnel syndrome (CTS) is the most common neuropathy seen in wheelchair users. The athlete with CTS typically presents with pain and paresthesias in the hand and wrist with activity and at night.[48] Median nerve damage has been attributed to the high-force, high-repetition wrist motions seen during wheelchair propulsion.[50] Boninger and his group were able to show a link between push-rim biomechanics and

Table 10.8   Musculoskeletal Causes of Shoulder Pain in Chronic SCI[42]

Impingement syndrome
Rotator cuff tendonitis and tendinosis
Bicipital tendonitis
Subacromial bursitis
Degenerative joint disease
Instability
Adhesive capsulitis
Myofascial pain syndrome
Osteolysis of the distal clavicle

Table 10.9   Factors Associated with Rotator Cuff Injury in SCI[42]

Extrinsic factors
Primary impingement
Frequent overhead activities
Secondary impingement
Glenohumeral instability
Muscle imbalances
Inflexibility
Upper limb weight bearing
Intrinsic factors
Overuse
Avascularity
Aging

Table 10.10   Musculoskeletal Causes of Wrist Pain[47]

Scaphoid impaction or fracture
Dorsal carpal capsulitis
Scapholunate interosseous ligament disruption
Occult dorsal carpal ganglion
Kienböck disease
Wartenberg syndrome

median nerve function.[51] They suggested that incorporating a smooth low impact stroke would reduce median nerve injury as well as reducing the rolling resistance by individuals losing weight. In a follow-up study, Boninger[52] was able to show a positive correlation between wrist range of motion and median and ulnar nerve function. Contrary to their hypothesis, subjects using a greater range of motion showed better nerve function, using less force and less strokes to propel their wheelchairs at a given speed. Changes to the wheelchair setup, including shortening the vertical distance between the wheelchair axle and the shoulder and a more forward axle position, were correlated with improvements in propulsion biomechanics and may be likely to reduce both shoulder and wrist injury.[53]

Lomond and Wiseman[54] have done an initial analysis of the propulsion techniques in sledge ice hockey which, like wheelchair propulsion, is a bilateral, simultaneous, repetitive motion of the upper limbs (Fig. 10.6). Smoothness of the movement, as a result of timing within the various phases, preparation, propulsion and recovery, may play a role in improving performance and reducing the risk for injury.

PRE-PARTICIPATION EVALUATION AND MANAGEMENT

Box 10.7: Key Points

- Medical history forms should be carefully reviewed to target onsite evaluations or testing.
- Pre-existing structural deformities and muscle imbalances may be directly and kinetically linked to recent or recurrent injuries.
- Return to play guidelines need not be altered for athletes with disabilities.

Jacob and Hutzler[55] describe a Sports-Medical Assessment Protocol (SMAP) for athletes with disability. The purpose of the protocol is to identify medical problems which can interfere with an athlete's performance, identify shortcomings in training and establish sport-specific goals, and to provide a baseline for ongoing follow-up. Many athletes with disabilities do not typically have access to adequate sports medicine resources during training or pre-competition. A sports medicine physician may meet the athletes just prior to an event or competition and there will be limited time to do a full and proper assessment.

As with the able-bodied athletes, the history is an extremely important part of the pre-participation exam.[56] Most event organizers will provide the sports medicine physician with copies of medical history forms completed in advance by the athletes or their primary physicians. These should be reviewed carefully to target additional on-site testing accordingly. Athletes with recent medical issues and those with tetraplegia, on multiple drug regimens for spasticity or epilepsy, should all be evaluated on site. Pre-existing structural deformities and muscle imbalances should be evaluated on all athletes with recent or recurrent injuries. Athletes with CP may have genu valgum and ankle hyperpronation, which can lead to increased biomechanical stress during intense sporting activities.[57] Athletes with short stature (dwarfism) may have postural abnormalities such as lordosis and scoliosis, gait disorders, decreased range of motion and bone deformities. Cervical spine disorders are also common among athletes with short stature. Athletes with tetraplegia, should have their bladder and bowel program reviewed and have baseline BP and heart rate recorded due to increased risk for AD. Lower extremity amputees should have their residual limbs examined for evidence of pressure ulceration due to inadequate suspension of the prosthesis.

Team physicians may be required to make return to competition decisions. Established return to play guidelines should not

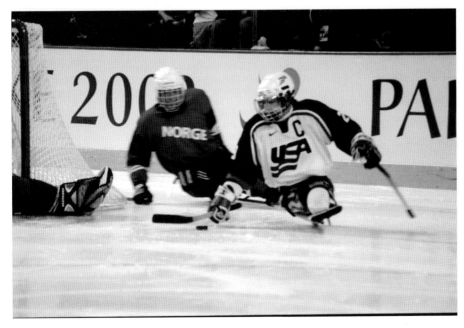

Figure 10.6 Sledge hockey.

require alteration for athletes with disabilities. Physicians may also be asked to render judgment on a particular athlete's level of participation. For example, I was asked to render an opinion of whether a young female swimmer with severe dystonia affecting the muscles of her jaw and neck should be allowed to dive into the pool in her swimming events. The athlete, her parents, her primary physician and coach were well aware of the potential risk to her condition. The athlete was also an experienced competitor and had developed specific techniques to minimize her risk sufficiently to be cleared for full participation.

Depending on the locale for the event or competition providing team members with pre-travel information as a form of prevention is also a recommended strategy. Physicians may need to consult a geographic medicine or infectious disease source to get the latest recommendation regarding immunization, risk and treatment for illnesses, food and air quality. Prevention of hepatitis A, 'traveler's diarrhea' and asthma can improve with athlete and coaching education.

'Having a physical disability is not the same as being disabled. Failing to make that distinction, we leave out the most important ingredient in human achievement, the desire in each of us to strive for the very best we can be. Everyone lives in age of opportunities and technological advances and yet, our most marvelous and moving experiences are still those victories of will and spirit against seemingly insurmountable odds'.

(Jean-Michel Cousteau: Handicapped Scuba Association)

REFERENCES

1 Nichols AW. Sports medicine and the Americans with Disabilities Act. Clin J Sports Med 1996; 6:190–195.

2 The Standard Rules on the Equalization of Opportunities for Persons with Disabilities. Adopted by the United Nations General Assembly, 48 Session, Resolution 48/96, annex, 20 December, 1993.

3 The European Union Disability Strategy. EU Commission on employment and social affairs, disability issues. Online. Available: http://europa.eu.int/comm/employment_social/disability/strategy_en.html

4 WHO. Towards a common language for functioning, disability and health, ICF. Geneva: WHO; 2002.

5 Heneban M, Shiple B, Coppola G. Nonsurgical sports medicine training in the US. A survey of sports medicine fellowship graduates. Clin J Sports Med 2003; 13:285–291.

6 International Paralympic Committee 2002. Online. Available: http://www.paralympic.org

7 Webborn ADJ. Fifty years of competitive sport for athletes with disabilities: 1948–1998. Br J Sports Med 1999; 33:138–139.

8 International Paralympic Committee. Paralympian 2004; 3.

9 Crandell DM. The development of a new Paralympic ice hockey program. VISTA Conference, Bollnäs, Sweden, 11–14 September 2003.

10 ESPN. Bristol, CT.

11 Nunn CJ. Coaching for Paralympic Gold. Experiences and future implications. VISTA Conference, Bollnäs, Sweden, 11–14 September 2003.

12 Heubner C. Malone LA. The Paralympic Academy: a national health promotion initiative for children with disabilities. VISTA Conference, Bollnäs, Sweden, 11–14 September 2003.

13 Lindstrom H. Doping Disables. ICSSPE Bull 2002; 35:34.

14 International Paralympic Committee. Anti-doping code, IPC Handbook. International Paralympic Committee; 2004.

15 Hedmon B. Classification in Paralympic sports. VISTA Conference, Bollnäs, Sweden, 11–14 September 2003.

16 Ferrara MS, Palutis GR, David RW. A longitudinal study of injuries to athletes with disabilities. Int J Sports Med 2000; 21:221–224.

17 Ferrara MS, Peterson CL. Injuries to athletes with disabilities; identifying injury patterns. Sports Med 2000; 30(2):137–143.

18 Crandell DM. Unpublished report. National wheelchair and amputee championships, 1995. Mexico City: US Team, Pan-Am Paralympic Games; 1999.

19 Hutzler Y, Felis O. Computerized search of scientific literature on sport for disabled persons. Percep Mot Skills 1999; 88:1189–1192.

20 Colliton J. Helmet use in disabled athletes. Safety in Disabled Athletes. Washington, DC: ASTM; 2004.

21 Silver JR. The history of Guttmann's and Whitteridge's discovery of autonomic dysreflexia. Spinal Cord 2000; 38:581–596.

22 Blackmer J. Rehabilitation medicine: 1. Autonomic dysreflexia. CMAJ 2003; 9:931–935.

23 Helkowski WM, Ditunno JF, Boininger M. Autonomic dysreflexia: incidence in persons with neurologically complete and incomplete tetraplegia. J Spin Cord Med 2003; 26:244–247.

24 Gao SA, Ambring A, Lambert G, Karlsson AK. Autonomic control of the heart and renal vascular bed during autonomic dysreflexia in high spinal cord injury. Clin Autom Res 2002; 12:457–464.

25 McGinnis KB, Vogel LC, McDonald CM, et al. Recognition and management of AD in pediatric SCI. J Spin Cord Med 2004; 27:61–74.

26 Frost F. Antihypertensive therapy, nifedipine and autonomic dysreflexia. Arch Phys Med Rehabil 2002; 83:1325–1326.

27 Esmail Z, Shalansky KF, Sunderji R, et al. Evaluation of captopril for the management of hypertension in autonomic dysreflexia: a pilot study. Arch Phys Med Rehabil 2002; 83:604–608.

28 Consortium for Spinal Cord Medicine. Acute management of autonomic dysreflexia: individuals with spinal cord injury presenting to health-care facilities. J Spin Cord Med 2002; 25(Suppl 1):67–88.

29 Webborn AD. 'Boosting' performance in disability sport. Br J Sports Med 1999; 33:74.

30 Coris EE, Ramirez AM, Van Durme DJ. Heat illness in athletes. The dangerous combination of heat, humidity and exercise. Sports Med 2004; 34:9–16.

31 Price MJ, Campbell IG. Thermoregulatory responses of spinal cord injured and able-bodied athletes to prolonged upper body exercise and recovery. Spinal Cord 1999; 37:772–779.

32 Price MJ, Campbell IG. Effects of spinal cord lesion level upon thermoregulation during exercise in the heat. Med Sci Sports Exerc 2003; 35:1100–1107.

33 Yaggie JA, Niemi TJ, Buono MJ. Adaptive sweat gland response after spinal cord injury. Arch Phys Med Rehabil 2002; 83:802–805.

34 Hagobian TA, Jacobs KA, Kiratli BJ, Friedlander AL. Foot cooling reduces exercise-induced hyperthermia in men with spinal cord injury. Med Sci Sports Exerc 2004; 36:411–417.

35 Maltais D. Thermoregulation in CP athletes. Unpublished thesis presented by O Bar-Or. VISTA Conference, Bollnäs, Sweden, 11–14 September 2003.

36 Bar-Or O. Physiologic responses to exercise with children and youths with a physical disability. CP athletes exercise in heat. Unpublished thesis by Maltais D. VISTA Conference, Bollnäs, Sweden, 11–14 September 2003.

37 McCann BC. Thermoregulation in spinal cord injury: the challenge of the Atlanta Paralympics. Spinal Cord 1996; 34:433–436.

38 Crandell D. When a DVT is not a DVT: atypical leg swelling in spinal cord injury: A case report and review. Am J PM&R 1999; 78:193.

39 Finnerup NB, Glydensted C, Fuglsang-Frederiksen A, Bach FW, Jensen TW. Sensory perception in complete spinal cord injury. Acta Neurol Scand 2004; 109:194–199.

40 Bruin ED de, Dietz V, Dambacher MA, Stussi E. Longitudinal changes in bone in men with spinal cord injury. Clin Rehabil 2000; 14:145–152.

41 Belanger M, Stein RB, Wheeler GD, Gordon T, Leduc B. Electrical stimulation: can it increase muscle strength and reverse osteopenia in spinal cord injured individuals? Arch Phys Med Rehabil 2000; 81:1090–1098.

42 Dyson-Hudson TA, Kirshblum SC. Shoulder pain in chronic spinal cord injury, Part I: Epidemiology, etiology, and pathomechanics. J Spin Cord Med 2004; 27:4–17.

43 Dalyan M, Cardenas DD, Gerard B. Upper extremity pain in spinal cord injury. Spinal Cord 1999; 37:191–195.

44 Mayer F, Bilow H, Orstmann T, et al. Muscular fatigue, a maximum strength and stress reactions of the shoulder musculature in paraplegics. Int J Sports Med 1999; 20:487–493.

45 Bernardi M, Castellano V, Ferrara MS, et al. Muscle pain in athletes with locomotor disability. Med Sci Sports Exer 2003; 35:199–206.

46 Curtis KA, Black K. Shoulder pain in female wheelchair basketball players. J Orthop Sport Phys Ther 1999; 29:225–231.

47 Finley MA, Rodgers MMJ. Prevalence and identification of shoulder pathology in athletic and non-athletic wheelchair users with shoulder pain: A pilot study. J Rehabil Res Dev May 2004; 41:395–402.

48 Groah S, Lanig IS. Neuromuscular syndromes in wheelchair athletes. Semin Neurol 2000; 20:201–208.

49 Hara Y. Dorsal wrist pain in tetraplegic patients during and after rehabilitation. J Rehabil Med Mar 2003; 35:57–61.

50 Vanlandewijck Y, Theisen D, Daly D. Wheelchair propulsion biomechanics. Implications for wheelchair sports. Sports Med 2001; 31:339–367.

51 Boninger ML, Cooper RA, Baldwin MA, Shimada SD, Koontz A. Wheelchair pushrim kinetics: body weight and median nerve function. Arch Phys Med Rehabil 1999; 80:91–115.

52 Boninger ML, Impink BG, Cooper RA, Koontz A. Relation between median and ulnar nerve function and wrist kinematics during wheelchair propulsion. Arch Phys Med Rehabil 2004; 85:1141–1145.

53 Boninger ML, Baldwin M, Cooper RA, Koontz A. Manual wheelchair biomechanics and axle position. Arch Phys Med Rehabil 2000; 81:608–613.

54 Lomond K, Wiseman R. Sledge hockey mechanics take toll on shoulders. Biomech 2003; Aug:71–76.

55 Jacob T, Hutzler Y. Sports-medical assessment for athletes with disability. Disabil Rehab 1998; 20:116–119.

56 Dec KL, Sparrow KJ, McKeag DB. The physically-challenged athlete: medical issues and assessment. Sports Med 2000; 29:1612–1642.

57 Rimmer JH. Physical fitness levels of persons with cerebral palsy. Dev Med Child Neurol 2001; 43:208–212.

CHAPTER 11

Special Considerations for Patients with Chronic Illness or Disease

Wayne E. Derman

INTRODUCTION

Chronic illness including chronic diseases of lifestyle will sadly affect most human beings at some point in their lifetime. Indeed, the burden of chronic illness and disability has a large global impact on health resources both with respect to financial and resource demand. Over the past 10 years, it has become apparent that chronic physical activity in the form of exercise training has not only the ability to prevent or delay the onset of illness and disease (primary prevention) but also forms an important part of the management of such illness (secondary prevention). The chronic medical conditions where exercise has been shown to be of benefit are listed in Table 11.1.[1]

With the advent of the data supporting physical activity in the management of chronic illness and the subsequent publication of official position stands and statements by numerous professional bodies advocating the use of physical exercise in the management strategies, so the growth of professionals in

the field of exercise science and sports medicine has occurred. Thus globally, sports physicians, physical therapists, biokineticists, exercise physiologists and athletic trainers have embraced this domain of intervention and from many postgraduate training programs have emerged teaching specific techniques and approaches to chronic illness management. Indeed, in many countries some aspects of exercise and positive lifestyle interventions have been included in the undergraduate training of primary care doctors.

While in-depth discussion and guidelines for exercise rehabilitation are beyond the scope of this chapter, the reader with an interest in this topic is referred to more detailed publications on this topic including *'ACSM's guidelines for exercise training for patients with chronic diseases and disabilities'* and available Position Statements from authoritative bodies.[2-6] The aim of this chapter is to outline some of the more common chronic illnesses where exercise plays an important role in the intervention and to advise the reader of how to formulate an exercise program for such patients, and provide some practical guidelines for exercise prescription and monitoring of such patients.

Table 11.1 Exercise in the Prevention and Management of Chronic Disease States

Exercise Aids in Prevention	Exercise Helps in Management
Coronary artery disease	Coronary artery disease
Hypertension	Heart failure
Obesity	Hypertension
Stroke	Obesity
Diabetes (Type I)	Diabetes (Type I)
Breast cancer	Diabetes (Type II)
Ovarian cancer	Osteoporosis
Cervical cancer	Rheumatoid arthritis
Colon cancer	Osteoarthritis
Osteoporosis	Depression
Depression	Pulmonary disease
Lower back pain	Lower back pain
	Chronic renal failure
	Acquired Immune Deficiency Syndrome
	Chronic fatigue syndrome and fibromyalgia

PATIENT ASSESSMENT, DEVELOPMENT OF A REHABILITATION PROGRAM AND PATIENT MONITORING

Box 11.1: Key Points

- Most patients with chronic disease should undertake some form of physical exercise.
- This exercise should take the form of an exercise prescription, detailing the intensity, duration, frequency and type of exercise.
- Patient evaluation and exercise prescription should follow a six step process.

As outlined above it is evident that many patients with chronic disease should undertake regular physical exercise instead of prolonged bed rest. Indeed, there are truly very few contraindications to participation in some form of regular physical exercise. However, prescribing exercise for patients with chronic disease can be very complex. The objective is to decrease physiological limitations and improve physical capacity through specific exercise therapy. The major dilemmas are not in determining which exercise therapies to use but in defining goals and choosing the appropriate training intensity, duration and frequency. It is important that the practitioner administers the appropriate exercise prescription for each disease and disability.

When considering the formulation of an exercise prescription for patients with chronic disease, one often has very little data on which to base decisions. Furthermore, restoring and maintaining functional capacity are very different goals from the prevention of disease. Unfortunately, exercise training to optimize functional capacity has not been well studied in the context of many chronic diseases and disabilities and as a result, many exercise professionals have used clinical experience to develop their own methods for prescribing exercise. Experience is an acceptable way to formulate an exercise prescription but a systematic approach would be better. Prescribing the correct dose of exercise is important as patients can suddenly become worn out, often by small amounts of exercise.

There are six practical steps to providing rehabilitation services and exercise prescriptions for any patient, regardless of the specific chronic disease: These are listed in Table 11.2.

Important considerations under each of these points will now be described.

Step 1: Take the patient history

- Uncover the nature of the problem as it relates to exercise. With regard to functional limitations, symptoms might include chest pain or palpitations during exercise, fatigue, shortness of breath, weakness, lower back pain, etc.
- Enquire about recent and past musculoskeletal injuries.
- Enquire about the patient's risk factors for both primary and secondary disease. A good rehabilitation program should incorporate risk reduction strategies, e.g. smoking cessation programs and management strategies for adverse blood lipid or homocysteine concentrations.
- Enquire about all medications and the doses of these medications. Many medications have the potential to interfere with the exercise prescription.

Table 11.2 Six Practical Steps to Providing Rehabilitation Services for Patients with Chronic Disease

1	Take a good history
2	Select an exercise test to gather objective data
3	Considerations when making an assessment
4	Developing an exercise program
5	Monitoring
6	Follow-up

- Enquire as to how the patient views exercise: What type of exercise does the patient desire to do? Has the patient attempted exercise training before? Was this successful? What were the reasons for previous non-compliance?
- Enquire as to the patient's access to exercise training facilities and formal rehabilitation programs.

Step 2: Select the appropriate exercise tests

- Select the group of exercise tests that is going to provide insight into the medical problem.
- Use modes and protocols of exercise testing that can be individualized.
- Use tests that will provide specific measures that either will further define the problem or determine specific aspects of the exercise program.
- Be aware of concomitant conditions and any specific circumstances, for example, a patient with pulmonary disease might also have severe osteoarthritis of the hip and be unable to walk on a treadmill.
- Specific exercise tests for cardiorespiratory endurance, muscle strength, muscle endurance, flexibility, coordination, proprioception and functional capacity during activities of daily living are outlined in the *ACSM's Guidelines for Exercise Testing and Prescription*.[7]

Step 3: Formulate the test results into an exercise prescription

- The exercise tests will have revealed the patient's functional limitations and will indicate where the practitioner should concentrate their efforts in rehabilitation.
- Select the groups and modes of exercises that best will treat the functional incapacity.
- The most important consideration is that the exercise program should be individualized to the patient's limitations and desires.
- Select goals that are realistically attainable to increase the chance of success.
- Start low and go slow! For example, for a patient in cardiac failure, the exercise stimulus might take the form of 20–30 s low-level aerobic exercise bouts separated by 3 min rest periods.
- Adjust exercise doses on the basis of exercise test measures, perceived exertion, intensity and fatigue threshold.
- Recommend frequency of training based on total exercise dosage and the adaptability of the patient.
- Consider the need for any need for prosthetic, orthotic or other assistive devices.
- Consider the potential interaction of the exercise and medications.

Step 4: Patient education and additional services

- Compliance with a rehabilitation program is improved in well informed and educated patients. Indeed, nearly all of the Position Statements referenced in this chapter advocate the implementation of educational programs and ancillary services in the form of dietary, psychological and other forms of counseling in the setting of an exercise rehabilitation program. Our education program includes aspects of normal anatomy and physiology, pathophysiology of the chronic diseases, medications and medication-exercise interactions, monitoring and self monitoring during rehabilitation.

Step 5: Patient monitoring

- Higher risk patients are generally monitored more intensely and frequently than low-risk patients.
- As the exercise specialist becomes more familiar with the individual patient, the nature of the required monitoring will become apparent.
- Be aware of a sudden onset of exhaustion as well as insufficient recovery and overtraining.
- Monitor stability of underlying medical problems and changes in medications.
- When in doubt about safety, if an activity causes discomfort, avoid it.
- When in doubt about progression, increase in very small increments.
- Do not encourage competition in the rehabilitation setting.

Step 6: Patient feedback and follow-up

- Patient follow-up should be at regular intervals where feedback is given to the patient regarding their progress or lack thereof. It is important to consider that some chronic conditions take a long time to respond to exercise training and indeed, in many patients the improvements are not witnessed in the form of improved exercise test parameters but in improved quality of life measures.
- Always follow-up on unresolved problems: most interventions take weeks or months to achieve benefit, and it is important that both the patient and the exercise specialist are patient.

Rehabilitation in patients with chronic cardiovascular, pulmonary and metabolic disorders are perhaps the most common and relatively well researched forms of exercise interventions, and therefore the remainder of this chapter will focus on those entities.

EXERCISE REHABILITATION PROGRAMS

Box 11.2: Key Points

- Exercise rehabilitation programs vary greatly.
- The optimal form of rehabilitation service provision is with the help of a multidisciplinary team.
- Due to high prevalence of co-morbidities, rehabilitation should focus on chronic disease rehabilitation rather than rehabilitation of only the primary illness.

Exercise rehabilitation programs throughout the world take on many different forms dependent on the demand for rehabilitation services, the expertise of the practitioners involved, refer-

ral patterns, available facilities and the socioeconomic status of the country, patients and practitioners. Thus, rehabilitation may be presented in the form of one-on-one training in an outdoor field setting, or may be presented in a complete multidisciplinary program. Therefore the programs need to be customized.

The authors have recently conducted an assessment of the clinical profiles of the patients enrolled in the cardiac rehabilitation program at the Sport Science Institute of South Africa. This study involved 275 patients enrolled in the program during 1996–1998. The findings of this descriptive study are shown in Figure 11.1.

The results of this study indicate that only 40% of patients in cardiac rehabilitation programs have cardiac pathology only, indeed, most patients have either an accompanying musculoskeletal injury or other chronic disease state that would require a modification of the routine exercise prescription.

Focus of cardiac rehabilitation programs should therefore be shifted to rehabilitation of patients with multiple chronic diseases and this has indeed become a modern trend in service provision. This would require the employment of appropriately skilled staff who are also able to prescribe exercise to patients with chronic musculoskeletal injury.

The findings of this study also indicate that the determination of cost saving of exercise rehabilitation in cardiac patients has in the past been underestimated, as the savings to finance 'spending' in areas other than cardiac consultations, medications and interventions has not been included. Images from our Chronic Disease Rehabilitation can be seen in Figure 11.2.

EXERCISE IN THE MANAGEMENT OF CARDIOVASCULAR AND CEREBROVASCULAR DISEASE

Cardiovascular disease

Cardiac rehabilitation services are comprehensive programs designed to limit the physiological and psychological effects of cardiovascular disease, control cardiac symptoms and reduce

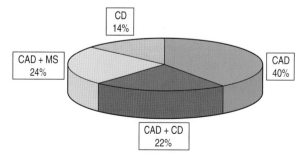

CAD = coronary artery disease only
CD = chronic disease other than CAD
MS = musculoskeletal condition requiring rehabilitation

Figure 11.1 Clinical profiles of patients enrolled into the Cardiac Rehabilitation Program of the Sports Science Institute of South Africa. CAD, coronary artery disease only; CD, chronic disease other than CAD; MS, musculoskeletal condition requiring rehabilitation.

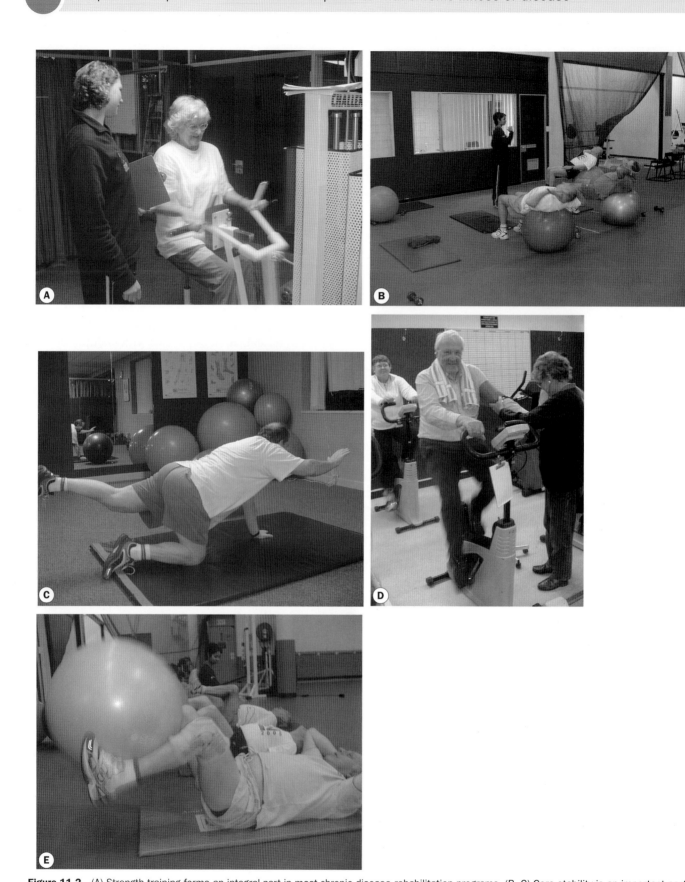

Figure 11.2   (A) Strength training forms an integral part in most chronic disease rehabilitation programs. (B, C) Core stability is an important part of physical fitness in patients with chronic disease. (D) Patient monitoring is important not only for patient safety, but also enhances compliance. (E) Many patients with chronic disease have orthopedic limitations to their participation, and rehabilitation must therefore include adaptation and specific rehabilitation of these conditions. The patient in (E) not only has cardiac disease, but also has osteoarthritis of the knee.

the risk of subsequent events by stabilizing or partially reversing the underlying atherosclerosis process through risk factor modification.[8]

A rehabilitation program may include patients who have had coronary artery disease, myocardial infarction, heart failure, bypass surgery, pacemaker implantation, cardiac transplantation, valve replacement, coronary angioplasty with or without stent placement, or who have other evidence of cardiovascular disease (including a positive stress test), angina pectoris or other evidence of disease from a radionuclide study or coronary catheterization.

Because there is diversity in the clinical spectrum of patients, there is as great diversity encountered in the rehabilitative needs of these patients.

Core components of cardiac rehabilitation programs

Recently, the American Heart Association and the American Association of Cardiovascular and Pulmonary Rehabilitation published a scientific statement regarding the core components of rehabilitation programs.[9] The statement recognizes that all rehabilitation programs should contain core components that aim to optimize cardiovascular risk reduction, reduce disability and foster healthy behaviors, including promotion of an active lifestyle for patients. Furthermore, the statement outlines the evaluation, interventions, and expected outcomes with respect to the core components of the programs listed in Table 11.3.

Current practice

In the last three decades, advances in the management of acute myocardial infarction, specifically the application of coronary thrombolysis with and without subsequent coronary angioplasty and stenting or coronary bypass surgery has led to a different pathophysiologic severity of the acute illness.

There is less myocardial necrosis, less residual ischemia and less resultant myocardial dysfunction. The patient has less disability, a greater chance of survival and a lower risk of early recurrent cardiac events. Therefore exercise rehabilitation can be initiated earlier and often at higher intensity. However, due to low post-infarction mortality and morbidity, it makes it difficult to demonstrate short-term survival or re-infarction benefits. Thus improvement in functional capacity and quality of life are increasingly considered as an important outcome measure for cardiac rehabilitation.

Physiological and health benefits of cardiovascular rehabilitation

Cardiovascular rehabilitation can be divided into early (Phase I) and later (Phase II and III) rehabilitation. If no contraindications to mild exercise exist, namely, stable cardiac parameters, absence of chest discomfort, cardiac failure, arrhythmias and dyspnea, rehabilitation can be initiated as soon as 48 h after the cardiac event or intervention procedure has occurred.

Rehabilitation in this phase is in the form of range-of-motion exercises, intermittent standing or sitting and walking. This phase of rehabilitation is usually conducted by a physiotherapist, exercise physiologist, or cardiac sister.

The benefits of early rehabilitation and mobilization for cardiac patients are listed in Table 11.4.

The benefits of chronic exercise training and participation in formal rehabilitation programs have been outlined in detail in various position statements and practice guidelines and are summarized in Table 11.5.[10–12]

It is thus clear that comprehensive cardiac rehabilitation seems to be successful with respect to: improvement in exercise tolerance, improvement in symptoms of cardiovascular disease, decreased cardiac arrhythmias, improvement in blood lipid concentrations, reduced blood pressure, improvement in insulin resistance and glucose intolerance, and reduced endothelial dysfunction of the coronary arteries.[12–15] Furthermore, reduction in cigarette smoking, reduced obesity, improvement in psychosocial well-being and reduction of stress/anxiety and a reduction in patient mortality and morbidity seem to be important patient benefits.[16–18] The magnitude of the effect of exercise training seems to be influenced by the nature of the exercise intervention, individual patient variation and whether the patient reduces body weight or alters body composition.

Table 11.3 Core Components of Cardiovascular and Pulmonary Rehabilitation Programs

Patient assessment
Nutritional counseling
Lipid management
Hypertension management
Smoking cessation
Weight management
Diabetes management
Psychosocial management
Physical activity counseling
Exercise training

Table 11.4 Benefits of Early Mobilization and Rehabilitation

Prevention of the detrimental effects of prolonged bed rest, namely:
decreased cardiorespiratory fitness
decreased blood volume
decreased red blood cell count
negative nitrogen and protein balance
decreased strength and flexibility
orthostatic hypotension
risk of thromboembolism
In those patients who have undergone coronary artery bypass grafting (CABG), physical activity decreases post-surgical stiffness and prevents complications of post-surgical atelectasis
Prevention of general de-conditioning
Promotion of psychological well-being
Decrease in incidence and severity of depression and anxiety
Provision of spiritual comfort
Decrease in length of hospital stay
Increased awareness of cardiac disease information and modes available for lifestyle alteration

Table 11.5 Summary of Evidence for Cardiac Rehabilitation Outcomes: Effects of Exercise Training

Outcome Measures	Strength of Evidence
Exercise tolerance	A
Exercise tolerance (strength training)	B
Exercise habits	B
Symptoms	B
Smoking	B
Lipids	B
Body weight	C
Blood pressure	B
Psychological well-being	B
Social adjustment and functioning	B
Return to work	A
Morbidity	A
Mortality	B
Pathophysiologic measures:	
Changes in atherosclerosis	A/B
Changes in hemodynamic measurements	B
Changes in myocardial ischemia	B
Changes in myocardial contractility, ejection fraction, and ventricular wall motion abnormalities	B
Heart failure patients	A
Cardiac transplantation patients	B
Elderly patients	B

Strength of evidence codes

A   Scientific evidence from well-designed and well-conducted controlled trials (randomized and non-randomized) provides statistically significant results that consistently support the guideline statement.

B   Scientific evidence is provided by observational studies or by controlled trials with less consistent results.

C   Guideline statements supported by expert opinion; the available scientific evidence did not present consistent results or controlled trials were lacking.

Adapted from Wenger et al. 1995.[11]

Practical recommendations for exercise training in patients with coronary artery disease

- Exercise training programs should be individualized and based on the patient's initial test of functional capacity.
- Tests of functional capacity should include an exercise stress electrocardiogram and a 6-min walk test.
- Exercise programming should include cardiovascular endurance, muscle strength, muscle endurance, flexibility and core stability exercises. The program should consist of a warm-up session, exercise training session and cool down.
- The patient's body composition and anthropometry should be measured before embarking on the program.
- Initiate the program at low level exercise and build up slowly as tolerated in single MET increments.
- Low-fit patients (functional capacity 5 METs) can often train at 40–50% VO_2 peak. However, 70% of VO_2 peak is appropriate for most low-moderate risk patients.
- Monitor patients at each exercise session for abnormal signs and symptoms including chest pain or pressure, dizzi-

ness and arrhythmias. Telemetry monitoring can be used on higher risk patients.

- High-intensity exercise may precipitate cardiovascular complications in post-myocardial infarction (MI) patients. Reserve high-intensity exercise for stable low-risk fit patients.
- Keep log books with a patient's attendance, medication changes, exercise frequency, intensity and duration, as well as recordable cardiovascular measurements. This alerts the practitioner to developing trends and enhances patient compliance.
- Medical supervision is suggested for moderate-to-high-risk patients, e.g. those with exercise-induced myocardial ischemia with possible ST-segment depression and/or angina pectoris and those with left ventricular ejection fraction <30%.
- Patients should be encouraged to exercise for at least 30 min on most days of the week.

Exercise rehabilitation in patients with hypertension

Hypertension is defined by the WHO as a sustained resting blood pressure above 140/90 mmHg (systolic/diastolic). Approximately 17% of the adult Westernized population suffers from this disease. In most cases (>90%) the cause is unknown and this is referred to as essential or primary hypertension. Untreated hypertension is associated with an increased risk of cerebrovascular disease (strokes), heart failure, kidney disease, and coronary artery disease. The importance of treating hypertension has been well established, particularly in reducing the risk of developing cerebrovascular disease. However, there is less evidence that treating the hypertension with drugs reduces the risk of developing coronary artery disease. This may be due to the negative effects that some antihypertensive agents have on other risk factors for coronary artery disease, including the lipid profile.

Regular exercise may also prevent the development of hypertension, and is useful in the treatment of hypertension.[19]

The benefits of regular exercise in hypertensive patients

Box 11.3: Key Points

- Exercise training provides substantial benefits with respect to symptom alleviation, improvement in risk factor profile and enhanced functional capacity in patients with chronic cardiovascular disease.
- Exercise training is beneficial in patients with controlled heart failure.
- Exercise training is effective in reducing both systolic and diastolic blood pressure in hypertensive patients through effects on numerous physiological systems.

Regular exercise has been shown to reduce the systolic blood pressure by an average of 7.4 mmHg and the diastolic blood pressure by an average of 5.8 mmHg in hypertensive patients.[20,21]

The effects of regular exercise appear to be more pronounced in certain sub-groups: (1) females, (2) patients with higher diastolic blood pressure, (3) patients with lower body weight, (4) patients who perform less strenuous exercise, and (5) patients who have made a long-term commitment to participate in regular exercise. Regular exercise is thus an essential adjunct to the non-pharmacological and the pharmacological management of hypertension, and may offset some of the negative effects that some anti-hypertensive medications may have on risk factors for coronary artery disease including lipoprotein metabolism. Patients should be followed-up on a regular basis as it is possible that antihypertensive medication may be reduced once the patient has become conditioned.

Mechanisms of blood pressure reduction through exercise in patients with hypertension

The mechanisms whereby regular exercise reduces blood pressure in hypertensive patients include neurohumoral, vascular and structural adaptations. Decreased circulation catecholamine concentrations, decreased total peripheral resistance, improved insulin sensitivity and alterations in vasodilators and vasoconstrictors as well as genetic factors are thought to explain the anti-hypertensive effects of exercise.[5]

Exercise prescription in hypertensive patients:

The first step in prescribing exercise to hypertensive patients is to ensure that the exercise is safe. It is recommended that the following subsets of patients undergo a medical evaluation (including a stress electrocardiogram, ECG) before embarking on an exercise program.

- males older than 45 years
- females older than 55 years
- any person with hypertension and another risk factor for coronary artery disease
- any person with hypertension who has symptoms suggestive of cardiopulmonary disease, metabolic disease or other major disease.

The second step is to educate patients with respect to aspects of safe exercise, in particular the symptoms and signs of an impending cardiac complication (chest pain, excessive shortness of breath, palpitations and dizziness).

The third step is to provide the patient with clear guidelines on the type, frequency, intensity and duration of exercise. Patients with no cardiac complications can exercise on their own, but patients with known heart disease (or other major disease) may require supervision as mentioned above.

The following exercise guidelines are currently recommended for patients with hypertension:

- *Type of exercise*: this should be predominantly endurance physical activity, including walking, jogging, cycling, swimming or dancing. This should be supplemented by resistance exercise which can be prescribed according to the ACSM or AHA guidelines[6]
- *Frequency of exercise*: most or preferably all days of the week
- *Intensity of exercise*: moderate intensity 40–60% of VO_2 peak

- *Duration of exercise*: more than 30 min continuous or accumulated moderate physical activity per day.

Anti-hypertensive medication and exercise

Anti-hypertensive medication, in particular non-selective and beta 1-selective beta-blockers decreases exercise tolerance. In active individuals who are also hypertensive, these drugs may not be ideal. Angiotensin converting enzyme (ACE) inhibitors, angiotensin II receptor blockers and calcium channel blockers may be better suited for these patients or athletes with hypertension.

Practical recommendations for exercise training in patients with hypertension

- Patients with uncontrolled hypertension should embark on exercise training only after evaluation and initiation of therapy. Patients should not exercise if resting systolic BP is 200 mmHg or diastolic BP >115 mmHg.
- Many patients with hypertension are overweight and should therefore be encouraged to follow a program that combines both exercise training and restricted calorie intake.[22]
- Beta-blockers and diuretics alter thermoregulation in hot environments and may provoke hypoglycemia. Patients using these medications should be educated with regard to exercising in the heat, clothing, the role of adequate hydration and methods to prevent hypoglycemia.[23,24]
- Vasodilators, calcium channel blockers and alpha blockers may cause hypotensive episodes on rapid cessation of exercise. A longer cool down period is therefore recommended.

Exercise training in patients with heart failure

Heart failure is defined as the condition in which abnormality of myocardial function is responsible for the ventricles' inability to deliver adequate quantities of blood to the metabolizing tissues at rest or during normal activity. The most common cause of heart failure is loss of cardiac muscle, secondary to ischemia on the basis of coronary artery disease. Viral and other cardiomyopathies are more common in younger patients. Heart failure can also occur in persons with poorly controlled blood pressure or with valvular heart disease.

Of the many symptoms experienced by patients with heart failure, dyspnea, fatigue and exercise intolerance are among the most common. The first indication of heart failure is a diminished tolerance to physical exercise. Functional capacity in patients with chronic heart failure is measured in terms of the four-tiered classification of breathlessness, which is subjective and only semi-quantitative. Only recently has exercise testing become more popular for the determination of functional capacity in patients with heart failure. Factors thought to limit exercise tolerance in patients with heart failure are listed in Table 11.6.

The role of exercise rehabilitation in patients with heart failure

A number of recent studies have assessed the role of exercise training in the management of patients with heart failure. Studies have varied in intensity, duration and frequency of the training stimulus; however, the majority of studies indicate

Table 11.6 Factors Thought to Limit Exercise Tolerance in Patients with Heart Failure

Cardiovascular factors
    Left ventricular systolic function altered
    Reduced cardiac output at rest and during exercise
    Impaired intrinsic contractility
    Elevated systemic vascular resistance
        Increased sympathetic activity
        Increased activity of the renin–angiotensin system
        Blunted peripheral arterial vasodilator response
    Myocardial ischemia (in some individuals)
    Mitral valve regurgitation (in some individuals)
    Altered distribution of cardiac output
    Altered pulmonary hemodynamics
Peripheral factors
    Abnormalities in blood flow
        Endothelial dysfunction
        Increased vascular stiffness
        Thickened capillary basement membranes
        Increased concentrations of endothelin
    Skeletal muscle abnormalities
        Structural skeletal muscle abnormalities
        Metabolic skeletal muscle abnormalities
    Abnormal ergoreflex activation
        From skeletal muscle
        From diaphragmatic muscle
    Increased concentrations of tumor necrosing factor alpha
Medication effects
Physical de-conditioning
Aging

that most patients demonstrate an improvement in functional capacity, increased duration of exercise and increased peak VO_2.[25] Only one study to date has noted worsening of ventricular ejection fraction in patients recovering from Q-wave anterior wall infarction randomized to exercise training compared with non-exercising controls.[26]

Physiological adaptations seen through exercise training include improvements in catecholamine concentrations; enhanced vagal control of heart rate variability; improvement in ventilatory mechanics and diaphragmatic function; decreased perceived dyspnea; improved endothelial function, blood flow and metabolism of skeletal muscles; improvement in myocardial and coronary vessel adaptations; improved stroke volume, cardiac output and peak ventricular filling rate.[27–30]

To date, large-scale randomized trials evaluating exercise training effects on patient survival rates have not been conducted and the results of such studies are keenly awaited. However, most (but not all) studies evaluating the effects of regular exercise training on quality of life indices in patients with stable heart failure have shown promising results.[31]

Practical recommendations for exercise training in patients with heart failure

- Use an individualized approach and be prepared to start at very low workloads after a long warm-up period.

- Interval training appears to be an effective form of cardiovascular endurance training. For example, some patients may only be able to manage an initial cycle workload of 15 W for a 20-s interval followed by a 2-min rest period. The exercise stimulus can be progressed by decreasing rest periods, increasing cycling intensity and finally increasing workload.
- Due to high use of beta-blockers in this patient population, both heart rate and ratings of perceived exertion should be monitored.
- For high risk patients, telemetry monitoring is recommended.
- Home-based programs may be suitable for selected stable and well-medicated, low-risk patients with heart failure.
- Patients should not exercise if they have uncontrolled edema, lung crackles and dyspnea, or new onset arrhythmias.
- Resistance training in the form of small free weights, elastic bands or circuit weight training can be prescribed in low-risk patients.

Exercise training for patients with peripheral vascular disease

Patients with peripheral vascular disease have a reduced exercise tolerance and walking distance due to calf claudication. Exercise training is an effective first line management for these patients. Indeed, patients with peripheral vascular disease have been able to increase their maximal walking distance by 122% and pain-free walking distance by 179% following exercise training and, in some instances, exercise seems to be more effective than pharmacological agents or angioplasty.[32,33]

Practical recommendations for exercise training in patients with peripheral vascular disease

- Interval walking and stair-climbing is the chosen mode of exercise training.
- Walking at an intensity that causes calf pain of a score of 3 on a 4-point scale should be undertaken with a full recovery between intervals.
- The initial program may start with 20 min exercise and should progress to over 30 min exercise at 50–70% of peak VO_2, most days of the week.
- Walking and stair-climbing should be supplemented with arm cranking exercise and resistance training, 2–3 times per week.
- As the patients exercise tolerance improves and greater work rates are achieved, coronary artery disease may be unmasked. Thus patients should be educated as to the symptoms of coronary artery disease.
- Because cold weather causes peripheral vasoconstriction, the warm-up period should be extended and the exercise session conducted indoors during cold winter months.
- Smoking cessation programs should be advised in this patient population.

Exercise rehabilitation for patients with cerebrovascular disease

Stroke continues to be the third leading cause of death in the US and a major cause of morbidity and mortality in other parts of the globe.[34] Patients presenting with stroke frequently have atherosclerotic lesions throughout their vascular system and therefore are at increased risk of comorbid cardiovascular disease. Thus, coronary artery disease and ischemic stroke share the same group of risk factors, including hypertension, smoking, abnormal blood lipids, sedentary lifestyle, diabetes and obesity. Modification of lifestyle-related risk factors, including exercise training, plays an important role for secondary prevention of recurrent strokes. Furthermore, improved short-term survival has resulted in a growing number of stroke survivors who have some form of disability or severe de-conditioning which may be improved through carefully directed exercise rehabilitation.

Rehabilitation of stroke survivors is difficult as the patient could present with hemiplegia, spasticity, aphasia, disorientation and impaired ability to perform daily functions and thus requires a specialist multidisciplinary team. While a detailed discussion of rehabilitation is beyond the scope of this chapter, the reader with an interest in this area is referred to a more detailed clinical guideline.[34]

Essentially, the benefits of exercise rehabilitation in stroke survivors include increased aerobic capacity and sensorimotor function, reduction in risk factors for cardiovascular and cerebrovascular disease and improved psychological function.[23,35–37]

Prior to exercise training, stroke survivors should undertake a medical evaluation and an exercise stress test to determine safety and effective exercise prescription. The exercise test may have to be modified according to the special needs of the patient.

The exercise prescription for patients with cerebrovascular disease

The elements of the exercise prescription are similar to exercise prescription in the other forms of cardiovascular disease, with certain individualized modifications for the stroke survivor. Exercise training should include aerobic training, muscle strength and endurance, flexibility and neuromuscular (coordination and balance activities).

Aerobic exercise in the form of walking, treadmill, cycling, arm ergometry or arm-leg ergometry should be performed at 40–70% of peak VO_2, most days of the week for a minimum of 30 min. Strength training in the form of free weights, or circuit weight training, 1–3 sets of 10–15 repetitions, 2–3 days per week should be encouraged. Stretching and coordination and balance activities should be added during the warm-up or cool down 2–3 days per week.

Practical recommendations for exercise training in patients with cerebrovascular disease

- Osteoarthritis particularly of the shoulder, hip and knee is common in stroke survivors; therefore the mode of exercise might have to be modified accordingly.
- Stroke patients may have pre-existing peripheral vascular disease which may impair the patient's ability to walk or cycle.
- Sensation and motor control of limbs may often be impaired, thus careful observation and modification of the exercise environment is necessary to avoid injury.

Risks of exercise training in cardiac patients

Exercise training in cardiac patients is a relatively safe endeavor and cardiac events are rare. The average incidence of cardiac arrest, non-fatal myocardial infarction and death is approximately 1 for every 117 000, 220 000 and 750 000 patient hours of participation, respectively.[38] The low ratio of cardiac arrest to death is thought to be due to resuscitation facilities and medical care on hand at these exercise programs.

EXERCISE REHABILITATION FOR PATIENTS WITH PULMONARY DISEASE

Box 11.4: Key Points

- Exercise training is effective in attenuating the symptoms of dyspnoea and fatigue in patients with COPD.
- Exercise training is effective in improving functional capacity and enhancing quality of life in these patients.

The goals of pulmonary rehabilitation are to reduce symptoms of dyspnea disability and improve functional capacity and quality of life in patients with lung disease.[39] While a relatively small number of studies have shown exercise training to be beneficial in chronic asthma, pulmonary fibrosis, cystic fibrosis and bronchiectasis, the vast majority of available data (and indeed rehabilitation participants) are from patients with chronic obstructive pulmonary disease (COPD). COPD is the term applied to a disease that is generally a result of emphysema, chronic bronchitis or a mixture of these two pathophysiological processes. COPD is characterized by gradual, largely irreversible chronic airflow limitation, a chronic cough, over-inflated lungs and impaired gaseous exchange.

In the US, COPD is reported to be the fourth highest cause of death, similarly in the European Union, it is the third highest cause of mortality. COPD is regarded as a largely irreversible disease. However, treatment of patients suffering from COPD focuses primarily on improvements in, or maintenance of, functional capacity. This is in an attempt to allow continued participation in activities of daily living by these patients.

Functional capacity of patients with COPD

Patients with COPD demonstrate marked exercise intolerance compared to healthy individuals, and typically present with exaggerated breathlessness, fatigue, muscle wasting and often malnutrition.

The causes of impaired exercise tolerance are listed in Table 11.7. It is of interest to note that COPD affects not only the respiratory system but also has a profound effect on the cardiovascular and musculoskeletal systems and the patient's psyche.

The effects of exercise training

Whereas 20 years ago many physicians generally counseled their patients with COPD to avoid physical exertion, nearly all pulmonary rehabilitation programs today place an important emphasis on exercise training. The importance of a multidisciplinary program comprising not only exercise training but also education, smoking cessation, nutritional counseling, occupational therapy, psychology and social support should be stressed.

Table 11.7   Postulated Causes of Impaired Exercise Tolerance in Patients with COPD

Ventilatory impairments
   Increased airways resistance
   Reduced lung compliance
   Increased work of breathing
   Ventilatory muscle weakness and fatigue
   Ventilatory inefficiency
   Ventilatory failure
Abnormalities of gaseous exchange
   Destruction on the capillary-alveolar membrane
   Ventilation/perfusion inequality
Cardiovascular impairments
   Cardiovascular de-conditioning
   Reduced pulmonary vascular conductance
Skeletal muscle impairments
   Peripheral muscle de-conditioning
   Diaphragmatic muscle abnormalities
   Skeletal muscle wasting and destruction
Psychological alterations
   Chronic anxiety
   Depression

Evidence exists that a multidisciplinary individually designed rehabilitation program should improve a patient's functional capacity and health status, reduce dyspnea, and have some economic advantages.[40,41]

In a review of exercise training studies, the vast majority showed increased exercise tolerance, reduction in hospital admission frequency, exacerbation rate and bronchodilator usage, after exercise rehabilitation programs both in the form of inpatient and outpatient programs.[41–43] The most dramatic improvements are often seen in the most severely impaired patients. A comprehensive rehabilitation practice guideline has been published by the ACCP/AACVPR.[44] The physiological benefits of exercise training for patients with COPD have been well documented and are detailed in Table 11.8.

It is of interest to note that many of these adaptations mentioned above which lead to increased functional capacity are in fact not due to pulmonary improvements. In fact, the diseased lung is not 'trainable' to the same extent as the peripheral muscles, respiratory muscles and cardiovascular system. Thus in

Table 11.8   The Benefits of Exercise Training in Patients with COPD

Improved ventilatory efficiency
Improved tolerance of dyspnea
Cardiovascular reconditioning
Improved skeletal muscle strength
Improved musculoskeletal flexibility
Improved body composition
Improved balance and proprioception
Improved body image

patients with COPD, exercise training does not appear to have a significant effect on lung function *per se*. Programs lasting 4–12 weeks have been shown to be effective and benefits of rehabilitation are seen up to 1 year, irrespective of attendance at a follow-up program.[45,46]

Practical recommendations for exercise rehabilitation in patients with COPD

- Patients with COPD who have significant disease severity should begin with a supervised rehabilitation program. The first step for any patient beginning an exercise program is a careful evaluation to assess cardiac risk and exercise capacity. Many patients also have some cardiac impairment, and an exercise intensity that will not induce arrhythmia, ischemia or hypoxia should be determined.

- Good tests of functional capacity in this group of patients include the 6-min walk test and the endurance shuttle walk.[47,48]

- Another appropriate form of testing is to use a treadmill or stationary cycle following a protocol that starts at a very low workload and is increased extremely slowly. A pulse oximeter should be used to monitor de-saturation.

- We find that stationary cycling is an extremely useful mode for exercise training in patients with COPD. Other cardiovascular exercise modalities including treadmill exercise, arm ergometry, walking, or stair-climbing are also acceptable.

- Patients should aim to exercise at 60% of their VO_2 peak or 60% of their maximal walking speed for 20–30 min, for a minimum of 3 days a week. But this goal may not be achievable for the first few months. The patient's exercise capacity should be your guide and most patients start with 2 min cycling intervals with zero load on the ergometer, followed by 3 min rest. Patients should then progress slowly; even small increments can make a significant difference in the quality of their lives.

- Progression of exercise can take the form of decreasing rest intervals, increasing duration of exercise or increasing work rate.[46,49]

- Upper and lower body strength training in the form of free or circuit weight programs are beneficial in this group of patients as skeletal muscle dysfunction may be reversed by training.[50,51]

- Many patients can graduate to an independent exercise program after 3 months of structured rehabilitation, but some will require a longer period in the supervised program, and some may always need some supervision.

- Patients with COPD generally require more monitoring and active encouragement and reassurance than do patients with other chronic disease. Anxiety and discomfort associated with shortness of breath are likely to be a problem, particularly at the initiation of exercise, and in the first few sessions, patients may require a substantial amount of education and encouragement.

- Psychological and nutritional counseling, as well as special exercises for the diaphragmatic and other respiratory muscles are seen as important aspects of the rehabilitation program for patients with COPD.

- Pursed lip breathing exercises have not shown to be effective in clinical trials, yet individual patients might respond well to this form of training.[52]
- Other modalities of treatment may be necessary for patients with COPD patients. Many patients who have significant COPD might require oxygen supplementation during exercise. This is particularly relevant to patients whose arterial oxygen tension falls to less than 55 mmHg or in those patients where oxyhemoglobin de-saturates to less that 88%. Most patients also require regular treatment with bronchodilators (sympathomimetic agonists), methylxanthines, glucocorticoids, mucolytics and anticholinergic agents.
- Increases in exercise tolerance and the patient's functional capacity for everyday tasks can be very slow and, if measured by conventional standards might seem somewhat unimpressive, but the impact of these seemingly small strides makes a big difference in quality of life for patients with COPD.
- Quality of life may be assessed by the Short Form-36 or the Chronic Respiratory Questionnaire (CRQ).[47,53]

EXERCISE REHABILITATION IN PATIENTS WITH DIABETES MELLITUS

Diabetes is one of the leading causes of death and disability with Type II diabetes accounting for up to 95% of cases.[54] While exercise rehabilitation has been shown to have a positive therapeutic effect with Type I and II diabetes mellitus and other specific diabetic conditions, including the metabolic syndrome, this section of the chapter will focus on Type II diabetes.[22] Type II diabetes mellitus is a metabolic disease typified by hyperglycemia. It is characterized by an insulin resistance syndrome or relative insulin deficiency, which is usually exacerbated by excess body fat. Patients with diabetes are at risk for developing sequelae of the disease, including either microvascular or macro-vascular pathology.[55] These complications may include autonomic and peripheral neuropathy, retinopathy, nephropathy and accelerated atherosclerosis.

Medications used in diabetes management not only include glucose-lowering agents, but may also include antihypertensives, lipid-lowering agents and pain medications. The effects of the glucose-lowering agents (oral hypoglycemic agents) on exercise testing and exercise training is important as these agents have the ability to cause hypoglycemia.

Exercise in the prevention and treatment of Type II diabetes mellitus

Regular physical activity is effective in the treatment and in some cases primary prevention of diabetes mellitus. The benefits of regular physical activity in patients with Type II diabetes include decreased risk of cardiac disease, reduction in body fat, improved glucose utilization, improved insulin sensitivity, enhanced socialization and stress reduction.

Benefits of exercise training in patients with Type II diabetes mellitus

- Decreased cardiac risk
  - Patients have a 2- to 4-fold increase in risk for cardiovascular disease. Contributing to this risk is

dyslipidemia. Exercise helps to alter favorably the lipid fractions which are: typically low HDL cholesterol, elevated triglycerides and in some cases high LDL cholesterol.[14,56]
  - Blood pressure decreases with exercise training.[20–22] High insulin concentrations cause hypertrophy of the media or smooth muscle of the vascular wall, and this hypertrophy is associated with sustained hypertension, common in Type II diabetes.[55]
  - Exercise increases insulin sensitivity (improved glucose tolerance), which may cause circulating insulin concentrations to decrease.[56,57] The hypertrophic effects are then lessened, potentially decreasing blood pressure.
- Reduction of body fat stores
  - Weight loss favorably alters insulin sensitivity and may allow patients with diabetes to reduce the amount of oral hypoglycemic agents needed. Exercise coupled with moderate caloric intake is considered the most effective way to lose fat and may be most beneficial early in the progression of Type II diabetes when insulin secretion is still adequate.[58,59]
- Improved glucose utilization
  - Glucose oxidation is enhanced through exercise and endogenous insulin is more effectively utilized in fitter diabetic patients.[60] Improvements in glucose tolerance have been shown in the Type II diabetic patients with as little as one week of aerobic training.[56] Improved glycogenic control reflected in lower glycosylated hemoglobin or fasting glucose measures, has also been documented after six to 12 weeks of an aerobic exercise program.[59,61] A single exercise session has been shown to increase insulin sensitivity for 16 hours or longer.[57]
- Enhanced fitness
  - Improvement in functional capacity, skeletal muscle hypertrophy and increases in VO_2max occur with exercise training.[3]
- Enhanced socialization
  - Exercise training and organized sports allow diabetic patients to participate in social activity, gain peer acceptance and enhanced self-esteem.[57]
- Stress reduction
  - Stress can affect diabetes control adversely by increasing counter-regulatory hormones, ketones, and free fatty acids. These findings make stress reduction an important benefit of exercise training and diabetes care.[62]

Exercise testing and prescription in patients with Type II diabetes mellitus
Exercise testing

As autonomic neuropathy may be associated with silent ischemia, postural hypotension or a blunted heart rate response to exercise, the primary objective for exercise testing in patients with diabetes is to identify the presence and extent of coronary artery disease, and to determine the appropriate intensity range for aerobic exercise training. Methods of exercise testing may require modification of standard protocols or require the use of arm ergometry depending on the patient's disability.

Exercise prescription

The exercise prescription for patients with diabetes must be individualized according to their medication schedule, presence and severity of diabetic complications, and goals and expected benefits from the exercise training program.

Choosing the appropriate mode of exercise

Diabetic patients are usually sedentary and de-conditioned at initial evaluation. Patients should therefore begin exercise by increasing their everyday activity, including using stairs instead of elevators, walking a few extra meters, or doing a few more minutes of housework. Walking is an excellent form of exercise in patients with Type II diabetes due to its low impact nature. Patients should gradually increase their walking distance and then perhaps advance to other forms of aerobic exercise including swimming, running, rowing, or cycling.

Exercise training should incorporate all components of a comprehensive program, including aerobic cardiorespiratory training, muscle strength, muscle endurance flexibility and core stability exercises.

Aerobic training

It is strongly recommended that patients with Type II diabetes expend a minimum cumulative total of 1000 kcal/wk in aerobic activity.[63] A workable goal for many patients is aerobic exercise at 40–70% of VO_2max for at least 30 min nearly every day of the week. Exercise sessions should begin with a gentle 5–10 min warm-up and stretching of the muscles to be exercised, and conclude with a 5–10 min cool-down period. Thus, the exercise session may last up to 60 min. Sustained aerobic activities, such as running, cycling, swimming, and aerobic dance, rely on a mix of aerobically processed fuels, but the major sources are fats and carbohydrates (both muscle glycogen and blood glucose fuels).

For exercise at higher intensities (70–85% of maximal aerobic capacity or higher), carbohydrates are the body's fuel of choice. Blood glucose utilization can become quite significant during these activities. As more glycogen is depleted, the risk of hypoglycemia increases. Hypoglycemia can be prevented by ingestion of adequate carbohydrate during exercise and/or modification of the dosage and timing of medication prior to the exercise bout.

If weight loss is a primary goal the intensity of aerobic exercise needs to be low–moderate (50% VO_2max) and the duration of the aerobic bout should be incrementally increased to approximately 60 min.

For prolonged exercise, including marathons, triathlons and long exercise periods, diabetic athletes must reduce their dose of oral hypoglycemic agents as increased carbohydrate intake by itself is not adequate to compensate for the accelerated glucose uptake during exercise

When considering types of exercise to prescribe, patients are most likely to continue in programs that involve activities they enjoy. Thus, working with patients to find activities that are pleasant and effective will encourage compliance.

Resistance training

> ### Box 11.5: Key Points
>
> - Regular physical exercise is important in the prevention of diabetes.
> - Exercise training is important in the management of both Type I and II diabetes mellitus and the metabolic syndrome.

Resistance training is effective in improving skeletal muscle strength and endurance, enhancing flexibility and body composition and decreasing risk factors for cardiovascular disease.[6] In both non-diabetic and diabetic subjects, resistance training has resulted in improved glucose tolerance and insulin sensitivity and may have a positive effect on intra-abdominal obesity.[64–66]

Patients with Type II diabetes mellitus should therefore incorporate strength training using light free weights or circuit stations of 8–10 different exercises using the major muscle groups, at least 2 days per week. Each exercise should consist of at lease one set of 10–15 repetitions, with the weight increased when the individual can complete 15 repetitions with ease. Increased resistance, additional sets or combinations of both of these may produce greater benefits and may be appropriate for selected patients. Caution should be used in patients with advanced retinal and cardiovascular complications. For these and older diabetic patients, more repetitions performed at a lower weight may be more suitable.

Flexibility and core stability training

Flexibility and core stability training should be incorporated into the overall fitness routine for a minimum of 2–3 days per week to develop and maintain joint range of motion, minimize the potential loss of flexibility which has been hypothesized to result from glycosylation of various joint structures and reduce the chances of developing lower back pain. Stretching for 5–10 min could be done either after the aerobic warm-up or following the completion of an exercise session. This may ease the transition between rest and exercise and help prevent muscle and joint injuries.

Monitoring of exercise in patients with Type II diabetes mellitus

Exercise intensity is typically prescribed and monitored using heart rate or a percentage of the maximal oxygen uptake (VO_2), which can be initially established during the exercise stress test. However, some patients can develop autonomic neuropathy which can affect the cardiovascular response to exercise and in such patients, exercise intensity can also be measured by rating of perceived exertion.

Blood glucose monitoring should be performed before and after physical activity to monitor the effect of the exercise on blood glucose concentration.

Supplemental carbohydrates are generally not needed in the patients with Type II diabetes; however, if patients are prone to hypoglycemia, they may require additional carbohydrates during and following exercise. A total of 1 h of exercise will require an additional 15 g of carbohydrate either before or after exercise. If exercise is vigorous or of longer duration, an additional 15–30 g of carbohydrate per hour may be required.

Practical guidelines regarding exercise in the patient with Type II diabetes mellitus

- Maintain adequate hydration before, during and after sustained exercise, particularly when exercising in the heat. Autonomic neuropathy may also disrupt thermoregulation in patients with Type II diabetes mellitus. Thus, it is important to avoid exercising in extreme heat and cold.
- Alcohol is a powerful inhibitor of gluconeogenesis, and the effects on hypoglycemia can persist 20 h after consumption. Patients with Type II diabetes mellitus should be advised not to drink alcohol at night if they plan to exercise the following morning.
- The pre-participation evaluation is a good time to ensure that patients with Type II diabetes mellitus select appropriate fitting shoes for exercise. Socks also should fit well and be made from material that absorbs moisture to keep the feet dry.
- When exercising, patients should wear a diabetes identification shoe tag or bracelet in such a way that it is clearly visible.
- Symptoms of dizziness, weakness, or shortness of breath should alert the physician to the possibility of cardiac disease. Such patients should undertake an exercise stress test and have monitored exercise sessions.
- Orthostatic hypotension is common in patients with autonomic dysfunction after upright exercise, thus cycling or swimming is more appropriate than running or brisk walking.
- Diabetic patients with retinopathy should be wary of high intensity activities that precipitate hemorrhage or retinal detachment. This warning applies particularly to activities that cause sudden increases in blood pressure, including weightlifting or sprinting.
- Non-weight-bearing activities or specially modified footwear should be considered for patients with peripheral neuropathy, so as to reduce trauma to the lower legs and feet.
- Patients with nephropathy should avoid strenuous activities which cause the systolic blood pressure to be increased above 200 mmHg. A low level program which does not increase the systolic blood pressure 20–30 mmHg above baseline should be prescribed for patients with Type II diabetes mellitus who have advanced retinopathy.

Precautions for exercising patients with Type II diabetes mellitus

- Measure blood glucose concentrations before, during and after exercise training. Blood glucose monitoring is an essential part of participating in exercise for the patient with Type II diabetes mellitus, particularly in the beginning stages of exercise. This approach has been shown to be effective particularly for diabetic athletes who engage in strenuous endurance exercise. According to the American Diabetes Association, patients should avoid exercise if blood glucose concentrations exceed 300 mg/dl (or 250 mg/dl with ketosis), and should ingest a carbohydrate snack before exercise if blood glucose concentrations fall below 100 mg/dl.
- Hypoglycemic reactions to exercise in patients with Type II diabetes mellitus are rare and mostly limited to those patients on oral sulphonylurea agents and/or insulin and occur mostly following very intense or prolonged exercise. Therefore, in most cases, there is no need for supplementary food intake before or after exercise unless the patient is undertaking extremes of physical activity.
- To avoid the occurrence of low blood sugar in some Type II diabetes patients the following advice may be beneficial:
  - Avoid exercise during periods of peak insulin activity. Meal timing is important. Exercise should be scheduled one to two hours after a meal, or exercise should be undertaken when circulating insulin concentrations are lower. Morning exercise usually produces a lower hypoglycemic effect than the same exercise done later in the day. This results from the effects of higher circulating cortisol other glucose-raising hormone concentrations early in the day (i.e. insulin resistance is generally greater in the morning), along with lower circulating concentrations of insulin. Conversely, evening exercise conveys the greatest risk for nocturnal hypoglycemia unless the patient makes changes to food intake or doses of medications.
- Unplanned prolonged exercise should be preceded by extra carbohydrates, e.g. 20–30 g of carbohydrates (CHO)/30 min of exercise.
- If exercise is planned, medication dosages may be decreased before and after exercise, according to the exercise intensity duration as well as the personal experience of the patient.
- During prolonged exercise, easily absorbable carbohydrates (6–8% as opposed to 13–14%) should be consumed, and after exercise, an extra carbohydrate-rich snack may be necessary.
- It is advisable to educate the diabetic patient to become knowledgeable of the signs and symptoms of hypoglycemia and always exercise with a partner.

THE EDUCATION COMPONENT OF CHRONIC DISEASE REHABILITATION PROGRAM

Regardless of the nature of the primary ailment that leads the patient to be referred to the rehabilitation program, it has been shown that patient education remains one of the most important aspects of the program. The components of the educational program presented to our patients are outlined in Table 11.9. The content is non-disease-entity-specific and can be customized for any chronic disease.

CONCLUSIONS

Exercise rehabilitation has become an accepted and integral part of the management of patients with chronic disease.

Table 11.9   Lecture or Note Outlines for Education of Patients with Chronic Disease

1	Anatomy and physiology of the affected organ system
2	Basic pathology and pathophysiology of the affected organ system
3	Understand the symptoms
4	Common pharmacological and non-pharmacological therapies
5	Benefits of exercise training in prevention and management of the chronic disease
6	Nutritional advice for optimal management of the chronic disease
7	Strategies for anxiety and stress management
8	Coping with setbacks
9	Identifying and challenging belief systems about disease- and health-related behavior
10	Goal setting, rewards and relaxation
11	Loving relationships and sexuality
12	Exercise and nutritional options while traveling

While the exercise training component forms the mainstay of chronic disease rehabilitation, programs should have a holistic approach and include nutritional, psychology and lifestyle counseling. Patient and spouse counseling and education forms an important part of the rehabilitation program.

While a comprehensive review of all the chronic diseases where exercise plays an important role in patient management is beyond the scope of this chapter, it is evident that more research is needed in certain areas, for example, the neurological conditions and the immunological/hematological disorders, where small patient numbers have prevented clear patient guidelines from being formulated. Nevertheless, the number of Position Statements and publications in this important area continues to grow rapidly.

With the growing evidence that exercise is an effective form of management for a wide range of different pathologies and medical conditions; and that medication dosages may often be reduced in exercising patients, there is an urgent need by the health insurance industry to quantify the cost savings which could be achieved through participation in regular exercise rehabilitation. There is no doubt that this important aspect of Sports Medicine will continue to flourish as more data become available regarding novel mechanisms of action of exercise training and as these findings are applied to a wider number of patients and chronic disease entities.

REFERENCES

1   Booth FW, Tseng BS. Exercise. In: Dulbecco R, ed. Encyclopedia of human biology, Vol. 3. 2nd edn. San Diego: Academic Press; 1997:853–863.

2   American College of Sports Medicine. ACSM's exercise management for persons with chronic diseases and disabilities. Champaigne, IL: Human Kinetics; 1997:1–269.

3   Albright A, Franz M, Hornsby G, et al. American College of Sports Medicine position stand. Exercise and type 2 diabetes. Med Sci Sports Exerc 2000; 32:1345–1360.

4   Kohrt WM, Bloomfield SA, Little KD, et al. American College of Sports Medicine Position Stand: physical activity and bone health. Med Sci Sports Exerc 2004; 36:1985–1996.

5   Pescatello LS, Franklin BA, Fagard R, et al. American College of Sports Medicine position stand. Exercise and hypertension. Med Sci Sports Exerc 2004; 36:533–553.

6   Pollock ML, Franklin BA, Balady GJ, et al. AHA Science advisory. Resistance exercise in individuals with and without cardiovascular disease: benefits, rationale, safety, and prescription: An advisory from the Committee on Exercise, Rehabilitation, and Prevention, Council on Clinical Cardiology, American Heart Association. Position Paper endorsed by the American College of Sports Medicine. Circulation 2000; 101:828–833.

7   American College of Sports Medicine. In: Franklin BA, ed. ACSM's guidelines for exercise testing and prescription. 6th edn. Philadelphia, PA: Lippincott Williams & Wilkins; 2000:1–368.

8   Leon AS. Exercise following myocardial infarction. Current recommendations. Sports Med 2000; 29:301–311.

9   Balady GJ, Ades PA, Comoss P, et al. Core components of cardiac rehabilitation/ secondary prevention programs: A statement for healthcare professionals from the American Heart Association and the American Association of Cardiovascular and Pulmonary Rehabilitation Writing Group. Circulation 2000; 102:1069–1073.

10   Balady GJ, Fletcher BJ, Froelicher ES, et al. Cardiac rehabilitation programs – A statement for health-care professionals from the American Heart Association. Circulation 1994; 90:1602–1610.

11   Wenger NK, Froelicher ES, Smith LK, et al. Cardiac rehabilitation as secondary prevention. Agency for Health Care Policy and Research and National Heart, Lung, and Blood Institute. Quick Ref Guide Clin 1995; 17:1–23.

12   Thompson PD, Buchner D, Pina IL, et al. Exercise and physical activity in the prevention and treatment of atherosclerotic cardiovascular disease: A statement from the Council on Clinical Cardiology (Subcommittee on Exercise, Rehabilitation, and Prevention) and the Council on Nutrition, Physical Activity, and Metabolism (Subcommittee on Physical Activity). Circulation 2003; 107:3109–3116.

13   Billman GE. Aerobic exercise conditioning: a nonpharmacological antiarrhythmic intervention. J Appl Physiol 2002; 92:446–454.

14   Leon AS, Sanchez OA. Response of blood lipids to exercise training alone or combined with dietary intervention. Med Sci Sports Exerc 2001; 33:502–515.

15   Hambrecht R, Wolf A, Gielen S, et al. Effect of exercise on coronary endothelial function in patients with coronary artery disease. N Engl J Med 2000; 342:454–460.

16   Ussher MH, West R, Taylor AH, et al. Exercise interventions for smoking cessation. CD002295. Cochrane Database Syst Rev; 2000.

17   Jolliffe JA, Rees K, Taylor RS, et al. Exercise-based rehabilitation for coronary heart disease. CD001800. Cochrane Database Syst Rev; 2001.

18   Belardinelli R, Paolini I, Cianci G, et al. Exercise training intervention after coronary angioplasty: the ETICA trial. J Am Coll Cardiol 2001; 37:1891–1900.

19   Paffenbarger RS Jr, Jung DL, Leung RW, Hyde RT. Physical activity and hypertension: an epidemiological view. Ann Med 1991; 23:319–327.

20   Halbert JA, Silagy CA, Finucane P, et al. The effectiveness of exercise training in lowering blood pressure: a meta-analysis of randomised controlled trials of 4 weeks or longer. J Hum Hypertens 1997; 11:641–649.

21   Fagard RH. Exercise characteristics and the blood pressure response to dynamic physical training. Med Sci Sports Exerc 2001; 33:484–492.

22   Carroll S, Dudfield M. What is the relationship between exercise and metabolic abnormalities? A review of the metabolic syndrome. Sports Med 2004; 34:371–418.

23   Franklin BA, Sanders W. Reducing the risk of heart disease and stroke. Physician Sportsmedicine 2000; 28:19.

24   Pescatello LS, Fargo AE, Leach CN Jr., et al. Short-term effect of dynamic exercise on arterial blood pressure. Circulation 1991; 83:1557–1561.

25   Pina IL, Apstein CS, Balady GJ, et al. Exercise and heart failure: A statement from the American Heart Association Committee on exercise, rehabilitation, and prevention. Circulation 2003; 107:1210–1225.

26   Jugdutt BI, Michorowski BL, Kappagoda CT. Exercise training after anterior Q wave myocardial infarction: importance of regional left ventricular function and topography. J Am Coll Cardiol 1988; 12:362–372.

27   Hambrecht R, Gielen S, Linke A, et al. Effects of exercise training on left ventricular function and peripheral resistance in patients with chronic heart failure: A randomized trial. JAMA 2000; 283:3095–3101.

28   Coats AJ, Adamopoulos S, Radaelli A, et al. Controlled trial of physical training in chronic heart failure. Exercise performance, hemodynamics, ventilation, and autonomic function. Circulation 1992; 85:2119–2131.

29   Gielen S, Erbs S, Schuler G. Exercise training and endothelial dysfunction in coronary artery disease and chronic heart failure. Minerva Cardioangiol 2002; 50:95–106.

30   Cheetham C, Green D, Collis J, et al. Effect of aerobic and resistance exercise on central hemodynamic responses in severe chronic heart failure. J Appl Physiol 2002; 93:175–180.

31   Tyni-Lenne R, Gordon A, Europe E, et al. Exercise-based rehabilitation improves skeletal muscle capacity, exercise tolerance, and quality of life in both women and men with chronic heart failure. J Card Fail 1998; 4:9–17.

32 Gardner AW, Poehlman ET. Exercise rehabilitation programs for the treatment of claudication pain. A meta-analysis. JAMA 1995; 274:975–980.

33 Whyman MR, Ruckley CV. Should claudicants receive angioplasty or just exercise training? Cardiovasc Surg 1998; 6:226–231.

34 Gordon NF, Gulanick M, Costa F, et al. Physical activity and exercise recommendations for stroke survivors: an American Heart Association scientific statement from the Council on Clinical Cardiology, Subcommittee on Exercise, Cardiac Rehabilitation, and Prevention; the Council on Cardiovascular Nursing; the Council on Nutrition, Physical Activity, and Metabolism; and the Stroke Council. Circulation 2004; 109:2031–2041.

35 Macko RF, Smith GV, Dobrovolny CL, et al. Treadmill training improves fitness reserve in chronic stroke patients. Arch Phys Med Rehabil 2001; 82:879–884.

36 Potempa K, Lopez M, Braun LT, et al. Physiological outcomes of aerobic exercise training in hemiparetic stroke patients. Stroke 1995; 26:101–105.

37 Franklin BA, Kahn JK. Delayed progression or regression of coronary atherosclerosis with intensive risk factor modification. Effects of diet, drugs, and exercise. Sports Med 1996; 22:306–320.

38 Franklin BA, Bonzheim K, Gordon S, et al. Safety of medically supervised outpatient cardiac rehabilitation exercise therapy: a 16-year follow-up. Chest 1998; 114:902–906.

39 Morgan MDL, Calverley PMA, Clark CJ, et al. Pulmonary rehabilitation. Thorax 2001; 56:827–834.

40 Davidson AC, Morgan MDL. A UK survey of the provision of pulmonary rehabilitation. Thorax 1998; 53:A86.

41 American Thoracic Society. Pulmonary rehabilitation, 1999. Am J Respir Crit Care Med 1999; 159:1666–1682.

42 Griffiths TL, Burr ML, Campbell IA, et al. Results at 1 year of outpatient multidisciplinary pulmonary rehabilitation: a randomised controlled trial. Lancet 2000; 355:362–368.

43 Guell R, Casan P, Belda J, et al. Long-term effects of outpatient rehabilitation of COPD: A randomized trial. Chest 2000; 117:976–983.

44 Ries AL, Carlin BW, Casaburi R, et al. Pulmonary rehabilitation: Joint ACCP/AACVPR evidence-based guidelines. Chest 1997; 112:1363–1396.

45 Criner GJ, Cordova FC, Furukawa S, et al. Prospective randomized trial comparing bilateral lung volume reduction surgery to pulmonary rehabilitation in severe chronic obstructive pulmonary disease. Am J Respir Crit Care Med 1999; 160:2018–2027.

46 Troosters T, Gosselink R, Decramer M. Short- and long-term effects of outpatient rehabilitation in patients with chronic obstructive pulmonary disease: a randomized trial. Am J Med 2000; 109:207–212.

47 Redelmeier DA, Guyatt GH, Goldstein RS. Assessing the minimal important difference in symptoms: a comparison of two techniques. J Clin Epidemiol 1996; 49:1215–1219.

48 Revill SM, Morgan MD, Singh SJ, et al. The endurance shuttle walk: a new field test for the assessment of endurance capacity in chronic obstructive pulmonary disease. Thorax 1999; 54:213–222.

49 Punzal PA, Ries AL, Kaplan RM, et al. Maximum intensity exercise training in patients with chronic obstructive pulmonary disease. Chest 1991; 100:618–623.

50 Simpson K, Killian K, McCartney N, et al. Randomised controlled trial of weightlifting exercise in patients with chronic airflow limitation. Thorax 1992; 47:70–75.

51 Clark AM, Barbour RS, McIntyre PD. Preparing for change in the secondary prevention of coronary heart disease: a qualitative evaluation of cardiac rehabilitation within a region of Scotland. J Adv Nurs 2002; 39:589–598.

52 Gosselink RA, Wagenaar RC, Rijswijk H, et al. Diaphragmatic breathing reduces efficiency of breathing in patients with chronic obstructive pulmonary disease. Am J Respir Crit Care Med 1995; 151:1136–1142.

53 Benzo R, Flume PA, Turner D, et al. Effect of pulmonary rehabilitation on quality of life in patients with COPD: the use of SF-36 summary scores as outcomes measures. J Cardiopulm Rehabil 2000; 20:231–234.

54 Harris MI. Classification, diagnostic criteria, and screening for diabetes. Publication No. 95-1468, 15–36. NIH; NIDDK; 1995.

55 McGavock JM, Eves ND, Mandic S, et al. The role of exercise in the treatment of cardiovascular disease associated with type 2 diabetes mellitus. Sports Med 2004; 34:27–48.

56 Rogers MA, Yamamoto C, King DS, et al. Improvement in glucose-tolerance after 1 wk of exercise in patients with mild NIDDM. Diabetes Care 1988; 11:613–618.

57 Schneider SH, Amorosa LF, Khachadurian AK, et al. Studies on the mechanism of improved glucose control during regular exercise in Type-2 (non-insulin-dependent) diabetes. Diabetologia 1984; 26:355–360.

58 Zierath JR, Wallberg-Henriksson H. Exercise training in obese diabetic patients. Special considerations. Sports Med 1992; 14:171–189.

59 Trovati M, Carta Q, Cavalot F, et al. Influence of physical training on blood glucose control, glucose tolerance, insulin secretion, and insulin action in non-insulin-dependent diabetic patients. Diabetes Care 1984; 7:416–420.

60 Wasserman DH, Zinman B. Exercise in individuals with IDDM. Diabetes Care 1994; 17:924–937.

61 Reitman JS, Vasquez B, Klimes I, et al. Improvement of glucose-homeostasis after exercise training in non-insulin-dependent diabetes. Diabetes Care 1984; 7:434–441.

62 Vasterling JJ, Sementilli ME, Burish TG. The role of aerobic exercise in reducing stress in diabetic patients. Diabetes Educ 1988; 14:197–201.

63 Fletcher GF, Blair SN, Blumenthal J, et al. Statement on exercise. Benefits and recommendations for physical activity programs for all Americans. A statement for health professionals by the Committee on Exercise and Cardiac Rehabilitation of the Council on Clinical Cardiology, American Heart Association. Circulation 1992; 86:340–344.

64 Eriksson J, Taimela S, Eriksson K, et al. Resistance training in the treatment of non-insulin-dependent diabetes mellitus. Int J Sports Med 1997; 18:242–246.

65 Fluckey JD, Hickey MS, Brambrink JK, et al. Effects of resistance exercise on glucose tolerance in normal and glucose-intolerant subjects. J Appl Physiol 1994; 77:1087–1092.

66 Treuth MS, Hunter GR, Kekes-Szabo T, et al. Reduction in intra-abdominal adipose tissue after strength training in older women. J Appl Physiol 1995; 78:1425–1431.

Principles of Injury Care and Rehabilitation

CHAPTER 12

Pre-Participation Evaluation

Thomas D. Rizzo, Jr

INTRODUCTION

Box 12.1: Key Points

- The pre-participation evaluation is a traditional component of athletic clearance before the beginning of the sports season.

- Standardized aspects of history taking and physical examination identify conditions that may make participation dangerous.

- Involvement of the team physician in the organizational process can build rapport with the athlete and coaching staff and ensure adequate time for rehabilitation or evaluation of any abnormalities.

- Questionable findings in the athlete's history or physical assessment should be addressed more thoroughly outside the screening process.

At the heart of the pre-participation examination is the goal of making athletic participation safe for the athlete. Athletic participation is desirable, but by its nature, it is physically demanding, stressful to the cardiovascular and musculoskeletal systems and potentially injurious. These risks are amplified in poorly prepared individuals and those with pre-existing, hidden disorders. In young people, their relative health and lack of medical history put them at risk for a severe condition manifesting through the rigors of athletic competition. Such an event can have devastating consequences.

There have been well-publicized instances of seemingly healthy athletes dying without warning. Many of these people were participating at an elite level and, presumably, had been evaluated and tested, formally and through the demands of their sport, without a hint of a health defect. Some of their deaths were due to a cardiac disorder, and, even though this is the most common cause of sudden death in the athlete, it is the hardest to detect on screening physical examination.

This chapter evaluates the mechanics of the pre-participation evaluation: why it is done, how it is done, what to look for and what to do once you find it.

WHY THE EXAMINATION IS DONE

In well-intentioned attempts to improve the health of athletes, pre-participation evaluations have become required, and the 'cattle call' of mass screening is a part of the preseason ritual. The American College of Sports Medicine has tried to help this process through position statements and guidelines for participation. The third edition of the pre-participation evaluation was published in 2005 through the joint efforts of the American Academy of Family Physicians, American Academy of Pediatrics, American College of Sports Medicine, American Medical Society for Sports Medicine, American Orthopedic Society for Sports Medicine, and the American Osteopathic Academy of Sports Medicine. It addresses the appropriate aspects of the history and physical examination for athletes of high-school or college age and those with special needs.[1]

The goals of the pre-participation evaluation are as follows:

1. To gather baseline data for future reference[2,3]
2. To detect manageable medical conditions that may interfere with sports participation[2,3]
3. To determine whether there are contraindications to participation[2,3]
4. To discover predispositions to injury, including previous athletic injuries from inappropriate conditioning programs[2,3]
5. To assess an athlete's current fitness level to help prevent injuries from inappropriate conditioning programs[2,3]
6. To fulfill legal and insurance requirements[2,3]
7. To provide an opportunity for health education[3]
8. To establish a doctor–patient relationship with the athlete, identifying the physician and training staff as part of the athletic team
9. To provide an opportunity for training programs to educate residents, student therapists, and medical students about aspects of the physical examination in healthy individuals.

Gather baseline data for future reference

One challenge for any rehabilitation team is knowing when an athlete is able to return to play. In a sports-specific evaluation, detailed testing can be done to establish a baseline level of objective performance. The training staff thus knows an athlete's pre-injury condition and will know when the injured athlete is approaching the pre-injury state. Grip strength test, single-leg-hop test, specific speed tests (e.g. the 40-yard dash) and strength tests (e.g. the bench press) have all been used. Their predictive value in determining sports performance is questionable, but they are reproducible and a functional screen of specific skills.

Similar injuries are rarely clustered on the same team. Maintaining data on injuries and sharing this information across teams in a league or on a nationwide basis may identify training errors or dangerous practices and lead to rule changes to make sports safer.

Detect manageable medical conditions that may interfere with sports participation

The cyclic nature of sports allows athletes to move from one activity to another during a calendar year. This change allows injured areas time to heal and become less painful. Unfortunately, this process is not the same as rehabilitation. Once an injury is asymptomatic, the athlete needs to regain flexibility and strength before resuming the dynamic components of a particular sport. An injured athlete who does not have rehabilitation may not have symptoms during the off season or while participating in another sport. Re-injury from season to season may actually be incomplete rehabilitation.

Sufficient time for rehabilitation dictates that the screening evaluation should occur well in advance of the onset of the sports season. Of course, ideally, injuries are identified and rehabilitation occurs soon after. Changes in schools, uncertainties about participation in the upcoming year and various external factors make the reality less than ideal.

The pre-participation evaluation should occur at least 6 weeks before pre-season practices. For some programs, this means that the evaluation should occur at the end of the school year, before the summer break.

Determine whether there are contraindications to participation

The key to the pre-participation evaluation is the athlete's medical history. Abnormal findings on physical examination may be subtle or related to vision, neuromusculoskeletal disorders, or cardiac concerns. Athletes are as likely to give a worrisome history (e.g. presyncope, syncope, exertional palpitations) as have physical abnormalities (e.g. hypertension, new murmur).[4] A typical pre-participation evaluation does not include objective testing beyond the physical examination to identify dangerous conditions: dilated cardiomyopathy, hypertrophic cardiomyopathy, neck instability, seizure disorders. Screening for these conditions is prohibitively expensive, and false-positive results add needless expense and anxiety to the process.

The nature of athletics, and childhood in general, can serve as a test of an individual's physiognomy. In an unstructured setting, a child or individual serves as his or her own regulator or monitor of exertion. It is not until there are external forces (coaches, peers or parents) that an individual is stressed to an extreme degree and puts himself or herself at risk. Obtaining an accurate and detailed history from the athlete and his or her parents can help identify risks and identify individuals in need of more detailed testing.

Discover predispositions to injury, including previous athletic injuries from inappropriate conditioning programs

Existing or 'leftover' injuries are a logistical problem that can be addressed with proper planning and timing, but not knowing is dangerous to the athlete. The athlete's medical history is essential (Table 12.1).

A family history of sudden death, shortness of breath, and syncope or presyncope (dizziness) should prompt a more thorough evaluation of the cardiac system. Other conditions that are not as dangerous may be problematic in certain sports. Hyperflexibility may seem to be advantageous for some sports (e.g. gymnastics) but may lead to pain and joint problems if the athlete has not developed the muscle to compensate for ligamentous incompetence.

Assess an athlete's current fitness level to help prevent injuries from inappropriate conditioning programs

The typical screening evaluation does little to directly assess cardiovascular fitness. The athlete's history gives some indication of ability to participate fully. The physical assessment suggests a level of fitness: resting pulse, blood pressure and body weight all may raise concerns about the athlete's level of fitness, although they are not direct measures of that fitness. Worrisome findings on the history or physical assessment should prompt referral and more in-depth evaluation by the athlete's primary care physician or a specialist.

Fulfill legal and insurance requirements

The frequency of pre-participation evaluations varies from state to state.[5] Many states require a physician's evaluation before the school year in anticipation of physical education class. Sport-specific evaluations may be required to identify sports-specific conditions or injuries peculiar to a particular activity.

Provide an opportunity for health education

In addition to screening for injuries and disqualifying conditions, the physician may have the opportunity to provide some counseling for the athlete. Unfortunately, the pre-participation evaluation has taken the place of the annual physical examination for some children. Athletes and their parents are not always aware that the pre-participation evaluation is a screening examination and not a comprehensive adolescent general medical examination. In some communities, the local primary care physician provides the pre-participation evaluation, an arrangement that can build on the rapport and trust between the physician and patient. Risk-assessment counseling and counseling regarding nutrition and skin care, including protection from sun exposure, can be a set part of the evaluation process or can occur informally during downtime or waiting periods between testing stations.

Table 12.1   Components of the History Taking in Pre-Participation Evaluations

History	Have you had a medical illness or injury since your last check-up or sports physical?
	Do you have an ongoing or chronic illness?
	Have you ever been hospitalized overnight?
	Have you ever had surgery?
Injury history	Do you use any special protective or corrective equipment or devices that are not usually used for your sport or position (e.g. knee brace, special neck roll, foot orthotics, retainer on your teeth, hearing aid)?
Performance-enhancing supplements	Are you currently taking any prescription or non-prescription (over-the-counter) medications or pills or using an inhaler?
	Have you ever taken any supplements or vitamins to help you gain or lose weight or improve your performance?
Pulmonary, allergies and asthma	Do you cough, wheeze, or have trouble breathing during or after activity?
	Do you have asthma?
	Do you have seasonal allergies that require medical treatment?
	Do you have any allergies (e.g. to pollen, medicine, food or stinging insects)?
	Have you ever had a rash or hives develop during or after exercise?
Cardiac and pulmonary	Have you ever passed out during or after exercise?
	Have you ever been dizzy during or after exercise?
	Have you ever had chest pain during or after exercise?
	Do you get tired more quickly than your peers do during exercise?
	Have you ever had racing of your heart or skipped heartbeats?
	Have you had high blood pressure or high cholesterol?
	Have you ever been told you have a heart murmur?
	Has a family member or relative died of heart problems or of sudden death before the age of 50?
	Have you had a severe viral infection (e.g. myocarditis or mononucleosis) within the last month?
	Has a physician ever denied or restricted your participation in sports for any heart problems?
Integument	Do you have any current skin problems (e.g. itching, rashes, acne, warts, fungus, or blisters)?
Neurologic	Have you ever had a head injury or concussion?
	Have you ever been knocked out, become unconscious, or lost your memory?
	Have you ever had a seizure?
	Do you have frequent or severe headaches?
	Have you ever had numbness or tingling in your arms, hands, legs, or feet?
	Have you ever had a stinger, burner, or pinched nerve?
Metabolic	Have you ever become ill from exercising in the heat?
Eyes	Have you had any problems with your eyes or vision?
	Do you wear glasses, contacts, or protective eyewear?
Musculoskeletal	Have you ever had a sprain, strain, or swelling after injury?
	Have you broken or fractured any bones or dislocated any joints?
	Have you had any problems with pain or swelling in muscles, tendons, bones, or joints?
Eating disorders	Do you want to weigh more or less than you do now?[a]
	Do you lose weight regularly to meet weight requirements for your sport?
Psychologic	Do you feel stressed out?
Public health	Record the dates of your most recent immunizations (shots) for tetanus, hepatitis B, measles, chickenpox
Gynecologic (females only)[a]	When was your first menstrual period?
	When was your most recent menstrual period?
	How much time do you usually have from the start of one period to the start of another?
	How many periods have you had in the past year?
	What was the longest time between periods in the last year?

Note: Various screening forms are available. The one endorsed by the major sports medicine groups is shown in Figure 12.1. Alternative questions are listed above.
[a]These questions also help to screen for persons at risk for the female athlete triad of amenorrhea, disordered eating and osteoporosis.

Establish a doctor–patient relationship with the athlete, identifying the physician and training staff as part of the athletic team

Other benefits of the pre-participation evaluation include establishing a relationship between the physician and athlete. This interaction is often strained and is related to the athlete's interaction with the physician in stressful and adversarial circumstances. If the athlete sees the physician only when an injury occurs and then only to hear bad news, the physician is unlikely to be regarded as a resource. The athletic trainers can be a valuable extension of the physician because they often have a better rapport with the athlete as a result of routine interaction. Subtle changes in condition can be discerned by the training staff and conveyed to the physician for further assessment. The pre-participation evaluation allows the team physician to participate with the team during a positive time of the year.

Provide an opportunity for training programs to educate residents, student therapists and medical students about aspects of the physical examination in healthy individuals

Another, less-often discussed benefit of the pre-participation evaluation is to the examiners. Rarely do physicians have the opportunity to see a range of healthy individuals in one place. Familiarity with normal examination findings makes any variation all the more obvious.

The physician, the athlete, the parents and the school should not expect too much from the evaluation. In essence, it is a screening method to identify athletes at risk for further or potential injury. It will not prevent injuries in healthy, asymptomatic individuals. It may not be the best setting for education and so may be only an opportunity to introduce certain topics.

COMPONENTS OF THE EVALUATION

Box 12.2: Key Points

There are different ways to complete the pre-participation evaluation, but basic components of the history and the physical examination should be included to identify athletes at risk for injury.

There are two basic approaches to the pre-participation evaluation. The first approach, the single-examiner system, is a focused general medical examination that includes all the components that need to be addressed before participation in the upcoming season. The history needs to consider the intense and risky nature of athletics. The history should identify clues that the individual could be at risk by participating. Single-examiner evaluations may be efficient and are valuable for promoting interaction with the primary care physician. Unfortunately, that format does not compensate for any diagnostic weaknesses of the examiner. A variation of the single-examiner method includes several examiners who do a complete examination on

a portion of the athletes being screened. This has the same limitations as the typical single-examiner examination, but it may be an efficient option when there are multiple examiners in similar specialties and space does not allow numerous stations.[4]

The second approach, the station approach, includes multiple examiners at multiple spots in a common area (office suite, gymnasium, locker room). It has the advantage of allowing specialists to focus on their area of expertise. This approach adds efficiency and is a great service to the athlete.

The subsequent description of the evaluation is based on the station approach and assumes that the physicians involved are either specialists who may be required to do screening in an area outside their specialty (e.g. a physiatrist listening to a murmur or discerning an arrhythmia) or generalists who are not an athlete's primary care physician. In these instances, the physician needs to understand what findings are disqualifying and what findings warrant further evaluation. In many instances, the worrisome finding is negative on review by a specialist or a physician who knows the patient. In others, the finding may be normal for a particular patient (e.g. hyperflexibility).

It is inappropriate for the screening physician to make the decision to disqualify a player when he or she is not comfortable doing so. It is probably best to refer the athlete for further evaluation by a specialist. This possibility is another reason to schedule the pre-participation evaluation with enough lead time to allow assessment of worrisome findings.

Table 12.2 provides one option for the station approach to the pre-participation examination. Ideally, the athlete and his or her parents complete the pre-participation evaluation history and physical examination forms (Figs 12.1, 12.2) before arriving at the assessment site. Non-physician staff can perform the initial assessment and ensure that the paperwork is complete; the heart, lung and visceral examination needs to be done by a physician. The musculoskeletal examination could be done by a skilled physical therapist but the results should be confirmed by a physician.

The order of the physical examination stations can vary. However, review of the findings at each of the stations and clearance to play should come from the lead or supervising physician at the last station. In some programs, there may be a preponderance of physicians. In those instances, it is reasonable to have physicians obtain vital signs and clarify the history. They can rotate into the evaluation stations as the athletes progress to other stations. It is important that the

Table 12.2 Example of the Station Approach to Pre-Participation Evaluation

Station	Activity	Suggested No. of Staff
1	Paperwork, height, weight	2
2	Vision screening	1
3	Blood pressure	1
4	HEENT, cardiopulmonary, skin, genitalia/hernia (males)	2 physicians
5	Neuromusculoskeletal	2 physicians
6	Review, disposition/follow-up, dietary, psychosocial counseling	2 physicians

HEENT, head, eyes, ears, nose, throat.
(From: Smith and Laskowski,[4] with permission.)

HISTORY FORM

DATE OF EXAM _____

Name _____ Sex _____ Age _____ Date of Birth _____
Grade _____ School _____ Sports _____
Address _____ Phone _____
Personal physician _____
In case of emergency, contact
Name _____ Relationship _____ Phone (H) _____ (W) _____

Explain "Yes" answers below. Circle questions you don't know the answers to.

	Yes	No		Yes	No
1. Has a doctor ever denied or restricted your participation in sports for any reason?	☐	☐	24. Do you cough, wheeze, or have difficulty breathing during or after exercise?	☐	☐
2. Do you have any ongoing medical condition (like diabetes or asthma)?	☐	☐	25. Is there anyone in your family who has asthma?	☐	☐
3. Are you currently taking any prescription or non-prescription (over-the-counter) medicines or pills?	☐	☐	26. Have you ever used an inhaler or taken asthma medicine?	☐	☐
			27. Were you born without or are you missing a kidney, an eye, a testicle, or any other organ?	☐	☐
4. Do you have allergies to medicine, pollens, foods or stinging insects?	☐	☐	28. Have you had infectious mononucleosis (mono) within the last month?	☐	☐
5. Have you ever passed out or nearly passed out DURING exercise?	☐	☐	29. Do you have any rashes, pressure sores or other skin problems?	☐	☐
6. Have you ever passed out or nearly passed out AFTER exercise?	☐	☐	30. Have you had a herpes skin infection?	☐	☐
7. Have you ever had discomfort, pain or pressure in your chest during exercise?	☐	☐	31. Have you ever had a head injury or concussion?	☐	☐
8. Does your heart race or skip beats during exercise?	☐	☐	32. Have you been hit in the head and been confused or lost your memory?	☐	☐
9. Has your doctor ever told you that you have (check all that apply):	☐	☐	33. Have you ever had a seizure?	☐	☐
☐ High blood pressure ☐ A heart murmur			34. Do you have headaches with exercise?	☐	☐
☐ High cholesterol ☐ A heart infection			35. Have you ever had numbness, tingling or weakness in your arms or legs after being hit or falling?	☐	☐
10. Has a doctor ever ordered a test for your heart? (for example, ECG, echocardiogram)	☐	☐	36. Have you ever been unable to move your arms or legs after being hit or falling?	☐	☐
11. Has anyone in your family died for no apparent reason?	☐	☐	37. When exercising in the heat, do you have severe muscle cramps or become ill?	☐	☐
12. Does anyone in your family have a heart problem?	☐	☐	38. Has a doctor told you that you or someone in your family has sickle cell trait or sickle cell disease?	☐	☐
13. Has any family member or relative died of heart problems or of sudden death before age 50?	☐	☐	39. Have you had any problems with your eyes or vision?	☐	☐
14. Does anyone in your family have Marfan syndrome?	☐	☐	40. Do you wear glasses or contact lenses?	☐	☐
15. Have you ever spent the night in a hospital?	☐	☐	41. Do you wear protective eyewear, such as goggles or a face shield?	☐	☐
16. Have you ever had surgery?	☐	☐	42. Are you happy with your weight?	☐	☐
			43. Are you trying to gain or lose weight?	☐	☐
			44. Has anyone recommended you change your weight or eating habits?	☐	☐

17. Have you ever had an injury, like a sprain, muscle or ligament tear, or tendonitis, that caused you to miss a practice or game? If yes, circle the affected area below:	☐	☐
18. Have you had any broken or fractured or dislocated joints? If yes, circle below:	☐	☐
19. Have you had a bone or joint injury that required x-rays, MRI, CT, surgery, injections, rehabilitation, physical therapy, a brace, a cast, or crutches? If yes, circle below:	☐	☐

45. Do you limit or carefully control what you eat? ☐ ☐
46. Do you have any concerns that you would like to discuss with a doctor? ☐ ☐

FEMALES ONLY

47. Have you ever had a menstrual period? ☐ ☐

Head	Neck	Shoulder	Upper arm	Elbow	Forearm	Hand/ fingers	Chest
Upper back	Lower back	Hip	Thigh	Knee	Calf/ shin	Ankle	Foot/ toes

48. How old were you when you had your first menstrual period? _____

49. How many periods have you had in the last 12 months? _____

Explain "yes" answers here: _____

20. Have you ever had a stress fracture?	☐	☐
21. Have you been told that you have or have you had an x-ray for atlantoaxial (neck) instability?	☐	☐
22. Do you regularly use a brace or assistive device?	☐	☐
23. Has a doctor ever told you that you have asthma or allergies?	☐	☐

_____
_____
_____
_____
_____

I hereby state, to the best of my knowledge, my answers to the above questions are complete and correct.
Signature of athlete _____ Signature of parent/guardian _____ Date _____

Figure 12.1 History form used for pre-participation evaluation. (With permission from American Academy of Family Physicians, American Academy of Pediatrics, American College of Sports Medicine.[1])

PHYSICAL EXAMINATION FORM

Name _____ Date of Birth _____

Height _____ Weight _____ % Body fat (optional) _____ Pulse _____ BP ___ / ___ (___ / ___ , ___ / ___)

Vision R20/ _____ L20/ _____ Corrected: Y   N   Pupils: Equal _____ Unequal _____

Follow-up questions on more sensitive issues

	Yes	No
1. Do you feel stressed out or under a lot of pressure?	☐	☐
2. Do you ever feel so sad or hopeless that you stop doing some of your usual activities for more than a few days?	☐	☐
3. Do you feel safe?	☐	☐
4. Have you ever tried cigarette smoking, even 1 or 2 puffs? Do you currently smoke?	☐	☐
5. During the past 30 days, did you use chewing tobacco, snuff, or dip?	☐	☐
6. During the past 30 days, have you had at least 1 drink of alcohol?	☐	☐
7. Have you ever taken steroid pills or shots without a doctor's prescription?	☐	☐
8. Have you ever taken any supplements to help you gain or lose weight or improve your performance?	☐	☐
9. Questions from the Youth Risk Behavior Survey (http://www.cdc.gov/Health Youth/yrbs/index.htm) on guns, seatbelts, unprotected sex, domestic violence, drugs, etc.	☐	☐

Notes: _____
_____

	NORMAL	ABNORMAL FINDINGS	INITIALS*
MEDICAL			
Appearance			
Eyes/ears/nose/throat			
Hearing			
Lymph nodes			
Heart			
Murmurs			
Pulses			
Lungs			
Abdomen			
Genitourinary (males only)**			
Skin			
MUSCULOSKELETAL			
Neck			
Back			
Shoulder/arm			
Elbow/forearm			
Wrist/hand/fingers			
Hip/thigh			
Knee			
Leg/ankle			
Foot/toes			

* Multiple-examiner set-up only
** Having a third party present is recommended for genitourinary examination

Notes: _____
_____

Name of physician (print/type) _____ **Date** _____
Address _____ **Phone** _____
Signature of physician _____ , MD or DO

Figure 12.2 Physical examination form used for pre-participation evaluation. (With permission from American Academy of Family Physicians, American Academy of Pediatrics, American College of Sports Medicine.[1])

physicians testing athletes feel comfortable with their component of the examination. In medical training programs, less experienced physicians may screen athletes for suspicious findings and more experienced physicians or specialists can confirm or clarify a confusing finding. This approach is efficient, improves the knowledge of the less experienced physicians, and may eliminate needless specialty consultations. Preferably, an athlete is examined thoroughly rather than allowed to play while there is uncertainty about the significance of a finding.

Ideally, the medical staff of the team or school is involved in the screening process. Their inclusion allows them to establish rapport with the team members and facilitates follow-up.

Specific considerations based on the history

> **Box 12.3: Key Points**
>
> Components of the history may not preclude athletic participation, but they often prompt further evaluation.

Hypertension
Athletes with a history of high blood pressure should be under the care of a physician. If there is no evidence of end-organ damage, they can compete in all sports. If they are older than 18 years and have a systolic blood pressure >159 mmHg or a diastolic blood pressure >99 mmHg, or have end-organ damage, they need to be treated[1] and should be held from activity until their blood pressure is controlled. Younger athletes are considered at risk on the basis of their blood pressure related to their sex, height and weight. A systolic blood pressure >130 mmHg or a diastolic blood pressure >90 mmHg needs to be evaluated. If values are close to these, the pressures need to be carefully re-determined and the appropriate tables consulted. Detailed tables can be found at: http://www.nhlbi.nih.gov/guidelines/hypertension/child_tbl.htm.[6]

Cardiovascular conditioning may be beneficial but should be prescribed on an individual basis. The athlete on a team is assumed to be able to participate fully and without restriction.

Diabetes mellitus
Athletes with diabetes who do not have complications should be allowed to participate in sports that do not constitute a high risk. The American Diabetes Association has guidelines for participation,[7] and the athlete should have a program established with his or her treating physician. Sports are considered high risk for athletes with diabetes according to the risk associated with a hypoglycemic episode (to the individual or their competition) or if they are solo endurance activities and so medical support may be problematic (Table 12.3).[8]

Heat illness
The deaths of athletes during exercise in the heat has directed attention toward heat-related illnesses. Obesity, deconditioning, sickle cell trait,[9] or febrile illness can put individuals at risk for a heat-related illness.[10–12]

Table 12.3 Sports that Pose a Risk for Athletes with Diabetes Mellitus

Risk of Hypoglycemia	Lack of Support	Risk to Competitors
Rock climbing	Ultramarathons	Motor sports
Skydiving	Cycling	
Scuba diving	Open-water swimming	

(Data from American Academy of Family Physicians et al.[1] and Draznin.[8])

Kidney abnormalities
Athletes with a single functioning kidney should not participate in contact-collision sports (see Table 12.8) until cleared by their urologist or nephrologist due to the consequences of the loss of this kidney.[1] Even though the risk of kidney loss is small, some experts believe that kidney abnormalities (e.g. hydronephrosis, multiple cysts) or malposition (e.g. iliac, pelvic) should disqualify athletes from contact-collision sports.[13]

Specific components of the physical examination

> **Box 12.4: Key Points**
>
> The purpose of the physical examination is to screen for abnormalities that may predispose to injury and to assess for pre-existing problems.

The physical examination is not the time to redo the history, but the examiner should review the athlete's forms to determine whether there are any pre-existing injuries or conditions that should be evaluated. In large programs or in a community setting, it may be possible to review the results of previous evaluations or injury records to ensure that components of the history or previous physical conditions have not been omitted. A systematic approach to the examination ensures efficiency and completeness. One approach is provided in Table 12.4 and Figure 12.3.

Height, weight and vital signs

> **Box 12.5: Key Points**
>
> Abnormal blood pressure readings necessitate repeated measurements several times during the testing session.

Abnormal blood pressure readings are common in pre-participation evaluations, and mildly increased blood pressures are not disqualifying for most sports.[1,14–17] Exercise is therapeutic

Table 12.4   Components of the Physical Examination in Pre-Participation Evaluations

Neuromusculoskeletal examination	
Instructions to the athlete	
(Athlete: stands facing the examiner)	Figure 3A
Look to the left and right	Figure 3B
Raise arms overhead	Figure 3C
Put arms behind neck	Figure 3D
Arms at sides, squat and walk forward 4 steps	Figure 3E
Stand up. Hop on right foot, hop on left	Figure 3F
Tandem walk to me	
Walk on heels	Figure 3G (right)
Squeeze my hands	
Shrug your shoulders	Figure 3H
Don't let me push down	Figure 3I
Don't let me push down	Figure 3J
Don't let me push up	Figure 3K
(May insert visceral examination here)	
Sit on table	
(Check biceps, triceps, patella and Achilles reflexes)	
Turn away	Figure 3L
Put arms behind back	Figure 3M
Arms straight ahead, palms together	
Flex at the waist	Figure 3N
Walk away on toes	Figure 3G (left)
Medical examination	
Instructions to the athlete:	
Follow my finger with your eyes	
(Rub fingers near each ear) – Can you hear this?	
(Tympanic membranes, optional for most, required for swimming)	
(Heart examination, listen for murmurs that change with inspiration or exertion)	
(Lung examination)	
Lie down	
(Feel for spleen and liver edge)	
(Genitalia examination, males: descended testicles, presence of a hernia)	

for adults with hypertension,[18] and thus participation should be encouraged for athletes with increased blood pressure. Resistance training should be avoided in athletes with significant essential (unexplained) hypertension (see Table 12.8). Stage 2 hypertension in children is defined as repeated systolic and diastolic pressures that are more than the 99th percentile values based on sex, height and age.[1] Detailed tables can be found at: http://www.nhlbi.nih.gov/guidelines/hypertension/child_tbl.htm.[6]

Table 12.5 lists systolic and diastolic blood pressures at the 99th percentile for boys and girls between the ages of 13 and 17 who are at the 50th percentile for height and the current recommendations for adults.

Blood pressure can normally be different in children to that in adolescents, but blood pressures more than 135/90 mmHg

warrant further evaluation. If blood pressure is increased, the athlete should sit quietly for 5 min before it is re-measured. The proper-sized cuff should be used because a small cuff on a large adolescent provides a falsely increased value. If the cuff size is correct and the pressure is still increased, the athlete should lie down for 15 min before the pressure is re-checked. Continued increased pressures require evaluation and treatment before clearance. Practically speaking, if an examiner obtains pressures close to these in a mass screening setting, the first step should be to repeat the test in a quiet part of the testing area. Repeated tests are necessary to diagnose hypertension, but they may not be possible at the evaluation. Athletes should be deferred from participation until evaluated by their primary care physician.

Height and weight are used to calculate the body mass index (BMI). Calculations are different for children and adults (defined as persons older than 20 years). In adults, a body BMI of 18.5–24.9 is considered normal, 25 is overweight, and 30 is obese.[19]

Children and adolescents are younger than 20 years, and they are considered underweight if the BMI is less than the 5th percentile for age and overweight if it is more than the 95th percentile.[20] Growth charts of BMI-for-age are age- and sex-specific.[20] Athletes who are underweight for their height and age may be at risk for disordered eating. These athletes may need more detailed questioning (Table 12.6).[21]

Head, eyes, ears, nose and throat

This part of the evaluation is considered one of the most straightforward components and is the part in which most of the abnormalities are discovered.[4] Visual acuity of 20/40 in one eye is considered adequate vision.[1] Athletes whose best visual acuity in one eye is worse than 20/40, even with correction, should be considered 'one-eyed'.[1,22] They would have a significant change in lifestyle if they lost the use of that eye.

The risks of eye injury by sport are listed in Table 12.7. Eye protection can help, but the consequences of an eye injury to an athlete with only one functioning eye need to be considered.

The build-up of cerumen may compromise hearing, but it may not be possible to correct it and re-assess during a large screening session. The athlete may need to return or see his or her primary care physician. Likewise, nasal polyps or a deviated septum does not affect clearance but should be noted. The athlete may need further treatment at the discretion of his or her primary care physician.[1]

Cardiovascular

> **Box 12.6: Key Points**
>
> Murmurs that increase with Valsalva maneuver or when changing position from sitting to standing need further evaluation.

The cardiovascular examination probably causes the greatest concern for the examining physician. The history provided by the athlete, whether a personal history of fainting, dizziness, loss of consciousness, seizure, or problems associated with physical

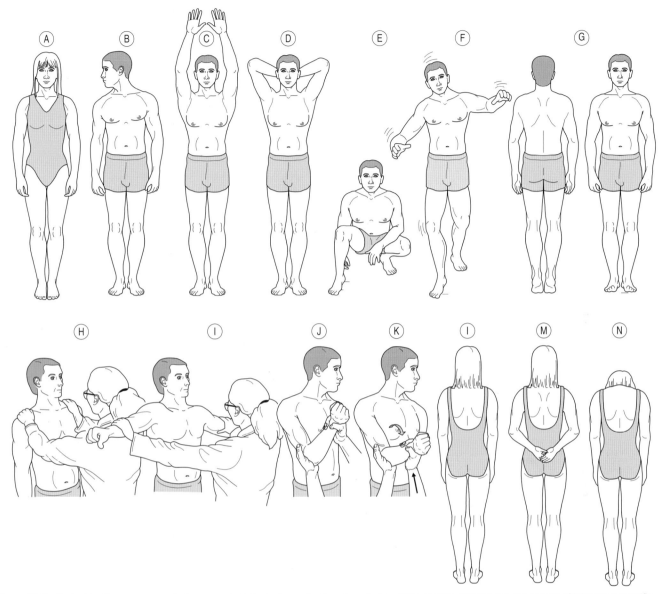

Figure 12.3 Typical testing maneuvers in the screening physical examination. Any abnormalities or asymmetries and any history of injury to a specific joint should be evaluated in more detail. (A) Inspection, athlete standing, facing examiner. (B) Neck rotation to right and left. (C) Arms overhead. (D) Shoulder external rotation and elbow range of motion. (E) 'Duck' walk. (F) One-legged hop (both sides should be tested). (G) Walk on heels and toes. (H) Resisted shoulder shrug (trapezius). (I) Resisted shoulder abduction (deltoid). (J) Resisted elbow flexion (biceps, brachialis). (K) Resisted elbow extension (triceps). (L) Inspection, athlete facing away from examiner. (M) Shoulder internal rotation and elbow range of motion. (N) Back flexion, knees straight.

exertion, is as telling as anything that will be discovered on the typical physical examination. More advanced testing has been proposed, but it has not been found to be cost-effective for screening a large number of asymptomatic individuals and may result in a significant number of false-positive results.[23] Lawless *et al.*[24] found that portable two-dimensional echocardiography was inexpensive and increased the number of students deferred until further evaluation from 3.9 to 4.95%. It is unclear how many of these subsequently were cleared to participate after further evaluation (e.g. false-positive rate). Cantwell[3] suggested screening electrocardiography on entry into high-school sports. Athletes with inappropriately high voltage or marked repolarization variation should have limited echocardiography to rule out hypertrophic cardiomyopathy.

Heart murmurs may be common in adolescents, but those that are loud (3/6 in intensity), any diastolic murmur, and a murmur that increases with Valsalva maneuver or on change in position from sitting to standing are signs of possible hypertrophic cardiomyopathy.[3,25] Non-cardiologists should refer such patients to a qualified internist or cardiologist for clearance.

Lungs

Both lungs should be evaluated for even air exchange without any wheezing. Athletes with wheezes, rubs, prolonged expiratory phase, or significant cough with forced expiration should be referred for further evaluation.[1] The most prevalent pulmonary problem in athletes is exercise-induced bronchoconstriction.[1,26]

Table 12.5 Systolic and Diastolic Blood Pressures at 99th Percentile for Boys and Girls at the 50th Percentile for Height

| Age (Years) | Blood Pressure (mmHg) | | | |
| | Boys | | Girls | |
	Systolic	Diastolic	Systolic	Diastolic
13	133	89	132	89
14	136	90	133	90
15	138	91	134	91
16	141	92	135	91
17	143	94	136	91
18 or older	160	100	160	100

(Modified from National Heart, Lung, and Blood Institute.[6])

Table 12.6 Questions Regarding Disordered Eating

1. How old were you when you had your first menstrual period?
2. How many periods have you had in the past 12 months?
3. Have you ever gone for more than 2 months without having a menstrual period?
4. How long do your periods last?
5. When was your last menstrual period?
6. Do you take birth control pills or hormones?
7. Have you ever been treated for anemia?
8. What have you eaten in the past 24 h?
9. Are there certain foods you refuse to eat? (e.g. meats, breads)
10. Are you happy with your present weight?
11. If not, what would you like to weigh?
12. Have you ever tried to control your weight with fasting? _____ vomiting? _____ laxatives? _____ diuretics? _____ diet pills? _____
13. Do you have questions about healthy ways to control weight?

(Modified from Johnson MD. Tailoring the pre-participation exam to female athletes. Phys Sports Med 1992; 20:60–72, with permission.)

Symptoms of exercise-induced bronchoconstriction include shortness of breath, wheezing, chest tightness and cough that occurs during or after exercise. These symptoms are more common in athletes participating in cold-weather sports.[27] Further testing is necessary. This testing can include spirometry and subsequent pulmonary function tests.[1] Participation is rarely restricted because of exercise-induced bronchoconstriction or asthma if proper treatment and monitoring are provided.

This part of the examination provides the opportunity to discuss the impact of smoking on athletic participation, particularly if there is an odor of tobacco about the athlete.[1] Any history of breathing difficulties during or immediately after exercise suggests exercise-induced asthma, and provocative testing may be needed.

Abdomen

In adults, we do not expect any organs to be palpable. Palpation of a liver or spleen tip is unexpected and should prompt referral back to the primary care physician. In a young person, particularly with a thin body habitus, this finding may not be unusual. However, masses, tenderness, rigidity, or enlargement of the liver or spleen or an abnormal kidney requires further evaluation.[1] Typically, the athlete's pediatrician can confirm such a finding from prior examinations, or an

Table 12.7 Risk of Eye Injury, by Sport

| Risk | | | |
High	Moderate	Low	Safe
Small, fast projectiles	Badminton	Bicycling	Gymnastics
Air rifle	Fishing	Diving	Track and field
BB gun	Football	Non-contact martial arts	
Paintball	Golf	Skiing (snow and water)	
Hard projectiles, 'sticks', close contact	Soccer	Swimming	
Baseball, softball	Tennis	Wrestling	
Basketball	Volleyball		
Cricket	Water polo		
Fencing			
Hockey (ice and field)			
Lacrosse			
Racquetball			
Squash			
Intentional injury			
Boxing			
Full-contact martial arts			

(From Vinger PF. A practical guide for sports eye protection. Phys Sports Med 2000; 28:49–69, with permission.)

athlete's choice of activities may not pose a greater risk. Patients with chronic hepatomegaly or splenomegaly should have their participation determined individually in consultation with their primary care physician.

In women, the lower abdomen can be palpated to determine the presence of a palpable (gravid) uterus.[1]

Tenderness to palpation is not normal and should prompt a further evaluation, as would a history that suggests a recent infectious process. Because of the risks of injury to affected organs, the athlete should not return to contact or collision sports until the inflammatory process has resolved.[28,29] This determination may require serial ultrasound evaluations to accurately assess the size of the spleen and liver.[30,31]

Genitalia

Inguinal hernias are traditionally assessed in men, although their presence does not preclude participation. Asymptomatic hernias should be monitored. Symptomatic hernias may require treatment at some time.[1] If the hernia affects participation, that decision may have to come before participation continues. Testicular disorders do not preclude participation.[32,33] A solitary testicle requires the use of a protective cup in contact or collision sports (Table 12.8). An undescended testicle should be referred for evaluation given the increased risk of testicular cancer.[1]

The female genitourinary examination should be done by the primary care physician.[1]

Skin

The skin examination should include attention to acne, evidence of sun damage, rashes, infections, marks of illicit drug use and infestations.[1] Suspicious lesions should be referred for further evaluation. Potentially contagious rashes such as herpes simplex, molluscum contagiosum, fungal infections, scabies and louse infestations should be evaluated and treated before the athlete continues contact with other athletes.[1,34-36]

Musculoskeletal

> **Box 12.7: Key Points**
>
> Previous injuries need to be assessed and rehabilitation completed before clearance for participation.

The key to an efficient neuromusculoskeletal examination is to make it performance-based and to look for asymmetry. Range of motion, strength and performance (e.g. hopping, grip strength) should be equal. Asymmetry should be explained (e.g. previous healed injury with a known deformity) and should be compatible with participation in the chosen activity or it will need more complete evaluation.

If the athlete has had an injury since the last evaluation or during the last sports season, he or she should be cleared by the physician who is treating that injury. If the general examination reveals any pain, joint instability, locking, weakness, or atrophy, a more detailed evaluation is indicated or the athlete should be referred to a specialist.[1]

Two findings on the musculoskeletal examination bear further discussion. Scoliosis in an adolescent may not have been determined at previous screenings. Scoliosis itself does not prevent athletic participation, but it should be followed to monitor any progression and to take necessary steps to prevent unwanted sequelae of developmental spinal deformities.[1] Hyperflexibility and characteristic morphologic features (long fingers, sunken chest) can be found in children with Marfan syndrome. There may be an aortic murmur. Because this condition can have catastrophic consequences, its suspicion should prompt a more thorough evaluation.

Neurologic

A performance-based musculoskeletal examination provides a good screening of the neurologic system. Checking the reflexes of the biceps, triceps, patella tendon and heel cord completes that aspect of the assessment of the peripheral nervous system (hearing and vision have already been screened). Asymmetry of strength or reflexes needs further assessment. Hyperreflexia also needs to be explored more fully through the history or detailed questioning about central nervous system injuries.[1]

Most worrisome neurologic conditions are described in the history. A history of pain in the arm associated with neck motion may be a burner or stinger. These may be benign but may indicate brachial plexus injury or cervical nerve root compression.[37] Transient quadriparesis is a controversial phenomenon that needs further evaluation. Evidence of instability or spinal cord injury requires treatment and likely will lead to exclusion from contact-collision sports. Congenital cervical stenosis also may predispose to transient quadripareses, but the disposition is less clear-cut.[38-41]

EDUCATION

> **Box 12.8: Key Points**
>
> The pre-participation evaluation is an opportunity to provide needed information to athletes and their parents on various topics.

During the pre-participation evaluation, the examiners may detect poor health practices in the athletes. Furthermore, the typical screening process tends to have a lot of downtime for the athletes. This is an opportunity to provide information in the form of charts, handouts, or other reading material to the athletes, coaches, or accompanying parents or guardians. Some topics to consider include nutrition and ergogenic aids and supplements, proper rest and hydration, cancer awareness from sun exposure and tobacco and general health and safety practices.

Nutrition

Updated information on a balanced diet for athletes can be provided during the screening program. It can be perused during waiting periods and brought home and used for reference. Diet information may help female athletes acquire a more appropriate attitude toward calorie intake as it relates to athletic performance.

Table 12.8 Medical Conditions and Sports Participation[a]

Condition	May Participate
Atlantoaxial instability (instability of the joint between cervical vertebrae 1 and 2)	Qualified yes
Explanation: Athlete needs evaluation to assess risk of spinal cord injury during sports participation.	
Bleeding disorder[b]	Qualified yes
Explanation: Athlete needs evaluation.	
Cardiovascular disease	
Carditis (inflammation of the heart)	No
Explanation: Carditis may result in sudden death with exertion.	
Hypertension (high blood pressure)	Qualified yes
Explanation: Those with significant essential (unexplained) hypertension should avoid weight and powerlifting, body building and strength training. Those with secondary hypertension (hypertension caused by a previously identified disease) or severe essential hypertension need evaluation. The National High Blood Pressure Education Working Group defined significant and severe hypertension.[c]	
Congenital heart disease (structural heart defects present at birth)	Qualified yes
Explanation: Those with mild forms may participate fully; those with moderate or severe forms or who have undergone surgery need evaluation. The 26th Bethesda Conference defined mild, moderate and severe disease for common cardiac lesions.[d]	
Dysrhythmia (irregular heart rhythm)	Qualified yes
Explanation: Those with symptoms (chest pain, syncope, dizziness, shortness of breath, or other symptoms of possible dysrhythmia) or evidence of mitral regurgitation (leaking) on physical examination need evaluation. All others may participate fully.	
Heart murmur	Qualified yes
Explanation: If the murmur is innocent (does not indicate heart disease), full participation is permitted. Otherwise, the athlete needs evaluation.	
Cerebral palsy[b]	Qualified yes
Explanation: Athlete needs evaluation.	
Diabetes mellitus	Yes
Explanation: All sports can be played with proper attention to diet, blood glucose concentration, hydration and insulin therapy. Blood glucose concentration should be monitored every 30 min during continuous exercise and 15 min after completion of exercise.	
Diarrhea	Qualified no
Explanation: Unless disease is mild, no participation is permitted, because diarrhea may increase the risk of dehydration and heat illness. (See 'Fever' below)	
Eating disorders	Qualified yes
Anorexia nervosa, bulimia nervosa	
Explanation: Patients with these disorders need medical and psychiatric assessment before participation.	
Eyes	Qualified yes
Functionally one-eyed athlete, loss of an eye, detached retina, previous eye surgery, or serious eye injury	
Explanation: A functionally one-eyed athlete has a best-corrected visual acuity of less than 20/40 in the eye with worse acuity. These athletes would suffer significant disability if the better eye were seriously injured, as would those with loss of an eye. Some athletes who previously have undergone eye surgery or had a serious eye injury may have an increased risk of injury because of weakened eye tissue. Availability of eye guards approved by the American Society for Testing and Materials and other protective equipment may allow participation in most sports, but this must be judged on an individual basis.	
Fever	No
Explanation: Fever can increase cardiopulmonary effort, reduce maximum exercise capacity, make heat illness more likely and increase orthostatic hypertension during exercise. Fever may rarely accompany myocarditis or other infections that may make exercise dangerous.	
Heat illness, history of	Qualified yes
Explanation: Because of the increased likelihood of recurrence, the athlete needs individual assessment to determine the presence of predisposing conditions and to arrange a prevention strategy.	
Hepatitis	Yes
Explanation: Because of the apparent minimal risk to others, all sports may be played that the athlete's state of health allows. In all athletes, skin lesions should be covered properly, and athletic personnel should use universal precautions when handling blood or body fluids with visible blood.	
Human immunodeficiency virus (HIV) infection	Yes
Explanation: Because of the apparent minimal risk to others, all sports may be played as the athlete's state of health allows. In all athletes, skin lesions should be covered properly, and athletic personnel should use universal precautions when handling blood or body fluids with visible blood.	

Table 12.8   Medical Conditions and Sports Participation[a]—Cont'd

Condition	May Participate
Kidney, absence of one	Qualified yes
Explanation: Athlete needs individual assessment for contact, collision and limited-contact sports.	
Liver, enlarged	Qualified yes
Explanation: If the liver is acutely enlarged, participation should be avoided because of risk of rupture. If the liver is chronically enlarged, individual assessment is needed before collision, contact, or limited-contact sports are played.	
Malignant neoplasm[b]	Qualified yes
Explanation: Athlete needs individual assessment.	
Musculoskeletal disorders	Qualified yes
Explanation: Athlete needs individual assessment.	
Neurologic disorders	
History of serious head or spine trauma, severe or repeated concussions, or craniotomy	Qualified yes
Explanation: Athlete needs individual assessment for collision, contact, or limited-contact sports and also for non-contact sports if deficits in judgment or cognition are present. Research supports a conservative approach to management of concussion	
Seizure disorder, well-controlled	Yes
Explanation: Risk of seizure during participation is minimal.	
Seizure disorder, poorly controlled	Qualified yes
Explanation: Athlete needs individual assessment for collision, contact, or limited-contact sports. The following non-contact sports should be avoided: archery, riflery, swimming, weight or powerlifting, strength training, or sports involving heights. In these sports, occurrence of a seizure may pose a risk to self or others.	
Obesity	Qualified yes
Explanation: Because of the risk of heart illness, obese persons need careful acclimatization and hydration.	
Organ transplant recipient[b]	Qualified yes
Explanation: Athlete needs individual assessment.	
Ovary, absence of one	Yes
Explanation: Risk of severe injury to remaining ovary is minimal.	
Respiratory conditions	
Pulmonary compromise, including cystic fibrosis	Qualified yes
Explanation: Athlete needs individual assessment, but generally, all sports may be played if oxygenation remains satisfactory during a graded exercise test. Patients with cystic fibrosis need acclimatization and good hydration to reduce the risk of heat illness.	
Asthma	Yes
Explanation: With proper medication and education, only athletes with the most severe asthma will need to modify their participation.	
Acute upper respiratory infection	Qualified yes
Explanation: Upper respiratory obstruction may affect pulmonary function. Athlete needs individual assessment for all but mild disease. (See 'Fever', earlier)	
Sickle cell disease	Qualified yes
Explanation: Athlete needs individual assessment. In general, if status of the illness permits, all but high exertion, collision and contact sports may be played. Overheating, dehydration and chilling must be avoided.	
Sickle cell trait	Yes
Explanation: It is unlikely that persons with sickle cell trait have an increased risk of sudden death or other medical problems during athletic participation, except under the most extreme conditions of heat, humidity, and, possibly, increased altitude. These persons, like all athletes, should be carefully conditioned, acclimatized and hydrated to reduce any possible risk.	
Skin disorders (boils, herpes simplex, impetigo, scabies, molluscum contagiosum)	Qualified yes
Explanation: While the patient is contagious, participation in gymnastics with mats; martial arts; wrestling; or other collision, contact, or limited-contact sports is not allowed.	
Spleen, enlarged	Qualified yes
Explanation: A patient with an acutely enlarged spleen should avoid all sports because of risk of rupture. A patient with a chronically enlarged spleen needs individual assessment before playing collision, contact, or limited-contact sports.	
Testicle, undescended or absence of one	Yes
Explanation: Certain sports may require a protective cup.	

[a]This table is designed for use by medical and non-medical personnel. 'Needs evaluation' means that a physician with appropriate knowledge and experience should assess the safety of a given sport for an athlete with the listed medical condition. Unless otherwise noted, this is because of variability in the severity of the disease, the risk of injury for the specific sports, or both.
[b]Not discussed in this chapter.
[c]Whelton PK, He J, Appel LJ, *et al*. National High Blood Pressure Education Program Coordinating Committee. Primary prevention of hypertension: clinical and public health advisory from the National High Blood Pressure Education Program. JAMA 2002; 288:1882-1888.
[d]26th Bethesda Conference: recommendations for determining eligibility for competition in athletes with cardiovascular abnormalities. January 6-7, 1994. Med Sci Sports Exerc 1994; 26(Suppl):S223-S283; Erratum in Med Sci Sports Exerc 1994; 26(12).
(Reproduced with permission from Pediatrics, Vol 107, pp.1205-1209, Copyright © 2001 by the AAP.)

Ergogenic aids and steroids

The mixed messages that adolescents receive regarding their appearance, the importance of sports performance, the misinformation regarding the safety of steroid use and the lack of oversight regarding the use of steroids require that information about these dangerous substances be available to young athletes. The medical community needs to continue to take a strong position against these substances to protect young athletes when they are most susceptible to the promise of an easy route to athletic success.

Rest

Adolescents need 8–10 h of sleep each night. Sports participation may provide the impetus to maintain a proper sleep routine, so as to not compromise performance.

Hydration

Several clusters of heat-related injuries and deaths highlight the importance of proper fluid intake during training sessions. Proper sodium intake is also important.

Sun exposure

Skin cancer due to sun damage is thought to be related to exposure that occurs before the age of 18 years. Therefore, children and adolescents should be counseled about the importance of using sunscreen whenever they are outdoors.

Health practice

As previously mentioned, the pre-participation evaluation may be the only opportunity to do health counseling with young athletes. Wearing seat belts while in a car and avoiding drug and alcohol use can be introduced or reiterated to the adolescent athlete during the pre-participation evaluation. Safe sexual practices, including abstinence, also can be addressed. Community standards and school district rules need to be considered in conjunction with this politically charged topic, and the team physician will have to assess his or her role in educating students in this regard.

DISPOSITION

Box 12.9: Key Points

The majority of athletes are cleared for play without restriction. Any concerns about safer participation should be deferred for further evaluation by a specialist or the primary care physician.

On the basis of the findings on the history and physical screening, the athlete can be cleared to play without restrictions, cleared to play with recommendations for further evaluation or treatment for specific conditions, not cleared for certain sports (e.g. no contact sports) (Tables 12.9, 12.10), or not cleared for any sport.[1] Because of possible confusion related to the mixed message of allowing participation but requiring fur-

Table 12.9 Classification of Sports by Extent of Contact

Extent of Contact		
Non-Contact	**Limited Contact**	**Contact-Collision**
Archery	Baseball	Basketball
Badminton	Bicycling	Boxing
Body building	Cheerleading	Diving
Canoeing/kayaking	Canoeing/kayaking	Field hockey
(flat water)	(white water)	Football
Curling	Fencing	Flag
Dancing	Field events	Tackle
Field events	High jump	Ice hockey
Discus	Pole vault	Lacrosse
Javelin	Floor hockey	Martial arts
Shot put	Gymnastics	Rodeo
Golf	Handball	Rugby
Orienteering	Horseback riding	Ski jumping
Powerlifting	Racquetball	Soccer
Race walking	Skating	Team handball
Riflery	Ice	Water polo
Rope jumping	In-line	Wrestling
Rowing	Roller	
Running	Skiing	
Sailing	Cross-country	
Scuba diving	Downhill	
Strength training	Water	
Swimming	Softball	
Table tennis	Squash	
Tennis	Ultimate Frisbee	
Track	Volleyball	
Weightlifting	Windsurfing, surfing	

ther evaluation, this category should be used for situations in which the condition that needs to be evaluated has little bearing on the athlete's ability to participate safely. For example, decreased hearing in a football player may not preclude safe participation but should be assessed by the primary care physician.

Because of the importance of athletic participation and as a result of epidemiologic research, conditions that were once thought to be disqualifying no longer are labeled as such. For example, the lack of a testicle was once disqualifying. However, the loss of a testicle in sports is infrequent, and contact and collision sports pose the greatest risk for this injury (Tables 12.8–12.10). Murmurs, organomegaly, joint laxity, or conditions that could lead to disqualification should be assessed and clearance withheld until given by a specialist who examines the athlete.

The pre-participation evaluation is an opportunity to identify problems that may have a significant impact on the long-term health of an athlete. Some of these findings are summarized in Table 12.11.

There are conflicting legal precedents to allowing or refusing an athlete's participation in organized sports based on perceived risk due to a medical condition. The federal court in Kansas sided with the University of Kansas and its medical staff in prohibiting participation by a football player with a congen-

Table 12.10   Classification of Sports by Dynamic and Static Status

Low Dynamic/ Low Static	Low Dynamic/ High Static	High Dynamic/ Low Static	High Dynamic/ High Static
Bowling	Archery	Badminton	Boxing
Cricket	Auto racing	Baseball	Cross-country
Curling	Diving	Basketball	skiing
Golf	Equestrian events	Field hockey	Cycling
Riflery	Field events (jumping, throwing)	Lacrosse	Downhill skiing
	Gymnastics	Orienteering	Fencing
	Karate, judo	Race walking	Football
	Motorcycling	Racquetball	Ice hockey
	Rodeo	Soccer	Rowing
	Sailing	Squash	Rugby
	Ski jumping	Swimming	Running (sprints)
	Water skiing	Table tennis	Speed skating
	Weightlifting	Tennis	Water polo
		Volleyball	Wrestling

itally narrowed cervical spine and an episode of transient paralysis. In Illinois, the federal court sided with two cardiologists and an athlete with an implanted cardioverter-defibrillator over his school, team physician and two other consultants, a decision that allowed the athlete to play basketball.[42]

A physician who allows an athlete to play because of the athlete's desire to play despite medical judgment to the contrary may be liable for malpractice.[43] It is inappropriate for the physician to allow clearance if an athlete offers to sign a liability waiver or threatens a lawsuit. The physician needs to make the judgment that he or she believes is medically appropriate. If there is a risk of life-threatening or permanently disabling harm, it is advisable to opt for caution and recommend against participation even though an athlete may legally challenge this recommendation.[42]

SPECIAL GROUPS AND CIRCUMSTANCES

Box 12.10: Key Points

Different groups may require specific components in the pre-participation evaluation in order to identify areas of concern.

Female athletes

There may be objection to addressing issues of female athletes separately. However, attention needs to be called to disordered eating and menstrual irregularities. Eating disorders may occur in 10% of female collegiate athletes.[21] An athlete's concerns about weight may require more detailed questioning. Similarly, a pattern of missed menstrual periods or long durations between periods (i.e. more than 2 months) should prompt closer scrutiny. Osteoporosis is not going to be detected on physical examination, but it may be inferred from a history of stress fractures in conjunction with amenorrhea.[21]

Weight certification

In some states, high-school wrestlers are certified at the beginning of the season as to their minimum wrestling weight for that season. Physicians involved in that process should familiarize themselves with the options available and any allowance for growth during the course of the season. Physicians should know that despite the lack of logic, wrestlers prefer to lose weight to compete at a lower weight class rather than gain weight and compete at a heavier class. Rapid weight loss is unsafe and is typically accomplished through dehydration. Matches, then, become contests between two dehydrated wrestlers. Less weight loss (or better hydration) leads to better performance. At the beginning of the season, the physician can consider the wrestler's age, competition weight from the previous year, and the time available to lose weight. In a 12-week season, it is inappropriate to allow an athlete to try to lose more than 24 pounds (2 pounds a week). Over time, it is hoped that wrestlers will be closer to their competition weight throughout the year and less likely to try to achieve an unrealistic and unhealthy weight. The American College of Sports Medicine recommends a minimum body fat of 7% in boys 16 years and 5% in those >16. Female wrestlers should have at least 12% body fat.[44]

Boxing

Despite condemnation of boxing by certain aspects of organized medicine, boxers may need to be cleared by a state commission before being allowed to fight professionally in a state. Again, the physician's job is to ensure the safety of the participant. Any neurologic abnormality, visual abnormality, or physical finding that would preclude strenuous activity could be fatal.

Several professional organizations have come out against boxing as a sport, particularly at the professional level, citing that one way to win is to render the opponent unconscious. Neurologic injury is an undesired occurrence in many sports, but because it is a desired option in boxing, the sport is

Table 12.11 Findings on History of Physical Examination and Suggested Actions[a]

Component of Examination or Specific Consideration	Point of Determination	Finding	Action
Heat illness	History	Possible disposing factors: obesity, history of febrile illness, medications, poor physical condition, sickle cell disease or trait	Refer for evaluation
Head, eyes, ears, nose, throat	History	High degree of myopia	Withhold clearance until evaluated by ophthalmologist
		Surgical aphakia	Withhold clearance until evaluated by ophthalmologist
		Retinal detachment	Withhold clearance until evaluated by ophthalmologist
		Eye surgery	Withhold clearance until evaluated by ophthalmologist
		Eye injury	Withhold clearance until evaluated by ophthalmologist
		Eye infection	Withhold clearance until evaluated by ophthalmologist
	Physical exam	Nasal polyps	Clear, F-U with primary care physician
		Deviated septum	Clear, F-U with primary care physician
		Visual acuity worse than 20/40 with correction, if available	Refer for evaluation and treatment
Cardiovascular	Physical exam	High blood pressure	Increased 3 times: withhold clearance until evaluated
		3/6 murmur or greater	Withhold clearance until evaluated
		Diastolic murmur	Withhold clearance until evaluated
		Murmur increases with Valsalva or change from sitting to standing	Withhold clearance until evaluated
Lungs	History	Breathing difficulty during or immediately after exercise	Provocative testing for exercise-induced asthma
	Physical exam	Wheezes	Refer for evaluation and treatment
		Rubs	Refer for evaluation and treatment
		Prolonged expiratory phase	Refer for evaluation and treatment
		Significant cough with forced expiration	Refer for evaluation and treatment
Abdomen	Physical exam	Mass	Withhold clearance until evaluated
		Tenderness	Withhold clearance until evaluated
		Rigidity	Withhold clearance until evaluated
		Enlarged liver	Withhold clearance until evaluated
		Enlarged spleen	Withhold clearance until evaluated
Skin	Physical exam	Suspicious nevi	Refer for evaluation and treatment
		Contagious rash (e.g. herpes)	Withhold clearance until evaluated and treated
Musculoskeletal	History	Previous injury	Clarify status of injury. May need clearance from treating physician
	Physical exam	Pain	Refer for evaluation and treatment
		Joint instability	Refer for evaluation and treatment
		Joint locking	Refer for evaluation and treatment
		Weakness	Refer for evaluation and treatment
		Atrophy	Refer for evaluation and treatment
		Excess ankle motion	Refer for evaluation and treatment
		Cavus foot	Refer for evaluation and treatment
		Rigid flatfoot	Refer for evaluation and treatment
		Toe deformities (e.g. bunions, contractures, calluses)	Refer for evaluation and treatment
		Generalized hypermobility of joints	Refer for evaluation and treatment
		Scoliosis	Refer for evaluation and treatment
Neurologic	History	Recurrent stingers or burners	Refer for evaluation and treatment
		Multiple or severe concussions	Refer for evaluation and treatment
		Transient quadriparesis	Withhold clearance until evaluated and treated
		Seizures	Withhold clearance until evaluated and treated

Exam, examination; F-U, follow-up.

[a]In a multistation evaluation in which various specialists are present, the evaluation and recommendations for treatment may occur during the pre-participation evaluation. The intent is not to avoid decisions about participation but to ensure that an appropriate specialist makes a confident decision.

thought by some physicians to be incompatible with their participation in the pre-fight assessment of boxers. These physicians should not participate in the pre-bout certification so as not to interject their anti-boxing bias into the approval (or disapproval) process. Accordingly, pro-boxing physicians need to maintain an objective approach to the process and act in the best interest of the athletes and their risk for injury.

Physically challenged athletes

The increase in sports participation for the physically challenged is a welcome phenomenon. One desire in sport is to allow fair competition between athletes of similar abilities. In able-bodied athletes, the reason for pre-competition and post-competition assessment (e.g. drug testing, gender testing) is to confirm that there has been no action on the athlete's part to hide his or her identity or to artificially enhance performance. In the physically challenged population, pre-participation assessments are performed to ensure that athletes compete against others with similar impairments. Physicians are often asked to certify a specific impairment in an athlete.[45] Athletes with a physical impairment should participate in the same sort of pre-participation evaluation as those without a known impairment. The answers to many of the screening questions will be positive and thus the process may take longer. Athletes with physical impairments may be susceptible to problems resulting from use of an assistive device (e.g. upper limb injuries due to wheelchair use).[45]

Regardless, the goal of pre-participation evaluation is to determine safety and risk and not to ascribe value to an individual's choice of sport or to hypothesize about whether an athlete with an impairment should participate in a particular activity. Presumably, a sport has rules and guidelines for participation. As long as these rules are met, the athlete should be cleared regardless of the examining physician's opinion on the value of the activity. Physicians who do not agree with a particular activity should not participate in clearing athletes in that activity rather than inject their own bias into the process (see Boxing above).

Special Olympians

Another group of athletes engaged in sports are those with cognitive or physical limitations. These events focus on participation and celebrate the camaraderie of competition rather than emphasize winning and losing. These are still strenuous activities, and athletes may need to be screened to participate. One area of particular concern is atlantoaxial instability in patients with trisomy 21 (Down syndrome) or connective tissue disease.[45]

Professional and elite athletes

The professional or elite amateur athlete poses a special problem for the examining physician. While maintaining the best interest of the patient, the examiner is assessing the athlete's health and fitness to participate in his or her chosen profession. The physician has an important role in determining whether an athlete is hired. In this setting, the physician has two duties: to ensure that the athlete is healthy and physically fit enough to participate fully in the sport and to collect objective data that may be used by team management in making a hiring decision. The physician needs to be objective in dealings with the athletes and coaching staff. Any compromise of integrity or principles of medical judgment will erode the doctor–patient relationship.

SUMMARY

The pre-participation evaluation is an opportunity to screen for medical conditions that would make athletic participation dangerous for an athlete. It should be done in a timely fashion so that any worrisome findings can be addressed or injuries rehabilitated. It should be efficient to respect the time of the healthcare professionals and the participants. It is not a substitute for a comprehensive examination done by a primary care physician. It is an opportunity to build rapport between the medical staff and the team and an opportunity for education.

As with any screening, it may not yield a diagnosis, but it may lead to more in-depth assessment to ensure safe participation. In sports, there are rarely worthwhile shortcuts to success. The pre-participation evaluation is no different, and the participants should understand that a conservative approach will lead to confidence in safe participation.

REFERENCES

1   American Academy of Family Physicians, American Academy of Pediatrics, American College of Sports Medicine, American Medical Society for Sports Medicine, American Orthopaedic Society for Sports Medicine, American Osteopathic Academy of Sports Medicine. Preparticipation physical evaluation. 3rd edn. New York: McGraw-Hill Professional; 2005.

2   Rice SG. Preparticipation physical examinations: giving an athlete the go-ahead to play. Consultant 1994; 34:1129–1144.

3   Cantwell JD. Preparticipation physical evaluation: getting to the heart of the matter. Med Sci Sports Exerc 1998; 30:S341–S344.

4   Smith J, Laskowski ER. The preparticipation physical examination: Mayo Clinic experience with 2,739 examinations. Mayo Clin Proc 1998; 73:419–429.

5   Wingfield K, Matheson GO, Meeuwisse WH. Preparticipation evaluation: an evidence-based review. Clin J Sport Med 2004; 14:109–122.

6   National Heart, Lung, and Blood Institute. Blood pressure tables for children and adolescents. Bethesda, MD: The Institute; 2004 (2005). Online. Available: http://www.nhlbi.nih.gov/guidelines/hypertension/child_tbl.htm

7   American Diabetes Association. Diabetes mellitus and exercise. Diabetes Care 2002; 25:S64–S68.

8   Draznin MB. Type 1 diabetes and sports participation: strategies for training and competing safely. Phys Sportsmed 2000; 28:49–56.

9   Martin TW, Weisman IM, Zeballos RJ, Stephenson SR. Exercise and hypoxia increase sickling in venous blood from an exercising limb in individuals with sickle cell trait. Am J Med 1989; 87:48–56.

10   NCAA. 2003–2004 Sports medicine handbook. Online. Available: http://www.ncaa.org/library/sports_sciences/sports_med_handbook/2003-04/2003-04_sports_med_handbook.pdf

11   Armstrong LE, De Luca JP, Hubbard RW. Time course of recovery and heat acclimation ability of prior exertional heatstroke patients. Med Sci Sports Exerc 1990; 22:36–48.

12   Epstein Y. Heat intolerance: predisposing factor or residual injury? Med Sci Sports Exerc 1990; 22:29–35.

13 Sharp DS, Ross JH, Kay R. Attitudes of pediatric urologists regarding sports participation by children with a solitary kidney. J Urol 2002; 168:1811–1814.

14 Goldberg B, Saraniti A, Witman P, Gavin M, Nicholas JA. Pre-participation sports assessment: an objective evaluation. Pediatrics 1980; 66:736–745.

15 Tennant FS Jr, Sorenson K, Day CM. Benefits of preparticipation sports examinations. J Fam Pract 1981; 13:287–288.

16 Lively MW. Preparticipation physical examinations: a collegiate experience. Clin J Sport Med 1999; 9:3–8.

17 DiFiori JP, Haney S. Preparticipation evaluation of collegiate athletes [abstract]. Med Sci Sports Exerc 2004; 36:S102.

18 Pescatello LS, Franklin BA, Fagard R, Farquhar WB, Kelley GA, Ray CA, American College of Sports Medicine. Exercise and hypertension. Med Sci Sports Exerc 2004; 36:533–553.

19 National Heart, Lung, and Blood Institute, National Institute of Diabetes and Digestive and Kidney Diseases. Clinical guidelines on the identification, evaluation, and treatment of overweight and obesity in adults: the evidence report. Bethesda MD: National Heart, Lung, and Blood Institute in cooperation with the National Institute of Diabetes and Digestive and Kidney Diseases; 1998 Report No. 98:4083.

20 Centers for Disease Control and Prevention. BMI – Body mass index: BMI for children and teens. Atlanta: CDCP; 2005. Online. Available: http://www.cdc.gov/nccdphp/dnpa/bmi/bmi-for-age.htm

21 Rumball JS, Lebrun CM. Preparticipation physical examination: selected issues for the female athlete. Clin J Sport Med 2004; 14:153–160.

22 Napier SM, Baker RS, Sanford DG, Easterbrook M. Eye injuries in athletics and recreation. Surv Ophthalmol 1996; 41:229–244.

23 Bonsell S, Grayburn PA. The accuracy of screening echocardiography in detecting hypertrophic cardiomyopathy in the preparticipation athletic physical [abstract]. Med Sci Sports Exerc 2004; 36:S102–S103.

24 Lawless CE, DeJong AC, DeJong JW, Joshi A, Panozzo J, Briner WW. Impact of preparticipation portable two-dimensional echocardiography in screening for cardiovascular disease in school-age athletes. Med Sci Sports Exerc 2003; 35:S316.

25 Andreoli TE, Carpenter CCJ, Griggs RC, Loscalzo J, editors. Cecil essentials of medicine. 6th edn. Philadelphia: Saunders; 2004.

26 Holzer K, Brukner P. Screening of athletes for exercise-induced bronchoconstriction. Clin J Sport Med 2004; 14:134–138.

27 Storms WW. Review of exercise-induced asthma. Med Sci Sports Exerc 2003; 35:1464–1470.

28 Maki DG, Reich RM. Infectious mononucleosis in the athlete: diagnosis, complications, and management. Am J Sports Med 1982; 10:162–173.

29 Farley DR, Zietlow SP, Bannon MP, Farnell MB. Spontaneous rupture of the spleen due to infectious mononucleosis. Mayo Clin Proc 1992; 67:846–853.

30 Johnson MA, Cooperberg PL, Boisvert J, Stoller JL, Winrob H. Spontaneous splenic rupture in infectious mononucleosis: sonographic diagnosis and follow-up. AJR Am J Roentgenol 1981; 136:111–114.

31 Dommerby H, Stangerup SE, Stangerup M, Hancke S. Hepatosplenomegaly in infectious mononucleosis, assessed by ultrasonic scanning. J Laryngol Otol 1986; 100:573–579.

32 McAleer IM, Kaplan GW, LoSasso BE. Renal and testis injuries in team sports. J Urol 2002; 168:1805–1807.

33 Committee on Sports Medicine and Fitness. American Academy of Pediatrics: medical conditions affecting sports participation. Pediatrics 2001; 107:1205–1209.

34 Bender TW III. Cutaneous manifestations of disease in athletes. Skin Med 2003; 2:34–40.

35 Brooks C, Kujawska A, Patel D. Cutaneous allergic reactions induced by sporting activities. Sports Med 2003; 33:699–708.

36 Metelitsa A, Barankin B, Lin AN. Diagnosis of sports-related dermatoses. Int J Dermatol 2004; 43:113–119.

37 Nissen SJ, Laskowski ER, Rizzo TD Jr. Burner syndrome: recognition and rehabilitation. Phys Sportsmed 1996; 24:57–64.

38 Torg JS. Cervical spinal stenosis with cord neurapraxia: evaluations and decisions regarding participation in athletics. Curr Sports Med Rep 2002; 1:43–46.

39 Fagan K. Transient quadriplegia and return-to-play criteria. Clin Sportsmed 2004; 23:409–419.

40 Castro FP Jr. Stingers, cervical cord neurapraxia, and stenosis. Clin Sportsmed 2003; 22:483–492.

41 Cantu RC. Cervical spine injuries in the athlete. Semin Neurol 2000; 20:173–178.

42 Mitten MJ. When is disqualification from sports justified? Medical judgment vs patients' rights. Phys Sportsmed 1996; 24:75–78.

43 Mitten MJ. Team physicians and competitive athletes: allocating legal responsibility for athletic injuries. U Pitt Legal Rev 1993; 55:129–169.

44 Oppliger RA, Case HS, Horswill CA, Landry GL, Shelter AC, American College of Sports Medicine. Weight loss in wrestlers. Med Sci Sports Exerc 1996; 28:ix–xii.

45 Boyajian-O'Neill L, Cardone D, Dexter W, et al. Working Group of the Preparticipation Physical Evaluation. 3rd edn. The preparticipation examination for the athlete with special needs. Phys Sportsmed 2004; 32:13–19, 42.

CHAPTER 13

Field Evaluation of the Injured Athlete

Kai-Ming Chan, Joseph Jeremy Hsi-Tse Chang and Fiona Chui-Yan Wong

INTRODUCTION

There has been a great upsurge in participation and public interest in sports in recent years. Consequently, the number of injuries due to sports participation has also been increasing. Tremendous resources have been put into understanding all aspects of medical management of athletic-related injuries and conditions. Although the majority of sports-related injuries are relatively minor, the potential for serious and possibly life-threatening injuries is constantly present. Therefore, the assessment of an injured athlete on the field is extremely important, since this is the first in a series of steps to provide proper care for an athletic injury, which is essentially the role of a team physician. This chapter provides a brief introduction to the evaluation and fieldside management of acute injuries encountered in sports medicine.

ROLE OF TEAM PHYSICIANS ON FIELD: MEDICAL AND LEGAL CONSIDERATIONS

In order to provide the best care to athletes on-field, team physicians should familiarize themselves with the sports they are covering, have the knowledge and skills necessary for assessing the condition of the athlete, and provide early stabilization and first-aid care if necessary.

When an athlete is injured, the priority of the team physician is to identify any life-threatening injuries. This can be achieved by the primary survey, with the recommended emergency protocol using the 'ABCDE' approach (Airway, Breathing, Circulation, Disability and Exposure), which will be further elaborated later in this chapter. Once the athlete is cleared from life-threatening conditions that require immediate transfer to an emergency medical facility, the team physician can start performing a detailed examination of the athlete as the secondary survey.

Upon completion of the secondary survey, the team physician may be required to perform a first-aid procedure to the athlete, or transfer the athlete to a medical center for more definitive care. As team physicians, they should at least comfortably provide certain essential first-aid care, however, they should also recognize their limitations in skills and resources.

The team physicians should transfer the athlete to a medical center for further care or investigations if they find uncertainties or difficulties in providing the most optimal first-aid care. Commonly useful first-aid skills on-field include suturing and wound dressing, application of pressure bandage, splinting and taping, application of ice or heat, massage, stretching and applying protective device and padding. Occasionally, reduction of a dislocated joint may be necessary, given that the physician is familiar with the diagnosis and treatments.

After assessment of the athlete's condition and provision of treatment on-field, the team physicians should decide if the athlete can return to play. They should discuss it with the athlete and the coach regarding the choice of return to play, observe on the sidelines for the athlete's potential to return to play, or withhold the athlete from continuing the game. To allow an athlete to return to play immediately, the team physician should determine if the athlete can be safe from further injury, efficient in participation and relatively pain-free. One of the ways to test whether the athletes are fit to return to play is to test the athlete functionally, by asking them to perform some sport-specific drills, and look out for any symptoms, pain and efficiency in playing. If athletes experience significant pain upon return to play, the team physician should seriously consider stopping the athletes from playing as the injury may be underestimated.

Having said all the necessary responsibilities that team physicians should take on-field, it is mandatory for them to take appropriate measures to avoid unnecessary legal actions. Possessing strict ethics on the safety and well-being of the athletes, team physicians should understand their limitations in knowledge, skills and resources. They should seek advice from other medical professionals whenever necessary to integrate and perfect their treatment. Moreover, it is also an obligation for team physicians to abide by the guiding regulations of the medical professional and the rules of the sport governing organizations. Team physicians must keep confidentiality of the athletes under all circumstances and undoubtedly must not benefit any secondary gain from the commercial body, for example, the mass media at the expense of the athletes' privacy. The use of illegal performance-enhancing drugs and other banned medications must be absolutely prohibited, unless indispensable in an emergency.[1] The team physicians should also make sure their own insurance schemes cover the cost of any legal actions that may arise during their duties in the team while in a foreign country. Moreover, the insurance scheme for the athlete should also be checked for details such as the minimum coverage allowed for further medical care, such as special medications or equipment in foreign countries, and the coverage for transfer back to their own countries.

Primary survey

Box 13.1: Key Points

- In evaluating the severity of injury, team physicians should identify life-threatening conditions which necessitate immediate hospital admission with primary survey.
- Primary survey with the 'ABCDE' approach (Airway, Breathing, Circulation, Disability and Exposure) is commonly adopted in the preliminary assessment. It serves to stabilize the patients' vitals and triage the patients for subsequent management.

Whether an injury is sports-related or not, any physician or paramedics attending an injured patient should begin with a primary survey by following 'ABCDE'. This algorithm, as introduced by the American College of Surgeons, provides a uniform examination of an injured patient: the airway and cervical spine; breathing; circulation; disability and exposure. Throughout the primary survey, the athletes should be left in the position in which they are found unless there is immediate danger or there is a serious injury that needs advanced intervention that can not be done in the field (Fig. 13.1).[2] The same principle holds true for an unconscious athlete; the 'ABCDE' approach is to determine and maintain the vitals and it is the first life-saving step for all injured athletes.

Airway

A top priority in management of the injured athlete is to establish an airway and maintain adequate ventilation. Airway compromise can result from occlusion of the air passages with fluid or solid substances, e.g. teeth, foreign bodies. The airway may also be obstructed due to the relaxation of pharyngeal soft tissue in an unconscious patient or soft tissue collapse from severe oral/facial trauma.

On the fieldside, a team physician should look for signs of airway obstruction. This could be presented as excessive use of accessory muscles, intercostals retractions, hoarseness, snoring, stridor and nasal alar flaring. Cyanosis is another sign to look out for, and the most common sites to assess are the nail beds and around the lips, where purplish discoloration may be present.

The first step to re-establish a patent airway is by manually removing any foreign body that is causing the obstruction. In the unconscious athlete, the attending physician should especially check for tongue relaxation that occludes the airway. If so, a chin lift and jaw thrust maneuver can be performed. The physicians place their index finger under the athlete's mandible and pull the lower lip down with the thumb, while the middle fingers are placed behind the angle of mandible and displacing the mandible forward. By doing so, the tongue will fall forward and thus relieve the obstruction. Note the neck should be maintained with in-line immobilization at all times while performing the maneuver as this may further damage any unstable cervical spine (Fig. 13.2).[2]

The survey is simpler in a conscious athlete. One simple test for checking the airway status in conscious athletes is by asking their name. If the athlete can respond clearly in sentence, the airway and breathing are usually secured. For an unconscious patient, the insertion of an oropharyngeal airway can be considered. Adult oropharyngeal airways come in three sizes: 8 cm (size 3), 9 cm (size 4) and 10 cm (size 5). The size of the airway is estimated by measuring the distance between the front of the teeth and angle of the jaw from the side. In most cases, the injured athlete should be able to ventilate with the

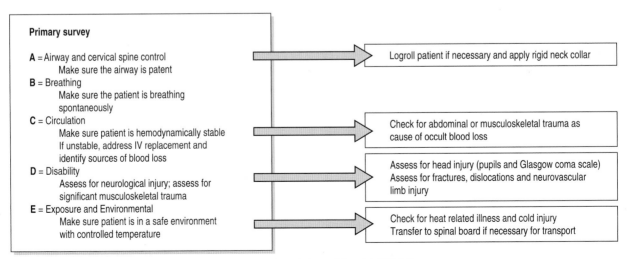

Figure 13.1 Primary survey: the 'ABCDE' approach. (Reproduced from Luke and Stanish 2001.[2])

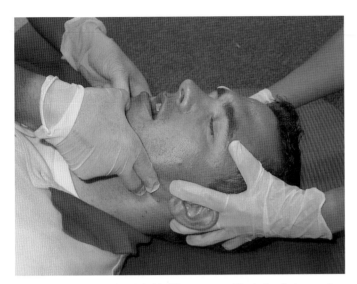

Figure 13.2 Jaw thrust and chin lift maneuver. The index fingers and middle finger lifts the angle of the jaw forward on each side while the thumbs pulls the lower lip and chin down opening the mouth. In-line immobilization of the neck should be maintained. (Reproduced from Luke and Stanish 2001.[2])

oropharyngeal airway and bag-valve-mask device, however if this fails, a definitive airway, e.g. orotracheal tube, nasotracheal tube, or tracheostomy may be required.

Cervical spine control Since injury to the cervical spine may lead to irreversible damage to the spinal cord, initial resuscitation must be conducted under the assumption that cervical spine injury exists until it is disproved radiographically. If unconscious, the player is also presumed to have an unstable fracture until proven otherwise. Hence, the injured athlete should be immobilized by manual in-line cervical control with neck in neutral position (Fig. 13.3).[2] A rigid neck collar is

indicated by significant trauma to the neck/upper back, head injury, post-traumatic loss of consciousness, post-traumatic shock, neurological deficits consistent with central nervous symptom dysfunction, intoxication or inability to speak.

Breathing

Optimal ventilation requires a patent upper and lower airway, along with the proper functioning thoracic wall, lungs and diaphragm. When assessing for adequate ventilation in an injured athlete, the following sequence can be adopted: 'look, listen and feel'. Respiratory compromise may present as tachypnea or bradypnea, paradoxical (see-saw movement) of the chest and abdomen indicating failure of normal diaphragmatic function. Check the trachea for any midline deviation, and auscultate each lung field for adequate air entry. If there is a decreased breath sound along with tracheal deviation to the contralateral side, then tension pneumothorax is highly suspected, and a large-bore needle/catheter should be inserted into the pleural cavity immediately through the second intercostal space in the mid-clavicular line anteriorly. Other life-threatening conditions such as flail chest, open pneumothorax, hemothorax, cardiac tamponade and penetrating wounds warrant immediate hospital care.

Athletes with inadequate ventilation can be supplemented with oxygen by a bag-valve-mask device on the fieldside until they are transferred to the nearest institute with oxygen supplement.

Circulation

Cardiogenic and hypovolemic shock are the most common problems encountered in sports medicine. Hypovolemic shock can arise among athletes with severe dehydration or when there is a continuous bleeding source; whereas a cardiogenic shock may arise among athletes with pre-existing cardiovascular diseases. Hence, it is important for the team physician to identify these signs. Clinical features of hypovolemic shock

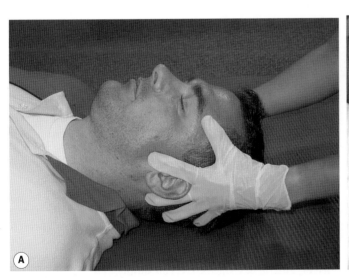

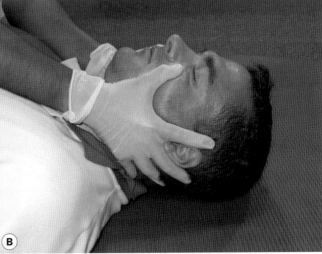

(A)   (B)

Figure 13.3 In-line immobilization techniques of the head and neck from (A) above and (B) below are shown. Hands should stabilize the head on both sides with the 4th and 5th fingers over the occiput. (Reproduced from Luke and Stanish 2001.[2])

include hypotension, tachycardia, pallor, sweaty cold and clammy extremities, delayed capillary refill (>2 s), low jugular venous pressure (JVP) or confusion. The clinical presentation of cardiogenic shock is similar to hypovolemic shock in its clinical presentation but with high JVP.

The cardiovascular system should initially be assessed by feeling for the carotid pulse. If the carotid pulse is not palpable on both sides along with the signs of shock, then cardiac arrest or arrhythmia is suspected. Hence, immediate cardiopulmonary resuscitation should be done. The rhythm can be determined with a portable defibrillation, and rhythm such as ventricular fibrillation or ventricular tachycardia can be converted to a stable rhythm by defibrillation. Time is precious in these conditions as for every minute of delay, there is a 10% decrease in survival.[3]

In the presence of shock, establishment of peripheral intravenous access with large bore cannula for volume resuscitation should commence as soon as airway and ventilation is secured. The principle for stabilizing an acutely injured athlete with 'ABC' should make no difference between conscious and unconscious athletes. Then the athlete should be transferred to the nearest medical center for further management. In the event of trauma, internal bleeding into third spaces such as the chest, abdomen or from fractures of long bones must be considered as a cause of hypovolemia. Therefore, look for any bruising and abdominal distention, and feel for any abdominal tenderness. Also, apply firm consistent pressure for any visible hemorrhage.

Disability

After securing 'ABC', the next step is to assess the athlete's level of consciousness. This can be done with the Glasgow coma scale (Table 13.1) by examining the athlete's speech, eye and motor responses to verbal command or pain.

Table 13.1 Glasgow Coma Scale

	Score
Eye opening	
Spontaneous	4
To voice	3
To pain	2
Nil	1
Verbal response	
Orientated	5
Confused	4
Inappropriate words	3
Incomprehensible sounds	2
Nil	1
Motor responses	
Obeys commands	6
Localizes pain	5
Withdraw	4
Flexion	3
Extension	2
Nil	1

Exposure or environment

The team physician should check for any imminent danger to the athletes during the assessment. Both the physician and the athlete should be moved to a safer environment if any other dangers are present. It is also necessary to adequately expose the athlete to check for any other sites of injury after the primary survey. In case of suspected heat stroke, any equipment or clothing that prevents the athlete from cooling down must be removed immediately.

Transportation

If the athlete is suspected of having vertebral column or spinal cord injury, he should be transported to an emergency department for the serial assessments. When it becomes necessary to move the athlete, the head and trunk must be moved in one unit. In most cases, that means the head and spine are repositioned into a neutral position, so that in-line stabilization can be accomplished with appropriate immobilization devices, although in some instances, it may be better for the head and neck to be immobilized in a position that the athlete is initially found. The appropriateness of repositioning should be assessed on individual basis. The athlete should be placed in a supine position with the spine safeguarded to a suitable backboard. Besides rigid neck collar, other methods of padding like towels or blanket rolls can be used to secure the head to the spine board. It has also been suggested that a cervical vacuum splint is an effective immobilizer in the athlete wearing protective equipment. And the application of spine board should always include straps to secure the pelvis, shoulders, legs and the head. For those who vomit or bleed from the oral cavity, they should be kept prone or placed on their side to prevent aspiration into the airway. However, this can be performed after immobilization and most preferably with suction apparatus being readily available. It should also be noted that the face-mask ought to be removed at the earliest convenience before transportation and regardless of current respiratory status. Due to the difficulty in attaining a definitive exclusion regarding the possibility of spinal injury in an on-field setting, the Inter-Association Task Force recommends that any suspected player should be evaluated in a controlled environment, and that any athlete with significant neck or spine pain, diminished level of consciousness, or significant neurological deficits, be transported to a medical facility with definitive diagnostic and medical resources. Athletes suspected of having a spinal injury should be transported by trained professionals in an ambulance. Transportation in a private vehicle should not be attempted. A transport team may include the team physicians, certified athletic trainers and the emergency medical service personnel. All medical or allied healthcare personnel arriving on the scene must receive a briefing of the situation. The coach, game official and administrative personnel can assist keeping the team-mates and family away from the injured athlete. Emergency equipment should include a spine board with straps, small garden pruners for removing face masks, screwdriver, emergency shears, oxygen supply, rigid cervical collars and suction apparatus, etc.

Secondary survey

> ### Box 13.2: Key Points
>
> - After initial resuscitation, a detailed head to toe survey should follow.
> - Neurological assessment includes the Glasgow Coma Scale, which covers the eye, verbal and motor responses. A more comprehensive examination with muscle tone, power, coordination, sensation and cranial nerve testing helps localize the lesion and give clues to the pathology.
> - Neck examination includes looking for any muscular or spinal asymmetry, feeling for any tenderness and muscle spasm, active and passive movement. All unconscious athletes are assumed to have an associated neck injury and should be immobilized until adequate radiological evaluation has been completed.
> - Chest, abdomen and pelvis examination should be followed.

Once the patient is stabilized with the initial resuscitation, a more detailed head to toe survey is carried out. The back and spine are examined by log-rolling the patients onto their side, looking for any localized tenderness, bruising or stepping. The secondary survey begins with assessment of the head and neck, followed by the chest, abdomen and pelvis, and then finally the rest of the musculoskeletal system, starting from the shoulder and down to the foot and ankle.

Head injury

The scope of head injury is immense, and it ranges from minor injuries such as concussion to more serious injuries, such as cerebral contusion or laceration. Hence, if there is a decreased level of consciousness following an impact to the head, an underlying head injury should be assumed. If the athlete has a declining level of consciousness, prolonged confusion, or post-traumatic seizure, then it may suggest a rapidly progressing head injury, and immediate intervention with neurological specialists in a nearby medical center must be done.

Before assessing for any neurological deficit, the ears, nose and the scalp should be inspected. Hemotympanum, ecchymosis over the mastoid process (Battle's signs) and periorbital ecchymosis (raccoon eyes) implicate basal skull fracture. Clear fluid coming out from the ear (otorrhea) or nose (rhinorrhea) indicates cerebrospinal fluid leak from a dural rent.

The Glasgow Coma Scale (Table 13.1) is a common system for grading the severity of head injury. The speech and cognitive function can be tested by asking the athlete a simple question such as 'What is your name?' 'What sport were you participating in before the injury', 'What is the name of your team?' During the eye examination, the physician should look for spontaneous eye movement, the size of the pupils, the reactivity of the pupils to light, and symmetry of extra-ocular movements. Any dilation or sluggish light response of one pupil suggests an intracranial injury, while asymmetrical extra-ocular movements suggest cranial nerve palsy or injury.

For motor response in a fully conscious patient, the tone, power and coordination are readily assessed in the standard manner. However, in an unconscious patient, the pattern of limb response to painful stimuli provides a useful indication of the conscious level.

If a subtle abnormality is suspected, the examination should include cranial nerve testing and muscle strength testing by asking the athletes to close their eyes and hold their arms outstretched, palm upwards for 1 min. Any pronation or downward drift on one side is indicative of brain injury. In addition, a mini mental status exam (MMSE) can be performed for testing the cognitive function. This includes the orientation to time, place and person; comprehension and short-term memory by asking the athlete to remember three words: apple, train, banana, and repeat them after a short while when they are asked after the concentration task which requires them to 'start at 100, subtract 7 and continue to subtract 7 from the remaining total'.

Neck injury

The usual mechanism in neck injury among sportsmen is an impact to the head with an axial load on cervical spine during collision or fall; others include a forceful flexion or extension of the head with or without rotation. All unconscious athletes are assumed to have an associated neck injury and should be immobilized until adequate radiological evaluation has been completed in a medical centre.

A thorough neurological examination from head to toe should be performed on any athlete suspected of neck injury. In conscious athletes, they may give a history of neck pain or stiffness, with or without neurological symptoms such as numbness, weakness and paralysis of the limbs. If any of the above symptoms has been present in their history, then the neck should be immobilized. On the fieldside, the stability of the neck should only be tested on an athlete with no complaints of neck pain or neurological symptoms. Otherwise, any tests should be withheld until further radiological evaluation.

While examining the neck, the sequence of 'look, feel and move' can be adopted. The physician should begin from the back of the neck, look for any muscular or spinal asymmetry, feel for any tenderness and muscle spasm. The alignment of the spine should be noted for any excessive curving of the C-spine. Ask the patient to actively test the flexion (from chin to chest), lateral flexion (ear to shoulder) and rotation (chin just before shoulder).

After checking for any structural abnormality, a thorough neurological exam should follow. This includes testing of the cranial nerves II–XII, both motor and sensory functions of the spinal roots. Details of the examination are listed in Table 13.2.[4]

There are no simple rules to determine return-to-play criteria after sustaining a cervical spine injury. Medical factors are undoubtedly important, although non-medical factors such as age of the athlete, level of competition, psychosocial issues do play a role. Some medical sequelae do represent absolute contraindications to return to contact sports, examples include neck injuries resulting in permanent central nervous system dysfunction, significant peripheral nerve injury, injuries resulting in spinal fusion at C4 level or above.

Table 13.2 Neurological Exam Maneuvers[a,4]

	Test
Cranial nerves	
II (optic nerve)	Visual acuity
III, IV, VI (extraocular nerves)	Extraocular movements
V	Sensation to the forehead, cheek, and lower jaw (check both sides)
VII	Facial muscles (look for symmetry with raising eyebrows, showing teeth)
VIII	Hearing
IX, X	Soft palate elevation (open mouth and say 'Aah')
XI	Trapezius elevation (test shoulder shrug strength)
XII	Tongue movement (stick out tongue – look for deviation)
Sensation/nerve root level tested	
C5	Lateral shoulder (deltoid area)
C6	Thumb
C7	Middle finger (3rd finger)
C8	Little finger (5th finger)
T4	Nipple line
T8	Lower border of the sternum
T10	Umbilicus
T12	Symphysis pubis
L4	Medial aspect of the lower leg
L5	Webspace between 1st and 2nd toes
S1	Lateral aspect of the foot
S3, S4, S5	Perianal area
Motor strength testing (nerve roots involved)[b]	
Axillary nerve (C5, C6)	Resisted shoulder abduction (deltoid)
Radial nerve (C5, C6)	Resisted wrist extension (extensor carpi radialis)
Median nerve (C6, C7, C8)	Resisted elbow extension (triceps) or thumb to little finger (opponens)
Ulnar nerve (C8, T1)	Resisted abduction or adduction of fingers (interossei)
Femoral nerve (L2, L3, L4)	Resisted knee extension (quadriceps)
Deep peroneal nerve (L4, L5)	Resisted ankle dorsiflexion (anterior tibialis)
Tibial nerve (S1, S2)	Resisted ankle plantarflexion (gastrocnemius, soleus)
Sciatic nerve (L5, S1, S2)	Resisted knee flexion (hamstrings)
Reflexes	
Upper extremity	Triceps, biceps, brachioradialis
Lower extremity	Knee, ankle, Babinski (soles of the feet)
Balance	
Romberg test	Have athlete stand with eyes closed, look for loss of balance
Coordination	
Finger–nose testing	Have athlete touch own nose, then the examiner's fingers, repeatedly
Tandem gait line	Heel-to-toe walking in a straight line

[a]These are some suggested maneuvers, however, the neurological examination may vary as clinically appropriate.
[b]Motor testing is graded on five levels: 5 = normal strength; 4 = active movement against resistance; 3 = active movement against gravity only; 2 = able to move limb with gravity eliminated; 1 = flicker of muscle contraction only; 0 = no contractions.

Chest, abdomen and pelvis injury

The chest assessment is similar to the primary survey, but it is more in-depth and it is in order to try to pick up any signs that might have been missed previously, e.g. a rib fracture. The abdomen is examined with each abdominal organ palpated carefully. More attention should be paid to the splenic region as a ruptured spleen might be deceptively silent, and signs such as tender, guarding and rigidity might be vaguely present. However, if there is a local collection of blood, the percussion note will be impaired on the left flank. The perineum is examined with a rectal examination. Signs that should be noted include the anal sphincter tone, the position of the prostate, any presence of blood, especially in cases suspected of internal bleeding or pelvic injury.

Shoulder injury

Box 13.3: Key Points

- Proper examination with observation, palpation and range of motion of shoulder region, followed by neurological assessment for associated brachial plexus and peripheral nerve injury is mandatory. Radiological confirmation is also important for making the diagnosis. Resting and immobilizing in an arm sling or splint with ice packing could be provided by team physicians on the sideline.

- Common shoulder injuries include rotator cuff strains or tears, biceps tendon ruptures and anterior shoulder dislocation. Acute elbow injuries commonly involve posterior elbow dislocation, distal humeral fracture. Hand injuries can be diversified as fracture, dislocation and soft tissue injuries. Fractures include boxer's fracture, Benett's fracture, Gamekeeper's thumb. Ligamental injuries presented as mallet finger and jersey fingers are also common.

Acute injuries of the shoulder frequently encountered on the fieldside include soft tissue injuries, including rotator cuff strains or tears and biceps tendon ruptures; dislocation of joints, like the glenoid-humeral joint, the acromion-clavicular joint and very rarely, the sterno-clavicular joint; and fractures around the shoulder region, including the clavicle, proximal humerus and less commonly the scapula.

The team physician should check the bones and joints in a systematic fashion. The sternoclavicular (SC) joint, clavicle, acromioclavicular (AC) joint, acromion process, coracoid process, the greater and the lesser tubercle of the humerus, should be inspected and palpated for deformity, asymmetry, edema, crepitus and tenderness, which are usually obvious in case of fracture or dislocation. For the later scenario, deformity is usually obvious, like squaring of the shoulder or anterior prominence in glenoid-humeral joint dislocation. For soft tissue injuries, most common signs are pain, swelling and local tenderness, while tests for individual muscle injuries on the field are neither specific nor sensitive because of pain.

Finally, obtain a general idea of the shoulder function with the active and passive range of movement, and never forget to perform a neurovascular examination at the end of assessment for associated brachial plexus and peripheral nerve injury. Nerves that should warrant special attention include the axillary nerve, musculocutaneous nerve, median, radial and ulnar nerve. The axillary nerve can be tested by asking the athlete to abduct their shoulder, but this will be difficult in a situation where there is a shoulder fracture. The so-called regimental badge area can be tested for sensation (Fig. 13.4).[5]

The motor supply of the musculocutaneous nerve can be tested by flexion of the elbow. Its sensory supply is along the lateral side of the forearm. The median, radial and ulnar nerve can be quickly assessed with the 'Stone, paper and scissors' movement of the hand/fingers. By asking the patients to flex their fingers and forming a firm grip (the 'stone' movement), this allow the physician to test the flexors of patients' hands, which is innervated by the median nerve (Fig. 13.5A). The radial nerve supplies the extensors of the hand, and this can be tested by asking the patients to extend their fingers

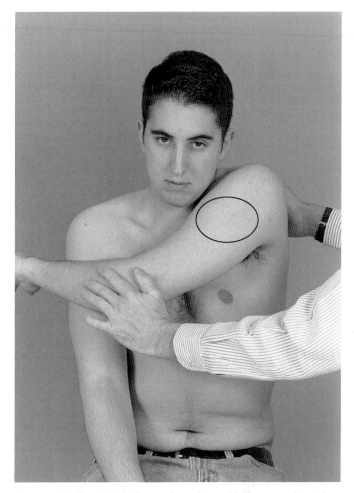

Figure 13.4 The circle indicates the regimental badge area; the region where the sensory part of the axillary nerve can be tested. (Reproduced from Gerbino 2001.[5])

(forming the 'paper') (Fig. 13.5B). Finally, the patient is asked to imitate the 'scissor movement' by abducting and adducting the fingers, this allows the testing of the ulna nerve (Fig. 13.5C). Note abduction of the thumb is performed by abductor pollicis brevis which is supplied by the median nerve.

In the case of suspected fractures, the injured limb should be supported with sling and applied with ice-packing. The athlete should be removed from play and sent for X-ray confirmation of fracture. In the case of a suspected joint dislocation, the joint should be rested with a sling and the athlete sent for further investigation. However, in the case of glenohumeral joint dislocation, reduction of the joint can be performed by a trained clinician with adequate muscle relaxant and analgesics. If there is a suspected posterior SC separation, an immediate cardiopulmonary assessment and treatment should be done because of its close relationship with the vital organs. The athlete may complain of dyspnea and there may be a plethora of ipsilateral extremity, face and neck as well as diminution of pulses on the affected side. If there are signs of ventilation compromise, an attempt should then be made to reduce the dislocation on the field by applying simple traction to the shoulder in a backward and outward direction with simultaneous outward

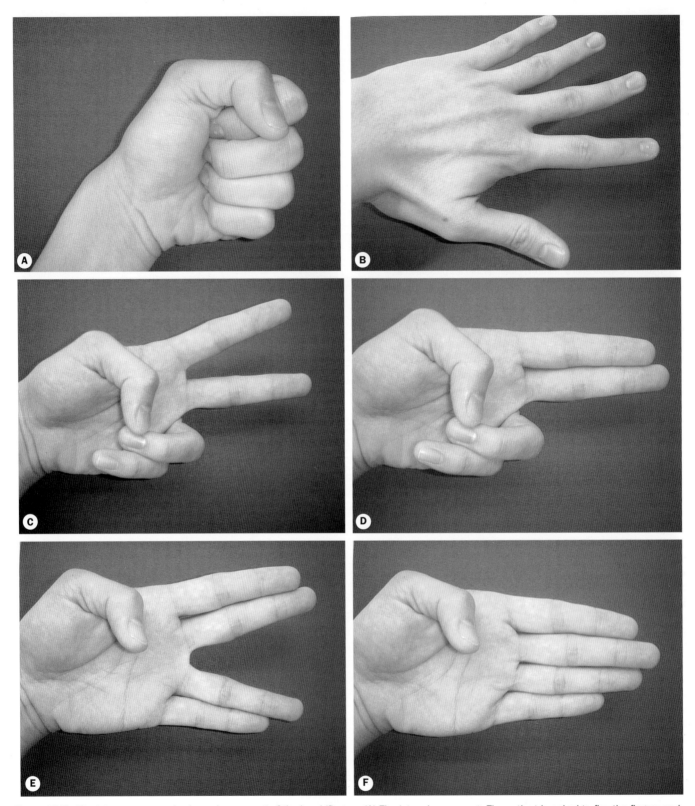

Figure 13.5 The 'stone, paper and scissors' movement of the hand/fingers. (A) The 'stone' movement. The patient is asked to flex the fingers and form a grip. The flexors are mainly innervated by the median nerve. (B) The 'paper' movement. By asking the patient to extend the fingers and form a 'paper', the extensors and the radial nerve are being tested. (C–G) The 'scissor' movement. This shows the abduction and adduction movement of the fingers, which imitates a 'scissor' movement. This abduction and adduction motion of the fingers is supplied by the ulnar nerve.

Continued

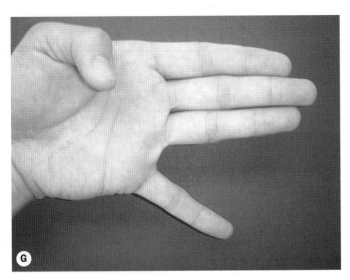

Figure 13.5 *Continued*

pressure on the inner end of the clavicle. Any athlete with a soft tissue injury should be rested with ice-packing, immobilized and protected from further injury. A magnetic resonance imaging (MRI) or ultrasound scan can be arranged for the athlete at a later stage.

Elbow injury

The elbow is likely to dislocate in a posterior direction when it is hyperextended in either abduction or adduction, causing ruptures of the collateral ligaments and anterior capsule. The athlete may give a history of severe elbow pain following a fall on an outstretched hand with the elbow fully extended. Distal humeral fracture is often seen after a fall or collision to the elbow, and it is relatively easy to diagnose on the fieldside. Usually the injured athlete complains of severe elbow pain together with a decreased range of movement which is then followed by rapid swelling of the elbow joint. Other fractures such as medial epicondyle avulsion fractures and olecranon fracture/epiphysis avulsion may be encountered and may have similar presentation. However, medial epicondyle avulsion fractures usually occur in young athletes following a hard throw. They will complain of sharp pain over the medial side of the elbow. Swelling is mild and localized over the medial epicondyle. The assessment is not complete without a neurovascular examination distal to the injury, as complications from irreversible nerve or blood vessels injury are not uncommon. Since all fractures have similar presentations, the exact site of injury must be confirmed by X-ray.

Treatment on the field includes applying splint or sling in the resting position of the elbow. The team physician should place ice over the swollen site, and then assist the athlete to the sideline for further evaluation. In case of close elbow dislocation, close reduction can be done on-field if the team physician is confident in the diagnosis and experienced in performing the maneuver. This can be done by gentle traction along the long axis of the forearm with the wrist and elbow in extension and the extremity slowly moves into flexion. The neurovascular status should be monitored especially if reduction is not successful, and the athlete should be taken to the hospital immediately for further management.

Forearm and wrist injury

Forearm fractures can result from a fall or direct blow on an outstretched arm, as in a missed wrestling or judo throw. The signs and symptoms of forearm fractures may include local tenderness, swelling, disability and crepitation. Whenever a fracture is suspected, a distal neurovascular examination should be done following the initial assessment. The limb should be splinted from the axilla to the mid-palm, and careful radiological evaluation must be made.

The most common wrist injuries include soft tissue strains, followed by fractures with or without dislocation of joints. Common soft tissue strains include collateral ligament sprains, flexor or extensor tendon injuries, and triangular-fibrocartilage complex (TFCC) injuries. Fractures around the wrist joints include the common distal radius fractures, ulnar styloid fractures, the easily missed scaphoid fractures, and less commonly the fracture dislocation of the carpal bones, like perilunate dislocation. The mechanism of injuries is mostly falls onto an outstretched hand or a direct blow, or wrist sprain in racket sports. The appearance may be normal, but usually there is pain, swelling and local tenderness at the injured area, such as at the base of the thumb and tenderness over the anatomical snuffbox for the scaphoid fractures.

For any injuries around the wrist, after on-field assessment, unless the team physician diagnoses it as a very minor injury, the wrist and thumb should be splinted, and arranged for further investigations and management.

Hand injury

Sports injuries of the hand and finger are quite diversified, and include fractures, dislocation, ligament and tendon injuries. The metacarpal bones are vulnerable to injury after a fall upon the hand or a direct blow with a closed fist or the so-called boxer's fracture. The usual sites of injury in boxer's fracture are the distal 4th and 5th metacarpophalangeal bones. While fracture of the base of the 1st metacarpal (Bennett's fracture) is also not uncommon, with the same mechanism of injury. The finger joints and bones are more prone to injury upon sudden hyperextension or hyperflexion, thus resulted in fractures of the phalanx, dislocations of the metacarpal or inter-phalangeal joint, or tendon ruptures. Gamekeeper's thumb (ulna collateral ligament sprain) occurs among athletes with a fall onto an outstretched hand with the thumb hyperabducted.

Physical examinations usually reveal localized pain, swelling and tenderness over the injured area, with deformity sometimes obvious. Mallet fingers (extensor tendon injuries) and jersey fingers (flexor tendon injuries) are usually presented with the inability to actively extend or flex the finger, respectively and local tenderness and swelling at the region of the distal phalanx.

In cases of joint dislocations, it is best to refer to a trained physician for reduction, no matter how minor the injury may seem. It is mandatory for the team physician to perform a neurovascular and motion assessment before any reduction is made. Closed reduction is done by progressive traction along the long axis of the dislocated bone, and then applying pressure to the proximal base of the dislocated unit in the direction opposite to the dislocating force. A click may be heard or palpated upon relocation. Whether or not the team physician decides to perform a closed reduction, any suspected dislocations, such as phalangeal fractures, can be managed on the field with a buddy splint, by strapping the injured finger to its neighboring finger. Similarly, mallet finger or jersey finger can be temporarily splinted and referred for further expert care.

Acute back injuries

> **Box 13.4: Key Points**
>
> - Common back injuries sustained during a game include muscle strains or sprain injuries, acute or chronic disc herniations, facet joints strains and fractures. 'Move in one piece' should always be the rule, with the neck supported during any rotation during the assessment. Presence of neurological symptoms and signs including muscle weakness, sensory loss and incontinence point to more serious injuries that require immediate transferal to a medical center.

Common back injuries sustained during a game include muscle strains or sprain injuries, acute or chronic disc herniations, facet joints strains, or less commonly fractures or fracture dislocations of spine (apart from cervical spine), with or without neurological complications.

Upon athlete-sustained injury to the back on-field, the team physician should always be aware of possible serious injuries that should not be overlooked initially, as serious consequences can result from initial improper management. Any history of pre-existing back problems will provide the clue to diagnosis, e.g. history of herniated disc. Any complaint of pain or stiffness in the back should be taken seriously, even if the athlete can walk without apparent difficulty. Ask about radicular pain, muscle weakness, numbness, paresthesia and urinary or fecal incontinence. Upon inspection, any bruises of the face, or a superficial abrasion of the forehead, should suggest a hyperextension injury. The limbs should be quickly examined for any evidence of neurological deficits like muscle weakness, sensory loss and asymmetrical reflexes. Bear in mind that examination of the back should be very cautious, as it requires turning of the patient onto one side, which should be done with extreme care. 'Move in one piece' should always be the rule, with the neck supported during any rotation. Any bruises or hematoma of the back are sinister features, and the level of the injury, as indicated by local tenderness and regional muscle spasm

always helps the team physician to better understand the pathology.

The presence of neurological symptoms and signs usually represent more serious injuries that may require proper immobilization and immediate transfer to a medical center for further management. Table 13.3 lists a summary of relations of neurological injuries and the corresponding suspicious levels.

As most of the cases are muscle strains or sprains, symptomatic treatment on-field followed by proper stretching may allow the athletes to return to play early, given that they are pain free and able to cope with the full demands of the specific sports. However, if there is severe pain persisting after a short period of rest, or when neurological complications arise, the athlete should be withdrawn from the game and further proper investigations and management in a medical center are crucial.

Acute hip, groin and pelvis injury

> **Box 13.5: Key Points**
>
> - Most lower limb injuries should initially be managed conservatively with the rest, ice, compression and elevation (RICE) principle on the sideline, followed by definite investigation, treatment and rehabilitation.
> - Acute hip injuries include adductor strains in hockey or skating, iliac crest contusions in contact sports, apophyseal avulsions in sprints.
> - In acute knee injuries, pivoting during soccer or skiing are prone to ACL, MCL and meniscus injuries. Direct posterior blow to anterior aspect of proximal tibia in a fixed leg may point to PCL injuries. Giving way of the knee cap from a sprain with a valgus or external rotation force may indicate patella dislocation.
> - The cardinal signs of ACL injuries include hemarthrosis, intensive painful swelling, locking, 'pop' sound, dead leg and inability to continue to play.
> - Acute ankle injuries commonly involve inversion sprain with anterior talofibular ligament injuries, ankle fractures and Achilles tendon rupture.

Commonly encountered hip, groin and pelvic injuries on-field include adductor or hamstring strains, iliac crest contusion (hip pointer), or avulsions of apophysis in adolescent athletes, like from the anterior superior iliac spine for the sartorius, anterior inferior iliac spine for the rectus femoris, and the ischial tuberosity for the hamstring. However, the external genitalia

Table 13.3   A Summary of the Relations of Neurological Injury and the Corresponding Suspicious Level

Level	Nerve Root	Sensory Loss	Motor Loss	Reflex Loss
L1–L3	L2, L3	Anterior thigh	Hip flexors	None
L3–L4	L4	Medial calf	Quadriceps, tibialis anterior	Knee jerks
L4–L5	L5	Lateral calf, dorsal foot	EDL, EHL	None
L5–S1	S1	Posterior calf, plantar foot	Gastrocnemius/soleus	Ankle jerks
S2–S3	S2, S3, S4	Perianal	Bowel/bladder	Cremasteric

should never be ignored, as improper early management can lead to serious sequelae.

Groin injuries during sports are commonly associated with direct contusion or avulsion fractures. Most of the time the athlete complains of sudden pain in the region involved, and indeed the athlete is usually able to indicate a specific point of pain, which can guide the physician to a diagnosis. Certain sports are particularly prone to certain injuries, e.g. adductor strains are more common in hockey or skating; iliac crest contusions are more common in contact sports such as soccer or rugby; while avulsions of apophysis are more common in running sports such as short distance sprints. Localized swelling, tenderness and muscle spasms around the injured area are quite typical, and usually the athlete is unable to continue the game. Most of these injuries require only conservative definite treatment, with application of the principle of 'RICE' in the acute phase on-field. Ice application and compression bandaging can significantly decrease the pain and swelling.

Unfortunately, although most of the definitive treatments for these injuries are conservative, the athletes are usually not able to return to play immediately after the injury. The treatment and rehabilitation usually takes at least 4–8 weeks before they can return to play.

Acute knee injuries

Commonly encountered acute knee injuries included quadriceps strains or contusions, hamstring strains, ligament injuries (mostly medial collateral ligament (MCL) or anterior cruciate ligament (ACL) ruptures), meniscus injuries, osteochondral or chondral fractures, patella dislocation, quadriceps or patella tendon ruptures, or less commonly fractures around the knee.

The mechanism of injury always helps the team physician with the diagnosis. Pivoting injuries during soccer or skiing are prone to ACL, MCL and meniscus injuries. Direct posterior blows to the anterior aspect of the proximal tibia in a fixed leg such as in a rugby game endanger posterior cruciate ligament (PCL) injuries. Sudden onset of giving way of the knee cap from a sprain with a valgus or external rotation force points to patella dislocation.

Physical examination gives further clues to the diagnosis. Presence of acute hemarthrosis indicates a very high chance of an ACL tear (75% of cases) (Fig. 13.6).[6] A positive Lachman test in a swollen knee is commonly illustrated in ACL injury (Fig. 13.7),[6] and this test is the most sensitive test in detecting acute ACL injury, compared with other tests (anterior drawer or pivot shift test) (Fig. 13.8).[6] Other cardinal signs of acute ACL injury include intensive painful swelling, locking or incomplete extension of the knee, feeling a 'pop' sound, a 'dead' leg, and finally the inability to continue to play. Local tenderness and pain in valgus stress are manifested in MCL sprain. Local joint line tenderness and pain with compression or rotation are suggestive of meniscal injury. Exquisite tenderness over the medial retinaculum of patella points to patella dislocation. But it is not uncommon that the aforementioned tests for ligamental laxities may not be elicited in the acute stage due to severe pain.

Application of the principle of 'RICE' is very helpful in the management of acute knee injuries on-field. Since most of these injuries require further investigation and management,

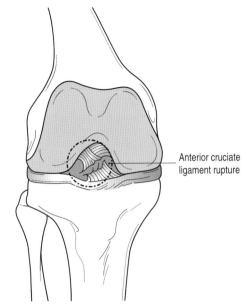

Figure 13.6 Anterior cruciate ligament (ACL) injury. (Reproduced from Rolf and Chan 2001.[6])

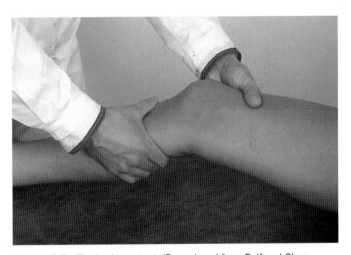

Figure 13.7 The Lachman test. (Reproduced from Rolf and Chan 2001.[6])

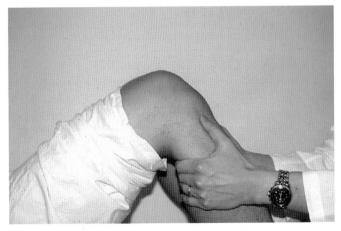

Figure 13.8 Anterior drawer test. (Reproduced from Rolf and Chan 2001.[6])

the patient should be referred to the medical center for further evaluation and definitive treatment.

Apart from minor muscle contusions, players sustaining other knee injuries are advised not to return to play immediately after assessment on-field. This is because the initial signs may not be obvious and are sometimes obscured by pain, so they will be more prone to subsequent injuries if they return to the game immediately, without detailed assessment.

Acute ankle injuries

Acute ankle injuries mainly revolve around ligament injuries, fractures of the ankles and Achilles tendon sprains or ruptures.

Inversion sprain injuries (Figs 13.9, 13.10),[7] being common in all athletes, usually result in anterior talofibular ligament injuries, with or without other lateral collateral ligament injuries. Other ligament injuries are not uncommon, like deltoid ligament injuries over the medial side, or anterior tibiofibular syndesmosis disruptions in 'high ankle sprains'. Local tenderness, swelling and deformities are usually the clues

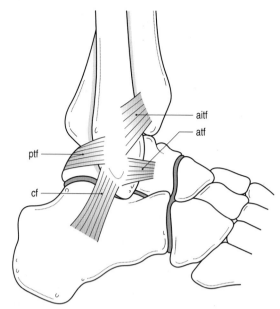

Figure 13.10   Lateral view of ankle ligaments. The lateral ligamentous complex of the ankle consists of the anterior talofibular (atf), calcaneofibular (cf) and posterior talofibular (ptf) ligaments. Aitf, anterior inferior tibiofibular ligament. (Reproduced from Olmedo and Per Renstrom 2001.[7])

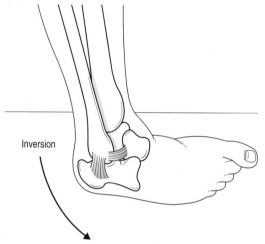

Figure 13.9   Inversion is the most typical injury mechanism in ankle sprain. (Reproduced from Olmedo and Per Renstrom 2001.[7])

to diagnosis, while those instability tests are neither sensitive nor specific early in the acute phase on-field.

Where fractures or dislocations cannot be ruled out, the ankle should be protected with temporary splintage, and the application of the principle of 'RICE' treatment. Apart from very minor inversion ankle sprains without much pain, the athlete should be directed for further investigations and treatment after first-aid care and protection.

Keys for return to play include being pain-free or having very mild pain, the absence of local tenderness or swelling, and the player's capability to perform sports specific drills.

REFERENCES

1   Stanish WD, Evans NA. The modern-day team physicians: roles, responsibilities, and required qualifications. In: Michell L, Smith A, Bachl N, et al., eds. FIMS team physician manual. Hong Kong: Lippincott Williams and Wilkins; 2001:4–10.

2   Luke A, Stanish WD. Fieldside assessment and triage. In: Michell L, Smith A, Bachl N, et al., eds. FIMS team physician manual. Hong Kong: Lippincott Williams and Wilkins; 2001:136–159.

3   Cummins RO, ed. Defibrillation. Textbook of advanced cardiac life support. Dallas: American Heart Association; 1994.

4   Luke A. Head and neck injuries. In: Michell L, Smith A, Bachl N, et al., eds. FIMS team physician manual. Hong Kong: Lippincott Williams and Wilkins; 2001:241–275.

5   Gerbino P. Shoulder injuries. In: Michell L, Smith A, Bachl N, et al., eds. FIMS team physician manual. Hong Kong: Lippincott Williams and Wilkins; 2001:278–298.

6   Rolf CG, Chan KM. Knee injuries. In: Michell L, Smith A, Bachl N, et al., eds. FIMS team physician manual. Hong Kong: Lippincott Williams and Wilkins; 2001:366–394.

7   Olmedo ML, Per Renstrom AFH. Foot and ankle injuries. In: Michell L, Smith A, Bachl N, et al., eds. FIMS team physician manual. Hong Kong: Lippincott Williams and Wilkins; 2001:406–427.

CHAPTER 14

Laboratory Tests and Diagnostic Imaging

William Micheo, Eduardo Amy and José Correa

INTRODUCTION

Laboratory and diagnostic testing are widely used in the practice of sports medicine. Clinical management guidelines for the sports medicine practitioner are similar to other medical disciplines in which the treating physician should be responsible for the ordering and interpretation of the diagnostic studies necessary for patient management.

Initially, the clinician should be guided by a detailed clinical history followed by a complete physical examination that allows the formulation of an orderly differential diagnosis. Once this step is completed, the physician can select the diagnostic and laboratory tests which can provide the most information to corroborate the presumptive clinical diagnosis. In addition, the sports medicine practitioner also needs to consider the cost effectiveness of the diagnostic work-up without sacrificing quality of care for the athlete. In the daily practice of sports medicine, laboratory and diagnostic tests can be used as part of a preventive medicine strategy or to plan appropriate treatment for illness or injury associated to sports or exercise participation.

This chapter will address some of the laboratory and diagnostic tests that are crucial in the management of medical and musculoskeletal conditions which are commonly encountered in sports medicine (Table 14.1). Also included in this chapter is an introduction to imaging with the emphasis on magnetic resonance imaging (MRI) as a diagnostic test for sport-associated musculoskeletal injuries, which hopefully will add knowledge about the proper indications and clinical use of this important, but sometimes over utilized study.

To discuss each laboratory and diagnostic study in detail is beyond our goals for this chapter, however, we expect readers to have a clinical understanding and practical approach to the use of laboratory and diagnostic studies in the management of common problems confronted daily in sport medicine practices.

PRE-PARTICIPATION EXAM SCREENING TESTING

The purpose of the pre-participation physical examination has been identification of conditions that may disqualify an athlete from competition or to fulfill a requirement for medical clearance prior to a competition. In recent years this philosophy has changed to one of using this exam for the prevention of common diseases, orientation of healthy athletes, who would otherwise not see a physician, and identification of high risk behaviors such as drinking and driving, abnormal eating patterns, as well as having unprotected sex.[1]

Many laboratories and screening test guidelines are based on the individual's age and disease risk profiles. Some of these, such as the one proposed by the US Preventive Services Task Force, are an effort to develop an evidence-based consensus of recommendations for preventive services. The recommendations include: clinical history, physical examination, immunizations, counseling, laboratories and screening tests for illnesses associated with different ages, levels of activity and sports participation.[2]

The sport medicine physician should apply these recommendations in pre-participation exams, especially in young individuals, who after 5 years of age are evaluated less frequently by physicians than other patient populations. Laboratory and diagnostic data that can be included in the examination, depending on the patient's age and health status, include urinalysis, complete blood count, electrolytes, creatinine, liver function tests, cholesterol, thyroid studies and an electrocardiogram.[3]

However, some clinicians advocate individualizing the exam, and not performing laboratory studies as part of every pre-participation examination because of the low yield of the testing and the possibility of false positive tests in asymptomatic individuals, such as the runner with normal kidneys who presents with hematuria or proteinuria.[4]

Table 14.1 Basic Diagnostic Studies in Sports Medicine

Laboratory Studies	Radiologic Studies
Blood hemogram	Conventional X-rays
Blood chemistries	Computed tomography (CT)
Urine analysis	Diagnostic ultrasound
Coagulation profile	Technetium bone scan
Muscle enzymes	Magnetic resonance imaging (MRI)
Electrocardiogram	CT/MRI arthrography

ENVIRONMENTAL PROBLEMS IN ATHLETES

Box 14.1: Key Points

Heat illness

- Basic tests
  - Initial rectal temperature
  - Clinical assessment, blood pressure and heart rate
- Emergency room
  - CBC, serum chemistries (electrolytes BUN/creatinine, phosphate, magnesium, calcium, CPK and liver enzymes), PT and PTT, INR, urinalysis and arterial blood gases
- Hospitalized athlete
  - Follow-up of above studies, electrocardiogram if there is electrolyte disturbances, fibrin split products if coagulopathy is suspected, brain MRI or CT scan if neurologic deficit appears.

Exertional heat illness/injuries

This illness is commonly seen in the summer and particularly in warm and humid climates. Heat illness can be classified in five exertional heat syndromes: heat edema, heat cramps, heat syncope, heat exhaustion and heat stroke.[5] In addition, slow runners or participants in long duration events such as ultramarathons may collapse from hyponatremia associated to over-zealous hydration.[6] Complications related to severe heat stroke are acute renal failure, disseminated intravascular coagulation, rhabdomyolysis, acute respiratory distress syndrome, acid base disorders and electrolyte disturbances. The prognosis for the patient is better when heat stroke is diagnosed early with appropriate studies and management with cooling measures and fluid and electrolytes replacement is started early. Prognosis is poor if treatment is started after 2 h of the initiation of symptoms.[7]

The initial evaluation of the athlete with suspected heat illness should include documentation of core temperature with a rectal probe, since tympanic membrane, oral or axillary temperatures do not correlate with core temperature. In addition, complete blood cell count (CBC), serum chemistries (electrolytes, blood urea nitrogen (BUN)/creatinine, phosphate, magnesium, calcium, creatine phosphokinase (CPK) and liver enzymes level), coagulation studies (prothrombin time (PT), partial thromboplastic time (PTT) and INR), urinalysis and arterial blood gases should be obtained.[8]

The initial abnormal findings may include elevated core temperature, as high as 104°F in the case of heat stroke, leuko-

cytosis or thrombocytopenia in the CBC, hypokalemia associated with catecholamine effects, hyperventilation and sweat losses, as well as physiologic hyperaldosteronism.[9]

After a few hours, hyperkalemia is found associated with sustained hyperthermia, hypoxia and hypoperfusion, hypocalcemia and elevated BUN and creatinine secondary to renal dysfunction. Other laboratory abnormalities will include hypophosphatemia due to an increase in glucose phosphorylation seen in alkalosis, hyperuricemia secondary to purine release from injured muscles, and an increase in liver enzymes AST, LDH and total bilirubin commonly seen associated with liver dysfunction. In severe cases of heat illness, a coagulation disorder with evidence of disseminated intravascular coagulation (DIC)/consumption coagulopathy can be seen with elevated fibrin split products, PT, PTT and INR. Muscle damage can be associated with rhabdomyolysis with elevated CPK and myoglobin casts in the urine.

Other ancillary diagnostic studies include an electrocardiogram which may show tachycardia, rhythm disturbances (atrial fibrillation, supraventricular tachycardia), conduction defects (right bundle branch block (RBBB), intraventricular conduction defect), prolongation of QT interval most common secondary to hypocalcemia, hypomagnesemia or hypokalemia, or ST changes of myocardial ischemia.

Neurological tests may be required in patients with central nervous system involvement associated with heat stroke. Neurological deficits are possibly secondary to metabolic changes, cerebral edema or ischemia. The cerebellum is the most susceptible area to heat illness and cerebellar atrophy can be found after several weeks.[9] Brain CT scans or MRI are indicated in patients with persistent neurologic deficit after heat stroke.

In exertional hyponatremia, usually the electrolyte tests will reveal sodium levels in the range of 110–130 mmol/l accompanied by symptoms of headache, nausea, dyspnea and muscle cramps. A high level of suspicion is required for this condition that affects particularly the slow runners in long distance events.[6]

Cold injuries

Box 14.2: Key Points

- Basic tests
  - Initial field clinical assessment, blood pressure and heart rate
  - Low reading rectal thermometer
- Emergency room
  - Serum electrolytes, arterial blood gases, CPK and electrocardiogram
- Hospitalized athlete
  - PT, PTT, INR, follow-up of emergency room laboratories.

Hypothermia usually occurs associated with exercise in the cold when the body temperature falls below 95°F (35°C). Mild hypothermia is seen when the body core temperature is 35°C or greater. Shivering, tachycardia, tachypnea and cool extremities are usual associated symptoms. Moderate hypothermia is seen when the body core temperature drops below 34°C. At this stage, there will be signs of CNS depression and the athlete is confused, displays gross incoordination, slurred speech, drowsiness and may become dehydrated. Shivering is diminished or may not be present at all.

In severe hypothermia, the body core temperature is less than 32°C. At this stage, the athlete displays marked cognitive impairment and may be comatose. The body is rigid, cool and there is no shivering. The athlete is hypotensive with bradycardia, and cardiac arrhythmias are commonly seen. Almost all mild hypothermic healthy athletes recover normally. In athletes with moderate to severe hypothermia, rates of recovery are lower with ventricular fibrillation being the most common cause of death.[10]

A low reading rectal thermometer should be available in the first aid kit to document low temperature during cold weather athletic events.[11] If this type of thermometer is not available, the core temperature can be grossly estimated by evaluating if the athlete is shivering, in which case the core temperature is usually >90°F (32°C), or if the athlete is obtunded and not shivering usually the core temperature is <90°F (32°C).

Laboratory studies should be performed after the patient arrives at a medical care facility and re-warming is started, and include serum electrolytes, a renal panel and arterial blood gases. An electrocardiogram should also be done. Abnormal findings include increased BUN-creatinine ratio associated with acute tubular necrosis, increased CPK associated with rhabdomyolysis, and fluctuating potassium (K+) levels. Arterial blood gases can show hypoxemia, carbon dioxide retention and acidosis. A coagulation panel can reveal abnormalities compatible with a self-limited coagulopathy.[12] The electrocardiogram can reveal atrial or ventricular fibrillation due to myocardial irritability. Sinus bradycardia is seen in mild hypothermia.

CARDIAC PROBLEMS IN ATHLETES

Box 14.3: Key Points

Cardiac diseases work-up
- Exertional syncope
  - EKG, exercise stress test, echocardiogram
- Exertional chest pain
  - Stress test, echocardiogram
- Marfan syndrome
  - Electrocardiogram, echocardiogram most important
- Coarctation of aorta
  - Electrocardiogram, echocardiogram, chest X-rays
- Athletes heart
  - Electrocardiogram
- Coronary artery anomalies
  - Electrocardiogram, echocardiogram, cardiac catheterization
- Hypertrophic cardiomyopathy
  - Electrocardiogram, echocardiogram
- Myocarditis
  - Electrocardiogram, CBC, ESR, cardiac enzymes, echocardiogram
- Aortic stenosis
  - Electrocardiogram, echocardiogram, stress test.

Sport medicine physicians should be familiar with the common cardiovascular diseases which can lead to sudden death. In patients <35 years old, hypertrophic cardiomyopathy, and in patients >35 years old, coronary artery disease are the most common causes of death.[13] Cardiovascular pre-participation evaluation remains a challenge, because potentially fatal abnormalities are uncommon and sometimes not detectable without sophisticated tests.[14] Exercise testing is recommended in males older than 40 and females older than 50 years of age and individuals with cardiac risk factors. Detailed recommendations for evaluation of particular cardiac diseases were reviewed and updated at the 26th Bethesda Conference for determining eligibility for competition.[15] Specific items that should be addressed in the pre-participation evaluation include a history of family members who died of heart problems or sudden death before the age of 50, or cardiac symptoms such as syncope or chest pain associated with exercise.

Examples of medical conditions that may require cardiovascular work-up to prevent morbidity and mortality associated with exercise and sports participation are briefly discussed in the following section.

Exertional syncope
Athletes with exertional syncope need evaluation to exclude coronary artery anomalies, dilated cardiomyopathy, long QT syndrome, aortic stenosis, hypertrophic cardiomyopathy, mitral valve prolapse, myocarditis, ventricular preexcitation, neurally mediated syncope and heart block.[16] The diagnostic work-up includes EKG, exercise testing, possibly echocardiography, and in rare instances, coronary arteriography to exclude coronary artery anomalies.

Exertional chest pain
The individual requires evaluation to exclude hypertrophic cardiomyopathy, mitral valve prolapse, coronary artery anomalies, myocarditis, Marfan syndrome, arrhythmogenic right ventricular dysplasia, and aortic stenosis.[17] The athlete will need exercise stress testing, an echocardiogram or nuclear imaging echocardiography to rule out cardiac pathology.

Marfan syndrome
The athlete who is suspected of having Marfan's syndrome should undergo cardiovascular evaluation because of the risk of sudden death. The EKG can be normal, but the echocardiogram can show aortic root dilatation, as well as mitral and aortic valve abnormalities.[18]

Coarctation of aorta
In coarctation of the aorta the EKG is usually normal but the echocardiogram may show left ventricular dilatation, hypertrophy, coarctation of the aorta with post-stenotic dilatation, and associated intracardiac abnormalities. A plain chest X-ray

may show cardiomegaly and reversed E sign along the lateral border of ribs from collateral vessels.[8,16]

Athlete's heart

The asymptomatic athlete may present some abnormalities known as athlete's heart. The EKG can show sinus bradycardia of 30–40 beats/minute and sinus arrhythmia, atrioventricular blocks the most common being first degree (PR interval >0.2 s) and second degree Mobitz I Wenckebach block. Other findings may include increased voltage without left axis, QRS prolongation, or left atrial enlargement. There may also be U waves, early repolarization changes and incomplete right bundle branch block in the EKG. Correct interpretation of these findings is necessary to avoid preventing individuals without cardiac disease from participating in sports.

Coronary artery anomalies

The EKG is usually normal, but may show evidence such as Q waves suggesting myocardial infarction. An echocardiogram may show anomalies in the origin of the coronary arteries. The thallium stress test may be abnormal with exercise but conventional stress tests are usually normal. Finally, cardiac catheterization is necessary to definitely identify anomalies of the coronary arteries.[8,16]

Hypertrophic cardiomyopathy

In hypertrophic cardiomyopathy, the EKG is abnormal in 95% of cases. The findings include a marked increase in voltage, prominent Q waves >0.04 s and deep negative T waves in two or more leads. The echocardiogram is the test of choice to diagnose this condition in adults and shows left ventricular wall thickening of more than 15 mm with an unusual distribution (concentric, asymmetrical septal or apical).[12]

Myocarditis

The patient with myocarditis has an EKG that shows diffuse low voltage, ST-T wave changes, heart block and ventricular arrhythmias. Laboratory tests may show a CBC with leukocytosis, eosinophilia, increased ESR and increased cardiac enzymes. Echocardiography will exhibit a dilated left ventricle, global hypokinesia, segmental wall abnormalities and decreased ejection fraction. An endocardial biopsy would help to confirm the diagnosis.[19]

Aortic stenosis

The EKG shows left ventricular hypertrophy and ST-T waves changes of left ventricular strain. An echocardiogram shows left ventricular hypertrophy, narrowing of the aortic valve with estimated gradient across the valve. Exercise testing may be needed to evaluate for evidence of ischemia, arrhythmia, and assess for exercise duration and blood pressure response.[8,16]

PULMONARY PROBLEMS IN ATHLETES

Exercise induced bronchospasm (EIB)

Box 14.4: Key Points

Exercise induced bronchospasm tests

- Peak flow meter before and after exercise
- Pulmonary function tests before and after exercise 1-3-5-10-15 min
- Eucapnic voluntary hyperventilation challenge with dry air [a]
- Methacholine inhalation challenge[a]

[a] Studies done only for investigation or as a last resort

EIB is one of the most common conditions in active children, adolescents and young adults. It develops when vigorous physical activity triggers airway narrowing in persons with heightened bronchial reactivity. EIB occurs after near maximum exercise for >5 min. The individual exercising experiences difficulty breathing with shortness of breath, coughing, chest tightness, wheezing and lack of energy. Physicians should have a high index of suspicion for this condition, particularly in children, since signs and symptoms are not a good predictor of EIB in kids with minimal complaints.[20,21]

A clinical trial with prophylactic medications such as inhaled beta agonists, cromolyn sodium, nedocromil sodium, theophylline, inhaled steroids, or ipratropium bromide can be used for diagnostic purposes. Although this is not a scientific method, it may aid in confirming the diagnosis, however, in patients with chronic asthma this technique may not permit physicians to differentiate this condition from EIB.[22]

The evaluation of EIB should include some of the following studies.

Initial evaluation can start with peak flow measurement before and after exercise. The baseline peak flow should be evaluated at rest, and following sustained vigorous exercise for 6–8 min with heart rate responses of >90% of predicted for age. Pulmonary function tests including forced expiratory volume (FEV), forced expiratory flow (FEF 25–75), peak expiratory flow rate (PEFR) can be measured before and after exercise at 1–3–5–10 to 15 min intervals while running on a treadmill or riding a bicycle ergometer.[8,23]

Different types of challenge tests can be performed when there is doubt of the diagnosis of EIB. A eucapnic voluntary hyperventilation (EVH) challenge with dry air has been shown to have high sensitivity and high specificity for EIB. However, this test is expensive and generally unavailable. The methacholine inhalation challenge has low sensitivity but high specificity in elite athletes, and is not recommend in the athlete with pure EIB. The osmotic challenge inhalation tests done with hypertonic saline or the inhaled dry powder mannitol challenge have both high sensitivity and specificity for EIB. They may be better alternatives than the EVH test to evaluate EIB.[24]

GASTROINTESTINAL PROBLEMS IN ATHLETES

Exercise induced diarrhea

Box 14.5: Key Points

Exercise induced diarrhea tests

- Stool samples for culture, ova and parasites, occult blood and leukocytes
- CBC, electrolytes, ESR, giardiasis
- Endoscopic studies.

Diarrhea is seen mostly in intense endurance training and most commonly in running (10–50% of runners). Proposed etiologies include anxiety, increased gastrointestinal motility (exercise increases secretion of gastrin, motilin and other hormones), dietary factors (high fiber, fruits, large doses of caffeine or vitamin C) and changes in the immune system.[8,25]

Initial laboratory and diagnostic tests are done based on the history, physical examination and stool evaluation (culture, ova and parasites, occult blood and leukocytes). These include tests for giardiasis, complete cell blood count, ESR and electrolytes. Initial treatment may include reduction of exercise intensity, followed by a gradual return to the previous level of training, dietary manipulation or antimotility agents.[26] If the diarrhea persists after the initial management endoscopic studies can help to rule out other etiologies such as colitis.

Lower gastrointestinal bleeding

Box 14.6: Key Points

Lower gastrointestinal bleeding

- Lower gastrointestinal endoscopy is the study of choice for persistent symptoms.

Mild exercise decreases intestinal perfusion by 40% and strenuous exercises may decrease it by 89%. This intestinal ischemia can cause focal areas of necrosis and ulceration with bleeding.[25] Other gastrointestinal pathology that causes bleeding such as colon cancer, hemorrhoids, and inflammatory bowel disease should be ruled out by endoscopic studies. In the case of bleeding associated with exercise, lower gastrointestinal endoscopic studies should be performed within 1–2 days of frank bleeding, since ischemic lesions could resolve after 2 days.

Upper gastrointestinal problems

Box 14.7: Key Points

- Some common gastrointestinal conditions are GERD, gastritis, PUD and delayed gastric emptying
- Upper gastrointestinal endoscopy is recommended if symptoms persist.

These problems include gastrointestinal reflux disease (GERD), peptic ulcer disease (PUD), gastritis and delayed gastric emptying. Upper endoscopy should be considered in patients that exhibit persistent symptoms after treatment trials with H_2 blockers, proton pump inhibitors and adequate dietary changes.

NEUROMUSCULAR PROBLEMS IN ATHLETES

Headache in athletes

The epidemiology of this common disorder is not clear, however it is frequently encountered by the sport medicine physician.[27] Most exertional headaches are benign but it is important to exclude secondary headache associated with serious conditions. Athletes should be evaluated for 'red flags' that indicate serious disease such as headache onset after the age of 50, sudden onset of headache, increased severity and frequency of headache with activity, new onset symptoms in the immunocompromised patient and headache associated with systemic illness. Other aspects of the history that are important include fever, neck stiffness, focal neurologic deficit, trauma, gait problems, amnesia, alteration of consciousness, early morning nausea, and vomiting (Table 14.2).[28]

Laboratory studies that should be performed include CBC, ESR, liver function tests and thyroid function tests to rule out metabolic pathology. Other diagnostic studies that may be required include cervical X-rays with flexion/extension views in patients with trauma to rule out cervical fracture and instability, head computer tomography (CT scan) without and with contrast in new onset exertional headache to rule out bleeding,

Table 14.2 Classification of Headache

Exertional Headache	Effort Headache	Post Traumatic Headache	Others
Occurs after strenuous activity (lifting weights or sprinting). Located on occipital cervical region. Brief duration.	Occurs after running for several hours. Initiated by aerobic activity and aggravated by dehydration, heat, fatigue, excessive exercise, alcohol, caffeine.	Headache occurring after head trauma.	Cervicogenic, trauma triggered migraine, and headache associated with altitude.

and magnetic resonance imaging (MRI) in patients with suspected arteriovenous malformation, tumor or posterior fossa lesions. Lumbar puncture can be performed to rule out subarachnoid hemorrhage from ruptured aneurysm since it can detect minor leaks in patients who can later have a rupture even with a negative CT scan.[28]

In the athlete with migraine, the American Academy of Neurology states that routine brain imaging is not warranted for adults with recurrent headaches that have been identified as migraine with no recent change in pattern, without history of seizures or other focal neurological sign or symptoms.[29]

Muscle weakness

Box 14.8: Key Points

- Initial laboratories
  - Serum chemistries electrolytes (calcium, magnesium, glucose), TSH, CPK, ESR, ANA.

Muscle weakness may be a complaint of an athlete presenting for clinical evaluation. A thorough clinical assessment is required to differentiate fatigue, focal weakness, or generalized weakness. Athletes may present with a medical condition associated with exercise or sport which results in weakness, or may have an underlying disease which is exacerbated by activity. The physician evaluating the patient with muscle weakness should try to identify if neurologic, endocrine, inflammatory, rheumatologic, genetic, metabolic, electrolyte-imbalance or drug-related conditions is what causes the individuals symptoms.[30]

If the cause of muscle weakness in unclear, serum chemistries (electrolytes, calcium, magnesium, glucose) and a thyroid-stimulating hormone assay should be obtained to evaluate for electrolyte disturbances and endocrine myopathies. Next, investigations looking for inflammatory, rheumatologic, or genetic myopathies can be performed. Although nonspecific, the creatine kinase (CK) level usually is normal in the electrolyte and endocrine myopathies with the possible exceptions of thyroid and potassium disorder myopathies. However, the CK level may be highly elevated (10–100 times normal) in the inflammatory myopathies and can be moderately to highly elevated in the muscular dystrophies.

In addition to CK, an erythrocyte sedimentation rate (ESR) and an antinuclear antibody (ANA) may help determine if a myopathy associated to rheumatic disease exists. If either the ESR or the ANA is positive, additional studies may be obtained, including rheumatoid factor looking for rheumatoid arthritis, anti-double-stranded DNA or antiphospholipid antibodies to evaluate for systemic lupus erythematosus, or anticentromere antibodies looking for scleroderma.[30] Nerve conduction and electromyography studies are a powerful tool for the diagnosis and localization of lesions within the lower motor neuron, neuromuscular junction, peripheral nerve and muscle. In addition, electrodiagnostic studies may help to establish the severity of lesion, prognosis for recovery, and help in making return to play decisions. Also, they may lead the clinician to order further studies including muscle or nerve biopsy.[31]

The application of molecular genetic techniques has resulted in significant gains in the understanding of the molecular and pathophysiologic bases of many neuromuscular diseases. In addition, molecular genetic studies aid in the diagnostic evaluation of dystrophin-deficient muscular dystrophies or hereditary neuropathies among other neuromuscular diseases that may present in athletes with complaints of weakness.[32]

Muscle pain

Box 14.9: Key Points

- Initial laboratories/studies
  - Serum electrolytes, CK, urinalysis, liver function tests, and coagulation studies.

The athlete who presents with muscle pain following activity needs to be evaluated for the possibility of muscle fiber damage. This could range in severity from delayed onset muscle soreness (DOMS) to rhabdomyolysis. Predisposition to muscle damage in the athlete may be related to poor conditioning, dehydration, underlying viral illness or medical condition, as well as intense eccentric exercise. Complications of rhabdomyolysis with severe muscle damage include renal failure, metabolic derangements, DIC and death.[33]

Initial studies in the athlete with suspected muscle injury associated to pain include serum electrolytes, CPK, urine analysis, liver function tests, and coagulation studies. Muscle injury seen in the individual with DOMS is usually associated to modest elevations of CPK while more severe injury is associated to high CPK, myoglobinuria, abnormal PT, PTT and fibrin split products.

HEMATOLOGIC PROBLEMS IN ATHLETES

Box 14.10: Key Points

Anemia

- Initial laboratories
  - CBC, peripheral smear, ferritin levels, vitamin B_{12} levels, folate levels

---

Anemia in athletes

Anemia is defined as a reduced number of circulating red blood cells (RBC) or reduced hemoglobin concentration. Hemoglobin or hematocrit levels cannot be used as the unique measure in the evaluation of anemia since both values do not indicate RBC mass. Anemia can be classified instead by RBC morphology (Table 14.3).

Table 14.3 Classification of Anemia

Microcytic	Macrocytic	Normocytic
Iron deficiency	Folate deficiency	Chronic disease
Thalassemia minor	Vitamin B_{12} deficiency	Hemolysis
Lead poisoning	Hypothyroidism	Rapid bleeding
Sideroblastic anemia	Drugs	Aplastic anemia

Dilutional pseudoanemia

Endurance athletes can present with hemoglobin levels 0.5 g lower and elite athletes 1 g lower than sedentary persons. Increases in plasma volumes of 10–20% lead to dilution of the measured hemoglobin level and has been named 'sports anemia' or dilutional pseudoanemia.[34] This condition does not seem to be pathologic but an adaptation to endurance training, and usually can revert to normal with training cessation of 3–5 days.[35] Although hemoglobin and hematocrit levels are lower, total RBC and RBC mass are increased with a normal morphology index (mean corpuscular volumes), so there is no need to treat this entity.[36]

Iron deficiency anemia

Iron deficiency is the most common etiology of anemia in athletes. Both inadequate iron intake and blood loss can be the cause. Iron deficiency anemia can be asymptomatic at rest with hemoglobin levels between 11–11.9 g/dl, but can affect athletic performance at high levels of intensity. Symptoms associated to lower hemoglobin levels can be weakness, lassitude, palpitations, shortness of breath and pica (craving for starch, or ice). Up to 20% of menstruating women may have iron deficiency anemia with low ferritin levels.[36] There is no clear evidence that athletes have a higher incidence of iron deficiency anemia than the general population.

Foot strike hemolysis

This diagnosis is one of exclusion seen in athletes after vigorous activity. It has been associated with high impact sports but has also been described in swimmers and rowers. There appears to be an association to increased temperature and flow dynamics in vigorous sports and not necessarily to impact as the cause of hemolysis.[37] However, significant hemolysis in athletes should make the physician search for other etiologies of hemolytic anemias.

The diagnostic work-up for all these hematologic conditions should start with a complete red blood cell count (CBC). In addition to hemoglobin and hematocrit levels, morphology indexes are obtained, which direct to the initial classification of anemia. Confirmation of anemia in adults (<12 g in women <14 g in men) can be done and further investigation for pseudoanemia can follow. There has been a controversy regarding the CBC as part of the screening laboratories performed in athletes in the pre-participation evaluation, but it is reasonable to do the test in any athlete who complains of a decrease in performance and may present other classic anemia symptoms. Finally, it is probably judicious to screen female

athletes after their menstruation starts to establish a baseline, even if the athlete does not present with symptoms or decreased performance.[38]

Ferritin level is the most commonly used indicator of body iron stores. Low ferritin levels (<12 µg/l) usually indicate exhausted iron reserves. However, normal or high ferritin level does not guarantee adequate iron stores since infection, inflammation, disorders of the liver, malignancies, and other conditions can cause increases in serum ferritin levels and mask potential iron depletion. Acute exercise and physical activity can be accompanied by an inflammatory like reaction which can cause an increase in ferritin levels for several days, and make an assessment of the iron stores difficult.[39]

Iron levels, total binding iron capacity (TIBC) and transferrin saturation can help the clinician when there is a suspicion that ferritin levels can be affected by other factors. If these are low, iron deficiency anemia can be the diagnosis.

Other diagnostic studies that can be considered include levels of vitamin B_{12}, folic acid or RBC folate, and thyroid function studies in the case of macrocytic anemia. LDH, haptoglobin, bilirubin levels, a direct Coombs' test, and cold agglutinins can be ordered if hemolytic anemia is suspected.

ENDOCRINE PROBLEMS IN ATHLETES

Exercise induced menstrual disorders

> **Box 14.11: Key Points**
>
> - Initial laboratories
>   - Pregnancy test, TSH and prolactin levels.

Irregular menses has been reported in 1–66% of athletes compared with 2–5% in the general population.[40] Menstrual disorders can be classified in five categories: delayed menarche, shortening of the luteal phase, anovulation, oligomenorrhea and amenorrhea. Amenorrhea has been described to be much more frequent in athletes than in non-exercising women. Menstrual dysfunction can lead to a decrease in bone mineral density particularly if the duration exceeds >1 year. Endocrine abnormalities such as a decrease in the pulsatile release of gonadotropin releasing hormone from the hypothalamus can lead to reduced levels of luteinizing hormone (LH) and follicle stimulating hormone (FSH).[41] This is apparently the result of reduced caloric intake and strenuous exercise, which leads finally to hypoestrogenism and subsequent amenorrhea (Table 14.4).[42]

The diagnostic work-up should include a pregnancy test, thyroid stimulating hormone (TSH) and prolactin levels. A progestin challenge test administering medroxyprogesterone (Provera 10 mg) orally for 5 days can also be performed to evaluate for anovulation, with absence of progesterone in the luteal phase, and adequate estrogen stores. In addition, evaluation of FSH/LH may reveal elevated levels in ovarian failure and low levels in athletic amenorrhea.

If the patient has a history of regular menses but becomes amenorrheic with increased training, a pregnancy test should

Table 14.4   Menstrual Abnormalities

Delayed Menarche	Amenorrhea	Anovulation	Oligomenorrhea
Absence of initial menstruation by age 16 years. Onset 1 year beyond average of mother and sisters.	Absence of 3-12 consecutive menstrual periods.	Younger women. Immature hypothalamic pituitary ovarian axis.	Irregular menstruation. 6-9 menstrual periods per year. Cycle length > 35 days and < 90 days.

be performed and if negative, amenorrhea can be considered to be due to training. If menstruation returns after reduction of training, no other work-up may be needed, however, hormone replacement therapy should be considered after 3–6 months of amenorrhea.

In the athlete with persistent amenorrhea and in particular the one with a stress fracture, bone densitometry testing with dual energy X-ray absorptiometry (DEXA) is the gold standard test to measure bone density to rule out osteopenia and osteoporosis.

DIABETIC ATHLETES

> **Box 14.12: Key Points**
>
> **Diabetes mellitus**
> - Pre-participation evaluation is essential
> - Initial laboratories
>   - FBS, HgbA$_1$C, renal function tests, urine microalbumin test, ketones.

Diabetic athletes on insulin or oral hypoglycemic agents are prone to hypoglycemia or hyperglycemia depending on glucose level before starting exercise. Athletes with type I diabetes mellitus (DM) who are insulin dependent are also at risk of developing ketoacidosis. The sport medicine physician must rely on laboratory testing to know which diabetic athlete should be cleared to do training. Physicians should instruct the patient to monitor the blood glucose prior to and after exercising to assess control and the response to specific training of different intensities.

Laboratory studies that should be performed in the diabetic athlete include fasting blood sugar, glycosylated hemoglobin (HgbA$_1$C) levels, renal function tests, and urine tests for microalbumin, as well as ketones.[43]

The diabetic athlete can be cleared to perform strenuous exercise when HgbA$_1$C is within 6–8%. Exercise tests to screen for coronary disease must be done for the diabetic individual >35 years of age who wants to start a program of moderate to vigorous exercises.

Renal function needs to be evaluated periodically, adequate hydration and restriction of anti-inflammatory agents (non-steroidal) in the diabetic training for long periods of time should be encouraged.[44]

At the time of starting exercise, if the blood sugar is <130 mg/d the athlete should consume 1–2 carbohydrate exchanges

per 30–45 min of light to moderate exercise. If the blood sugar is 130–180 mg/dl he/she should consume one carbohydrate exchange per 30–45 min of heavy exercise. In the case of levels of 180–240 mg/dl the individual should not take food before exercise. If the blood sugar level is >250 mg/dl urine ketones should be checked and exercise may be permitted if no ketones are present.

GENITOURINARY PROBLEMS IN ATHLETES

Hematuria

> **Box 14.13: Key Points**
>
> - Initial laboratories
>   - Urinalysis, repeated at 48–72 h post exercise.

Hematuria can be macroscopic associated with trauma in contact sports or microscopic (>3 RBC/HPF) and seen in non-contact sports. It usually resolves within 48–72 h but in some cases of prolonged exercise, it may be present up to 7 days. Exercise-induced hematuria can originate from the kidney, bladder, urethra or prostate.

Hematuria of renal origin can be caused by either ischemia (non-traumatic) or direct as well as indirect (traumatic) renal injury. Hematuria can also be caused by repetitive trauma to the bladder posterior wall against its base in long distance events.[45]

Some athletes that present with hematuria may have underlying medical problems such as urinary tract infection, nephrolithiasis, tumor, coagulopathies and rhabdomyolysis. In the individual with persistent painless hematuria, identification of factors associated with malignancy should be addressed (Table 14.5).

Table 14.5   Factors Associated with Genitourinary Malignancy

Smoking history
Occupational exposure to chemicals or dyes
History of gross hematuria
Age >40 years
History of irritative voiding symptoms
History of urinary tract infections
Analgesic abuse
History of pelvic irradiation

The diagnostic studies include a urinalysis, which may show microhematuria of three or more red blood cells per high power field on microscopic evaluation of urinary sediment from two of three properly collected urine specimens. In the athlete, hematuria persisting after 48–72 h post-exercise should lead to other studies which help to rule out associated diseases.

A microscopic urine analysis could be done to assess mean corpuscular volume and red blood cell morphology to search the origin of bleeding. If mean corpuscular volume (MCV) >72 its origin is from a non-glomerular site and if MCV <72 it is from glomerular origin.[46] Urine culture and sensitivity tests are done to rule out infection, serum chemistry including blood urea nitrogen, creatinine and electrolytes to assess renal function, CPK levels if rhabdomyolysis is suspected, LDH is done for hemolysis and PT, PTT, INR to rule out coagulopathy.[47]

Other considerations include performing a sickle cell test and urine cytology in cases where sickle cell anemia is suspected, renal ultrasound, for detection, characterization of renal cysts and identification of hydronephrosis. Intravenous urography (IVU) is considered to be the best initial study for evaluation of the urinary tracts. It is widely available and it is cost effective, however it has limitations in detecting small renal masses and differentiating solid from cystic masses. Computed tomography is the preferred modality for detection and characterization of solid renal masses, with detection rates comparable with that of magnetic resonance imaging. CT is the best modality for evaluation of urinary stones, renal and perirenal infections, with a sensitivity of 94–98% for detection of renal stones compared with 52–59% for intravenous urography and 19% for ultrasonography.[12] If the above tests are normal, a cystoscopy or voiding cystourethrogram, especially in patients >40 years of age, can be performed to rule out neoplasia.

Hematuria is probably not secondary to exercise if it persists after 24–72 h, if there is the presence of gross hematuria, if the athlete is older than 40 years, if it is recurrent, or if it is not associated with intense or prolonged exercise. Distance running athletes have been shown to have post-exercise hematuria at least once, specially after a workout run at 110% of VO$_2$max over short to moderate distances, but in general, cases resolve within 2 h of recovery.[48]

Proteinuria

Box 14.14: Key Points

- Initial laboratories
- Urinalysis, urine dipstick at 24–48 h post-exercise.

Increased protein in the urine is present in up to 70% of athletes after exertion. Normal protein excretion is 30–45 mg/day and exertional proteinuria ranges from 100–300 mg/day, which usually occurs within 30 min of exercise and decreases in 24–48 h. It is more commonly seen in strenuous and prolonged exercise but mostly directly related to intensity.[49]

Studies have shown that albumin contributes more than other proteins in exercise induced proteinuria, which is probably from glomerular and tubular origin in the kidney, and this change is usually reversible. A urine dipstick method to detect protein is good for screening but does not detect the microalbuminuria seen in diabetics. In the athlete, a dipstick urine and urinalysis should be performed 24–48 h after exercise, if looking for persistent proteinuria associated to renal disease, diabetes mellitus, hypertension or orthostatic proteinuria.[50]

Renal trauma

Renal trauma can occur secondary to a direct blow or from a high speed collision. The patient can present with pain, tenderness, ecchymosis and hematuria. A correlation with the amount of hematuria and the severity of injury is not reliable and the patient can be seen with hypotension from bleeding. Abdominal CT scan with intravenous and oral contrast can evaluate for contusion and localize an injury which can lead to surgery.[45]

DIAGNOSTIC IMAGING

Diagnostic imaging in athletic injuries has taken an increasingly important role in the management of such injuries. The higher level of competitiveness and the urgency to return to competition demands a faster diagnosis in order to make a therapeutic decision. There is also an increasing role for accurate diagnostic tests in the prevention of new injuries, or the exacerbation of existing ones.

Although the progress of diagnostic imaging techniques has been impressive, these tests are not a substitute but a complement to a good history, a careful physical exam and an extensive differential diagnosis which continue to be the mainstay of musculoskeletal diagnosis.

The most common imaging techniques used in sports medicine are conventional radiography, magnetic resonance imaging, radio nuclide imaging and diagnostic ultrasonography. A brief review of these will be covered in the following section.

Radiography

Box 14.15: Key Points

- Conventional radiography remains the standard in the diagnosis of fractures.
- High sensitivity in fractures and availability in the case of emergencies.
- Important in the follow-up of fracture treatment to document healing.

X-ray diagnosis has been extensively used and is a safe, proven and inexpensive diagnostic test. Plain X-ray can be used in virtually all bone injuries and because of its high sensitivity, as well as relative availability, it remains as the standard in the diagnosis of fractures.[51] These include all long bones as well as tarsal and axial skeletal bones.

In the management of traumatic injury, it is important to order at least two radiographic views of the injured part, perpendicular to each other, and in the child athlete with open growth plates, it may be necessary to compare the films with the uninvolved extremity. In the individual with overuse injury, the use of plain radiographs is less common; however, plain films can still be used to identify anatomical variants, tumors, signs of degenerative joint disease and sub-acute or chronic changes of a stress fracture.

In addition, radiographic evaluation is important after treatment of a fracture to ensure proper post-reduction alignment and to document healing. Also, conventional radiographs aid in the diagnosis of certain complications, such as infection, avascular necrosis, or post-traumatic osteoarthritis.

Computed tomography (CT)

Box 14.16: Key Points

- Image slices of variable thickness can be used to depict bone details.
- Allows identification of intraarticular and stress fractures, which may be missed in conventional radiographs.
- May be combined with contrast enhancement.

Computerized axial tomography uses X-ray generating tubes and image detectors to produce images in the transverse, sagittal and coronal planes. Image slices can vary in thickness from 1–10 mm and can be used to depict bone detail. Conventional CT consists of a rotating X-ray tube emitting a collimated radiation beam and multiple detectors to measure transmission through a stationary patient. A computer then processes the data to provide a two-dimensional or simulated three-dimensional image.[52] The use of a CT scan allows the identification of intraarticular fractures, stress fractures and others which may be missed in conventional radiographs. In addition, CT can be used with contrast enhancement, which can be of benefit in particular clinical scenarios, such as the athlete with shoulder instability and a suspected labral lesion.[53]

The athlete with head or spine trauma may require the use of CT which is an excellent diagnostic modality to evaluate intracerebral bleeding and for vertebral fractures which should be considered for emergency treatment. In the individual with back pain the use of thin cuts across the pars interarticularis may allow for the identification of spondylolysis and performing images across the disc or facet joints may help to diagnose discogenic disease or spinal stenosis.[54]

Magnetic resonance imaging (MRI)

MRI has revolutionized diagnostic imaging of the musculoskeletal system. Non-invasive direct visualization of bone, marrow and supporting soft tissue structures are clearly obtained via this technology.

The principles of nuclear magnetic resonance were originally described in 1946 by two independent researchers who

Box 14.17: Key Points

- MRI has the ability to display excellent soft tissue contrast.
- Different imaging sequences can be used to study anatomic detail or to diagnose injury.
- MRI is highly sensitive in the diagnosis of meniscal and anterior cruciate ligament injuries.

were awarded the Nobel Prize. These principles were applied to MRI in 1973 for medical use. By 1980, it was widely used for the diagnosis of neurological diseases and since then it has been widely used in the musculoskeletal system.

MRI is a tomographic multiplanar technique with the ability to display outstanding soft tissue contrast. It works by detecting the relaxation times of hydrogen atoms. The human body is placed in a strong magnetic field usually 1.5 T (Tesla) provided most commonly by an electromagnet, energized in a super conductor state cooled by liquid helium, and nitrogen to 4° above absolute zero. Hydrogen protons in the body will spin and align themselves with the direction of the external magnetic field and reach a state of equilibrium. This is followed by the emission of energy by the machine in the form of radio wave frequencies. This energy is absorbed by the hydrogen protons, which exist in all tissues. Upon discontinuation of the radio waves, the excited protons lose this extra energy through T1 (longitudinal) relaxation and T2 (transverse) relaxation mechanisms. The intensity of the magnetic resonance signal that results is chiefly determined by these two relaxation patterns as well as the proton density. This minute amount of energy released by the resonating hydrogen protons is picked up by coil antennas placed around the extremity.

This recorded energy signal is taken through a mathematical process (Fourier) and the computer forms the image. The body is not exposed to ionized radiation but rather to magnetic and radio frequency energy. TR stands for repetition time, the time between successive excitation pulses. The TE stands for echo time, the time that an echo is formed.[55]

Three basic sequences are used, T1-weighted, T2-weighted and proton density sequences, because tissues in the body emit different intensity signals in T1, T2 and proton density images. For example, fat will look bright in T1-weighted images, and fluid will look dark. However, the opposite is true for T2-weighted images. T2 images will show, fluid, soft tissue edema, bone marrow edema and bone contusion as a bright signal (Table 14.6).[56]

Most acute traumatic injuries will be dramatically revealed in the T2-weighted sequence. Therefore T2 tends to be more of a pathology sequence, while T1 tends to be more of an anatomy sequence. T2 is determined by a long TR >1500 μs and TE >60 μs, while a T1 image is determined by a short TR <400 μs. A third type of image commonly used is determined by a long TR and short TE referred to as a proton density image T2 (Table 14.7).[55, 56]

Table 14.6 MRI Tissue Signal Intensities

	T1-Weighted	T2-Weighted	T2-Proton Density
Cortical bone	Low	Low	Low
Marrow edema	Low	High	Intermediate
Hyaline cartilage	Intermediate	Intermediate	Intermediate/high
Meniscus	Low	Low	Low
Meniscal tear	High	Intermediate	High
Ligament	Low	Low	Low
Tendon	Low	Low	Low
Fluid	Low	High	High
Fat	High	Intermediate	Low
Blood – acute	Low/Intermediate	Low	Mixed

(Modified from Miller et al. 1997.[57])

MRI is very useful in the diagnosis of bone and soft tissue injuries including ligamentous injuries, meniscal injuries, and injuries to tendon and muscle. MRI will reveal structural changes such as fractures and ligament tears as well as physiologic changes related to injury such as bone marrow edema in bone contusions. This technique can be used in virtually every tissue in the body. For example, it is very useful in the diagnosis of shoulder injuries including rotator cuff tears, as well as labral tears where imaging can be enhanced with intraarticular gadolinium.[52]

Gadolinium, a rare earth element, chelates into the vascular and interstitial compartments and works by altering the magnetic environment facilitating T1 and T2 relaxation, shortening times. The net effect is that of producing high contrast images in demarcation of cysts, edema and meniscal re-tears and infection. Gadolinium is safer as a contrast when compared with iodine, since it is not nephrotoxic and allergic reactions are rare.[57]

MRI is especially useful in the diagnosis of ligamentous knee injuries in children where damage to the growth plate is always a possibility and it is enhanced by the presence of edema on T2 sequences.[58]

MRI enhances the appearance of fractures including stress fractures on T2-weighted images, since bone edema will be very bright and has been considered by some clinicians as the study of choice in the management of this condition.[59, 60] Chondral lesions and bone bruises are highlighted by subchondral edema on T2 images. Other conditions where MRI is very useful include osteochondritis dissecans, meniscal cysts, popliteal cysts, pathologic plicae and neoplastic lesions.

MRI in meniscus injury
MRI is a valuable tool for meniscal tear diagnosis. Its accuracy ranges between 90–95%, depending on the level of competence of the individual reading the study and the quality of the images.[61,62]

Classification systems have been developed to describe the appearance of a meniscal lesion in MRI and allow clear communication between the clinician and the radiologists. Intrasubstance signals of the meniscus classified as Grade I globular in appearance, which do not intercept the superior or inferior articular surfaces of the meniscus are thought not to represent a tear. A Grade II intrasubstance signal is linear in appearance, does not intersect the superior or inferior articular surface of the meniscus and does not represent a tear. A Grade III signal intersects the superior and/or the inferior articular surface of the meniscus and represents a tear. Grade I and Grade II represent either meniscal degeneration called myxoid degeneration, or in the young athlete vascular proliferation where a Grade III always represents a tear (Fig. 14.1).

MRI in ACL injury
ACL tears are frequently seen in athletes. MRI is very useful and has been shown to be cost-effective if used appropriately in the evaluation of these injuries. The accuracy of MRI ranges from 90 to 95% in the acute injury. However, it is less accurate in partial tears of ACL, and chronic ACL insufficiency (Table 14.8).[56,63] In the case of the patient with a previous history of knee surgery, the use of MRI with contrast has improved the evaluation of the residual meniscus and the anterior cruciate ligament graft.[64]

Table 14.7 MRI Imaging: Clinical Advantages and Disadvantages

Sequence	Advantages	Disadvantages
Spin echo T1	Anatomic detail. Evaluates subacute hemorrhage, meniscal, and marrow pathology. May be used with gadolinium enhancement.	Poor detection of soft tissue edema and other T2-sensitive pathology. Not as sensitive as STIR or fast spin echo-T2 with fat saturation for marrow pathology.
Proton density T2	Anatomic detail. Meniscal pathology.	Poor detection of fluid and marrow pathology. Long imaging times.
Fast spin echo Proton density T2	Anatomic detail. T2 contrast obtained with shorter imaging times. Detection of marrow pathology combined with fat saturation. Good in patients with metal hardware.	Potential blurring artifact can lead to missing meniscal tears. Poor detection of marrow pathology when not combined with fat saturation.
Gradient echo T2	Evaluates ligaments and tendons acute pathology. Loose bodies and subtle hemorrhage 3D imaging.	Poor detection of marrow pathology at high field strengths. Metallic hardware (artifacts due to susceptibility effects).
STIR	Marrow and soft tissue pathology.	Should not be used with gadolinium.

(Modified from Kaplan et al. 2001.[55])

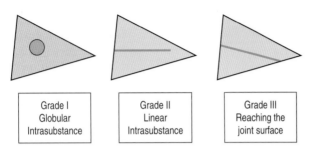

Figure 14.1 MRI meniscal signal system classification.

Table 14.9   Contraindications for MRI

Cardiac pacemakers
Ferromagnetic aneurysmal clips
Cochlear implants
Metallic foreign bodies in the eyes
Implanted neurostimulants
Although not proven unsafe, not recommended in the first trimester of pregnancy
Coronary stents first 6 months after implantation

MRI safety

MRI is generally a very safe procedure, however some patients may suffer from claustrophobia when placed in the machine, but this can be managed with sedation (Table 14.9).

Technetium scintigraphy

Box 14.18: Key Points

- Bone scan can provide physiologic information about changes in living tissues.
- Highly sensitive technique but not specific with positive scans in infections, tumors and fractures.

Technetium scan or bone scan as it is more commonly known is a safe, cost-effective and highly sensitive imaging method, although not as specific as MRI. Different from MRI, radiography and sonography which provide structural information; a technetium scan provides a physiologic insight into what is happening in living tissues. In the standard study, 20 mCi of technetium-99 (a gamma photon-emitter) is injected by intravenous route to the patient. The technetium is attached to methylene diphosphonate, a compound readily absorbed to metabolically active bone. A gamma camera and computer system provide reflecting images of the human body.[65] The first phase of a three phase uptake study is done immediately and reflects the arterial flow of the extremity. The second phase, taken a few minutes later, provides the venous pooling phase of the scan and a third phase of delayed static images reflects the relative distribution of the technetium in the body taken up by metabolically active new bone formation. Phases one and two demonstrate increased uptake in conditions like sympathetic dystrophy and infection, however phase three demonstrates bone pathology in its active repair phase.[66] Single-photon emission computed tomography (SPECT) is a technique to more accurately reflect the technetium distribution to a specific anatomic region within a bone or joint and has been used for evaluation of suspected spondylolysis.[67] The bone scan is highly sensitive, poorly specific and will be positive for infections, tumors and fractures alike. However, it is very useful in the diagnosis of stress fractures in the athlete.[68] Another important concept is that of increased osseous metabolic activity (IOMA), demonstrated by positive bone scan. IOMA demonstrated by positive scan can be seen in conditions of repetitive submaximal loading such as early stress fractures, as well as meniscus pathology and ACL insufficiency.[69,70] These bone scan changes however can be reversed with the correction of the pathology or abnormal mechanical loading in the athlete's sports technique or training.[71]

Diagnostic ultrasound

Box 14.19: Key Points

- Musculoskeletal ultrasound can be used for dynamic imaging of soft tissues including tendons and ligaments but requires a skilled examiner.
- Can be used safely in special populations such as children and pregnant women.

Musculoskeletal sonography has been shown to be effective for many applications related to sports medicine. Some advantages of sonography over MRI include portability, accessibility, high

Table 14.8   MRI Signs of ACL Disruption

Direct	Indirect
Discontinuity of fibers	Bone contusion of lateral femoral condyle and posterior lateral tibial plateau
Abnormal slope of ACL	Deep sulcus sign on lateral terminal condyle >2 mm deep with marrow edema on T2 image
Non-visualization of ACL fibers in both sagittal and coronal planes	Segond's capsular avulsion fracture of the lateral tibial plateau
Avulsion of anterior tibial spine	Anterior displacement of the tibia on the femur

resolution and relative lower cost. More importantly, dynamic imaging under sonographic visualization allows the clinician to make diagnoses that cannot be made with other diagnostic imaging studies.[72] Sonography is universally tolerated across a broad patient population, including pediatric and pregnant patients and those in whom traditional magnetic resonance imaging is not an option, because of absolute or relative contraindications.[73]

Ultrasound refers to energy above the perceptible range of frequencies (20 Hz–20 kHz). The frequencies used for diagnostic ultrasound range from 2 to 10 MHz. Ultrasound waves are directed to the tissues and as these bounce back from the tissues their echo is received by sensor and interpreted by a computer and an image is constructed.[52] It is especially useful in the diagnosis of acute tendon ruptures, muscle tears and muscle hematomas, and avulsion fractures. It appears to be safe, sensitive and specific in the hands of a skilled examiner. However, in chronic cases of tendinopathy such as the one affecting the Achilles tendon, only moderate correlation with clinical assessment has been found by some researchers.[74]

CONCLUSION

Laboratory and diagnostic studies are very important for the clinician treating individuals with exercise or sports related illness or injury. Sports medicine physicians should feel comfortable in ordering specific diagnostic tests for commonly encountered medical conditions and should be able to interpret the results as well as use them to plan an appropriate treatment program.

Basic studies that should be available to the sports medicine team include blood hemogram and chemistries, urine analysis, coagulation profiles, muscle enzymes and electrocardiograms. More advanced studies may be required in particular instances of individuals with underlying medical problems and who participate in sports. These include cardiovascular studies such as echocardiography and coronary angiography.

Radiologic studies are also part of the basic diagnostic armamentarium that should be available for the sports medicine practitioner. Clinicians who treat athletes should understand the indications and be able to interpret basic as well as advanced imaging studies.

REFERENCES

1 Koester MC, Amudson CL. Pre-participation screening of high school athletes: are recommendations enough? Phys Sports Med 2003; 31:35-38.
2 US Preventive Task Force. Guide to clinical preventive services. 2nd edn. Washington DC: US Department of Health and Human Services Office of Disease Prevention and Health Promotion; 1998.
3 Mellman MF, Podesta L. Common medical problems in sports. Clin Sports Med 1997; 16:635-662.
4 Grafe MW, Paul GR, Foster TE. The pre-participation sports examination for high school and college athletes. Clin Sports Med 1997; 16:569-591.
5 Barrow MW, Clarck KA. Heat-related illness. Am Fam Phys 1998; 58:749-758.
6 Cianca JC, Roberts WO, Horn D. Distance running: Organization of the medical team. In: Connor FG, Wilder RP, Nirschl R, eds. Textbook of running medicine. New York: McGraw-Hill; 2001:489-503.
7 Yeo TP. Heat stroke: a comprehensive review. AACN Clin Issues 2004; 15:280-293.
8 Mellion MB, Shelton GL. Safe exercise in the heat and heat injuries. In: Mellion MB, Walsh WM, Madden C, et al., eds. Team physician's handbook. 3rd edn. Philadelphia: Hanley & Belfus; 2002:133-143.
9 Grogan H, Hopkins PM. Heatstroke implications for critical care and anesthesia. Br J Anaesth 2002; 88:700-707.
10 Halperin JS, Khan K. Environmental injuries. In: O'Connor FG, Wilder RP, Nirschl R, eds. Textbook of running medicine. New York: McGraw-Hill; 2001:405-417.
11 McCullough L, Arora S. Diagnosis and treatment of hypothermia. Am Fam Phys 2004; 70:2325-2332.
12 Mustafa S, Shaikh N, Gowda RM, et al. Electrocardiographic features of hypothermia. Cardiology 2005; 103:118-119.
13 Hipp AA, Heitkamp HC, Rocker K, et al. Hypertrophic cardiomyopathy – sports related aspects of diagnosis, therapy and sports eligibility. Int J Sports Med 2004; 25:641-642.
14 Seto CK. Pre-participation cardiovascular screening. Clin Sports Med 2003; 22:23-25.
15 Maron BJ, Isner JM, McKenna WJ. Recommendations for determining eligibility for competition in athletes with cardiovascular abnormalities. Task Force 3: hypertrophic cardiomyopathy, myocarditis and other myopericardial diseases and mitral valve prolapse. 26th Bethesda Conference. J Am Coll Cardiol 1994; 24:880-885.
16 Magalski GO. The athletes heart. In: Mellion MB, Walsh WM, Madden C, et al., eds. Team physician's handbook. 3rd edn. Philadelphia: Saunders; 2001:265-277.
17 Firoozi S, Sharma S, McKenna J. Risk of competitive sport in young athletes with heart disease. Heart 2003; 89:710-714.
18 Glorioso J Jr, Reeves M. Marfan syndrome: Screening for sudden death in athletes. Curr Sports Med Rep 2002; 1:67-74.
19 Brennan FH Jr, Stenzler B, Oriscello R. Diagnosis and management of myocarditis in athletes. Curr Sports Med Rep 2003; 2:65-71.
20 De Baets F, Bodart E, Dramaix-Wilmet M, et al. Exercise-induced respiratory symptoms are poor predictor of bronchoconstriction. Pediatr Pulmonol 2005; 39:301-335.
21 Storms WW. Asthma associated with exercise. Immunol Allergy Clin North Am 2005; 25:31-43.
22 Hermansen CL, Kirchner JT. Identifying exercise induce bronchospasm: Treatment hinges on distinguishing it from chronic asthma. Postgrad 2004; 115:15-16, 21-25.
23 Kobayashi RH, Kobayashi AD. Exercise-induced bronchospasm, anaphylaxis, and urticaria safe exercise in the heat and heat injuries. In: Mellion MB, Walsh WM, Madden C, et al., eds. Team physician's handbook. 3rd edn. Philadelphia: Saunders; 2001:287-293.
24 Hulzer K, Brunkner P. Screening of athletes for exercise induced bronchoconstriction. Clin J Sport Med 2004;. 14:134-138.
25 Natarajan B, Torres JL, Mellion MB. Gastrointestinal problems safe exercise in the heat and heat injuries. In: Mellion MB, Walsh WM, Madden C, et al., eds. Team physician's handbook. 3rd edn. Philadelphia: Saunders; 2001:244-248.
26 Butchers JD. Runners diarrhea and other intestinal problems of athletes. Am Fam Phys 1993; 48:623-627.
27 McCrory P. Headaches and exercise. Sports Med 2000; 30:221-229.
28 Putukian M. Headaches in athlete safe exercise in the heat and heat injuries. In: Mellion MB, Walsh WM, Madden C, et al., eds. Team physician's handbook. 3rd edn. Philadelphia: Saunders; 2001:299-311.
29 Report of the Quality Standards Subcommittee of the American Academy of Neurology Practice Parameter. The utility of neuroimaging in the evaluation of headache in patients with normal neurologic examinations. Neurology 1994; 44:1353-1354.
30 Saguil A. Evaluation of the patient with muscle weakness. Am Fam Phys 2005; 71:1327-1336.
31 Krivickas LS. Electrodiagnosis in neuromuscular diseases. Phys Med Rehab Clin N Am 1998; 9:83-114.
32 McDonald CM. Clinical approach to the diagnostic evaluation of progressive neuromuscular disease. Phys Med Rehab Clin N Am 1998; 9:9-48.
33 Adams WB. Hematologic concerns in the runner. In: Connor FG, Wilder RP, Nirschl R, eds. Textbook of running medicine. New York: McGraw-Hill; 2001:325-340.
34 Bartsch P, Mairbaurl H, Friedmann B. Pseudoanemia caused by sports. Ther Umsch 1998; 55:251-255.
35 Shaskey DJ, Green GA. Sports haematology. Sports Med 2000; 29:27-38.
36 Chatard JC, Mujika I, Guy C, et al. Anaemia and iron deficiency in athletes. Practical recommendations for treatment. Sports Med 1999; 27:229-240.
37 Smith JA, Martin DT, Telford RD, et al. Greater erythrocyte deformability in word-class endurance athletes. Am J Physiol 1999; 45:2188-2193.
38 Rowland TW. Iron deficiency in the adolescent athlete. In: Bar-Or O, ed. The encyclopaedia of sports medicine an IOC Medical Commission Publication: The child and adolescent athlete. Germany: Blackwell Science; 1996:274-286.
39 Fallon KE. Utility of hematological and iron related screening in elite athletes. Clin J Sport Med 2004; 14:145-152.

40 Kimberley G, Harmon MD. Evaluating and treating exercise-related menstrual irregularities. Phys Sports Med 2002; 30:29–35.

41 Warren MP, Goodman LR. Exercise induced endocrine pathologies. J Endocrinol Invest 2003; 26:873–878.

42 Warren MP, Perlroth NE. The effects of intense exercise on the female reproductive system. J Endocrinol 2001; 170:3–11.

43 Albright A, Franz M, Hornsby G, et al. American College of Sports Medicine position stand: Exercise and type 2 diabetes. Med Sci Sports Exerc 2000; 32:1345–1360.

44 Bhaskarabhatla KV, Birrer R. Physical activity and Type 2 diabetes. Phys Sport Med 2004; 32:13–17.

45 Holmes FC, Hunt JJ, Sevier TL. Renal injury in sport. Curr Sports Med Rep 2003; 2:103–109.

46 Kallmeyer JC, Miller NM. Urinary changes in ultra long distance marathon runners. Nephron 1993; 64:119–121.

47 Jones GR, Newhouse I. Sport-related hematuria: A review. Clin J Sport Med 1997; 7:119–125.

48 Grossfeld GD, Wolf JS, Litwin MS, et al. Asymptomatic microscopic hematuria in adults: Summary of the AUA best practice policy recommendations. Am Fam Phys 2001; 15:6.

49 Gerth J, Ott U, Funfstuck R, et al. The effect of prolonged physical exercise on renal function, electrolytes balance and muscle cell breakdown. Clin Nephrol 2002; 57:425–431.

50 Clerico A, Giammattei C, Cecchini L. Exercise-induced proteinuria in well-trained athletes. Clin Chem 1990; 36:562–564.

51 Tung GA, Brody JM. Contemporary imaging of athletic injuries. Clin Sports Med 1997; 16:393–471.

52 Sanders TG, Fults C. Imaging techniques. Imaging of sports related injuries. In: DeLee JC, Drez D, Miller MD, eds. Orthopaedic sports medicine: principles and practice. Philadelphia: Saunders; 2003:557–596.

53 Lehmann M, Kreitner KF, Kirschner P, et al. Possibilities of computerized arthrotomography in the diagnosis of shoulder instabilities. Unfallchirug 1990; 93:228–231.

54 Hollenberg GM, Beitia AO, Tan RF, et al. Imaging of the spine in sports medicine. Curr Sports Med Rep 2003; 2:33–40.

55 Kaplan PA, Helms CA, Dussault R, et al. Musculoskeletal MRI. Philadelphia: Saunders; 2001.

56 Sanders TG, Miller MD. A systematic approach to magnetic resonance imaging interpretation of sports medicine injuries of the knee. Am J Sports Med 2005; 33:131–148.

57 Miller MD, Osborne JR, Warner JJ, et al. MRI arthroscopy correlative atlas. Philadelphia: Saunders; 1997.

58 Gross GW. Imaging techniques. Differences between the immature and mature skeleton. In: DeLee JC, Drez D, Miller MD, eds. Orthopaedic sports medicine: Principles and practice. Philadelphia: Saunders; 2003:597–614.

59 Bruker P, Bennell K. Stress fractures in female athletes: Diagnosis, management and rehabilitation. Sports Med 1997; 24:410–429.

60 Batt ME, Ugalde V, Anderson MW, et al. A prospective controlled study of diagnostic imaging for acute shin splints. Med Sci Sports Exerc 1998; 30:1564–1571.

61 Mandelbaum BR, Finerman GA, Reicher MA, et al. Magnetic resonance imaging as a tool for evaluation of traumatic knee injuries: anatomical and pathoanatomical correlations. Am J Sports Med 1986; 14:361–370.

62 Reicher MA, Hartzman S, Bassett LW, et al. MRI imaging of the knee. Traumatic Disord Radiol 1987; 162:547–551.

63 Carrino JA, Shweitzer ME. Imaging of sports related knee injuries. Radiol Clin North Am 2002; 40:181–202.

64 McCauley TR. MRI evaluation of the postoperative knee. Radiology 2005; 234:53–61.

65 Rosenthall L, Hill RO, Chuang S. Observation on the use of 99m Tc-phosphate imaging in peripheral bone trauma. Radiology 1976; 119:637–641.

66 Martin P. Bone scanning of trauma and benign conditions. In: Freeman LM, Weissman HS, eds. Nuclear medicine annual. New York: Raven Press; 1982:81–118.

67 Gregory PL, Batt ME, Kerslake RW, et al. Single photon emission computerized tomography and reverse gantry computerized tomography findings in patients with back pain investigated for spondylolysis. Clin J Sport Med 2005; 15:79–86.

68 Sterling JC, Edelstein DW, Calvo RD, et al. Stress fractures in the athlete. Diagnosis and management. Sports Med 1992; 14:336–346.

69 Bauer HC, Persson PE, Nilsson OS. Tears of the medical meniscus associated with increased radionuclide activity of the proximal tibia: Report of three cases. Int Orthop 1989; 13:153–155.

70 Mooar P, Gregg J, Jacobstein J. Radionuclide imaging in internal derangement of the knee. Am J Sports Med 1987; 15:132–137.

71 Dye SF, Chew M, McBride JT, et al. Restoration of osseous homeostasis of the knee following meniscal surgery. Ortho Trans 1992; 16:725.

72 Jacobson JA. Ultrasound in sports medicine. Radiol Clin North Am 2002; 40:363–386.

73 Sofka CM. Ultrasound in sports medicine. Semin Musculoskelet Radiol 2004; 8:17–27.

74 Khan KM, Forster BB, Robinson J, et al. Are ultrasound and magnetic resonance imaging of value in assessment of Achilles tendon disorders? A two year prospective study. J Sports Med 2003; 37:149–153.

CHAPTER 15

Prescribing Medications for Pain and Inflammation

Julio A. Martinez-Silvestrini

PAIN IN SPORTS

Pain is defined as a localized sensation of discomfort, distress or agony, resulting from the stimulation of specialized nerve endings.[1] The stimulation of these nerve endings, known as C fibers and A delta fibers, is caused by tissue damage, which releases a variety of mediators such as histamine, peptides, prostaglandins and serotonin. The resulting impulse from the interaction of these chemicals with the pain fibers is transmitted to the dorsal horn of the spinal cord and via the spinothalamic tract to the ventroposterolateral and posterior thalamus.[2] The final pain perception depends on the balance between exciting and inhibitory effects, which modulate the pain transmission.[3]

The inciting factor for musculoskeletal pain in athletes may be a sports-related injury or delayed onset muscle soreness (DOMS). A sports injury arises from acute macrotrauma, chronic repetitive microtrauma or an acute exacerbation of a chronic injury[4]; the sources of pain may be muscular, vascular, cutaneous, visceral, osseous, ligamentous, neuropathic, or a combination of the above. DOMS is described as muscle tenderness and pain that occur following introduction for the first time to certain types of activities (as eccentric biased muscle contractions) in an athlete's training. Six hypotheses try to explain the mechanisms of DOMS, including muscular lactic acidosis, muscle spasm, connective tissue injury, muscular micro-injury, inflammation and enzyme efflux theories.[5] It is believed that DOMS may affect athletic performance by causing reduction in joint range of motion, shock attenuation and peak torque, as well as by altering the muscle sequencing and recruitment patterns, which may result in increased stress to ligaments and tendons.[5] Multiple treatment strategies have been attempted to alleviate the severity and limit the duration of DOMS, including massage, cryotherapy, stretching, ultrasound, electrical stimulation and medications. While most of these measures have been proven ineffective, massage, exercise and medications may have a role treating DOMS, although they only provide temporary relief.[5] If not controlled, pain may promote compensatory mechanisms affecting the athlete's technique, performance, and potentially promote further injury at the same site or other areas of the kinetic chain. Careful history and examination of the possible pain genera-

tors will help the clinician to determine the possible sources of pain. These sources of pain, as well as the general health status of the athlete, are important considerations for the initiation of medications as a part of the treatment plan.

INFLAMMATION

Kibler[4] categorizes pain as a component of the 'clinical symptom complex' of athletic injuries, while inflammation is part of the anatomic alterations observed, or 'tissue injury complex'. Inflammation is a localized protective response elicited by injury or destruction of tissues, which contributes to the destruction, dilution or sequestration of the injured tissue. An early inflammatory response is the first step of tissue healing, characterized by pain, increased temperature, erythema, swelling and loss of function.[1] After an acute injury, a cascade of events, including hematoma formation, inflammatory cell reaction and tissue necrosis will be elicited.[6] Increased dilation of arterioles, capillaries and venules will follow, resulting in increased permeability, blood flow, exudation of fluids and plasmatic proteins, as well as hormonal responses and leukocyte (neutrophils, monocytes) and fibroblasts migration.[6,7] All these events contribute to the classical signs of inflammation (Table 15.1). Coupled with pain, the inflammatory response limits the use of the injured structure, thereby avoiding the possibility of further injury to the affected tissue.

The inflammatory response phase is followed by regeneration of the injured tissue (reparative phase), and scar formation, remodeling and maturation (remodeling phase). Excessive hematoma formation or inflammatory response may interfere with adequate tissue regeneration or scar formation, promoting poor quality healing or a 'failed healing response', which is one of the theories for recurrent musculoskeletal injuries, such as tendinopathies.[8]

SELECTION OF MEDICATIONS

Control of pain and inflammation, as well as tissue healing promotion, are the goals of the initial or acute phase of rehabilitation.[4] Medications, splinting, modalities, and in some

Table 15.1   Classical Signs of Inflammation

Latin Term	English Translation
Dolor	Pain
Calor	Heat
Rubor	Redness
Tumor	Edema
Functio Laesa	Loss of function

cases surgical management, are important treatment components during this phase. But the decision regarding which medication to recommend for an individual patient is not an easy task. The necessity of the drug, its side-effects, and its potential to be banned by a sports governing organization, should be considered prior to the prescription of any agent.[9]

In most cases, there are no clear guidelines to assist in the selection of the most appropriate agent, but one of the considerations should be compliance. Medication compliance improves dramatically as prescribed dose frequency decreases. Compliance may be as low as 59% of daily dosages on a three times a day regimen, and improves to 83.6% on a once a day regimen.[10] More recently, Claxton,[11] in his systematic review on associations between doses and compliance recommends simpler, less frequent dosing regimens, which result in better compliance. Low medication compliance has been associated with lack of motivation,[12] significant side-effects, complexity and organization of the treatment regimen (including daily multiple doses or multiple agents), cost and low perceived benefits.

Box 15.1: Key Points

Factors affecting medication compliance

- Presence and severity of symptoms
- Number of medications
- Side-effects
- Dosing frequency
- Length of treatment
- Motivation for treatment
- Costs

PAIN LADDER

As described by Leadbetter,[13] 'If pain and signs of inflammation are persistent, repeated efforts to turn off the body's alarm is not a substitute for finding the cause of the fire. Indeed to remove the "fire alarm" of pain from the onset of an injury can clearly place the athlete in great jeopardy with respect to tissue overload and failure'. It is important to control pain and inflammation with either physical or pharmacologic measures, but these interventions are not a substitute for proper medical care and rehabilitation. The World Health Organization

(WHO) designed a three-step 'ladder' for pain relief in cancer patients (Fig. 15.1).[14] This 'pain ladder' has been used more recently with success for non-malignant and musculoskeletal-related pain,[15] as well as in the pediatric population.[16] It may be appropriate to use as a tool for initial selection of medications in the athletic population, as well as to guide pharmacotherapeutic regimen changes, if needed. The administration of medications to control pain consists of scheduled, 'by the clock' rather than 'as needed' or 'on demand' doses. The clinician needs to know the pain severity experienced by the patient, prior to selecting which 'pain ladder' step to start the treatment plan. Pain is considered to be mild when rated between 1 and 4 on the visual analog scale, moderate when rated 5 or 6 and severe when described as 7 to 10.

The first step of the ladder is the use of non-opioid medications, such as non-steroidal anti-inflammatories, acetaminophen or aspirin, for the treatment of patients with pain of mild to moderate intensity. Patients with persistent mild to moderate pain despite the use of first step medications benefit from adding a second step drug, such as codeine, hydrocodone or oxycodone.[17] Tramadol has been considered a possible alternative as a second step drug.[18] The third step medications, which include morphine, hydromorphone, fentanyl and high doses of oxycodone, are reserved for patients with moderate to severe pain refractory to step 2 medications or that cannot take oral medications, as in patients with acute severe trauma, in which intramuscular or intravenous administration may be more appropriate. This pharmacotherapeutic regimen is considered to be relatively inexpensive and 80–90% effective.[17] Adjuvant agents, such as anticonvulsants or antidepressants, are recommended to treat concurrent symptoms that exacerbate pain and may also enhance the effect of the primary steps medication. These adjuvant agents may be used in any of the steps of the 'pain ladder' (Fig. 15.1).

When implementing the use of this tool, it is important to emphasize that pain perceptions in athletes seem to be decreased, compared to non-exercising subjects. Although

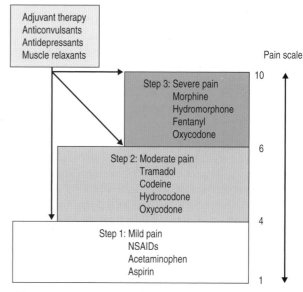

Figure 15.1   Analgesic pain ladder. (Modified from WHO 1990.[14])

most research studies confirm this observation, the reason for this is unknown. Multiple theories had been postulated for decreased pain perception in athletes, including the presence of high levels of endogenous opiates, such as beta-endorphin and beta-lipotropin, in response to training and acute exercise, stress induced growth hormone, catecholamine and corticosteroid release,[19] the presence of a baseline higher pain threshold which increases even more after physical activity,[20] motivational factors,[21] and enhanced pain tolerance.[22] Besides pain perception, other factors that may influence pain management in athletes is their initiative to seek medical care. Staes observed that although 17.8% of adolescents with back pain reduced or stopped their sports activities and 13.1% reported that their pain intensity was high enough to seek medical attention, only 8.5% received medical consultation or treatment.[23] Reduction of sports participation or medical interventions were observed in subjects with statistically significant higher pain levels (5.5–6/10) compared with their peers (3–5.5/10).

MEDICATIONS

Non-steroidal antiinflammatory drugs

The group of drugs known as non-steroidal anti-inflammatories (NSAIDs) is one of the most commonly used classes of medications worldwide. It is estimated that 30 million people take NSAIDs daily,[24] and there are 20–24 million NSAIDs prescriptions written in the UK each year.[25] NSAIDs are known for their anti-inflammatory, antipyretic and analgesic effects.[26] These effects are mediated by inhibition of the cyclooxygenase enzyme (COX), which results in decreased prostaglandin production (Fig. 15.2).[27] Prostaglandins promote the initial inflammatory response and sensitize nerves by increasing the nervous membrane permeability to sodium and calcium. The antipyretic

effect of NSAIDs is mediated through vasodilation of peripheral vessels, enhancing heat dissipation. Older NSAIDs and salicylates are believed to inhibit both COX-1 and COX-2. COX-1 is a constitutive enzyme which has a role in the regulation of the gastric mucosa, vascular homeostasis, renal function and platelet aggregation.[28] COX-2 is an inducible enzyme, also present in brain, kidney and bone in small amounts, but the expression increases during inflammation. In theory, selective inhibition of COX-2 will inhibit the inflammatory effects of prostaglandins, with minimal adverse effects.

NSAIDs also have an inherent capacity to inhibit a number of cellular processes. These include disruption of protein to protein interactions, decreased neutrophil endothelial adherence, reduction of superoxide generation, uncoupling of oxidative phosphorylation, inhibition of phospholipase C activity and reduction of glycosaminoglycan synthesis.[26] They may also have a role on attenuation of muscle protein synthesis after 24 h of high-intensity eccentric resistance exercise.[29] NSAID use for brief periods of time has shown to be beneficial for short-term recovery of muscle function after exercise-induced muscle injuries.[30]

There are no guidelines to assist in selecting the most appropriate NSAID. Selection should be based on the athlete's previous experience and convenience, clinical experience, side-effects and costs. Knowing the NSAIDs used by the patient in the past, as well as their perceived benefits and adverse effects, may help the clinician in the selection process. Once a patient has failed to respond to one NSAID, some investigators have found that the likelihood of benefiting from another agent in the class is low.[31] However, although NSAIDs share the same basic mode of action, there is evidence suggesting that in equipotent doses, individual responses are highly variable.[32] These differences may be secondary not only to compliance, but to several functional, biochemical and physiological indicators,[33] including enantiomeric forms, protein binding capacity, half-lives, synovial fluid kinetics, metabolism, chronobiology, adverse effect profile and other drug interactions.[32] Thus it may be a reasonable therapeutic option[34] to substitute one NSAID for another of a different class in patients with refractory pain (Table 15.2).

When prescribing NSAIDs, the clinician needs to consider the potential of drug interactions or current over-the-counter NSAID use. Mahler[35] observed that 5–10% of endurance athletes use NSAIDs prior to athletic event participation. As some athletes may not perceive over-the-counter drugs as medications, it is important to ask the athlete about current medication or supplement use. Other considerations should include the age of the athlete, as only four NSAIDs have been approved by the United States Food and Drug Administration (FDA) for use in children. These include aspirin, ibuprofen, naproxen and tolmetin. However, recommended doses, efficacy and toxicity for non-FDA approved NSAIDs, are available.[34] Also one needs to take in consideration the drug compliance when prescribing a NSAID. To promote better compliance and adherence to the treatment regimen, once- or twice-a-day drugs are recommended (Table 15.3).

The use of NSAIDs in patients with chronic tendon injuries or tendinosis may be considered inappropriate by some clinicians, since inflammation has not been observed in pathologic

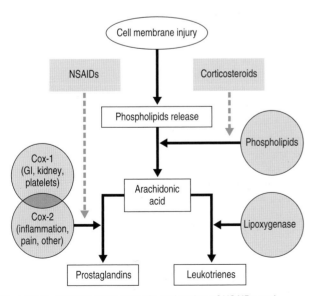

Figure 15.2 Inflammatory cascade and action of NSAIDs and corticosteroids. Cellular membrane injury will promote the release of phospholipids. By influence of phospholipase, phospholipids will convert into arachidonic acid which in turn converts to prostaglandins or leukotrienes mediated by cyclooxygenase or lipoxygenase, respectively.

Table 15.2   Non-Steroidal Anti-Inflammatory Drug Classes

Class	Drug	Daily Maximal Dosage (mg)
Acetic acids	Diclofenac	150
	Etodolac	1200
	Indomethacin	200
	Sulindac	600
	Tolmetin	2400
Carboxylic acids	Aspirin	6000
	Diflunisal	1500
	Salsalate	3000
	Trisalicylate	3000
COX-2 inhibitors	Celecoxib	400
	Etoricoxib[a]	
	Lumiraxcoxib[a]	
	Parecoxib[a]	
	Rofecoxib[b]	50
	Valdecoxib[c]	20
Enolic acids	Meloxicam	30
	Piroxicam	20
	Phenylbutazone	600
Fenamates	Meclofenamate	400
	Mefenamic acid	1000
Naphthylamines	Nabumetone	1500
Propionic acids	Fenoprofen	2400
	Flurbiprofen	300
	Ibuprofen	3200
	Ketoprofen	225
	Naproxen	1000
	Oxaprozin	1200

[a]Not available in the US. [b]Removed from US market due to increased risks of cardiovascular and cerebrovascular events. [c]Removed from US market due to increased risks of cardiovascular and serious skin reactions.

studies.[8] Nevertheless, most studies showed improved pain scores at final follow-up in patients with chronic tendon injuries who have used NSAIDs. In an animal study, Virchenko[36] observed that NSAIDs may have a detrimental effect during early surgical tendon repairs, if used in the first 5 days after tendon injury. However, if used after 5 days, NSAIDs seems to promote a more efficient healing response,

Table 15.3   Non-Steroidal Anti-Inflammatories: Frequency of Dosage

Once a Day[a]	Twice a Day	Three Times a Day
Celecoxib	Diclofenac	Ibuprofen
Ketoprofen	Etodolac	Indomethacin
Meloxicam	Fenoprofen	Meclofenamate
Nabumetone	Flurbiprofen	Phenylbutazone
Oxaprozin	Naproxen[b]	Tolmetin
Valdecoxib	Sulindac	Carboxylic acids

[a]Most of them may be given twice a day. [b]Available as a once a day preparation.

decreasing the cross-sectional area of the tendon and increasing the maximum stress tolerance capacity. This supports the concept that uncontrolled inflammatory response may interfere with the normal reparative phase of the normal healing response. As long-term prospective studies in patients with tendon injuries are not available, it remains to be determined whether NSAIDs change the natural history of the injury or merely have some analgesic action in these injuries.

Other NSAID subclasses
Salicylates

Aspirin (acetylsalicylic acid) and other salicylates are usually defined as NSAIDs, as their mechanism of action includes COX inhibition. The biotransformation of aspirin yields salicylate, which has similar anti-inflammatory potency as aspirin, but lacks its inhibitory effect on the COX enzyme. At present there is no common agreement about the anti-inflammatory mechanism of action of salicylates, independent from COX inhibition or expression. The postulated mechanisms include activation of mitogen-activated protein kinases, inhibition of nuclear transcription factors, antioxidant properties, adenosine release and lipoxin formation.[37]

Peripherally acting NSAIDs

Bromfenac and ketorolac tromethamine are peripherally acting NSAIDs indicated for short-term management of moderate to severe pain, requiring analgesia at the opiate level. The use of these drugs is limited to up to 5 days in adults. These drugs may potentially be used in the treatment of acute musculoskeletal injuries although no studies are available for this indication.[26]

COX-2 inhibitors (Coxibs)

COX-2 selective inhibitors were introduced to the market as a possible alternative for patients unable to take conventional NSAIDs secondary to their GI adverse effects. But recently, this class of drugs has come under intense scrutiny owing to reported increased risk of cardiovascular and cerebrovascular events.[38,39]

The heightened risk of these serious adverse effects may relate to the ability of these drugs to suppress prostaglandin I_2.[38] Suppression of prostaglandin I_2 formation might be expected to elevate blood pressure, accelerate atherogenesis and predispose patients to an exaggerated thrombotic response to the rupture of an atherosclerotic plaque.[39] In 2003, Fowles recommended the addition of aspirin for patients with cardiovascular risk who are prescribed a COX-2 selective inhibitor; aspirin's inhibition of COX-1 leads to decreased platelet aggregation and vasoconstriction.[40] Given the current controversy around COX-2 inhibitors, most now advocate the use of nonselective NSAIDs, which are more cost effective. COX-2 inhibitors may be considered in patients with a low risk of cardiovascular or cerebrovascular events.

Adverse effects

One of the limitations of the use of NSAIDs is their analgesic ceiling effect. Doses above a certain level produce no additional analgesia but may incur additional toxicity. It is important to emphasize that for some NSAIDs, the analgesic ceiling effect is significantly lower than the anti-inflammatory ceiling dosage.[27] In athletes with pain and minimal or no inflammation, lower doses of NSAIDs may be used, limiting the potential of adverse effects. The maximal daily doses of the most commonly used NSAIDs are listed in Table 15.2. The NSAIDs cause considerable morbidity and mortality related to gastrointestinal adverse effects, and may contribute to 2600 deaths annually.[41] Proton pump inhibitors (PPI), hydrogen receptor (H_2) blockers and Misoprostol,[42] a prostaglandin E_1 analog, has shown to be effective in preventing NSAID induced gastrointestinal ulcerations and dyspepsia. PPI have been useful for gastric ulceration,[43] while H_2 blockers have been effective in duodenal ulcers.[44] The selective COX-2 inhibitors (Table 15.2), inhibit 200–300 times the COX-2 isoform over COX-1. They may have fewer gastrointestinal adverse effects, with a risk of gastrointestinal bleeding lower, but similar to the use of a combination of nonselective NSAIDs and omeprazole.[45] This protective effect may be eliminated with the concomitant use of low dose aspirin[46] or corticosteroids. Although dyspepsia and other gastrointestinal adverse effects are notoriously attributed to NSAIDs, less than 3% of patients treated with ibuprofen will develop gastrointestinal symptoms.[27]

Box 15.2: Key Points

Non-steroidal anti-inflammatories
- Most commonly used pain analgesic
- Have anti-inflammatory, antipyretic and analgesic effects
- Multiple classes available
- Have analgesic ceiling effect
- Hepatic and liver function should be followed closely
- Most common adverse effect: GI toxicity.

Other adverse effects of NSAIDs include renal toxicity, dehydration, electrolyte disturbances, hepatic injury, skin reactions, elevated cardiovascular and cerebrovascular events risk[38,47] and drug-induced aseptic meningitis. They may be relatively contraindicated in patients with platelet dysfunction, bleeding disorders, renal or hepatic insufficiency. Also, this group of medications should be used carefully in patients with allergy to aspirin, while celecoxib and valdecoxib should not be used in patients allergic to sulfa drugs.

Acetaminophen

The medication acetaminophen, also known as N-acetyl-P-aminophenol (APAP), is indicated for the treatment of mild to moderate pain. Although also an antipyretic drug, APAP does not have anti-inflammatory effects. APAP should be considered as the first line of treatment for athletes allergic to aspirin or NSAIDs, or when inflammation is not a pre-

dominant component of the 'tissue injury complex'. The mechanism of action of APAP is poorly defined, but it is believed to interrupt prostaglandin synthesis within the central nervous system (CNS), with minimal effect in the peripheral tissue, which may explain its analgesic and antipyretic effects, as well as the absence of peripheral antiinflammatory action. The recommended adult dosage is 325–650 mg every four to six hours or up to 1000 mg four times a day. One gram of APAP is considered the analgesic ceiling dosage. In children younger than 12 years old, the recommended dose is 10–15 mg/kg per dose, without exceeding 2.6 g in 24 h. APAP may be delivered orally or rectally with an onset of action of less than 1 h. If needed, APAP may be used in combination with other agents, as NSAIDs or opiates, for a synergistic analgesic action.

Box 15.3: Key Points

Acetaminophen
- Available in combination with other pain medications (opiates, tramadol)
- Analgesic and antipyretic effects
- Has analgesic ceiling effect
- May cause severe hepatic dysfunction in acute or chronic overdosage.

Adverse effects

APAP is mainly metabolized by the liver to sulfate and glucuronide metabolites, while approximately 5% is metabolized by the cytochrome P-450 system to N-acetyl-p-benzoquinone, which is conjugated to glutathione, inactivated and excreted by the kidneys.[48] Hepatotoxicity may occur with doses of >4 g a day or acute overdosage. In these settings, glutathione conjugation becomes insufficient, resulting in the accumulation of acetylimidoquinone, a metabolite of acetaminophen, which may cause hepatic cell necrosis. The used of ethanol or other medications metabolized by the liver should be limited while using this drug. APAP is also present in combination with other medications and is available without prescription, increasing the potential risk of concomitant use of agents containing acetaminophen and increasing the risk of overdose. Other adverse effects observed include rash, electrolyte disturbances, anemia, blood dyscrasias and nephrotoxicity. Hypersensitivity reactions are rare.

Opiates

Since its discovery, morphine has been considered the gold standard for pain control. Currently, multiple opiate derivatives are available (Table 15.4). They are classified as agonists, mixed agonist-antagonists, or partial agonists, based upon their activity at opiate μ- and/or κ-receptors.[27] But due to their high potency and risk of physical dependence, potential for abuse and significant side-effects, the use of opiates should be limited to

Table 15.4   Opiates, Time to Onset and Equivalent Doses

Drug	Oral Onset (min)	Oral: Equivalency between Opiates (μg)[a]
Codeine	10–30	200
Hydromorphone	15–30	7.5
Levorphanol	30–90	4
Meperidine	10–45	300
Methadone	30–60	20
Morphine sulfate	15–60	30
Oxycodone	15–30	30
Propoxyphene	30–60	200

[a]Oral equivalency between opiates. The doses on this column are equivalent doses between opiates. For example, 200 mg codeine is equivalent to approximately 7.5 mg hydromorphone.

Table 15.5   Opioids Banned by the World Anti-Doping Agency

Buprenorphine
Dextromoramide
Heroin
Fentanyl and derivatives
Hydromorphone
Methadone
Morphine
Oxycodone
Oxymorphone
Pentazocine
Pethidine

athletes with moderate to severe pain levels, and for short periods of time, until the primary treatment of the injury is completed and the pain has diminished. A large number of commercial compounded analgesics are available, combining an opiate (such as hydrocodone, oxycodone or codeine) with acetaminophen or ibuprofen. These preparations are prescribed frequently for the management of acute or chronic pain. For example, hydrocodone combined with acetaminophen is the most common of the compounded analgesics prescribed for acute pain management in the US.[27] When prescribing these combination products, the clinician must pay particular attention to the amount of acetaminophen or ibuprofen in these preparations, when used separately, to avoid surpassing the ceiling dosage. The primary objective while using opiates is to achieve an acceptable balance between analgesia and adverse effects. Specifically, in opioid-naive patients, short acting, low potency agents should be started and advanced gradually. It is recommended prescribing stool softeners and antiemetics to minimize adverse effects that may jeopardize compliance. In athletes with a history of severe chronic pain, as in other patients with chronic pain, the optimal maintenance regimen will be focused in long-acting opiates, with short acting agents utilized for breakthrough pain. One of the virtues of opioid use for pain management is the absence of maximal dosage, which permits the dose to be increased until relief is obtained or limiting side-effects develop.[27]

Relative contraindications for opiate prescriptions include a history of substance abuse or substance abusers in the patient's household, psychiatric illnesses, non-compliance with treatment regimen and borderline or antisocial personality disorders. Healthy subjects demonstrated decrements in reaction time and task tracking in simple hand–eye coordination.[49] These decrements in function may adversely affect athletic performance.

Other considerations

The World Anti-doping Agency prohibits the use of multiple narcotics (Table 15.5).[50] The use of these substances may result in fines and suspension of the athlete, coach, clinicians and/or team. Prior to use or prescription of these substances, or participation in competition while using these prohibited substances, communication with the appropriate anti-doping organization is strongly recommended.

Box 15.4: Key Points

Opiates

- Gold standard for pain control
- Limited use in sports injuries
- Indicated for moderate to severe pain control
- Prohibited by the World Anti-doping Agency.

Tramadol

Tramadol is a central analgesic with binary action, indicated for moderate to severe pain. This agent acts as a weak opioid μ-receptor agonist, as well as a re-uptake inhibitor of norepinephrine and serotonin. It is considered to be more appropriate than NSAIDs for patients with gastrointestinal or renal disease. The analgesic property of tramadol is greater than that of NSAIDs and weak opiates, such as codeine and dextropropoxyphene. Tramadol is also considered to have fewer side-effects compared with opiates.[51] Tramadol has been used alone and in conjunction with NSAIDs in the management of musculoskeletal pain, including back pain and breakthrough pain.[18] The combination of tramadol and NSAIDs is synergistic, producing central analgesia and peripheral prostaglandin synthesis inhibition. A recent report[52] concluded that tramadol is an effective treatment for the management of neuropathic pain. It can also be used in combination with acetaminophen, with a more rapid onset of action and greater efficacy than tramadol alone, without an apparent increase in adverse effects.[53] Tramadol and acetaminophen compounded tablets are available and provide similar onset of action and pain relief when compared with codeine and acetaminophen combined capsules. Although a compounded combination of acetaminophen and tramadol may be practical and convenient, the increased cost of this preparation compared with single agent tramadol and acetaminophen tablets may be an obstacle for some patients. Dosage recommendations are 50–100 mg every 4–6 h, without exceeding 400 mg/day. Tramadol is metabolized by the liver, via demethylation, glucuronidation and sulfation;

however, this is one of the few medications that can be used in patients with hepatic impairment, with a recommended dose of 50 mg every 12 h.

Adverse effects
Adverse effects include dizziness, coordination impairment and somnolence. Tramadol should be used carefully in patients using other medications that may cause somnolence. Constipation, nausea, agitation, anxiety, rash, abdominal pain and dry mouth may also be observed. Slow dose escalation (25–50 mg every 6–8 h) may improve the tolerability and decrease the onset of adverse effects. Allergic reactions are rare. This medication may decrease the seizure threshold in patients requiring dosages higher than 400 mg daily or with concomitant use of antidepressant drugs (tricyclic antidepressants or selective serotonin reuptake inhibitors) or amphetamines. Tramadol should be used carefully in athletes with a history of seizure disorder or in those requiring antidepressants.

Box 15.5: Key Points

Tramadol

- Central analgesic with bimodal action
- May be used in athletes with renal or liver insufficiency
- May cause somnolence
- Decreases the seizure threshold.

Anticonvulsants
Evidence from neuropathic pain animal models suggests that many pathophysiologic and biochemical changes occur in the peripheral nerve and central nervous system, which have similarities with seizure activity models. This evidence justifies the use of anticonvulsants in the symptomatic management of neuropathic pain, trigeminal neuralgia, diabetic neuropathy, postherpetic neuralgia, HIV neuropathy, central or thalamic pain syndrome and complex regional pain syndrome.[54] Anticonvulsants may also be useful as prophylactic agents in athletes with migraine headaches. The mechanisms of action of anticonvulsants include effects on the voltage-gated sodium and calcium channels and inhibition promotion by affecting the gamma-aminobutyric acid (GABA)-A receptors.[55] There is no role for anticonvulsant use in musculoskeletal disorders, unless associated neuropathic pain or injury is present. These medications may take several days to weeks to have a beneficial effect. For instance, the use of concomitant fast-acting agents, such as APAP, tramadol or NSAIDs, is recommended. The effectiveness of anticonvulsants correlates with their serum levels. In addition, older agents, such as carbamazepine or phenytoin, have a narrow therapeutic serum level range, thus requiring close monitoring. Rapid dose escalation may increase the serum levels of these drugs, but may result in more adverse effects or toxic levels. Newer anticonvulsants (such as lamotrigine, gabapentin, topiramate and zonisamide) appear to

have better tolerability and drug interaction profile;[56] with these agents, monitoring serum levels is not necessary.

Box 15.6: Key Points

Anticonvulsants

- Multiple drugs available
- Indicated for neuropathic pain
- Neuropathic pain use may be an off-label use for certain drugs
- Newer drugs do not need serologic monitoring.

Carbamazepine
Phenytoin and carbamazepine are medications widely and commonly used in the treatment of seizure disorders. In contrast to phenytoin, in which the evidence supporting its use in neuropathic pain is conflicting,[54] the efficacy of carbamazepine for pain syndromes is widely known. The medical literature supports the use of carbamazepine in patients with trigeminal neuralgia, diabetic neuropathy, postherpetic neuralgia, central pain and chronic pain.[54,57] Dosages used for these pain syndromes range from 300 to 1000 mg/day. Multiple mechanisms of action for analgesia have been postulated including a reduction of sodium and potassium conductance, neuron activity inhibition, upregulation of GABA receptors, reduction of N-methyl-D-aspartate induced depolarization at lower concentrations, potentiation of opioid induced behaviors and antidepressant effects.[57]

Adverse effects
The most common adverse effects include dizziness, nausea and vomiting, which usually subside 1 week after starting treatment or with dose reductions. Bone marrow suppression occurs rarely, but may be serious. Severe dermatologic reactions may also be observed rarely, requiring discontinuation of therapy. Hepatic and renal toxicity have also been reported. Consequently, complete blood counts, hepatic and renal function tests should be done prior to treatment, followed by repeated tests, including carbamazepine levels, at regular intervals. As the chemical conformation of this drug is similar to tricyclic antidepressants, this drug should be used with caution in patients with adverse reactions to tricyclics.

Gabapentin
Gabapentin is approved by the Food and Drug Administration of the United States as an adjunct treatment for seizure disorders, postherpetic neuralgia and bipolar disorders, although popular off label uses with significant literature supporting them include migraine prophylaxis and neuropathic pain. Efficacy in the pediatric population has been suggested, with case series describing the drug utility in athletes with complex regional pain syndrome[58] and patients with phantom limb pain.[59] Gabapentin was designed as a GABA agonist, but its mechanism of action for pain control is postulated to result from its effect as a ligand at the alpha 2 delta subunits of

voltage-related calcium channels.[60] The dosage range for treatment of neuropathic pain is 900–3600 mg daily, administered in three divided doses. Gabapentin needs to be adjusted in patients with renal impairment, but may be used in patients on hemodialysis. Adverse effects include somnolence, edema, depression, nervousness, nausea and weight gain.

Lamotrigine

As a phenyltriazine derivative, lamotrigine blocks voltage-gated sodium channels and inhibits glutamate release. This drug has been used in the treatment of trigeminal neuralgia, HIV associated painful neuropathy, central post-stroke pain and a variety of neuropathic pain conditions. In doses from 50 to 400 mg/day, lamotrigine has demonstrated efficacy in relieving pain in patients with some types of neuropathic and central pain,[54] but has adverse effects which include dizziness, ataxia, constipation, nausea and somnolence, which can be a limiting factor in the use of this drug.

Topiramate

This drug was first licensed in the UK in 1995 for adjunctive treatment of patients with intractable partial seizures. There are preliminary data to support its role as a potential treatment for neuropathic pain, while there are at least three ongoing international placebo-controlled multi-centered trials. The postulated modes of action of topiramate include modulation of voltage-gated sodium and calcium ion channels, potentiation of GABA inhibition, blockage of excitatory glutamate neurotransmission and inhibition of carbonic acid anhydrase. Most of the information about the pharmacology of topiramate is collected from studying hippocampal preparations, but may be useful to understand the molecular behavior of this drug on the peripheral nerves. Studies for the treatment of neuropathic pain in patients with diabetic neuropathy, trigeminal neuralgia, intercostal neuralgia and other neuropathic pain syndromes, including complex regional pain syndrome and other peripheral neuropathies are available. The use of this drug for neuropathic pain management is a not approved by the Food and Drug Administration of the United States.[61]

Zonisamide

Zonisamide is believed to block the sodium and T type calcium channels and to increase GABA release. In a 10-week open label study involving subjects with diabetic neuropathy, peripheral neuropathy, complex regional pain syndrome, postlaminectomy syndrome, and radiculopathies zonisamide recipients showed marginally improved pain scores: Mean Neuropathic Pain and Mean Investigator Global Assessment scores.[54]

Antidepressants

The effects of the antidepressants occur at the level of the nerve synapse. They modulate pain by altering the magnitude of the effects of neurotransmitters at these synapses,[62] either by blockage of neurotransmitter uptake, or by blocking certain receptors.

Tricyclic antidepressants (TCA)

TCA are used as the first line of adjuvant therapy for neuropathic pain and may also improve underlying depression and insomnia. The mechanism of action is the reuptake of norepinephrine and serotonin at nerve endings. Amitriptyline has been the most widely used drug of this type, but it has dose limiting sedating and anticholinergic adverse effects. Nortriptyline and desipramine may cause fewer of these adverse effects, facilitating upward titration. Low doses of any of these drugs (10–25 mg) should be administered at night and titrated upward every few days as needed, while monitoring pain relief and adverse effects. Night administration may help to normalize the sleep pattern, due to the sedative properties of this drug class. In healthy young patients, starting with 25 mg daily may facilitate the titration with good tolerability. Usually the dose for clinical response in patients with neuropathic pain is lower than the needed to treat depression. Tricyclic antidepressants should be used with caution in patients with glaucoma, urinary retention or cardiac disease.

Selective serotonin reuptake inhibitors (SSRI)

The antidepressants known as SSRI have been used commonly in patients with the classic presentation of pain and dysthymic or depressive disorders. The mechanism of action of the SSRI consist of elevation of serotonin in the neuron synapse, followed by desensitization and down regulation of serotonergic, somatodendritic and presynaptic inhibitory autoreceptors, increasing both synthesis and release of serotonin.[62]

Nemoto and colleagues[63] studied the regional cerebral blood flow and subjective pain and hot sensation during laser evoked pain and heat sensation before and after administration of fluvoxamine for 7 days. They concluded that fluvoxamine reduces activation of multiple brain areas and subjective pain scores in comparison with placebo, with no significant change in the sensory threshold, suggesting a possible mechanism of action for SSRI in pain modulation.

Other agents
Muscle relaxants

The medications known as muscle relaxants or relaxers have been used frequently for patients with muscular type pain, although their use is somewhat controversial. This group of drugs is very heterogeneous if we take into consideration their mechanisms of action, which range from centrally acting agents to calcium ion release blockage at the sarcoplasmic reticulum level (Table 15.6). The muscle relaxants as a class, seem to be effective in both acute and chronic neck and back pain.[5] Although the mechanism of actions of each of these agents is different, no significant differences in outcomes were found between agents when comparing them in the treatment of musculoskeletal disorders. They are used with the goal of reducing muscular tension or stiffness and the resulting pain associated with injury. The muscle relaxants are also believed to control hypertonicity and promote muscle relaxation. These medications may be used safely in combination with NSAIDs and APAP. The most common adverse effects of this drug class include anticholinergic effects, weakness, drowsiness or dizziness, as well as a risk of dependence even after 1 week of use.[5]

Table 15.6   Mechanism of Action of Muscle Relaxants

Muscle Relaxant	Mechanism of Action
Baclofen	Presynaptic inhibition by GABA β-receptor activation
Carisoprodol	Blocks interneural activity at descending reticular formation and spinal cord
Cyclobenzaprine	Central acting agent; reduction of tonic somatic motor activity
Dantrolene	Blocks release of calcium from sarcoplasmic reticulum
Diazepam	Central acting agent; facilitates post synaptic effects of GABA
Metaxalone	Unknown; possibly CNS depression
Methocarbamol	Central acting agent
Orphenadrine	Unknown
Tizanidine	Alpha 2 agonist

These medications should be used with caution in patients using other medications that may cause sedation, such as tramadol or opiates, and while operating motor vehicles or participating in activities requiring fast responses, such as combat sports. Muscle relaxers do not have a defined role in the WHO 'pain ladder', but may be used as adjuvant therapy, if needed (Fig. 15.1).

Box 15.7: Key Points

Muscle relaxants

- Heterogeneous drug class
- Multiple modes of action
- May cause somnolence.

Do muscle relaxants interfere with sports performance?

Although in theory, the sedation caused by these agents may negatively affect sports performance, no data was found confirming this hypothesis. Nevertheless, there is a reported case of post-triathlon delirium in an athlete taking muscle relaxers (cyclobenzaprine and benzodiazepines), cocaine, barbiturates and marijuana.[64] Muscle relaxer classes should not be combined, unless: (1) the agents are considered necessary for treatment, (2) optimal trials have been attempted unsuccessfully (maximal dosages and adequate frequency, for reasonable time periods, e.g. 2–4 weeks), (3) Patients need to have close medical monitoring, (4) Adverse effect potentiation and drug interactions need to be monitored and avoided. One group of athletes that may benefit from multiple muscle relaxer agents are patients with upper motor neuron syndromes, as spinal cord injury or brain injured athletes.

Glucosamine and chondroitin

Glucosamine and chondroitin are natural compounds found in healthy cartilage, which lately have been used and studied frequently in both human and veterinary medicine. They are extracted from animal products and have been used in Europe for more than a decade. Because of their safety, these remedies would have great appeal for the treatment of primary osseous musculoskeletal conditions, such as osteoarthritis, even if they were only modestly effective.[65] These supplements are used in an attempt to modulate the glycosaminoglycan and proteoglycan constituents of the articular cartilage. Although more than 500 studies have been done with these supplements, most of them contain design flaws. Trials of glucosamine and chondroitin preparations collectively demonstrate moderate to large treatment effects on symptoms, but detailed methodological analysis suggests that the actual efficacy of these products is likely to be substantially more modest.[65]

Both supplements appear to be similar in effectiveness and have a minimum onset of action of 2 weeks,[66] while the full therapeutic benefit may take longer than 1 month.[65] Although the role of glucosamine or chondroitin as analgesics is not completely known, as most studies allowed NSAID rescue doses, the combination of any of these supplements with NSAIDs have been observed to be superior to NSAIDs alone. However, considering the low dose of the rescue medications utilized, it is unlikely that rescue medication use affected the pain relieving effect of these two supplements.[66] Regarding the use of combined glucosamine and chondroitin preparations, no studies were found that compared the combination of both supplements *versus* glucosamine or chondroitin alone. Numerous studies using combination therapy have been reported, with similar results to those that used glucosamine or chondroitin alone. For this reason, the National Institute of Health in the United States has initiated an ongoing, four arms, multi-year study to compare glucosamine and chondroitin in combination with both agents alone and with placebo in the treatment of knee osteoarthritis.

Box 15.8: Key Points

Glucosamine and chondroitin

- Natural component of cartilage
- May decrease pain and prevent progression of osteoarthritis
- Minimal adverse effects.

Glucosamine and chondroitin are considered dietary supplements in the US and their use is regulated by the Dietary Supplement Health Education Act, rather than by the United States Food and Drug Administration Regulation. In Europe, however, they are licensed as pharmaceuticals. Dietary supplements are not required to meet the same standards of purity and labeling as other prescription medications or over-the-counter drugs.[67] When recommending any dietary supplement to patients, the clinician should take into account the purity of the ingredients, reputation of the manufacturer and the molecular weight of glucosamine and/or chondroitin supplied.[67] No major adverse effects and drug interactions had been observed with these supplements.

Glucosamine sulfate

Glucosamine sulfate is a normal component of glycosaminoglycans in the cartilage matrix and synovial fluid. This salt may have a role in slowing cartilage breakdown. The mechanisms of action for glucosamine include maintaining elasticity, strength and resilience of the cartilage, the inhibition of proteolytic enzymes (elastase, hyaluronidase) and promotion of glycosaminoglycan and proteoglycan synthesis. Other mechanisms of action include mRNA transcriptional effects, anti-inflammatory, immunosuppressive and anticatabolic properties.[67] Studies have shown the effectiveness of this supplement in decreasing joint space narrowing, and in slowing the degenerative process of the articular cartilage.[66] Although no significant drug interactions have been reported, glucosamine containing supplements are believed to alter the glucose regulation and insulin sensitivity. However, Scroggie and colleagues[68] concluded that oral glucosamine-chondroitin supplementation does not result in clinically significant alterations in glucose metabolism in patients with type II diabetes mellitus. The dosage recommended for glucosamine sulfate is 1500 mg/day.

Chondroitin sulfate

The predominant glycosaminoglycan found in articular cartilage is chondroitin sulfate. It is composed of multiple units of glucuronic acid and galactosamine sulfate. The effectiveness of chondroitin in pain relief compared with placebo has been observed to be statistically significant, while there is no difference between placebo and chondroitin in adverse effects. The mechanism of action is postulated to be water absorption, which increases cartilage thickness, compressibility and load absorption. It may have a role in proteolytic enzymes inhibition. Chondroitin also has anticoagulant effects, which may be one possible mechanism of action. Platelets secrete glycosaminoglycans, including chondroitin, as part of the normal control of coagulation. With aging, the amount of chondroitin secreted diminishes, promoting possible bone microthrombosis. Chondroitin may improve the microcirculation to subchondral bone, synovium and other tissues.[67] Although it may have a role in symptom modification, there is no literature supporting the use of chondroitin to slow or prevent joint space narrowing.[66] The suggested dosage for this supplement is 880–1200 mg/day. Due to the possible anticoagulant effects, this supplement should be used carefully in patients with blood dyscrasias or using anticoagulant drugs.

Glucocorticoids

The adrenal cortex synthesizes and secretes the corticosteroid hormones. These hormones include the mineralocorticoids, androgenic hormones and glucocorticoids. The glucocorticoids have potent anti-inflammatory and immunomodulating effects. At the molecular level, glucocorticoids bind to intracytoplasmic receptors, cross the nuclear membrane and interact with the cell DNA, modulating the production of mRNA. These actions change the rate of protein synthesis and lysosomal stability,[69] and induce apoptosis in cells of the hematopoietic system. Amsterdam[70] observed that glucocorticoids protect glandular cells and fibroblasts from signals evoked by cytokines, cyclic AMP, tumor suppressors and death genes, suggesting a bimodal, complementary mechanism of action: inducing death of inflammation promoting cells while protecting resident cells of the inflamed tissue by arresting apoptotic signals.

The glucocorticoids also decrease vascular permeability, and decrease activity, number, chemotactic attraction and tran-

sit of neutrophils and monocytes. They also block the production of prostaglandins, by blocking the biosynthesis of COX 2,[69] and inhibit the production of immunoglobulins, and leukotrienes (Fig. 15.2). Glucocorticoids inhibit phospholipase A2 by induction of the production of macrocortin and lipomodulin.[26] There is limited evidence supporting the use of oral corticosteroids for acute injuries, most of it in acute nerve injuries and low back pain.[71]

Adverse effects Glucocorticoid toxicity is related to both the average dose and cumulative duration of use, although for most toxicities a 'threshold' dose or duration has not been established. It is clear that even low dose corticosteroids (≥5 mg/day) for periods of 1 year or more may result in significant adverse effects, including fractures, infections, gastrointestinal ulcers or bleeding, and cataracts.[72] The naturally occurring cortisone and hydrocortisone, as well as the synthetic prednisone and prednisolone have both glucocorticoid and mineralocorticoid effects (salt retaining properties). These salt retaining properties promote the development of hypertension, fluid retention, hypokalemia and weight gain (which may be problematic for athletes that compete in weight divisions, such as combat sports or Olympic-style weightlifting). Thus, synthetic compounds, with marked glucocorticoid activity and no salt retaining effects, such as triamcinolone, betamethasone, dexamethasone or methylprednisolone, are preferred.

The glucocorticoids may also decrease the systemic immune response if taken orally, limiting the capacity of the athlete to mount an adequate defense mechanism against infections. Other potential adverse effects include skin thinning, changes in corporal hair distribution, acne, cataracts, increased intraocular pressure, dyspepsia, gastrointestinal bleeding, decreased fertility, menstrual abnormalities, osteoporosis and osteonecrosis.

Considering the possible systemic effects of oral administration, *versus* the limited absorption with local administration, local therapy is generally preferred, either topical or injected. Corticosteroids may be used topically, delivered by iontophoresis or phonophoresis. Injections may be recommended in selected cases, for subacute or chronic intra-articular or soft tissue injuries. Each corticosteroid has a specific plasma half-life and potency which should be considered prior to topical administration or injection (Table 15.7). Please refer to Chapter 16 for a discussion of topical corticosteroid use (iontophoresis and phonophoresis) and to Chapter 23 for an extensive discussion of the indications and use of corticosteroid injections.

Other considerations

All glucocorticoids are prohibited by the World Anti-doping Agency when administered orally, rectally, intravenously or intramuscularly. Their use requires a therapeutic use exemption approval by the appropriate anti-doping organization. Athletes are particularly susceptible to unintentional anti-doping rule violations with multiple substances, including glucocorticoids. A doping violation for glucocorticoid use may result in a reduced sanction provided that the athlete can establish that the use was not intended to enhance sports performance.[50]

Table 15.7 Glucocorticoid Equivalency and Plasma Half-Life

Glucocorticoid	Equivalent Potency (mg)	Half-Life
Cortisone	25	30
Hydrocortisone	20	80–118
Prednisone	5	60
Prednisolone	5	115–212
Triamcinolone	4	>200
Methylprednisolone	4	78–188
Dexamethasone	0.75	110–210
Betamethasone	0.75	>300

Box 15.9: Key Points

Corticosteroids

- Dramatic anti-inflammatory effects
- Limited use by oral route
- Topical or injectable preparations are recommended for athletic injuries.

TOPICAL AGENTS

Topical agents have been used to decrease pain and inflammation. The possible mechanisms of action include decreasing local irritation, local agent absorption,[73] blood-borne delivery,[74] and the rubbing action during agent application.[75] Most of these drugs are available without prescription and advertised for acute and chronic condition management.

Salicylates

Salicylic acid derivatives, although frequently defined as NSAIDs, and included in this chapter in this group, do not seem to have the same mechanism of action of this medication group.[37] Although the available literature on topical salicylates use is limited by small size, inadequate design and validity, these topical agents have been demonstrated to be significantly superior to placebo in acute and chronic musculoskeletal pain. However, the best assessment of the limited available information suggests that topical salicylates may be efficacious in acute pain and moderately to poorly efficacious in chronic musculoskeletal pain.[73] One of the limitations of studies for chronic conditions is that the longest trial lasted only 28 days. Local adverse effects seem to be seen in only 2% of subjects and without significant difference between treatment and placebo groups. Adverse effects associated to prolonged use of these topical agents in unknown.

NSAIDs

Topical NSAIDs have been widely used in Europe for decades. Preparations available include felbinac, ibuprofen, indomethacin, ketoprofen, naproxen and piroxicam. Following topical NSAID administration, levels of the drug are found in muscle and subcutaneous tissue, while serum concentrations are less than 10% compared with oral administration.[76] These drugs produce an improvement in pain scores and range of motion, and a decrease in subjective complaints.[26] A quantitative systemic review showed that topical NSAIDs are significantly more effective than placebo for pain relief, independent from the rubbing effect during application.[25] In a double blind study, naproxen gel was superior to placebo, with significant improvement of symptoms in 3 days.[77] However, the efficacy of topical NSAIDs appears to be of short duration. There is evidence suggesting pain relief and functional improvement for up to 2 weeks, with no apparent benefit after the third or fourth week.[77] This route is very promising, as the medication is administered to the site of injury, with minimal systemic absorption and decreased adverse effects. Adverse effects of this class are minimal and limited to mostly topical symptoms, such as itching,[77] rash or burning.[78] Local reactions are seen in approximately 3.6% of patients, while systemic effects are even rarer (<0.5%) and comparable with those seen in placebo recipients.[25] Head to head comparisons of topical *versus* oral NSAID administration are available, but limited by trial size and lack of comparison between the same drug given by different routes.[78] Topical NSAID administration may be an alternative for athletes with poor tolerance to oral NSAIDs or when the oral route is undesirable. The long-term (>1 month) efficacy and adverse effects of these agents after prolonged use are unknown, as studies for more than 1 month are not available.

Capsaicin

This topical agent is derived from chili peppers, and is available in preparations of 0.025% and 0.075%. The mechanism of action is depletion, inhibition of synthesis and transport of substance P, decreasing local discomfort. Capsaicin has been used successfully in the management of neuropathic and rheumatologic conditions, but some patients cannot tolerate the drug due to intense itching and burning. One third of patients may experience some local irritation and up to 10% may even stop treatment.[79] To avoid these symptoms, broken or irritated skin should be avoided and a four times a day application is important, to achieve maximal substance P depletion. Patients should wear gloves to apply capsaicin, and should avoid touching any mucosal membranes or eyes. Following application, they need to wash their hands with soap and water to avoid local absorption of the drug in other areas.

Lidocaine patch

Lidocaine patches of 5% are approved by the FDA for the treatment of post-herpetic neuralgia. The mechanism of action is skin diffusion and binding to sodium channels in the nociceptors and sensory nerve fibers. The amount of lidocaine that penetrates the skin is sufficient to cause analgesia without anesthesia. Only 3% of the lidocaine dose is systemically absorbed. The patch can only be applied on intact skin and a maximum of three patches can be used for 12 h in a 24 h period (12 h on/ 12 h off). There is a one patient, open-label case report that suggests that lidocaine patches may have a role in the treatment of myofascial pain, instead of trigger point injections.[80] There are also small uncontrolled reports of lidocaine patch use with benefits in painful neuropathies, such as polyneuropathies, meralgia paresthetica and complex regional pain syndrome.[81] These uses are off-label and not FDA approved. No randomized controlled studies examining the utility of lidocaine patches in sports-related injuries or musculoskeletal injuries are available.

Adverse effects

Local reactions, such as erythema, edema, itching or cold sensation may be experienced after patch application. These reactions are usually mild and transient. The delivery device should be used with caution in patients with severe hepatic disease, those using Class 1 antiarrhythmic drugs (such as tocainide) or during the use of other local anesthetics, as the risk of toxic lidocaine levels in these patients is higher.

CONCLUSIONS

Medications for pain and inflammation control may be useful tools for the treatment of acute or chronic injuries. The use of

---

Box 15.10 Key Points

Topical Agents

- Promising route of administration
- Limited systemic effects
- May be effective for short periods of time.

---

medications is not a replacement for rehabilitation, but may be an important tool for symptom modification during the rehabilitation process. The selection of these agents may be a difficult task. Tools that may help guide drug selection include the past medical history of the athlete, previous or current medication or supplement use, and the medication adverse effects profile. Drugs that may be considered illegal by sports governing organizations should be avoided, if possible. Close monitoring, dose adjustment and the addition or substitution of medications, using tools such as the WHO 'pain ladder', is strongly recommended.

REFERENCES

1   Dorland's illustrated medical dictionary. 30th edn. Philadelphia: Saunders; 2003.
2   Hendler N. Concepts in pain, suffering and behavior. The challenge of pain. Postgrad Healthcare 1996; 2:3.
3   Guirimand F. Recent data on the physiology of pain. Nephrologie 2003; 24:401–407.
4   Kibler WB. A framework for sports medicine. Phys Med Rehab Clin North Am 1994; 5:1–8.
5   Hansen TM, Stothard D, Stothard J. Musculoskeletal disorders. In: Goddle F, ed. Clinical evidence. 2004:12. Online. Available: www.clinicalevidence.org
6   Jarvinen TAH, Kaarianen M, Jarvinen M, Kalimo H. Muscle strain injuries. Curr Opin Rheum 2000; 12:155–161.
7   Gallin JL, Goldstein IM, Snyderman R, eds. Inflammation: Basics principals in clinical correlates. New York: Raven; 1992:1–4.
8   Almekinders LC, Temple JD. Etiology, diagnosis and treatment of tendonitis: an analysis of the literature. Med Sci Sports Exerc 1998; 30:1183–1190.
9   Henderson JM. Therapeutic drugs: What to avoid with athletes. Clin Sports Med 1998; 17:229–243.
10 Eisen SA, Miller DK, Woodward RS, et al. The effect of prescribed daily dose frequency on patient medication compliance. Arch Int Med 1990; 150:1881–1884.
11 Claxton AJ, Cramer J, Pierce C. A systematic review of the associations between dose regimens and medication compliance. Clin Ther 2001; 23:1296–1310.
12 Williams GC, Grow VM, Freedman ZR, et al. Motivational predictors of weight loss and weight-loss maintenance. J Pers Soc Psychol 1996; 70:115–126.
13 Leadbetter WB. Anti-inflammatory therapy in sports injury. The role of nonsteroidal drugs and corticosteroid injection. Clin Sports Med 1995; 14:353–410.
14 WHO. Cancer pain relief and palliative care: report of a WHO expert committee. WHO Tech Rep Ser 1990; 804:1–73.
15 Cohen RI, Chopra P, Upshur C. Guide to conservative, medical, and procedural therapies. Geriatrics 2001; 56:38–42.
16 McGrath PA. Development of the World Health Organization Guidelines on cancer pain relief and palliative care in children. J Pain Symp Manage 1996; 12:87–92.
17 Levy MH. Pharmacologic treatment of cancer pain. N Engl J Med 1996; 335:1124–1132.
18 Reig E. Tramadol in musculoskeletal pain – a survey. Clin Rheum 2002; 21:S9–S11.
19 Haber VJ. Sutton JR. Endorphins and exercise. Sports Med 1984; 1:154–171.
20 Guien R, Blin O, Pouget J, Serratrice G. Nociceptive threshold and physical activity. Can J Neurol Sci 1992; 19:69–71.
21 Fuller AK, Robinson ME. A test of exercise analgesia using signal detection theory and a within-subjects design. Percept Mot Skills 1993; 73:1299–1310.
22 Pain perception in competitive swimmers. Brit Med J Clin Research Ed 1981; 283:91–93.
23 Staes F, Stappaerts K, Lesaffre E, Vertommen H. Low back pain in Flemish adolescents and the role of perceived social support and effect on the perception of back pain. Acta Paediatr 2003; 92:444–451.
24 Singh G, Triadafilopoulus G. Epidemiology of NSAID induced gastrointestinal complications. J Rheum 1999; 56:18–24.
25 Moore R, Tramer MR, Carroll D, et al. Quantitative systematic review of topically applied non-steroidal antiinflammatory drugs. BMJ 1998; 316:333–338.
26 Stanley KL, Weaver JE. Pharmacologic management of pain and inflammation in athletes. Clin Sports Med 1998; 17:375–392.
27 Phero JC, Becker DE, Dionne RA. Contemporary trends in acute pain management. Curr Opin Otol and Head and Neck Surg 2004; 12:209–216.
28 Meade EA, Smith WL, DeWitt DL. Differential inhibition of prostaglandins endoperoxide synthase (cyclooxygenase) isoenzyme by aspirin and other nonsteroidal anti-inflammatory drugs. J Biol Chem 1993; 268:6610–6614.
29 Trappe TA, White F, Lambert CP, et al. Effect of ibuprofen and acetaminophen on post-exercise muscle protein synthesis. Am J Physiol Endocrinol Metab 2002; 282:551–556.
30 Baldwin LA. Use of nonsteroidal anti-inflammatory drugs following exercise-induced muscle injury. Sports Med 2003; 33:177–185.
31 Khaund R, Henderson J. Switching from one NSAID to another: Myth or madness. (unpublished research). Columbus, GA: Hughston Sports Medicine Foundation; 1997.
32 Furst DE. Are there differences among non steroidal antiinflammatory drugs? Comparing acetylated salicylates, nonacetylated salicylates, and nonacetylated nonsteroidal antiinflammatory drugs. Arthritis Rheum 1994; 37:1–9.
33 Walker JS, Sheather-Reid RB, Carmody JJ, et al. Nonsteroidal antiinflammatory drugs in rheumatoid arthritis and osteoarthritis: support for the concept of "responders" and "nonresponders". Arthritis Rheum 1997; 40:1944–1954.
34 Lovell DJ, Gianni EH, Brewer EJ. Time course of response to nonsteroidal antiinflammatory drugs in juvenile rheumatoid arthritis. Arthritis Rheum 1984; 27(1443):1443–1447.
35 Mahler N. Misuse of drugs in recreational sports. Ther Umsch 2001; 58(4):226–231.
36 Virchenko O. Parecoxib impairs early tendon repair but improves later remodeling. Am J Sports Med 2004; 32:1743–1747.
37 Amann R, Peskar BA. Anti-inflammatory effects of aspirin and sodium salicylate. Eur J Pharm 2002; 447:1–9.
38 FitzGerald GA. COX-2 and beyond: Approaches to prostaglandin inhibition in human disease. Nat Rev Drug Discov 2003; 2:879–890.
39 FitzGerald GA. Coxibs and cardiovascular disease. N Engl J Med 2004; 351:1709–1711.
40 Fowles RE. Potential cardiovascular effects of COX-2 selective nonsteroidal antiinflammatory drugs. J Pain Palliative Pharm 2003; 17:27–50.
41 Gabriel SE, Jaakilimanen L, Bombardier C. Risk of serious gastrointestinal complications related to nonsteroidal antiinflammatory drugs: a meta-analysis. Ann Int Med 1991; 115:787.
42 Silverstein FE, Graham DY, Senior JR, et al. Misoprostol reduces serious gastrointestinal complications in patients with rheumatoid arthritis receiving nonsteroidal anti-inflammatory drugs. Ann Int Med 1995; 123:241–249.
43 Ekstrom P, Carling L, Wetterhun S, et al. Prevention of peptic ulcer and dyspeptic symptoms with omeprazole in patients receiving continuous nonsteroidal anti-inflammatory drug therapy. Scand J Gastroenterol 1996; 31:753–758.
44 Robinson MG, Griffin JW, Bowers J, et al. Effect of Ranitidine on gastroduodenal mucosal damage induced by nonsteroidal anti-inflammatory drugs. Dig Dis Sci 1989; 34:424–428.

45   Chan FK. Hung LC, Suen BY, et al. Celecoxib versus diclofenac and omeprazole in reducing the risk of recurrent ulcer bleeding in patients with arthritis. N Engl J Med 2002; 347:2104.

46   Cryer B. Second-generation cyclooxygenase-2 specific inhibitors. Clin Perspect Gastroenterol 2002; 122

47   Bombardier C, Laine L, Reicin A, et al. Comparison of upper gastrointestinal toxicity of rofecoxib and naproxen in patients with rheumatoid arthritis. N Engl J Med 2000; 343:1520-1528.

48   Bartlett D. Acetaminophen toxicity. J Emerg Nurs 2004; 30:281-283.

49   Allen GJ, Hartl TL, Duffany S, et al. Cognitive and motor function after administration of hydrocodone bitartrate plus ibuprofen, ibuprofen alone, or placebo in healthy subjects with exercise-induced muscle damage: a randomized, repeated-dose, placebo-controlled study. Psychopharmacology 2003; 166:228-233.

50   World Anti-doping Agency. The 2005 Prohibited list. World Anti-doping code: International Standard. World Anti-doping Agency. Online. Available: www. wada-ama. org/rtecontent/document/list_2005.pdf 27 Jan 2005.

51   Wilder-Smith CH, Schimke J, Osterwalder B, et al. Oral tramadol , a μ-opioid agonist and monoamine reuptake-blocker, and morphine for strong cancer-related pain. Ann Oncol 1994; 5:141-146.

52   Duhmke RM, Cornblath DD, Hollingshead JR. Tramadol for neuropathic pain. CD-ROM. Cochrane Database Syst Rev 2004; 4.

53   Medeve RA, Wang J, Karim R. Tramadol and acetaminophen tablets for dental pain. Anesth Prog 2003; 48:79-81.

54   Backonja MM. Use of anticonvulsants for treatment of neuropathic pain. Neurology 2002; 59:S14-S17.

55   Rogawski MA, Loscher W. The neurobiology of antiepileptic drugs for the treatment of nonepileptic conditions. Nat Med 2004; 10:685-692.

56   Spina E, Perugi G. Antiepileptic drugs: indications other than epilepsy. Epileptic Disord 2004; 6:57-75.

57   Kudoh A, Ishihara H, Matsuki A. Effect of carbamazepine on pain scores of unipolar depressed patients with chronic pain: a trial of off-on-off-on design. Clin J Pain 1998; 14:61-65.

58   Martinez-Silvestrini JA, Micheo WF. Complex regional pain syndrome in pediatric sports: A case series of 3 young athletes. Arch Phys Med Rehabil 2001; 82:1295.

59   Rusy LM, Troshynski TJ, Weissman SJ. Gabapentin in phantom limb pain management in children and young adults: report of seven cases. J Pain Symptom Manage 2001; 21:78-81.

60   Stahl SM. Anticonvulsants and the relief of chronic pain: pregabalin and gabapentin as alpha (2) delta ligands at voltage-gated calcium channels. J Clin Psych 2004; 65:596-597.

61   Chong MS, Libretto SE. The rationale and use of topiramate for treating neuropathic pain. Clin J Pain 2003; 19:59-68.

62   Richelson E. Pharmacology of antidepressants. Mayo Clin Proc 2001; 76:511-527.

63   Nemoto H, Toda H, Nakajima T, et al. Fluvoxamine modulates pain sensation and affective processing of pain in human brain. Neuroreport 2003; 14:791-797.

64   Stephen JM, Ghezzi KT, Bailey K, et al. Post-triathlon delirium. J Emerg Med 1991; 9:265-269.

65   McAlindon TE, LaValley MP, Gulin JP, et al. Glucosamine and chondroitin for treatment of osteoarthritis: a systematic quality assessment and meta-analysis. JAMA 2000; 283:1469-1475.

66   Richy F, Bruyere O, Ethgen O, et al. Structural and symptomatic efficacy of glucosamine and chondroitin in knee osteoarthritis: a comprehensive meta-analysis. Arch Med 2003; 163:1514-1522.

67   Hungerford MW, Valaik D. Chondroprotective agents: glucosamine and chondroitin. Foot Ankle Clin 2003; 8:201-209.

68   Scroggie DA, Albright A, Harris MD. The effect of glucosamine-chondroitin supplementation on glycosylated hemoglobin levels in patients with type 2 diabetes mellitus: a placebo-controlled, double-blinded, randomized clinical trial. Arch Int Med 2003; 163:1587-1590.

69   Szczepanki A, Moatter T, Carley W, et al. Induction of cyclooxygenase II in humans synovial microvessel endothelial cells by interleukin-1: Inhibition by glucocorticoids. Arthritis Rheum 1994; 37:495-503.

70   Amsterdam A, Sasson R. The anti-inflammatory action of glucocorticoids is mediated by cell type specific regulation of apoptosis. Mol Cell Endocrinol 2002; 189:1-9.

71   Jonsson E. Back pain, neck pain: An evidence based review. Summary and conclusions. The Swedish Council on Technology Assessment in Health Care; 2000:1-30.

72   Saag KG, Koehnke R, Caldwell JR, et al. Low dose long-term corticosteroid therapy in rheumatoid arthritis: an analysis of serious adverse events. Am J Med 1994; 96:115-123.

73   Mason L, Moore RA, Edwards JE, et al. Systematic review of efficacy of topical rubefacients containing salicylates for the treatment of acute and chronic pain. BMJ 2004; 328:995-997.

74   Cooper C, Kelsey M. Topical NSAIDs in osteoarthritis. 2004; 329:304-305.

75   Vaile JH, Davis P. Topical agents for musculoskeletal conditions. A review of literature. Drugs 1998; 56:783-799.

76   Heynemann CA. Topical nonsteroidal anti-inflammatory drugs for acute soft tissue injuries. Ann Pharmacother 1995; 29:780-782.

77   Thorling J, Linden B, Berg R, Sandahl A. A double-blind comparison of naproxen gel and placebo in the treatment of soft tissue injuries. Curr Med Res Opin 1990; 12:242-248.

78   Lin J, Zhang W, Jones A, Doherty M. Efficacy of topical non-steroidal anti-inflammatory drugs in the treatment of osteoarthritis: meta-analysis of randomised controlled trials. BMJ 2004; 329:324.

79   Mason L, Moore RA, Derry S, Edwards JE, McQuay HJ. Systematic review of topical capsaicin for the treatment of chronic pain. BMJ 2004; 328:991-994.

80   Dalpiaz AS, Dodds TA. Myofascial pain response to topical patch therapy: case report. J Pain Palliative Care 2002; 16:99-104.

81   Galer BS. Topical lidocaine patch relieves a variety of neuropathic pain conditions: An open-label pilot study. Presented at Am Acad Neurology, Seattle, WA, 6-13 May 1995.

CHAPTER 16

Physical Modalities

Joel M. Press and Deborah A. Bergfeld

INTRODUCTION

This chapter provides a fundamental overview of various physical modalities. It addresses their use as adjuncts in the treatment of sports related injuries and musculoskeletal complaints with an emphasis on current literature pertinent to each individual modality. However, studies regarding the use of physical modalities are often conflicting and a review of such literature leaves the clinician with a sense of ambiguity as to the effectiveness of these treatments. In addition, many studies are performed in patients with arthritis and undifferentiated back pain syndromes. Therefore, the evidence-based use of modalities in clinical sports medicine must be extrapolated from these other patient populations as well.

Physical modalities, when used in the appropriate setting, may help minimize time lost due to an injury or facilitate progress in a rehabilitation program, but they are not without some degree of risk. A survey of athletic trainers using physical modalities found a reported complication rate of 26%.[1] The most common complications are skin irritation, burns, intolerance to treatment and pain with treatment. That being said, by understanding the basic physiology as well as indications and contraindications for these modalities, a safe and rational prescription can be formulated.

It cannot be emphasized enough that it is the duty of every practitioner to recognize that physical modalities should not be used in isolation. They should be part of a comprehensive rehabilitation program with the patient's eventual goals (i.e. return to sport) and individual response to the overall treatment plan kept in mind.

CRYOTHERAPY (COLD THERAPY)

Cold application produces a variety of physiologic effects. Cold diminishes muscle spindle activity. This may assist in breaking the pain-spasm cycle by decreasing muscle spasticity and muscle guarding.[2,3] It also slows nerve conduction velocity, possibly affecting the firing patterns of peripheral sensory pain fibers. It causes decreased local metabolism and minimizes enzymatic activity, decreasing the subsequent demand for

Box 16.1: Key Points

- Cryotherapy is most effective in the treatment of acute injuries and postoperatively.
- It is contraindicated in ischemic areas, cold intolerance and insensate skin.
- The cold is usually applied for 20–30 min sessions multiple times per day to avoid unwanted complications.

oxygen.[4,5] Cold application produces vasoconstriction with vasodilation following reflexively. Cryotherapy, as opposed to therapeutic heat, increases connective tissue stiffness and muscle viscosity, thereby diminishing flexibility.

Based on these various effects, cryotherapy is most commonly used during the first 48 h of an acute musculoskeletal injury. Hocutt *et al.*[6] demonstrated that early cryotherapy (started within 36 h of injury) allowed patients with ankle sprains to reach full activity in 13.2 days. This number was in comparison to 30.4 days using cryotherapy initiated at >36 h and 33.3 days using heat therapy. Use beyond the acute phase is justified for continued pain control, muscle re-education, and control of swelling when utilized with compression.[7,8]

Contraindications for cryotherapy include ischemia, cold intolerance, Raynaud's phenomenon, cold allergy, inability to communicate and insensate skin. Care must be taken when using cold therapy over nerves due to the potential development of neuropraxia (conduction block). Recommendations to minimize this complication include limiting ice application to less than 30 min and protecting any peripheral nerves in the region.[9]

Techniques of application

Ice packs, iced compression wraps, slushes, ice massage, ice whirlpool, and vapocoolant sprays are some methods of cold application (Fig. 16.1).[10] Regardless of the method used, there is a rapid drop in skin temperature with a delayed effect on muscle. This effect on muscle depends on the amount of overlying subcutaneous tissue with maximum cooling occurring to a

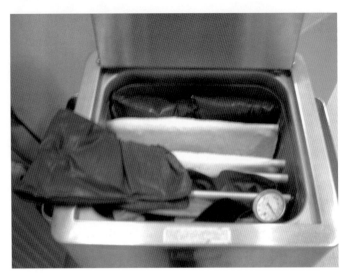

Figure 16.1   Cold packs.

muscle depth of 1–2 cm.[11] MacAuley[12] reviewed 45 textbooks and found considerable variation in the recommended duration and frequency of ice. Although there is no definitive recommendation regarding the duration of treatment, cryotherapy is typically used for a period of 20–30 min at a time.

In a comparison of various application techniques, a 20 min application of a 454 g packet of frozen peas was more effective than a frozen gel pack in achieving a mean skin temperature adequate to induce localized skin analgesia, to reduce localized nerve conduction velocity and to reduce metabolic enzyme activity to clinically relevant levels.[13] As well, care must be taken when using chemical or gel packs due to poor control of temperature and risk of skin irritation should the envelope break and the chemical come in contact with the individual's skin.

Cryostretch and cryokinetics refers to the use of cryotherapy to facilitate joint movement. Decreasing pain and muscle guarding may lead to improved flexibility and muscle function.[11,14] An additional method of cryotherapy involves the use of vapocoolant sprays (fluori-methane and ethyl chloride), which provide very effective cutaneous local anesthesia and are commonly used to treat myofascial trigger points. The use of cryotherapy in this context promotes normal muscle resting length by a 'spray and stretch' technique rather than by cooling the muscle itself.[15] Fluori-methane is less explosive, less flammable and produces less cooling than ethyl chloride.[16] Concerns, however, have been raised regarding the destruction of the ozone layer by the use of vapocoolant sprays, some of which are considered chlorofluorocarbons.[17,18]

The effectiveness of cryotherapy

Many studies on the effects of postoperative cryotherapy have been performed. Ohkoshi et al.[19] attempted to show a relationship between cryotherapy, intra-articular temperature changes and pain relief in patients having undergone anterior cruciate ligament (ACL) reconstruction. A total of 21 patients undergoing ACL reconstruction were randomized into three groups: cryotherapy at 5°C, cryotherapy at 10°C, and no

cryotherapy for the first 48 postoperative hours. A temperature probe was placed intraoperatively in the suprapatellar pouch and the intercondylar notch through arthroscopic portals. Both cryotherapy groups had a triphasic temperature curve. A low temperature phase occurred immediately and lasted approximately 2 h. This was followed by a temperature rising phase, and finally, a thermostatic phase. The control group, however, went immediately to a thermostatic phase. During the low temperature phase, the cryotherapy groups' suprapatellar pouch temperatures were significantly lower than the intercondylar notch temperatures with both sites being significantly lower than body temperature. Only the suprapatellar pouch temperature remained significantly lower than body temperature during the thermostatic phase. Although the numbers were not large in this interesting study, it helps to link objective intraarticular temperature changes to clinical outcomes. The cryotherapy groups reached 120° of knee flexion 4 days sooner than controls. The 10°C group had significantly lower pain scores and analgesic use as compared with the control group. Similarly, Lessard et al.[20] showed decreased pain scores and analgesic use following arthroscopic knee surgery in a randomized, blinded, controlled study of 45 patients using cryotherapy. Levy and Marmar[21] reported less swelling, less pain and better range of motion with the use of cryotherapy in patients following total knee arthroplasty. Unlike the previous studies, pain scores were reported in a randomized, controlled study of cryotherapy in 50 postoperative shoulder patients done by Speer et al.[22] The cryotherapy group reported decreased pain frequency and intensity, less need to use medication, better sleep, less swelling, and less pain with shoulder movement.

On the flip side, in a randomized, controlled study, Konrath et al.[23] did not find significant differences in medication usage or range of motion in 100 postoperative anterior cruciate ligament reconstruction patients treated with cryotherapy. Levy et al.[24] studied the effect of cryotherapy on temperatures in the glenohumeral joint and the subacromial space following shoulder arthroscopy in 15 patients. They found no significant differences in temperatures as compared to control. The effect of cryotherapy on pain scores was not recorded in either study.

Paddon-Jones and Quigley[25] and Yackzan et al.[26] did not find cryotherapy to be effective in treating delayed onset muscle soreness. In a study of rats, Fu et al.[27] found that post-endurance training cryotherapy may actually be deleterious by causing histologic myofibril damage.

Contrast baths

Contrast baths, which alternate the use of heat and cold, have been described as a form of 'vascular exercise' due to alternating dilation and constriction of blood vessels. By alternating cycles of heat and cold, a hyperemic response may by created, thereby improving circulation and assisting in the healing response. More specifically, contrast baths are used to improve range of motion, control swelling and provide pain control. Contraindications include those discussed for therapeutic heat and cold, particularly active bleeding and vascular insufficiency. A protocol commonly used is as follows[4,11]:

1 Affected region is submerged in a warm bath of 38–43°C for 10 min
2 Cold bath of half ice/half water at 13–18°C for 1 min
3 Warm bath for 4 min
4 Cold bath for 1 min
5 Steps 3 and 4 are then alternated for a total treatment cycle of 20–30 min
6 The sequence ends with cold.

Exercising the area may occur during the heating phase with rest during the cooling phase.

Frequently in the management of ankle injuries, contrast baths have been used for the treatment of an unchanging effusion, with the alternating cycle of hot and cold being used to create a cycle of alternating vasodilation and vasoconstriction.[28]

However, Myrer and Safran[29] in their study of contrast therapy, found that 20 min of contrast therapy had no effects on the temperature of the gastrocnemius muscle as measured 1 cm below subcutaneous fat with a microprobe.

THERAPEUTIC HEAT MODALITIES

Box 16.2: Key Points

- Heat is indicated in the more subacute to chronic phases of injury and healing.
- Contraindications to the use of heat include: sensory deficits, peripheral vascular disease, bleeding diathesis, malignancy and acute stages of trauma or inflammation.

To best utilize therapeutic heat modalities, an understanding of the physiologic effects of heat is necessary. Heating can create changes, which are both local and distant, with the far-field effects being less pronounced. A consensual response may also be seen whereby heating one part of the body creates an increase in blood flow to other regions. As heat is applied to a body surface, circulatory changes occur. Because of increased metabolic tissue demands with heat, a subsequent increase in blood flow occurs. This leads to the arrival of various leukocytes, improved delivery of oxygen, increased capillary permeability and hyperemia. Diffusion across membranes occurs more effectively and can lead to edema formation, especially with acute injuries.[30]

Additional physiologic effects of heat include pain control during the later stages of healing. Vasodilation leads to improved tissue blood flow and increased removal of pain-causing inflammatory substances such as bradykinins, prostaglandin and histamine substrates. Heat also acts directly on free nerve endings and provides muscle relaxation by decreasing the muscle spindle's sensitivity to stretch via the gamma system.[31] Inhibitory pathways can be activated by the use of heat modalities with subsequent muscle relaxation. Central processes may also provide for sedation and decreased pain awareness. Thus, therapeutic heat assists in altering the pain-muscle guarding (spasm) cycle.[32]

Other useful effects of therapeutic heat include improved collagen flexibility (especially when accompanied by prolonged stretching) and a subjective decrease in joint stiffness. Lehmann et al.[33] showed that tendon lengthening and decreasing tendon tension occurred most effectively when the tendon was loaded in an elevated temperature bath of 45°C as compared to that at 25°C. Furthermore, only when stretch was applied in conjunction with heat, did lengthening occur.[34,35] There are some studies, however, that do not support this. In a small study of 24 subjects, Taylor et al.[36] showed that application of heat or cold modalities made no significant difference in hamstring length when used in conjunction with a sustained hamstring stretch.

Based on the physiologic effects of therapeutic heat, general indications for heat modalities in the athlete include pain, muscle spasm, contracture, bursitis, and tenosynovitis. Contraindications for heat include: sensory deficits, peripheral vascular disease (due to the inability to meet the demands of increased blood flow and metabolism), bleeding diathesis, malignancy, acute stages of trauma and acute inflammation.[10]

Therapeutic heat, like other modalities, can often provide short-term relief, but there is little evidence to support long lasting effects. Timm[37] studied 250 subjects who had persistent low back pain following an L5 laminectomy in a randomized, controlled trial. The subjects were randomized into five groups including control, manipulation, simple home exercise program, supervised exercise program, and physical agents, including hot packs, ultrasound, and transcutaneous electrical nerve stimulation (TENS) (Fig. 16.2). The physical agent group did no better than the control group on the functional Oswestry scale, but was the most costly of all groups (US$1,842 per subject). The exercise groups had the most improvement in the Oswestry disability scores and had fewer recurrences of low back pain The simple home exercise program was the most economical (US$1,392 per subject).

Techniques of application
Heat can be transferred to tissue in three ways.

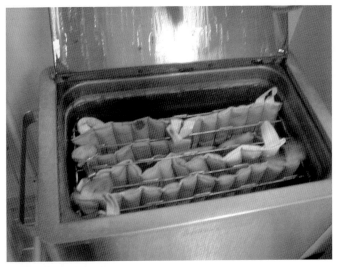

Figure 16.2 Hot packs.

Conduction

Direct heat transfer from one surface to another due to direct contact. This is a form of superficial heat. Examples include hydrocollator packs, paraffin baths, electric heating pads and hot water bottles.

Convection

Heat transfer due to the movement of air or water across a body surface. This, too, is a form of superficial heat. Examples include hydrotherapy and fluidotherapy.

Conversion

Transfer of heat due to a change in the form of energy. Examples of superficial heat conversion include radiant energy such as that produced by infrared lamps. Deep heating, also known as diathermy, is due to conversion through the use of short waves, electromagnetic microwaves and ultrasound.

Superficial heat modalities

The common denominator of superficial heat modalities is direct heat penetration. Penetration is greatest within 0.5 cm from the skin surface, depending on the amount of adipose tissue present.[38,39] The more commonly used modes for sports rehabilitation are hydrocollator packs, whirlpool and contrast baths. Other forms of superficial heat include infrared lamps, paraffin baths, fluidotherapy and moist air.

Hydrocollator packs

Hydrocollator packs serve to transfer heat via conduction. These packs come in three standard sizes and are heated in stainless steel containers containing water at temperatures between 18 and 32°C. After appropriate heating, toweling is applied to the packs in order to minimize burning of the skin and to maintain heat insulation. The highest temperatures produced by the hydrocollator packs are at the skin surface. The pack is able to maintain heat for approximately 30 min with treatment sessions lasting 20–30 min.

Other heating packs are also available and include hot water bottles, electric heating pads, and chemical packs. The major disadvantage of using these devices is limited temperature control.

Hydrotherapy: exercise in water

Hydrotherapy is a term that can describe two distinct entities: warm water immersion and exercise performed in the water. Warm water immersion will be discussed in the next section.

A patient exercising in the water can get the therapeutic benefit of exercise while using the buoyancy principles of water to decrease the biomechanical stresses on the musculoskeletal system. The temperature of the water can be modified to individual needs. Patients with acute injuries and pregnant women are typically treated in cooler pools of 28°C, whereas subacute or chronic injuries are treated in warmer temperatures of 33–34°C.[40] Water exercises can also be used to cross-train patients who require weight-bearing restrictions, such as those with stress fractures. Buoyancy-assisting devices can be used to allow patients to run in water (cooler temperatures of 29–30°C) and maintain cardiovascular fitness.[40] Hall et al.[41] compared water-based exercise, land-based exercise, seated water immersion, and progressive relaxation in 139 chronic rheumatoid arthritis patients in a randomized trial. At 3 months, the water-based exercise group maintained the most improvement in emotional and psychological scales. In a comparison study of electroacupuncture versus hydrotherapy in the treatment of hip osteoarthritis, Stener-Victorin et al.[42] showed that hydrotherapy reduced pain, improved disability rating scores and improved quality of life measurements for 3–6 months post-treatment. Norton et al.[43] showed that after anterior cruciate ligament repair, patients had quicker range of motion gains with water-based exercise when compared to conventional land-based therapy.

Regardless, the goal of water-based therapy is often to prepare the body for improved function on land. Therefore, for anyone being treated in the water, incorporation of a land-based exercise program is an integral part of a rehabilitation program.

Hydrotherapy: warm water immersion

Heating through the use of submersion in water is a form of convection. Whirlpools are used when a small area of the body is to be heated, such as a part of the upper or lower extremity, while Hubbard tanks are used to treat larger surface areas. The Hubbard tank, due to its larger size, also allows for range of motion maneuvers. Since larger body areas are exposed to heat during hydrotherapy, there is an increased risk of elevation in core body temperature. Therefore, water temperature rarely exceeds 40°C for total body immersion, whereas temperatures as high as 43°C may be used for partial limb immersion. As larger areas of the body are immersed in the heated water, diminished regulation of core body temperature occurs, as sweating and heat exchange can only occur in the non-immersed portions.[44] As an area with poor circulation is exposed to heat, a greater demand for blood supply is created due to increased metabolic needs. However, this demand for increased circulation may not be adequately met, leading to ischemic results. Therefore, in addition to contraindications for superficial heat, warm water immersion should not be used for pregnant patients and those with cardiovascular disease.

The benefits of whirlpool treatment stem from the principle of buoyancy, in which a gravity-eliminated environment assists the patient in upward movement. An additional benefit comes from the resistance to flow, which provides low resistance for muscle strengthening and training. Agitation created by the water flow provides sensory input to the skin, assisting with pain control as well as maintaining appropriate water temperature.

DIATHERMY/DEEP HEATING MODALITIES

Diathermy utilizes the principle of conversion to heat deeper tissues. The most commonly used deep heating agents include ultrasound, phonophoresis, shortwave diathermy and microwave diathermy. The general indications and contraindications are similar to those already discussed for superficial heat. However, specific clinical uses and precautions will be presented.

Ultrasound

Box 16.3: Key Points

- Ultrasound provides the deepest penetration of all heating modalities since most of the energy conversion takes place at the bone interface.

- A continuous, rather than stationary, application of ultrasound is most often used.

- General indications for the use of ultrasound are similar to those for other therapeutic heat modalities.

- Additional precautions include: using ultrasound over laminectomy sites, fluid filled cavities or in pregnancy (over the uterus).

- Phonophoresis is the use of ultrasound to increase the percutaneous absorption of a drug for the management of pain and inflammation.

Ultrasound is defined as sound waves with frequencies higher than the audible acoustic spectrum (above 20 000 Hz) (Fig. 16.3). It is unique among diathermy modalities in that the production of heat is due to a high-frequency alternating electric current (0.8–1.0 MHz), which is converted via a crystal transducer to acoustic vibrations rather than to electromagnetic energy. Energy transfer occurs due to the piezoelectric effect whereby the crystal undergoes changes in shape when voltage is applied. By altering the crystal's configuration, vibrations are created which then pass through the tissues being treated. The heating effects depend on the absorption and reflection of ultrasonic energy which, in turn, is based on differences in the acoustic impedance at different tissue interfaces. Selective heating is greatest when acoustic impedance is high, such as at

the bone-muscle interface. On the other hand, ultrasonic energy is readily conducted through homogeneous structures such as subcutaneous fat or metal implants with minimal thermal effects due to the rapid removal of heat energy. Thus, ultrasound can be safely used in the presence of most metal implants. However, in the presence of methyl methacrylate and high-density polyethylene, which may be used in total joint replacements, a greater amount of ultrasound energy will be absorbed with the potential for overheating.[44] Significant heating can occur to depths up to 5 cm below the skin surface, thereby providing therapeutic effects to bone, joint capsule, tendons, ligaments and scar tissue.[45] In summary, ultrasound provides for the deepest penetration of all heating modalities since minimal energy is converted to heat in subcutaneous fat or muscle with most of the conversion occurring at the bone interface.

In addition to the above noted thermal effects, ultrasound also has non-thermal effects, which do not relate to tissue temperature elevation but rather to molecular vibration. Although heat can increase membrane permeability, diffusion can also occur due to the non-thermal streaming/stirring effect of fluids created by the ultrasonic field. Gaseous cavitation is also a non-thermal ultrasonic event. Gas bubbles are created as a result of acoustic rarefaction and compression causing subsequent enlargement in bubble size and pressure changes within the tissues. As the gas-filled cavity vibrates due to alternating compression and rarefaction, surrounding fluid movement occurs with the potential for cell destruction. Cavitation can be minimized by the application of external pressure and the use of a stroking, rather than a stationary technique, which will be discussed shortly.

Application methods for ultrasound

Two primary methods of ultrasound application may be used: continuous and stationary. A coupling medium, such as mineral oil/gel or water for irregular surfaces is utilized to ensure adequate transmission of sound energy.[35,46] With the continuous method, the ultrasound head is moved in a stroking fashion over the area being treated. This provides for safer, more uniform heating. The size of the applicator head should be larger than the treatment field with common sizes ranging from 5 square cm to 10 square cm. The stationary method, as the name implies, does not involve the continuous movement of the applicator head. Since a rapid rise in temperature is produced over a localized area with increased risk of burning and gaseous cavitation, this method is less commonly used. When the stationary technique is employed, intensity output is reduced.

Dosimetry is measured in W/cm^2, which reflects the applicator output divided by the surface area of the applicator. Intensities of $1.0 W/cm^2$–$4.0 W/cm^2$ are most commonly used for the continuous method. Treatment often begins at $0.5 W/cm^2$ and the total output gradually increases. When using the stationary head, a safe range would be $0.1 W/cm^2$–$1.0 W/cm^2$.[31] The duration of most treatments is 5–10 min per site based on the size of the treatment area, with 10–12 treatments per series. As with all therapeutic modalities, the patient's subjective response to heating with ultrasound is the best guide for proper dosing.

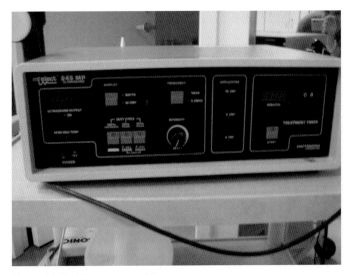

Figure 16.3 Ultrasound machine.

Pulsed application is a method of administering ultrasound waves whereby the energy produced is intermittent. The purpose is to produce the mechanical, non-thermal reactions of ultrasound by allowing for rest periods and subsequent cooling.[47] However, evidence is lacking that the non-thermal effects produced by pulsing have any advantage over the similar results produced by the continuous method.[31]

Ultrasound in musculoskeletal conditions

General indications and contraindications for ultrasound are the same as for therapeutic heat. Additional precautions include using ultrasound over laminectomy sites, the heart, brain, cervical ganglia, tumors, acute hemorrhage sites, pacemakers, infection sites and fluid filled cavities such as the eyes.[10] Its use is also contraindicated in pregnant women, over the uterus.

In general, ultrasound may be effective as a therapeutic modality in subacute and chronic inflammation. There is evidence to suggest that the use of ultrasound during acute inflammation may be detrimental to healing. Leung et al.[48] found increased levels of inflammatory mediators (PGE_2 and LTB_4) when ultrasound was used 2 days post-injury in rats with medial collateral ligament transections.

Pain control may occur by both thermal and non-thermal effects. Various studies have shown alteration in nerve conduction velocity after diathermy application, with the changes appearing to be related to energy intensity of the ultrasound field.[49–52] The presumption is that by altering the conduction velocity in the peripheral nervous system, analgesic effects may be obtained.

Studies have also documented increased levels of cortisol following ultrasound application to peripheral nerves. This release may provide increased anti-inflammatory effects.[53] However, Gnatz[54] found that ultrasound applied to the backs of two patients with documented lumbar disc herniation caused increased pain in a radicular pattern. Thus, any pain-relieving effects secondary to cortisol release may be overcome by the increased edema due to the deep heating effects of ultrasound.

The effectiveness of ultrasound

As with many of the physical modalities discussed in this chapter, the literature is unclear and often conflicting in regards to the effectiveness of ultrasound in treating a variety of musculoskeletal conditions.

Gam et al.[55] studied the effects of ultrasound, massage, and exercise in 58 patients with neck and shoulder myofascial trigger points. The first group received all three treatments. The second group received massage, exercise, and sham ultrasound. And, the third group was a control group receiving no treatment. Both of the treatment groups had significantly improved number of myofascial trigger points compared to the non-treatment control group, but there was no difference between the therapeutic ultrasound and the sham ultrasound groups.

van Der Heijden et al.[56] studied 180 patients with soft tissue shoulder disorders in a randomized, blinded, controlled trial comparing bipolar interferential electrotherapy to ultrasound as adjuvants to a supervised exercise program. All 180 subjects received exercise therapy: 73 subjects received active treatments, 72 subjects received dummy ultrasound and interferential electrotherapy, and 35 subjects received no adjuvants. At 6 week and 12-month follow-up, there was no apparent benefit seen in the ultrasound and electrotherapy groups *versus* the exercise program alone.

The effect of ultrasound on the treatment of calcific rotator cuff tendonitis has been studied by multiple groups. In a randomized, double-blinded, sham controlled study, Ebenbichler et al.[57] studied ultrasound therapy in 54 patients with radiographically confirmed calcific rotator cuff tendonitis. Thirty-two shoulders were treated with ultrasound and 29 shoulders were treated with sham ultrasound 5 times a week for the first 3 weeks, followed by 3 times a week for the following 3 weeks. At 6 weeks, the treatment group reported greater improvement in pain and quality of life; however, there was no significant difference at 9-month follow-up. Interestingly, 42% of the ultrasound treated shoulders demonstrated resolution of calcium deposits and 23% showed improvement. In contrast, the sham group showed calcium deposit resolution in only 8% and improvement in only 12% of subjects ($p = 0.002$). Perron and Malouin[58] however, did not find improvement with ultrasound and acetic acid iontophoresis above control for their smaller group of 22 patients with calcific shoulder tendonitis. Nykanen[59] also found no benefit in using ultrasound over sham ultrasound in 72 in-patients with shoulder pain in a randomized, double-blinded, sham controlled study. In a double-blinded, sham controlled study of ultrasound use for patients with subacromial bursitis, Downing and Weinstein[60] also found no significant benefit from treatment with ultrasound.

For a variety of other clinical entities, the evidence is again inconclusive. Binder et al.[61] studied the use of ultrasound *versus* sham ultrasound in the treatment of lateral epicondylosis. A total of 38 patients underwent ultrasound treatments (1 MHz, 1–2 W/cm^2) *versus* 38 patients receiving sham ultrasound for a diagnosis of lateral epicondylosis. There was a significant difference reported between the two groups. Twenty-four subjects in the treatment group *versus* only 11 in the sham group reported improvement. Other studies evaluating ultrasound as a treatment for lateral epicondylosis do not confirm such satisfactory results.[62–66] In addition, a focused review of four placebo controlled trials and the use of ultrasound in ankle sprains by Van der Windt et al.[67] does not support the use of ultrasound for acute ankle sprains. In this review, the magnitude of most treatment effects was small and of questionable clinical importance.

Regarding muscle pain and injury, Tiidus[68] reviewed the literature and found little data to support the use of ultrasound for postexercise muscle damage. However, there is conflicting evidence regarding whether ultrasound may be beneficial for delayed onset muscle soreness.[69,70] In addition, Wilkin et al.[71] studied the use of ultrasound in rats with a muscle contusion injury and found that ultrasound did not improve or hasten the regeneration of skeletal muscle following such an injury. In a similarly focused human study, Rantanen et al.[72] found ultrasound had no significant effect on the overall morphology of muscle regeneration following contusion injuries.

There is some evidence to suggest that ultrasound may hasten bone and tendon healing. Ramirez et al.[73] performed work with ultrasound and Achilles tendon injuries in neonatal rats.

They suggest that ultrasound stimulates collagen synthesis in tendon fibroblasts and stimulates cell division during phases of rapid cell growth. Jackson et al.[74] also found that ultrasound facilitated the rate of rat Achilles tendon repair by promoting synthesis of collagen which also proved to have a greater breaking strength. Enwemeka[75] found similar increased tensile strength in Achilles tendons of rabbits that were treated with ultrasound. In an attempt to determine whether ultrasound dosing impacted these findings, Ng et al.[76] found that both high and low dose ultrasound accelerated the healing process of ruptured Achilles tendons in rats.

In regards to bone healing, it has been reported that low-intensity pulsed ultrasound (LIPUS) at less than 0.1 W/cm, can reduce fracture healing times by between 30–38% as well as stimulate healing and union in up to 86% of non-united fractures.[77] Kristiansen et al.[78] studied 61 distal radius fractures in a multicenter, prospective clinical trial comparing low intensity, non-thermal pulsed ultrasound versus a placebo device. The ultrasound group experienced significantly faster radiographic fracture healing (mean of 61 days in treatment group versus 98 days in the placebo group). Brand et al.[79] used LIPUS in the treatment of eight patients with radiographically confirmed tibial stress fractures. The authors concluded that daily low-intensity pulsed ultrasound for 4 weeks was effective in improving pain relief and expediting early vigorous return to activity without bracing for posterior-medial stress fractures. This was not the case, however, for one anterior tibial stress fracture that required intramedullary nailing.

Multiple authors, through a review of the literature, conclude that there is little evidence to support the efficacy of ultrasound in the treatment of musculoskeletal disorders.[68,80–83] Taking the available literature as a whole, there is some evidence to support the use of ultrasound to improve tendon and bone healing. Less convincing evidence suggests a modest benefit of ultrasound in rotator cuff calcific tendonitis and lateral epicondylosis.

Phonophoresis

Phonophoresis is the use of ultrasound to increase the percutaneous absorption of a drug, usually an anti-inflammatory or anesthetic agents, for the management of pain and inflammation in musculoskeletal/sports-related injuries.

There are few randomized, controlled clinical trials documenting the effectiveness of phonophoresis. Initial experiments demonstrated that it is possible to drive cortisol ointment onto pig skin in situ with penetration into underlying muscle using ultrasonic energy at levels within the clinical range.[84] Newman et al.[85] reported that hypospray injection of cortisol followed by local application of ultrasonic energy showed an improvement in symptoms of shoulder bursitis compared with the use of ultrasound alone. Davick et al.[86] demonstrated that ultrasonically treated topical application of tritiated cortisol can lead to significant increases in cortisol penetration beyond the stratum corneum and into the viable epidermis as compared with topical cortisol alone. They concluded that once beyond the stratum corneum, the cortisol may penetrate over time and be absorbed into the deep soft tissue structures. Cagnie et al.[87] confirmed by biopsy (of knee

synovial and adipose tissue) that ketoprofen phonophoresis achieved higher local tissue concentration of the medication by using continuous or pulsed ultrasound with negligible systemic plasma levels.

Clinically, when comparing phonophoresis with iontophoresis of naproxen in treating lateral epicondylitis, there were significant improvements in pain scores and grip strength after treatment, but no significant differences were noted between the two groups.[88]

Despite the paucity of literature on phonophoresis, there are studies that call into question its effectiveness either alone or in comparison to other treatment modalities. Klaiman et al.[89] studied phonophoresis versus ultrasound in 49 patients with various soft tissue injuries in a randomized, double-blinded, uncontrolled trial. Each group underwent treatments 3 times a week for 3 weeks. Both treatment groups had decreased pain levels at the end of 3 weeks, but there was no significant difference between the treatment groups. Kozanoglu et al.[90] studied the effects of ibuprofen phonophoresis versus traditional ultrasound in patients with knee osteoarthritis. They found that both modalities were generally well tolerated and effective but that there was no significant difference in improvement rates between the two groups.

Other deep heating modalities

Other heat modalities not frequently used today include radiant heat, shortwave diathermy, and microwave diathermy. They will not be covered here, but are mentioned for historical reference.

THERAPEUTIC ELECTRICITY

Box 16.4: Key Points

- Electrical stimulation can be used to promote tissue healing, to stimulate muscle for edema reduction or muscle re-education, to slow muscle atrophy, to improve strength gains and to stimulate nerves for pain reduction.
- Contraindications to the use of therapeutic electricity include: use over cardiac pacemakers, electrical implants, carotid sinus, epiglottis, abdomen, gravid uterus, anesthetic areas, recent scars, areas where metal is embedded.

The use of therapeutic electricity dates back many centuries. One of the earliest accounts of the use of electricity for a musculoskeletal problem occurred in 1747, when a man with rheumatoid arthritis and involvement of the small joint in his hands received marked relief of his pain symptoms through the use of electricity.[91] Today, different forms of therapeutic electricity are used in the treatment of musculoskeletal and sports injuries. Electrical currents are used to promote healing of injured tissue, to stimulate muscles, to stimulate sensory nerves in treating pain, or to create an electrical field on the skin surface to drive ions beneficial to the healing process into or through the skin. This section will describe different forms of therapeutic electricity, the scientific basis for their use, their indications and contraindications, briefly describe the techniques used in their applications and elaborate on their use in sports medicine.

Electrical devices can put out either alternating current (AC or faradic), which is usually found in household appliances, or direct current (DC or galvanic), which is found in a generator or battery. Direct current can be continuous or intermittent, and can have different waveforms, frequencies, duration and amplitudes. Adjustments in any or all of these parameters will have an effect on the quality, type and form of stimulation received by the patient. Details of these parameters can be found in cited texts.[47]

It is important to note that muscle and nerve responses to electricity vary. Nerve tissue accommodates rapidly to current. Nerve stimulation requires a current which rises rapidly to maximum intensity. High frequencies and short durations are used. Sensory nerves respond to 100–150 cycles/s with a stimulus duration of 100 μs or shorter. Motor nerves respond to short duration (<500 μs) simulation of 25 cycles/s. Muscle tissue does not accommodate as rapidly. Muscle can be stimulated with very slowly rising currents. Lower frequency and longer duration stimulus are used in stimulating muscle as compared to nerve.

There are a number of contraindications to the use of electrical current in sports rehabilitation. Contraindications of electrical therapy include stimulation over cardiac pacemakers, electrical implants, carotid sinus, epiglottis, abdomen and gravid uterus.[10] Treatment should be avoided over any area that is anesthetic to avoid local burns. Recent scars in the area to be treated should also be avoided because of the potential for wound dehiscence. Any area where metal is embedded close to the skin in the area to be treated should be avoided for fear of concentrating the heat source at the metal surface. Any form of electricity should be avoided near an area of acute injury if active bleeding is still present to prevent worsening of the hemorrhage.

Electrical stimulation to promote tissue healing

Medical galvanism, or the use of galvanic stimulation, uses direct current modalities that deliver a unidirectional, uninterrupted current flow within the tolerance of the patient and without the destruction of tissue. This type of modality can be used to directly stimulate muscle following a nerve injury, to produce ionic changes within the tissues and decrease edema, or to introduce topically applied medications into the skin (iontophoresis).[92] The purpose of this electrical stimulation is primarily for the vasomotor effects, i.e. increased circulation. Under the electrodes, ions accumulate in the skin. The sensation experienced acts as a physiological stimulus to the sensory nerve endings, producing reflex vasodilatation.[93] These vasomotor effects can assist in resolution of inflammation, relief of pain, and reduction of interstitial edema through electro-osmosis and the shifting of water toward the electrical cathode.[47]

Direct, uninterrupted electric current tends to be quite uncomfortable and may cause superficial skin burns. For this

reason, a modification of the technique has been developed whereby the current is applied in an alternating or 'pulsed' manner, termed high voltage pulsed galvanic stimulation (HVPGS). Although the main use of HVPGS in sports rehabilitation is for relief of pain, it can also be used to aid in tissue healing.[94]

Electrical stimulation of muscle

Electrical stimulation of muscle is accomplished with either direct or alternating current, or a combination of the two. Alternating current is usually preferred to direct current because of greater patient comfort.[92] Muscles are stimulated for one of four reasons: (1) to aid in muscle pumping for edema reduction and tissue healing; (2) to re-educate muscle; (3) to retard atrophy in immobilized or partially denervated muscle; and (4) to enhance strength.

Certain general principles need to be adhered to when performing electrical stimulation of muscle.[95] Good contact should be maintained between the skin and the electrodes. The active electrode should be placed over the motor point of the muscle. The two electrodes used should generally be placed on the same side of the body. Finally, since denervated muscle does not have a motor point, the active electrode may be placed at the point that gives the best motor response, or the two electrodes may be placed, one at each end of the muscle so that the current will pass through the muscle and stimulate all of it.

Electrical stimulation for edema reduction and tissue healing

Electrically induced muscle contraction, such as that obtained with direct current or HVPGS, can be used to duplicate regular muscle contractions. These contractions help stimulate circulation by pumping blood through venous and lymphatic channels after acute injuries, when fluid accumulation is significant. Intermittent muscle contraction, which permits increased blood flow, may also produce relaxation of the muscles. Electrical stimulation of muscle contractions can allow resolution of inflammatory fluid, while keeping an injured joint protected. There has also been some suggestion that neuromuscular electrical stimulation can help in controlling edema after injury.[96–98] In order to be successful in reducing swelling, the current intensity must be high enough to provide a strong, comfortable muscle contraction. Therefore interrupted or surge type pulses must be used.[47]

Electrical stimulation for muscle re-education

Electrical muscle stimulation can be used for muscular re-education after sports injuries.[99] Muscular inhibition is quite common after traumatic injuries or surgery. Central nervous system inhibition is often the cause, as muscle contraction causes pain. The ultimate result is immobilization of the affected muscle. The injured patient or athlete may have a difficult time initiating contraction of an injured muscle because of the pain associated with movement and the lack of sensory input from that muscle due to disuse. Forcing the muscle to contract through electrical stimulation causes an increase in the sensory input from the muscle, allowing the patient to see the muscle contract. The patient then attempts to duplicate this muscular response.[47] The focus of this type of training is on kinetic training and the sensory awareness of muscular contraction. For muscle re-education to occur, the current intensity must be adequate for a muscle contraction, but not too uncomfortable for the athlete. High voltage galvanic stimulation or high frequency alternating current may be most effective.[47] Although the clinical implications are not clear, electrical muscle stimulation has been shown to selectively increase strength when applied to the abdominal muscles,[100] triceps brachii,[101] and erector spinae[102] and to improve motor performance in the deltoid, the pectoralis major and the abductor hallucis.[103,104]

Muscle stimulation for retardation of atrophy

Electrical muscle stimulation may help prevent strength losses as well as prevent muscular atrophy which occurs when a limb is immobilized. Stanish et al.[105] and Eriksson et al.[106] have shown that the biomechanical changes occurring in the muscles of immobilized limbs are retarded by electrical muscle stimulation. Eriksson and Haggmark[107] showed better muscle function in a group of patients after reconstruction of the anterior cruciate ligament when treated with electrical muscle stimulation and isometric exercise than with isometric exercise alone. In a study of rats and prevention of atrophy after 1 week of disuse, Yoshida et al.[108] found that twitch electrical stimulation was effective in preventing deterioration of maximum tension and oxidative capacity.

In general, it is agreed that electrical muscle stimulation programs are more effective than no exercise program, but not more effective than traditional strengthening exercise programs.[109–114] Snyder-Mackler et al.[115] showed there may be some additional benefit from using high intensity muscle stimulation in addition to an exercise program. They studied 110 patients following anterior cruciate ligament reconstruction and randomized them to receive high intensity neuromuscular electrical stimulation, high level volitional exercise, low intensity neuromuscular electrical stimulation, or combined high and low intensity neuromuscular stimulation in addition to a standard closed kinetic chain strengthening program. At 4 weeks, the high intensity stimulation group enjoyed the best quadriceps strength gains of 70% of the uninvolved side, as opposed to 57% in the high level volitional exercise group. Long-term benefits and other functional outcomes were not studied. Paternostro-Sluga et al.[116] also studied electrical stimulation after anterior cruciate ligament surgery. Postoperatively, patients received either neuromuscular stimulation treatment and early exercise therapy or an early exercise program alone. The researchers found no difference in measured isometric strength and isokinetic torque in both knee flexor and extensor muscle groups up to 52 weeks out from treatment.

While electrical stimulation retards denervation atrophy, its effect depends on the pulse duration, the frequency and intensity of current, the placement of the stimulating electrode, the duration and number of treatment sessions, the rest periods between the treatment sessions, and the resting length of the muscle during the stimulation. Further discussion of these parameters is beyond the scope of this chapter, but is well described by Licht.[91] Gibson et al.[117] suggest that electrical stimulation seems to prevent the fall in muscle protein synthesis that is related to immobility. Cabric et al.[118] found that lower frequency electrical stimulation (50 Hz) of muscle increased muscle fiber size which was thought to be correlated to proliferation of muscle cell nuclei.

Muscle stimulation for strength gains

In order to improve strength under any circumstance, either by electrically stimulating muscle or through voluntary contraction, maximal or near maximal contractions must occur to the point of muscle fatigue. Electrical stimulation is achieved by stimulating the motor nerve to a muscle by means of electrodes placed on the skin. Electrical stimulation can either increase the maximum contractile force in the muscle or it can recruit more fibers to contract with a given stimulus, thereby enhancing the strength of contraction.[119] When done via electrical stimulation, tetanic contractions (achieved at pulse rates above 20–30/s) are required for maximum muscle contraction. The discomfort of the stimulation remains a major limitation.[120] Most research to date indicates that, with few exceptions, maximal contractile forces can be produced by voluntary contractions as well.[119]

Significant strength gains in normal muscles have been described by Kots.[121] Kots' 'Russian' stimulation used an alternating type current of high pulse rate and high intensity to produce strong, involuntary muscle contraction with associated stimulation of local blood flow.[92] Perez et al.[122] reported biopsy proven changes in normal, healthy subjects who received short-term (6 weeks) electric stimulation to quadriceps muscles. Such changes included an increase in the muscle's oxidative capacity, changes in myosin heavy chain (MHC) composition, and a mean increase in the number of capillaries for fast twitch (type II) fibers with minimal muscle fiber hypertrophy. Whole body aerobic performance was not altered by electric stimulation. Yanagi et al.[123] performed a study in 12 healthy individuals. Training consisted of elbow flexion and extension exercises whereby volitional movements were countered by electrically stimulated antagonists. Controls received electrical stimulation without performing volitional muscle contraction. Elbow extension torques increased significantly in the limbs trained against electrically stimulated antagonists. Elbow flexion torques improved in both groups but did not reach statistical significance.

In summary, the literature suggests that electrical muscle stimulation may be helpful in strengthening normal muscle, preventing loss of muscle bulk and strength associated with immobilization, selective strengthening, enhancing motor control, and controlling edema after injury.[124] Again, individual clinical scenarios and desired outcomes must be weighed when deciding to use electrical muscle stimulation in the treatment of an injured athlete.

Electrical stimulation of nerves

The use of alternating and direct current for pain reduction via nerve stimulation is commonly used in the rehabilitation of

Box 16.5: Key Points

- Transcutaneous electrical nerve stimulation (TENS) is commonly used in sports rehabilitation for pain control. Electrodes can be applied around any painful area including: over specific dermatomes, myotomes or sclerotomes, close to specific spinal cord segments and over trigger points or acupuncture points.

- High frequency or low frequency TENS can be used. Each is thought to be effective by different pathways.

- No serious complications have been noted with the use of TENS.

- Interferential current is used in pain relief and is believed to allow for deeper tissue penetration.

- Percutaneous electrical nerve stimulation (PENS) is a technique where small gauged needles are placed in superficial tissue and muscle followed by stimulation with electrical impulses.

- Iontophoresis uses direct current to drive medicinal ions locally into the skin and mucous membranes.

sports injuries. The goal of nerve stimulation is to stimulate sensory nerves to change the patient's perception of a painful stimulus coming from an injured area. Nerves, being more sensitive to electrical current than muscle, are usually stimulated at high frequency and short duration. Three theories have been put forth to explain the analgesic effects of electrical stimulation: the gate-control theory, the central biasing theory and the opiate pain control theory.

Melzak and Wall proposed the gate-control theory in 1965.[125] It postulates that when large diameter afferent nerve fibers are electrically stimulated, painful stimuli arriving at the spinal cord through small fibers at the dorsal horn are blocked from transmission to the central nervous system where pain is perceived. By this mechanism, stimulation of these large fibers allows the 'gate' of painful signal transmission to be closed.

The central biasing theory also uses the idea of gating impulses. In this model, intense stimulation of smaller fibers (C fibers or pain fibers) at peripheral sites, for short periods, causes stimulation of descending neurons. These neurons effect further transmission of pain information by closing the gate at the spinal cord level.[47]

The opiate pain control theory is founded on the premise that endogenous opiates (enkephalins and β-endorphins) exist in our body systems. Electrical stimulation of peripheral sensory nerves may stimulate the release of these compounds from local sites throughout the central nervous system, providing pain relief.

A recent study also suggests that specific neurotransmitters, namely glycine and glutamate, may contribute to the effects of electrical nerve stimulation and perceived pain relief from such interventions.[126]

Transcutaneous electric nerve stimulation

Transcutaneous electric nerve stimulation (TENS) is defined as the application of electrical current therapy through the skin to a peripheral nerve or nerves for the control of pain.[119] TENS units are very commonly used in sports rehabilitation (Figs 16.4, 16.5). There are a number of advantages to using TENS. It is comfortable, fast-acting, can be used continuously, and can be used in a variety of pain syndromes. However, disadvantages do exist. Carry-over is often variable and adaptations may need to be made for continued benefit, i.e. increasing the pulse width or amplitude.

There are two major forms of TENS: high frequency and low frequency. High frequency TENS stimulates sensory nerves and causes an increase in pain threshold, although it does not stimulate the release of endorphins. Low frequency TENS will cause pain relief, which can be blocked by administration of opiate antagonists, implicating the opiate theory of pain control. It is sometimes likened to acupuncture. Walsh et al.[127] found that low frequency TENS (4 Hz) was the best in decreasing immediate pain visual analog scores for ischemically induced pain when comparing 4 Hz TENS, 110 Hz TENS, placebo and no treatment.

When applying electrodes for either type of TENS, electrodes may be placed on or around the painful area; over specific dermatomes, myotomes or sclerotomes that correspond to the painful area; close to the spinal cord segment that innervates a painful area; over trigger points or over acupuncture points. Chesterton et al.[13] studied normal subjects and their pain pressure thresholds in response to TENS. Volunteers were randomized into one of six experimental groups, a SHAM group or control. Two TENS frequencies (110 Hz or 4 Hz) and two intensities (strong but comfortable and highest tolerable) at a fixed duration (200 µs) were applied at three sites relative to a measurement site (segmentally, extra-segmentally or a combination of these). They found that high frequency, high intensity, segmental and combined stimulation groups showed significant hypoalgesic responses. The effect was sustained for 20 min post-stimulation. All other TENS intervention groups reached a level of hypoalgesic response similar to the sham group.

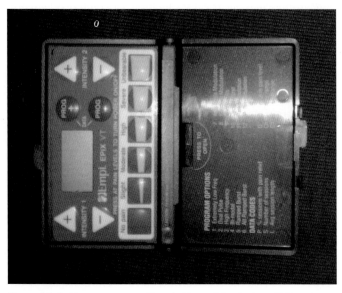

Figure 16.4 Transcutaneous Electric Nerve Stimulation (TENS) unit.

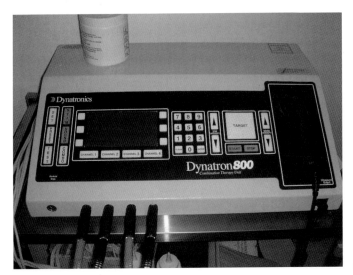

Figure 16.5 Combination ultrasound and stimulation unit.

No serious complications have been observed from the use of TENS.[91] Hypersensitivity of the skin has been observed in up to 10% of the patients, either due to the electrode or the electrode jelly. Minor burns were observed when high-frequency stimulation and high intensity stimulation were used at the same time. TENS should not be used in patients with pacemakers, stimulation should not be applied over the carotid sinus, and it should probably not be used during pregnancy, as the effects are unknown.[119]

The effectiveness of TENS

The efficacy of TENS is not clear-cut.[91,128] Thorsteinsson et al.[129] studied 93 patients with various disorders in a double blind, randomized, sham controlled, crossover study. A total of 49% of the TENS group *versus* 32% of the sham group reported partial or complete pain relief, but this difference was not statistically significant.

Ordog[130] studied 100 patients with acute traumatic disorders, including sprains, fractures, and contusions, in a randomized study comparing four groups: (1) active TENS plus acetaminophen/codeine, (2) sham TENS plus acetaminophen/codeine, (3) active TENS and (4) sham TENS. Pain levels in 2 days dropped 63% in the active TENS plus drug, 58% in the sham TENS plus drug, 45% in the active TENS and 17% in the sham TENS group. There was no statistical difference between the active TENS and the sham TENS plus drug suggesting that TENS may be as effective as acetaminophen/codeine for acute traumatic disorders.

The use of TENS in the treatment of back pain has been extensive, yet inconclusive. Lehmann et al.[131] studied 54 patients with chronic low back pain in a randomized study of active subthreshold TENS, sham TENS or electroacupuncture. They found that although all groups improved from baseline, there were no statistically significant differences between the groups at 6 months. Deyo et al.[132] studied 145 volunteers with chronic low back pain in a randomized trial comparing four groups: (1) active TENS, (2) sham TENS, (3) active TENS with exercise and (4) sham TENS with exercise. At 8 weeks following the 4-week treatment period, there were no significant differences between the active TENS groups and the sham TENS groups.

Marchand et al.[133] studied 43 patients with chronic low back pain in a randomized sham TENS (placebo) and no intervention ('nocebo') controlled study. Immediately after two treatments of 30 min each a week, the active TENS group showed a 43% reduction of pain intensity compared with a 17% reduction in the sham TENS group; this finding was statistically significant. Active TENS patients maintained significantly decreased pain intensity scores at 1 week compared with sham TENS patients. Both sham and active TENS groups' pain intensity scores were significantly better than the no treatment group at 3- and 6-month follow-ups, but there was no statistically significant difference between the sham TENS and active TENS groups.

Herman et al.[134] studied 58 work-related acute low back injuries of 3–10 weeks' duration in a randomized study of active TENS *versus* sham TENS. Both groups received the same exercise program. Outcome measures showed the active TENS group produced a drop in visual analog pain scores immediately after TENS, but showed no difference in disability, return to work rates, or pain scores at the 4-week follow-up.

In a study of chronic knee osteoarthritis pain, there were no significant differences noted in pain scores between groups receiving TENS, TENS with an exercise program, and an isometric exercise program alone after 4 weeks. However, in longer-term follow-up, reduction of knee pain was maintained in the TENS group but not in the exercise-alone group.[135]

Other groups have studied the effectiveness of TENS on post-procedural pain. TENS can be helpful for postoperative pain. Jensen et al.[136] showed that a group of patients treated with TENS following arthroscopic surgery experienced less pain, required less narcotics and regained strength more quickly than the control group. Sluka et al.[137] studied high intensity TENS and found it to be more effective in providing immediate pain relief than low intensity TENS for knee pain following injection. Likar et al.[138] studied the immediate, short-term use of TENS following shoulder surgery. The use of TENS had no significant impact on patients' reported pain with rest or activity, but there was clearly reduced analgesic consumption in the TENS group for the first 72 h postoperatively.

There is conflicting evidence about the use of TENS for relief of delayed onset muscle soreness.[139–142]

Overall, clinical experiences seem to show that TENS appears to give the best benefit in the treatment of early postoperative pain or pain from acute injuries. However, the response can be variable, unpredictable and short lived. It appears that TENS is not harmful, may sometimes provide pain relief above placebo response, is more effective in acute pain relief with short-term benefit, and is more effective at higher stimulation intensities.[128]

Interferential current

Interferential current (IFC) is another type of electrical stimulation that is used to control pain. Electric signals from two sets of electrodes with the same waveform are applied so that they arrive at the point to be stimulated from two directions. The area where the current overlaps is called the interference pattern, and the intensity summates in a manner that can be effective in modifying pain.[119] The frequency obtained at the interference pattern, through cancellation of some waveforms, allows stimulation of local muscle and nerve at a greater depth than if applied only from the surface at that point. Thus, interferential current uses high frequency carrier circuits to afford deeper penetration. The main use of interferential currents in sports is for pain reduction. Other clinical applications do include muscle stimulation, increased blood flow, and reduction of edema.

The effectiveness of interferential current

Minder et al.[143] studied the effects of interferential current on delayed onset muscle soreness (DOMS) and found no beneficial effects from the use of interferential current at different frequencies. Bircan et al.[144] studied the use of interferential current and low-frequency currents on quadriceps strengthening in healthy subjects. They found statistically significant increases in isokinetic quadriceps muscle strength in both groups as compared to controls. This increase did not differ between the two groups receiving electrical stimulation. In a study in 2003, home interferential current (IFC) therapy was used in patients having undergone anterior cruciate ligament reconstruction, meniscectomy, or knee chondroplasty versus a placebo group.[145] Outcomes were measured at 24, 28 and 72 h postoperatively as well as 1–8 weeks postoperatively. All IFC subjects reported significantly less pain with greater range of motion at all postoperative time points. ACL and meniscectomy IFC subjects experienced less edema at all time points while chondroplasty subjects also experienced less edema but not until 4 weeks postoperative.

Percutaneous electrical nerve stimulation

Percutaneous electrical nerve stimulation (PENS) combines the therapeutic effects of TENS and electroacupuncture. It is performed by placing small gauge needles (32 gauge) 2–4 cm into soft tissues and muscles, in a dermatomal distribution, followed by subsequent stimulation with electrical impulses (<25 mA at a frequency of 4 Hz).

The effectiveness of PENS

Ghoname et al.[146] investigated the efficacy of PENS. They studied 60 patients with stable, chronic, non-radicular low back pain from radiographically-confirmed degenerative disc disease in a randomized, single-blinded, sham controlled, crossover study. Each subject received all of the following four treatments in random order: sham-PENS, PENS, TENS, and exercise. Sham-PENS consisted of needle placement but no electrical stimulation. In the exercise-only group, patient's performed spinal flexion and extension while sitting in a chair. At 24 h, the PENS group showed significant improvements on pain, activity, sleep, sense of well-being, and narcotic usage scores as compared with the other three groups. Some 91% identified the PENS treatment as the preferred pain therapy and 81% identified it as a treatment for which they would be willing to pay extra. However, these results were short-lived and people returned to their baseline levels of pain, activity, sleep quality and oral analgesic use after 1 week without

treatment.[147] Ghoname et al.[146] also found that a stimulus frequency of alternating 15/30 Hz is more effective than 4 Hz or 100 Hz, implying that mixed high and low frequency treatment was more effective than either end-range alone. In addition, based on another study, this same group found that 30-min treatment sessions provided optimal results.[148]

Most other recent studies have also focused on the use of PENS in the treatment of low back pain. Hsieh et al.[149] found that a simple one-shot treatment with PENS and TENS in combination with oral analgesics provided similar immediate relief from low back pain complaints. In addition, no further differences between the two treatment groups appeared to emerge at 3 days to 1 week post-treatment. In a study of community-dwelling, older adults (age >65) with chronic low back pain, Weiner et al.[150] found that PENS plus PT resulted in a reduction in pain intensity and self-reported disability versus PT with sham PENS. These effects were maintained for the PENS plus PT group at the 3-month follow-up. Yokoyama et al.[151] studied PENS versus TENS in the treatment of chronic low back pain. They found that repeated PENS was more effective than TENS in achieving analgesia in chronic low back pain patients but that these effects gradually faded after the treatment was terminated. Their treatment effects were not sustained at the 2-month follow-up.

Iontophoresis: driving ions with electrical stimulation

Iontophoresis uses direct current to drive medicinal ions locally into the skin and mucous membranes (Fig. 16.6). Ions of the medicinal compounds are absorbed subcutaneously. This absorption occurs slowly into the local soft tissue, while some is ultimately absorbed systemically. Evidence for penetration much beyond the skin is variable and may depend on the particular substance.[152] James et al.[153] showed that percutaneous iontophoresis of 1% prednisolone sodium phosphate through human skin and nails gives peak plasma levels of about one third that produced by oral ingestion of 10 mg prednisolone. Similarly, Zankel et al.[154] showed that the absorption of the

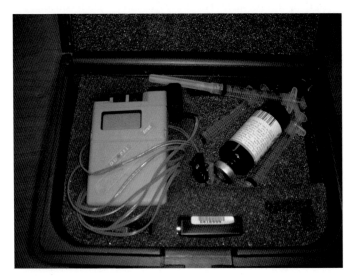

Figure 16.6 Iontophoresis unit.

negative ion I[131] through unbroken skin only occurred in those conditions which included iontophoresis. Bertolucci,[155] in a double blind study, found that patients below the age of 45 years with shoulder dysfunction related to primary tendonitis responded well to iontophoresis steroid administration, whereas the placebo group received no benefit from the iontophoretic treatment with sodium chloride. However, Chantraine et al.[156] in studies done both *in vivo* and *in vitro* failed to demonstrate the transcutaneous migration of corticosteroids with iontophoresis.

Iontophoresis has been used to drive multiple substances into the skin, some of which include calcium chloride, hydrocortisone, lithium chloride, lidocaine, and acetic acid. Theoretically, acetic acid replaces carbonate in calcium carbonate to become calcium acetate, which is blood soluble, thereby leaching the calcium away from the site of bony spur and inflammation. Japour et al.[157] reported very encouraging results using acetic acid iontophoresis in 35 patients with chronic heel pain in an uncontrolled case series. After only an average of 5.7 sessions over an average 2.8-week treatment period, 94% of patients reported relief of heel pain. Pain scores decreased from 7.5 to 1.8, and remained low at 27-month follow-up. Without a control group, however, it is not known whether these encouraging results are from treatment effect or the natural course of heel pain. Gudeman et al.[158] studied 0.4% dexamethasone iontophoresis in the treatment of 40 feet with plantar fasciitis in a randomized, double-blinded, placebo controlled trial. After six treatments over 2 weeks, the treatment group significantly improved, but were no different from placebo at one month follow-up. Taniguchi et al.[159] reported significantly increased pain threshold in 30 healthy volunteers with clonidine iontophoresis, as compared to amitriptyline and imipramine iontophoresis. The clinical implications of this finding are not known. Hasson et al.[160] studied 18 females with delayed onset muscle soreness with dexamethasone iontophoresis, placebo iontophoresis, and no treatment. Perceived muscle soreness was significantly less in the treatment group 48 h later, but no change in strength was noted.

The clinical effectiveness of iontophoresis is still debatable. Perron and Malouin[58] did not find improvement with ultrasound and acetic acid iontophoresis above controls in 22 patients with calcific shoulder tendonitis. Some of the claimed benefits for pain relief may be due to the effects of the direct current used as opposed to the medicinal compounds purportedly driven into the circulation. Few side-effects have been described other than drug sensitivity and sensitive skin.

TRACTION

Traction is the technique in which a distractive force is applied to a part of the body to stretch soft tissues and to separate joint surfaces or bone fragments.[161] Cyriax popularized traction in the 1950s as a treatment for lumbar disc lesions. Prior to that, traction was mainly used in the treatment of fractures. Over the years, traction has gained some popularity in the field of sports rehabilitation, particularly with respect to cervical and lumbosacral spine injuries.

Box 16.6: Key Points

- Traction uses a distraction force to stretch soft tissues and separate joint surfaces for pain relief.
- Cervical traction can be used for a number of cervical spine injuries including: cervical herniated nucleus pulposus, radiculopathy, zygapophyseal joint syndromes and myofascial pain.
- Contraindications to the use of cervical spine traction include: an unstable spine, ligamentous instability, vertebrobasilar artery insufficiency, atlantoaxial instability, rheumatoid arthritis, osteomyelitis, cauda equina syndrome and myelopathy.
- Lumbar spine traction is more challenging since the necessary traction load to achieve vertebral separation is much greater than in the cervical spine.

Cervical traction

Cervical traction is used for a number of cervical spine injuries including cervical herniated nucleus pulposus, radiculopathy, strains, zygapophyseal joint syndromes and myofascial pain (Fig. 16.7). The main reason for its use is relief of pain. Pain relief may occur through one of several mechanisms, including: rest through immobilization and support of the head, distraction of the zygapophyseal joints and associated improved

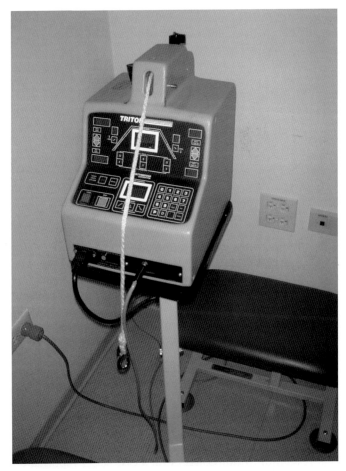

Figure 16.7 Office cervical traction machine.

nutrition to the articular cartilage, tightening of the longitudinal ligament and decreasing intradiscal pressure (both of which press a bulging disc more centrally), relieving nerve root pressure via increased foraminal diameter, improving head posture, and elongating muscles to improve blood flow and reduce spasm.

Determination as to whether the patient has any contraindications to cervical traction is the first step in its administration. Contraindications to the use of spinal traction include an unstable spine, ligamentous instability, vertebrobasilar artery insufficiency, atlantoaxial instability, rheumatoid arthritis, osteomyelitis, discitis, neoplasm, severe osteoporosis, untreated hypertension, severe anxiety, cauda equina syndrome and myelopathy.[162] Before it is prescribed, the examiner may find it helpful to first try manual traction to better predict the therapeutic response they can expect.

To achieve separation of spinal segments, a force of significant magnitude and duration must be exerted. Traction can be delivered manually, through weights and pulleys or via a mechanical device. The direction of pull can be vertical, horizontal or at an angle. Traction can be performed while the patient is standing, sitting, lying on a horizontal or inclined plane, or in the prone or supine position. Traction can be continuous, sustained, intermittent or intermittent-pulsed. Surface resistance to traction is dependent on the weight of the body or body segment undergoing traction and the size, quality, contour and texture of the two surfaces in contact.[161]

With cervical traction, the optimal angle of pull (to obtain the most distractive force with the least weight) is 20–30° of head flexion. The supine position may be more effective than sitting, as it allows more relaxation. In the supine position, the force must be sufficient enough to overcome friction and must have a pull of at least half the weight of the head. Eight to ten pounds is a usual starting point. In sitting, the pull must be sufficient to support the head. Usually 25–40 pounds is necessary.

Cervical traction can be continuous or intermittent. Continuous traction will allow quieting of the stretch reflex and decrease muscle guarding. It will also allow separation of the posterior structures (zygapophyseal joints) if maintained for at least 7 s at a time. Intermittent traction is believed to act by cyclically causing muscle contraction and relaxation thereby increasing blood flow in a 'massage-like' action.

The effectiveness of cervical traction

Zylbergold and Piper[163] studied 100 patients with disorders of the cervical spine in a randomized, controlled trial comparing static traction, intermittent traction, manual traction, and no traction. At 6 weeks, all groups improved significantly compared to baseline, but the intermittent traction group scored significantly better than the no traction group in pain and cervical range of motion measures. In a retrospective study, Swezey et al.[164] showed that 81% of their 58 patients with cervical spondylosis had symptomatic relief with home cervical traction. In a small case series of four patients with large volume cervical disc herniations and symptoms of radiculopathy, Constantoyannis et al.[165] treated them with home intermittent cervical traction. All four patients experienced complete symptom resolution within 3 weeks. In a case series reported by Moeti and Marchetti in 2001,[166] patients with cervical radicu-

lar symptoms of <12 weeks' duration demonstrated a reduction in pain and perceived disability in response to intermittent cervical traction.

Lumbar traction

The traction load necessary to produce vertebral separation in the lumbar spine is much greater than that required to produce vertebral separation in the cervical spine. de Seze and Levernieux[167] estimated that a tractive force of 730 pounds was required to obtain a separation of 1.5 mm at the L4–5 vertebral level and that 810 pounds were required to obtain a separation of 2 mm at the L3–4 level. Numerous other studies confirm the need for great force to obtain even a small separation in the lumbar spine.[168,169] Clinically, lumbar traction functions to significantly limit the activity of the patient. It may assist to decrease muscle spasm by forcing rest. There is no evidence that lumbar traction facilitates nuclear migration of the disc.

The set up for lumbar traction is similar to cervical traction except that a corset, rather than a head halter, is used. Several types of lumbar traction are described including gravity inversion traction, gravity lumbar reduction and auto-traction. Inversion traction must be avoided in patients with hypertension or retinal problems because of the potential for increasing blood pressure and retinal pressures. Generally, at least one-quarter of the body weight must be used just to overcome the friction of lumbar traction. The maximum force that a patient can tolerate is often used.[161] Meszaros et al.[170] attempted to determine the effects of three different amounts of force (10%, 30% and 60% body weight) on pain free mobility as measured by a straight leg raise (SLR) test. The mean SLR measurements significantly increased from pre-traction levels for both the 30% and 60% of body weight traction groups but not the 10% body weight group.

Although ample experimental evidence that a traction force of sufficient magnitude and duration applied to the spine produces separation of the vertebrae and zygapophyseal joints and increases the size of the foramen, no clear scientific evidence of its therapeutic value has been reported in the few controlled studies to date.[161] Christie's[171] controlled study of traction in the treatment of acute and chronic lumbar pain – with and without root signs – showed that traction, when effective, was most useful in patients with chronic backaches with root signs. Weber's[172] double-blinded, controlled study of patients with sciatica from a prolapsed disc treated with traction or simulated traction failed to show any significant difference in pain, mobility of the lumbar spine, or the presence of neurologic signs in either group. Beurskens et al.[173] studied 151 patients with nonspecific low back pain in a randomized, sham controlled trial and showed no difference between the treatment and control groups. van der Heijden et al.[174] reviewed only randomized clinical trials studying traction. Beneficial effects of lumbar traction were suggested in only 3 of 14 randomized studies and in only 1 of the 11 studies that the authors considered to be of better quality. They concluded that there was no evidence to support or refute the use of traction. In a study of lumbar traction combined with physical therapy versus physical therapy alone, Borman et al.[175] did not find any significant difference in global improvement, improvement in disability scores or improvement in pain scores between the two groups.

Although hard data supporting the use of traction is not available, many clinicians and patients will speak of its many benefits. Some of these positive experiences may be related to enforced bed rest or the effects of some active intervention for their back complaints. Cheatle and Esterhai[176] surveyed 369 orthopedic surgeons and 165 physiatrists about their use of pelvic traction. A total of 28% of the responding physicians said they would prescribe traction. The chief rationale (54% of respondents) of this prescription is to ensure bedrest.

MAGNETIC THERAPY

Box 16.7: Key Points

- Magnetic therapy is used by many athletes for pain relief.

- Studies have suggested that it may also be useful for delayed bone healing.

- Contraindications include: use in patients with allergies to metals, use in patients with a pacemaker and use in patients with implanted defibrillators.

For centuries, magnetic therapy has been used for pain relief and is replete with anecdotal successes. The strongest scientific evidence in support of the therapeutic use of magnetic fields in treating musculoskeletal disorders involves using pulsating magnetic fields of strengths over 10 gauss. The World Health Organization reported that there is no available evidence to show adverse effects on humans exposed to static magnetic fields up to two Tesla, which is equal to 20 000 gauss. Typically, most over-the-counter magnets that are purchased by patients generate a magnetic field of 250–500 gauss.

Regarding the therapeutic effectiveness of magnets, the mechanism of action is unknown.[177] Increased peripheral blood flow has been proposed as a mechanism of action.[178–180] The increased blood flow may also be associated with changes in fibroblast concentration, fibrin fibers, and collagen at wound sites.[181] Other postulates include blockage of action potentials such as those that transmit pain signals,[182] the role of water,[183] resonance, ions, induction, subatomic magnetic field interactions and closed electrical circuits within endothelium.[184]

Contraindications to magnetic therapy include use in patients with a pacemaker or implanted defibrillator and in those with an allergy to metals. Some practitioners recommend not using magnets near the abdomen before one hour after eating, since the magnets may affect the blood flow in the digestive tract. As well, some people have reported feeling light-headed when wearing magnets placed near the carotid arteries.

The effectiveness of magnetic therapy

Pulsating electromagnetic field therapy has shown some promise in the treatment of osteoarthritis of the knee and spine.[185,186] Trock et al.[186] studied 86 subjects with knee osteoarthritis and 81 subjects with cervical spondylosis in a randomized, double-blinded, placebo controlled trial. The group treated with pulsating electromagnetic fields (10–20 gauss) showed significant changes from baseline at a follow up interval of one month. This change was not seen in the placebo group. Foley-Nolan et al.[187] studied the use of pulsating electromagnetic therapy in acute whiplash syndrome. Twenty patients wore active pulsed electromagnetic therapy collars and 20 patients wore placebo collars for 8 h a day. The treatment group had significantly improved pain complaints at 2 and 4 weeks compared with placebo. Pujol et al.[188] randomized a small group of 30 patients to receive 40 min of real or sham current magnetic coil stimulation over localized tender body regions. Post-procedure pain scores decreased by 59% in the treatment group versus 14% in the sham group. This finding reached statistical significance. Gross et al.[189] reviewed the use of electromagnetic therapy in the treatment of mechanical neck disorders. The studies that they reviewed suggested that the daily (8 h) use of electromagnetic therapy for 3–4 weeks produced significant reductions in pain complaints.

The healing rate of non-union fracture can be improved with pulsating high magnetic fields.[190,191] Sharrard et al.[192] studied electromagnetic therapy in the treatment of delayed union tibial shaft fractures using active electromagnetic stimulation units in 20 patients versus dummy control units in 25 patients. Nine subjects in the treatment group and only three subjects in the control group showed union of the fracture, which was a statistically significant finding.

Not all studies support the use of magnet therapy in musculoskeletal disorders. In a study of magnet therapy and wrist pain attributed to carpal tunnel syndrome, Carter et al.[193] found that use of a 1000 gauss magnet worn over the carpal tunnel area for 45 min was no more effective than placebo in decreasing pain, numbness, burning or tingling when compared with placebo. Collacott et al.[194] reported on the use of bipolar magnets in 20 patients with chronic low back pain in a randomized, double-blind placebo controlled crossover study. They did not find any significant difference in pain complaints nor lumbar range of motion in either the real or sham magnet group.

There are fewer studies to support the use of static magnets. Washnis[195] cites a multitude of studies using static magnets, but few have been randomized, double-blinded, placebo-controlled trials appearing in peer-reviewed journals.[196]

In general, the literature on the use of magnets in sports-related injuries and musculoskeletal care is sparse and conflicting. Nonetheless, as clinicians we are obligated to know about this highly sought after treatment as it continues to be a popular adjunct treatment by many lay people that we treat.

ACUPUNCTURE

Although not thought of as a physical modality in the traditional sense, acupuncture is an enduring alternative medical treatment utilized by many throughout the world. Acupuncture is commonly sought as a treatment for acute and chronic musculoskeletal disorders to provide pain relief, improve quality of life, reduce the use of medications, avoid surgery and maintain health and fitness.[197,198] Williamson et al.[198] surveyed older adults (age >65) on their use of complementary and alternative medicine. Acupuncture was among the most commonly used therapies (33%) in addition to massage, chiropractic treatment and herbal medications.

Multiple schools of thought regarding acupuncture exist, but the most prominent and well-established are the Chinese, Japanese and French teachings. The theory behind traditional Chinese acupuncture lies in the concept of Qi, a 'life force' which circulates through meridians (acupuncture channels) to nourish and protect the body. If the Qi is out of balance, then pain and disease results. Therefore, the goal of acupuncture is to rebalance Qi to promote healing. Many traditional Chinese practitioners believe that in order for acupuncture to be effective, one must obtain a sensation known as 'de Qi' when the needles are inserted. It is a subjective sensation of the 'muscle grabbing onto the needle' that signals when the body's energy has been contacted.[199]

For musculoskeletal pain, acupuncture treatment typically consists of using needles (typically 32 gauge) in precise points that lie along meridians or points that are painful to palpation (Ah Shi points). The needle are stimulated by manual manipulation, electrical stimulation (electroacupuncture (EA)), or heat to promote the movement of energy in order to rebalance Qi.[199]

The mechanism of action behind acupuncture is unclear. Evidence exists to support both endorphin release as well as engagement of descending inhibitory pathways as contributing mechanisms for pain relief.[199] Regarding electroacupuncture, there is also an involvement of humeral factors, as suggested by cross-perfusion experiments; involvement of endorphins as suggested by the prevention of EA-induced analgesia by naloxone; and the release of endorphins into the CSF as shown in both human and animal models.[200] As well, with electroacupuncture, different frequencies result in the release of different neuropeptides. Low frequencies result in a release of enkephalin, β-endorphin and endomorphin while high frequency electric stimulation results in a more selective release of dynorphin. However, using the two frequencies in combination can result in the simultaneous release of all four opioid peptides, theoretically leading to maximal therapeutic affect.[201] Some researchers have attempted to study the central effects of electro-acupuncture. Zhang et al.[202] studied EEG changes before, during and after electric acupoint stimulation and found a modulation in multiple ipsi- and contralateral cortical areas compared with controls. Using functional MRI to study central responses to real and sham electroacupuncture, Wu et al.[203] also found multiple cortical and sub-cortical areas that were activated. Both sham (stimulation at non-meridian points) and real electroacupuncture activated a reported 'pain neuromatrix'; however, real electroacupuncture elicited significantly higher activation of the hypothalamus and primary somatosensory-motor cortex with deactivation of the anterior cingulated cortex. Therefore, the hypothalamic-limbic system seems to be significantly modulated by EA at acupoints rather than at non-meridian points. Of note, there is some feeling that PENS should be considered, at most, a variation of electroacupuncture rather than a novel form of therapy. This stems from the fact that electroacupuncture and PENS share

similarities including stimulation parameters, the selection of treatment points and reported efficacy.[204]

Auricular acupuncture is a more contemporary practice, which involves the placement of needles at non-meridian points on the ear. It is based on a somatotopic system organized on the external ear which reflects innervation of different regions of the body. It can be used alone or in combination with meridian-based treatment to augment the potency of the latter.[199]

Effectiveness of acupuncture treatments

Sator-Katzenschlager et al.[205] in a study of auricular electroacupuncture in the treatment of chronic cervical pain found significant reduction in pain scores as well as improvement in psychological well-being, activity and sleep in those patients receiving electrical simulation of auricular acupuncture points versus those undergoing manual auricular acupuncture. A similar study by Sator-Katzenschlager et al.[206] looked at the use of continuous low frequency auricular acupuncture versus manual auricular acupuncture in patients with chronic low back pain and inadequate relief on oral medications. Again, pain relief was significantly better in the group receiving electroacupuncture during the study and during the 3-month follow-up period. The consumption of analgesic rescue medications and the number of patients who returned to work was improved in the electroacupuncture group as well.

In a small, evaluator-blinded study of patients with chronic low back pain (>6 weeks duration), Tsukayama et al.[207] found electroacupuncture to be more effective at short-term pain relief than TENS after a 2-week trial period. During this study, all patients received 'conservative orthopedic treatment' (COT), which included physical therapy, back school and diclofenac. In addition, one group was treated with acupuncture and another group with sham needling. In the whole sample, there was an overall improvement in pain relief of >50% on visual analogue scales (VAS) at the end of the treatment protocol. There was a significant difference between the two treatment groups, however. The acupuncture + COT group had a change of 65% on VAS while sham + COT group reported improvement in pain relief scores of 34%.

Carlsson and Sjolund[208] studied the long-term effect of acupuncture (both electroacupuncture and manual acupuncture) on chronic low back pain. They found long-term improvement (at 6 months follow-up) in patients that received both forms of acupuncture in comparison with controls.

In a randomized trial studying the effects of massage and acupuncture in the treatment of chronic low back pain, Kalauokalani et al.[209] found that patient expectations seems to influence clinical outcomes independent of the treatment itself. Patients who expected a greater benefit from massage than from acupuncture were more likely to experience better outcomes with massage than with acupuncture and vice versa. On a greater scale, these expectations likely confound most studies where a specific intervention or treatment is involved and highlights the need to control for the non-specific 'placebo' effect.

Green et al.[210] reviewed the use of acupuncture in treating lateral elbow pain and found that there was inconclusive evidence in the literature to support or refute the use of acupuncture in treating lateral elbow pain. Two small trials, which could not be combined for meta-analysis, showed short-term benefits not lasting >24 h. Tsui and Leung[211] studied manual acupuncture *versus* electroacupuncture in a similar population with chronic 'tennis elbow'. Subjects received either of the two treatments 3 times per week for 2 weeks. After the 2 weeks, there was significantly greater pain relief (as measured by VAS) and pain free hand grip strength in the electroacupuncture group compared with the manual acupuncture group.

Kleinhenz et al.[212] studied 52 athletes with rotator cuff tendonitis. The treatments included acupuncture with penetration of the skin *versus* a placebo needling. The acupuncture group showed significant improvement after eight treatment sessions in comparison with the control groups.

Koo et al.[213] studied an animal model of ankle sprain and the effect of electroacupuncture on this model. Electro-acupuncture produced a 40% recovery in stepping force of the sprained foot. This improvement was interpreted as an analgesic effect since this same improvement was noted with systemic administration of 2 mg/kg of morphine.

In an interesting study undertaken by Akimoto et al.[214] the physiological and psychological effects of acupuncture were studied in elite female soccer players during extended competition. Subjects were divided into a treatment group (those who received acupuncture) and a control group. In the treatment group, acupuncture stimulus was applied at four specific points 4 h after each game during a competition period. Measured outcomes included cortisol levels in the saliva, salivary secretory immunoglobulin A (SIgA) levels, subjective ratings of physical well-being and a profile of mood status. They found that exercise induced changes such as decreased SIgA and increased salivary cortisol were inhibited by acupuncture. Subjects also reported improved subjective ratings of muscle tension and fatigue.

As with many other modalities highlighted in this chapter, the evidence as to the effectiveness of acupuncture is inconclusive at times. In general, the use of acupuncture can be considered a reasonable adjuvant in the treatment of musculoskeletal pain complaints, especially since it is a treatment that is generally well-tolerated with few adverse side-effects.

CONCLUSION

The use of therapeutic modalities is commonplace in the treatment of both acute and chronic musculoskeletal injuries. The rational use of such physical modalities within a comprehensive rehabilitation program requires an understanding of their proposed mechanism of action as well as indications and contraindications for each. Effectiveness of these passive approaches is highly variable. The individual patient and their response to any given individual treatment program is the best guide to their use.

REFERENCES

1 Nadler SF, Prybicien M, Malanga GA, Sicher D. Complications from therapeutic modalities: results of a national survey of athletic trainers. Arch Phys Med Rehabil 2003; 84:849-853.

2 Chambers R. Clinical uses of cryotherapy. Phys Ther 1969; 49:245-249.

3 McMaster W. Cryotherapy. Phys Sportsmed 1982; 10:112-119.

4 Lehmann J, de Lateur B. Cryotherapy. In: Lehmann J, ed. Therapeutic heat and cold. Baltimore: Williams & Wilkins; 1982:563-602.

5 Ork H. Uses of cold. In: Kuprian W, ed. Physical therapy for sports. Philadelphia: Saunders; 1982:62-68.

6 Hocutt JE, Jr. Cryotherapy. Am Fam Physician 1981; 23:141-144.

7 Quillen W, Rouillier L. Initial management of acute ankle sprains with rapid pulsed pneumatic compression and cold. J Orthop Sports Phys Ther 1982; 4:39-43.

8 Sloan J, Giddings P, Hain R. Effects of cold and compression on edema. Phys Sportsmed 1988; 16:116-120.

9 Drez D, Faust DC, Evans JP. Cryotherapy and nerve palsy. Am J Sports Med 1981; 9:256-257.

10 Basford J. Physical agents. In: DeLisa J, Gans B, eds. Rehabilitation medicine principles and practices. Philadelphia: Lippincott-Raven; 1998:483-520.

11 Halvorson G. Principles of rehabilitating sports injuries. In: Teitz C, ed. Scientific foundations of sports medicine. Toronto: Decker; 1989:345-371.

12 MacAuley D. Do textbooks agree on their advice on ice? Clin J Sport Med 2001; 11:67-72.

13 Chesterton LS, Foster NE, Wright CC, Baxter GD, Barlas P. Effects of TENS frequency, intensity and stimulation site parameter manipulation on pressure pain thresholds in healthy human subjects. Pain 2003; 106:73-80.

14 Roy S, Irvin R. Sports medicine prevention, evaluation, management and rehabilitation. Englewood Cliffs: Prentice Hall; 1983.

15 Mennell JM. The therapeutic use of cold. J Am Osteopath Assoc 1975; 71:1146-1158.

16 Travell J, Simons D. Myofascial pain and dysfunction: The trigger point manual. Baltimore: Williams & Wilkins; 1983.

17 Simons D, Travell J, Simons L. Protecting the ozone layer. Arch Phys Med Rehabil 1990; 71:64.

18 Vallentyne SW, Vallentyne JR. The case of the missing ozone: are physiatrists to blame? Arch Phys Med Rehabil 1988; 69:992-993.

19 Ohkoshi Y, Ohkoshi M, Nagasaki S, et al. The effect of cryotherapy on intraarticular temperature and postoperative care after anterior cruciate ligament reconstruction. Am J Sports Med 1999; 27:357-362.

20 Lessard LA, Scudds RA, Amendola A, Vaz MD. The efficacy of cryotherapy following arthroscopic knee surgery. J Orthop Sports Phys Ther 1997; 26:14-22.

21 Levy A, Marmar E. The role of cold compression dressings in the postoperative treatment of total knee arthroplasty. Clin Orthop Relat Res 1993; 297.

22 Speer K, Warren R, Horowitz L. The efficacy of cryotherapy in the postoperative shoulder. J Bone Jt Surg 1996; 77:62-68.

23 Konrath GA, Lock T, Goitz HT, Scheidler J. The use of cold therapy after anterior cruciate ligament reconstruction. A prospective, randomized study and literature review. Am J Sports Med 1996; 24:629-633.

24 Levy A, Kelly B, Lintner S, Speer K. Penetration of cryotherapy in treatment after shoulder arthroscopy. Arthroscopy 1997; 13:461-464.

25 Paddon-Jones DJ, Quigley BM. Effect of cryotherapy on muscle soreness and strength following eccentric exercise. Int J Sports Med 1997; 18:588-593.

26 Yackzan L, Adams C, Francis KT. The effects of ice massage on delayed muscle soreness. Am J Sports Med 1986; 12:159-165.

27 Fu FH, Cen HW, Eston RG. The effects of cryotherapy on muscle damage in rats subjected to endurance training. Scand J Med Sci Sports 1997; 7:358-362.

28 Safran MR, Zachazewski JE, Benedetti RS, Bartolozzi AR 3rd, Mandelbaum R. Lateral ankle sprains: a comprehensive review part 2: treatment and rehabilitation with an emphasis on the athlete. Med Sci Sports Exerc 1999; 31:438-447.

29 Myrer JW, Draper DO, Durrant E. Contrast therapy and intramuscular temperature in the human leg. J Athl Training 1994; 29:318-325.

30 Cox J, Andrish J, Indelicato P, Walsh W. Heat modalities. In: Drez D, ed. Therapeutic modalities for sports injuries. Chicago: Year Book Medical Publishers; 1986:1-23.

31 Lehmann J, de Lateur B. Therapeutic heat. In: Lehmann J, ed. Therapeutic heat and cold. Baltimore: Williams & Wilkins; 1982:404-562.

32 Fountain F, Gersten J, Sengir O. Decrease in muscle spasm produced by ultrasound, hot packs, and infrared radiation. Arch Phys Med Rehabil 1960; 41:293-298.

33 Lehmann J, Masock A, Warren C, Koblanski J. Effect of therapeutic temperatures on tendon extensibility. Arch Phys Med Rehabil 1970; 51:481-486.

34 Warren CG, Lehmann JF, Koblanski JN. Elongation of rat tail tendon: effect of load and temperature. Arch Phys Med Rehabil 1971; 52:465-474.

35 Warren CG, Koblanski JN, Sigelmann RA. Ultrasound coupling media: their relative transmissivity. Arch Phys Med Rehabil 1976; 57:218–222.

36 Taylor B, Waring C, Brachear T. The effects of therapeutic application of heat or cold followed by static stretch on hamstring muscle length. J Orthop Sports Phys Ther 1995; 21:283–286.

37 Timm KE. A randomized-control study of active and passive treatments for chronic low back pain following L5 laminectomy. J Orthop Sports Phys Ther 1994; 20:276–286.

38 Lehmann JF, Silverman DR, Baum BA, Kirk NL, Johnston VC. Temperature distributions in the human thigh, produced by infrared, hot pack and microwave applications. Arch Phys Med Rehabil 1966; 47:291–299.

39 Michlovitz S. Biophysical principles of heating and superficial heat agents. In: Michlovitz S, Wolf S, eds. Thermal agents in rehabilitation. Philadelphia: FA Davis; 1986:99–118.

40 Konlian C. Aquatic therapy: Making a wave in the treatment of low back injuries. Orthop Nurs 1999; 18:11–20.

41 Hall J, Skevington SM, Maddison PJ, Chapman K. A randomized and controlled trial of hydrotherapy in rheumatoid arthritis. Arthritis Care Res 1996; 9:206–215.

42 Stener-Victorin E, Kruse-Smidje C, Jung K. Comparison between electro-acupuncture and hydrotherapy, both in combination with patient education and patient education alone, on the symptomatic treatment of osteoarthritis of the hip. Clin J Pain 2004; 20:179–185.

43 Norton C, Shaha S, Stewart L. Aquatic versus traditional therapy: contrasting effectiveness of acquisition rates. Salt Lake City: Orthopedic Specialty Hospital; 1996.

44 Lehmann J, de Lateur B. Diathermy and superficial heat and cold therapy. In: Kottke F, Stillwell G, Lehmann J, eds. Krusen's handbook of physical medicine and rehabilitation. Philadelphia: Saunders; 1982:275–350.

45 Santiesteban A. Physical agents and musculoskeletal pain. In: Gould J, Davies G, eds. Orthopedic and sports physical therapy. St Louis: Mosby; 1985:199–211.

46 Balmaseda MT Jr, Fatehi MT, Koozekanani SH and Lee AL. Ultrasound therapy: a comparative study of different coupling media. Arch Phys Med Rehabil 1986; 67:147–150.

47 Prentice W. Therapeutic modalities in sports medicine. St Louis: Times Mirror/Mosby College Publishing; 1986.

48 Leung MC, Ng GY, Yip KK. Effect of ultrasound on acute inflammation of transected medial collateral ligaments. Arch Phys Med Rehabil 2004; 85:963–966.

49 Currier DP, Greathouse D, Swift T. Sensory nerve conduction: effect of ultrasound. Arch Phys Med Rehabil 1978; 59:181–185.

50 Halle JS, Scoville CR, Greathouse DG. Ultrasound's effect on the conduction latency of the superficial radial nerve in man. Phys Ther 1981; 61:345–350.

51 Madsen P, Gersten J. The effect of ultrasound in conduction velocity of peripheral nerve. Arch Phys Med Rehabil 1961; 42:645–649.

52 Zankel HT. Effect of physical agents on motor conduction velocity of the ulnar nerve. Arch Phys Med Rehabil 1966; 47:787–792.

53 Griffin J, Touchstone J, Liu A. Ultrasonic movement of cortisol into pig tissues, II. Movement into paravertebrae nerve. Am J Phys Med Rehabil 1965; 41:20–25.

54 Gnatz SM. Increased radicular pain due to therapeutic ultrasound applied to the back. Arch Phys Med Rehabil 1989; 70:493–494.

55 Gam AN, Warming S, Larsen LH, et al. Treatment of myofascial trigger-points with ultrasound combined with massage and exercise – a randomised controlled trial. Pain 1998; 77:73–79.

56 Van Der Heijden GJ, Leffers P, Wolters PJ, et al. No effect of bipolar interferential electrotherapy and pulsed ultrasound for soft tissue shoulder disorders: a randomised controlled trial. Ann Rheum Dis 1999; 58:530–540.

57 Ebenbichler GR, Erdogmus CB, Resch KL, et al. Ultrasound therapy for calcific tendinitis of the shoulder. N Engl J Med 1999; 340:1533–1538.

58 Perron M, Malouin F. Acetic acid iontophoresis and ultrasound for the treatment of calcifying tendinitis of the shoulder: a randomized control trial. Arch Phys Med Rehabil 1997; 78:379–384.

59 Nykanen M. Pulsed ultrasound treatment of the painful shoulder a randomized, double-blind, placebo-controlled study. Scand J Rehabil Med 1995; 27:105–108.

60 Downing DS, Weinstein A. Ultrasound therapy of subacromial bursitis. A double blind trial. Phys Ther 1986; 66:194–199.

61 Binder A, Hodge G, Greenwood AM, Hazleman BL, Page Thomas DP. Is therapeutic ultrasound effective in treating soft tissue lesions? BMJ 1986; 290:512–514.

62 Halle J, Franklin R, Karalfa B. Comparison of four treatment approaches for lateral epicondylitis of the elbow. J Orthop Sports Phys Ther 1986; 8:62–69.

63 Lundeberg T, Abrahamsson P, Haker E. A comparative study of continuous ultrasound, placebo ultrasound and rest in epicondylalgia. Scand J Rehabil Med 1988; 20:99–101.

64 Haker E, Lundeberg T. Pulsed ultrasound treatment in lateral epicondylalgia. Scand J Rehabil Med 1991; 23:115–118.

65 Vasseljen O. Jr, Hoeg N, Kjeldstad B, Johnsson A and Larsen S. Low level laser versus placebo in the treatment of tennis elbow. Physiotherapy 1992; 78:37–42.

66 Pienimaki T, Tarvainen T, Siira P, Vanharanta H. Progressive strengthening and stretching exercises and ultrasound for chronic lateral epicondylitis. Physiotherapy 1996; 82:522–530.

67 van der Windt DA, van der Heijden GJ, van den Berg SG, ter Riet G, de Winter AF, Bouter LM. Ultrasound therapy for acute ankle sprains. [update of Cochrane Database Syst Rev. 2000;(2):CD001250; PMID: 10796428]. Cochrane Database Syst Rev 2002; 2:CD001250.

68 Tiidus PM. Massage and ultrasound as therapeutic modalities in exercise-induced muscle damage. Can J Appl Physiol 1999; 24:267–278.

69 Hasson S, Mundorf R, Barnes W, Williams J, Fujii M. Effect of pulsed ultrasound versus placebo on muscle soreness perception and muscular performance. Scand J Rehabil Med 1990; 22:199–205.

70 Plaskett C, Riidus P, Livingston L. Ultrasound treatment does not affect postexercise muscle strength recovery or soreness. J Sports Rehabil 1999; 8:1–9.

71 Wilkin LD, Merrick MA, Kirby TE, Devor ST. Influence of therapeutic ultrasound on skeletal muscle regeneration following blunt contusion. Int J Sports Med 2004; 25:73–77.

72 Rantanen J, Thorsson O, Wollmer P, Hurme T, Kalimo H. Effects of therapeutic ultrasound on the regeneration of skeletal myofibers after experimental muscle injury. Am J Sports Med 1999; 27:54–59.

73 Ramirez A, Schwane JA, McFarland C, Starcher B. The effect of ultrasound on collagen synthesis and fibroblast proliferation in vitro. Med Sci Sports Exerc 1997; 29:326–332.

74 Jackson BA, Schwane JA, Starcher BC. Effect of ultrasound therapy on the repair of Achilles tendon injuries in rats. Med Sci Sports Exerc 1991; 23:171–176.

75 Enwemeka CS. The effects of therapeutic ultrasound on tendon healing. A biomechanical study. Am J Phys Med Rehabil 1989; 68:283–287.

76 Ng CO, Ng GY, See EK, Leung MC. Therapeutic ultrasound improves strength of Achilles tendon repair in rats. Ultrasound Med Biol 2003; 29:1501–1506.

77 Warden SJ. A new direction for ultrasound therapy in sports medicine. Sports Med 2003; 33:95–107.

78 Kristiansen TK, Ryaby JP, McCabe J, Frey JJ, Roe LR. Accelerated healing of distal radial fractures with the use of specific, low-intensity ultrasound. A multicenter, prospective, randomized, double-blind, placebo-controlled study. J Bone Jt Surg 1997; 79A:961–973.

79 Brand JC Jr, Brindle T, Nyland J, Caborn DN and Johnson DL. Does pulsed low intensity ultrasound allow early return to normal activities when treating stress fractures? A review of one tarsal navicular and eight tibial stress fractures. Iowa Orthop J 1999; 19:26–30.

80 van der Windt DA, van der Heijden GJ, van den Berg SG, ter Riet G, de Winter AF, Bouter LM. Ultrasound therapy for musculoskeletal disorders: a systematic review. Pain 1999; 81:257–271.

81 Baker KG, Robertson VJ, Duck FA. A review of therapeutic ultrasound: biophysical effects. Phys Ther 2001; 81:1351–1358.

82 Robertson VJ, Baker KG. A review of therapeutic ultrasound: effectiveness studies. Phys Ther 2001; 81:1339–1350.

83 Gam AN, Johannsen F. Ultrasound therapy in musculoskeletal disorders: a meta-analysis. Pain 1995; 63:85–91.

84 Griffin J, Touchstone J. Ultrasonic movement of cortisol into pig tissues, I. Movement into skeletal muscle. Am J Phys Med Rehabil 1963; 42:72–85.

85 Newman M, Kill M, Frampton G. Effects of ultrasound alone and combined with hydrocortisone injections by needle or hypospray. Am J Phys Med Rehabil 1958; 37:206–209.

86 Davick JP, Martin RK, Albright JP. Distribution and deposition of tritiated cortisol using phonophoresis. Phys Ther 1988; 68:1672–1675.

87 Cagnie B, Vinck E, Rimbaut S, Vanderstraeten G. Phonophoresis versus topical application of ketoprofen: comparison between tissue and plasma levels. Phys Ther 2003; 83:707–712.

88 Baskurt F, Ozcan A, Algun C. Comparison of effects of phonophoresis and iontophoresis of naproxen in the treatment of lateral epicondylitis. Clin Rehabil 2003; 17:96–100.

89 Klaiman MD, Shrader JA, Danoff JV, et al. Phonophoresis versus ultrasound in the treatment of common musculoskeletal conditions. Med Sci Sports Exer 1998; 30:1349–1355.

90 Kozanoglu E, Basaran S, Guzel R, Guler-Uysal F. Short term efficacy of ibuprofen phonophoresis versus continuous ultrasound therapy in knee osteoarthritis. Swiss Med Wkly 2003; 133:333–338.

91 Licht S. History of electrotherapy. In: Stillwell G, ed. Therapeutic electricity and ultraviolet radiation. Baltimore: Williams & Wilkins; 1983:8–21.

92 Hillman SK, Delforge G. The use of physical agents in rehabilitation of athletic injuries. Clin Sports Med 1985; 4:431–438.

93 Marino M. Principles of therapeutic modalities: Implications for sports injuries. In: Nicholas J, Herschmena E, eds. The lower extremity and spine in sports medicine. St Louis: Mosby; 1986:195–244.

94 Ross C, Segal D. High voltage galvanic stimulation – an aid to post-operative healing. Curr Podiatry 1981; 34:19.

95 Stillwell G. Electrotherapy. In: Kottke F, Stillwell G, Lehmann J, eds. Krusen's handbook of physical medicine and rehabilitation. Philadelphia: Saunders; 1982:360–371.

96 Gould N, Donnermeyer D, Gammon GG, Pope M, Ashikaga T. Transcutaneous muscle stimulation to retard disuse atrophy after open meniscectomy. Clin Orthop Relat Res 1979; 178:190–197.

97 Lake D. Increases in range of motion of the edematous hand with the use of electro-mesh glove. Phys Ther Forum 1989; 8:6.

98 Griffin JW, Newsome LS, Stralka SW, Wright PE. Reduction of chronic posttraumatic hand edema: a comparison of high voltage pulsed current, intermittent pneumatic compression, and placebo treatments. Phys Ther 1990; 70:279–286.

99 Amrein L, Garrett TR, Martin GM. Use of low-voltage electrotherapy and electromyography in physical therapy. Physiother Can 1971; 51:1283–1287.

100 Alon G, McCombe S, Koutsantonis S, Stumphauzer L, Burgwin K. Comparison of the effects of electrical stimulation and exercise on abdominal musculature. J Orthop Sports Phys Ther 1987; 8:567–573.

101 Snyder-Mackler L, Celluci M, Lyons J, Magno J. Effects of duty cycle of portable neuromuscular electrical stimulation on strength of the non-dominant triceps brachii. J Orthop Sports Phys Ther 1988; 68:833–839.

102 Kahanovitz N, Nordin M, Verderame R, et al. Normal trunk muscle strength and endurance in women and the effect of exercises and electrical stimulation. Part 2: Comparative analysis of electrical stimulation and exercises to increase trunk muscle strength and endurance. Spine 1987; 12:112–118.

103 Fleury M, Lagasse P. Influence of functional electrical stimulation training on premotor and motor reaction time. Percept Mot Skills 1979; 48:387–393.

104 LeDoux J, Quinones M. An investigation of the use of percutaneous electrical nerve stimulation in muscle reeducation. Abstract R183. Phys Ther 1981; 61:737.

105 Stanish WD, Valiant GA, Bonen A, Belcastro AN. The effects of immobilization and of electrical stimulation on muscle glycogen and myofibrillar ATPase. J Can Sci Appl Sport 1982; 7:267–271.

106 Eriksson E, Haggmark T, Kiessling KH, Karlsson J. Effect of electrical stimulation on human skeletal muscle. Int J Sports Med 1981; 2:18–22.

107 Eriksson E, Haggmark T. Comparison of isometric muscle training and electrical stimulation supplementing isometric muscle training in the recovery after major knee ligament surgery. A preliminary report. Am J Sports Med 1979; 7:169–171.

108 Yoshida N, Sairyo K, Sasa T, et al. Electrical stimulation prevents deterioration of the oxidative capacity of disuse-atrophied muscles in rats. Aviat Space Environ Med 2003; 74:207–211.

109 Currier DP, Lehman J, Lightfoot P. Electrical stimulation in exercise of the quadriceps femoris muscle. Phys Ther 1979; 59:1508–1512.

110 Currier DP, Mann R. Muscular strength development by electrical stimulation in healthy individuals. Phys Ther 1983; 63:915–921.

111 Halbach J, Straus D. Comparison of electro-myo stimulation to isokinetic power of the knee extensor mechanism. J Orthop Sports Phys Ther 1980; 2:20–24.

112 Kramer J, Mendryk S. Electrical stimulation as a strength improvement technique: a review. J Orthop Sports Phys Ther 1982; 4:91–98.

113 Kramer J, Semple J. Comparison of selected strengthening techniques for normal quadriceps. Physiother Can 1983; 35:300–304.

114 Kubiak R, Whitman K, Johnston R. Changes in quadriceps femoris muscle strength using isometric exercise versus electrical stimulation. J Orthop Sports Phys Ther 1987; 8:537–541.

115 Snyder-Mackler L, Ladin Z, Schepsis AA, Young JC. Electrical stimulation of the thigh muscles after reconstruction of the anterior cruciate ligament. Effects of electrically elicited contraction of the quadriceps femoris and hamstring muscles on gait and on strength of the thigh muscles. J Bone Jt Surg 1995; 77:1025–1036.

116 Paternostro-Sluga T, Fialka C, Alacamliogliu Y, Saradeth T, Fialka-Moser V. Neuromuscular electrical stimulation after anterior cruciate ligament surgery. Clin Orthop Relat Res 1999; 368:166–175.

117 Gibson JN, Smith K, Rennie MJ. Prevention of disuse muscle atrophy by means of electrical stimulation: maintenance of protein synthesis. Lancet 1988; 2:767–770.

118 Cabric M, Appell HJ, Resic A. Effects of electrical stimulation of different frequencies on the myonuclei and fiber size in human muscle. Int J Sports Med 1987; 8:323–326.

119 Singer K, D'Ambrosia A, Graf B. In: Drez D, ed. Therapeutic modalities for sports injuries. Chicago: Year Book Medical Publishers; 1989:

120 Currier D. Neuromuscular electrical stimulation for improving strength and blood flow, and influencing changes. In: Nelson R, Currier D, eds. Clinical electrotherapy. Norwalk, Stamford: Appleton and Lange; 1991:35–103.

121 Kots Y. Electrostimulation. Canadian Soviet Exchange Symposium, Concordia University, December 1977.

122 Perez M, Lucia A, Rivero JL, et al. Effects of transcutaneous short-term electrical stimulation on M. vastus lateralis characteristics of healthy young men. Pflugers Archive-European. J Physiol 2002; 443:866–874.

123 Yanagi T, Shiba N, Maeda T, et al. Agonist contractions against electrically stimulated antagonists. Arch Phys Med Rehabil 2003; 84:843–848.

124 Lake D. Neuromuscular electrical stimulation: an overview and its application in the treatment of sports injuries. Sports Med 1992; 13:320–336.

125 Melzak R, Wall PD. Pain mechanisms: A new theory. Science 1965; 150:971–979.

126 Somers DL, Clemente FR. The relationship between dorsal horn neurotransmitter content and allodynia in neuropathic rats treated with high-frequency transcutaneous electric nerve stimulation. Arch Phys Med Rehabil 2003; 84:1575–1583.

127 Walsh DM, Liggett C, Baxter D, Allen JM. A double-blind investigation of the hypoalgesic effects of transcutaneous electrical nerve stimulation upon experimentally induced ischaemic pain. Pain 1995; 61:39–45.

128 Robinson AJ. Transcutaneous electrical nerve stimulation for the control of pain in musculoskeletal disorders. J Orthop Sports Phys Ther 1996; 24:208–226.

129 Thorsteinsson G, Stonnington HH, Stillwell GK, Elveback LR. Transcutaneous electrical stimulation: a double-blind trial of its efficacy for pain. Arch Phys Med Rehabil 1977; 58:8–13.

130 Ordog GJ. Transcutaneous electrical nerve stimulation versus oral analgesic: a randomized double-blind controlled study in acute traumatic pain. Am J Emerg Med 1987; 6:6–10.

131 Lehmann TR, Russell DW, Spratt KF, et al. Efficacy of electroacupuncture and TENS in the rehabilitation of chronic low back pain patients. Pain 1986; 26:277–290.

132 Deyo RA, Walsh NE, Martin DC, Schoenfeld LS, Ramamurthy S. A controlled trial of transcutaneous electrical nerve stimulation (TENS) and exercise for chronic low back pain. N Engl J Med 1990; 322:1627–1634.

133 Marchand S, Charest J, Li J, et al. Is TENS purely a placebo effect? A controlled study on chronic low back pain. Pain 1993; 54:99–106.

134 Herman E, Williams R, Stratford P, Fargas-Babjak A, Trott M. A randomized controlled trial of transcutaneous electrical nerve stimulation (CODETRON) to determine its benefits in a rehabilitation program for acute occupational low back pain. Spine 1994; 19:561–568.

135 Cheing GL, Hui-Chan CW, Chan KM. Does four weeks of TENS and/or isometric exercise produce cumulative reduction of osteoarthritic knee pain? Clin Rehabil 2002; 16:749–760.

136 Jensen JE, Conn RR, Hazelrigg G, Hewett JE. The use of transcutaneous neural stimulation and isokinetic testing in arthroscopic knee surgery. Am J Sports Med 1985; 13:27–33.

137 Sluka KA, Bailey K, Bogush J, Olson R, Ricketts A. Treatment with either high or low frequency TENS reduces the secondary hyperalgesia observed after injection of kaolin and carrageenan into the knee joint. Pain 1998; 77:97–102.

138 Likar R, Molnar M, Pipam W, et al. Postoperative transcutaneous electrical nerve stimulation (TENS) in shoulder surgery (randomized, double blind, placebo controlled pilot trial). Schmerz 2001; 15:158–163.

139 Denegar C, Huff C. High and low frequency TENS in treatment of induced musculoskeletal pain: a comparison study. Athletic Train 1988; 23:235–237.

140 Denegar C, Perrin D, Rogoi A, Rutt R. Influence of transcutaneous electrical nerve stimulation on pain, range of motion and serum cortisol concentration in females experiencing delayed muscle soreness. J Orthop Sports Phys Ther 1989; 11:100–103.

141 Denegar C, Perrin D. Effect of transcutaneous electrical nerve stimulation, cold, and a combination treatment on pain, decreased range of motion, and strength loss associated with delayed onset muscle soreness. J Athletic Train 1992; 27:200–206.

142 Craig JA, Cunningham MB, Walsh DM, Baxter GD, Allen JM. Lack of effect of transcutaneous electrical stimulation upon experimentally induced delayed onset muscle soreness in humans. Pain 1996; 67:285–289.

143 Minder PM, Noble JG, Alves-Guerreiro J, et al. Interferential therapy: lack of effect upon experimentally induced delayed onset muscle soreness. Clin Physiol Funct Imaging 2002; 22:339–347.

144 Bircan C, Senocak O, Peker O, et al. Efficacy of two forms of electrical stimulation in increasing quadriceps strength: a randomized controlled trial. Clin Rehabil 2002; 16:194–199.

145 Jarit GJ, Mohr KJ, Waller R, Glousman RE. The effects of home interferential therapy on post-operative pain, edema, and range of motion of the knee. Clin J Sport Med 2003; 13:16–20.

146 Ghoname EA, Craig WF, White PF, et al. Percutaneous electrical nerve stimulation for low back pain: a randomized crossover study. JAMA 1999; 281:818–823.

147 Berkman R. Percutaneous electrical nerve stimulation for treatment of low back pain. JAMA 1999; 282:941–942.

148 Ghoname ES, Craig WF, White PF, et al. The effect of stimulus frequency on the analgesic response to percutaneous electrical nerve stimulation in patients with chronic low back pain. Anesth Analg 1999; 88:841–846.

149 Hsieh RL, Lee WC. One-shot percutaneous electrical nerve stimulation vs. transcutaneous electrical nerve stimulation for low back pain: comparison of therapeutic effects. Am J Phys Med Rehabil 2002; 81:838–843.

150 Weiner DK, Rudy TE, Glick RM, et al. Efficacy of percutaneous electrical nerve stimulation for the treatment of chronic low back pain in older adults. J Am Geriatr Soc 2003; 51:599–608.

151 Yokoyama M, Sun X, Oku S, et al. Comparison of percutaneous electrical nerve stimulation with transcutaneous electrical nerve stimulation for long-term pain relief in patients with chronic low back pain. Anesth Analg 2004; 98:1552–1556.

152 O'Malley E, Oester Y. Influence of some physical chemical factors on iontophoresis using radioisotopes. Arch Phys Med Rehabil 1955; 36:310–316.

153 James M, Graham R, English J. Percutaneous iontophoresis of prednisolone – a pharmacokinetic study. Clin Exp Dermatol 1986; 11:54–61.

154 Zankel H, Cress R, Kamin H. Iontophoresis studies with radioactive tracer. Arch Phys Med Rehabil 1959; 40:193–196.

155 Bertolucci L. Introduction of antiinflammatory drugs by iontophoresis: a double blind study. J Orthop Sports Phys Ther 1982; 4:103–108.

156 Chantraine A, Ludy JP, Berger D. Is cortisone iontophoresis possible? Arch Phys Med Rehabil 1986; 67:38–40.

157 Japour CJ, Vohra R, Vohra PK, Garfunkel L, Chin N. Management of heel pain syndrome with acetic acid iontophoresis. J Am Podiatr Med Assoc 1999; 89:251–257.

158 Gudeman SD, Eisele SA, Heidt RS Jr, Colosimo AJ, Stroupe AL. Treatment of plantar fasciitis by iontophoresis of 0.4% dexamethasone. A randomized, double-blind, placebo-controlled study. Am J Sports Med 1997; 25:312–316.

159 Taniguchi K, Yoshitake S, Iwasaka H, Honda N, Oyama T. The effects of imipramine, amitriptyline and clonidine administered by iontophoresis on the pain threshold. Acta Anaesthesiol Belg 1995; 46:121–125.

160 Hasson SM, Wible CL, Reich M, Barnes WS, Williams JH. Dexamethasone iontophoresis: effect on delayed muscle soreness and muscle function. Can J Sport Sci 1992; 17:8–13.

161 Hinterbucher C. Traction. In: Basmajian J, ed. Traction and massage. Baltimore: Williams & Wilkins; 1985:172–200.

162 Rechtein J, Andary M, Holmes T, Wietig M. Manipulation, massage and traction. In: DeLisa J, Gans B, eds. Rehabilitation medicine principles and practices. Philadelphia: Lippincott-Raven; 1998:521–552.

163 Zylbergold RS, Piper MC. Cervical spine disorders. A comparison of three types of traction. Spine 1985; 10:867–871.

164 Swezey RL, Swezey AM, Warner K. Efficacy of home cervical traction therapy. Am J Phys Med Rehabil 1999; 78:30–32.

165 Constantoyannis C, Konstantinou D, Kourtopoulos H, Papadakis N. Intermittent cervical traction for cervical radiculopathy caused by large-volume herniated disks. J Manipulative Physiol Ther 2002; 25:188–192.

166 Moeti P, Marchetti G. Clinical outcome from mechanical intermittent cervical traction for the treatment of cervical radiculopathy: a case series. J Orthop Sports Phys Ther 2001; 31:207–213.

167 de Seze S, Levernieux J. Pratique rheumatologie des tractions vertebrales. Sem Hop Paris 1951; 27:2085.

168 Frazer E. The use of traction in backache. Med J Aust 1954; 41:694.

169 Lawson G, Godfrey C. A report on studies of spinal-traction. Med Services J Can 1958; 14:762.

170 Meszaros TF, Olson R, Kulig K, Creighton D, Czarnecki E. Effect of 10%, 30%, and 60% body weight traction on the straight leg raise test of symptomatic patients with low back pain. J Orthop Sports Phys Ther 2000; 30:595–601.

171 Crisp EJ, Cyriax JH, Christie BG. Discussion on the treatment of backache by traction. Proc R Soc Med 1955; 48:805–814.

172 Weber H. Traction therapy in sciatica due to disc prolapse. J Oslo City Hosp 1973; 23:167.

173 Beurskens AJ, de Vet HC, Koke AJ, et al. Efficacy of traction for nonspecific low back pain. 12-week and 6-month results of a randomized clinical trial. Spine 1997; 22:2756–2762.

174 van der Heijden GJ, Beurskens AJ, Koes BW, et al. The efficacy of traction for back and neck pain: a systematic, blinded review of randomized clinical trial methods. Phys Ther 1995; 75:93–104.

175 Borman P, Keskin D, Bodur H. The efficacy of lumbar traction in the management of patients with low back pain. Rheumatol Int 2003; 23:82–86.

176 Cheatle MD, Esterhai JL. Pelvic traction as treatment for acute back pain. Efficacious, benign, or deleterious? Spine 1991; 16:1379–1381.

177 Ayrapetyan S, Avanesian R, Avetisian T. Physiological effects of magnetic fields may be mediated through actions of the state of calcium ions in solutions. In: Carpenter DO, Ayrapetyan S, eds. Biological effects of electric and magnetic fields – Sources and mechanisms. San Diego: Academic Press; 1994:181–192.

178 Erdman W. Peripheral blood flow measurement during application of pulsed high frequency currents. Am J Orthop 1960; 2:196–197.

179 Fenn J. Effect of pulsed electromagnetic energy (Diapulse) on experimental hematomas. Can Med Assoc J 1969; 100:251–254.

180 Ross J. Biological effects of PEMFs using Diapulse. In: Connor M, Bentall R, Monahan J, eds. Emerging electromagnetic medicine. New York: Springer; 1990:269–282.

181 Goldin JH, Broadbent NR, Nancarrow JD, Marshall T. The effects of Diapulse on the healing of wounds: a double-blind randomised controlled trial in man. Br J Plast Surg 1981; 34:267–270.

182 McLean MJ, Holcomb RR, Wamil AW, Pickett JD, Cavopol AV. Blockade of sensory neuron action potentials by a static magnetic field in the 10 mT range. Bioelectromagnetics 1995; 16:20–32.

183 Carpenter D, Ayrapetyan S. Biological effects of electric and magnetic fields – sources and mechanisms. San Diego: Academic Press; 1994.

184 Hazlewood C, VanZandt R. A hypothesis defining an objective end point for the relief of chronic pain. Med Hypotheses 1995; 44:63–65.

185 Miner WK, Trock DH, Bollet AJ, Dyer RH Jr, Fielding LP, Markoll R. A double-blind trial of the clinical effects of pulsed electromagnetic fields in osteoarthritis. J Rheumatol 1993; 20:456–460.

186 Trock DH, Bollet AJ, Markoll R. The effect of pulsed electromagnetic fields in the treatment of osteoarthritis of the knee and cervical spine. Report of randomized, double blind, placebo controlled trials. J Rheumatol 1994; 21:1903–1911.

187 Foley-Nolan D, Moore K, Codd M, et al. Low energy high frequency pulsed electromagnetic therapy for acute whiplash injuries. A double blind randomized controlled study. Scand J Rehabil Med 1992; 24:51–59.

188 Pujol J, Pascual-Leone A, Dolz C, et al. The effect of repetitive magnetic stimulation on localized musculoskeletal pain. Neuroreport 1998; 9:1745–1748.

189 Gross AR, Aker PD, Goldsmith CH, Peloso P. Physical medicine modalities for mechanical neck disorders. Cochrane Database Syst Rev 2000; 2:CD000961.

190 Bassett A. Therapeutic uses of electric and magnetic fields in orthopedics. In: Carpenter DO, Ayrapetyan S, eds. Geological effects of electric and magnetic fields. San Diego: Academic Press; 1994:13–48.

191 O'Connor M, Bentall R, Monahan J. Emerging electromagnetic medicine. New York: Springer; 1990.

192 Sharrard W. A double-blind trial of pulsed electromagnetic fields for delayed union of tibial fractures. J Bone Jt Surg Br 1990; 72:347–355.

193 Carter R, Aspy CB, Mold J. The effectiveness of magnet therapy for treatment of wrist pain attributed to carpal tunnel syndrome. J Fam Pract 2002; 51:38–40.

194 Collacott EA, Zimmerman JT, White DW, Rindone JP. Bipolar permanent magnets for the treatment of chronic low back pain: a pilot study. JAMA 2000; 283:1322–1325.

195 Washnis G. Discovery of magnetic health: A health care alternative. New York: Health Research Publishers; 1998.

196 Vallbona C, Richards T. Evolution of magnetic therapy from alternative to traditional medicine. Phys Med Rehabil Clin North Am 1999; 10:729–754.

197 Cassidy S, Nielsen D. Cardiovascular response of healthy subjects to calisthenics performed in land versus water. Phys Ther 1992; 72:81–88.

198 Williamson AT, Fletcher PC, Dawson KA. Complementary and alternative medicine. Use in an older population. J Gerontol Nurs 2003; 29:20–28.

199 Weiner DK, Ernst E. Complementary and alternative approaches to the treatment of persistent musculoskeletal pain. Clin J Pain 2004; 20:244–255.

200 Ulett GA, Han S, Han JS. Electroacupuncture: mechanisms and clinical application. Biol Psychiatry 1998; 44:129–138.

201 Han JS. Acupuncture and endorphins. Neurosci Lett 2004; 361:258–261.

202 Zhang W, Luo F, Qi Y, et al. Modulation of pain signal processing by electric acupoint stimulation: an electroencephalogram study. Beijing Xua Xue Bao 2003; 35:236–240.

203 Wu MT, Sheen JM, Chuang KH, et al. Neuronal specificity of acupuncture response: a fMRI study with electroacupuncture. Neuroimage 2002; 16:1028–1037.

204 Cummings M. Percutaneous electrical nerve stimulation – electroacupuncture by another name? A comparative review. Acupunct Med 2001; 91:32–35.

205 Sator-Katzenschlager SM, Szeles JC, Scharbert G, et al. Electrical stimulation of auricular acupuncture points is more effective than conventional manual auricular acupuncture in chronic cervical pain: a pilot study. Anesth Analg 2003; 97(5):1469–1473.

206 Sator-Katzenschlager SM, Scharbert G, Kozek-Langenecker SA, et al. The short- and long-term benefit in chronic low back pain through adjuvant electrical versus manual auricular acupuncture. Anesth Analg 2004; 98:1359–1364.

207 Tsukayama H, Yamashita H, Amagai H, Tanno Y. Randomised controlled trial comparing the effectiveness of electroacupuncture and TENS for low back pain: a preliminary study for a pragmatic trial. Acupunct Med 2002; 20:175–180.

208 Carlsson CP, Sjolund BH. Acupuncture for chronic low back pain: a randomized placebo-controlled study with long-term follow-up. Clin J Pain 2001; 17:296–305.

209 Kalauokalani D, Cherkin DC, Sherman KJ, Koepsell TD, Deyo RA. Lessons from a trial of acupuncture and massage for low back pain: patient expectations and treatment effects. Spine 2001; 26:1418–1424.

210 Green S, Buchbinder R, Barnsley L, et al. Acupuncture for lateral elbow pain. Cochrane Database Syst Rev 2002; 1:CD003527.

211 Tsui P, Leung MC. Comparison of the effectiveness between manual acupuncture and electro-acupuncture on patients with tennis elbow. Acupunct Electro Ther Res 2002; 27:107–117.

212 Kleinhenz J, Streitberger K, Windeler J, et al. Randomised clinical trial comparing the effects of acupuncture and a newly designed placebo needle in rotator cuff tendinitis. Pain 1999; 83:235–241.

213 Koo ST, Park YI, Lim KS, Chung K, Chung JM. Acupuncture analgesia in a new rat model of ankle sprain pain. Pain 2002; 99:423–431.

214 Akimoto T, Nakahori C, Aizawa K, et al. Acupuncture and responses of immunologic and endocrine markers during competition. Med Sci Sports Exerc 2003; 35:1296–1302.

CHAPTER 17

Exercise in the Rehabilitation of the Athlete

Sheila A. Dugan

INTRODUCTION

Exercise is the mainstay in rehabilitating athletes to return to sport. Restoration of functional strength, flexibility, conditioning and neuromuscular coordination for athletic performance guides the exercise prescription. Deficits in one or more of these areas may have led to the original injury, especially in the setting of overuse injuries, or may result from direct tissue damage at the time of acute injury or from immobilization prescribed to enhance healing. Principles of training, such as specificity and overload, direct the progression of exercise while sports specific activities are incorporated to facilitate motor relearning. Multiplanar functional training is crucial in returning to the field of play where an extensive array of movements beyond unidirectional planes is required. Exercise professionals must recognize that muscles rarely act in isolation and that strength or flexibility deficits or maladaptive movement patterns anywhere along the loaded or unloaded limb and trunk can lead to re-injury.

STAGES OF REHABILITATION

The stages of tissue healing and repair must be considered as one plans and executes the rehabilitation exercise program. For instance, the magnitude and direction of tensile load is gauged based on tissue recovery. Wolff's law states that changes in form or function of a bone are followed by certain, definitive changes in the bone structure. Hence, it is imperative that bone and other connective tissues be loaded in the appro-

priate direction and with appropriate force to optimize recovery without compromising healing. Additionally, attention to the overall level of cardiovascular fitness and flexibility continues throughout the rehabilitation process.

Three stages have been defined to guide the rehabilitation of injured athletes: acute stage, recovery stage and functional stage.[1] See Table 17.1 for examples of exercise by type and indication during the three stages.

Acute stage

The acute stage of rehabilitation is focused on moderating the inflammatory response and decreasing symptoms.[2] Preserving strength and mobility of the injured limb is important but may be forfeited temporarily if immobilization is required. Uninvolved segments of the injured limb should be exercised in conjunction with an overall cardiovascular fitness program. Isometric exercise (in which there is no change in muscle length and no movement of the limb segment) can be utilized to maintain a controlled contraction. Gentle stretching and range of motion exercises are instituted, guided by discomfort. With multidirectional stretching, the practitioner may discover that particular planes are better tolerated than others.

Recovery stage

The recovery stage of rehabilitation begins as tissue healing is nearly complete. The focus during the recovery stage of rehabilitation is functional improvement by restoration of joint range of motion, soft tissue flexibility, and strength, then rebuilding endurance and recovering proprioception. It is generally the longest stage. Protected mobility may continue to be necessary but multiplanar re-mobilization drives the flexibility program. A gradated progression in force generation and degrees of freedom is necessary. The athlete must be closely monitored for response to exercise and any resumption of the inflammatory response signifies a need to reduce the level of rehabilitation activities. Any setbacks can delay this stage of rehabilitation. Medications, modalities and therapy techniques are constantly re-evaluated and minimized as active exercise becomes the main feature of this stage of rehabilitation.

Box 17.1: Key Points

Exercise may be progressing too rapidly and the program should be re-evaluated when:

- Pain increases
- Swelling increases
- Joint range of motion declines.

Table 17.1   Exercise by Rehabilitation Stage

Intervention	Example	Indication
Exercise in acute stage	Static strengthening (isometrics)	Reduce atrophy and weakness
	Gentle static stretching	Limit loss of range of motion
Exercise in recovery stage	Contract relax stretching	Improve flexibility
	Closed kinetic chain exercise	Improve limb strength and co-contraction
	Open kinetic chain exercise	Improve strength
	Medicine ball	Prepare for sports specific activity
	Physioball	Improve trunk strength
Exercise in functional stage	Balance board	Improve balance
	Mini trampoline	Increase proprioception
	Figure of 8 drills	Improve agility and foot placement
	Jump training	Improve tensile strength of muscle-tendon unit and ligaments
		Improve force production
		Regain sports specific neuromuscular control
	Overhead throwing	Maintain proximal stability and alignment
	Progress physioball program	Prevent future injury

Later in the chapter, specific types of exercises will be reviewed. In general, the exercise prescription must be selected carefully to address impairments. The SAID (Specific Adaptation to Imposed Demand) principle necessitates that the effects of training are velocity, joint angle and site specific.[3] The overload principle requires that a muscle must be worked at a level higher than it is accustomed in order to increase strength. The exercise workload can be varied to meet a particular goal. For example, exercising with low resistance and higher numbers of repetition builds endurance. Low repetition, high resistance training builds strength. Trunk or core stabilization exercises are an important part of the rehabilitation process and will be reviewed below. When one considers the kinetic chain and the transmission of forces from the distal extremity to the proximal extremity to the trunk, it is key to maintain or increase proximal stability while training for mobility.

Box 17.2: Key Points

The Specific Adaptation to Imposed Demand (SAID) Principle states that training effects of an exercise program are specific to:

- Speed
- Joint position
- Muscles included.

Functional stage

The functional stage of rehabilitation commences once range of motion is normal and pain-free and the athlete is tolerating a progressive exercise program. The focus of this stage of rehabilitation includes improved neuromuscular control, sports specific and multiplanar activity and cessation of maladaptive behaviors that could lead to a future injury. The athlete completes this stage when he or she can meet the return to play criteria. Therapeutic modality and medication use is infrequent related to symptom exacerbations. An exercise program including flexibility, strengthening and proprioception is well established. Progression of sports specific activity is very important to allow successful return to play. The focus on correct technique will prevent future injury. Chapter 20 will focus on returning to training and competition.

APPLIED EXERCISE PHYSIOLOGY

Principles of exercise physiology and conditioning have been previously reviewed (see Chapter 2, in the section on general scientific and medical concepts). These principles are directly applied in the rehabilitation exercise program. Appropriate incorporation of specific types of muscle contractions and functional positions guides the execution of the program. The exercise prescription includes intensity, duration, frequency and mode of exercise (Table 17.2) Objective outcomes include strength, power, endurance, flexibility, motor control and functional performance. One cannot discount subjective complaints about pain or instability. This feedback provides valuable input on tissue healing and helps direct progression of training, for example in the setting of stress fractures.[4]

THE EXERCISE PRESCRIPTION

The exercise prescription is based on the particular goals of the athlete. Exercises are selected to meet the desired training effect.

Intensity

Intensity of exercise describes the difficulty level of the exercise. The major muscle groups are trained with one or multiple (up to 3) sets of 8–12 repetitions. Once the athlete can perform 12–15 repetitions with ease, the resistance is increased.

Table 17.2   The Exercise Prescription

Element	Definition	Common Programs
Type or mode of exercise	Specific activity the athlete will engage in	Resistance training Cardiovascular training
Frequency	No. of times per week	3–5 times per week (more often in season)
Duration	For strength training:	
	No. of repetitions per set OR	6–10 repetitions per set OR
	No. of sets per session	3 sets per session
	For endurance training:	
	Total number minutes	30–60 min
Intensity	For strength training:	
	% of repetition maximum	50–100% of 6–10 repetition max
	For endurance training:	
	No. of repetitions	100% of 15–30 repetition max
	% VO_2 OR	40–85% VO_2
	% maximum heart rate	55–90% maximum heart rate

Resistance or strength training intensity has its roots in the DeLorme method.[5] In this schema, a 10-repetition maximum weight was established at the outset of the training program and then weekly. The individual performed 10 repetitions of a weight 50% the 10-repetition maximal weight, followed by 10 repetitions of a weight 75% the 10-repetition maximal weight, and finally 10 repetitions of a weight 100% the 10-repetition maximal weight. The Oxford technique trained in an opposite manner, with the athlete starting at 10 repetitions of a weight 100% the 10-repetition maximal weight, then 75% and finally 50% the 10-repetition maximum.[6] Other techniques, utilizing 6- to 10-repetition maximum weight to develop the progressive-resistance training program, have been used over the past several decades.[7]

Alternatively, intensity can be approached with higher repetition, submaximal resistance sets, which are employed during the acute and recovery stages of rehabilitation.[8] This type of resistance training increases endurance. Cardiovascular training intensity is gauged by: percentage of VO_2 maximum (40–85%); percentage of calculated maximal heart rate (55–90%); or rating of perceived exertion (14 on the RPE scale).[9]

Duration

Duration of exercise describes the timeframe of the exercise sessions. In general, 30–60 min is the target. Intensity and time of performance of exercise are inversely proportional. Metabolic demand and substrate utilization varies depending on duration of exercise. High intensity exercise is limited by lactic acid build-up; exercise for >1 h performed at low intensity promotes more efficient utilization of free fatty acids.[10] The duration of training should mimic the sport participant's functional needs. In the acute stage, duration may be limited. However, alternative methods, such as upper body ergometry

in an athlete with a lower extremity injury, may increase duration. Many sports, such as soccer and basketball, require both short bursts of high intensity anaerobic power in addition to a solid aerobic base. Interval training is one means of providing training for both the anaerobic (work periods) and aerobic systems (relief periods).[11] There are many different protocols for interval training.

Frequency

Frequency of exercise indicates how often the exercise is performed. This can vary depending on if the athlete is in or out of season. Generally, injured and non-injured athletes in season exercise 5–7 days per week. During a given week, game participation substitutes for a training session. In particular sports, athletes may rest on the day after the game. The resistance training component of the rehabilitation program is usually done on an every other day basis to allow for intervals of rest. It will generally take about six weeks for strength improvements.

Mode

Mode of exercise includes the type of exercise performed. It should mimic the type of sport the rehabilitating athlete participates in. It can be varied to provide the broadest coverage of muscle groups and to remediate conditioning deficits.

TYPES OF MUSCLE CONTRACTION

Box 17.3: Key Points

Isometric contractions
- Hold for 5–10 s
- Performed at multiple joint angles.

Isometric

Isometric (fixed muscle length) contraction is most useful in the acute stage when mobilization of injured tissue may be contraindicated. Isometric contractions can generate significant force and are crucial in many sports. For instance, gymnasts must maintain fixed postures during floor exercise, bars and rings. Isometric co-contraction would be included in the gymnastic exercise prescription throughout all three rehabilitation stages, as this type of contraction is very functional for the athlete. The athlete is typically told to hold the maximal contraction for 5–10 s. The contraction is repeated at multiple joint angles.

Concentric

Concentric contraction involves shortening of the muscle with requisite movement of the origin or insertion and limb translation.[9] Athletes use concentric contractions to counter a load. They are used to accelerate the distal segment of the limb and attached equipment, such as a racquet or ball. With skill training, the ball can be released with kinetic energy at the appropriate time or toward the appropriate target. Initial concentric exercise training can be done using only the resistance of the limb mass against gravity or in a gravity-assisted or gravity-eliminated position. Progressive resistance can be advanced using a variety of equipment, including flexible cords, weighted balls, hand weights or resistance training equipment. Body positioning can be manipulated to provide for more functional alignment. In regard to rehabilitating athletes, one must remember that these concentric contractions are not performed in isolation and occur with a host of biomechanical challenges brought about by changes in trunk alignment or surface of play, just to name a few.

Isotonic

Isotonic exercise includes contraction against a constant external resistance. The resistance can be manual or mechanical. Isokinetic is the term used to describe contractions that take place at a constant velocity. Isokinetic contractions do not occur *in vivo*. However, computerized exercise equipment can provide constant resistance or constant velocity. Variable resistance machines have been developed to provide resistance that matches the torque curves produced by particular muscle groups. Isokinetic data has been used to follow post-surgical patients and in research studies but has limited clinical application. Most equipment tests uniplanar movements, limiting its functional applicability.

Box 17.4: Key Points

Closed kinetic chain (CKC) exercises
- Fixed distal limb

Open kinetic chain (OKC) exercises
- Freely moving distal limb.

Moving beyond therapeutic exercise regimens limited to one muscle, joint or direction, the sport rehabilitation exercise program includes the entire kinetic chain (or linked segments of the limbs and trunk and the muscles that co-contract around them). Open kinetic chain (OKC) exercise is one in which the distal limb segment is not fixed and able to move freely. Closed kinetic chain (CKC) exercise is one in which the distal limb segment is fixed or in contact with a ground reaction force. Different muscle activation patterns are seen between OKC and CKC exercises. Knee extension and flexion CKC exercise with mini-squats co-activates the quadriceps and hamstrings (Fig. 17.1).[12] Muscle activation may also be impacted by proximal or distal joint positioning, such as performing the leg press exercise with the hips flexed versus extended (Fig. 17.2).

Biomechanical deficits in joints outside of the injured limb can lead to re-injury. In fact, these deficits in the kinetic chain may have led to the current injury. For example, a baseball pitcher transmits forces from the lower limbs via the trunk to augment force production in the upper limb. Therefore,

identifying and treating flexibility and strength deficits in the lower limbs and trunk are an important part of the rehabilitation program of a throwing athlete with an upper limb injury. Motion analysis using videotaping can also be helpful in reinforcing correct movement patterns once biomechanical deficits have been addressed. This should be done prior to return to play when ingrained maladaptive movement patterns are likely to resurface.

While kinetic chain consideration has expanded the repertoire of exercise in the rehabilitation of the athlete, functional rehabilitation has moved to another level. Most fundamental is the acknowledgement that sports-related function is dictated by forces of gravity, momentum, and ground reaction in multiple planes of motion.[13] Research in the arena of non-contact ACL injuries demonstrates the utility of this multidirectional and functional consideration. Multiplanar control at the knee may be directly impacted by foot position, ligamentous laxity, muscle fatigue after repetitive eccentric contractions or knee joint positioning that inhibits rather than recruits the optimal muscle co-contraction patterns; therefore, all these areas are being studied in conjunction with the increase in non-contact ACL injuries in girls and women compared to boys and men.[14] The goals of rehabilitating (and likewise prehabilitating) athletes at risk for ACL injury is to provide exercise training that simulates sports-related activities in order to expand the biomechanical and neurophysiological repertoire of the athlete. This expanded repertoire can then be called into action on the field of play to enhance performance and reduce injury rate. Most crucial to this functional training is expansion of eccentric muscle control. In keeping with the tradition of kinetic chain principles, lower limb performance demands that the joints of the entire lower limb, pelvis and trunk make appropriate adaptations to the forces of gravity, momentum and ground reaction in multiple planes of motion. Eccentric muscle contractions are paramount to regulate limb and body movement.

An eccentric muscle contraction generates muscle tension while a muscle is lengthening (muscle origin and insertion are moving away from one another). Eccentric contractions are crucial in slowing or decelerating segments of the body that have acquired kinetic energy, such as the lower limbs in running. Eccentric contractions are associated with delayed onset muscle soreness and microscopic trauma.[15] Soft tissue injuries, such as hamstring strains, have been linked to this microscopic damage.[16] The microscopic area of damage may progress to a muscle tear with ongoing eccentric contractions. Further research is needed to guide practitioners in prescribing eccentric exercise, especially in the acute stage of rehabilitation. Currently, eccentric training starts at low levels with gradual progression to higher intensity and frequency.

Eccentric training is important as it mirrors the physiologic manner in which human muscle performs, in particular the lower limbs. Running has been described as a series of lower limb pronations (during loading) and supinations (during unloading and swing).[13] The pronation phase, or first half of stance, involves mostly eccentric contraction to provide for joint control and shock absorption. The supination phase, or second half of stance and early swing, involves mostly concentric contractions. Eccentric training of the lower limbs is employed using various heights and planes of movement from

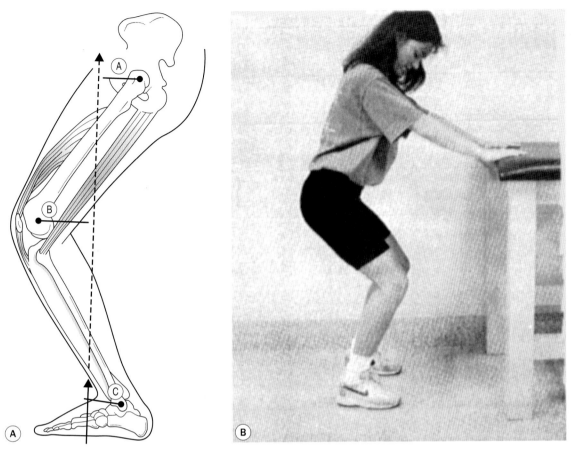

Figure 17.1 Closed kinetic chain (CKC) exercise with a mini-squat. Hamstring and gastrocnemius-soleus contraction is created by flexion moments at the (A) hip, (B) knee and (C) ankle. (From Prentice WE. Rehabilitation techniques in sports medicine. 2nd edn. St Louis, MO: Mosby; 1994:100–101.)

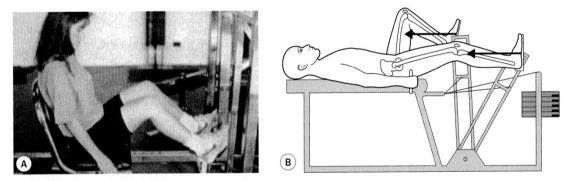

Figure 17.2 Leg press exercise performed with the hips flexed in standard position (A) and hips extended with modified position (B). The hip extended position provides a more functional pattern of contraction. (From Prentice WE. Rehabilitation techniques in sports medicine. 2nd edn. St Louis, MO: Mosby; 1994:102.)

which the athlete controls loading and unloading (Fig. 17.3). Step up and downs can be done in the frontal, sagittal or transverse plane training both concentric and eccentric lower extremity musculature in a functional way.

Plyometric

Plyometric training describes rapid eccentric loading followed by an explosive concentric contraction.[17] The extent of viscoelastic stretching and joint load varies and must be

---

Box 17.5: Key Points

Plyometric exercises

- Rapid eccentric load followed by explosive concentric contraction
- Moderated by varying height, speed and vigor of contraction
- Carefully progressed to avoid tissue overload and re-injury.

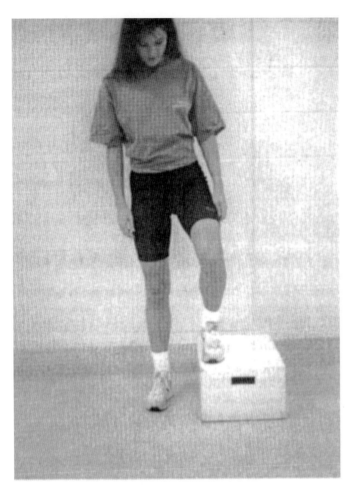

Figure 17.3 Step up exercises performed in the frontal plane. Variations incorporating diagonal patterns and upper limb reaching can incorporate the sagittal and transverse planes. (From Prentice WE. Rehabilitation techniques in sports medicine. 2nd edn. St Louis, MO: Mosby; 1994:103.)

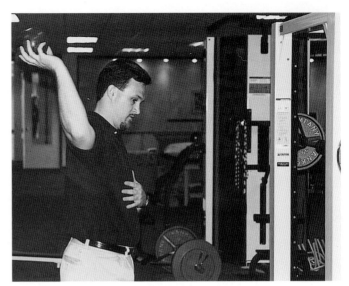

Figure 17.4 Upper extremity plyometric exercise with weighted ball. The exercise can be progressed by speed, weight and number of repetitions. (From Paine RM, Johnson RM. Open and closed chain exercises; Non-weight-bearing and weight-bearing exercises. In: DeLee JC, Drez D, Miller MD, eds. DeLee & Drez's orthopaedic sports medicine: principles and practice, Vol 1. 2nd edn. Philadelphia: Saunders; 2003:347.)

Power and endurance

Power and endurance are also important considerations for the training program. Muscle power is the product of force and velocity and represents the amount of work a muscle can produce per unit of time. Power can be trained with a periodized progressive exercise program, or one that manipulates training variables such as speed, repetitions, and sets over time. Endurance relates to the muscles' ability to sustain contraction or perform repeated contractions. Endurance training impacts the aerobic pathways, most typically via low load, high repetition exercise. Conditioning with treadmills or elliptical trainers develops muscular and cardiovascular endurance. Workload can be advanced via changing the grade, resistance, speed or duration of workout on the equipment.

CORE STRENGTHENING

Exercise to increase trunk stability, or 'core strengthening', is included in almost all sports rehabilitation programs. The 'core' is defined by the diaphragm superiorly, pelvic floor inferiorly, abdominals anteriorly and lumbar extensors posteriorly.[18] While application of core strengthening may be obvious in athletes with low back pain, it is thought to play an integral role in rehabilitating athletes with limb injuries, in particular in the throwing athlete. Co-contraction of the trunk muscles provides active stiffening and reduces spinal loading while connecting the upper and lower limbs via the abdominal fascial system.[19] In particular, the posterior layer of the thoracolumbar fascia is crucial in supporting the lumbar and abdominal muscles. The aponeurosis of the latissimus dorsi muscles forms the superficial layer of the posterior thoracolumbar fascia and the transversus abdominus has extensive attachments to the

carefully titrated to avoid re-injury. One can manipulate height from which the athlete drops and speed and vigor of contraction. While plyometric training has been used informally for many decades, it has become a mainstay in rehabilitating athletes and preparing them for return to sports. Lower extremity plyometric exercises can be advanced from tuck jumping to drop jumping (dropping to the ground from a raised height then immediately jumping). Upper extremity plyometric training can be done with press-ups and hand claps or using equipment such as a medicine ball or weighted ball (Fig. 17.4).

Agility drills

Agility drills are dynamic exercises that combine plyometric training with coordination, proprioception and neuromuscular control. The shuttle run, for example, is the ultimate kinetic chain activity, requiring coordination of upper and lower body movement, controlling eccentrically the force of gravity and momentum, while challenging aerobic capacity and joint load tolerance. Agility drills are incorporated as part of the sport specific training in the functional stage of rehabilitation.

middle and posterior thoracolumbar fascia, thereby connecting the upper and lower limbs.[20] The hip girdle musculature plays an integral role in stabilizing the lumbar spine and pelvis, especially in ambulatory activities.[21]

Box 17.6: Key Points

Muscle groups included in a core strengthening program

- Transversus abdominus
- Multifidis
- Lumbar paraspinals
- Gluteus maximus and medius
- Pelvic floor.

Core strengthening programs incorporate specific exercises, some that isolate and others that combine the muscular activation of the core. It is described extensively and is the moniker used to label a wide-variety of exercise programs. The muscles most frequently targeted include the transverses abdominus, multifidus, lumbar paraspinals, gluteus maximus and medius, and the pelvic floor musculature.

While theoretically aimed to prevent and treat musculoskeletal injuries in athletes, there have been no randomized controlled studies of core strengthening in sports medicine rehabilitation. Core strengthening has been studied in regards to preventing low back injuries and improving sports performance.[22] There may be some inherent risks to at least the spine with some core strengthening programs and further study is warranted. Particular exercises, such as the Roman chair extensor training, are considered unsafe by some researchers.[23]

Many core strengthening programs have their grounding in dynamic lumbar stabilization exercises.[24] The beginning exer-

cises include the curl-up, side bridge and bird dog (Fig. 17.5).[25] Exercise progression includes addition of the physioball or other labile surfaces and upright positioning. Many programs do not include the transverse plane, or rotational movements, so pertinent to athletic function.[25]

FLEXIBILITY TRAINING

Flexibility is the total achievable excursion of a body part through its potential range of motion.[26] Flexibility relates to tissue extensibility to allow for normal motion while laxity describes excessive tissue extensibility to allow for abnormal motion of a joint. Static factors in flexibility include collagen type or inflammation. Dynamic factors include motor control or pain. The goal of flexibility training is adequate flexibility without injury or excessive joint laxity. Joint mobility plays a role in flexibility and must be evaluated by a trained manual therapist. Stretching denotes applying a deforming force along the joint and muscles. Deficits in capsular mobility must be treated at the outset of the flexibility program. Application of an oscillatory or sustained force distally while stabilizing the joint proximally mobilizes the joint. Historically, stretching has focused on end range, single plane force. More recently, functional programs are moving beyond single plane, end range focused stretching programs.[13] This is in keeping with the multiplanar muscle, joint and fascial planes.

Stretching before sports participation is a routine activity, endorsed by coaches, trainers, and team physicians. Athletes are typically told to warm up to begin to sweat prior to stretching. While stretching is believed to prevent muscle soreness and injury and enhance performance, several reviews of the medical literature have concluded there is insufficient evidence to support these claims.[27-29] In many studies, the major

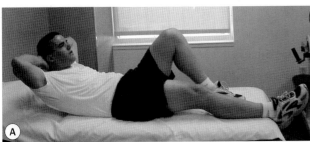
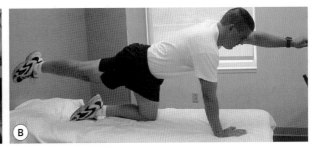
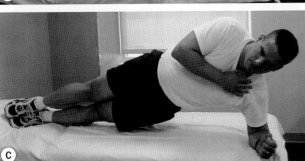

Figure 17.5 Basic exercises for spine stabilization programs include (A) the curl-up, (B) the side bridge and (C) the bird dog. These exercises can be performed with a physioball or other labile surface to increase difficulty. (From Akuthota and Nadler 2004.[25])

predictor of joint injury was previous injury and joint laxity, not necessarily inadequate flexibility.[30,31]

Stretching is employed in the exercise program of injured athletes after evaluation reveals flexibility deficits. There are many types of stretching exercises used by therapists and trainers and taught to rehabilitating athletes (Table 17.3). Historically, ballistic (bouncing) stretching including rapid, repetitive jerking motions was employed; it has fallen from favor due to concerns of soft tissue injury.[32] Passive stretching includes slow sustained external force applied by another individual. Proprioceptive neuromuscular facilitation or PNF may require another individual providing isometric or isotonic resistance followed by passive muscle lengthening.[33] PNF relies heavily on the neurophysiological principles of reciprocal inhibition and the stretch reflex in its attempt to impact the muscle spindles and Golgi tendon organs.

Table 17.3 Types of Stretching

Method	Typical Requirements
Passive stretching	Partner for external force
	Slow sustained stretch
Static stretching	Self imposed force
	Hold for 15–60 s
	2 sets for each muscle group
Ballistic stretching	Repetitive jerking movement
	Rapid movements
	Possibly injurious
Proprioceptive	Partner for external force
neuromuscular	Immediate application of force after contract
facilitation (PNF)	isometrically (contract-relax stretching)
Functional stretching	Self imposed stretch
	Apparatus for positioning
	Incorporation of all 3 planes of cardinal
	movement (frontal, sagittal and
	transverse)

Typical patterns of inflexibility are observed in the sports medicine clinic, reflecting similar patterns in the population at large. The major muscle groups are typically targeted along with the injured limb or area. The stretches for the major muscle groups are generally described with unidirectional, end range focus.[34] It is not clear if this type of end range stretching is functional as most athletes do not move at the end range or in one particular plane; rather, they work in midranges with a combination of frontal, sagittal and transverse planes. Several PNF patterns reflect this multiplanar joint movement pattern. There is contradictory research on increased flexibility and performance, with some showing enhancement and others with adverse effects.[27] These studies include exercise interventions with the uniplanar, end range stretching described above.

It is not clear how to educate and counsel athletes with regard to stretching. Knowledge of the biomechanics of the athletes' sport will direct one to obligate movement patterns she will engage in. Directing the stretching program to prepare the athlete for these movement patterns is logical. In addition, incorporating multiplanar directionality to the stretch should be useful. For instance, rather than having the athlete stretch the psoas muscle with a sagittal plane, end range stretch, the addition of the frontal and transverse plane is much more in keeping with sports activity required for rebounding in basketball.

CONCLUSION

Exercise is the keystone in sports medicine and rehabilitation. It provides a practical means of restoring injured and deconditioned tissue to function, in the case of the athlete, for sport. The exercise building blocks required include strength, cardiovascular fitness, neuromuscular coordination and flexibility. A thorough understanding of the specific sport the athlete competes in allows one to tailor the program to meet the needs of that athlete. The utilization of plyometrics, core strengthening, multiplanar stretching and other novel techniques require further innovative research.

REFERENCES

1 Kibler WB. A framework for sports medicine. Phys Med Rehabil Clin North Am 1994; 5:1.

2 Herring SA, Kibler WB. A framework for rehabilitation. In: Kibler WB, Herring SA, Press JM, eds. Functional rehabilitation of sports and musculoskeletal injuries. Gaithersburg: Aspen; 1998:1–8.

3 Sale D, MacDougall D. Specificity in strength training: a review for the coach and athlete. Can J Appl Sports Sci 1981; 6:87.

4 Brukner P, Khan K. Clinical sports medicine. Sydney: McGraw-Hill; 1997:404–416.

5 DeLorme T, Watkins A. Technics of progressive resistance exercise. Arch Phys Med Rehabil 1948; 29:263.

6 Vinowieff AN. Heavy resistance exercise: the Oxford technic. Br J Phys Med 1951; 14:129.

7 Knight KL. Knee rehabilitation by the daily adjustable progressive resistance exercise technique. Am J Sports Med 1979; 7:336–337.

8 Childs JD, Irrgang JJ. The language of exercise and rehabilitation. In: DeLee JC, Drez D, Miller MD, eds. DeLee & Drez's orthopaedic sports medicine: principles and practice, Vol 1. 2nd edn. Philadelphia: Saunders; 2003:319–335.

9 Young JL, Press JM. The physiologic basis of sports rehabilitation. Phys Med Rehabil Clin North Am 1994; 5:9–36.

10 McArdle WD, Katch FI, Katch VL. Exercise physiology: energy, nutrition, and human performance. 3rd edn. Philadelphia: Lea & Febiger; 1991.

11 Astrand PO, Rodahl K. Textbook of work physiology. New York: Mc-Graw Hill; 1986.

12 Draganich LF, Jaeger RJ, et al. Coactivation of the hamstrings and quadriceps during extension of the knee. J Bone J Surg Am 1989; 71:1075–1081.

13 Gray G. Course notes, Functional issues. Chicago, IL: 2004.

14 Dugan SA. Sports-related knee injuries in female athletes: what gives? Am J Phys Med Rehabil 2005; 84:122–130.

15 Proske U, Morgan DL. Muscle damage from eccentric exercise: mechanism, mechanical signs, adaptation and clinical application. J Physiol 2001; 537:333–345.

16 Brockett CL, Morgan DL, Proske U. Predicting hamstring injury in elite athletes. Med Sci Sports Exerc 2004; 36:379–387.

17 Sharkey BJ. Training for sport. In: Cantu RC, Michelli LJ, eds. ACSM's guidelines for the team physician. Philadelphia: Lea & Febiger; 1991:34–47.

18 Richardson C, Jull G, et al. Therapeutic exercise for spinal segmental stabilization in low back pain: scientific basis and clinical approach. Edinburgh: Churchill Livingstone; 1999.

19 Konin JG, Beil N, Werner G. Functional rehabilitation. Facilitating the serape effect to enhance extremity force production. Athl Ther Today 2003; 8:54–56.

20   Vleeming A, Pool-Goudzwaard AL, et al. The posterior layer of the thoracolumbar fascia. Its function in load transfer from spine to legs. Spine 1995; 2:753-758.

21   Lyons K, Perry J, et al. Timing and relative intensity of hip extensor and abductor muscle action during level and stair ambulation. An EMG study. Phys Ther 1983; 63:1597-1605.

22   Nadler SF, Malanga GA, et al. Hip muscle imbalance and low back pain in athletes: influence of core strengthening. Med Sci Sports Exerc 2002; 34:9-16.

23   McGill S. Low back disorders: evidence-based prevention and rehabilitation. Champaign: Human Kinetics; 2002.

24   Saal JA, Saal JS. Nonoperative treatment of herniated lumbar intervertebral disc with radiculopathy. An outcome study. Spine 1989; 14:431-437.

25   Akuthota V, Nadler SF. Core strengthening. Arch Phys Med Rehabil 2004; 85:86-92.

26   Saal JS. Flexibility training. In: Kibler WB, Herring SA, Press JM, eds. Functional rehabilitation of sports and musculoskeletal injuries. Gaithersburg: Aspen; 1998:85-97.

27   Thacker SB, Gilchrist J, et al. The impact of stretching on sports injury risk: a systematic review of the literature. Med Sci Sports Exerc 2004; 36:371-378.

28   Weldon SM, Hill RH. The efficacy of stretching for prevention of exercise-related injury: a systematic review of the literature. Man Ther 2003; 8:141-150.

29   Herbert RD, Gabriel M. Effects of stretching before and after exercising on muscle soreness and risk of injury: a systematic review. BMJ 2002; 325:468-470.

30   Godshall R. The predictability of athletic injuries: an eight year study. J Sports Med 1975; 3:50-54.

31   Keller C, Noyes F, Buchner R. Sports traumatology series: the medical aspects of soccer injury epidemiology. Am J Sports Med 1987; 15:230-237.

32   DeVries H. Prevention of muscular distress after exercise. Res Q 1961; 32:177-185.

33   Knott M, Voss D. Proprioceptive neuromuscular facilitation patterns and techniques. New York: Harper & Row; 1968:72-73.

34   Anderson B, Burke ER. Scientific, medical, and practical aspects of stretching. Clin Sports Med 1991; 10:63-86.

CHAPTER 18

Proprioception and Coordination

Emin Ergen and Bülent Ulkar

INTRODUCTION

From the sports medicine point of view, the coordination of a movement is mainly the internal organization of the optimal control of the motor system and its parts.[1] The basis of coordinative capabilities lies in the highest levels of the central nervous system (CNS) and sensory motor subsystems. Thus, the coordination can be regarded as an umbrella term embracing the concept of optimization for intramuscular and intermuscular coordination and cooperation for a given task including internal and external feedback mechanisms. These mechanisms are disrupted in case of an injury and the continuation of information processing is ceased which would lead to performance deteriorations and re-injury.

Sometimes the proper management of sport injuries can be complex and challenging for the sports medicine clinician. In order to prevent athletic injuries and program the rehabilitation after a joint lesion, understanding the role of proprioception is essential. Therefore, the terms 'proprioceptive deficit', 'proprioceptive training', and 'proprioceptive rehabilitation' are being used increasingly in sports medicine.[2]

DEFINITIONS

Coordination has been defined as a cooperative interaction between the nervous system and skeletal muscles.[1] The optimal development of coordinative capability serves as the basis for successful motor learning in every sport and the eventual performance of movements and sport skills at the highest levels of mastery. This is particularly important for the prevention of injuries in a risky sports situation such as cutting, dribbling, jumping and landing. Coordination therefore encompasses the proprioceptive abilities. With regard to proprioception, many researchers have defined it as the afferent input of joint position sense (i.e. awareness of position or movement), whereas others consider proprioception in a broader sense that includes neuromuscular control. Most contemporary authorities define proprioception as a specialized variation of the sensory modality of touch that includes the sensation of joint movement (kinesthesia) and joint position (joint position sense).[3]

During any voluntary movements or perturbations occurring during walking, running or jumping, due to rapid responses of lower and to some extent upper extremities, the musculature of these parts play an important role in maintaining the desirable posture. Postural control is dependent on reflex mechanisms that maintain the body's center of mass over the feet (a static or dynamic balance). Any sudden change of the foot or feet position stimulates a sequence of muscle firing that is dependent upon central generators and programs interacting with peripheral reflexes. Afferent information for necessary fine tuning of movements is provided by proprioceptive, visual, vestibular, and somatosensorial receptors (Fig. 18.1).

Somatosensorial receptors are located in muscles, tendons, joints, and other tissues. Classically, three types of somatic senses are described: pain, thermo-receptivity, and mechano-receptivity. Proprioception relates primarily to the mechano-receptive sensation which includes tactile and position sense.

Proprioception encompasses two aspects of position sense: static and dynamic. Static sense gives conscious orientation of one body part with respect to another. Dynamic sense provides the neuromuscular system feedback about the rate and direction of a movement. Thus, proprioception can be thought of as a complex neuromuscular process that involves both afferent input and efferent signals and allows the body to maintain stability and orientation during both static and dynamic activities.[4]

There are also two levels of proprioception: conscious (voluntary) and unconscious (reflex initiated). Conscious proprioception enables proper joint function in sports, activities, and occupational tasks. Unconscious proprioception modulates muscle function and initiates reflexive stabilization of joints by way of the muscle receptors.[5]

PROPRIOCEPTIVE ORGANS – MECHANORECEPTORS

Two-way communication between sensory and motor systems is crucial for normal motor control. Visual input is one of the most important aspects in proprioception. Information from the vestibular apparatus about head position in relation to gravity and to head movements is also important. The other

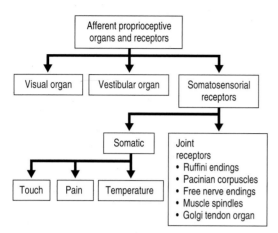

Figure 18.1 Afferent proprioceptive organs and receptors.

important body sense is obtained through somatosensory receptors. The sensory receptors for proprioception that are found in the skin, muscles, and joints as well as in ligaments and tendons all provide input to the CNS regarding tissue deformation.[6]

Specialized nerve endings and proprioceptive mechanoreceptors (Pacinian corpuscles, Ruffini endings, Golgi tendon organ like endings) have been histologically identified in the knee joint in the capsule,[7–9] in the anterior cruciate ligament (ACL),[10–12] posterior cruciate ligament (PCL),[13] meniscus,[14] lateral collateral ligament[15] and infrapatellar fat pad.[16]

Box 18.1: Key Points

Proprioceptive mechanoreceptors are present in articular and muscular structures

Articular mechanoreceptors

- Type I: Ruffini endings (SA)

- Type II: Pacinian corpuscle (QA)

- Type IV: Unmyelinated free nerve endings

Muscular mechanoreceptors

- Type III: Golgi-organ tendon (SA)

- Muscle spindle (SA)

(SA: Slow adapting, QA: Quick adapting).

The role of mechanoreceptors

Mechanoreceptors are specialized neurons that transmit mechanical deformation information (e.g. joint rotation due to positional change and motion) into electrical signals.[17,18] Stimulation of these receptors results in reflex muscle contraction about the joint as an adaptive control to sudden movements of acceleration or deceleration.[9]

Each of the above mentioned five mechanoreceptor types responds to different stimuli and transmits specific afferent information that modifies neuromuscular function. All receptors need a stimulus to change their membrane potential caus-

ing an action potential to travel to the CNS. For example, it is speculated that longitudinal tension on a ligament results in compression of the connective tissue that stimulates the mechanoreceptors.[19] Mechanoreceptors can also be stimulated by muscle-length change, including the rate of change in tension and length. The mechanical deformation of a receptor stretches the membrane and opens the ion channel. This allows positively charged ions (Na^+) into the cell, which creates a net depolarizing effect that generates a nerve receptor potential. Mechanoreceptors detect deformation of the receptor itself or of cells adjacent to the receptor.[20]

Mechanoreceptors demonstrate different adaptive characteristics related to their response to a stimulus. Quick-adapting (QA) mechanoreceptors (Pacinian corpuscle), decrease their discharge rate to extinction within milliseconds of the onset of a continuous stimulus. Slow-adapting (SA) mechanoreceptors (Ruffini ending and the Golgi tendon organ), remain discharging in response to a continuous stimulus. QA mechanoreceptors are very sensitive to changes in stimulation and are therefore considered to mediate the sensation of joint motion QA mechanoreceptors may be more important in some sports characterized with sudden directional changes like pivoting, shifting, tackling etc. SA mechanoreceptors are maximally stimulated at certain joint angles, and thus a continuum of SA receptors is thought to mediate the sensation of joint position.[21,22] Stimulation of these receptors results in reflex muscle contraction about the joint.[9,23] When there is no capsuloligamentous strain (or load) on the joint (midrange of position), afferent neurons are not active and they do not play a role in proprioception. Rather, many studies argue that joint afferents (especially Ruffini corpuscle) are limit detectors.[24]

The muscle spindle receptor is a complex, fusiform, SA receptor located within skeletal muscle. Via afferents and efferents to intrafusal muscle fibers, the muscle spindle receptor can detect muscle tension over a large range of extrafusal muscle length. The monosynaptic stretch reflex involves muscle spindle receptor connecting I-a nerve fibers as well as Golgi tendon organs connecting to I-b fibers. During rapid perturbation such as tripping or falling, monosynaptic reflexes are absent and compensation occurs as a result of transmission along group II and III afferent fibers from secondary muscle spindles. These connect through a polysynaptic reflex system to generate an appropriate response. The contribution of vestibular and visual input to these reflexes is minimal. Gravity and pressure on joints and on the plantar skin surface may be critical to these reflexes.[25]

CLINICAL IMPORTANCE OF PROPRIOCEPTION

In any specific situation there are gravity, inertia and reaction forces creating a specific external load upon musculoskeletal structures. This load is counteracted by the internal forces and the internal forces balance the external. Good proprioception and coordination means that all the components of musculoskeletal fitness are in balance to overcome any overloading on structures and this is important in maintaining dynamic joint stability.[26]

Dynamic joint stability can be defined as the ability of appropriately activated muscles to stabilize a joint together with the support of mechanical stabilizers (Fig. 18.2). In essence, dynamic joint stability is the 'product' of the proprioceptive system.[2]

In relation to dynamic (functional) joint stability, cognitive programming also plays a role in the neuromuscular control mechanism which involves the highest level of CNS function (motor cortex, basal ganglia, and the cerebellum). This function refers to voluntary movements that are repeated and stored as central commands. The awareness of body position and movement allows various skills to be performed without continuous reference to consciousness.[27] As defined earlier, proprioceptive feedback is crucial in the conscious and unconscious awareness of a joint or limb in motion. Therefore, enhancement of dynamic (functional) joint stability is important both in prevention and rehabilitation of athletic injuries. This requires a constant and appropriate flow of sensory information, integrated with motor output, in a coordinated manner.[28]

Trauma to tissues may result in partial deafferentation by causing mechanoreceptor damage, which can lead to proprioceptive deficits. Consequently, susceptibility to re-injury may become a possibility because of this decrease in proprioceptive feedback. However, studies have shown at least partial restoration of kinesthesia and joint position sense in surgically reconstructed shoulders and knees after rehabilitation.[29,30]

The effect of ligamentous trauma resulting in mechanical instability and proprioceptive deficits contributes to functional instability, which could eventually lead to further microtrauma and re-injury. Achieving functional and sport-specific activities following musculoskeletal trauma and rehabilitation can be established significantly if proprioception is addressed and instituted early in the treatment program.

ANKLE PROPRIOCEPTION

Functional instability of the ankle is one of the most common residual disabilities after an acute ankle sprain. Ankle joint instability can be defined as either mechanical or functional instability. Mechanical instability refers to objective measurement of ligament laxity, whereas functional instability is defined as the feeling of giving way. Casual factors include a proprioceptive deficit, muscular weakness, and/or absent coordination.[31]

Ankle instability as a result of partial deafferentation of articular mechanoreceptors with joint injury was first postulat-

ed by Freeman (1965).[32] They observed that a decrease in the ability to maintain a one-legged stance occurred in the sprained ankle versus the contralateral uninjured ankle. Konradsen and Ravn (1990) attributed the cause of functional instability to both mechanical and functional causes in stating that functional instability results from 'damage to mechanical receptors in the lateral ligaments or muscle/tendon with subsequent partial de-afferentiation of the proprioceptive reflex'.[33]

Glencross and Thornton (1991) reported deficits in the ability to actively replicate passive ankle and foot positioning while testing the sprained ankle versus the contralateral uninjured ankle.[34] Gross (1987) also revealed that an increased probability of re-injury occurs as a result of a decrease in sensory input from joint.[35]

Konradsen and Ravn (1990) found that chronic ankle instability resulted in a prolonged peroneal reaction time in response to a sudden inversion stress when compared with age matched controls.[33] Partial deafferentation resulting in diminished reflex joint stabilization may contribute to these findings.

No increases in postural sway were observed by Tropp and Odenrick (1988) when comparing a group of soccer players with previous ankle sprains to a control group of uninjured soccer players.[36] However, significant increases in postural sway were observed by Cornwall and Murrell (1991) when comparing patients with acute ankle sprains with uninjured controls as long as 2 years after their injuries.[37]

Muscle reaction time

In terms of lateral foot and ankle perturbations, several authors have evaluated the timing and power of neuromuscular response in the lower leg muscles. A significantly faster reflex time has been found in the peroneal muscles compared with the quadriceps and hamstring.[25] Peroneal reaction time has been found significantly shorter in mechanically stable ankles.[38] However, all these studies have been conducted on subjects in a standing position with lower extremity muscles at rest. In an action like walking, running or jumping, a considerable preactivation of related muscles prior to touchdown exist.[25] Therefore, exercises including perturbations on wobble board may increase ankle stability both for preventive and rehabilitative purposes.

Taping

It has been postulated that ankle taping induced prophylaxis is associated with sensory feedback. By uniting the skin of the leg with the plantar surface of the foot, Robbins et al. (1995) suggested that the sensory cues to plantar surface of the foot are increased, thereby allowing a more accurate foot placement and reducing the changes of excessive ligamentous strain.[39] Karlsson and Andreasson (1992) concluded that tape may help patients with unstable ankles by facilitating proprioceptive and skin sensory input to the central nervous system.[38] Therefore, taping or using lace-up brace may contribute proprioception with sensory stimulation. There are some studies emphasizing that ankle taping rapidly loses its initial level of resistance, nevertheless restraining effect on extreme ankle motion has not been eliminated by prolonged activity as well.[40,41]

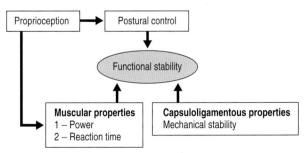

Figure 18.2 Factors effecting functional stability.

KNEE PROPRIOCEPTION

The presence of neuroreceptors in the human knee joint had been described by Rauber over a hundred years ago, whereas the presence of numerous mechanoreceptors in the human ACL was well documented in the 1980s.[42]

The afferent innervation of joints is based on peripheral receptors located in articular, muscular, and cutaneous structures. Articular receptors include nociceptive free nerve endings and proprioceptive mechanoreceptors. Mechanoreceptors which have been identified histomorphologically in the ACL, PCL, meniscus, lateral collateral ligament and infrapatellar fat pad are Ruffini endings, Pacinian corpuscles, and Golgi tendon organs.[43]

Knee joint proprioception which is essential for adequate joint movement and stability, arises from receptors located in muscles, tendons, skin and joint structures. Sensory information from the knee joint receptors affects the activity of the gamma-motor neurons which in turn affect the muscle spindle afferents. The joint receptors are thereby participating in the continuous regulation of muscle stiffness around the joint; thus theoretically, defective proprioception may lead to instability of the joint.[44]

Proprioception may play a protective role in acute knee injury through reflex muscular splinting. Kennedy *et al.* (1982) hypothesized that loss of mechanoreceptor feedback from torn knee ligaments contributed to a vicious cycle of loss of reflex muscular splinting, repetitive major and minor injury and progressive laxity.[10]

The protective reflex arc initiated by mechanoreceptors and muscle spindle receptors occurs much more quickly than the reflex arc initiated by nociceptors (70–100 m/s *versus* 1 m/s). Thus, proprioception may play a more significant role than pain sensation in preventing injury in the acute setting.[45]

Mechanoreceptors found in the ACL together with the mechanoreceptors in the PCL and collateral ligaments, is a very important factor in the complicated neural net of proprioception. After an ACL injury, the gait patterns of the ACL-deficient knee are altered, probably due to changes in proprioception. Proprioceptive deficits after ACL rupture can predispose to other injury and may contribute to causing degenerative joint disease by pathological wearing of the cartilage because of the altered gait patterns of a joint with poor sensation.[46]

In addition to mechanical disruption of articular structures following injury, the loss of proprioception may have a profound effect on neuromuscular control and the activities of daily living. It appears that neurological feedback mechanisms originating in articular and musculotendinous structures provide an important component for the maintenance of functional joint stability.[47] Articular deafferentation results following the injury to capsuloligamentous structures. This contributes to alterations in kinesthesia and joint position sense and further degenerative changes in the joint, as the spinal reflexive pathway may be impaired.[47]

Most clinical studies about knee joint proprioception have dealt with ACL deficient or ACL reconstructed knee joints. There is one unequivocal result of these studies; even when totally different methods of evaluating the proprioceptive capabilities are applied, patients suffering from an ACL rupture have significantly worse knee joint proprioception than healthy groups.[48]

Safran *et al.* (1999) have demonstrated that isolated PCL deficiency in the human knee does result in reduced kinesthesia, as tested by the threshold to detect passive positioning and enhanced reproduction of passive positioning (RPP).[43] On the other hand, proprioceptive deficits in studies of patients with ACL disruption reveal greater proprioceptive deficits, both in magnitude and over a greater range of motion, than the findings presented by Safran *et al.* (1999) for PCL deficiency.[43]

Disruptions in the afferent pathway which are mediated partly by articular mechanoreceptors may also contribute significantly to an insidious pattern of microtrauma and reinjury.[47] Beard *et al.* (1994) demonstrated the inhibition of reflex arc, which leads to reductions in reflex muscular stabilization resulting from ACL deficiency.[49] Partial restoration of kinesthetic awareness on patients who had undergone anterior cruciate ligament reconstruction by a modified MacIntosh-Jones method has been demonstrated by Barrett (1991).[50] This study indicates that proprioception, together with the clinical excellence of the repair and re-establishing the stability, is another important factor in the outcome of anterior cruciate ligament reconstruction.

It has been proposed that loss of the proprioceptive feedback after an ACL rupture contributes to the progressive instability and disability that occurs in a high percentage of ACL deficient knee joints.[3,46,51] Reconstruction of the ruptured ACL does not always result in the expected successful outcome. Success after ligament reconstruction may depend not only on the tightness or strength of the reconstruction but also on the quality of recovery of proprioception.[50,52] Correct stability seems to be the basis for later ligamentization and recovery of proprioception.[46]

SHOULDER PROPRIOCEPTION

Positioning the hand is a necessary motion during activities of daily living in addition to sport-specific patterns. Joint position sensibility not only plays an important role in the maintenance of dynamic shoulder stability but also shows alterations after injury. Ligaments around the shoulder joint are in action during normal kinematics and also provide neurological feedback mediating muscular reflex inhibition. Shoulder articulation is not constrained to a large extent, therefore a coordinated dynamic control of muscles about the joint is necessary for stabilizing the arm during motion. The ligamentous structures function only at extreme positions of rotation to prevent excessive translation or rotation of the humeral head on the glenoid. In the midranges of rotation, the capsuloligamentous structures are relatively lax and joint stability is attained with dynamic action of the rotator cuff and biceps tendons. Contraction of these muscle tendon units generates joint compression and increases the concavity compression fit of the humeral head into the glenoid cavity. In addition, a coordinated, synergistic contraction of the rotator cuff and biceps may protect the ligamentous structures from injury by increasing torque resistance against excessive rotation and preventing excessive translations of the humeral head.[53]

Proprioceptive ability does not show a difference between the dominant and non-dominant shoulder, but in unstable shoulders this has been found to be significantly decreased.[3,54] Several studies have demonstrated deficits in shoulder kinesthesia and joint position sense in male non-athletes subjects with unilateral, traumatic, recurrent anterior shoulder instability and proprioceptive deficits have also been observed in the pathologic shoulder as compared with the contralateral normal shoulder.[3,55] Reduction in neuromuscular activation of the pectoralis major, subscapularis, and latissimus dorsi muscles was shown to contribute to anterior instability through a decrease in the normal internal rotation force necessary for this motion. Compensatory increases in biceps and supraspinatus muscle activity were also discovered in an attempt to restore anterior stability. This loss in the normal synchronization of neuromuscular firing patterns in the unstable shoulder has been attributed to altered joint kinematics resulting in repetitive microtrauma. Surgical intervention (capsulolabral reconstruction) has been shown to partially restore joint proprioception through the repair of traumatized tissue.[3] The authors have commented that the procedure modifies soft tissue dissection and a minimal loss of intact mechanoreceptors and a promotion of re-population were observed. In addition, the use of the capsular shift in these shoulder instability cases, which tightens the capsule, 're-tensions' the soft tissue and most likely facilitates proprioception function. It may be through this procedure of re-tensioning that mechanoreceptor-containing shoulder capsuloligamentous structures send afferent information at a more functional level regarding joint position sensibility. Restoring dynamic neuromuscular control of the unstable or postoperative shoulder is of primary importance for returning to functional activity.

MEASUREMENT OF PROPRIOCEPTION

The assessment of neuromuscular control includes the measurement of cortical, spinal reflex, and brainstem pathways. The evaluation of this complex neuromuscular system as different components allows a more detailed explanation of afferent control mechanisms.[3]

Kinesthesia and joint position sensibility are the two major assessment methods of joint proprioception. Kinesthesia is assessed by measuring threshold to detection of passive motion (TTDPM), while joint position sense is assessed by measuring reproduction of passive positioning (RPP) and reproduction of active positioning (RAP). These tests are performed at slow angular velocities (0.5–2.5°/s) to selectively stimulate Ruffini or Golgi-type mechanoreceptors, and because the test is performed passively, it is believed to maximally stimulate joint receptors while minimally stimulating muscle receptors.[47]

Several methods and devices have been described to test proprioceptive status of healthy and injured people. Studies that have investigated the proprioceptive ability of ACL-deficient and reconstructed knees have primarily relied on measurement of TTDPM and reproduction of knee joint angles.[45,47,56]

Box 18.2: Key Points

Measurement Methods of Proprioception

Measurement of kinesthesia and joint position sense

- Special devices developed for this purpose (PTD)
- Isokinetic dynamometers
- Goniometers, inclinometers
- Motion analysis systems

Measurement of balance and postural control

- Stabilometers
- Force plates

Measurement of muscular latency

- Electromyographic analyses

Non-instrumented methods

- Limb matching tests
- Hop tests.

Several researchers utilized proprioception testing devices (PTDs) similar in action and design.[51,56–58] These devices have moving arms rotating the limbs through the axis of the joint. A rotational transducer interfaced with a digital microprocessor counter provides the angular displacement values. Pneumatic compression cuffs are placed on each limb distal to the tested joints to reduce cutaneous input. The subjects are blindfolded to eliminate visual cues and headphones with white noise are used to eliminate auditory cues. The subjects are holding an on-off switch to press when they detect the threshold of passive motion or the pre-positioned angle. Some of these devices are designed to perform measurements both on knee and shoulder joints (Figs 18.3, 18.4).[51,57–59] Friden et al. (1996, 1997, 1998, 1999) reported several studies conducted with a

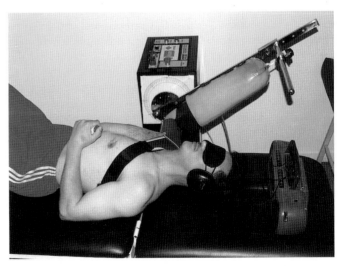

Figure 18.3 Threshold to detection of passive motion (TTDPM) and position sense measurement device with shoulder apparatus. (Prosport 1000 HMS, Tümer Engineering Co. Ltd., Ankara, Turkey.)

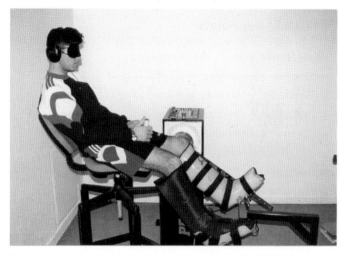

Figure 18.4 Threshold to detection of passive motion (TTDPM) and position sense measurement device with knee apparatus. (Prosport 1000 HMS, Tümer Engineering Co. Ltd., Ankara, Turkey.)

PTD which measured the threshold for detecting a passive motion of knee joint in lateral decubitus position.[60–63]

The abilities of position replication on subjects' joints are performed by using isokinetic dynamometers as well.[57,64–66] Some researchers use modified isokinetic devices to record the changes in positioning.[67] Active reproduction of joint position was another way of assessing joint position sense using an electromagnetic tracking device and an isokinetic dynamometer.[57,66]

Photographic record of the position-matching test with goniometric measurements is useful to investigate the accuracy in position-matching.[68] A simple inclinometer may be used for joint position sense (JPS) testing besides range of motion (ROM) measurements.[69]

In recent years, motion analysis systems have been used to record target joint angles, calculate reproduced angles (e.g. angle velocity reproduction test-AVRT) and to test dynamic sensorimotor abilities of joints.[57,70–72]

For the determination of the combination of peripheral, vestibular and visual contributions to neuromuscular control; postural sway and balance are evaluated. Functional assessment of the combined peripheral, vestibular and visual contributions to neuromuscular control is best accomplished through the use of balance and postural sway measurements for the lower extremity. The availability of stabilometric methods and instrumentation can provide a relatively accurate index for these measures.[73–76]

Balance stabilometry provides a specialized mode of assessment for the overall contribution of these various neural afferent signals to maintain upright standing posture. Postural balance and sway measurements are conducted using various types of force platform devices. Postural control is assessed by measuring changes in the center of pressure signal provided by a force plate during tests of limb standing balance.[75,77–81]

The assessment of the spinal reflex pathway is conducted to determine the latency of muscular activation to involuntary perturbations. Electromyographic (EMG) analysis has been utilized extensively to examine the role of this neuromuscular pathway during movements that place functional loads on the ankle and knee joint.[47] The assessment of reflex capabilities is

usually performed using EMG interpretation of firing patterns those muscles crossing the respective joint.

The delay between the initiating stimulus and the onset of the peroneal muscle reflex response is defined as the peroneal latency. Electromyographic studies that investigate muscle onset-latency alterations that develop after an ankle sprain have typically used a simulated inversion ankle sprain perturbation in association with surface EMG to record peroneal muscle onset latencies. The electromechanical delay (EMD) was defined as the time interval between the onset of the peroneus longus electromyogram detected by surface electrodes and the onset of the lateral ground reaction force (Fy) measured on a force plate. Mora *et al.* (2003) investigated ankle instability by measuring the electromechanical delay of the peroneal muscles (foot pronators).[82]

Non-instrumented, clinically applicable tests to assess neuromuscular and functional deficits, are reliable and valid for both research and clinical purposes.[83] Limb matching tasks are examples to evaluate proprioception without utilizing an electromechanical device. Providing different angles joint movements, the patients are asked to reproduce the given angle with the other limb.[84] Although various hop tests have been used to measure the lower limb power and functional ability of the athletes, they are assumed to be useful in the evaluation of proprioceptive status of the injured athlete at the end of the rehabilitation periods. These tests are performed either for distance or time to evaluate lower extremity symmetry.[85,86]

PROPRIOCEPTIVE TRAINING FOR PREVENTION AND REHABILITATION

The concept of doing proprioceptive exercises to regain neuromuscular control initially was introduced in rehabilitation programs (see Progression of a Proprioception Exercise Program, Figs 18.5–18.17 and Table 18.1).[87] It was considered that because mechanoreceptors are located in ligaments an injury to a ligament would alter afferent input. Training after an injury, would be needed to restore this altered neurologic function. Neuromuscular conditioning techniques have also been advocated for injury prevention. Increased postural and movement accuracy increases the consistency with which activities can be performed safely.[26]

An intervention program consisting of injury awareness information, specific technical training and a program of proprioceptive training for players with a history of ankle sprains, demonstrated a 47% reduction in the incidence of ankle sprains in the course of single season.[88] Studies have also shown that proprioceptive training not only reduces the risk of re-injury, but also the incidence of acute lateral ankle sprain if used prophylactically.[88]

Proprioceptive or 'kinesthetic' awareness is one aspect of rehabilitation obtained through specific exercises. The objectives of proprioceptive rehabilitation are to retrain altered afferent pathways to enhance the sensation of joint movement. Proprioceptively-mediated neuromuscular control of joints comes into action at three distinct levels of motor activation within the CNS.[89]

Table 18.1 Progression of a Program Should be Designed to Proceed from Easy to More Difficult Movements as the Pain During the Exercises is Tolerated[91]

Easy	Difficult
Double leg	Single leg
Standing position (on the floor)	Moving platforms and different surfaces (e.g. pneumatic or foam pads)
Single direction (e.g. rocker board, ankle inversion-eversion boards, ankle flexion-extension boards)	Multidirection (e.g. ankle disk, mini trampoline)
Eyes open	Eyes shut
Free hands	Fixed arms (crossed over the chest)
Straight leg	Flexed knee
Fewer repetitions and sets	More repetitions and sets
Simple drills (e.g. walking, stepping down and up)	Complicated drills (e.g. hops, jumps, perturbations, and plyometrics)

1 Reflexes at the spinal level mediate movement patterns that are received from higher levels of the nervous system. This action provides reflex for joint stabilization during conditions of excessive stress around the articulation and has significant implications for rehabilitation.

2 The second level of motor control, located within the brainstem which receives information from joint mechanoreceptors, vestibular system, and visual input from the eyes to maintain posture and balance of the body. Reactivated neuromuscular actions allowing this pathway to process input from the aforementioned forms of afferent stimuli can be used to enhance brainstem function.

3 The highest level of CNS function (motor cortex, basal ganglia, and cerebellum) obtains cognitive awareness of body position and movement in which motor commands are initiated for voluntary movements. Use of the cortical pathway allows movements that are repeated and stored as central commands to be performed without continuous reference to consciousness. Kinesthetic and proprioception training are such types of activity that can develop this function.

Incorporating the three levels of motor control into activities to address proprioceptive deficiencies should be started in the early phases of rehabilitation program. Encouraging maximum afferent discharge to the respective CNS level should be the target in stimulating joint and muscle receptors. To stimulate reflex joint stabilization, which emanates from the spinal cord, activities must focus on sudden changes in joint positioning that necessitate reflex neuromuscular control. Development of motor function at the brainstem level can be gained by performing balance and postural activities, both with and without visual input. Maximally stimulating the conversion of conscious to unconscious motor programming can be achieved by performing joint positioning activities, especially at joint end ranges. Simple tasks such as balance training and joint repositioning should begin early in the rehabilitation program and should become increasingly more difficult as the patient progresses.[27] Some authors believe that adaptations that occur during rehabilitation are mediated by feed-forward processing and are less a function of enhanced afferent pathways.[3] This theory suggests that fast movements are controlled by advance information known about the task, while concurrent proprioceptive feedback is relatively less important. Feedback is used primarily at the cortical level to determine the success or failure of that movement and to a lesser extent at the subcortical level for directing the movement. With repetition, the cerebral cortex can determine the most effective motor pattern for a given task, based on the proprioceptive information of previous attempts. Biofeedback training appears to use the feed-forward learning process.[90]

PROPRIOCEPTIVE TRAINING FOR THE SHOULDER

Proprioception training of the upper extremity has been incorporated into the rehabilitation program to a lesser extent than that of the lower extremity. Because the primary sport-specific activity of the upper extremity is the throwing motion, refined joint positioning and repositioning of the shoulder is vital. Therefore, mechanoreceptor activity plays an important role in both performance and dynamic shoulder stabilization. The following progression of activities is conducted to allow an athlete returning to functional levels[91]:

1 joint position sense and kinesthesia
2 dynamic joint stabilization
3 reactive neuromuscular control and
4 functionally specific activities.

Such a progression allows the rehabilitation program to integrate spinal reflex, cognitive, and brainstem pathways focusing on scapular stabilization, glenohumeral stabilization, humeral motion, and neuromuscular control. Position sensibility activities are designed to restore joint position sense and kinesthesia. These exercises stimulate cognitive level processing through the use of such an exercise as glenohumeral repositioning both with and without visual input and proprioceptive neuromuscular facilitation patterns performed with manual resistance. Dynamic stabilization activities are designed to stimulate muscular coactivation. In the shoulder, such activities include axial loading of the glenohumeral joint promote coactivation of the glenohumeral and scapulothoracic force couples. Ultimately, plyometrics can be used for the integration of both spinal and cognitive levels. Shoulder plyometric exercises stimulate reflexive activity through the facilitation of the myotactic reflex via the release of stored elastic energy. Such activities stimulate reflex joint stabilization, which are critical to the overhead athlete. Once joint sensibility and dynamic muscle joint stabilization are restored, functionally specific activities can be accomplished.[91]

PROPRIOCEPTIVE TRAINING FOR THE KNEE

Reconstructing the ACL seems to improve afferent input needed for functional joint stability, and histologic studies have shown a re-population of mechanoreceptors in ACL graft tissue.[28] Exercises to enhance motor control therefore are essential after an anterior cruciate ligament reconstruction. In the past several years, there also has been a heightened awareness of the need for preseason sport conditioning to focus on lower extremity balance and conditioning to attempt to diminish the incidence of knee ligament injuries. Neuromuscular training incorporating plyometrics and agility drills and stressing the need for proper technique for pivoting, shifting, and landing, has been advocated to decrease the incidence of ACL injuries. Griffis (quad-cruciate interaction), Henning Sportsmetrics (a three-part prevention consisting of stretching, plyometrics, and strengthening drills), Caraffa (a five-phase progressive skill acquisition program) and Santa Monica by Mandelbaum (a five-part program designed to improve strength, flexibility, injury awareness, plyometrics and agility skills) are some of the program examples successfully implemented in rehabilitation.[28]

PROPRIOCEPTIVE TRAINING FOR THE ANKLE

Freeman (1965), has first recognized the importance of afferent input in neuromuscular coordination and the significant consequences that result when such input is disrupted.[32] He has analyzed previously injured patients following a training period and revealed that such exercises can help to achieve less functional instability than patients not trained in this manner.

Tropp (1986) found that 10 min daily wobble board training during a 10-week period could improve pronator muscle strength in patients with functional instability.[92] Further training has not been found to give any added effect. Wester *et al*. (1996) have conducted a similar study on 48 patients (24 training and 24 no-training group) with residual functional instability due to Grade II.[93] ankle sprain. Comparing with no training group, 12-week training group showed significantly fewer recurrent sprains in a 230 days follow-up period. Eils and Rosenbaum (2001) have studied the effects of a 6-week multistation proprioceptive exercise program.[31] Joint position sense, postural sway and muscle reaction times showed significant improvements following this multi-station training program consisting of 12 different exercises (on mat, swinging platform, air squab, eversion-inversion boards, ankle disc, mini trampoline, step, uneven walkway, hanging and swinging platforms, and with exercise bands). The program has been conducted in a way that each exercise was performed for 45 s followed by a 30 s break where subjects move over to the next station.

FOCUS ON THE BACK

The lower back is often considered the 'weak link' in the kinetic chain. Dynamic lumbar muscle stabilization has become a popular method of proprioceptive training for the low back. This involves coordinated strengthening of the abdominal, back, and trunk muscles in functional movement planes. Dynamic lumbar stabilization exercises are designed to progressively challenge this segment to promote successive adaptation, with an emphasis on balanced load distribution via a neutral pelvis, optimal skeletal alignment, and balanced strength.[2]

PROPRIOCEPTIVE EXERCISES

Although many companies sell fairly complex computerized equipment to help improve proprioceptive input and balance, such training can also be accomplished through various simple drills done on various surfaces with eyes open and eyes shut, progressing from a double to a single limb stance. However, if available, such technologically advanced devices can also be used in proprioceptive training and rehabilitation programs. Exercises should include repetitive, consciously mediated movement sequences performed slowly and deliberately as well as sudden, externally applied perturbations of joint position to initiate reflex, 'subconscious' muscle contraction.[20]

In injury, 'pain free' does not necessarily mean 'completely treated or rehabilitated' and unless the full proprioceptive ability is restored, rehabilitation has not been accomplished. In addition, correction of a damaged static restraint (e.g. surgical correction of mechanically disrupted tissue) may not be sufficient to maximize the afferent neuromuscular input needed to enhance dynamic joint stability.

Balance training

One major category of proprioceptive exercise is balance training. These exercises help to train the proprioceptive system in a mostly static activity. In the lower extremities, activities can include one-legged standing balance exercises, progressive use of wobble board exercises, and tandem exercises in which a postural challenge (e.g. perturbations) can be applied to the individual by the therapist.

Plyometric exercises

Plyometric exercises incorporate an eccentric preload (a quick eccentric stretch) followed by a forceful concentric contraction. This exercise technique is thought to enhance reflex joint stabilization and may increase muscle stiffness. It has become increasingly popular as an example of neuromuscular control exercise that integrate spinal and brain stem levels and has been effective addition to upper and lower extremity conditioning and rehabilitation programs.[26] As with the ankle and knee, plyometric exercises are added after near-normal strength in all targeted muscles has been achieved. In the shoulder, plyometrics are performed using the balls with known weight, thrown or bounced and caught at various angles using stable and unstable rebounding boards or tossed at varying speeds by a physiotherapist.[28]

Isokinetic exercises

Isokinetic exercises can be performed to enhance joint position sense using isokinetic devices. The athlete places his/her extremity in a predetermined position and is asked to reproduce this position, initially with the eyes open and then with eyes shut to block visual cues that might aid in neuromuscular control. This exercise can be performed with and without eccentric and/or concentric loads.

Closed and open kinetic chain exercises

Closed-kinetic-chain exercises challenge the dynamic and reflexive aspects of proprioception in the legs and feet. During a closed-chain movement at one joint, a predictable movement at other joints is produced, usually involving axial forces. The lower extremities function in a closed-chain manner during sports and daily life activities, so these exercises will facilitate to regain the proper neuromuscular patterns.

Leg press, squat, circle running, figure eights, single-leg hops, vertical jumps, lateral bounds, one-legged long jumps, and carioca (crossover walking) are some examples. In the upper extremities, physiotherapist application of graded, multi-directional manual resistance can provide proprioceptive feedback in a closed-chain fashion. Open-chain manual resistance exercises with rhythmic stabilization (rapid change in direction of applied pressure) are also considered proprioceptively useful. In either case, resistance can be modified, depending on pain tolerance, as the patient progresses.

Reaction time

The length of reaction time indicates that motor activity cannot be regarded solely in response to environmental stimuli. In order to prevent injuries, a stored set of muscle commands is necessary. This motor programming allows the initiation of activity on exposure to unfolding event. The repetition of such

exercises also contributes the cerebral cortex to determine the most effective motor pattern for that task and potentially decrease the response time.[26]

Sport-specific maneuvers

The final phase of any functional rehabilitation or conditioning program must include exercises that mimic those the athlete does in daily sport activities. This specificity of training improves feed forward mechanism and reflex and consciously controlled motor functions.[28] Sport-specific exercises will serve to 'hard wire' the proprioceptive pathways and solidify a neuromuscular engram specific to these activities. Rehabilitation will then be completed as maneuvers specific to the sport and the athlete's position in the sport can be performed maximally and without pain or loss of function. These skills should be tested in the clinic, laboratory or field before the patient returns to competition.

In summary, for constructing programs with the aim of conditioning and rehabilitation, one should incorporate exercises that improve joint motion sense, increase awareness of joint motion, enhance dynamic joint stability, and improve reactive neuromuscular control.

Under the light of present literature, an exercise prescription for a proprioceptive training can be seen in Table 18.2. It is generally recommended to continue such a program for at least 6–10 weeks in order to improve proprioceptive abilities, *especially during preseason*. It should also be remembered that proprioceptive exercises should incorporate with other specific training items such as strength, flexibility, agility etc. during workouts.

Table 18.2 Program for Proprioceptive Training

Number of exercises	2-5 (to be chosen from the figures)
Number of repetitions of exercises	10-15
Number of sets	1-3
Duration of total proprioceptive training	5-15 min (shorter for prevention, longer for rehabilitative purposes), preferably training every day (at least 3-5 days a week)

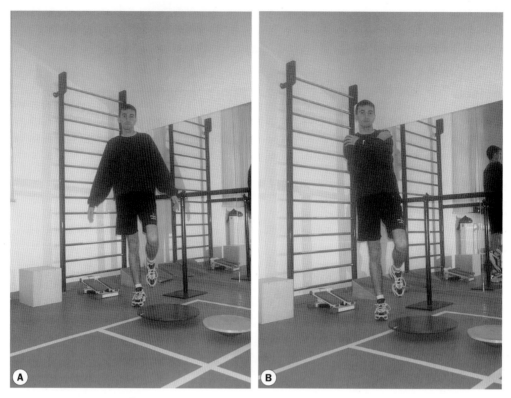

Figure 18.5   Flat surface single leg exercises (A) hands free, (B) fixed.

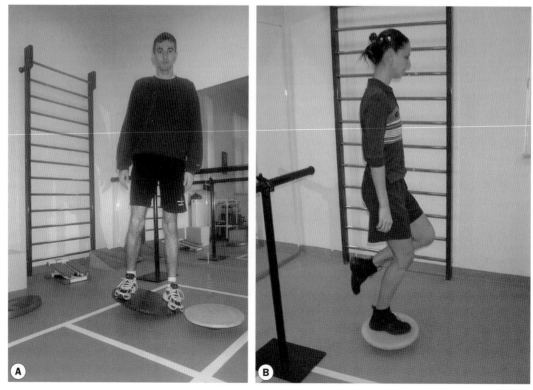

Figure 18.6   Ankle disk/wobble board (A) double leg, (B) single leg.

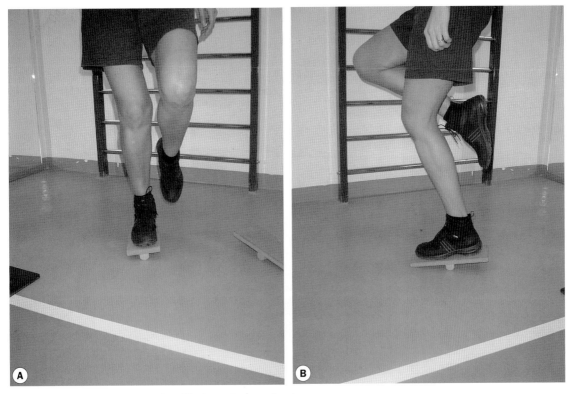

Figure 18.7   Ankle boards, (A) inversion-eversion, (B) plantar flexion-extension.

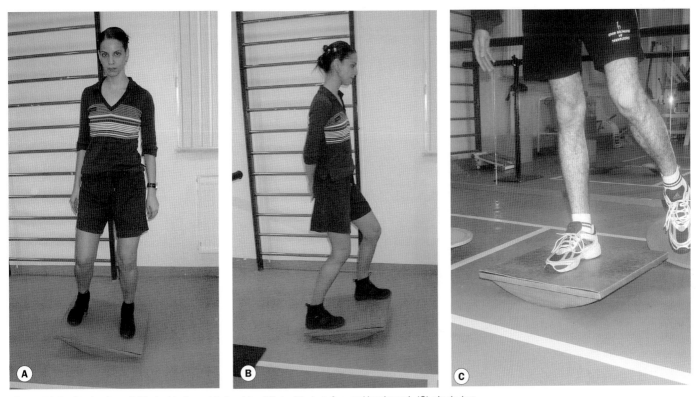

Figure 18.8   Rocker board (A) double leg, side-to-side, (B) double leg, forward-backward, (C) single leg.

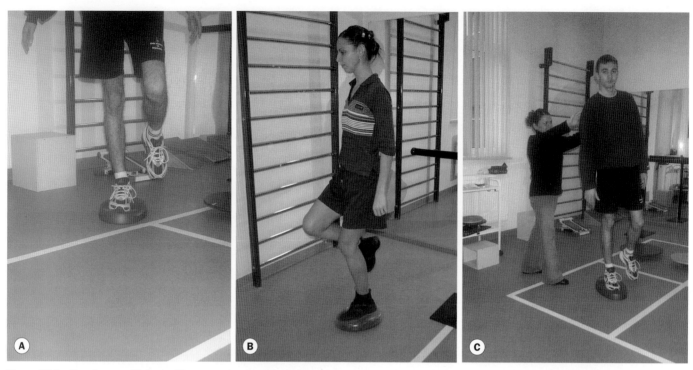

Figure 18.9   Exercises on (A) foam, (B) pneumatic pad, (C) perturbated exercise.

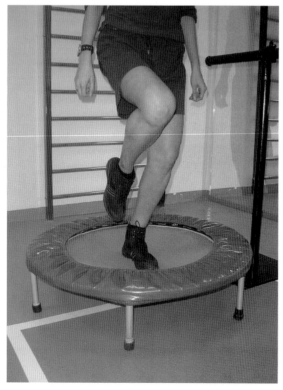

Figure 18.10   Mini trampoline exercises.

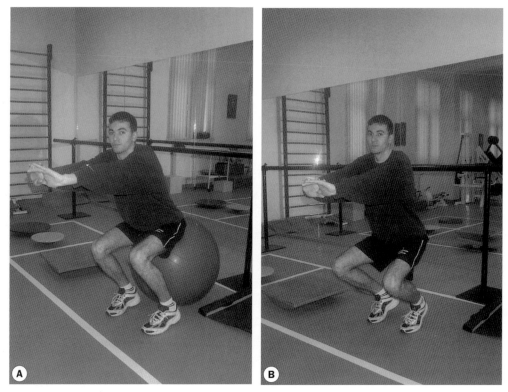

Figure 18.11   Knee bends (A) with and (B) without gym ball.

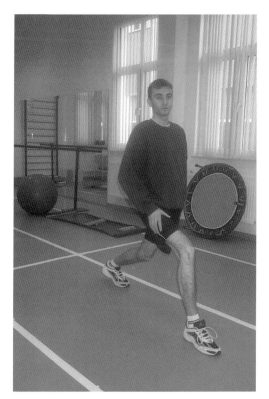

Figure 18.12   Walk with deep knee bends.

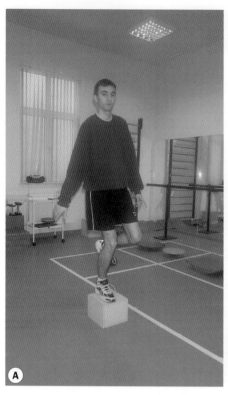
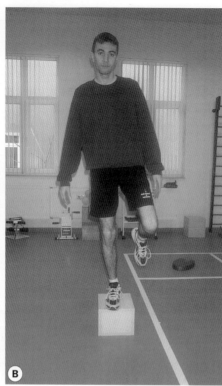
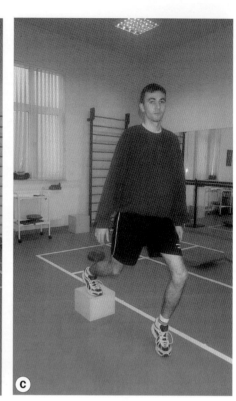

Figure 18.13 (A–C) Step up and down.

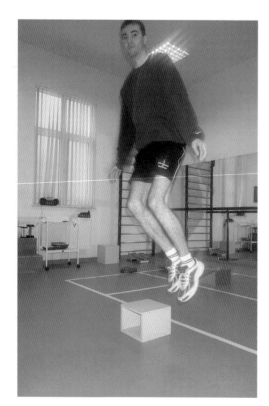

Figure 18.14 Double leg hops.

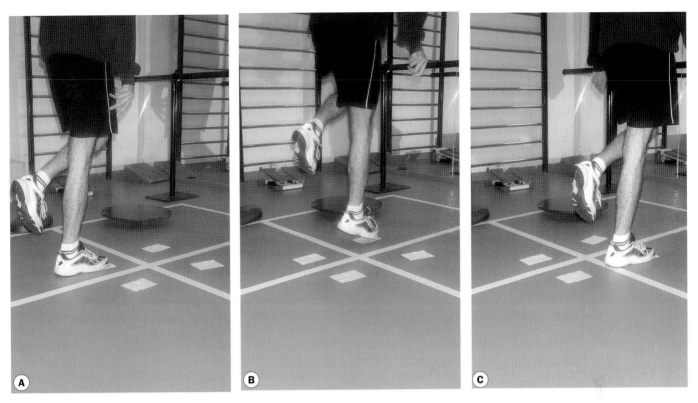

Figure 18.15 (A–C) Single leg hops (patterned).

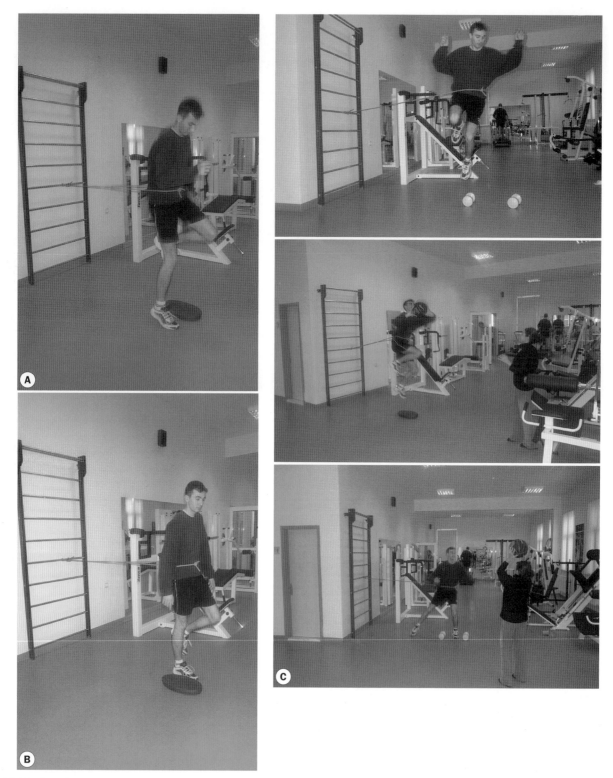

Figure 18.16 Complex perturbated (with elastic band) lateral jumps. (A) elastic tube resisted forward-backward, (B) elastic tube side to side jumps, (C) same exercise complicated with ball catch and throw.

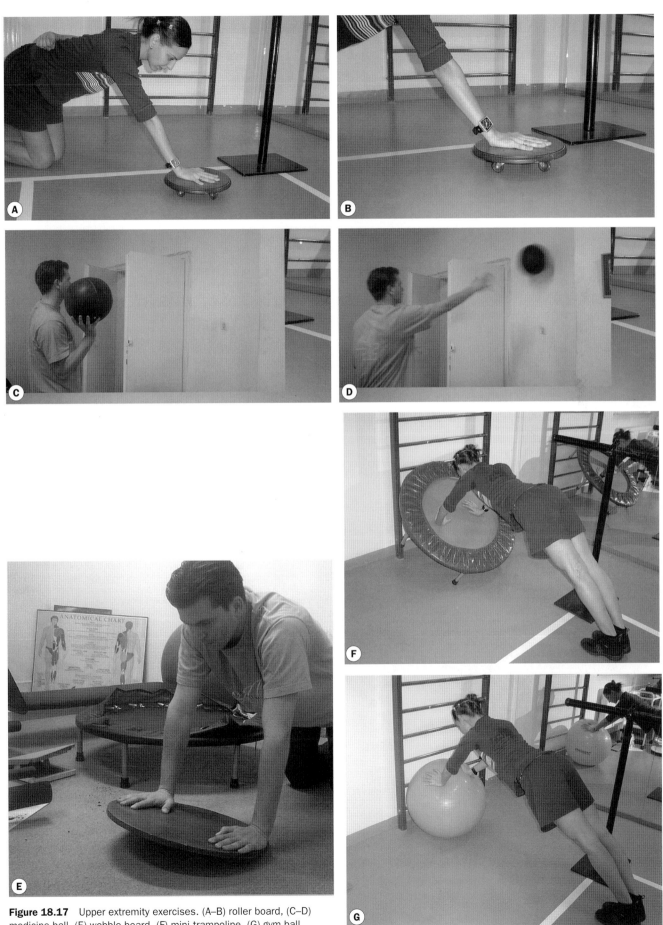

Figure 18.17 Upper extremity exercises. (A–B) roller board, (C–D) medicine ball, (E) wobble board, (F) mini trampoline, (G) gym ball.

REFERENCES

1 Tittel K. Coordination and balance. In: Dirix A, Knuttgen HG, Tittel K, eds. Encyclopedia of sports medicine, Vol.1. London: Blackwell; 1988:194–211.

2 Laskowski ER, Newcomer-Aney K, Smith J. Refining rehabilitation with proprioception training: Expediting return to play. The physician and sports medicine. Online. Available: http://www.physsportsmed.com/issues/1997/10oct/laskow.htm 1997.

3 Lephart SM, Pincivero DM, Giraldo JL, et al. The role of proprioception in the management and rehabilitation of athletic injuries. Am J Sports Med 1997; 25:130–137.

4 Bunton EE, Pitney WA, Kane AW, et al. The role of limb torque, muscle action and proprioception during closed kinetic chain rehabilitation of the lower extremity. J Athletic Train 1993; 28:10–20.

5 Snyder-Mackler L, Fitzgerald GK, Bartolozzi AR, et al. The relationship between passive joint laxity and functional outcome after anterior cruciate ligament injury. Am J Sports Med 1997; 25:191–195.

6 Grigg P. Peripheral neural mechanism in proprioception. J Sports Rehab 1994; 3:2–17.

7 Barrack RL, Skinner HB, Brunet ME, et al. Joint kinesthesia in the highly trained knee. J Sports Med Phys Fitness 1983; 24:18–20.

8 Barrett DS, Cobb AG, and Bentley G. Joint proprioception in normal, osteoarthritic, and replaced knees. J Bone Jt Surg (Br) 1991; 73:53–56.

9 Sojka P, Sjolander P, Johansson H, et al. Influence from stretch sensitive receptors in the collateral ligaments of the knee joint on the gamma-muscle spindle systems of flexor and extensor muscles. Neurosci Res 1991; 11:55–62.

10 Kennedy JC, Alexander IJ, Hayes KC. Nerve supply of the human knee and its functional importance. Am J Sports Med 1982; 10:329–335.

11 Schultz RA, Miller DC, Kerr CS, et al. Mechanoreceptors in human cruciate ligaments: A histological study. J Bone Jt Surg 1984; 66A:1072–1076.

12 Schutte MJ, Dabezies EJ, Zimny ML, et al. Neural anatomy of the human anterior cruciate ligament. J Bone Jt Surg 1987; 69A:243–247.

13 Katonis PG, Assimakopoulos AP, Agapitos MV, et al. Mechanoreceptors in the posterior cruciate ligament. Histologic study on cadaver knees. Acta Orthop Scand 1991; 62:276–278.

14 Zimny ML, Albright DJ, Dabezies E. Mechanoreceptors in the human medial meniscus. Acta Anat 1988; 133:35–40.

15 DeAvila GA, O'Connor BL, Visco DM, et al. The mechanoreceptor innervation of the human fibular collateral ligament. J Anat 1989; 162:1–7.

16 Krenn V, Hofmann S, Engel A. First description of mechanoreceptors in the corpus adiposum infrapatellare of man. Acta Anat 1990; 137:187–188.

17 Grigg P, Hoffman AH. Properties of Ruffini afferents revealed by stress analysis of isolated sections of cat knee capsule. Journal of Neurophysiology 1982; 47:41–54.

18 Grigg P, Hoffman AH. Calibrating joint capsule mechanoreceptors as in vivo soft tissue load cells. J Biomechanics 1989; 22:781–785.

19 Michelson JD, Hutchins C. Mechanoreceptors in human ankle ligaments. J Bone Jt Surg (Br) 1995; 77:219–224.

20 Hoffman M, Payne VG. The effects of proprioceptive ankle disk training on healthy subjects. J Orthop Sports Phys Ther 1995; 21:90–93.

21 Heetderks WJ. Principal component analysis of neural population responses of knee joint proprioceptors in cat. Brain Research 1978; 156:51–65.

22 Johansson H, Sjolander P, Sojka P. Receptors in the knee joint ligaments and their role in the biomechanics of the joint. Crit Rev Biomed Eng 1991; 18:341–368.

23 Johansson H, Sjolander P, Sojka P. Activity in receptor afferents from the anterior cruciate ligament evokes reflex effects on fusimotor neurons. Neurosci Res 1990; 8:54–59.

24 Grigg P. Articular neurophysiology. In: Zachazewski JE, Magee DJ, Quillen WS, eds. Athletic injuries and rehabilitation. Philadelphia: Saunders; 1996:152–169.

25 Richie DH. Functional instability of the ankle and the role of neuromuscular control: A comprehensive review. Journal of Foot and Ankle Surgery 2001; 40:240–251.

26 Tropp H, Alaranta H, Renström A. Proprioception and coordination training in injury prevention. In: Renström PAFH, ed. Sports injuries basic principles of prevention and care. Oxford: Blackwell Science; 1992:277–288.

27 Tyldesling B, Greve JI. Muscles, nerves anti movement: kinesiology in daily living. Boston: Blackwell Science; 1998:26, 34, 284.

28 Griffin LYE. Neuromuscular training and injury prevention in sports. Clin Orthop Rel Res 2003; 409:53–60.

29 Lephart SM, Kocher MS, Fu FH, et al. Proprioception following anterior cruciate ligament reconstruction. J Sport Rehabil 1992; 1:188–196.

30 Lephart SM, Warner JP, Borsa PA, et al. Proprioception of the shoulder in normal, unstable and post-surgical individuals. J Shoulder Elbow Surg 1994; 3:371–380.

31 Eils E, Rosenbaum D. A multi-station proprioceptive exercise program in patients with ankle instability. Med Sci Sports Exerc 2001; 33:1991–1998.

32 Freeman MA. Instabilities of the foot after lateral ligament injuries of the ankle. J Bone Jt Surg 1965; 47:669–677.

33 Konradsen L, Ravn JB. Ankle instability caused by prolonged peroneal reaction time. Acta Orthop Scand 1990; 61:388–390.

34 Glencross D, Thornton E. Position sense following joint injury. J Sports Med Phys Fitness 1991; 21:23–27.

35 Gross MT. Effects of recurrent lateral ankle sprain on active and passive judgments of joint position. Phys Ther 1987; 67:1505–1509.

36 Tropp H, Odenrick P. Postural control in single-limb stance. J Orthop Res 1988; 6:833–839.

37 Cornwall MW, Murrell P. Postural sway following inversion sprain of the ankle. J Am Podiatr Med Assoc 1991; 81:243–247.

38 Karlsson J, Andreasson GO. The effect of external ankle support in chronic lateral ankle joint instability: An electromyographic study. Am J Sports Med 1992; 20:257–261.

39 Robbins S, Waked E, Rappel R. Ankle taping improves proprioception before and after exercise in young men. Br J Sports Med 1995; 29:242–247.

40 Myburgh KH, Vaughan CL, Isaacs SK. The effects of ankle guards and taping on joint motion before, during, and after a squash match. Am J Sports Med 1984; 12:441–446.

41 Manfroy PP, Ashton-Miller JA, Wojtys EM. The effect of exercise, prewrap, and athletic tape on the maximal active and passive ankle resistance of ankle inversion. Am J Sports Med 1997; 25:156–163.

42 Barrack RL, Lund PJ, Skinner HB. Knee joint proprioception revisited. J Sport Rehabil 1994; 3:18–42.

43 Safran MR, Allen AA, Lephart SM, et al. Proprioception in the posterior cruciate ligament deficient knee. Knee Surg Sports Traumatol Arthroscopy 1999; 7:310–317.

44 Roberts D, Ageberg E, Andersson G et al. Effects of short-term cycling on knee joint proprioception in ACL-deficient patients. Knee Surg Sports Traumatol Arthroscopy 2004; 12:357–363.

45 Lephart S. Reestablishing proprioception, kinesthesia, joint position sense and neuromuscular control in rehabilitation. In: Prentice WE, ed. Rehabilitation techniques in sports medicine. St Louis, MO: Mosby; 1994:118–137.

46 Georgoulis A, Pappa L, Moebius U et al. The presence of proprioceptive mechanoreceptors in the remnants of the ruptured ACL as a possible source of re-innervation of the ACL autograft. Knee Surg Sports Traumatol Arthroscopy 2001; 9:364–368.

47 Lephart SM. Proprioception of the ankle and knee. Sports Med 1998; 25:149–155.

48 Jerosch J, Prymka M. Proprioception and joint stability. Knee Surg Sports Traumatol Arthroscopy 1996; 4:171–179.

49 Beard DJ, Kyberd PJ, O'Connor JJ, et al. Reflex hamstring contraction latency in anterior cruciate ligament deficiency. J Orthop Res 1994; 12:219–228.

50 Barrett DS. Proprioception and function after anterior cruciate ligament reconstruction. J Bone Jt Surg (Br) 1991; 73:833–837.

51 Borsa PA, Lephart SM, Irrgang JJ, et al. The effects of joint position and direction of joint motion on proprioceptive sensibility in anterior cruciate ligament-deficient athletes. Am J Sports Med 1997; 25:336–340.

52 Ochi M, Iwasa J, Uchio Y, et al. The regeneration of sensory neurons in the reconstruction of the anterior cruciate ligament. J Bone Jt Surg (Br) 1999; 81:902–906.

53 Warner JJP, Lephart S, Fu FH. Role of proprioception in pathoetiology of shoulder instability. Clin Orthop Relat Res 1996; 330:35–39.

54 Aydin T, Yildiz Y, Yanmis I, et al. Shoulder proprioception: a comparison between the shoulder joint in healthy and surgically repaired shoulders. Arch Orthop Trauma Surg 2001; 121:422–425.

55 Smith RL, Brunolli J. Shoulder kinesthesia after anterior glenohumeral joint dislocation. Phys Ther 1989; 69:106–112.

56 Barrack RL, Skinner HB, Buckley SL. Proprioception in the anterior cruciate deficient knee. Am J Sports Med 1989; 17:1–6.

57 Lephart SM, Myers JB, Bradley JP, et al. Shoulder proprioception and function following thermal capsulorraphy arthroscopy. J Arthroscopic Relat Surg 2002; 18:770–778.

58 Ulkar B, Kunduracioglu B, Cetin C, et al. Effect of positioning and bracing on passive position sense of shoulder joint. Br J Sports Med 2004; 38:549–552.

59 Beynnon BD, Ryder SH, Konradsen L, et al. The effect of anterior cruciate ligament trauma and bracing on knee proprioception. Am J Sports Med 1999; 27:150–155.

60 Friden T, Roberts D, Zatterstrom R, et al. Proprioception in the nearly extended knee. Measurements of position and movement in healthy individuals and in symptomatic anterior cruciate ligament injured patients. Knee Surg Sports Traumatol Arthroscopy 1996; 4:217–224.

61 Friden T, Roberts D, Zatterstrom R, et al. Proprioception after an acute knee ligament injury: a longitudinal study on 16 consecutive patients. J Orthop Res 1997; 15:637–644.

62 Friden T, Roberts D, Movin T, Wredmark T. Function after anterior cruciate ligament injuries. Influence of visual control and proprioception. Acta Orthop Scand 1998; 69:590–594.

63 Friden T, Roberts D, Zatterstrom R, et al. Proprioceptive defects after an anterior cruciate ligament rupture: the relation to associated anatomical lesions and subjective knee function. Knee Surg Sports Traumatol Arthroscopy 1999; 7:226–231.

64 Janwantanakul P, Magarey ME, Jones MA, et al. Variation in shoulder position sense at mid and extreme range of motion. Arch Phys Med Rehabil 2001; 82:840–844.

65 Swanik KA, Lephart SM, Swanik B, et al. The effects of shoulder plyometric training on proprioception and selected muscle performance characteristics. J Shoulder Elbow Surg 2002; 11:579–586.

66 Lee HM, Liau JJ, Cheng CK, et al. Evaluation of shoulder proprioception following muscle fatigue. Clin Biomechanics 2003; 18:843–847.

67 Edmonds G, Kirkley A, Birmingham TB, et al. The effect of early arthroscopic stabilization compared to nonsurgical treatment on proprioception after primary traumatic anterior dislocation of the shoulder. Knee Surg Sports Traumatol Arthroscopy 2003; 11:116–121.

68 Ramsey JRE, Riddoch JM. Position-matching in the upper limb: professional ballet dancers perform with outstanding accuracy. Clin Rehabil 2001; 15:324–330.

69 Dover G, Powers ME. Cryotherapy does not impair shoulder joint position sense. Arch Phys Med Rehabil 2004; 85:1241–1246.

70 Hopper DM, Creagh MJ, Formby PA, et al. Functional measurement of knee joint position sense after anterior cruciate ligament reconstruction. Arch Phys Med Rehabil 2003; 84:868–872.

71 Jerosch J, Brinkmann T, Schneppenheim M. The angle velocity reproduction test (AVRT) as sensorimotor function of the glenohumeral complex. Arch Orthop Traumatol Surg 2003; 123:151–157.

72 Barden JM, Balyk R, Raso JV, et al. Dynamic upper limb proprioception in multidirectional shoulder instability. Clin Orthop 2004; 420:181–189.

73 Berg KO, Wood-Dauphinee SL, Williams JI, et al. Measuring balance in the elderly: validation of an instrument. Can J Public Health 1992; 83:S7–S11.

74 Hansen MS, Dieckmann B, Jensen K, et al. The reliability of balance tests performed on the kinesthetic ability trainer (KAT 2000). Knee Surg Sports Traumatol Arthroscopy 2000; 8:180–185.

75 Ageberg E, Roberts D, Holmström E, et al. The effect of short-duration sub-maximal cycling on balance in single-limb stance in patients with anterior cruciate ligament injury: a cross-sectional study. BMC Musculoskeletal Disord 2004; 5:44.

76 Arnold BL, Schmitz RJ. Examination of balance measures produced by the Biodex Stability System. J Athletic Train 1998; 33:323–327.

77 Adlerton AK, Moritz U, Nilssen RM. Force plate and accelerometer measures for evaluating the effect of muscle fatigue on postural control during one-legged stance. Physiother Res Int 2003; 8:187–199.

78 Fuchs S, Tibesku CO, Frisse D, et al. Clinical and functional comparison of uni and bicondylar sledge prostheses. Knee Surg Sports Traumatol Arthroscopy 2004: 24. Online. Available: http://www.springerlink.com.

79 Gosselin G, Rassoulian H, Brown I. Effects of neck extensor muscles fatigue on balance. Clin Biomechanics 2004; 19:473–479.

80 Madeleine P, Prietzel H, Svarrer H, et al. Quantitative posturography in altered sensory conditions: a way to assess balance instability in patients with chronic whiplash injury. Arch Phys Med Rehabil 2004; 85:432–438.

81 Kovacs EJ, Birmingham TB, Forwell L, et al. Effect of training on postural control in figure skaters a randomized controlled trial of neuromuscular versus basic off-ice training programs. Clin J Sports Med 2004; 14:215–224.

82 Mora I, Quinteiro-Blondin S, Pe'rot C. Electromechanical assessment of ankle stability. Eur J Appl Physiol 2003; 88:558–564.

83 Gribble PA, Hertel J, Denegar CR, et al. The effects of fatigue and chronic ankle instability on dynamic postural control. J Athletic Train 2004; 39:321–329.

84 Bäthis H, Perlick L, Blum C, et al. Midvastus approach in total knee arthroplasty: a randomized, double-blinded study on early rehabilitation. Knee Surg Sports Traumatol Arthroscopy. Online. Available: http://www.springerlink.com 2005.

85 Noyes FR, Barber SD, Mangine RE. Abnormal lower limb symmetry determined by function hop tests after anterior cruciate ligament rupture. Am J Sports Med 1991; 19:513–518.

86 Risberg MA, Ekeland A. Assessment of functional tests after anterior cruciate ligament surgery. J Orthop Sports Phys Ther 1994; 19:212–217.

87 Unver F. The effects of proprioceptive training on ankles with inversion injuries. Doctoral thesis, Hacettepe University Institute of Health Sciences, Ankara, 2004.

88 Bahr R. Injury prevention. In: Reeser JC, Bahr R, eds. Volleyball; Handbook of sports medicine and science. Madlen: Blackwell Science; 2003:94–106.

89 Guyton AC. Textbook of medical physiology. 6th edn. Philadelphia: Saunders; 1981:122–137, 534–536, 562–564, 588–595, 629.

90 Dunn TG, Gillig SE, Ponsor SE. The learning process in feedback: Is it feed forward or feedback? Biofeedback Self Regul 1986; 11:143–156.

91 Lephart SM, Henry TJ. The physiological basis for open and closed kinetic chain rehabilitation for the upper extremity. J Sport Rehabil 1996; 5:71–87.

92 Tropp H. Pronator muscle weakness in functional instability of the ankle joint. Int J Sports Med 1986; 7:291–294.

93 Wester JU, Jespersen SM, Nielsen KD, et al. Wobble board training after partial sprains of the lateral ligaments of the ankle: a prospective randomized study. J Orthop Sports Phys Ther 1996; 23:332–336.

CHAPTER 19

Aquatic Rehabilitation

Anton Wicker

INTRODUCTION

Water is an essential therapeutic medium in rehabilitation programs. The concept of underwater therapy offers many possibilities to develop and specify the rehabilitation of injuries. Several metabolic and kinetic factors can be influenced by utilizing various effective elements of water such as buoyancy, temperature, resistance, hydrostatic pressure and electrolyte content.

Patients after injuries, have limited joint motion, pain, edema after surgery, weakness, poor coordination, balance and stamina are all benefit from aquatic rehabilitation concepts. It is the reduced weight of the human body in water that makes it possible to produce motions like walking, jumping and other movement patterns, even though an injured joint cannot be subjected to normal stress.

The various kinetic factors affected by the injury and by surgical trauma undergo a phase of repair,[1] during which certain reactions are set in motion. These reactions have major effects on the mobility, the loading capacity and the strength of the joints. An additional cumulative effect of the above-mentioned factors is that the central regulation of motion is altered. The patient loses confidence and starts to feel afraid. Fear essentially influences the course of motion, in particular the timing of motion.[2]

The consequences of fear can be immediately observed at a clinical level. The dynamic-motor stereotype of motion, including that of automatized patterns of motion, such as ordinary walking, undergoes marked changes.

Reducing stress on the body helps to reduce fear. Fear disturbs the rhythm of motion and rhythm is the primary criterion for the evaluation of motion.[3]

Additional criteria are flow, precision, stability, force, speed and extent of motion. A summation of these factors causes what is known as the harmony of motion.

As an exercise medium, water is very beneficial for those who understand its principles and properties. All aquatic exercise therapy concepts must address two important factors: the body's physiologic response to being immersed in water and the physical properties of water. By considering these two parts, a special rehabilitation program which is safe and effective can be designed.

PRINCIPLES AND PROPERTIES OF WATER

Buoyancy

The principle of Archimedes states that when a body is fully or partially submerged in a fluid at rest, it experiences an upward thrust equal to the weight of the fluid displaced. Thus, an object with a relative density less than one will float because the weight of the object is less than the weight of the water displaced.[4]

The heavier the weight of the displaced material, the larger is the buoyancy. The body in the water is more supported by the buoyancy as the water is heavier. An increase of the weight of the water like a water with many minerals leads to an increase of buoyancy. For example, the buoyancy of a human body in the Dead Sea is so big that the body is not able to sink.

Water usually used for rehabilitation purposes has a relative density of one. The relative density of an object is the ratio of the weight of an equal volume of water.[5] If this value is greater than one, the object will sink; if it is less than one, the object will float. If the value is exactly one, the object will float just below the surface of the water.

The specific gravity also indicates the portion of a body's volume that will be floating underwater. For example, if a floating person's specific gravity is 0.98, 2% of the body will be above the surface of the water and 98% will be below the surface.

The relative density of a body depends on its composition. The specific gravities of fat is 0.8; of bone about 1.8 and of lean muscle about 1.1. Consequently, lean people tend to sink and obese people tend to float.

If rehabilitation is done with patients with congenital or traumatic loss of limbs, we have to handle unequal relative densities between the two sides of the body. The side with the higher relative density tends to sink and the other side to float, producing instability in the water. Flotation devices can be used to alter the position of the centre of buoyancy and maintain a vertical position. Buoyancy and relative density are very closely related. Buoyancy can be used in rehabilitation in three ways: assistive, resistive and supportive. This force assists any movement toward the surface of the water and resists any movement down the surface. When buoyancy equals the force of gravity, any horizontal movement is supported (Fig. 19.1).

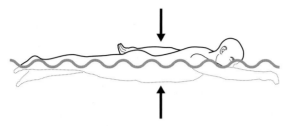

Figure 19.1 Equality of buoyant force and weight of the water displaced by the swimmer (Principle of Archimedes).

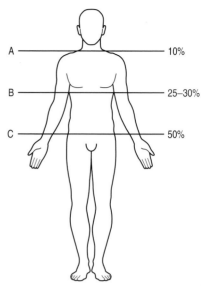

Figure 19.3 Percentage of body weight at various water depths (A) at the neck (C7), (B) the chest (xiphoid process) and (C) the pelvis (anterior superior iliac spine).

With floating devices one can influence the force of gravity and the buoyant force and use these effects in designing the rehabilitation plan (Fig. 19.2).

One of the main advantages of underwater therapy is the reduction in weight-bearing forces. Patients exercising in water feel lighter, have a decrease of pain, move more easily, without fear and feel less weight in their joints because of the buoyancy. On land, the center of gravity of a body is just in front of the sacrum. In the water, the center of gravity is located at the level of the lungs.[6] Hence, the degree of partial weight bearing varies with pool depth (Fig. 19.3).

Water content

The usual buoyancy can be increased by using water with a high content of minerals, such as seawater or special types of natural mineral waters. Salt water is more dense than fresh water and besides influencing buoyancy, the diuretic effect of fluid shifting slightly increases.[7]

The diuretic response to head-out immersion in hydrated subjects is greater than in dehydrated subjects. The main diuresis-inducing factor during water immersion may be the suppression of antidiuretic hormone.[8] The increase of the diuresis induces a fluid shift in the body and in combination with the hydrostatic pressure, edema, caused by the injury or postoperatively decreases. These effects are supported by hydrodynamic-buoyancy processes.

The term 'hydrodynamic buoyancy' means water in motion in the therapy pool. Water in motion becomes a complex physical substance. When water is moving smoothly inside a pool, with all layers moving at the same speed and parallel, the water is said to be in 'laminar flow'. Typically, laminar flow rates are slow. When water moves rapidly, even minor oscillations

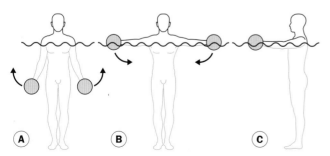

Figure 19.2 A hand-fixed flotation device can be (A) assistive during shoulder abduction, (B) resistive during shoulder adduction and (C) supportive during horizontal anteversion on the surface of the water.

create uneven flow and parallel paths are knocked out of alignment. When this happens, another type of pattern occurs called 'turbulent flow'.[9] Within the mass of water, flow patterns arise that run dramatically out of parallel and may even set up paths running in opposite directions. Artificially these 'turbulent flows' are built in whirlpools and they cause massage effects and also lead to an increase of buoyancy in its special form, called 'hydrodynamic-buoyancy'. Aquatic rehabilitation uses these phenomena to reduce pain, muscle soreness and edema.

Resistance

The resistance to movement through water is caused by friction between the molecules of the fluid and is known as viscosity. This resistance is usually ignored when the medium is air. In water, however, there are several forces that come into play. Cohesion is the force of attraction between neighboring molecules of the same type of matter. Surface tension is the force of attraction between the surface molecules of a fluid. This is not a factor if the moving body part is completely submerged in water, but it is a significant factor when a limb breaks the surface of the water.[10]

Viscosity acts as a resistance to movement because molecules of a fluid tend to adhere to the surface of a body moving through it. This force of resistance is known as 'drag' and it should be considered during development of an aquatic rehabilitation program.

The amount of drag that an object experiences as it moves through water depends on a number of factors.

The first factor that must be considered is that the movement can be either streamlined or turbulent. The resistance to turbulent flow is greater than the resistance to streamline flow (Fig. 19.4).

The velocity at which the object is moving through the water and frontal area is a very important variable. From the

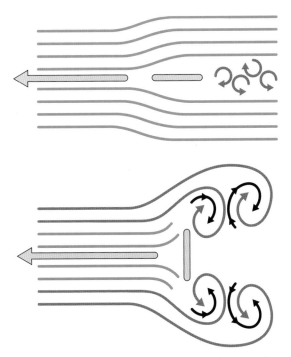

Figure 19.4 The movement of a paddle perpendicular to the flow of water produces a turbulence flow.

equation, it can be seen that the drag force is proportional to the square of the velocity. Therefore, if the velocity of a moving limb is doubled, the drag force is multiplied by a factor of four. The fact that frontal area is directly proportional to drag force means that it has a significant effect on the resistance of a given aquatic exercise. So for example, it can be said that doubling the frontal area doubles the drag.

With upper limb exercises, the area of the hand can be effectively increased, simply by separating the fingers slightly. This occurs because the 'boundary layer' of fluid moving around an object, such as a finger, is greater in water than in air. When the fingers are slightly separated, their boundary layers overlap.[11]

It is important to understand, however, how small changes in the size, shape and velocity of resistance devices like paddles or fins can affect exercises performed in the water. The fact that an object is buoyant implies that it will assist movement, but its size and shape may produce a drag force that resists movement. The net effect of the device on the limb's movement must be considered.

The combined total of a moving limb's velocity, the body's velocity and the water's velocity also affects the drag force during exercise. If the patient is walking forward and also moving the arm forward, the two velocities must be added together to determine the arm's velocity relative to the water. Any movement of the water, such as that produced during alternating reciprocal movements, also affects the drag. For example, abduction of the arm causes the water to move in the same direction as the arm. If the arm movement is suddenly reversed, the arm will be moving against the flow of water. The result is a dramatic increase in drag and this increases the resistance of the exercise. Conversely, any movement that occurs in the same direction as moving water will encounter less drag than if it were occurring in stationary water.

In addition to increasing the drag forces, reversing the direction of movement adds the work of having to overcome inertia. In order to stop a moving limb, the appropriate muscles must produce the force necessary to decelerate both the mass of the limb and the mass of the water that is moving behind it.

Hydrostatic pressure

Pascal's law states that fluid pressure is exerted equally on all surfaces of an immersed body at a given depth. The pressure is directly proportional to both the depth and the density of the fluid. From a baseline of about 15 psi (atmospheric pressure – pounds per square inch) at the surface, fluid pressure of water increases by 0.43 psi per foot of depth.[12] This implies that hydrostatic pressure opposes the tendency of blood to pool in the lower portions of the body, which helps to reduce the post-traumatic or postoperative swelling in injured patients. Hydrostatic pressure helps also to stabilize unstable joints.

Thus a body immersed to a depth of 48 inches is subjected to a force slightly greater than diastolic pressure. This is the force that aids the resolution of edema but this is also the reason that it is not advisable to put patients with heart diseases or with chronic obstructive pulmonary diseases into a pool at 75% immersion. Such patients may have difficulty breathing because the pressure of the water resists the chest wall expansion. In the worst case scenario, this may be end in death by pulmonary edema.

Specific heat of water

One important physical property of water is that of its specific heat. This is defined as the amount of energy required to raise the temperature of 1 g of water by 1°C. The specific heat of water is several thousand times that of air and heat loss to water is 25 times that to air at a given temperature.

The therapeutic utility of water depends greatly on both its ability to retain heat and its ability to transfer heat energy. Exchange of energy in the form of heat occurs in three ways: conduction, convection and radiation. Conduction may be defined as heat transfer through individual molecular collisions occurring over a small distance. Convection transfers heat through the mass movement of large numbers of molecules over a large distance. Liquids and gases in general are poor conductors but good convectors. Radiation transfers heat through the transmission of electromagnetic waves. Water and metals tend to conduct heat well; air and gas-containing materials, like wood, cork, etc. conduct heat poorly. Water is an efficient conductor of heat and transfers heat 25 times faster than air. Heat transfer increases as a function of velocity. Thus, a swimmer loses more heat when swimming rapidly through cold water than a person standing still in the same water.

Consequently, both the temperature of the water and the amount of heat produced by the body must be considered when determining a comfortable water temperature in which to exercise. Vigorous exercise performed in warm water (33°C and more) results in an increase in core temperature and premature fatigue. Vigorous exercise in cold water (20°C and below) leads to a drop in core temperature and an inability to contract muscles. The ideal temperature for aquatic rehabilitation exercises should be kept about 32°C. In rehabilitation concepts of high level athletes, where vigorous exercises are done, it is suggested that the temperature of the therapeutic pool should be kept about 30°C.[13]

AQUATIC EQUIPMENT

Water therapy is becoming more and more popular in the rehabilitative and conditioning environment. Healthcare professionals are becoming interested, educated and skilled in the field of aquatic exercise and rehabilitation.

Water's physical properties alone provide an environment for exercise in which there is little need for elaborate or expensive equipment. With greater understanding of these properties and hydrodynamics, this unique medium offers many possibilities to improve the quality of rehabilitation and helps the patients to return to their normal daily activity and in case of high level athletes to their usual training units, earlier.

Pools

Aquatic equipment used for exercise and rehabilitation can range from a custom-designed swimming pool to a wide array of accompanying equipment. The basis for high quality aquatic rehabilitation is an in-ground swimming pool, minimum range 4–5 m, with a depth between 1.2 m and 1.4 m. Where there is no access to a full sized swimming pool, a customized therapy pool is an alternative, but always second choice.

For working with groups of patients (*n* 3–10) a pool minimum 8–10 m is necessary.

For offering aqua-jogging and special aquatic exercises, a second pool with a depth of more than 10 m should be used.

The author's standard pool for aquatic rehabilitation is an in-ground swimming pool with a range of 5–6 m and a common depth of 1.3 m. The depth can be changed from 1 m to 1.5 m. The wall of the pool towers 1 m above the floor. When entering the pool one has first to go upstairs on to the top of the pool wall, then downstairs into the water. Wheelchair and other handicapped patients are able to use a lift to enter the water. In one of the pool walls there is an integrated window of double glass in which a video-camera is located. Inside the walls of the pool, 30 cm down the edge is a hand-rail surrounding the pool. Integrated into the pool walls and at the bottom of the pool there are buckles into which ropes and sport cords can be fixed. Also integrated in the bottom of the pool and in every pool wall, are two jets in order that drag forces can be created by moving water. The room in which the pool is located has an air temperature of 26–27°C. Fixed on the ceiling is one moveable video-screen, so that the patients can observe themselves during exercises. The water temperature in the pool is about 31–32°C. If specific sports rehabilitation with a high level athlete is required, a temperature of about 30°C is used.

Access equipment

Many manufacturers of aquatic equipment are designing devices to be used in aquatic rehabilitation. The most popular

devices in flotation equipment are swim bars, the WetVest®, AquaJogger®, kick boards, water tires, webbed gloves, fins and tubes (Fig. 19.5). Weights, like dumbbells, weight belts, ankle and hand weights are often used in the pool for traction or strengthening. These weights must be of a type designed for water exercise. Devices to force coordination and balance, such as wobble boards, trampolines, swing boards and therapy-discs must also be designed for being used in water.

REHABILITATION

Box 19.1: Key Points

- Begin aquatic rehabilitation as early as possible after the injury.
- Water reduces stress and consequently reduces pain to a great extent.
- Water is an ideal medium for improvement of mobility in the whole body.
- Strengthen and stabilize the body core at a very early stage.

Because of the unique properties of water, aquatic rehabilitation offers advantages over land-based rehabilitation. It is imperative that the clinician applies aquatic principles appropriately when designing a rehabilitation program for an injured patient.

Buoyancy decreases weight bearing and joint compressive forces and this allows an early process with closed chain kinetics in usual movement patterns like walking. The patient may also perform sport-specific rehabilitation exercises, mimicking the weight bearing activity.

Similar to those of land-based programs, the principles of tissue healing and exercise progression must be considered when an aquatic-based rehabilitation program is designed. Based upon functional limitations, impairments and disabilities

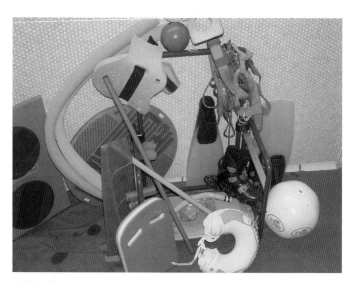

Figure 19.5 Flotation equipment (balls, elastic bands, tubes, ropes, AquaJogger®, chest belts, inline skates, fins, resistive paddles, kickboards, trampoline, swing board).

identified in the examination, a specific program can be created with the patient's goals in mind.

The stages of healing must be taken into account to prevent delayed healing and further injuries.

Beginning aquatic rehabilitation

Aquatic rehabilitation should begin as soon as possible after the injury, because the period of immobilisation of a body or a joint should be kept to a minimum. Immobilization reduces the functional reserve of the musculoskeletal system, resulting in weakness, atrophy and poor endurance.[14]

After surgery, it is usual to begin therapy as soon as the wound is healed. High level athletes may begin aquatic therapy 1 week after surgery, without concern of infection.[15]

Reducing fear

Owing to mechanical and nociceptive stimulation of sensory nerve endings (Pacini's, Ruffini's, Golgi's organs, free nerve endings and muscle spindles) from the injury as well as from surgical trauma, the activity of motor neurons and the strength of the joint muscles are downregulated, such that these factors adjust to and protect the weakened tissue.[16] Disturbances of this magnitude cause the patient to alter his or her movement pattern, for example in an injured lower limb, the gait is altered. In order to relieve the leg of stress, the patient will assume a limp. This so-called 'stereotyped limp' may become automatic in the presence of prolonged irritation. Subsequently, 'learning to forget' such stereotyped habits will prove difficult and will require a lot of time; a fact that has been known to significantly prolong the time required for complete rehabilitation (i.e. complete fitness).

Water reduces stress and consequently reduces pain to a great extent. Moreover, it reduces the inhibitory factors in those sections of the central nervous system that are responsible for the regulation of motor functions. Hence, the development of a 'stereotyped limp' can be effectively counteracted by this concept of treatment. Therefore, at the start of the rehabilitation, the patient is trained to move around in the water as he would if there was no injury. The execution of this movement should result in symmetric motions. Since stress is reduced, the muscles and the psyche relax, which helps to reduce fear. Fear disturbs the rhythm of motion. Rhythm is a most important criterion in exercises. The patient also experiences less pain and consequently, a normal gait is achieved early in the water; a fact that counteracts the development of stereotyped patterns of motion. For example, when a patient who has sustained injury of the knee joint and has undergone surgery of the anterior cruciate ligament consistently trains to walk in water during the first 4 weeks following surgery, the following results will be achieved:

1   Fear is reduced and this permits rhythm training and has a favorable effect on the timing of motion.
2   Training of symmetry is easily accepted and there is a less pronounced tendency to develop stereotyped patterns of motion.
3   The water supports the coordination of the trunk, arms and legs, and thus makes it possible to drill the entire chain of motion.

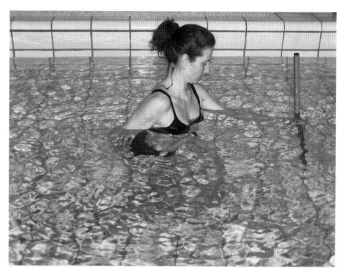

Figure 19.6   Walking in chest high water.

4   Buoyancy of the body in water; the resistance of water permits safe enhancement of kinesthetic perception.
5   The water permits early commencement of proprioceptive training (position, flexion, extension, direction, speed, acceleration and position of body parts in space) and favorably influences the sense of equilibrium.
6   Improvement of the elasticity and the sensitivity of the entire musculature of the trunk and the legs.

Aquatic rehabilitation should always be started with walking in water. This is the base of all exercises; the patient learns to move in this new therapy-medium, feels quite relaxed and pain and fear are reduced (Fig. 19.6).

Mobility

Mobility may be impaired after an injury or surgery. Mobility can also result from pain of overuse of tendons, ligaments and muscles. A goal of rehabilitation is to restore normal osteokinematics and joint arthrokinematics. Water is an ideal medium for improvement of mobility in the whole body. For example, the upward movement of the glenohumeral joint is assisted by buoyancy and the patient may discover that normal shoulder movement patterns occur earlier in the pool than on land.

The athlete can position himself in his sport-specific position, resulting in the restoration of familiar muscle length-tension relationship in the extremities and the trunk.

Buoyant equipment may assist the movement initially and may be discontinued as active and resistive range of motion exercises begin (Fig. 19.7).

Water with a temperature of 30–32 °C provides a relaxing environment, which may allow for increased soft tissue extensibility. Stretch techniques are used in two ways: (1) Active stretching done by the athlete himself. The duration of the stretch can vary. To promote tissue elongation and permanent structural changes, a low intensity stretch with long duration (about 30 s) should be tackled. (2) Passive stretching is done by the therapist. The duration is about 30 s. This type of stretching is often combined with manual techniques, like tractions and joint mobilizations. It is important to work in closed chain kinetics, to restore

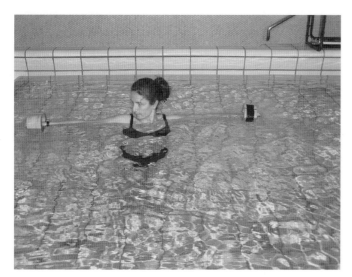

Figure 19.7 Assisted elevations of the upper limbs.

the initial movement patterns. PNF (proprioceptive-neuro-muscular-facilitation) techniques can also be used to this aim.

Trunk stabilization

Trunk stability and postural control are essential for any kind of exercises and sport. For example, basketball players must be able to transfer kinetic energy from the lower limb to the upper limb via their trunk.

In all kind of movements, it is necessary and very useful, first to strengthen and stabilize the body core. The stability of the trunk correlates with the stability of the peripheral joints.[17]

In all sporting activities, the trunk musculature performs as a dynamic stabilizer. Aquatic rehabilitation offers many possibilities for performing body core stability at a very early stage after the injury.

The first step is walking and marching in the pool. Forward walking in the sagittal plane – standing upright, flex one hip and knee – extend the leg and dorsiflex the ankle, landing on the heel – roll forward onto the toes and push off – repeat with the opposite leg and increase velocity of walking – water resistance is increasing – always walk in upright position – trunk muscles and the muscles of the lower limbs are well trained.

Marching in the sagittal plane – standing upright – hip and knee are flexed to 90° – the leg is brought down and the opposite hip and knee are flexed in a marching action.

The second step is jumping in high duck position: Stretched lower limbs with light flexion in knee and hips – similar to floating squats – jumping forward, sideways and backward and sometimes circle around – 180° left, then 180° right – extend the arms at the side (Fig. 19.8).

The third step is arm circling and straight arm pulls: Standing upright – circle both arms forward 90° until the surface of the water is reached – then push down and backwards at about 60°. Step-by-step, the velocity of these exercises should increase (Fig. 19.9). Straight arm pulls – keeping the elbow straight – supinate one hand (palm up) and push the arm in front of the body – at the same time pronate the other hand (palm down) and push the arm behind the body – repeat switching arms.

The fourth step is arm supported open chain hip, knee and ankle flexion and extension in backward position: First, sitting in the water – straighten the body in backward position to the surface of the water, supported by the arms and open chain

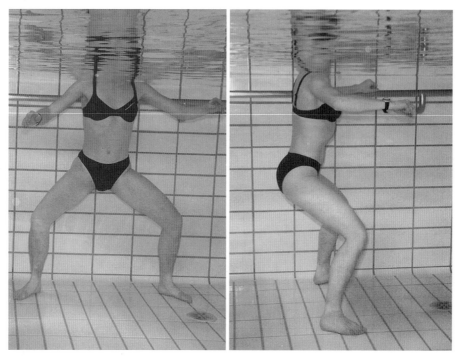

Figure 19.8 High duck position frontal and sagittal.

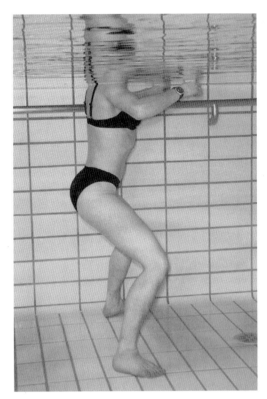

Figure 19.9 Standing position.

hip, knee and ankle flexion and extension (similar to crawling backwards) is done – stabilized by the trunk

The fifth step is arm supported open chain hip, knee and ankle flexion and extension in forward position: First, standing in the water – the body is straightened in the forward position to the surface of the water – supported by the arms and open chain hip, knee and ankle flexion and extension (similar to crawling forwards) is done – stabilized by the trunk (Fig. 19.10).

The sixth step is aqua jogging in deep water: Assume a vertical position – alternately flex and extend the hips and knees, performing a walking action – allow the arms to swing diametrical to the legs (Fig. 19.11).

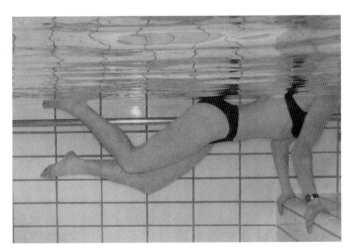

Figure 19.10 Arm supported crawling forwards.

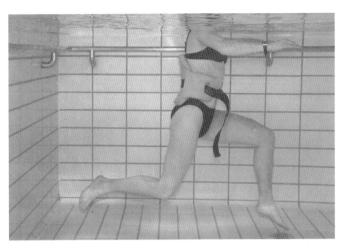

Figure 19.11 Aqua jogging.

Functional progression and training of the upper extremity

Shoulder-strengthening exercises that are performed on land can also be performed in the pool. For example, glenohumeral abduction/adduction, flexion/extension from 0 to 90°, outside/inside rotation in shoulder-deep water, horizontal abduction/adduction, elbow flexion and extension can be restored.

In addition, diagonal patterns such as those utilized in proprioceptive neuromuscular facilitation may be used. As with stretching activities, resistive exercises can be performed, if indicated, only through a partial range of motion. Another consideration for upper extremity training is that the mechanics are different for some water exercises, compared with their land-based counterparts. For example, in the water, shoulder horizontal abduction and adduction performed at 90° abduction are resisted in the transverse plane, but supported in the sagittal plane. That is, the athlete no longer has to hold the arm abducted against gravity while performing the horizontal component of the exercise.

Overhead activities can also be very well performed in the pool in the supine position or in the prone position by using a snorkel.

Resistive tubing may be used in the pool just as it is on land. It can be incorporated as a part of a total training program that is to be performed in one location. In addition, the water will provide additional resistance to the body core.[18] For example, a patient may practice the motion of a tennis serve while standing in shoulder-deep water and using resistive bands. The water is providing core body resistance, while the band resists arm movement.

A wide range of activities can be performed in these positions in the pool, but it is necessary that the clinician must be cognizant of these changes in order to appropriately utilize the principles of aquatics.

Functional progression and training of the lower extremity

Performing in lower extremity functions can also be done in both, the open and the closed chain kinetics. In water, lower extremity strengthening exercises can be performed completely non weight bearing in the open chain. For example, running in deep water with the 'AquaJogger®' or the 'WetVest®' includes trunk stabilization, hip flexion/extension, abduction/adduction and knee and ankle flexion/extension. These exercises are helping to increase mobility and muscle endurance. Kicking in the prone or supine position with fins is another excellent exercise for increasing muscle endurance of the lower limb.

In neck-deep water weight bearing walking can begin; weight bearing can be increased by reducing the depth or by using weight belts during walking exercises and accelerates the velocity.

To strengthen the gluteals and the quadriceps in closed chain kinetics, exercises such as squats, lunges and step downs should be incorporated.

Resistive boots can increase the resistance as much as 4-fold and exercises using boots are useful in sports requiring explosive power, such as figure skating and gymnastics.[19,20]

Lower extremity balance and proprioception are important to any athlete and a well-designed rehabilitation program should address all balance impairments. Balance is controlled by sensory input, central processing and neuromuscular responses.[21] Proprioception is defined as position sense that orients the body or specific body parts to space or other objects.[2] Any self perturbation activity, such as hip flexion/extension or circumduction in chest-deep water while standing on one leg will challenge balance. Balance devices like the mini-trampoline, wobble boards, swing boards, therapy discs and so on can be used. Additionally the patient may close the eyes, relying more heavily on neuromuscular rather than visual input. When more impact is required for return to daily activities or sport, jumping and hopping drills may be introduced in the pool.

ENDURANCE TRAINING

Endurance training and cardiovascular conditioning is a key component of a high quality rehabilitation program. In addition to being suitable for training coordination of motion, water is eminently suitable for training stamina.

One focus of an aquatic rehabilitation program is to preserve the athlete's basic stamina. The movements designed for this purpose can be performed in water for a long period without experiencing pain and without subjecting the injured joint or the injured structures of the body to stress or tensile load. Basic stamina training improves and/or preserves the capacity and the performance of the cardiovascular, respiratory, metabolic and the immune systems. Simultaneously, it supports local adjustment processes in the musculature such as capillarity, and increases the number and size of mitochondria. Moreover, it activates the enzymes involved in aerobic metabolism and increases the intramuscular glycogen store.

While carrying out basic stamina training in water, various aids can be used. One such aid is a life jacket provided with rubber bands. These rubber bands are fixed to the edge of the pool such that the athlete is forced to swim against insurmountable resistance. The patient floats on his back and perform backstrokes, primarily using his arms if suffering a lower limb injury and using his legs if suffering an upper limb injury (Fig. 19.12).

The injured extremities are not stressed during the first weeks. Later, once the symptoms have subsided, the athlete may practice kicking injured limbs upwards and downwards. This movement may be performed more intensively, in various rhythms of coordination. Rubber fins may also be used as an additional aid.

Depending on the individual performance, the heart rate may vary from 130 to 150 beats/min. One training unit should range from 20 to 40 min and in high level athletes, up to more than 1 h/day. These prolonged training units are entailing continuous cyclic motion of the arms or the legs in water. Its intensity will be determined by the patient's heart rate. Although this information regarding intensity is rather imprecise, it is adequate for rehabilitation, because the main purpose of the first postoperative weeks is to preserve the athlete's endurance.

As time progresses, especially in high level athletes, a carefully regulated training program, involving measurement of lactate, urea and ammonia levels and the application of tests, such as the Conconi test, is offered. By increasing intensity, the training units can also be performed in the interval method (extensive and intensive interval training).[23]

In high level athletes, we found that the training unit fitted best with the total daily treatment and rehabilitation program, when it was carried out in the early hours of the evening. The reason is that a lymphatic drainage (special massage technique) of the injured extremity can be performed immediately thereafter, and the resulting vagus impulse and hypotonus of the musculature allow for general relaxation and create favorable conditions for regeneration (Tables 19.1–19.3).

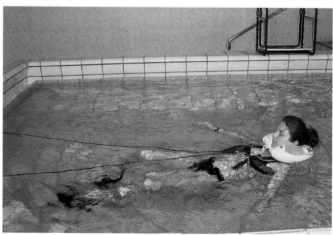

Figure 19.12 Swimming against insurmountable resistance.

Table 19.1   Sample Training Program for Back Injury

Area of focus	Activity
Trunk stabilization	Walking (forward, backward, sideways) in chest-deep water
	Pelvic movements (slightly knee bent; moving the hips in sequence forward, backward, right side, left side)
	Straight arm pulls
	Side to side steps
	Duck jumps
	Ball push downs
	Marching
	Deep-water jogging with WetVest® or AquaJogger®
Balance training	Eyes closed hip flexion/extension
	Eyes closed hip abduction/adduction/circumduction
	Stand upright on wobble boards, therapy discs, trampoline and swing board
	One leg stand (up to toes – down to heel – repeating)
Upper extremity training	Standing shoulder horizontal abduction/adduction
	Standing rows
	Pendulum exercises of the arms
	Straight arm pulls
	Cross country walking with hand-fins
Lower extremity training	Walking with tray
	Duck jumps
	Standing buoyancy resisted knee extension/flexion
	Standing hip adduction, abduction and circumduction
	Vertical kicking with fins
Endurance training	Walking in chest-deep water
	Rope fixed swimming
	Deep water walking or running in cross country style

Table 19.2   Sample Training Program for Shoulder Injury

Area of focus	Activity
Trunk stabilization	Walking in chest-deep water (forward, backward, sideways)
	Floating squats
	Duck jumps with rotation
	Deep water walking with flotation aids
Balance training	Single leg standing on heels (up to toes – back to heels – repeat)
	Single leg standing like above with eyes closed
	Stand upright position on unstable devices (e.g. therapy disc)
	Lunge jumps forward
	Straddle split jumps
Upper extremity training	Pendulum exercises always symmetric
	Standing abduction/adduction with gloves
	Standing flexion/extension of the elbow with gloves
	Standing kickboard plows (scapular protraction/retraction)
	Standing wall push-ups
	Shoulder press down and pull up with flotation devices
	Cross country walking
Lower extremity training	Walking (forward, backward, sideways)
	Walking with knee stiff
	Floating squats
	Resisted double/single leg jumping all planes
	Resisted hip flexion/extension, abduction/adduction
Endurance training	Walking in hip-deep water
	Crawling backwards only with the legs (body is fixed by ropes at the WetVest® in supine position)
	Aqua jogging in deep water

SPORT SPECIFIC AQUATIC REHABILITATION CONCEPT IN HIGH LEVEL ATHLETES

Sport specific aquatic rehabilitation in elite skiers after ACL reconstruction

---

Box 19.2: Key Points

- Trust in the body is synonymous with trust in oneself.
- Athletes can execute motion patterns pertaining to the relevant type of sport.
- Structure of motion is a unit of spatial-temporal and temporal-dynamic impulse elements.
- Training consists of motion patterns with full concentration by performing imitative exercises.
- Mimicking skiing motions in the pool by use of videotapes.

Introduction

For elite competitive athletes, injury is associated with enormous economic pressures, as well as with public pressure. This is particularly true in major competitive events. In such cases, the athlete's foremost desire is to return to competition or training as soon as possible. The desire is countered by the medical expert, who is forced to place time restraints, depending on the type of injury and the specific problems associated with it.

The medical expert's foremost principle should be not to permit an athlete to re-enter a competition unless he is healthy and able to sustain stress.

Injured tissue does not repair faster in competitive athletes than in average human beings. Hence, it has become necessary to improve the quality of rehabilitation by developing and applying rehabilitation techniques specifically designed to treat the injury sustained by the athlete. In spite of the injury, the athlete should be able to train as intensively as possible.

The following three aspects should be in harmony:

1   The injured structure of the body should be given specific treatment.

2   Attention should be given to the position of the injured anatomic structure in the chain of motion pertaining to the specific type of sport.

Table 19.3   Sample Training Program for Knee Injury

Area of focus	Activity
Trunk stabilization	Walking (forward, backward, sideways)
	Floating jumps in duck position (forward, backward, sideways and with rotation)
	Arm supported open chain hip, knee and ankle
	Flexion/extension in floating supine and prone position
Balance training	Single leg standing on heels (up to toes – down to heels – repeat)
	Single leg standing like above with eyes closed
	Floating single leg squats (forward, backward, sideways and rotating)
Upper extremity training	Resistive shoulder flexion and extension
	Pendulum exercises
	Cross body pull
	Straight arm pull
	Combination arm movements
Lower extremity training	Walking (forward, backward, sideways)
	Marching
	Resistive knee flexion/extension
	Proprioceptive training on unstable devices
	Single leg squats
	Lunges
	Single leg heel raises
	Stork stand
	Step ups
Endurance training	Swimming backwards only with the arms (body is fixed by ropes at the WetVest®) in supine position
	Walking in deep water with the AquaJogger® in intervals (extensive/intensive intervals)

3   It should be ensured that the athlete's stamina is not overly impaired, especially in terms of strength, speed and endurance. A training program specifically designed to maintain the athlete's stamina should be pursued, as far as possible, even while the athlete is affected by the injury.

It should be remembered that the athlete is injured, but still in training. In modern rehabilitation centers, an important aspect of treatment is the personality of the injured athlete. This specifically concerns the patient's ability to learn.[24] The treatment should include conscious visualization of the motion pertaining to the specific type of sport. Ski-specific technical motions can be recalled in the present time and made directly available to the patient at the therapeutic pool (by means of modern videotaping techniques). This is one of several aspects of so-called mental training. The major prerequisites for treatment of this type are high motivation, a good mental state of the patient and a clearly specified goal. Notwithstanding his injury, the skier should remain in close contact with his colleagues who are in regular training.

Although the incidence of injury to the anterior cruciate ligament has markedly increased among alpine skiers and has become a controversial issue in modern skiing, there are diverse opinions regarding postoperative rehabilitation measures following injury of this type. All specialists agree that functional treatment should be started as early as possible. However, opinions diverge widely with regard to the type of functional treatment, the steps of treatment, and, last but not least, the temporal sequence of treatment in terms of how much stress is permissible.

The goal of treatment after surgical reconstruction of the cruciate ligament may be summarized as follows:

- Swift and painless stress-bearing capacity
- Passive as well as active stability
- Passive and active mobility
- A feeling of confidence with regard to the knee joint.

Confidence in the strength of the knee joint is known to be an absolute prerequisite for optimum skiing performance. Once these results are achieved, it may be assumed that the injury has probably healed. From a medical (ethical) point of view, there should be no objection to subjecting the joint to normal stress.

The treatment of complex mobility disorders, such as those encountered after knee surgery, necessitates the application of educational and scientific training principles to a much greater extent than has been done so far, especially if the injured person is an elite athlete.

A rehabilitation program for a ski racer should be based on the principles of training and motion. The program should include exercises, training instructions and corrective measures specially adapted to the sport and the specific injury.

Water is an excellent therapeutic medium for this purpose, because underwater therapy takes the reduced weight bearing capacity of the injured knee into account and yet permits the patient to drill motion patterns that are characteristic for skiing.

Inner training

Water may be an entirely new world of experience for the patient. Underwater therapy may be regarded as a step towards so called 'inner training'.

The method of inner training originates from ancient Asian religions. It is based on a practical philosophy whose aim is to arouse and enhance spiritual and creative abilities by meditation and by perfecting the execution of physical exercises.[25]

An important aspect of inner training is trust in the human body. The human body is an intricate, computer-like organism that regulates itself in a predetermined rhythm. In the final analysis, trust in the body is synonymous with trust in oneself.

Accepting a situation for what it is may prove to be a practical way of approaching it and may be of great psychological help. The patient who goads himself to make maximum use of the rehabilitation will not achieve maximum benefit from the program. Rather, the patient who consistently pursues the program but also realizes that the injury is an integral aspect of his being will be happy and will rapidly achieve success. Awareness of this fact will help the athlete to accept the injury and will make it easier for him to develop a positive attitude towards it.

So-called inner training is a valuable adjunct to conventional training and treatment, because it takes not only external aspects, but also the athlete's subjective world of experience into account.

Inner training enhances the ability to relax, to regenerate and reduces the subjective stress associated with training and treatment.

Ski-specific imitative training

In the treatment of sports injury, a lot of attention has been given to the injured part of the body. The fact that every aspect of the body is an integral part of a kinematic chain that is indispensable for the execution of any sport or, for that matter, any motion, is not given enough attention. If it were possible for the athlete to execute the complete sequence of a complex motion even with a knee joint that is, in fact, not capable of sustaining normal stress levels, it would mean less loss of coordination during the rehabilitation period.

The neurologist Jackson[26] came to the conclusion that the brain does not know anything about the existence of muscles. Rather, the brain is only aware of motion patterns. Hence, the major goal of rehabilitation should be purposeful application of water in a manner that would enable the athlete to execute motion patterns pertaining to his daily life as well as specific motions associated with his kind of sport.

The buoyancy of the human body in water makes it possible to perform natural motions which are executed in three-dimensional fashion, in a spiral pattern and via several joints, in spite of the fact that the knee joint is too weak to sustain ordinary stress levels (Fig. 19.13).[27]

As far as the execution of movements is concerned, the same neuromuscular principles that apply to motion outside water apply to motion inside water. However, the stress level is highly reduced because water relaxes both the body and the psyche.

While the athlete drills skiing movements in water, he is surrounded by a sum of spatial and temporal motion-related stimuli. In our rehabilitation program, many of these stimuli are specifically related to the sport. Drilling this type of motion makes the athlete aware of his potential abilities, which, owing to the injury, are temporarily passive. Functionally significant patterns of motion can be drilled in this environment (Fig. 19.14).

The term spatial summation here refers to the sum of stimuli that may be released by various factors such as extension, physical contact and resistance.

Thus, performing specific skiing movements in water permits early commencement of a training program designed on the basis of motion techniques that are specifically adapted to the injury. Moreover, the program is designed such that it favorably influences neuromuscular patterns of motion.

Timing

Successful motor execution of motions related to any type of sport consists of the following:

Application of the right measure of strength, a high degree of coordination and exact timing
The motion of elite skiers is characterized by certain uniformity in terms of specific accentuated muscular contraction. The rehabilitation program, proposed here, is designed such that this uniformity is preserved to a great extent. This is achieved by a high level of task-oriented and target-oriented coordination while mimicking specific skiing motions (Fig. 19.15).

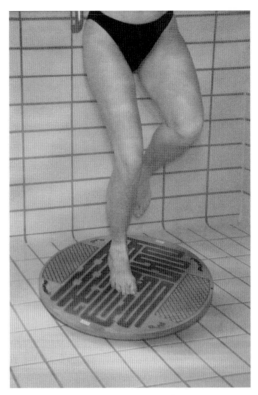

Figure 19.13 Proprioceptive training by increased ordinary stress levels.

The structure of a motion may be defined as a unit of spatial-temporal as well as temporal-dynamic impulse elements
In other words, the structure of the program of a motion is the rhythm of the motion and the rhythm of the program of motion, which may also be interpreted as the personality or the character of a motion.[28]

For execution of imitative exercises whose purpose is optimum rehabilitation, it is not the activity of a specific muscle that is of prime importance but the structural program of a motion. This structure should be preserved. The structure of the program is determined by and is the expression of the interaction of various impulses.

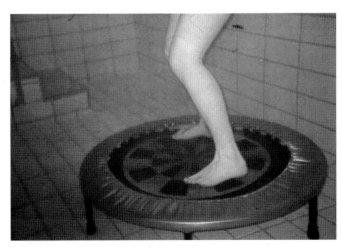

Figure 19.14 Transferring weight by a swinging motion similar to skiing.

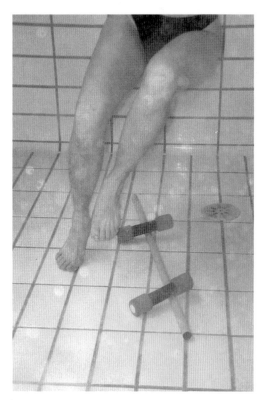

Figure 19.15 Mimicking parallel swinging.

The inter-relationship between the following aspects is of decisive importance:

1 Time interval (beginning of the impulse)
2 Duration (length of the impulse) and
3 Muscular intensity (extent of intensity of the impulse).

These temporal and dynamic aspects determine the structure of the program. Owing to these factors, the program acquires form-related elements and spatial implications.

Moreover these factors determine the quality of an observable motion pattern. The quality of coordination of the three factors mentioned above (the beginning, duration and extent of the impulse) within the structure of a motion is known as the impulse timing of a motion.[29]

The unity of temporal-spatial and temporal-dynamic impulse elements may also be summarized as 'the rhythm of motion'. A characteristic aspect of rhythm is that it retains its individual structure and nature even it is performed at a different (fluctuating) speed, i.e. at a speed that denotes a deviation from the norm.

A thorough understanding of these aspects is highly significant for preserving consolidated motion programs during rehabilitation. These aspects may be summarized as follows:

1 The essence of a motion pattern is expressed by its rhythm, i.e. by its temporal and dynamic determinants.
2 If the preservation of a program is defined as the preservation of motion and technique, it may be argued that the preservation of motion and technique is, in fact, synonymous with the preservation of rhythm (because the essence of motion is rhythm).

3 A basic guideline for learning motion is that initially the motion should be precisely acquired in the phase of learning. After it has been learned, it may be performed swiftly. This principle could be applied in a converse manner for rehabilitation. In this context, it may be interpreted as follows: *Motion patterns that cannot be performed swiftly and under full stress (because of injury) can be repeated slowly and precisely by maintaining a rhythm that may be modified to suit the specific conditions, and can be conserved by being performed in water).*

Several skiing techniques can be drilled in water at various degrees of skill, in a highly realistic fashion, without subjecting the knee to high levels of stress. The movements related to a specific kind of sport are stored in the athlete's motor memory. These programs of motion can be recalled at various degrees of proficiency, with the help of interpretation and decoding systems, and the programs can be used for specific training. These systems of interpretation and decoding may be presented in verbal (words, sentences) and/or visual (videos, diagrams, pictures, demonstrations) form.

The use of imagination in water

An athlete's imagination permanently influences his performance, both consciously and unconsciously. If the athlete's idea of a situation matches with the challenge the situation actually poses, the idea will help him to preserve the stored structure of a motion in his motor memory. The more precisely the steps of motion are processed in the athlete's imagination, the more effectively can the proposed rehabilitation plan (whose major goals are minimum loss of the skiing feeling and maximum preservation of the skiing technique) be realized.

Owing to the fact that elite athletes undergo several years of intensive training, they are highly proficient in their kind of sport. Hence, during rehabilitation, they are much superior to persons who do not practice sports and even to those who pursue sports in terms of a hobby.

We apply athlete's imagination in consciously regular, controlled and targeted manner. The athlete is made to train motion patterns with full concentration by performing imitative exercises, the basic pattern of which is similar to that of the skiing techniques performed on snow. This specific imitative training for skiers may be regarded as a special type of training.

Specific aspects of so-called mental training are combined with certain technical elements of so-called 'regular training on the skiing piste'. The chain of motion, although executed under less pressure, is carried out in the correct rhythm, and what is more in three-dimensional fashion.

With regard to mental training, this training program offers the following possibilities:

1 Subvocal training
   a The athlete is trained to repeat the training sequences in the form of a monologue.
2 Concealed perception training
   b This involves looking at a film on the execution of a motion (that the athlete is accustomed to perform) through the 'mental eye'. To put it more simply, one

imagines one's movement with the help of video recordings. In our setting, the athlete takes on the role of an observer, i.e. he looks at himself from an exterior point of view.

3   Ideomotor training

   c   In contrast to concealed perception training, ideomotor training is an interior process. From an interior perspective, the athlete vividly recalls the motion and re-experiences it in the present. He imagines himself performing the motion and tries to experience the mental processes that usually take place when he performs the motion (for instance, he may recall a cut swinging motion in the under-surface of his foot).

Various techniques of regular training are transferred to water and mimicked in this setting.

The following motions can be drilled well in chest-high water without putting too much stress on the injured knee joint:

- Parallel swinging motion
- Transferring weight by a swinging motion
- Canting techniques
- Sliding motions.

In order to train motion in an even more realistic fashion, the athlete is asked to wear inline skates (mimicking the feeling of the canting process in skiing) while performing some of the underwater training techniques in the therapeutic pool (Fig. 19.16).

These above-mentioned aspects of training are combined such that they form a harmonious unit, whose application in rehabilitation has proved to be of great value for ace skiers. There are two reasons why this aquatic training program succeeds. First, athletes are familiar with mental training and second, water is a convenient medium and does not pose any major problems for drilling ski-specific motion patterns. It is interesting to note how swiftly top competitive athletes adapt to motion conditions that are initially unusual for them. When the athlete drills skiing techniques in chest-high water in a pool with a flat ground, it is obvious that external factors, such as speed, the inclination of the slope, the texture of snow and centrifugal forces do not exist. Hence, the steering phase of a swinging motion cannot be mimicked at all.

Balancing and turning skills can be drilled to an extent that certain aspects of the kinematic chain of skiing may be reproduced on a neuromuscular level. Consequently, these skills are not jeopardized as much as they would be if the athlete did not train at all.

Once the knee joint is trained such that it is capable of sustaining more stress, and once the athlete feels fit to advance from skill drills to full participation (training on actual skis), he will be able to start at a higher level than he would have done without this training. Thus, the program shortens the total time needed for rehabilitation, i.e. from the time of the injury or surgery until complete fitness for participating in a competition.

Use of videotapes to train motion in the pool

Sport-motor-video-training is defined as video-based learning of motor skills in the context of sports training.[30] It is a process

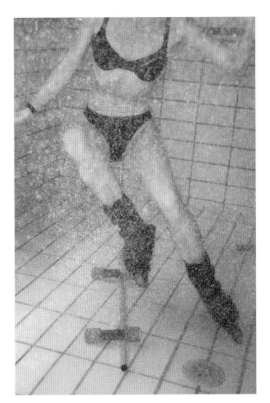

Figure 19.16   Inline skates in water.

regulated by information and its aim is to achieve maximum approximation of a realistically performed motion to a pre-given, kinematically defined ideal technique.[31] Sport-motor video training is based on the fact that one of the basic prerequisites for the acquisition of specific motor skills[32] is the creation of an internal representation of a motion, which, in this context, is based on the characteristic kinetic conditions of perception and execution of motion in video training.[33]

The creation and preservation of this representation of motion are based on the processing of information.

The information obtained by video documentation has two aspects:

1   The ideal technique is presented and is intended to communicate what exactly should be done (video instruction).
2   The presentation informs the observer about what he has actually done (video feedback).

We do not use video training to learn sport-motor-skills. Rather, we use it as a means to transfer actual skiing conditions to this specially designed rehabilitation training. In the pool, we try to create an environment that is similar to the environment on the skiing slope.

A major goal of video training is the conservation of training and motion patterns during rehabilitation. A further goal is to ensure that the injured athlete is in close contact with the remaining team members who are in training or are participating in the competition.

Evidently, when the athlete is able to mentally participate in the regular training program of his team, his motivation is significantly enhanced. These factors increase the efficiency of the training and rehabilitation.

One of the essential principles of modern rehabilitation *'injured but still in training'* is expressed in this program in an excellent manner. Almost all elite athletes have been filmed in action at some time or other. Video tapes of excellent quality are available from regular training as well as from television broadcasts of major competitions. These films can be intensively used for the program.

In any kind of training, but particularly in rehabilitation training, there should be a great deal of emphasis on attention. During video training, the tasks should be demonstrated and reproduced accurately. And this is possible only if the athlete applies full concentration.

Mentally, the rehabilitation training program should be carried out as if the techniques were being performed during regular training on snow. In other words, the athlete should carry out the training program with total concentration and with his entire attention directed towards the motion patterns and the training conditions.

Possibilities of video training While using video-taped documentation, the following three types of video recordings can be used in the training setting (Fig. 19.17):

1 *Video recordings of the training runs, performed by the athlete himself*: The athlete can analyze his own runs and train these motions in the therapeutic swimming pool by mimicking the skiing motions in a slower rhythm, without subjecting the injured knee joint to high stress. This will make it possible for him to consciously examine his own technique. He may discover technical errors that may have become automatic and can discuss these with his trainer and he could learn to conceal or rectify these errors by mentally rehearsing the correct pattern of motion.

2 *Video-taped recordings of training with one's own team or with opposing teams*: In spite of being in rehabilitation, the injured athlete will be able to participate actively in the regular training program of his team by watching these video films. Provided all members of the team cooperate, it will be quite easy to make the most recent training videotapes available to the athlete. This, in turn, will enable him to be in close contact with this team. This will also enhance his

motivation and will help him to better accept the treatment and the training program. Moreover, it will favorably influence the outcome of the therapeutic measures.

3 *Video-taped recordings of alpine ski slopes*: Video-taped recordings could also provide the athlete with valuable information about alpine ski slopes and racing pistes. The athlete would be able to carefully observe the downhill run of well-known slopes, such as the 'Hahnenkamm' ('cockscomb') slope in Kitzbühel in the Austrian Alps.

While mimicking skiing motions in the pool, the skier could mentally run the downhill slope such that his motor memory is trained and the information is stored.

When the athlete is capable of sustaining full stress, he will have the racing piste well stored in his motor memory and will be able to adjust better and more swiftly to the competition.

Training (mimicking) ski-specific motion in deep water

It has been proven that the AquaJogger® is very useful for mimicking ski-specific motions in deep water. This accessory ensures buoyancy and enables the athlete to move freely, with a slight forward inclination of 10° when he is in neck-high water.

The skier has to stabilize his body by using the muscles of his trunk. In this position and using the AquaJogger®, he will be able to mimic all the ski-specific exercises that he practiced in chest-high water, with the additional advantage of having no contact with the ground.

The same applies to video training. The only difference is that in video training there is absolutely no ground contact, a fact that further reduces stress on the injured joint. However, the neuromuscular aspects of motion can be practiced several times and the rhythm of ski-specific imitative exercises can be preserved. This is highly valuable when the athlete transfers the skills acquired during rehabilitation to the actual training environment in the piste.

CONCLUSION

It has been shown that applying various possibilities of modern underwater therapy and combining these techniques with a rehabilitation concept specifically designed to suit the type of injury and the injured athlete improves the quality of rehabilitation and helps the skier to return early to competitive training after surgery of the anterior cruciate ligament.

SUMMARY OF AQUATIC REHABILITATION

Principles of aquatics
Buoyancy

The submerged body loses weight equal to the weight of the water displaced (Principle of Archimedes) – thus resulting in less stress and pressure on the body.

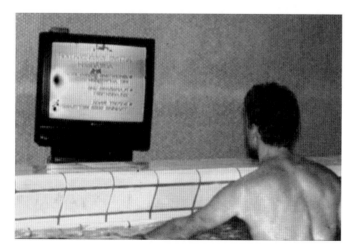

Figure 19.17 Video training.

Hydrostatic pressure

Hydrostatic pressure is proportional to depth and equal in all directions. It increases the venous return to the heart and also assists resolution of edema related to musculoskeletal injuries.

Viscosity

Viscosity acts as a resistance to movement of a body. This resistance is proportional to the effort exerted and allows the aquatic environment to be used as an effective strengthening medium.

Temperature

The aquatic environment allows regulation of the temperature during exercise and can have a significant effect on heart rate response and on the mobility of the tendons and muscles.

Biologic and physiologic effects

Aquatic immersion has profound biologic effects on the circulatory, the pulmonary, renal, the musculoskeletal and the nervous system.[34] These effects are both immediate and delayed, and allow water to be used with therapeutic efficacy in a great variety of rehabilitative problems.

Therapeutic medium

Water is an essential therapeutic medium in rehabilitation programs. The concept of underwater therapy offers many possibilities to develop and specify the rehabilitation of injuries, especially of sports-injuries.

As an exercise medium, water is very beneficial for those who understand its principles and properties. All aquatic exercise therapy concepts must address two important factors: the body's physiologic response to being immersed in water and the physical properties of water. By considering these two parts, a special rehabilitation program, which is safe and effective, must be designed and then the outcome will be optimized.

REFERENCES

1   Frank CB. Pathophysiology and healing of ligament injuries. In: Zachazewski JE, Magee DJ, Quillan WS, eds. Athletic Injuries and Rehabilitation. Saunders; 1998.

2   Hotz A. Techniklernen als Programm – und Rhythmuslernen, Traineracademy, Fachschriftenreihe des Österreichischen Schiverbandes. Innsbruck; 1998.

3   Meinel K, Schnabel G. Bewegungslehre. Berlin: Volk und Wissen; 1997.

4   Edlich RF, Towler MA, Goitz RJ, et al. Bioengineering principles of hydrotherapy. J Burn Care Rehabil 1978; 8:580–584.

5   Giancoli DC. Physics. Principles with applications. 2nd edn. Englewood Cliffs: Prentice Hall; 1985.

6   Bates A, Hanson N. Aquatic exercise therapy. Philadelphia, PA: Saunders; 1996.

7   Routi RG, Morris DM, Cole A. Aquatic rehabilitation. Philadelphia, PA: Lippincott; 1997.

8   Tajima F, Sagawa S, Iwamoto J, Miki K, Claybaugh RH, Shiraki K. Renal and endocrine responses in the elderly during head-out water immersion. Am J Physiol 1988; 254:977–983.

9   McMurray RG, Fieselman CC, Avery KE, Sheps DS. Exercise hemodynamics in water and on land in patients with coronary artery disease. Cardiopulm Rehabil 1988; 8:69–75.

10   Jamison L, Ogden D. Aquatic therapy using PNF patterns. Tucson, AZ: Therapy Skill Builders; 1994.

11   Bolton E, Goodwin D. An introduction to pool exercises. 2nd edn. London: E & S Livingstone; 1962.

12   Die Physik. Lehrbuch. Bertelsmann Verlagsgruppe International GesmbH. München; 1986.

13   Wicker A. Neue Wege in der Rehabilitation nach Sportverletzungen. Spektrum der Sportwissenschaften 1992; 4:2.

14   Clark LP, Dion DM, Barker WH. Taking to bed. Rapid functional decline in an independently mobile older population living in an intermediate-care facility. J Am Geriatr Soc 1990; 38:967–972.

15   Wicker A. Sportartspezifische Rehabilitation nach verletzungen des vorderen kreuzbandes bei alpinen spitzenschiläufern. Habilitationsschrift. Salzburg; Juni 1997.

16   Freiwald J, Srarischka S, Engelhardt M. Rehabilitatives krafttraining. Deutsche Zeitschrift für Sportmedizin 1993; 44:376.

17   Nashner L. Practical biomechanics and physiology of balance. In: Jacobson G, Newman C, Kartush J, eds. Handbook of balance, function and testing. St Louis, MO: Mosby Year Books; 1993:261–279.

18   Thein-Nissenbaum JM. Aquatic rehabilitation. In: Andrews JR, Harrelson GL, Wilk KE, eds. Physical rehabilitation of the injured athlete. 3rd edn. Philadelphia, PA: Saunders; 2004:295–313.

19   Frey LA, Smith GL. Underwater forces produced by the Hydro-Tone bell. J Orthop Sports Phys Ther 1996; 23:267.

20   Visnic MA. Aquatic physical therapy comes of age. Aqua Phys Ther Rep 1994; 1:6.

21   Wegener L, Kisner C, Nichols D. Static and dynamic balance responses in persons with knee osteoarthritis. J Orthop Sports Phys Ther 1997; 25:13–18.

22   Anderson MA, Foreman TL. Return to competition: Functional rehabilitation. In: Zachazewski JE, Magee DJ, Quillen WS, eds. Athletic injuries and rehabilitation. 1st edn. Philadelphia, PA: Saunders; 229.

23   Harre D. Trainingslehre. Einführung in die theorie und methodik des sportlichen trainings. Berlin: Sportverlag; 1983.

24   Pöhlmann R. Motorisches Lernen, 3. Auflage. Berlin: Sportverlag.

25   Willimczik K, Roth K. Bewegungslehre. Grundlagen – methoden – analysen: Berlin: Rowohlt-Verlag; 1991:2.

26   Jackson JH. Willkürbewegungen und linkshemisphärisches Bewusstsein. In: Birbaumer N, Schmidt FR, eds. Biologische psychologie. Berlin: Springer Verlag; 1996:3.

27   Knott M, Voss D. Komplexbewegungen im sport. Stuttgart: Gustav Fischer Verlag; 1970.

28   Hotz A. Praxis der trainings und Bewegungslehre. 1. Auflage. Frankfurt am Main: Sauerländer Verlag; 1991:57–76.

29   Roth K. Die Impuls – timing – hypothese. In: Röthig P, Grössing ST, eds. Wiesbaden: Bewegungslehre; 1990:9–54.

30   Olivier N, Blischke K, Daugs R, Müller H. Visuelle selektion beim sportmotorischen videotraining. Psychol Sport 1994; 4:140–141.

31   Daugs R, Blischke K, Marschall F, Müller H. Videotechnologien für den spitzensport. Leistungssport 1990; 20:12–17.

32   Müller H, Olivier N, Blischke K, Daugs R. Visuelle selektion beim sportmotorischen videotraining. Psychol Sport 1994; 4:1.

33   Prinz W. Wahrnehmung. In: Spada H Huber, ed. Berne: Allgemeine Psychologie; 1992.

34   Wilder PR, Cole AJ, Becker BE. Aquatic strategies for athletic rehabilitation. In: Kibler BW, Herring StA, Press JM, Lee PA, eds. Functional rehabilitation of sports and musculoskeletal injuries. Gaithersburg, Maryland: Aspen; 1998.

CHAPTER 20

Functional Restoration: Return to Training and Competition

W. Ben Kibler and Christopher J. Standaert

INTRODUCTION

Box 20.1: Key Points

- Optimal athletic function results from the coordinated interaction of anatomic, physiologic and biomechanical factors that generate forces and actions.

- The athlete presents to the sports medicine clinician because of dysfunction.

Athletes desire optimal athletic function. This requires three inter-related components: anatomy, physiology and mechanics. Optimal athletic function is the result of physiological motor activations creating specific biomechanical motions and positions using intact anatomical structures to generate forces and actions. The athlete presents to the sports medicine clinician because of dysfunction. This alteration in or deviation from normal function in the sport may be due to pain, injury, or decreased performance. Dysfunction may involve pathoanatomy, pathophysiology, or pathomechanics. The goal of function-based rehabilitation programs is the return of the athlete to optimum athletic function. To accomplish this goal, the athlete should be treated so that they can return to function in a specific sport or activity.

Sport-specific function occurs when the activations, motions and resultant forces are specific and efficient for the needs of that sport. We use the 'critical point' framework (Fig. 20.1) to understand sport specificity. Every sport has metabolic, physiological and biomechanical demands inherent in the way the sport is played, at whatever level of skill or intensity. Every athlete brings a specific musculoskeletal base to interact with the demands. Performance in the sport and risk of injury are the results of the interaction. The initial phase of the functional restoration program should include the assessment of the inherent demands of the sport and a complete evaluation of the musculoskeletal alterations that are associated with the presenting dysfunction. After this assessment, rehabilitation should be instituted in organized protocols or structures that are designed to protect healing tissues while maximizing functional capacity. The rehabilitation protocols

should merge into *pre*-habilitation, a phase which is preparatory for return to play. Finally, return-to-play decisions should be based on the achievement of optimal anatomy, physiology and mechanics in preparation for the sport-specific demands. This chapter will discuss sport-specific demands, musculoskeletal base assessment, rehabilitation protocols, prehabilitation, and return-to-play criteria.

SPORT-SPECIFIC DEMANDS

Box 20.2: Key Points

- Each sport has its own specific set of inherent demands, and these demands may change with the level of skill, intensity, or frequency with which the sport is played, or with the position played or event performed in a given sport.

- An evaluation system that profiles the physiological requirements and the biomechanical kinetic chains necessary to play the sport can allow good discrimination between sports.

There are many similarities in the demands sporting activities in general place on athletes. Most sports require some level of energy expenditure to generate the forces necessary to move the body, ball, or other object toward a certain goal. Most require some stability of one part of the body to achieve some movement of another part. Most require some degree of flexibility of some body parts and some degree of aerobic fitness. However, each sport has its own specific set of inherent demands, and these demands may change with the level of skill, intensity, or frequency with which the sport is played, or with the position played or event performed in a given sport.

The specificity of the physiological variables required for sports performance is reflected in the specificity with which the body adapts to training and physiologic demands. Numerous examples of this are documented in the medical literature. Although there are clearly limitations to the value of isokinetic training, studies performed using isokinetic dynamometry at different velocities generally show velocity-specific improvements in performance.[1] Immobilization of a limb has

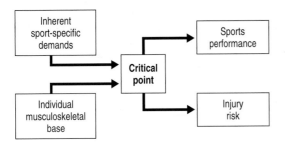

Figure 20.1 The 'critical point' framework showing the relationship between sports demands and the musculoskeletal base in determining performance and injury risk.

been shown to result in a decrease in the area of the motor cortex associated with the activation of the specific muscles affected, a process which reversed with subsequent movement of the limb.[2] Overall, there are a variety of means by which the body responds to training, including neural adaptations, cardiovascular changes, direct changes in muscle volume and structure, and alterations in the viscoelastic properties of soft tissues.[3,4] These factors are all affected by injury and disuse and can all potentially be addressed by specific methods of training. Training is clearly associated with a host of specific physiologic changes that may both directly impact the efficiency, speed, control, or force with which a certain complex motion is performed and have more broad effects on general physical performance. In designing a rehabilitation program for an injured athlete, therefore, it is important to understand the actual physiological effects of training maneuvers and to be able to coordinate the use of a variety of techniques in an appropriate manner to optimize functional outcome for the performance of a given task. In order to accomplish this, therapists and doctors need to know the parameters involved in a sport in order to prehabilitate the athlete properly for that sport.

Many different systems may be set up to profile sports and their demands. They may be based on anatomical requirements (range of motion required, strength required), metabolic requirements (aerobic or anaerobic activity) or amount of contact (collision, frequent contact, or minimal contact). We use an evaluation system that profiles the physiological requirements and the biomechanical kinetic chains necessary to play the sport.[5] This method allows good discrimination between

sports and generates enough information about the specific sport to plan an adequate prehabilitation program that will be sufficiently specific for the sport.

Box 20.3: Key Points

- The kinetic chain is a coordinated sequencing of activation, mobilization, and stabilization of body segments to produce an athletic activity.
- Athletic performance is dependent upon appropriate functioning of the individual components of the kinetic chain and appropriate coordination of the individual segments.
- Dysfunction of a particular segment in the chain can result in either altered performance or injury to a more distal segment.

The five physiological parameters we use are flexibility, strength, power (force × distance per unit of time), anaerobic capacity and aerobic endurance. We grade each sport from 1 to 3 based on the parameter's importance in the sport:
1 The parameter is important for general body fitness (e.g. aerobic endurance in golf)
2 The parameter is important in performance or injury risk reduction (e.g. flexibility in tennis or basketball)
3 The parameter is essential for maximum performance (e.g. aerobic endurance in running, strength in weightlifting).

Each sport will then have a profile that can be used to help an athlete meet the demands of that sport. Table 20.1 lists some sports and their resulting profiles.

Similarly, each sport can be characterized by the kinetic chains necessary to perform the sport. The kinetic chain is a coordinated sequencing of activation, mobilization and stabilization of body segments to produce an athletic activity.[6] Body segments have been described according to the Hanavan model as major bone and the joints on each end (Fig. 20.2). Kinetic chain activities have been grouped into open and closed chains.[7] Characteristics of open chains generally include free movement of the terminal segment, large terminal segment velocities and relatively many degrees of freedom in the proximal segments. Characteristics of closed chains generally include fixed or minimal movement of the terminal segment,

Table 20.1 Individual Sport Profile

	Flexibility	Strength	Power	Anaerobic	Aerobic
Basketball	2	2	3	3	3
Tennis	3	2	3	3	2
Golf	3	2	3	1	1
Soccer	2	2	3	3	3
Swimming	2	2	3	3	3
Running	2	1	2	1	3
Sprinting	3	2	3	3	1
Bicycling	2	2	3	3	3
Volleyball	2	2	3	3	1

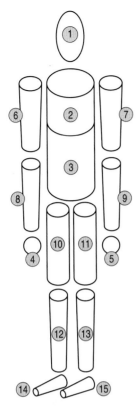

Figure 20.2 The Hanavan model of body segments. (Redrawn with permission from Hanavan EP. Mathematical model of the human body. AMRL-TR 1964; 18:1–149.)

substantial angular velocities seen at the shoulder during throwing; the force is largely generated by the more proximal segments of the lower extremities and trunk.[6,8,9] The substantial forces that are transferred to, and subsequently reabsorbed by, the distal segments at the shoulder and arm during throwing leave these segments vulnerable to injury.[10] Rehabilitation of the injured athlete must address the performance and kinematics of the entire kinetic chain.

General descriptions of kinetic chains have been demonstrated for many sports and activities. The kinetic chains represent general patterns that appear to be reproducible for a specific activity with some variation between individuals doing the activity.[11,12] Table 20.2 lists some of the most common sports and their predominant kinetic chain patterns.

When the physiological and biomechanical requirements of the sport or activity are categorized, exercises and progressions of load and intensity can be employed to prepare the body for the sport. A runner will need back and leg flexibility exercises, progressive aerobic training with longer duration of training bouts, and eccentric strength training of the legs to absorb the closed chain loads in the stance phase. An ice hockey player will need anaerobic training for short bursts of activity and power training in both the arms and legs. A baseball pitcher will need appropriate arm and back flexibility, lower body strength, power training to develop force, and eccentric training for the arm to control deceleration loads.

low terminal segment velocities, minimal degrees of freedom and coupling of movements of the segments. Many kinetic chains exhibit both closed and open chain activity.

Box 20.4: Key Points

- Kinetic chain activities can generally be characterized as either open or closed chain.

- Open chain activities include free movement of the terminal segment, large terminal segment velocities, and relatively many degrees of freedom in the proximal segments.

- Closed chain activities include fixed or minimal movement of the terminal segment, low terminal segment velocities, minimal degrees of freedom and coupling of movements of the segments.

- Closed chain activities may be particularly helpful in the rehabilitation of an injured athlete.

- Many functional kinetic chains exhibit both closed and open chain activity.

Athletic performance is dependent upon appropriate functioning of the individual components of the kinetic chain and appropriate coordination of the individual segments. Dysfunction of a particular segment in the chain can result in either altered performance or injury to a more distal segment. For example, the muscles of the shoulder girdle are not capable of generating the

MUSCULOSKELETAL ASSESSMENT

Box 20.5: Key Points

- Evaluation of injured athletes using the kinetic chain approach should take into account the broad scope of causative and contributing factors that may exist in addition to the clinical symptoms

- These factors include deficits in joint flexibility, relative muscle weakness or lack of endurance, sub-optimal mechanics, and any other biomechanical deficits that may be present

- The frequent association of distant tissue alterations with clinical symptoms can lead to a 'victims and culprits' approach to evaluation and treatment of sports medicine injuries, especially overload or chronic injuries, where the 'victim' is the site of clinical symptoms, and the 'culprits' are the distant alterations.

Table 20.2 Sport Kinetic Chains

Running	Ground → Leg → Hip/trunk → Opposite leg → Ground
Throwing	Ground → Leg → Hip/trunk/opposite leg → Shoulder → Arm
Serving	Ground → Legs → Trunk → Shoulder → Arm
Golf	Ground → Legs → Trunk → Shoulder/arm → Wrist
Kicking	Ground → Plant leg → Trunk/opposite hip → Kick leg → Ball
Swimming	Water → Hand/wrist → Arm/shoulder → Trunk/legs → Arm → Water
Shooting ball	Ground → Legs → Arm/wrist → Ball

Any system of evaluating injuries using the kinetic chain approach should take into account the broad scope of causative and contributing factors that may exist in addition to the clinical symptoms. These include deficits in joint flexibility, relative muscle weakness or lack of endurance, sub-optimal mechanics, and any other biomechanical deficits that may be present.

The frequent association of distant tissue alterations with clinical symptoms can lead to a 'victims and culprits' approach to evaluation and treatment of sports medicine injuries, especially overload or chronic injuries.[13] This approach allows a broad-based perspective on the pathophysiology underlying these injuries and an extensive clinical evaluation of all the physiological and biomechanical alterations that may be associated with the injury. The 'victim' is the site of clinical symptoms, and the 'culprits' are the distant alterations. For example, patellar tendinopathy may be associated with hip inflexibility or hip abductor weakness, and 'tennis elbow' (lateral elbow tendinosis) may be associated with posterior deltoid weakness.

Our evaluation is based on a framework in which most of the factors related to an injury or dysfunction are categorized into five main areas, called complexes.[14] These complexes interact with each other in the causation of micro-traumatic injuries, can be present as a result of macro-traumatic injuries, and are detectable on a clinical level. These complexes are composed of the following:

- *Clinical symptom complex*: that group of overt symptoms and signs that clinically characterize the injury
- *Tissue injury complex*: that group of anatomic structures that have overt pathological change
- *Tissue overload complex*: that group of structures that have non-symptomatic but clinically detectable changes
- *Functional biomechanical deficit complex*: alterations in biomechanics due to injury or overload
- *Subclinical adaptations*: substitute actions that the athlete uses to compensate for altered mechanics to maintain performance.

These complexes interact in a negative feedback vicious cycle to cause or maintain a soft tissue injury (Fig. 20.3).[14] In micro-trauma cases, an athlete may 'cycle' as a 'susceptible' athlete for some time before overt clinical symptoms appear. Most acute injuries exhibit relatively fewer tissue overloads and biomechanical deficits, but some of these may occur as a result of treatment, such as loss of endurance, lower extremity strength, and ankle range of motion following immobilization after Achilles tendon surgery. In this model, clinical symptoms are a relatively small part of the entire pathophysiologic picture. These obviously require treatment, but it is also important to emphasize restoration of function encompassing all of the physiological and biomechanical alterations, rather than only resolution of symptoms.

The medical history should include questions about previous injury, either local to or distant from the present injury. Examples include inquiring about previous ankle injury (present ankle injury or knee injury), previous hip injury (present knee pain, low back pain, or shoulder injury), previous back pain (present knee pain, low back pain, or shoulder injury), and previous shoulder injury (present shoulder injury or elbow injury). Also, one should ask questions about the exact nature of any treatment and rehabilitation of previous injury as both prior injury and inadequate rehabilitation of a prior injury have been suggested as risk factors for further injury.[15,16]

The physical exam should include not only standard peripheral joint and neurologic examinations but also some functional screening tests for distant parts of the kinetic chain to highlight deficits. Good screening tests include standing posture evaluation from front and back, the 'one-leg stability series' of one-leg stance and one-leg squat, sit and reach for lumbar flexibility, repetitive arm elevation/depression for scapular stability, and glenohumeral rotation off a stabilized scapula.[7,17,18] Further evaluation can take place if the screening exam shows alterations.

EXAMPLES OF KINETIC CHAIN-BASED EVALUATION AND TREATMENT

This section gives examples of the assessment of specific conditions utilizing the approach described above. Evaluation and treatment in this manner may result in a more thorough clinical evaluation and, subsequently, a more efficacious rehabilitation program. Each condition is covered more extensively in other sections of the book.

Plantar fasciitis
Plantar fasciitis is exacerbated by loss of dynamic protraction control of the foot and ankle. Several kinetic chain alterations may be present. Factors evident in the complexes include the following:

- *Clinical symptoms*: point tenderness over plantar fascial insertion into calcaneus, stiffness in the morning or upon standing after sitting
- *Tissue injuries*: plantar fascia, short flexors
- *Possible tissues overloaded*: gastrocnemius/soleus complex, Achilles tendon, gluteal muscles
- *Functional biomechanical deficits*: look for decreased active ankle dorsiflexion, decreased foot pronation/supination

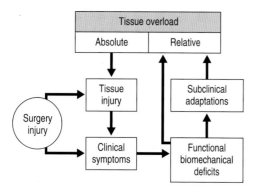

Figure 20.3 The negative feedback vicious cycle.

control or positive Trendelenburg sign with one-leg stance, or both; decreased strength in toe-off
- *Subclinical adaptations*: look for shorter stride on affected leg, look for leg external rotation with stance.

Chronic hamstring muscle strain

Chronic hamstring strain results from repeated episodes of re-injury. Each re-injury creates more deficits and adaptations.
- *Clinical symptoms*: point tenderness and pain localized along the course of the muscle, possibly a defect (tear) or a palpable knot (scar), pain when running, stiff at rest
- *Tissue injury*: hamstring at muscle–tendon junction
- *Possible tissues overloaded*: adductors, hip extensors
- *Functional biomechanical deficits*: look for excessive hip flexion and knee flexion in stance or running, a positive Trendelenburg sign on one-leg stability testing
- *Subclinical adaptations*: shortened stride on injured leg, no pivoting on injured leg

Rotator cuff tendonitis

Rotator cuff injury has obvious local causative factors (poor intrinsic blood supply, subacromial abrasion, direct or indirect trauma), but also may be associated with many kinetic chain alterations.
- *Clinical symptoms*: pain over anterior or lateral acromion; (+) impingement testing; pain and weakness with horizontal abduction, forward flexion, external rotation; pain at night
- *Tissue injury*: rotator cuff tendon, partial or complete
- *Possible tissues overloaded*: shoulder capsule, scapular stabilizing muscles
- *Functional biomechanical deficits*: look for glenohumeral internal rotation deficit, scapular dyskinesis with lower trapezius weakness, upper trapezius hyperactivation and acromial depression
- *Subclinical adaptations*: look for shoulder shrug with arm elevation, thoracic kyphosis, dropping the arm below shoulder elevation in throwing or serving.

Lateral elbow tendonitis

Lateral elbow tendonitis (misnamed lateral epicondylitis, more properly named lateral elbow tendinosis) is common in older athletes and is commonly associated with mechanical kinetic chain deficits.
- *Clinical symptoms*: point tender pain over lateral epicondyle and extensor carpi radialis brevis; pain with grip; pain with one-hand backhand tennis stroke
- *Tissue injury*: extensor carpi radialis brevis, occasionally extensor carpi radialis longus or joint capsule
- *Possible tissues overloaded*: biceps, shoulder external rotators, lateral epicondyle
- *Functional biomechanical deficits*: look for scapular dyskinesis, alterations in scapular position and motion that affect scapular roles in activity, deficits in strength of shoulder external rotation
- *Subclinical adaptations*: look for alterations in hitting mechanics, including leading with the elbow, hitting the ball behind the body, or trying to swing the racquet using the wrist extensors.

REHABILITATION AND PREHABILITATION

Box 20.6: Key Points

- Our rehabilitation approach includes three phases:
  - Acute
  - Recovery
  - Functional.
- Different levels of exercises may be used in the early (acute) phase, the intermediate (recovery) phase and the late (functional) phase of rehabilitation.
- The functional phase marks a transition between *rehabilitation* and *prehabilitation*, which can be defined as conditioning strategies in the formerly injured athlete to prepare him or her for the stresses and demands inherent in the sport, and which must be faced in return to sport.
- The functional progressions in a rehabilitation program should simulate the actual activities required in the sport.

Rehabilitation protocols are structured around frameworks of progressions of exercises, loads, and applied and generated forces as the athlete improves his or her ability to generate and control sport-specific forces. Our rehabilitation approach includes three phases: acute, recovery and functional (Fig. 20.4).[14] The patient progresses through each phase in a 'flow' dependent upon reaching certain criteria of injury healing and achievement of control of certain physiological and biomechanical functions.

The acute phase is a broad, relatively non-specific phase with goals of:
1 protection or healing of injured tissues
2 improvement of general flexibility and strength
3 improvement in function of the distant links in the kinetic chains involved in the sport or activity.

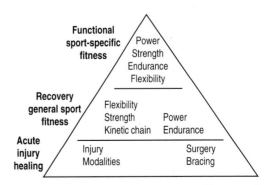

Figure 20.4 Phases of the rehabilitation process. The start of rehabilitation includes all causes of injury, but the end focuses on return to function.

The recovery phase is a relatively long phase with goals of:
1 preparation for maximum physical activity
2 improvement in kinetic chain linkage sequencing
3 normalization of any distant kinetic chain dysfunction such as inflexibility or strength imbalance
4 setting up the strength and power base for sport-specific progressions.

The functional phase is a focused phase, with the goals of:
1 obtaining sport-specific flexibility and strength
2 optimization of sport-specific physiological activations and biomechanical motions
3 sport-specific functional progressions.

Our experience has led us to favor closed-chain rehabilitation protocols for most of our patients. Closed-chain rehabilitation protocols have beneficial characteristics that are associated with functional physiology and biomechanics. Closed kinetic chain exercises, in general, may simulate functional tasks more effectively, provide more appropriate proprioceptive feedback, and protect joint surfaces through co-contraction and more 'physiologic' loading of joint structures when compared to open chain exercise.[19] They may be utilized early in the rehabilitation sequence to protect the injured area and to prepare the entire kinetic chain for function.

Different levels of exercises may be used in the early (acute or healing) phase, the intermediate (recovery) phase, and the late (functional) phase of rehabilitation, depending on the degree of tissue healing, the possible positions of the extremity, and the amount of load and the range of motion that are allowed.[20,21]

Knee and leg rehabilitation
Closed-chain rehabilitation techniques have been utilized to accelerate and improve functional restoration after ACL injury and reconstruction.[22–24] These techniques create weight-bearing forces across the joint that increase local agonist–antagonist muscle co-activation, decrease joint shear, minimize joint displacement and ACL strain, and reproduce proprioceptive stimuli. In addition, they activate the kinetic chains of weightbearing, running, and jumping. This reproduces the normal biomechanics of the entire leg, allowing hip-muscle activation to increase quadriceps and hamstring force output by transferring muscle work to these biarticular muscles and by creating a hip moment that is a major contributor to the knee moment.[25,26] Hip-muscle activation and work output create load-absorbing capacity that can compensate for a low load-absorbing capacity in the knee so that the entire leg functions at an acceptable level early in rehabilitation.[26] Closed-chain exercises also reproduce the physiologic length-dependent patterns for hip- and knee-joint stability, as well as force-dependent patterns of coordination of hip, knee, and ankle joint motion. The effect that closed-chain exercises have on the entire kinetic chain is more functionally important than the effect on the knee joint alone.

Closed-chain techniques are also useful in rehabilitation of the patient with patello-femoral pain, largely due to the same factors of joint position control, larger improvements in the strength of the entire kinetic chain, and alteration of the magnitude and position of applied forces. Increased total leg stiffness, with resultant knee joint control, is achieved by activating the hip muscles concurrently with the knee muscles.[25,27] Closed-chain exercises have been shown to produce greater improvements in quadriceps strength and leg performance than open-chain exercises.[28] When compared with open-chain exercises, closed chain exercises of the quadriceps muscles have also been shown to result in more simultaneous activation of the different components of the quadriceps with more effective motor-unit synchronization.[19,29] Closed-chain exercises produce lower patello-femoral joint stresses in the functionally and symptomatically important arc of motion from extension to 45° of flexion than do open-chain exercises.[30]

Shoulder rehabilitation
On superficial analysis, it would appear that closed-chain rehabilitation would have little application for the shoulder and arm. The hand is moving in an open-chain fashion in throwing and serving, and the arm assumes a weight-bearing position only in gymnastics and blocking in football. However, shoulder position, motion and force transfer fit the physiologic and biomechanical requirements of closed-chain activities. In throwing and serving, the scapula and shoulder display intersegmental coordination, with coupled movements that are predictable on the basis of arm position.[31,32] The shoulder acts as a stable funnel, transferring and regulating forces in the kinetic chain from the legs to the hand.[6,33] The shoulder muscles are activated in mainly co-contraction length-dependent patterns to stabilize the joint.[25,32–34] Proprioception plays a major role in controlling and activating muscle patterns.[35] In swimming, weightlifting, and playing on the offensive or defensive line in football, the hand meets considerable resistance but still moves, creating mobile end-external load conditions at the distal end of the extremity.

Closed-chain exercises should, therefore, be utilized in shoulder and scapula rehabilitation for functional return to most athletic activities from all types of shoulder injuries. Rehabilitation protocols for tendonitis, postoperative instability and postoperative labral injuries are basically the same in the acute phase and in the early functional phase.[20,36] Postoperative rotator cuff protocols should vary with the integrity of the repair, but can also benefit from the proximal activation and low shear characteristics associated with closed-chain activities. Just as in knee and leg rehabilitation, closed-chain exercises may be used in the early stages of rehabilitation, and emphasis should be placed on involving all of the joints of the kinetic chain.

Functional progression
The functional progressions in a rehabilitation program should simulate the actual activities required in the sport. Return-to-play criteria are based on successful completion of the functional phase goals. The functional phase marks a transition between *re*habilitation and *pre*habilitation, which can be defined as conditioning strategies in the formerly injured athlete to prepare him or her for the stresses and demands inherent in the sport, and which must be faced in return to sport.[37] Prehabilitation focuses on sport-specific musculoskeletal areas that have been shown to be weak or susceptible to injury, or have actually been injured, in a specific sport.[38]

Functional musculoskeletal prehabilitation exercises can be strenuous as they replicate the motions, positions, forces, intensities and muscle activations inherent in the sport. The athlete's body should have enough general athletic fitness to allow these vigorous activities without undue injury risk. The anatomical lesion should be healed. The physiological muscle activations, flexibility and endurance capabilities should be capable of withstanding the strength and power exercises.

The physician and therapist should monitor and test for these parameters as rehabilitation progresses and as the athlete goes into the prehabilitation protocols. For throwing athletes, the general criteria should include hip and trunk control over the planted leg, trunk rotational flexibility and strength, control of scapular elevation and protraction, functional glenohumeral internal rotation, and rotator cuff co-contraction strength.[39] For running athletes, general criteria should include appropriate gastrocnemius, quadriceps and hamstring flexibility, hip and trunk control over the planted leg, trunk extensor strength and aerobic capacity.

As noted previously, athletes frequently have areas of inflexibility and weakness in other parts of the kinetic chain that may contribute to the injury or to decreased performance, and these issues should be addressed in the prehabilitation exercises. The frequency of these distant alterations may be as high as 50–85% in association with injury.[18,40–43] A thorough evaluation of the entire kinetic chain involved in sports performance should result in the identification of these functional and biomechanical alterations.

SPECIFIC EXAMPLES: PREHABILITATION PROTOCOLS

The prehabilitation protocols should be based on progressions of flexibility, strength exercises, increasing loads and durations and progress from closed-chain to open-chain configurations. This is illustrated by specific protocols for: (1) tennis/baseball, for overhead activities; (2) running, for long distances and for a long duration; and (3) soccer, for high-intensity power running and jumping.

Tennis/baseball
Prehabilitation plan
The athlete should begin a shoulder flexibility and strengthening program focusing on increasing the internal rotation range of motion and external rotation strength. Flexibility exercises are performed after the throwing activity is complete for the day. Due to the high tensile loads developed in the shoulder external rotators and due to the inflexibility of the athlete in this area, a flexibility program is warranted. For strengthening, the goals of the training program are to increase the strength of the scapular stabilizers and shoulder external rotators, while maintaining explosiveness in those muscles. Plyometric/agility drills are incorporated into the prehabilitation program as they may reduce the risk of injuries related to these ballistic movements. In addition to the prehabilitation program, it is assumed the athlete participates in a general resistance training program two or three times per week.

At this stage of healing and rehabilitation, physical therapy modalities (heat, ice, ultrasound, stimulation) are usually not indicated. Very little tissue alteration is expected at this stage of healing that would be modified by these modalities. Some heat may be used to help in increasing tissue pliability before the exercise bout, and cold may occasionally be used if there is some swelling postexercise (Table 20.3)

Table 20.3 Tennis/Baseball Prehabilitation Program

Weeks 1–2	
Flexibility (daily, after activity):	
Cross body stretch, scapula stabilized	3×30 s
Internal rotation, scapula stabilized	3×30 s
Triceps stretch	3×30 s
Racquet stretch	3×30 s
Strength (3–5 × week):	
Shoulder external rotators/scapula retraction with tubing	3×25 reps (moderate speed)
Rows with dumbbells/tubing, elbows down	3×15 reps
Reverse flies with dumbbells/tubing	3×15 reps
Plyometric/agility (3–5 × week):	
5-dot drill (Fig. 20.5)	2×20 foot contacts
Hexagon drill (Fig. 20.6)	3×15 s, double leg
Line drill (Fig. 20.7)	2×20 double leg foot contacts
	2×20 single leg foot contacts
Footwork ladder, bounding	2×20 double leg foot contacts
	2×20 single leg foot contacts
Footwork ladder, quick feet	4×20 low-intensity foot contacts
Footwork sprints (carioca, shuffle, back pedal, cross-over step, skip, high knee, etc.)	5–8×9 meters
Weeks 3–4	
Flexibility (daily, after activity):	
Cross body stretch, scapula stabilized	2×30 s
Internal rotation, scapula stabilized	2×30 s
Triceps stretch	2×30 s
Racquet stretch	2×30 s
Strength (3–5 × week):	
Shoulder external rotation/scapula retraction with tubing	4×25 reps (high speed)
Rows with dumbbells/tubing, elbows down	4×25 reps (high speed)
Shoulder internal rotators with tubing	4×25 reps (high speed)
Medicine ball forehand	2×25 reps
Medicine ball backhand	2×25 reps
Medicine ball serve	2×25 reps
Plyometric/agility:	
5-dot drill	2×20 foot contacts
Hexagon drill	4×10 s, single and double leg
Line drill	2×20 double leg foot contacts
	2×20 single leg foot contacts
Footwork ladder, bounding	2×20 double leg foot contacts
	2×20 single leg foot contacts
Footwork ladder, quick feet	3×20 low-intensity foot contacts

Continued

Table 20.3 Tennis/Baseball Prehabilitation Program—Cont'd

Footwork sprints (carioca, shuffle, back pedal, cross-over step, skip, high knee, etc.)	10–15 × 4.5 meters
Weeks 5–6	
Flexibility (daily, after activity):	
Internal rotation, scapula stabilized	2 × 30 s
Racquet stretch	2 × 30 s
Strength (2–4 × week):	
Shoulder external rotation/scapula retraction with tubing	2 × 25 reps (high speed)
Shoulder internal rotation with tubing	2 × 25 reps (high speed)
Plyometrics/agility:	
5-dot drill	2 × 20 foot contacts
Hexagon drill	5 × 10 s, single and double leg
Line drill	2 × 20 double leg foot contacts
	2 × 20 single leg foot contacts
Footwork ladder, bounding	2 × 20 double leg foot contacts
	2 × 20 single leg foot contacts
Footwork ladder, quick feet	3 × 20 low-intensity foot contacts
Footwork sprints (carioca, shuffle, back pedal, cross-over step, skip, high knee, etc.)	10 × 4.5 meters

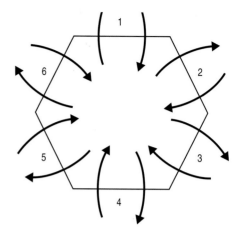

Figure 20.6   The hexagon drill. Do in the sequence shown and repeat three times.

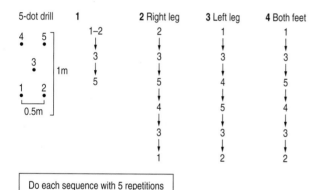

Do each sequence with 5 repetitions

Figure 20.5   The 5-dot drill. Each sequence should be done in the order listed and completed five times. (Redrawn with permission from Kibler WB, Chandler TJ. Functional rehabilitation and return to training and competition. In: Frontera WR, ed. Rehabilitation of sports injuries: Scientific basis. Oxford: Blackwell Science; 2003:288–300.)

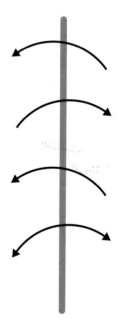

Figure 20.7   The line drill. Jump back and forth across a line, which could be a tennis court sideline, baseball foul line, soccer touch line, etc. Land on both feet (double leg) or one foot (single leg).

Soccer
Prehabilitation plan

Soccer requires aerobic endurance, anaerobic capacity and power. It is common that injuries may recur if prehabilitation is not complete, because of the varied and large loads inherent in the demands (Table 20.5)

Running
Prehabilitation plan

It is suggested that the athlete should start prehabilitation on a more forgiving surface for training purposes whenever possible, such as grass or a rubber track. The main goal of the prehabilitation program is to allow the athlete to progress at 10–25% increases in work load, which are usually safe progressions. Strengthening the ankle while trying to improve ankle range of motion is warranted. Flexibility of the hamstrings and gastrocnemius is stressed. Low-intensity plyometric and eccentric activities may help prepare the athlete to withstand the repetitive loads of running, as well as improve explosiveness for the kick at the end of the race (Table 20.4).

CRITERIA FOR RETURN TO SPORTS

Box 20.6: Key Points

- The injured athlete must be anatomically healed and must complete all of the rehabilitation stages to be considered for return to sport.

- All injured athletes must complete sport-specific functional progressions of activities, demonstrating that they have the physiology and biomechanics necessary to withstand the inherent demands of the sport, before returning to sports competition.

Table 20.4   Running Prehabilitation Program

Weeks 1–4: The athlete is running 1.6–4.8 km, 3–4 days per week		Strength (2–3 × week):		
Flexibility (daily, after activity):		Squats (light resistance)	3 × 10 reps	
Lying hamstring stretch	3 × 30 s	Lunges with light dumbbells	3 × 10 reps	
Standing quadriceps stretch	3 × 30 s	Weighted heel raise	3 × 10 reps	
Leg twists for iliotibial band	3 × 30 s	Plyometrics/agility (non-running days		
Wall calf stretch	3 × 30 s	on grass):		
Trunk sit and reach	3 × 30 s	5-dot drill	2 × 20 foot contacts	
Strength (4–5 × week):		Line drill	2 × 20 single leg foot contacts	
Squats (light resistance)	3 × 20 reps	Bounding drill	2 × 10–15 foot contacts	
Lunges with light dumbbells	3 × 20 reps	Weeks 9–10: The athlete is running		
Weighted heel raise	3 × 20 reps	8–16 km on Monday and Wednesday		
Plyometrics/agility (3 × week,		and 16–24 on Saturday		
non-running days on grass):		Flexibility (daily, after activity):		
5-dot drill	3 × 30 foot contacts	Lying hamstring stretch	2 × 30 s	
Line drill	3 × 30 double leg foot contacts	Standing quadriceps stretch	2 × 30 s	
Weeks 5–8: The athlete is running		Wall calf stretch	2 × 30 s	
4.8–8 km on Monday and		Strength (2 × week):		
Wednesday and 8 km on Friday		Squats (light resistance)	2 × 10 reps	
and Saturday		Lunges with light dumbbells	2 × 10 reps	
Flexibility (daily, after activity):		Weighted heel raise	2 × 10 reps	
Lying hamstring stretch	3 × 30 s	Plyometrics/agility (non-running		
Standing quadriceps stretch	3 × 30 s	days on grass):		
Leg twists	3 × 30 s	Fartlek progressions: alternating	20 meter jog → 10 meter	
Wall calf stretch	3 × 30 s	low-intensity and high-intensity	run → 10 meter sprint	
Trunk sit and reach	3 × 30 s	running bouts		

Table 20.5   Soccer Prehabilitation Program

Weeks 1–3		Plyometrics/agility (3 × week):	
Flexibility (daily, after activity):		5-dot drill	2 × 30 foot contacts
Lying hamstring stretch	2 × 30 s	Line drill	2 × 20 double leg foot contacts
Standing quadriceps stretch	2 × 30 s		2 × 20 single leg foot contacts
Leg twists	2 × 30 s	Footwork ladder, bounding	2 × 20 double leg foot contacts
Wall calf stretch	2 × 30 s		2 × 20 single leg foot contacts
Trunk sit and reach	2 × 30 s	Footwork ladder, quick feet	4 × 30 low-intensity foot contacts
Strength (3 × week, body weight as resistance):		Footwork springs (carioca,	5–8 × 18 meters
Squats	2 × 20 reps	shuffle, back pedal,	
Forward lunges	2 × 20 reps	cross-over step, skip,	
Side step/cross step lunges	2 × 20 reps	high knee, etc.)	
Heel raise	2 × 20 reps	Weeks 7–10	
Plyometrics/agility (3 × week):		Flexibility (daily, after activity):	
5-dot drill	2 × 20 foot contacts	Lying hamstring stretch	2 × 30 s
Line drill	2 × 20 double leg foot contacts	Standing quadriceps stretch	2 × 30 s
Footwork ladder, bounding	2 × 20 double leg foot contacts	Wall calf stretch	2 × 30 s
Footwork ladder, quick feet	3 × 30 low-intensity foot contacts	Standing knee to chest	2 × 30 s
Weeks 4–6		Strength (3 × week, medicine ball or dumbbells as resistance):	
Flexibility (daily, after activity):		Squats	2 × 10 reps
Lying hamstring stretch	2 × 30 s	Forward lunges	2 × 10 reps
Standing quadriceps stretch	2 × 30 s	Side step/cross step lunges	2 × 10 reps
Wall calf stretch	2 × 30 s	Heel raises	2 × 10 reps
Standing knee to chest	2 × 30 s	Plyometrics/agility (3 × week):	
Strength (medicine ball or dumbbells as resistance):		5-dot drill	2 × 20 foot contacts
Squats	3 × 15 reps	Line drill	2 × 20 double leg foot contacts
Forward lunges	3 × 15 reps		2 × 20 single leg foot contacts
Side step/cross step lunges	3 × 15 reps		
Heel raises	3 × 15 reps		

The injured athlete must be anatomically healed and must complete all of the rehabilitation stages to be considered for return to sport. Understanding the inherent demands of the sport allows for an objective set of criteria for return. Throwers must have sport-specific functional range of motion of arm joints, stable scapula, trunk/core stability and plyometric power development in the leg, no matter where their original injury occurred. Runners must have leg flexibility, trunk/core stability and aerobic endurance, no matter where their original injury occurred.[39] All injured athletes must then complete sport-specific functional progressions of throwing, running, jumping, kicking or swimming. These exercises demonstrate that the athlete has the physiology and biomechanics necessary to withstand the inherent demands of the sport.

Some authors have advocated return to sport based on quantitative criteria such as quadriceps/hamstring ratios in run-

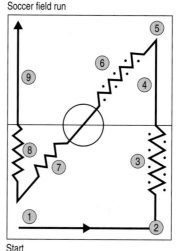

Soccer field run

1 Sprint
2 Jump and head a ball
3 Run around cones
4 Run backwards
5 Pick up soccer ball
6 Dribble around cones
7 Three running jumps
8 Plyometric jumps over lines
9 Sprint

Start

Figure 20.8 Return to soccer functional program. The drill encompasses all of the soccer-specific demands. (Redrawn with permission from Kibler WB, Chandler TJ. Functional rehabilitation and return to training and competition. In: Frontera WR, ed. Rehabilitation of sports injuries: Scientific basis. Oxford: Blackwell Science; 2003:288–300.)

Table 20.6   Interval Throwing Program Starting off the Mound

Stage 1: Fastball only	
Step 1: Interval throwing	Use interval throwing to 120 ft
15 Throws off mound 50%	phase as warm-up
Step 2: Interval throwing	
30 Throws off mound 50%	
Step 3: Interval throwing	All throwing off the mound
45 Throws off mound 50%	should be done in the
Step 4: Interval throwing	presence of your pitching
60 Throws off mound 50%	coach to stress proper
Step 5: Interval throwing	throwing mechanics
30 Throws off mound 75%	
Step 6: 30 Throws off mound 75%	
45 Throws off mound 50%	
Step 7: 45 Throws off mound 75%	Use speed gun to aid in effort
15 Throws off mound 50%	control
Step 8: 60 Throws off mound 75%	
Stage 2: Fastball only	
Step 9: 45 Throws off mound 75%	
15 Throws in batting practice	
Step 10: 45 Throws off mound 75%	
30 Throws in batting practice	
Step 11: 45 Throws off mound 75%	
45 Throws in batting practice	
Stage 3	
Step 12: 30 Throws off mound 75%	Warm-up
15 Throws off mound 50%	Breaking balls
45–60 Throws in batting practice	Fastball only
Step 13: 30 Throws off mound 75%	
30 Breaking balls 75%	
30 Throws in batting practice	
Step 14: 30 Throws off mound 75%	
60–90 Throws in batting practice 25%	Breaking balls
Step 15: Simulated game: Progressing	
by 15 throws per workout	

ners or internal rotation/external rotation ratios in throwers. These ratios are usually based on isokinetic data, which have not been conclusively shown to be associated with true muscle capability.[1] These ratios can be helpful in determining weaknesses, but do not represent total capabilities, and should not be used as sole determinants of return to play. It is more important to know if the athlete can do all of the functions required in play, rather than if the athlete can generate torque at one joint.

It may appear that the criteria for return to sport are rigid or easily determined. Actually, the criteria should be employed with some leeway, based on the athlete and the situation. The athlete should not be allowed to 'play yourself into shape', with no guidelines or input. This allows deleterious kinetic chain substitutions and increases the chances of reinjury.[44] The athlete also should not be 'rushed' through the prehabilitation protocol, because the sport-specific exercises do impose significant demands, once again increasing the chances of re-injury.

Experience has taught us the value of gradual return to play, with emphasis on steady progression of exercises, strict attention to the preparedness of the musculoskeletal base for new exercises, involvement of the kinetic chain, and resolution of both the local and distant alterations that may exist in association with the injury.[14,41]

Return to play is completed by sport-specific functional progression of doing the specific activity. Table 20.6 illustrates a sport-specific throwing progression, while Figure 20.8 illustrates a sport-specific soccer progression.[45,46]

REFERENCES

1 Cronin JB, McNair PJ, Marshall RN. Is velocity-specific strength training important in improving functional performance? J Sports Med Phys Fitness 2002; 42:267–273.

2 Liepert J, Tegenthoff M, Malin JP. Changes of cortical motor area size during immobilization. Electroencephalogr Clin Neurophysiol 1995; 97:382–386.

3 Grimby G, Thomee R. Strength and endurance. In: Frontera WR, ed. Rehabilitation of sports injuries: Scientific basis. Oxford: Blackwell Science; 2003:258–273.

4 Schwellnus M. Flexibility and joint range of motion. In: Frontera WR, ed. Rehabilitation of sports injuries: Scientific basis. Oxford: Blackwell Science; 2003:232–257.

5 Kibler WB. The sports preparticipation exam. Champaign, IL: Human Kinetics; 1990.

6 Putnam CA. Sequential motions of body segments in striking and throwing skills: Descriptions and explanations. J Biomech 1993; 26:125–135.

7 Kibler WB, Livingston BP. Closed chain rehabilitation for the upper and lower extremity. J Am Acad Orthop Surg 2001; 9:412–421.

8 MacWilliams BA, Choi T, Perezous MK, Chao EY, McFarland EG. Characteristics of ground reaction forces in baseball pitching. Am J Sports Med 1998; 26:66–71.

9 Press JM, Young JL. The role of the spine in the throwing athlete. SpineLine 2000; September/October:21–23.

10 Fleisig GS, Barrentine SW, Escamilla RF, Andrews JR. Biomechanics of overhand throwing with implications for injuries. Sports Med 1996; 21:421–437.

11 Hirashima M, Kadota H, Sakurai S, Kudo K, Ohtsuki T. Sequential muscle activity and its functional role in the upper extremity and trunk during overarm throwing. J Sports Sci 2002; 20:301–310.

12 Marshall RN, Elliott BC. Long axis rotation: The missing link in proximal to distal segmental sequencing. J Sports Sci 2000; 18:247–254.

13 MacIntyre JG, Lloyd-Smith DR. Overuse running injuries. Sports injuries, principles of prevention and care. London: Blackwell Scientific; 1993.

14 Kibler WB, Chandler TJ, Pace BK. Principles of rehabilitation after chronic tendon injuries. Clin J Sports Med 1992; 11:661–673.

15 Emery CA. Risk factors for injury in child and adolescent sport: A systematic review of the literature. Clin J Sports Med 2003; 13:256–268.

16 Standaert CJ, Herring SA, Cole AJ, Stratton SA. The lumbar spine and sports. In: Cole AJ, Herring SA, eds. The low back pain handbook. Philadelphia: Hanley & Belfus; 2003:385–404.

17 Kibler WB, McMullen J. Scapular dyskinesis and its relation to shoulder pain. J Am Acad Orthop Surg 2003; 11:142–152.

18 Burkhart SS, Morgan CD, Kibler WB. Shoulder injuries in overhead athletes: The 'dead arm' revisited. Clin Sports Med 2000; 19:125–159.

19 Stensdotter A, Hodges PW, Mellor R, Sundelin G, Hager-Ross C. Quadriceps activation in closed and in open kinetic chain exercises. Med Sci Sports Exerc 2003; 35:2043–2047.

20 Kibler WB, Livingston B, Bruce R. Current concepts in shoulder rehabilitation. Adv Oper Orthop 1995; 3:249–300.

21 Nichols TR. A biomechanical perspective on spinal mechanisms of coordinated muscular action: An architecture principle. Acta Anat (Basel) 1994; 151:1–13.

22 Shelbourne KD, Nitz P. Accelerated rehabilitation after anterior cruciate ligament reconstruction. Am J Sports Med 1990; 18:292–299.

23 Bynum EB, Barrack RL, Alexander AH. Open versus closed chain kinetic exercises after anterior cruciate ligament reconstruction: A prospective randomized study. Am J Sports Med 1995; 23:401–406.

24 Beynnon BD, Johnson RJ. Anterior cruciate ligament injury rehabilitation in athletes: Biomechanical considerations. Sports Med 1996; 22:54–64.

25 Umberger BR. Mechanics of the vertical jump and two-joint muscles: Implications for training. Strength Cond 1998; 10:70–74.

26 DeVita P, Hortobagyi T, Barrier J. Gait biomechanics are not normal after anterior cruciate ligament reconstruction and accelerated rehabilitation. Med Sci Sports Exerc 1998; 30:1481–1488.

27 Thomeé R, Augustsson J, Karlsson J. Patellofemoral pain syndrome: A review of current issues. Sports Med 1999; 28:245–262.

28 Augustsson J, Esko A, Thomeé R, Svantesson U. Weight training of the thigh muscles using closed vs. open kinetic chain exercises: A comparison of performance enhancement. J Orthop Sports Phys Ther 1998; 27:3–8.

29 Mellor R, Hodges PW. Motor unit synchronization of the vasti muscles in closed and open chain tasks. Arch Phys Med Rehabil 2005; 86:716–721.

30 Steinkamp LA, Dillingham MF, Markel MD, Hill JA, Kaufman KR. Biomechanical considerations in patellofemoral joint rehabilitation. Am J Sports Med 1993; 21:438–444.

31 Zattara M, Bouisset S. Posturo-kinetic organization during the early phase of voluntary upper limb movement. I. Normal subjects. J Neurol Neurosurg Psychiatry 1988; 51:956–965.

32 Happee R, Helm FCT Van der. The control of shoulder muscles during goal-directed movements: An inverse dynamic analysis. J Biomech 1995; 28:1179–1191.

33 Kibler WB. Biomechanical analysis of the shoulder during tennis activities. Clin Sports Med 1995; 14:79–85.

34 Kibler WB. The role of the scapula in athletic shoulder function. Am J Sports Med 1998; 26:325–337.

35 Lephart SM, Pincivero DM, Giraldo JL, Fu FH. The role of proprioception in the management and rehabilitation of athletic injuries. Am J Sports Med 1997; 25:130–137.

36 Lephart SM, Henry TJ. The physiological basis for open and closed kinetic chain rehabilitation for the upper extremity. J Sports Rehab 1996; 5:71–87.

37 Kibler WB, Chandler TJ. Sports specific conditioning. Am J Sports Med 1994; 22:424–432.

38 Chandler TJ. Exercise training for tennis. Clin Sports Med 1995; 14:33–46.

39 Kibler WB, McMullen J, Uhl TL. Shoulder rehabilitation strategies, guidelines, and practice. Oper Tech Sports Med 2000; 8:258–267.

40 Ekstrand J, Gilquist J. The frequency of muscle tightness and injuries in soccer players. Am J Sports Med 1982; 10:75–78.

41 Kibler WB, Goldberg C, Chandler TJ. Functional biomechanical deficits in running athletes with plantar fasciitis. Am J Sports Med 1991; 19:66–71.

42 Knapik JJ, Bauman CL, Jones BH, et al. Preseason strength and flexibility imbalances associated with athletic injuries in female college athletes. Am J Sports Med 1991; 19:76–81.

43 Warner JJP, Micheli L, Arslenian LE, et al. Scapulothoracic motion in normal shoulders and shoulders with glenohumeral instability and impingement syndrome. Clin Orthop Relat Res 1992; 285:199–210.

44 Devlin L. Recurrent hamstring symptoms in rugby. Sports Med 2000; 29:279–287.

45 Andrews JR, Wilk KE. Throwing progressions for return to baseball. Birmingham, Alabama: American Sports Medicine Institute; 1996.

46 Kibler WB, Naessens GC. Soccer pre-participation physical exam. In: Garrett WE, Kirkendall DT, Contigulia SR, eds. The US soccer sports medicine book. Chicago, IL: US Soccer Federation; 1996:147–167.

CHAPTER 21

Common Injections in the Injured Athlete

Ted A. Lennard

INTRODUCTION

Today's athlete has come to expect aggressive treatment for complex as well as self-limiting injuries. This expectation is driven, in part, by the desire to maintain their competitive edge, team pressures, and, in the case of the professional athlete, financial renumeration. As a result, numerous strategies and techniques have been developed to effectively treat the athlete injured with soft tissue disorders, intrinsic joint dysfunction and spinal injuries. The treatments include minimally invasive surgery, exercise programs, manual medicine techniques, medications and injections. This chapter will focus on injections and is divided into two basic sections,[1] basic principles of injections in the athletic population and[2] specific injection techniques for disorders arising from the soft tissue, joints and spine. Details of common injection procedures will be covered for joint and soft tissue injuries. An overview of spine injections will be discussed, but details of these advanced procedures will be left to other texts.[3–5]

BASIC PRINCIPLES OF INJECTIONS IN THE ATHLETIC POPULATION

Injections are commonly performed to reduce, eliminate, or diagnose a painful stimulus originating from the soft tissue, joint, nerve, or spinal disc. These procedures should be utilized within the framework of broader goals of recovery and rarely in isolation to cure or repair a disorder. For example, the tennis player with lateral epicondylitis should undergo careful scrutiny of their technique, i.e. grip position, racket weight, string tension, handle diameter, etc., all known biomechanical factors in the development of lateral epicondylitis.[6,7] This analysis should be implemented simultaneously with a supervised therapy program that emphasizes modalities, stretching and progressive exercises. Only when progress stagnates should an injection be considered.[8] The response to the injection should be noted for confirmation of the working diagnosis. Any interval improvement can be used to advance their therapeutic exercise program.

Box 21.1: Key Point

- Injections should be utilized within the framework of broader goals of recovery and rarely in isolation to cure or repair a disorder.

Prior to an injection, a thorough medical history is required. One should inquire about drug allergies, current medications and medical conditions. The use of injections in patients on blood thinners such as coumadin, aspirin, or other anti-platelet drugs should be approached with caution, but are not contraindicated in superficial injections, but should be avoided in deep injections such as spinal blocks.[9] Injections are contraindicated in patients who have local infections or an immunosuppressed condition. Diabetics should be cautioned about a transient elevation of their blood glucose when corticosteroids are used. Adequate skin prep with Betadine or Hibiclens is usually recommended and reduces the chance of local infections.[10,11] Common sense precautions should be adhered to regarding numbers of injections and placement of injections. One should avoid intratendinous needle placement,[12] advancing into the periosteum of local bone, or injecting into vascular or neural structures.

Medications

Most injections consist of a mixture of anesthetics and corticosteroids. The specific concentrations and types of these drugs injected varies among practitioners' preferences and is dependent on their intended use. For example, a single subacromial injection for a clear diagnosis of subacute bursitis may consist of a short acting corticosteroid, i.e. triamcinolone, and a short acting anesthetic, i.e. 1% lidocaine. By comparison, the athlete with a complex shoulder and neck injury with diffuse shoulder and neck pain, may benefit from a single diagnostic subacromial anesthetic injection, i.e. 2% lidocaine, without corticosteroid. The response to the injection would be closely monitored to help differentiate the possible pain generators within the neck and shoulder complex. Other injectables such as normal saline or sterile water can be used when one needs to expand the volume injected without risking possible side-effects such as anesthetic toxicity. In cases when proliferation therapy is considered, dextrose, glycerin, phenol or sodium morrhuate may be used.[13]

Corticosteroids

Corticosteroids produced by the adrenal cortex can be classified as androgenic or estrogenic, salt-retaining (mineralocorticoids) and anti-inflammatory (glucocorticoids).

The glucocorticoid class is commonly used in injections for the treatment of inflammatory disorders. The primary glucocorticoid produced in humans is cortisol (hydrocortisone). Cortisol and other synthetic glucocorticoids possess varying degrees of anti-inflammatory and salt-retaining properties. It is these properties that dictate which glucocorticoid should be injected (Table 21.1).[14–17]

Box 21.2: Key Point

- Corticosteroids commonly cause subcutaneous fat atrophy. Flush the needle with anesthetic or sterile water during withdrawal.

Anesthetics

Most physicians are familiar with common anesthetics, such as lidocaine or Marcaine®. The pain within a joint, tendon, or nerve can be reduced or eliminated when these drugs are used to provide temporary anesthesia. This change in their condition assists the physician in the ultimate diagnosis. There are two common classes of anesthetics: esters and amides. Table 21.2 outlines the differences and compares individual anesthetic drugs.[16,18,19]

SOFT TISSUE INJECTIONS

Myofascial trigger point injections

Myofascial trigger points (Tp) are localized tender spots within taut bands of skeletal muscle located within the muscle or fas-

Table 21.2 Comparison of Common Anesthetics[16,18,19]

	Onset (min)	Duration (min)[a]	Equal concentration	Toxicity[b]
Esters				
Procaine (Novocaine)	5	30–60	2	6
Tetracaine	6–12	30–60	2	7
Chloroprocaine	15	175	0.25	1
Amides				
Lidocaine	0.5–1	100	1	5
Bupivacaine	5	120–240	0.25	2
Mepivacaine	3–5	100	1	4
Etidocaine	5	120–240	0.25	3

[a]Varies with method of administration.
[b]Approximate ranks among the anesthetics listed (1, most toxic; 7, least toxic).
(Adapted from Lennard 1995.[16])

cial tissue (Fig. 21.1). These points can be found in other tissue such as periosteum, joint capsules, ligaments and tendons. Characteristically, trigger points refer pain to distant locations also known as reference pain zones.[20–22] Autonomic phenomenon and changes in proprioception may often accompany this referred pain.

Tender points, like trigger points, have areas within the taut bands of skeletal muscle that cause pain. These spots, however, do not refer pain or cause other symptoms such as

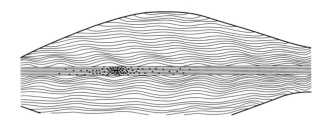

Figure 21.1 Trigger point within a taut band of muscle fibers.

Table 21.1 Comparison of Commonly Used Glucocorticoid Steroids[14–17]

Agent	Anti-Inflammatory Potency[a]	Salt Retention Property	Plasma Half-Life (min)	Equivalent Oral Dose (mg)
Hydrocortisone (cortisol)	1	2+	90	20
Cortisone	0.8	2+	30	25
Prednisone	4–5	1+	60	5
Prednisolone	4–5	1+	200	5
Methylprednisolone (Medrol, Depo-Medrol)	5	0	180	4
Triamcinolone (Aristocort, Kenalog)	5	0	300	4
Betamethasone	25–35	0	100–300	0.6
Dexamethasone (Decadron)	25–30	0	100–300	0.75

[a]Relative to hydrocortisone
(Adapted from Lennard 1995.[16])

proprioceptive abnormalities or autonomic dysfunction, but rather cause isolated and well localized areas of discomfort within muscle.

The anatomic components of trigger points are not entirely understood. Travell and Simons propose that muscle strain leads to isolated fiber overload, which leads to muscle fiber damage. This event results in elevated calcium levels, which, in combination with adenosine triphosphate, cause sustained isolated fiber contraction, increased metabolism, and local base constriction. Nearby muscle fibers shorten independently and result in taut fibers.[21]

Myofascial trigger point injection techniques

Various needle sizes, techniques and injected medication have been well discussed in the literature.[2,20,21,23–27] The most important factor in myofascial trigger point injections appears to be the mechanical disruption of abnormal tissue, rather than the actual solution injected. The primary purpose of the injection is to disrupt the sensitized abnormal tissue mechanically by the repeated probing of a needle. The injection of solution such as an anesthetic tends to increase the mechanical disruption during the procedure. Typically, a needle ranging from 25–27-gauge in diameter is required to facilitate this mechanical disruption (Fig. 21.2). Once the examiner has identified a trigger point within a taut band of muscle tissue, a needle is introduced through the skin, fatty tissue and fascia directly into the muscle. The needle is directed toward the fibrotic tissue previously noted on manual examination. The needle is redirected along the taut band and within the myofascial trigger point itself. The solution injected into each area requires a volume of 1–3 cc. The resistance is reduced when one has penetrated through the taut band of a myofascial trigger point as well as at the edges superior to the band and trigger point. A trigger point injection could theoretically be performed in any specific muscle or muscle group that is found to have trigger points as described above. The example below demonstrates the technique in the trapezius muscle.

Trapezius muscle trigger point injection

Athletes who present with diffuse neck and shoulder pain may be candidates for Tp injections. Localized areas of tenderness within taut bands of the trapezius muscle that when palpated

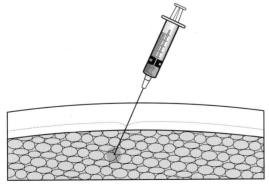

Figure 21.2 Trigger point injection. The needle tip is shown in the trigger point.

Box 21.3: Key Point

- The most important factor in myofascial trigger point injections is the mechanical disruption of abnormal tissue rather than the actual solution injected.

radiate pain in well-defined areas may confirm one's suspicion of the diagnosis of Tp. The physician should be keenly aware of the differential diagnosis of neck and shoulder pain in the athlete including primary pathology within the shoulder joint or cervical spine.

The patient is placed in a relaxed prone position and the trapezius muscle is palpated. Many practitioners use some type of lubricant such as soap or gels to improve their tactile abilities. Once a trigger point is located, the skin is cleaned with alcohol, and a 25–27-gauge needle is inserted into the trigger point. Using a repetitious insertion and withdrawal of the needle through the trigger point, but not out of the muscle, the Tp is mechanically disrupted. Small amounts of anesthetics (1–3 cc of 0.5% or 1% lidocaine) can be injected during this mechanical disruption as one option for treatment. As long as one's needle stays within the trapezius muscle, few complications are likely to occur. However, caution should be exercised if the needle tip is allowed to advance too deeply and possible complications may arise depending on the segment of muscle that is being injected. For example, if the thoracic portion of the trapezius muscle is the target site, the deep structures including the intercostal space and underlying thorax should be noted. However, if the upper cervical portion of the trapezius muscle is being injected, cervical spinal structures including the nerve roots and vertebral artery should be remembered.

Bursa injections

The bursa is a fluid filled sac located between tendons and/or bony prominences that act to reduce friction. These synovial lined sacs secrete fluid that when injured by overuse or trauma can swell and be a source of pain in the athlete. Often other structures, i.e. tendons, ligaments, etc., are injured and act as a co-existing source of pain. Most bursa are located adjacent to joints and can be easily and safely injected. Below is a list of the more commonly injected bursa.

Box 21.4: Key Point

- An injection into the bursa may help differentiate various pain syndromes.

Trochanteric bursa injection

Inflammation of this bursa is located in the proximal lateral femur over the greater trochanter adjacent to the attachment of the gluteus maximus muscle and under the iliotibial band from the tensor fascia. Characteristic findings of trochanteric bursitis include pain at the proximal lateral thigh on manual palpation typically directly over the greater trochanter. At

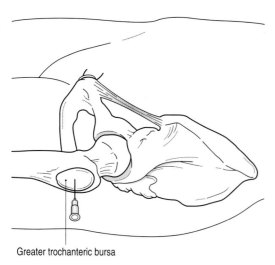

Figure 21.3 Trochanteric bursa injection. The needle tip is placed inside the bursa.

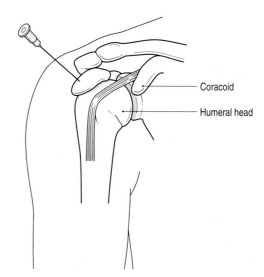

Figure 21.4 Subacromial bursa injection. The needle is inserted through the deltoid muscle and adjacent to the acromion.

times, it radiates along the lateral thigh to the knee. Injection into the trochanteric bursa is common. The examiner should palpate the superior and posterior surface of the greater trochanter directed adjacent to these landmarks (Fig. 21.3). Typically, a 22–27-gauge needle will be utilized injecting volumes ranging between 5 and 8 cc of anesthetic and corticosteroid mixture. Some have proposed the use of fluoroscopy for this injection to confirm proper needle placement.[28] If the needle trajectory is placed superiorly, an intraarticular injection may occur. One should also be cautious as the needle tip advances past the bone of the greater trochanter.

Subacromial bursa injection

The subacromial bursa is located on the superior aspect of the humerus and appears as a 'cap' in this region. The bursa's medial extension is seen under the acromion, coracoacromial ligament, and coracoid process and further extends inferiorly under the proximal bicipital tendon and bicipital groove. An injection into this bursa may reduce or eliminate shoulder pain, and can allow the physician to better differentiate bursitis, rotator cuff tears or tendonitis. A 25 or 27-gauge 1.5–2 in needle is inserted after a Betadine prep. The insertion point is usually anterolateral or posterior under the acromion (Fig. 21.4). The accuracy rates of these approaches are not significantly different.[29] Inferior traction on the arm can increase the acromiohumeral space and make the injection easier. The needle is advanced approximately 1.5–2 in and a 4–8 cc volume containing an anesthetic and corticosteroid solution injected. If the needle tip is advanced too far medially or inferiorly, an intraarticular injection may occur. If the needle tip is too superficial or directed superiorly, a subcutaneous fat or muscular injection will occur.

Pes anserine bursa injection

The pes anserine bursa is located on the proximal medial tibia at the insertion site of the sartorius, gracilis and semitendinosus muscles. Deep to this bursa lies the medial collateral ligament of the knee and the medial joint space. Clinical suspicion should remain high for other etiologies that mimic pes anserine bursitis such as meniscal and ganglion cysts and other benign or malignant soft tissue tumors.[30] On clinical examination, a focal area of tenderness can be palpated at the insertion site of the above noted muscle groups. Injection utilizing a 25–27-gauge needle and 2–5 cc of corticosteroid and anesthetic at the point of maximum tenderness within the bursa is identified by palpation and the needle advanced to the bursa (Fig. 21.5). The physician should be aware of the superficial nature of this injection and the injection may penetrate the articular space of the knee joint.

Tendon injections
Bicipital tendonitis
Bicipital tendonitis of the shoulder is characterized by proximal anterior arm pain and is made worse with resisted

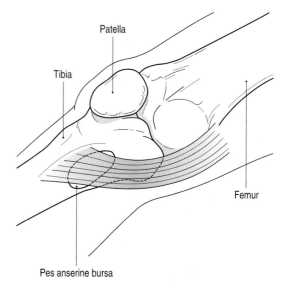

Figure 21.5 Pes anserine bursa injection.

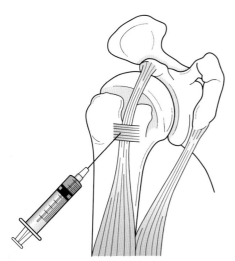

Figure 21.6   Bicipital tendon injection. The needle is placed parallel to the tendon.

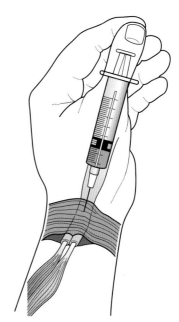

Figure 21.7   De Quervain's injection. The needle is placed parallel to the extensor pollicis tendons within the tendon sheath.

shoulder flexion. Focal tenderness can be palpated along the tendon proper between the greater and lesser tuberosities along the proximal humerus.

An injection adjacent to the biceps tendon can be performed by palpating the greater tuberosity of the proximal humerus and by locating and injecting the needle just inferior to the point of directing the needle cephalad in a parallel fashion to the tendon itself (Fig. 21.6). One should be careful not to penetrate the tendon with the needle tip. A 25–27-gauge needle can be used with an anesthetic and steroid mixture between 2 and 5 cc of volume.

It is important to recognize the greater tuberosity of the humerus and the easily palpable long head of the biceps brachii muscle when using the anterior approach. The border of the deltoid muscle can be sometimes mistaken for the bicep's tendon, especially in overweight or large patients. Superficially, the cephalic vein can be found adjacent to the deltopectoral groove, although usually this vein is medial to the entry point of the injection. If the needle trajectory is too far laterally, conceivably the axillary nerve could be encountered.

Box 21.5: Key Point

- The border of the deltoid muscle can be mistaken for the bicep's tendon, especially in large patients.

De Quervain's tenosynovitis

Tendonitis involving the abductor pollicis longus or the extensor pollicis brevis tendons is generally known as stenosing tenosynovitis or de Quervain's tenosynovitis. Clinically, the patient has focal tenderness over these tendons at the dorsoradial aspect of the wrist and pain is reproduced with a provocative maneuver known as Finkelstein's test (thumb abduction in flexion with the wrist deviated to the ulnar side). Prior to injection, the abductor pollicis long and extensor pollicis brevis tendons are palpated. Utilizing a small needle ranging from 25–27-gauge in diameter,

the physician inserts the needle adjacent to the tendon proper into the tendon sheath and advanced parallel to the tendon (Fig. 21.7).

One should avoid direct penetration into the tendon with the needle tip. A volume of 2–5 cc of injectate utilizing a corticosteroid and an anesthetic mixture is normally used. If the trajectory of the needle deviates into the anatomic snuffbox, potentially the radial artery could be penetrated. The physician should also be aware of the location of the superficial radial sensory nerve that crosses the extensor pollicis tendon in the distal forearm.

Box 21.6   Key Point

- Avoid injections directly into the tendon.

Lateral epicondylitis

Lateral epicondylitis, often referred to as 'tennis elbow', is often treated with local corticosteroid injection. The hallmark of this diagnosis is well localized tenderness directly over the lateral epicondyle of the distal humerus. Reproduction of pain in this region is often noted with resistance to wrist extension and gripping activities. Typically a 25–27-gauge diameter needle is directed at the point of maximum tenderness in the region of the lateral epicondyle. The needle traverses the skin, subcutaneous fat, and into the substance of the common extensor tendon from the extensor compartment of the forearm. Then the needle tip strikes the lateral edge of the bony end of the lateral epicondyle (Fig. 21.8). Small volumes of injectate ranging from 2–5 cc is typically required. The injection is typically quick and simple if the practitioner is well versed in the regional anatomy. If the needle were to stray medially to the inferior portion of the cephalic vein at its

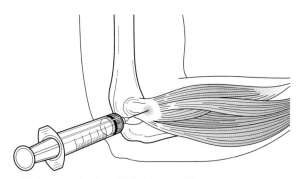

Figure 21.8 Lateral epicondylitis injection. The needle is injected at the site of maximal tenderness at the lateral epicondyle and extensor mass.

juncture with the median cubital vein or the lateral ante-brachial cutaneous nerve may be encountered. If the needle strays deep in the medial direction, one could potentially encounter the radial nerve. Post-injection, subcutaneous atrophy could occur in this region and cause cosmetic deformity if the physician who injects fails to flush the corticosteroid from the needle prior to withdrawing through the subcutaneous fat.

Medial epicondylitis

Medial epicondylitis, commonly referred as golfer's elbow, can be diagnosed in patients who present with isolated tenderness over the medial epicondyle of the distal humerus. This condition can be found in athletic sports that require prolonged or resisted wrist flexion with supination, such as golf. Patients may also experience pain in the proximal forearm or distal arm. This condition is amenable to injection using a similar technique to that described for the lateral epicondylitis. Using aseptic technique, the point of maximum tenderness is located and a 25 or 27 gauge needle injected and advanced to this point usually along the medial epicondyle. A total of 2–5 cc of a corticosteroid/anesthetic mixture can be injected. The physician should be aware of the proximity of the medial epicondyle to the ulnar nerve in the cubital tunnel during the injection.

Box 21.7 Key Point

- Be aware of the proximity of the ulnar nerve to the medial epicondyle during the injection.

JOINT INJECTIONS

Glenohumeral joint

The glenohumeral joint can be injected from a superior, anterior, or posterior approach.[1,31] All three injection approaches are relatively safe, though of the three, the anterior approach is closer to larger neurovascular structures. Regardless of the approach used, each joint is injected with strict aseptic technique, with Betadine prep and a total volume of 5–10 cc of anesthetic and corticosteroid mixture. The superior approach[32] can be performed when the needle is inserted just anterior to the acromioclavicular (AC) joint, lateral to the

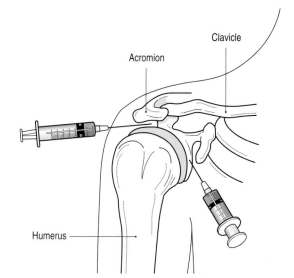

Figure 21.9 Glenohumeral joint injection. This diagram demonstrates the anterior and lateral approach.

coracoid process, and advanced inferiorly into the glenohumeral joint (Fig. 21.9). The needle trajectory is through the deltoid muscle. When the physician advances the needle medial to the AC joint, he or she should avoid the coracoacromial ligament. The acromial branches of the thoracoacromial artery usually lie anterior and just inferior to the coracoid process with no other significant vascular structures nearby. The musculocutaneous and axillary nerves are the largest nerves in the region; each are inferior to the coracoid process and are rarely at risk with the superior approach.

When a physician uses the anterior approach to the glenohumeral joint, he or she should insert the needle 1–2 cm lateral to the lateral tip of the coracoid process. Needle insertion is advanced laterally and then inferior to the coracoid process passing through the coracobrachialis and subscapularis muscles until the needle tip is advanced through the glenohumeral ligaments. One should be aware of the axillary sheath containing the axillary artery and vein in the region, this sheath maintains its greatest distance from the coracoid process with the patient's arm adducted to their side.

Box 21.8 Key Point

- The axillary sheath can be avoided during the anterior approach if the patient's arm is placed in adduction.

The thoracoacromial artery branches anteriorly off the axillary artery just above the coracoid process. The smaller acromial branch from the thoracoacromial artery travels laterally, superficial to the upper border of the glenohumeral joint. The needle tip should be kept lateral and inferior to the coracoid process to avoid this portion of the arterial branch. Furthermore, the brachial plexus travels adjacent to the axillary sheath at the level of the glenohumeral joint. This is commonly found approximately 5–6 cm medial and caudal to the

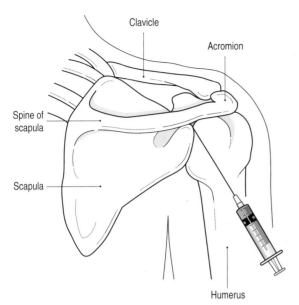

Figure 21.10 Glenohumeral joint injection. This diagram demonstrates the posterior approach.

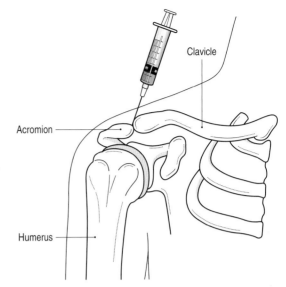

Figure 21.11 Acromioclavicular (AC) joint injection.

coracoid process. The musculocutaneous nerve exits the lateral cord at the level of the coracoid process closest to the anterior glenohumeral joint. The posterior approach to the gleno-humeral joint requires that the needle be placed approximately 3 cm below the posterior lateral angle of the acromion. The needle should be advanced anteromedially toward the cora-coid process (Fig. 21.10). One should be aware of the supra-scapular nerve and artery, which lie close to the injection site or typically medial to this injection approach.

Box 21.9 Key Point

- The suprascapular nerve and artery lie close to the entry point of the posterior injection approach.

Acromioclavicular joint

The acromioclavicular joint is located along the superior medi-al aspect of the shoulder complex. This joint is comprised of the distal portion of the clavicle and the acromion and is a small superficial, easily palpable joint. This joint is commonly injured when athletes fall directly on the shoulder, which often results in separations. The joint is injected with the patient either in the supine or sitting position. The examiner palpates along the distal portion of the clavicle until the end of clavicle can be palpated and the adjacent acromion noted. Following Betadine prep, a small gauge (25 or 27-gauge) needle is quickly and easily inserted into the joint from a superior approach (Fig. 21.11). Small volumes are usually injected of an anesthet-ic and/or corticosteroid mixture between 2 and 5 cc. One can inject this joint successfully by tapping the tip of the needle along the distal portion of the clavicle with a sudden 'give way' with gentle advancing pressure on the needle tip. If one keeps the needle tip at the edge of the distal clavicle and acromion, very little room for complication can occur.

Hip joint

The hip joint can be injected from either an anterior or lateral approach. The anterior approach poses more potential for injury because of significant neurovascular structures injury.[33] Gatter recommends inserting the needle at the intersection of a vertical line extending from the anterior superior iliac spine (ASIS) with a horizontal line even with the trochanter. He notes that the femoral artery is usually about two finger-breadths medial to this point. The needle is directed postero-medially toward the umbilicus, angled at 60° from the frontal plane. Others have recommended inserting the needle 2–3 cm lateral to the femoral artery pulse and 2–3 cm inferior to the ASIS and directing the needle 60° from the frontal plane.[34,35]

The femoral sheath is located just below the inguinal liga-ment and contains, from lateral to medial, the femoral artery, vein and lymph vessels. These vessels should pose minimal risk during hip injection if the femoral pulse is palpable as a land-mark. The only arteries and veins in close vicinity of the needle path are the superficial and deep circumflex iliac arteries and veins branching laterally from the femoral artery heading supe-riorly and laterally. Typically, these vessels are represented by small branches at a level 2 cm inferior to the ASIS. The femoral nerve is located just lateral to the femoral sheath. The main trunk of this large nerve usually is safe if the needle is inserted 2–3 cm lateral to the adjacent femoral artery. Two primary cutaneous nerves travel superficial to the anterior hip joint.

The lateral femoral cutaneous nerve (LFCN) of the thigh typically passes about 2–3 cm medial to the ASIS beneath the inguinal ligament and continues on an inferior slightly lateral course. Also at this point, the LFCN is usually divided into three or four branches. A needle placed into the hip joint at this level passes within 2–4 mm of the medial branches. A small femoral branch of the genitofemoral nerve lies superficially and directly above the anterior hip joint and can pass directly through the field of the injection.

For the lateral approach, the needle is inserted just anterior or posterior to the greater trochanter and advanced in a medial and slightly cephalad direction.[35,36] The needle passes through

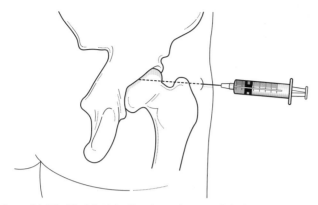

Figure 21.12 Hip joint injection. Lateral approach is demonstrated.

the iliotibial band and usually through the gluteus medius muscle before entering the thick iliofemoral ligament just superficially to the joint capsule (Fig. 21.12). The lateral approach to the hip joint places no significant vascular structures at risk. The superior gluteal nerve travels in a posterior/anterior direction across the deep surface of the gluteus medius and is located an average of 4.4 cm superior to a probe directed into the lateral hip joint described above.[37]

Box 21.10 Key Point

- The lateral approach to the hip joint places no significant vascular structures at risk.

Knee joint

The knee joint is the most commonly injected joint in the body. The approaches commonly used are the lateral or medial approach (Fig. 21.13). In both cases, the patient is placed in a supine position with a pillow or plinth placed under the knee joint with the knee in a flexed position. Betadine prep is utilized prior to the injection and typically 10–15 cc of volume is injected with a combination of corticosteroid and anesthetic.[38]

The lateral approach to the knee is quick and easy. This approach has been reported as being less reliable with low volumes because smaller volumes result in an intraarticular delivery less than half the time with a high incidence of soft tissue infiltration.[39] The knee is in slight flexion, approximately 10°, the patella is manually displaced laterally to enlarge the distance between the femur and the patella in this lateral position. Local anesthetic is usually applied and the needle is injected midway between the upper pole of the patella and the midbody of the patella lateral and inferior to the patella. The needle is advanced in an inferior medial trajectory. If aspiration is desired, the needle is advanced and one aspirates with the syringe. Furthermore, if aspiration is desired a large bore needle is placed such as an 18- or 20-gauge.

The medial approach is also felt to be quick and simple. The practitioner places slight lateral pressure on the patella subsequently increasing the space between the patella and the femur medially. The needle is injected at the level of the midportion of the patella just medial to the patella between the

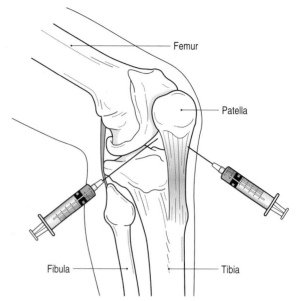

Figure 21.13 Knee joint injection. The medial and lateral approach is shown.

medial border of the patella and the femur. After the injection, an anesthetic is given to the skin. As described above, if aspiration is desired, a larger bore 18–20-gauge needle is advanced while aspirating with a syringe.

Ankle joint

The ankle can be injected at the medial tibiotalar, lateral tibiotalar (talofibular), or the subtalar articulation (Fig. 21.14).[35,36] The tibiotalar joint is injected from an anterior medial or anterior lateral approach, depending on the origin of pain and injury. The anterior medial approach involves needle insertion either just medial to the tibialis anterior tendon[35] or between the tibialis anterior (TA) and extensor hallucis longus (EHL) tendons.[36] The anterior tibial artery is typically located just lateral to the EHL tendon and then travels distally into the foot as the dorsalis pedis artery. Near the level of the tibiotalar joint, the medial

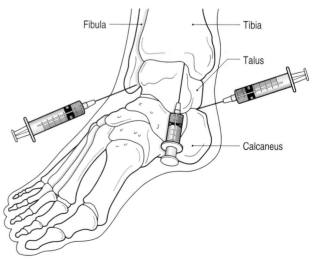

Figure 21.14 Ankle joint injection. Medial, lateral, and posterior sites for injection are demonstrated.

malleolar artery branches medially from the anterior tibial artery through the interval between the EHL and TA tendons. The great saphenous vein lies between the TA tendon and the medial malleolus, usually along the anterior edge of the anterior malleolus, and in some patients may make the approach just lateral to the TA tendon preferable. The deep peroneal nerve lies beside the anterior tibial artery and is often medial to the artery just lateral to the EHL tendon. The saphenous nerve is located immediately anterior and lateral to the saphenous vein and is best avoided by needle insertion just medial to the TA tendon.

The anterolateral approach to the tibiotalar joint involves needle entry just medial to the distal fibula and lateral to the digitorum extensor tendons.[36] The lateral anterior malleolar artery typically runs along the anterior medial aspect of the fibula at this level. The cutaneous branch of the superficial peroneal nerves traverse the anterior lateral ankle. At the level of the tibiotalar joint, the larger sensory branch of the superficial peroneal nerves is the medial dorsal cutaneus nerve, which lies about midway between the medial and lateral malleoli. The smaller branch, named the lateral dorsal cutaneus nerve, lies one third of the distance from the lateral to the medial malleolus and is more at risk from the anterolateral approach.[40]

The subtalar articulation accessible to injection is the posterior talocalcanean joint or facet, whereas the anterior medial calcanean facets are relatively inaccessible to injection.

The posterior subtalar joint is injected by inserting the needle midway between the anterior tip of the lateral malleolus and the Achilles tendon and progressing in the medial direction.[35,36] Immediately posterior to the lateral malleolus is a common tendon sheath containing the peroneus brevis and longus tendons, with the peroneus longus tendon most posterior and nearest the injection site. Deeper at the injection site lies the calcaneal fibular ligament connected at the posterior tip to the lateral malleolus to the calcaneus. The vascular structures in this region include the small branches of the lateral calcanean artery, a continuation of the peroneal artery. The small saphenous vein and its branches are usually slightly lateral to the injection site described above and located just posterior to the lateral malleolus. The small lateral calcaneal branch of the sural nerve lie adjacent and usually medial to the small saphenous venous network and may traverse the injection site.

SPINE INJECTIONS

Spinal injections are an important part of the treatment algorithm in the evaluation and management of spinal disorders in the athlete. When these injections are used in a judicious manner, they can eliminate a painful stimulus or confirm a working diagnosis. As noted above with other forms of injections, the athlete should be involved in an active rehabilitation program when the consideration of an injection is given.[41–46]

Box 21.11 Key Point

- Spinal injections are an important part in the treatment algorithm in the management of the athlete with spinal pain.

Preparation for a spinal injection

Specialized training is required to become proficient in spinal injections. The physician who performs these injections should be confident in radiographic, surface and spinal anatomy, well versed in the treatment of spinal disorders, educated on proper patient selection and be able to recognize and treat any complications that may arise from the procedure. A procedure room should be properly staffed with experienced assistants and have equipment available for patient monitoring and resuscitation. The spinal injection suite should also contain high quality fluoroscopy. The use of fluoroscopy allows the physician to accurately place the needle tip into the desired target location which can then be confirmed with contrast dye.

Box 21.12 Key Point

- The use of fluoroscopy is essential in proper needle placement.

Patient selection

As noted earlier in this chapter, injections should be performed within the framework of broader rehabilitation goals. A sport specific exercise program should be incorporated within the treatment algorithm and every opportunity to improve without injections should be encouraged. When an injection is contemplated, X-rays and imaging studies should be performed to eliminate the possibility of the unexpected fracture, infection, or tumor. Advanced imaging studies such as MRI, can be used, along with the physical examination, to determine what specific type and location the injection should be performed. For example, the middle-aged softball player who reports a twisting injury and presents with unilateral right sided lumbar pain that extends into the buttock and proximal posterior thigh appears to have injured his right sided lumbar facet joints. On physical examination the patient's pain is reproduced with manual palpation along the right-sided lumbar paraspinals and the pain is aggravated with extension and twisting maneuvers. In addition, the neurological exam remains normal. This clinical presentation suggests the lumbar facet joints as the primary pain generator. In this case, lumbar facet injections would be the procedure of choice. If however, MRI reveals a L5–S1 herniated disc, a lumbar epidural steroid injection may be indicated. Combined injections may become necessary if the earlier selected location is unsuccessful.[47,48] The spine can be divided into three sections: anterior (intervertebral disc and vertebral body), neuroaxial (neural structures and epidural space) and posterior (zygapophyseal (z or facet) joints). Injections into the epidural space are typically used to treat disorders within the anterior or neuroaxial compartments, while injections directed into the spinal facet joints are used to treat disorders of the posterior compartment.

Epidural injections

Injections into the epidural space can be performed from a midline, paramedian, transforaminal, or caudal approach. The specific approach to the epidural space is usually dependent on the underlying spinal pathology or the physician's preference.

Midline epidural approach

A midline epidural approach is normally used for primary discogenic pain. This technique has been used for decades for spine pain and continues to be in common use.

This procedure is performed with the patient in the prone position. The spinous processes of the vertebral body of the vertebrae above and below the affected disc level is marked on the skin under fluoroscopy. In addition, the inferior border of the lamina of the most cephalad vertebrae and the superior border of the lamina of the most caudad vertebrae are also marked on the skin. The skin is scrubbed with Betadine and 3–5 cc of 1% lidocaine are used to anesthetize the skin, subcutaneous tissue, and interspinous ligaments. Once proper anesthesia is obtained, an 18-gauge Tuohy needle is advanced through the interspinous ligament using the loss of resistance technique (Fig. 21.15). A small skin puncture can be made with an 18-gauge needle for the anticipated entry point for the Tuohy needle. Once the 18-gauge Tuohy needle has penetrated the ligamentum flavum the epidural space will be entered. It is helpful to check lateral views under fluoroscopy to monitor depth of penetration especially in larger patients. One should be cautious to avoid aggressive advancement of the needle to avoid penetration of the dural sac. Contrast is injected under fluoroscopy to confirm proper epidural spread and to avoid vascular uptake. A test dose of lidocaine with epinephrine may also be given and the patient monitored for changes in heart rate and blood pressure. Once confirmation is definitively determined, a solution of corticosteroid and anesthetic can be injected.

Paramedian epidural approach

Similar to the midline approach, the paramedian approach utilizes loss of resistance technique. Landmarks are identified as noted above including the spinous processes and lamina that border the discs that are the purported pain generator. Utilizing

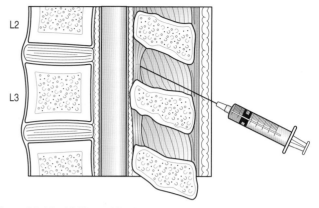

Figure 21.15 Midline epidural injection. The needle tip is located in the interspinous ligament and adjacent to the ligamentum flavum.

an 18-gauge Tuohy needle, the needle entry point is lateral to midline outside the interspinous ligaments through the paraspinal muscles. The Tuohy needle is advanced to the upper edge of the lamina in the most inferior marked vertebrae. The tip of the Tuohy needle is felt to tap the lamina and slowly 'walked off' in a cephalad direction until entering the ligamentum flavum (Fig. 21.16). Once again, the needle is slowly advanced into the epidural space and when one senses loss of resistance the epidural space has been entered. Aggressive advancement of the needle tip may risk dural puncture. Proper needle localization can be identified with contrast. Corticosteroid and anesthetic solution can then be injected.

Transforaminal epidural approaches

Perhaps the most difficult of the epidural approaches is that of the transforaminal injection. This requires proper needle trajectory and depth of needle placement under fluoroscopic

Figure 21.16 Paramedian epidural injection. This AP radiograph (A) demonstrates a typical contrast dye pattern following a paramedian lumbar epidural injection. The needle tip is located in the epidural space. (B) Lateral X-ray demonstrating contrast in the epidural space. (With permission from Woodward, J, Herring, S, Windsor, RE. Epidural procedures in spine pain management. In: Pain procedures in clinical practice. Lennard T, ed. Philadelphia: Hanley & Belfus; 2000 and courtesy of Paul H Dreyfuss, MD.)

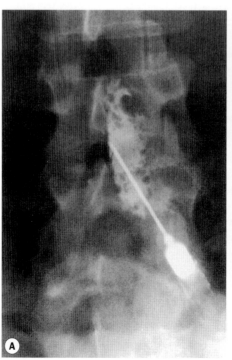

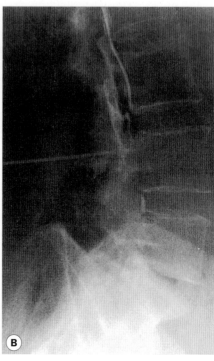

guidance. The foramen to be injected based on the probability of specific radicular symptoms is correlated with imaging studies. In the case of lumbar foraminal injections, the superior and inferior transverse process above and below the foramen and the lateral portion of the lamina are identified and marked on the skin. In the lower lumbosacral level, the upper margins of the sacrum are identified. For example, when one is to perform a L5 transforaminal epidural injection, the L5 transverse process, upper border of the sacrum, and the lateral lamina of the L5 vertebrae are identified and marked on the skin. The area is scrubbed with Betadine and the patient is dressed in the routine sterile fashion. A total of 3–5 cc of 1% lidocaine can be used to anesthetize the skin and subcutaneous tissue, fascia, and paraspinal muscles. Once proper anesthesia is obtained, a 22-gauge spinal needle (some physicians prefer other needle sizes) is inserted inferior to the L5 transverse process and slowly advanced in a superior medial trajectory just inferior to the pedicle. It may take several adjustments of the needle tip under fluoroscopy prior to proper needle placement. Contrast is injected, and with proper needle placement, can be seen to flow under the pedicle and into the epidural space (Fig. 21.17).

Once needle placement is confirmed, a solution of 3–5 cc of a corticosteroid and anesthetic mixture can be injected. This same technique can be utilized at other spinal levels despite changes in the regional anatomy. In the case of an S1 transforaminal injection, the S1 foramen is the target site.

Caudal epidural approach

The use of caudal epidural steroid injections is limited to those patients with lower lumbosacral disc disease. This approach has less risk of dural puncture since the dural sac typically terminates at the second sacral segment.

Box 21.13 Key Point

- Caudal epidurals are limited to patients with lower lumbo-sacral pain.

Landmarks for a caudal injection include the sacral hiatus and sacral cornu. These structures can be palpated with the patient in the prone position. Large individuals will require extra tactile pressure in this region to localize these landmarks. It helps if the patient internally rotates both hips to aid in the relaxation of the buttock muscles. Once located a sterile prep is performed and the skin is anesthetized with 1% lidocaine. A 22-gauge, 3.5 in spinal needle can then be inserted into the sacral hiatus. The initial needle entry point is positioned at a 30° angle to the sacrum and once the needle tip penetrates the hiatus, the needle is lowered and advanced parallel to the sacrum. The tip of the needle can be advanced about 2 cm, when the epidural space is commonly encountered. Contrast dye is injected to confirm needle placement which creates a typical 'Christmas tree' pattern that outlines the lower sacral nerve roots (Fig. 21.18).

Contrast is also used to avoid injection into vascular structures. A corticosteroid and lidocaine solution is then injected in volumes ranging from 10–20 cc. Some physicians prefer the use of sterile water rather than large volumes of anesthetic. During the injection, patients may feel pressure in their sacrum

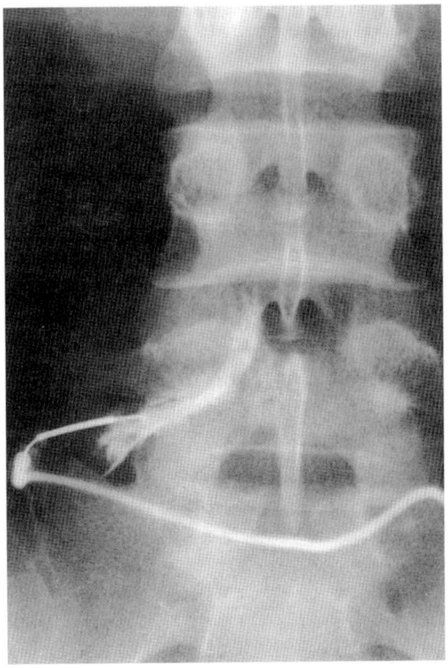

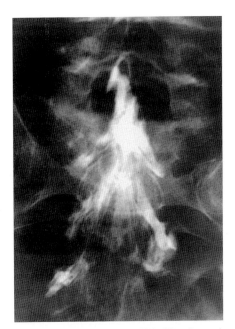

Figure 21.17 Transforaminal epidural injection. This AP radiograph demonstrates contrast dye adjacent to the L5 nerve root. The thin radiopaque structure that crosses the midline is tubing attached to the needle. (With permission from Woodward J, Herring S, Windsor RE. Epidural procedures in spine pain management. In: Pain procedures in clinical practice. Lennard T, ed. Philadelphia: Hanley & Belfus; 2000.)

Figure 21.18 Caudal epidural injection. This AP radiograph demonstrates a typical 'Christmas tree' pattern of contrast dye. Note the needle tip in the mid-lower portion of the radiograph. (With permission from Woodward J, Herring S, Windsor RE. Epidural procedures in spine pain management. In: Pain procedures in clinical practice. Lennard T, ed. Philadelphia: Hanley & Belfus; 2000.)

and buttocks region and at times tingling into the lower extremities.

Facet joint injections

Facet joint injections can be performed in the cervical, thoracic or lumbar regions and are considered the gold standard in diagnostic evaluation for posterior element pain.[49] The facet joint nerve (medial branch of the posterior ramus) can be temporarily anesthetized (medial branch block or MBB) or solution can be placed within the joint (intraarticular or IA). The diagnostic MBB is often performed as a prelude to a medial branch rhizotomy. These techniques are well described in the literature.[3–5] The intraarticular approach can be performed for diagnostic and therapeutic reasons.

Box 21.14 Key Point

- Facet injections are the gold standard for the diagnosis of posterior element pain.

Intraarticular lumbar facet joint injection

Intraarticular facet injections are commonly performed throughout the spinal axis. Variation in regional anatomy within the cervical, thoracic, or lumbar spine requires minor adjustments in technique and awareness of potential complications. IA facet injections require fluoroscopy to visualize each joint prior to injection. In general, these procedures are technically easy to perform in comparison to epidural injections, but can be time consuming, especially when multiple joints are to be injected. In the lumbar spine, these joints are best visualized with the patient in a prone-oblique position. Using fluoroscopy, the target joints are identified and marked on the skin. At times, the position of either the patient or C-arm fluoro unit must be adjusted to locate the joint. If the L5–S1 joint is targeted, an oblique approach may be difficult due to the height of the iliac crest and therefore a direct posterior approach may be required. The patient is scrubbed with Betadine and dressed in the routine sterile fashion and 3–5 cc of 1% lidocaine are used to anesthetize the skin, subcutaneous tissue, fascia, and muscle overlying the injection target. Using a 22- or 25-gauge 3.5 in spinal needle and fluoroscopic guidance, the needle is slowly advanced to the joint. The needle tip can be felt to tap the adjacent articulating process as a sudden 'give way' is felt as the joint is penetrated. This can be confirmed under fluoroscopy and with the injection of contrast dye (Fig. 21.19). The contrast can be aspirated and 0.5–2 cc of corticosteroid-anesthetic solution injected.

Sacroiliac joint injection

Intraarticular sacroiliac (SI) joint injections are technically easy to perform with fluoroscopic guidance. The patient is placed in the prone position and under fluoroscopy, the lower third of the sacroiliac joint is identified and marked on the skin. The patient is scrubbed with Betadine and dressed in a routine sterile fashion. The skin and subcutaneous tissue are anesthetized

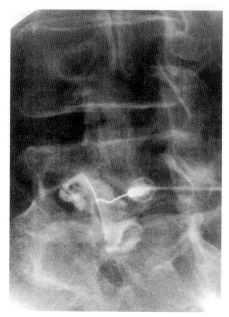

Figure 21.19 Intraarticular facet injection. This oblique radiograph demonstrates contrast dye in the L5–S1 facet joint. The superior and inferior capsular recesses are demonstrated. (With permission from Dreyfuss P, Kaplan M, Dreyer S. Zygapophyseal joint injection techniques in the spinal axis. In: Pain procedures in clinical practice. Lennard T, ed. Philadelphia: Hanley & Belfus; 2000.)

with 3–5 cc of 1% lidocaine. Once proper anesthesia is obtained, a 22- or 25-gauge 3.5 in spinal needle can be slowly inserted into the lower portion of the joint. Slight changes in the needle trajectory are often required under fluoroscopy. As the needle advances, the tip usually taps the joint margin and can be felt to 'walk off' into the joint. This can be visualized under fluoroscopy which makes this technique quite simple (Fig. 21.20). Contrast can reconfirm needle placement within the joint. A solution of corticosteroid and anesthetic can then be injected.

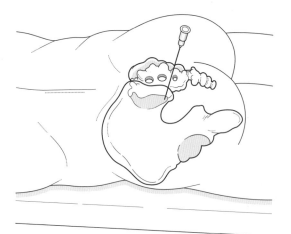

Figure 21.20 Sacroiliac joint injection. This diagram depicts the needle entry point into the lower portion of the sacroiliac joint. (Redrawn with permission from Fortin J, Sehgal N. Sacroiliac joint injection and arthrography with imaging correlation. In: Pain procedures in clinical practice. Lennard T, ed. Philadelphia: Hanley & Belfus; 2000.)

Box 21.15 Key Point

- The entry point for a sacroiliac joint injection is in the lower third of the joint.

the sports medicine physician to become experienced with soft tissue and joint injections as described in this chapter. A solid understanding of the benefits and pitfalls of spinal injections is also helpful when determining which athletes need procedures. Injections clearly expand one's treatment options and ultimately improve outcomes.

CONCLUSIONS

The athlete in pain can be treated successfully with injections when used within a broader scope of rehabilitation. It behoves

REFERENCES

1 Arroll B, Goodyear-Smith F. Corticosteroid injections for painful shoulder: a meta-analysis. Br J Gen Pr 2005; 55:224.

2 Baldry P. Management of myofascial trigger point pain. Acupunct Med 2000; 20:2–10.

3 Fenton DS, Czervionke LF. Image-guided spine intervention. Philadelphia: Saunders; 2002.

4 Lennard TA. Pain procedures in clinical practice. Philadelphia: Hanley & Belfus; 2000.

5 Renfrew DL. Atlas of spine injections. Philadelphia: Saunders; 2003.

6 Boyer MI, Hastings H. Lateral tennis elbow: 'Is there any science out there?' J Shoulder Elbow Surg 1999; 8:481–491.

7 Whaley AL, Baker CL. Lateral epicondylitis. Clin Sports Med 2004; 23:677–691.

8 Newcomer KL, Laskowski ER, Idank DM, McLean TJ, Egan KS. Corticosteroid injection in early treatment of lateral epicondylitis. Clin J Sport Med 2001; 11:214.

9 Thumboo J, O'Duffy JD. A prospective study of the safety of joint and soft tissue aspirations and injections in patients taking warfarin sodium. Arthritis Rheum 1998; 41:736.

10 Unglaub F, Guehring T, Fuchs PC, et al. Necrotizing fasciitis following therapeutic injection in a shoulder joint. Orthopaedics 2005; 34:250.

11 Hofmeister E, Engelhardt S. Necrotizing fasciitis as complication of injection into greater trochanteric bursa. Am J Orthop 2001; 30:426.

12 Hugate R, Pennypacker J, Saunders M, et al. The effects of intratendinous and retrocalcaneal intrabursal injections of corticosteroid on the biomechanical properties of rabbit Achilles tendons. J Bone Jt Surg Am 2004; 86:794–801.

13 Dagenais S, Haldeman S, Wooley JR. Intraligamentous injection of sclerosing solutions (prolotherapy) for spinal pain: a critical review of the literature. Spine J 2005; 5:310–328.

14 Celeste C, Ionescu M, Robin Poole A, et al. Repeated intraarticular injections of triamcinolone acetonide alter cartilage matrix metabolism measured by biomarkers in synovial fluid. J Orthop Res 2005; 23:602.

15 Cole BJ, Schumacher HR Jr. Injectable corticosteroids in modern practice. J Am Acad Orthop Surg 2005; 13:37–46.

16 Lennard TA. Fundamentals of procedural care. In: Lennard TA, ed. Physiatric procedures in clinical practice. Philadelphia: Hanley & Belfus; 1995:5–6.

17 Olin BR. Adrenal cortical steroids. In: Olin BR, ed. Drug facts and comparisons. St Louis: Facts & Comparisons; 1993:465–466.

18 Covino BG. Clinical pharmacology of local anesthetic agents. In: Cousins MJ, Bridenbaugh PO, eds. Neural blockade in clinical anesthesia and management of pain. 2nd edn. Philadelphia: Lippincott; 1988:111–144.

19 Olin BR. Local anesthetics. In: Olin BR, ed. Drug facts and comparisons. St Louis: Facts & Comparisons; 1993:2654–2665.

20 Fisher AA. Trigger point injection. In: Lennard TA, ed. Physiatric procedures in clinical practice. Philadelphia: Handley and Belfus; 1995:28–35.

21 Travell JG, Simons DJ. Myofascial pain and dysfunction: The Trigger Point Manual. Baltimore: Williams & Wilkins; 1983.

22 Wheeler AH. Myofascial pain disorders: theory to therapy. Drugs 2004; 64:45–62.

23 Garvey TA, Marx MR, Wiesel SW. Perspective randomized double blind evaluation of trigger point injection therapy for back pain. Spine 1989; 14:962–964.

24 Ingber RS. Shoulder impingement in tennis/racquetball players treated with subscapularis myofascial treatments. Arch Phys Med Rehabil 2000; 81:679–682.

25 Iwama H, Akama Y. The superiority of water-diluted 0.25% to near 1% lidocaine for trigger-point injections in myofascial pain syndrome: a prospective, randomized, double-blinded trial. Anesth Analg 2000; 91:408.

26 Iwama H, Ohmori S, Kaneko T, Watanabe K. Water-diluted local anesthetic for trigger-point injection in chronic myofascial pain syndrome: evaluation of types of local anesthetic and concentrations in water. Reg Anesth Pain Med 2001; 26:333–336.

27 Hong CZ, Hsueh TC. Difference in pain relief after trigger point injections in myofascial pain patients with and without fibromyalgia. Arch Phys Med Rehabil 1996; 77:1161.

28 Cohen SP, Narvaez JC, Lebovits AH, et al. Corticosteroid injections for trochanteric bursitis: is fluoroscopy necessary? A pilot study. Br J Anaesth 2005; 94:100.

29 Matthews PV, Glusman RE. Accuracy of subacromial injection: anterolateral versus posterior approach. J Shoulder Elbow Surg 2005; 14:145–148.

30 Koh WL, Kwek JW, Quek ST, Peh WC. Clinics in diagnostic imaging. Pes anserine bursitis. Singapore Med J 2002; 43:485–491.

31 Buchbinder R, Green S, Youd JM. Corticosteroid injections for shoulder pain. Cochrane Database Syst Rev 2003; 1:CD004016.

32 Micheo WF, Rodriguez RA, Amy E. Joint and soft tissue injections of the upper extremity. Phys Med Rehab Clin North Am 1995; 6:823–840.

33 Gatter RA. Arthrocentesis technique and intrasynovial therapy. In: McCarty DJ, ed. Arthritis and allied conditions, a text book of rheumatology. Philadelphia: Lea and Fibiger; 1989:646–656.

34 Resnick D. Arthrography, tenography, bursography. In: Resnick D, Niwayma G, eds. Diagnosis of bone and joint disorders. Philadelphia: Saunders; 1988:302–440.

35 Millard RS, Dillingham MF. Peripheral joint injections: lower extremity. Phys Med Rehab Clin North Am 1995; 6:841–849.

36 Obermiller JP, Locks MD. Peripheral joint injections. In: Lennard TA, ed. Physiatric procedures in clinical practice. Philadelphia: Handley and Belfus; 1995:14–27.

37 Byrd JW, Pappas JN, Pedley MJ. Hip arthroscopy: An anatomic study of portal placement in relationship to the extraarticular structures. Arthroscopy 1995; 11:418–423.

38 Bellamy N, Campbell J, Robinson V, et al. Intraarticular corticosteroid for treatment of osteoarthritis of the knee. Cochrane Database Syst Rev 2005; 2:CD005328.

39 Wind WM Jr, Smolinski RJ. Reliability of common knee injection sites with low-volume injections. J Arthroplasty 2004; 19:858–861.

40 Blaire JM, Botte MJ. Surgical anatomy of the superficial peroneal nerve of the ankle and foot. Clin Orthop Relat Res 1994; 305:229–238.

41 Tong HC, Williams JC, Haig AJ, et al. Predicting outcomes of transforaminal epidural injections for sciatica. Spine J 2004; 4:605–606.

42 Weinstein SM, Herring SA. Lumbar epidural steroid injections. Spine J 2003; 3:37–44.

43 Vad VB, Bhal AL, Lutz Ge, et al. Transforaminal epidural steroid injections in lumbosacral radiculopathy: a prospective randomized study. Spine 2002; 27:11–6.

44 Papagelopoulos PJ, Petrou HG, Triantafyllidis PG, et al. Treatment of lumbosacral radicular pain with epidural steroid injections. Orthopedics 2001; 24:145.

45 Lutz GE, Vad VB, Wisneski RJ. Fluoroscopic transforaminal lumbar epidural steroids: an outcome study. Arch Phys Med Rehabil 1998; 79:1362.

46 Botwin KP, Gruber RD, Bouchlas CG, et al. Fluoroscopically guided lumbar transforaminal epidural steroid injections in degenerative lumbar stenosis: an outcome study. Am J Phys Med Rehabil 2002; 81:898–905.

47 Butterman GR. Lumbar disc herniation regression after successful epidural steroid injection. J Spinal Discord Tech 2002; 15:469–476.

48 Michel JL, Lemaire S, Bourbon H, et al. Fluoroscopy guided L5-S1 transforaminal injection as a treatment for S1 radiculopathy. J Radiol 2004; 85:1937–1941.

49 Bogduk N. International Spinal Injection Society guidelines for the performance of spinal injection procedures. Part I: Zygapophysial joint blocks. Clin J Pain 1997; 13:285–302.

CHAPTER 22

Orthotic Devices for Injury Prevention and Rehabilitation

Karl B. Fields and Katherine M. Walker

INTRODUCTION

Shoe inserts are one type of orthotic device designed to correct skeletal abnormalities, provide cushioning, correct gait abnormalities, stimulate sensory feedback and decrease injury rates.[1-5] Over the past five decades orthotic devices have become part of the treatment of multiple diagnoses including plantar fasciitis, Achilles tendonitis, patello-femoral disorders, metatarsalgia and 'shin splints'.[1,6-8] In addition, orthotic devices often are prescribed for individuals with specific skeletal abnormalities including leg length inequality, cavus feet, Morton's foot and pes planus. The typical gait problems modified by orthotic use include excessive pronation, excessive supination and forefoot varus.

Box 22.1: Key Points

Orthotic devices

Orthotic devices are shoe inserts designed to:

- correct skeletal abnormalities
- provide cushioning
- correct gait abnormalities
- stimulate sensory feedback
- decrease injury rates.

Physicians utilize many different types of orthotic devices including 'off the shelf' brands and custom made inserts molded from the patient's foot. Numerous techniques and materials exist for the manufacture of custom orthoses. Currently, no randomized controlled trials demonstrate an unequivocal benefit of orthotic devices. Blinding patients to the use of orthotic devices poses logical difficulties. Some studies seek to compare 'off the shelf' *versus* custom-made products or products using different materials. However, the literature remains of limited value since even these studies cannot control for the marked differences in the types of devices used. Nonetheless, a number

of studies show a high degree of patient satisfaction with the devices.[6-8] The authors reviewed 100 patients with 1–3 years of usage and found that 90% continued wearing prescribed custom-made full-length orthotic devices. Of these, 50% found complete relief from the diagnosed condition; 25% significant improvement; 15% felt more comfortable in them even though the original problem had not responded; and 10% found they were not helpful. These response rates are similar to those reported by others.

Traditionally, orthotic devices were thought to work by changing skeletal alignment, however, recent research questions this theory. Some studies show patient improvement with orthotic devices despite minimal change in the biomechanical problems suspected of causing the injury. Kannus described the classical theory of prescribing orthotics:

> 'In treatment of athletes' overuse injuries it should be kept in mind that custom-made, expensive orthotics should not be prescribed for overuse symptoms without obvious malalignment, for asymptomatic athletes with a malalignment, or for symptoms in which a causal relationship between the biomechanical abnormality and symptoms is difficult to see.'[9]

To illustrate the point made by Kannus, an individual with pes planus would not necessarily need orthotic devices unless the history and physical exam suggests that the flat feet contribute to a physical symptom that could be improved by mechanical correction. This was a departure from earlier clinical thinking that suggested that anatomical changes alone, such as pes planus, were sufficient to predict injury. During the Second World War, the US military considered the diagnosis of pes planus a sufficient risk marker to merit disqualification from active duty. Studies by Ifeld and others discovered that more than 15% of the military population had asymptomatic flat feet.[10,11] In addition, during the 1930s, military physicians like Ifeld and Bingham began to note higher rates of foot and lower extremity injury in soldiers with cavus feet *versus* flat feet.[11,12] More recent studies indicate limited risks for pes planus but substantial increased injury rates for pes cavus. Cowan found a relative risk of 6.1 for lower extremity injury in individuals having a navicular soft tissue arch height >3.15 cm (highest 20% of individuals.) Other authors found an association of cavus feet with recurrent stress fractures and with patello-femoral syndrome.[10,13] While pes planus may not be enough of an anatomical problem to merit treatment for all affected individuals with orthotics, perhaps the same will not hold true with pes cavus. Additional research is needed to define the magnitude and type of static anatomical and dynamic biomechanical problems that may pose a risk for injury. Since orthotic devices also seem to work well in individuals without obvious anatomical or biomechanical problems, newer theories have emerged to help explain the beneficial effect of the devices.[2–3]

Nigg's research[2] shows differences in muscular work when individuals wear orthotic devices. Changing the sequence of muscle firing or reducing the workload of individual muscle groups has the potential of changing injury risk through modulating both the impact and the pattern of stress throughout the lower extremity. In addition, coupling anatomical changes with gait analysis to see if the anatomy affects the function may be more beneficial than relying on static examination. Individuals make significant form compensations for anatomical variations that may effectively reduce the risk that the anatomical change would imply. Gait analysis demonstrates whether a given abnormality translates to a specific breakdown of form that would affect injury risk.

PHYSICAL EXAMINATION

Box 22.2: Key Points

Physical examination

Inspection

- calluses
- Morton's foot (longer 2nd metatarsal)
- cavus foot
- leg length inequalities
- forefoot varus and valgus
- first metatarsal insufficiency

Gait analysis

- symmetry of motion
- pronation or supination
- foot strike and orientation
- body position
- limb swing patterns.

Physical examination of the foot should begin with inspection. A normal foot bears approximately 50% of weight at the heel, 35% at the first metatarsophalangeal (MTP) joint and 15% at the 5th MTP joint. Typically, skin calluses should not occur under other metatarsal heads, as they are a part of the transverse arch. Skin callous patterns provide clues as to where the patient's foot has broken down and to the location of excessive plantar surface pressure.

A Morton's foot (2nd metatarsal longer than 1st metatarsal) is particularly noteworthy because of its long-term association with injuries such as metatarsalgia and Morton's neuroma. Two distinct patterns often get labeled as Morton's foot. The first

actually results from a first metatarsal significantly shorter than the second metatarsal. This pattern more correctly described as first metatarsal insufficiency affects the ability of the great toe and first metatarsal to act as a counter to prevent excessive pronation in the toe-off phase of the gait cycle. This has the potential to lead to stresses that cause hallux valgus (bunion) formation or midfoot and longitudinal arch breakdown. Oftentimes, the first metatarsal-cuneiform joint is hypermobile as well. A second pattern, the classic Morton's foot, consists of long thin metatarsals in which the second metatarsal is longer than a normal length first metatarsal. This foot type is at risk for Morton's callous (thick callousing under second metatarsal head), metatarsalgia, stress fracture and Morton's neuroma. The thin first metatarsal recruits the second metatarsal for more effective function during the toe-off phase of gait (Figs 22.1, 22.2).

A second foot type that has a strong association with injury is the cavus foot deformity. A cavus foot can be measured using a bony arch index, a ratio of the navicular height to foot length measured from the heel to the first metatarsal phalangeal joint.[10] A high ratio indicates a cavus foot. Another measure of cavus change is the distance from the floor to the soft tissue arch height of the navicular. The examiner palpates the surface anatomy of the navicular prominence and measures at this level. Arch height in this location greater than 3 cm suggest cavus deformity (Fig. 22.3). In cavus feet, the relative weight bearing shifts forward to the forefoot. Since form follows function, the examiner typically sees a broad forefoot and a narrow heel. More narrow heels may also point to extreme restriction of dorsiflexion of the foot and a shortened Achilles tendon as the heel rarely strikes the ground in these 'toe runners'. Excessive transverse width at the forefoot identifies strong impact to this region and increases the likelihood of specific forefoot injuries such as hallux rigidus, bunionettes (5th MTP varus subluxation) and sesamoid stress fractures. While clinical studies have not established standard anthropomorphic measures for the foot, the author's clinical experience suggests that ratios of forefoot width (measured at the 1st and 5th MTPs) to heel width at the mid-portion of the calcaneus typically average 1.6 to 1 or less. Width ratios >1.8:1 have strong association with forefoot breakdown in our clinics.

Leg length inequalities are usually evaluated by measuring the distance between the anterior superior iliac spine and the

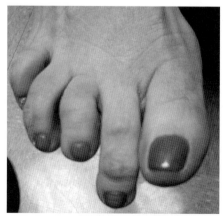

Figure 22.1 Morton's toe.

toe being elevated. Measurements can be done standing or in the non-weight bearing position. For the supine patient, the examiner places the calcaneus in the sub-talar neutral position and the angle between the 1st and 5th metatarsals is measured. For extreme forefoot varus, when the patient lies prone with knees flexed at 90° the examiner cannot return the foot to a neutral position.

Gait analysis is needed to assess pronated or supinated foot strike. However, the examiner can estimate static degrees of pronation/supination by observing patients standing and then flexing their knees to 45 degrees while their feet are flat on the ground. The pronated foot causes the medial malleoli to move inward and downward during knee flexion, whereas little change occurs in a supinated foot. On observation, an excessively pronated foot will show malalignment of the midfoot making it more prominent than the medial malleolus. Pronation beginning at the rear foot also shows calcaneal valgus on inspection from the rear (Figs 22.4, 22.5). Walking and running gait either demonstrates an exaggeration of the static observation or will show that the athlete can compensate for the static anatomy with form changes. This gives the examiner a better idea of the dynamic function of the feet. Asymmetry of foot strike ('toeing-in or toeing-out'), unequal knee lift, upper body lean, a limp or an unbalanced arm swing are findings that merit analysis to understand why the gait pattern is altered. Comparison of the gait analysis to the wear pattern of the athlete's shoes often helps confirm impression of form change and excessive pressure patterns at foot strike.

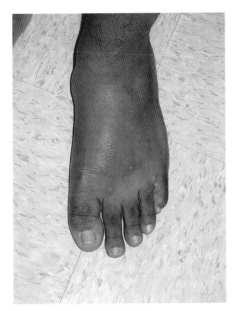

Figure 22.2 Metatarsal insufficiency. (It is the authors' experience that individuals with first metatarsal insufficiency often have a ratio of the length of the 2nd metatarsal to the 1st metatarsal of 1.6:1 or greater).

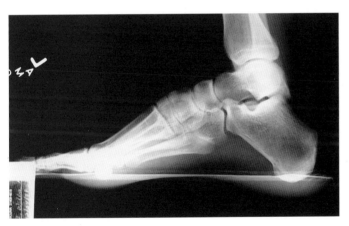

Figure 22.3 X-ray extreme cavus foot.

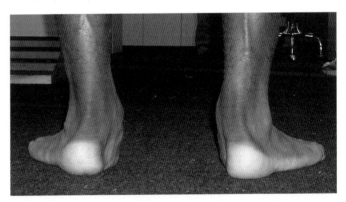

Figure 22.4 Calcaneal valgus.

medial malleolus. The examiner measures the individual lying and sitting. An apparent leg length difference that reverses from lying to sitting may indicate a pelvic rotation or fixed sacroiliac joint. When questions arise, a standing evaluation allows the examiner to compare relative heights of the iliac crests; length from the umbilicus to each medial malleolus and other confirmatory maneuvers to evaluate leg length inequality. Another examination method is to place blocks of wood with different widths underneath the suspected shorter leg. Once the width of the block exceeds the leg length inequality, the patient starts to feel the lift. When problematic, differences >5 mm should be measured via standing AP radiograph that include the lower extremities and pelvis.

Forefoot varus and forefoot valgus can be measured standing by placing the patient in a subtalar neutral position. If the great toe is elevated off the ground, the forefoot is in some degree of varus. Forefoot valgus is indicated by the 5th

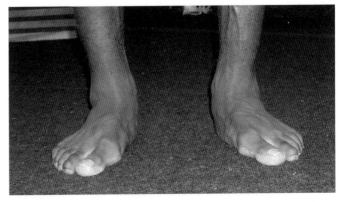

Figure 22.5 Pronated foot with pes planus.

Evaluation of the remainder of the lower extremity and foot and ankle flexibility are also important in the examination. Full range of motion at each joint allows the individual to have a balanced gait pattern. For example, when individuals return to running after piriformis syndrome or any injury to the external rotators of the hip, a decrease in internal rotation triggered by some contracture of the hip rotators often occurs. The corresponding gait observation may be external rotation ('toeing-out') of the foot on the affected side. Similarly, an iliopsoas strain may leave residual weakness and contracture of the hip flexors. The corresponding gait change likely would be uneven lift of the knees. Knee examination looks for genu varum/valgum as this correlates with changes in foot strike or gait and dictates changes in the preparation of the orthotic.

TYPES OF ORTHOTIC DEVICES/FABRICATION

Box 22.3: Key Points

General types of orthotic shoe inserts

Three primary types

- *Rigid*: typically used in industrial settings and for post surgery correction
- *Semi-rigid*: most commonly used by athletes
- *Soft*: most commonly used for neurological injury (i.e. diabetic patients).

There are three main types of orthotic devices: rigid, semi-rigid and soft. Rigid orthotic devices are made of acrylic plastics and thermoplastic polymers which makes them more durable and supportive. While some athletes prefer these, they find most usage in industrial settings and for individuals who need correction post surgery. Soft orthotic devices are commonly composed of polyethylene foams and provide cushion, flexibility and the most padding. Soft orthotic devices are beneficial for those patients with neurological injury that decreases the normal sensation of the feet. Diabetics frequently use these in combination with high volume shoes. They also help athletes recovering from stress fractures, surgery and other injuries in which the need for the orthotic is felt to be temporary and not permanent. For example, runners with plantar fasciitis who seem to have developed the injury from overtraining as opposed to other possible causes may use these until symptoms resolve.

Semi-rigid orthotic devices are the type used most commonly by athletes and are sometimes marketed under the term 'athletic orthotics'. These inserts have cushioned upper surfaces made of leather, urethanes, ethyl vinyl acetate polymers, high-density rubber compounds and similar materials. Their interior has a thermolabile plastic that becomes moldable when heated and gives enough support to maintain the correction applied for the athlete. Styrofoam, plastic and cork bases stabilize the base and provide protection of the upper materials from impact and wear and tear. The combination of padding and support provide both theoretical benefits that orthotic devices accomplish: impact protection and biomechanical correction.[1]

Once the material is selected, there are various mechanisms for custom molding the orthotic. Plaster-cast molds sent to an orthotic fabrication laboratory have been the most common method employed in past years. These have lost popularity to newer processes such as standing impressions of the feet with a crushable foam box or a similar technique using wax impressions. Newer technology includes CAD/CAM (Computer-Aided Design/Computer-Aided Manufacture) in which a digitalized foot pressure pattern drives the formation of the orthotic.[1,14] The authors use a system where patients stand in a semi weight bearing position on heated orthotic blanks. The base employs cushions with memory foam so that once the individual is correctly positioned the orthotic molds into the desired shape. Regardless of the fabrication method, the patients' feet are placed in the subtalar neutral position. This position aligns the foot, ankle and lower extremity and is believed to be the most efficient for running and walking. Removing anatomical rotations and malalignments puts less stress on the surrounding ligaments, tendons and muscles.[1,8]

Subtalar position is found by placing one's thumb and forefinger on the talus, while pronating and supinating the foot. If the foot is hyperpronated, the talus will be more prominent on the medial side and with supination, the talus will be felt more on the lateral side. The subtalar neutral position is when the talus is felt equally on both sides. Corresponding physical findings include a vertical Achilles tendon and a level tibiotalar articulation. Since the subtalar joint is not palpable, these techniques at best approximate true subtalar neutral position but have been correlated by X-ray imaging.

With the plaster casting technique, the foot is held in the subtalar neutral position and the cast is formed. Once it has hardened, a positive mold can be made from the negative mold and the orthotic constructed from this positive mold.[8] Positive molds can also be generated from foam or wax impression boxes. The CAD/CAM method cuts down on the storage space of the plaster casts or box molds and uses a digitized computer image of the foot to manufacture the orthotic.[1,14]

With the weight bearing method, using crushable foam pillows, the orthotic blank is heated in a convection oven and then placed under the patients' feet. An orthotic stand allows positioning of the patient in semi weight bearing at 10–15° of knee flexion and 5–10° of ankle dorsiflexion. (This simulates late stance phase, before push-off, when maximum muscle stresses occur and when patients typically increase their pronation.) The patient is then placed in the subtalar neutral position and arch support can be molded. It takes approximately 4 min for the orthotic to mold and harden. Once the orthotic is molded, a base is applied to level the insole platform for impact, increase cushioning and prevent movement within the shoe. The base is glued onto the bottom of the orthotic and a grinder is used to help with custom fitting. Other adjustments to the orthotic such as adding a metatarsal pad to help those with metatarsalgia or adding a medial post for hyperpronators will be described in the following section (Figs 22.6–22.8).

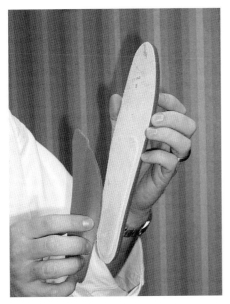

Figure 22.6   Orthotic materials.

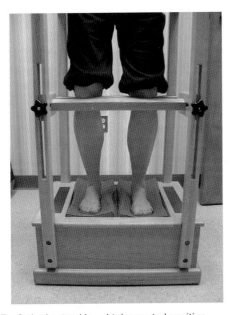

Figure 22.7   Orthotic stand in subtalar neutral position.

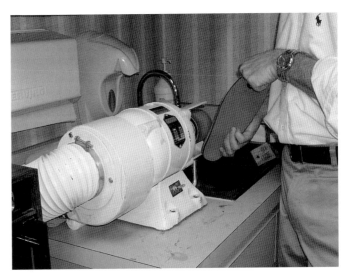

Figure 22.8   Grinding the orthotic.

SPECIAL CONSIDERATIONS AND ORTHOTIC ACCOMMODATION

Orthotic devices can be modified to treat various types of foot abnormalities. For example, in patients with a Morton's foot, a first ray extension post (cushioned material) added to the bottom of the orthotic allows the first metatarsal to bear more weight. This theoretically lessens the burden on the other metatarsals and reduces the risk of transverse arch breakdown.[1] In patients with metatarsalgia, a metatarsal pad can be added that takes pressure off the metatarsal heads. If a leg length discrepancy is detected, a lift can be added to the base of the orthotic. Metatarsal stress fractures can be managed by making a cutout under the involved metatarsal. Heel spurs can be treated with heel spur cutouts. A forefoot medial wedge is commonly added in the case of forefoot varus. In hyperpronation, some advocate a medial extension and accommodation of the first ray to allow for a kinetic wedge.[15] Also, a higher heel cup may prevent excessive motion of the rearfoot.

Box 22.4: Key Points

Special adjustments to orthotic devices

- first ray extension posts
- metatarsal padding and cutouts
- medial or lateral wedges
- heel cup
- heel lift.

Achilles and posterior tibialis tendinosis are examples of specific conditions in which adjustments to the orthotic help treat an acute condition. The posterior tibialis is a major inverter/plantar flexor of the foot and is a key muscle for the toe-off phase of gait. Valgus stance and excessive pronation place increase stress on the posterior tibialis. Since injury and inflammation of this tendon dramatically alters function of the foot, special support may be needed to help the athlete return to normal gait. Supporting the medial aspect of the orthotic with additional longitudinal arch support lessens pronation and the stress this tendon undergoes during toe-off. This may be an essential type of splinting to help athletes recover from this condition. In addition, those athletes with anatomical or functional excess pronation may need the orthotic correction on a permanent basis.[1]

Modification of the orthotic for Achilles tendinosis includes incorporating a heel lift or additional cushion which theoretically decrease the stress on the Achilles tendon during eccentric contraction.[1,16] Achilles tendon injury risk increases for individuals with a rigid, high-arched cavus foot so this seems a logical intervention. Other anatomical changes such as the foot with a plantar flexed first metatarsal and forefoot valgus may respond to application of lateral wedging and padded support of the first metatarsal head. Lateral foot instability such as that found in a runner with recurrent pain over the lateral aspect of the foot and suspected peroneal-cuboid syndrome warrants treatment with a lateral extension post.[15]

DO ORTHOTIC DEVICES DECREASE INJURY RATES?

Few prospective randomized controlled trials address the benefit of orthotic devices in injury prevention. A recent Cochrane review of interventions for preventing and treating stress fractures and stress reactions of bone of the lower limbs in young adults included a few studies of orthotic use in military recruits.[17] A study done by Schwellnus et al. showed that neoprene insoles were associated with a decrease in overuse injuries suffered by military recruits.[18] Smith et al. compared two different types of insoles: Spenco (a closed cellular neoprene polymer) and Poron (cellular polyurethane). The greatest number of injuries occurred in the control group (no insoles), followed by the individuals using Poron insoles and then the group using Spenco insoles. Most of the injuries prevented were less severe than stress fractures and included plantar fasciitis, metatarsalgia, callus, and blister formation.[19]

Not all studies show benefits of orthotic inserts. A study done by Gardner et al. showed no significant differences in stress reactions among 3025 marine recruits using an elastic polymer insole versus the standard mesh insoles during a 12-week intensive training program.[20] Similarly, Andrish et al. prospectively followed first-year midshipmen on five different shin splint prophylactic protocols. One of these groups incorporated a heel pad for running activities and this type of intervention did not decrease the incidence of shin splints.[21] Thus, studies looking at any of the types of shoe inserts showed mixed results.

Research design demonstrates limitations that lessen the clinical conclusions one can draw from studies of orthotic inserts. The studies cited above involved asymptomatic individuals and were used as primary prevention. Most clinicians prescribe orthotic devices for situations in which they feel the athlete has a biomechanical or symptomatic structural abnormality. Thus high satisfaction rates by users and reports of good clinical outcomes are comparing symptomatic and asymptomatic individuals and would be expected to show differences. In addition, studies use a wide range of materials and devices most of which were not customized for the individual users as would typically be done in an office setting. No specific method has arisen which blinds users to orthotic inserts, thus making double blinded trials impractical.

A study by Simkin et al. addressed the relationship between specific foot structure abnormalities, foot orthotics and stress fracture patterns. Tibial and femoral stress fractures were more common in those with high arched feet, while metatarsal stress fractures were more common in those with low arches.

Orthotic devices did decrease the rate of femoral stress fractures with cavus feet and metatarsal stress fractures with flat feet. While the rate of injury was decreased, the mechanism by which it occurred remained unclear.[22]

There are a number of non-randomized observational studies that examine the benefit of orthotic devices by patient questionnaires. Gross et al. received 347 questionnaire responses from long distance runners and found that >75% of the patients reported either complete resolution or great relief of their symptoms. The most common diagnoses for orthotic devices in this population were excessive pronation, leg length discrepancy, patello-femoral disorders, plantar fasciitis, Achilles tendonitis and shin splints. Over 90% of the patients continued to wear their orthotic devices even after their symptoms had resolved indicating a high level of patient satisfaction.[6] Donatelli et al. also reported a high level of patient satisfaction in non-athletes with the use of custom-made orthotic devices. Some 96% of patients reported pain relief with the orthotic devices and 94% were still wearing their orthotic at the time of follow-up (3 months to 2 years). A total of 76% were able to return to their previous level of activity and 52% would not leave home without their orthotic devices.[23] Eggold et al. surveyed 146 runners who were prescribed orthotic devices for knee pain, plantar fasciitis/heel spurs, arch pain, Achilles tendonitis, and shin splints. Approximately 75% of respondents obtained at least 80% pain relief or better.[7] D'Ambrosia prescribed orthotic devices for 200 runners at Louisiana State University Runners' Clinic, with posterior tibial syndrome being the most common diagnosis. Some 70% of the men and 83% of the women improved. A cavus foot deformity was less common (13 out of 200 runners), however orthotic devices only improved 25% of these patients. This data may be misleading in that a three-quarter length orthotic was used, which would not be ideal for the cavus foot deformity.[8]

Fauno et al. published one primary prevention study that showed potential benefit. They evaluated the incidence of soreness in the lower extremities and back in soccer referees with the use of shock absorbing heel inserts. A total of 91 asymptomatic referees were randomly assigned to either a control group or to receive shock-absorbing inserts during a 4-day period of refereeing 4–5 games per day. Those referees who wore the shock absorbing insoles reported less soreness in the back, calves and Achilles tendons.[24] Considering the studies done to date, the effect of orthotic devices for primary prevention is uncertain. Stronger evidence does show that the use of orthotic devices has resulted in a high degree of patient satisfaction, continued use and symptom resolution. Weaker data suggests use of orthotics for specific foot types and injuries.

HOW DO ORTHOTIC DEVICES WORK?

One of the proposed mechanisms through which orthotic devices work is by better alignment of the skeleton for a more efficient gait and decreased impact forces. Nigg et al. challenged this hypothesis by citing a number of studies that show that orthotic devices have not resulted in predictable changes in biomechanics. He studied four different types of shoe inserts (full medial, full lateral, half medial and half lateral compared to neutral insert) in 15 subjects to study whether kinematics, center of pressure, and leg joint movements could be predictably altered. For the most part, the subjects' responses to the various orthotic devices were not consistent and occasionally counterintuitive to what the researchers expected. For example, the full lateral insert resulted in a shift of the center of pressure laterally and not medially as was expected.[5]

Williams *et al.* recently studied inverted orthoses (a more aggressive type of orthotic in which there is more lateral tilt) to evaluate whether they changed biomechanics. While there was no change in rearfoot eversion, there was a decrease in measures of peak rearfoot inversion and a change in biomechanics at the knee.[25] Since the orthotic may increase the load on lateral structures of the knee, this type of intervention merits caution until data indicates whether the risk of knee injuries is affected. A recent study examined the effect of orthotic devices on postural sway in asymptomatic soccer players. The results revealed that the addition of an orthotic to a soccer shoe did not affect postural sway.[26] Others have shown that orthotic devices are helpful in improving balance in those with a history of an ankle injury.[27,28]

Nigg has proposed a new theory on the function of orthotic devices. The skeleton has a preferred movement for a task. If an orthotic intervention can support that movement, then muscle activity is reduced. A reduction in muscle work would theoretically be perceived as more comfortable and result in a delayed onset of fatigue. Therefore, if muscle activity is minimized, performance should improve. Nigg has shown some evidence with a small sample size that subjects running in comfortable shoes used less of their max VO_2 than those wearing a shoe that was uncomfortable. Another study showed that orthotic comfort is related to a series of kinematic, kinetic and electrodiagnostic variables.[3] This study found some objective correlation of comfort with various biomechanical variables. Certainly, more studies are required to confirm this hypothesis.

CONCLUSION

Box 22.5: Key Points

- Good response rates in non-randomized clinical trials.
- No prospective randomized clinical trials demonstrate benefits.
- Favorable review by Cochrane for prevention and treatment of stress fractures in lower limbs (moderate strength evidence).
- No strong evidence for primary prevention in asymptomatic individuals.

Orthotic devices have become a standard part of the treatment approach for running athletes. High levels of patient satisfaction, symptom relief and continued usage drive the prescribing patterns of sports medicine physicians. Nevertheless, the scientific support for their use remains at best limited.

The fabrication of orthotic devices is an art, thus those with more experience will construct or prescribe devices that would be expected to have better results. The wide variety of methods, materials and practice experience of the various physicians, orthotists, athletic trainers, and physical therapists utilizing orthotic inserts makes comparison of clinical results complex. Even the basic mechanisms through which orthotic devices work warrant additional scientific scrutiny. A completely new understanding of the beneficial effects of orthotic devices; whether they can be used for primary or secondary prevention; their role in the treatment of specific injuries; and identification of patients most likely to benefit from their prescription; holds the promise of improving their utilization in the care of athletes.

REFERENCES

1 Goodman A. Foot orthoses in sports medicine. South Med J 2004; 97:867–870.
2 Nigg BM, Nurse MA, Stefanyshyn DJ. Shoe inserts and orthotics for sport and physical activities. Med Sci Sports Exerc 1999; 31:421–428.
3 Nigg BM. The role of impact forces and foot pronation: A new paradigm. Clin J Sports Med 2001; 11:2–9.
4 Mundermann A, Nigg BM, Humble RN. Stefanyshyn. Orthotic comfort is related to kinematics, kinetics, and EMG in recreational runners. Med Sci Sports Exerc 2003; 35:1710–1719.
5 Nigg BM, Stergiou P, Cole G.S, Mundermann A, Humble N. Effect of shoe inserts on kinematics, center of pressure, and leg joint moments during running. Med Sci Sports Exerc 2003; 35:314–319.
6 Gross ML, Davlin LB, Evanski PM. Effectiveness of orthotic shoe inserts in the long-distance runner. Am J Sports Med 1991; 19:409–412.
7 Eggold JF. Orthotics in the prevention of runners' overuse injuries. Physician Sports Med 1981; 9:125–128.
8 D'Ambrosia RD. Orthotic devices in running injuries. Clin Sports Med 1985; 4:611–618.
9 Kannus VPA. Evaluation of abnormal biomechanics of the foot and ankle in athletes. Br J Sp Med 1992; 26:83–89.
10 Fields KB. Flatfeet become respectable. Arch Fam Med 1993; 2:723–724.
11 Ilfeld FW. Pes planus military significance and treatment with simple arch support. JAMA 1944; 124:281–283.
12 Bingham R. Painful feet. JAMA 1944; 124:283–286.
13 Cowan DN, Jones BH, Robinson JR. Foot morphologic characteristics and risk of exercise-related injury. Arch Fam Med 1993; 2:773–777.

14 Staats TB, Kriechbaum MP. Computer aided design and computer aided manufacturing of foot orthoses. J Prosthet Orthotics 1989; 1:182–186.
15 Subotnick SI. Foot orthotics. In: O'Connor FG, Wilder RP, eds. Textbook of running medicine. New York: McGraw-Hill; 2001:595–603.
16 McLauchlan GJ, Handoll HHG. Interventions for treating acute and chronic Achilles tendonitis. Issue 4. The Cochrane Library; 2004.
17 Gillespie WJ, Grant I. Interventions for preventing and treating stress fractures and stress reactions of bone of the lower limbs in young adults. Issue 4. The Cochrane Library; 2004.
18 Schwellnus MP, Jordan G, Noakes TD. Prevention of common overuse injuries by the use of shock absorbing insoles. Am J Sports Med 1990; 18:636–641.
19 Smith W, Walter J, Bailey M. Effects of insoles in coast guard basic training footwear. J Am Podiatr Med Assoc 1985; 75:644–647.
20 Gardner LI, Dziados JE, Jones BH, et al. Prevention of lower extremity stress fractures: a controlled trial of shock absorbing insole. Am J Public Health 1988; 78:1563–1567.
21 Andrish JT, Bergfeld JA, Walheim J. A prospective study on the management of shin splints. J Bone Jt Surg 1974; 56:1697–1700.
22 Simkin A, Leichter I, Giladi M, Stein M, Milgrom C. Combined effect of foot arch structure and an orthotic device on stress fractures. Foot Ankle 1989; 10:25–29.
23 Donatelli R, Hurlbert C, Conaway D, St. Pierre R. Biomechanical foot orthotics: A retrospective study. J Ortho Sports Phys Ther 1988; 10:205–212.
24 Fauno P, Kalund S, Andreasen I, Jergensen U. Soreness in lower extremities and back is reduced by use of shock absorbing heel inserts. Int J Sports Med 1993; 14:288–290.
25 Williams DS, Davis IM, Baitch SP. Effect of inverted orthoses on lower-extremity mechanics in runners. Med Sci Sports Exerc 2003; 35:2060–2068.

26 Percy ML, Menz HB. Effects of prefabricated foot orthoses and soft insoles on postural stability in professional soccer players. J Am Podiatr Med Assoc 2001; 91:194-202.

27 Orteza LC, Vogelbach WD, Denegar CR. The effects of molded and unmolded orthotics on balance and pain while jogging following inversion ankle sprain. J Athl Train 1992; 27:80.

28 Guskiewicz K, Perrin D. Effect of orthotics on postural sway following inversion ankle sprain. J Orthop Sports Phys Ther 1996; 23:326.

CHAPTER 23

Complementary and Alternative Medicine and the Athlete

Joseph F. Audette and Allison Bailey

INTRODUCTION

In recent years, the popularity of complementary and alternative medicine (CAM) has been increasing. A 1993 survey found that 33% of adult Americans had used some sort of CAM therapy in the previous year.[1] In 1998, the percentage had increased to 42%.[2] It has been estimated that Americans made 629 million visits to CAM providers in 1997, exceeding the total number of visits to primary care physicians. The same survey estimated that US$27 billion was spent on CAM that year, comparable to the out-of-pocket expenditures for all physician services in the US in 1997.[2] The most common diagnoses for which patients sought CAM in these surveys were back pain, headache, depression and anxiety.

The most comprehensive information on CAM use was gathered by the National Center for Health Statistics (NCHS) as part of the National Health Interview Survey (Fig. 23.1).[3] As part of this study, tens of thousands of Americans were interviewed about their experiences with health and illness. The 2002 version, which was completed by 31 044 adults, included detailed questions on CAM. This survey found that 36% of adult Americans had used some form of CAM, excluding megavitamins and prayer for health reasons, in the last 12 months. People who were more likely to use CAM included women greater than men, those with higher educational levels, those who had been hospitalized in the last year, and former smokers more than current or never smokers.

One difficulty in surveys of CAM use is that the definition of CAM may vary. The National Center for Complementary and Alternative Medicine (NCCAM) has defined CAM as diverse healthcare systems, practices and products that are not currently considered to be part of conventional medical training and practice.[4] While scientific evidence has begun to accumulate regarding some CAM therapies for certain diagnoses, important questions regarding most of these approaches remain unanswered. The list of treatments that are considered to be CAM will continue to shift as certain CAM therapies are shown to be effective and are accepted into mainstream practice.

Despite the strong interest in CAM therapies among the general population, the numbers of athletes who make use of CAM are not known. There have been no large-scale observational studies of CAM use by athletes published in the medical literature. The few small surveys available have focused on specific CAM modalities, such as nutritional supplementation and chiropractic care, rather than on more general information relating to CAM use.

There are many reasons, however, why athletes may be interested in CAM therapies. Athletes may be willing to try new and unproven treatments as they seek new methods by which to gain a competitive advantage over their opponents. They are frequently vulnerable to injury as they challenge themselves to perform at high levels for long periods of time, and when an injury has occurred, they will often try any means to hasten their recovery and return to their sport promptly. The conditions for which athletes may seek CAM are numerous. These include hastening recovery from fatigue and muscle soreness after intense athletic competitions and training sessions, treatment of acute injuries, and help with recovery from chronic, overuse or over-training injuries. CAM strategies may also be used generally for overall enhancement of athletic performance.

For the purposes of this chapter, some of the major CAM therapies that may be used by athletes will be reviewed briefly. The scope of this chapter does not permit an in-depth review of each of these therapies. In many cases, CAM treatments may overlap with areas no longer considered 'alternative'. For example, sports nutritionists are now recognized as vital members of the treatment team involved in the care of elite athletes. The importance of proper nutrition to athletic performance is well accepted. However, many athletes use nutritional supplements that are not well proven with the intention of improving sports performance. The use of nutritional supplements in sport has been covered in depth in Chapter 3 of this text.

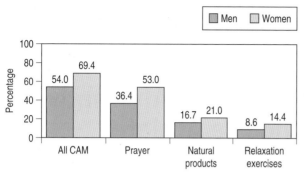

Figure 23.1 Percentage of adults aged ≥18 who used complementary and alternative medicine (CAM) for health reasons during the preceding 12 months, by gender in the US in 2002. (Modified from the National Center for Health Statistics.)

BODY-ORIENTED/MANUAL THERAPIES

Box 23.1: Key Points

- There are a number of different types of massage practices from classical methods such as Swedish massage to methods based on acupuncture theory such as shiatsu.

- Massage has not proven effective for the treatment of delayed onset muscle soreness.

- There is evidence in the literature that massage is safe, and may be a cost effective treatment for low back pain and other soft tissue injuries, however, better studies are needed within the athletic population.

Massage

Massage is the manipulation of body tissues using rhythmically applied strokes with varying amounts of pressure and stretching. The classical or Swedish system of massage uses strokes such as effleurage, pétrissage, friction and tapotement. Effleurage is the deep or superficial stroking of the skin, which produces various therapeutic effects depending on the amount of pressure applied. Pétrissage, the lifting and kneading of the skin, stretches and separates the underlying muscle fibers and is thought to be helpful in breaking up underlying scar tissue. Friction, or deep tissue massage, involves the application of deep transverse or circular friction to a small area of tissue with the thumbs or fingertips in order to stimulate an inflammatory response and increase healing. Tapotement, also known as percussion, involves tapping or pounding of the skin to promote relaxation and desensitize nerve endings.[5]

There are many additional forms of massage therapy. Some of the more popular include myofascial release, a technique used to relieve hyperirritable foci within taut bands of skeletal muscle, known as myofascial trigger points; acupressure, which is based on Chinese acupuncture theory and involves the application of circular friction to acupuncture points; and shiatsu, a Japanese technique that also employs acupuncture principles.[5]

The purported positive effects of massage include increased blood flow in muscles, increased lymph flow, a relaxing effect on the central nervous system and loosening and prevention of adherent scar tissue. Massage has also been used to increase flexibility and coordination; increase pain threshold; decrease neuromuscular excitability; stimulate circulation, thus improving energy transport to the muscle; restore joint range of motion; and to relieve post-exercise muscle soreness by removing lactic acid from tissues. Like many complementary therapies, the evidence regarding many of these purported effects of massage is lacking. The limitations of studying such a technique are numerous and include the wide variation in technique, experience of the practitioner, and frequency, timing, and duration of treatment used in the available studies, making comparison between studies difficult.

Massage has been utilized for its therapeutic effects in the context of athletics since early civilization.[6] The use of sports massage has remained popular, despite the above mentioned research difficulties. The treatment of delayed onset muscle soreness (DOMS) is among the most common uses of massage by athletes. Studies examining the effect of massage on DOMS have shown varying results. The proposed benefit of massage in the treatment of DOMS is felt to be due to increased blood flow to the injured area. However, studies examining the effect of massage on blood flow have been equivocal. Some researchers reported an increase in local blood flow during massage.[7] Conversely, a study by Tiidus showed no difference in arterial or venous blood flow during effleurage of the quadriceps.[8] However, reductions in serum CK levels have been noted in study participants who were massaged for 15 min or 30 min, both 2 h following exercise.[9] Despite these encouraging results, other studies have found no differences in soreness levels or force deficits between the massaged or control limb with an 8-min massage following high intensity exercise.[10] If some of the effects of massage can be explained by central mechanisms, the use of the contralateral limb as control in these studies could explain the negative findings.

Massage is often used prior to sporting activities to enhance performance, although scientific evidence has not supported this use. No significant changes in VO_2max, cardiac output, heart rate, blood pressure, or lactic acid levels were noted in studies of pre-exercise massage in 10 healthy men.[11] Another study examined the effects of massage *versus* warm-up and stretching on joint range of motion. Warm-up and stretching significantly increased range-of-motion at all joints examined. Massage and warm-up, both separately and in combination, increased ankle range of motion only. It was concluded that warm-up and stretching were more effective than massage at increasing flexibility.[6]

Massage may also be used as part of a rehabilitation treatment plan after an injury has occurred. Athletic activities often require the repetitive use of one group of muscles more than others, which may result in strength imbalances and compensatory strain patterns in other areas of the body. Massage is often used to treat this kind of soft tissue dysfunction. Although it has not been studied specifically in athletes, some evidence has accumulated for the use of massage to treat non-specific low back pain. A randomized control trial comparing therapeutic massage, acupuncture and self-care education for persistent low back pain showed that massage was superior to self-care in terms of symptoms and disability reduction and superior to acupuncture in terms of disability reduction at 10 weeks. At 1 year, massage was no better than self-care but better than acupuncture. The massage group used the least medications and had the lowest cost of subsequent care.[12] In a review of massage for low back pain, three randomized clinical trials were identified that reported effectiveness of massage for treating chronic or subacute low back pain.[13]

In clinical practice, the type, frequency and duration of massage will vary according to the goals of treatment. Massage given for the general purpose of relaxation or stimulation can be given as often as needed with durations ranging from several minutes to an hour. When performed for edema reduction, daily massage lasting 5–10 min is generally recommended. Likewise, friction massage should be performed on a daily basis for approximately 5 min. Caution should be used whenever massage is performed early after an injury, as it may potentiate the inflammatory response. Absolute contraindications to massage include deep venous thrombosis, malignancy, atherosclerotic plaque, unhealed fractures, and infection. Relative contraindications include anticoagulation, acute soft tissue injury and skin grafts.[14]

Acupuncture

Box 23.2: Key Points

- There is strong pathophysiological evidence in the literature that acupuncture can modulate pain, reduce inflammation, and promote tissue healing via central neuromodulatory and hormonal mechanisms.
- The clinical evidence suggests that acupuncture is safe and may be helpful for the treatment of tendonitis of the elbow and shoulder, osteoarthritis of the knee, and hasten recovery from shoulder surgery. These studies need to be repeated in the athletic population.

Acupuncture is part of a complex system of health care, known as traditional Chinese medicine that has been practiced throughout Asia for at least 2000 years (Fig. 23.2). Interest in acupuncture in this country has been growing since the opening of China in the 1970s. Today, acupuncture is practiced to a great extent in this country by both physician and non-physician practitioners. A National Institutes of Health (NIH) consensus development panel that convened in 1997 found good evidence to support the use of acupuncture for postoperative and chemotherapy related nausea and vomiting, nausea of pregnancy, and postoperative dental pain.[15] The panel also found evidence to support the use of acupuncture as an adjuvant treatment for addiction, stroke rehabilitation, headache, dysmenorrhea, lateral epicondylitis, fibromyalgia, low back pain, carpal tunnel syndrome and asthma.

The use of acupuncture by athletes to treat acute injuries is very common in Asia and Eastern Europe and is increasingly becoming an option in many Western nations. International exposure came at the Winter Olympics in Japan in 1998 when an acupuncturist in Nagano offered treatments to Olympic athletes and officials, emphasizing that it is a drug-free way to treat injuries. The public was stunned by the near miraculous recovery of the Austrian, Hermann Maier in response to acupuncture. Maier won the gold medal in the giant slalom and super G, 3 days following a dramatic fall that occurred during the downhill competition. Maier attributed his quick recovery from shoulder and knee injuries sustained in that fall to his treatments with acupuncture.

Over the last 30 years, a great deal of scientific evidence has accumulated to substantiate that acupuncture stimulation (AP) and electroacupuncture stimulation (EA) have physiological effects that strongly influence the neurohumoral systems that modulate pain. The evidence for the release of endogenous opioids with AP and EA goes back to the seminal work of

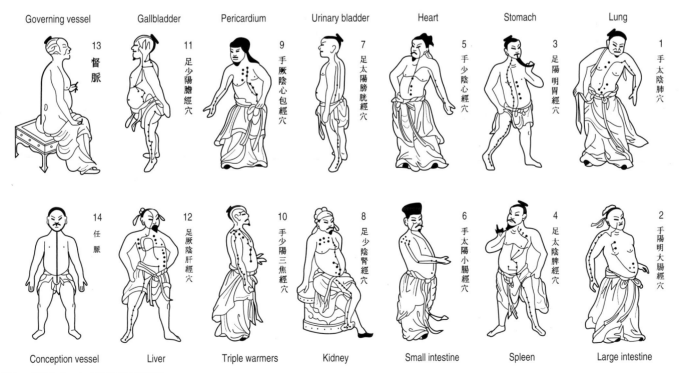

Figure 23.2 Acupuncture meridians.

Pomeranz in animals and Mayer in humans in the early 1970s.[16,17] We now know that acupuncture causes the release of endorphins and enkephalins in the CNS and that these neuropeptides play a significant role in its analgesic efficacy.

There is growing evidence that the descending inhibitory control system also plays a role in acupuncture analgesia. This involves the activation of serotonergic neurons in the midbrain that in turn act to inhibit the transmission of nociceptive information at the level of the dorsal horn (Fig. 23.3). Release of 5-hydroxytryptamine (5-HTP) in the raphe nucleus of the midbrain has been shown with both EA and AP, and acupuncture analgesia is attenuated with the injection of a serotonin antagonist such as parachlorophenylalanine.[18]

Acupuncture has been shown in animal models to strongly influence the pituitary-hypothalamic system as well. The arcuate nucleus of the ventromedial hypothalamus contains the β-endorphin-producing cells and lesions of this nucleus abolish acupuncture analgesia in rats.[18] The hypothalamus secretes β-endorphin into the bloodstream, consistent with the elevated blood levels of endorphin found with both AP and EA. Concurrent with the release of β-endorphin is the secretion of adrenocorticotrophic hormone (ACTH) with acupuncture, which in turn stimulates adrenal secretion of cortisol causing a general anti-inflammatory effect.[19] Given that peripheral opioid receptors have been found to be present on C-fibers in inflammatory conditions,[20] the elevation of systemic beta-endorphin with acupuncture may exert both an analgesic and an anti-inflammatory effect in sports injuries.

Recent studies indicate that acupuncture also influences the release of immune modulating cytokines from the hypothalamus such as interleukin 1B and 6 during experimental models of fever.[21] The rise of blood β-endorphin with acupuncture also influences peripheral cytokine production in the spleen by causing increases in interferon-gamma and reduction of natural killer cell activity.[22] These early data suggest that acupuncture has physiological effects that go far beyond the release of endorphins in the CNS, and has important immune-modulating effects that may prove to be important in the recovery from injury.

The use of acupuncture for acute injuries has not been studied extensively in athletes. However, a study of rotator cuff tendonitis in subjects with sports-related injuries found that true acupuncture needling was significantly superior when looking at both its analgesic effects as well as strength, range of motion and functional scores when compared with a placebo needling group. Treatment consisted of using a combination of points in the hands and feet, based on Chinese acupuncture principles, together with meridian-based local points around the shoulder based on tenderness. Subjects received two 22-min treatments/week for 4 weeks and had follow-up assessments at the end of the treatment period and again at 4 months.[23]

Another study has shown that acupuncture hastens recovery from arthroscopic acromioplasty performed for impingement syndrome. Subjects in this study were randomized to treatment with either real or sham acupuncture beginning 3–8 days following arthroscopic acromioplasty. Subjects in the real acupuncture group had significantly lower pain intensity scales, less analgesic use, and improved range of motion for abduction than the sham acupuncture group at all follow-up visits through the four month follow-up period.[24]

There is also strong evidence to suggest that acupuncture is effective in short-term relief of lateral epicondyle pain. Haker and Lundeberg randomized 86 patients to receive either real or sham acupuncture treatments for lateral epicondylitis. Patients underwent 10 treatment sessions. At initial follow-up, the real acupuncture group had significantly less pain complaints than the sham group. However, these differences did not remain significant at either 3-month or 1-year follow-up.[25] In a separate study, 48 patients with lateral epicondylitis were also randomized to real versus sham acupuncture treatments. A single 20 min treatment was given using only one point near the fibular head (gallbladder 34) on the leg ipsilateral to the elbow pain. The treatment group had significantly greater acute pain relief following this treatment.[26]

Acupuncture has also shown some efficacy in the treatment of knee osteoarthritis (OA). The risk for knee OA is elevated in athletes with histories of knee injuries, such as those commonly incurred in American football and soccer. One of the most thorough systematic reviews of acupuncture examined its efficacy in knee OA. A major strength of this review was that it rated seven different clinical trials on how closely they conformed to guidelines put forth by acupuncture experts. These guidelines included (1) an average of 10 treatment sessions for a chronic condition, (2) stimulation of at least eight points per session, (3) elicitation of the De Qi sensation, and (4) use of a combination of high and low frequency stimulation, when used, to avoid accommodation to the impulse.[27] The meta-analysis found four of the seven studies to have a positive effect on pain and three of the seven studies were neutral.[28] None of these studies followed all four treatment guidelines. However, the most important of these

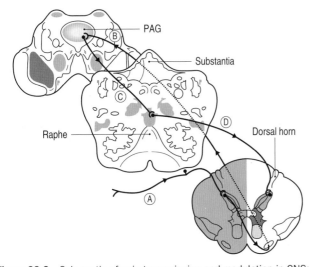

Figure 23.3 Schematic of pain transmission and modulation in CNS: (A) Nociceptive input into the dorsal horn. (B) Ascending pain pathway via the spinothalamic tract with synapse in the peri aqueductal grey area (PAG) in mesencephalon. (C) Descending, excitatory pathway to raphe magnus in rostral medulla. (D) Serotonergic descending pain modulating tract has inhibitory action on Dorsal horn.

Body oriented/manual therapist **311**

guidelines is felt to be treatment duration for a chronic condition, such as knee OA. The three studies that administered the minimum of 10 treatments all had positive results. Supporting the importance of treatment length, a recent large NIH supported randomized controlled trial assessed the effect of acupuncture as an adjuvant treatment for knee OA. This trial compared 24 acupuncture sessions over 26 weeks with sham acupuncture or arthritis education in 570 patients with osteoarthritis of the knee. Acupuncture led to greater improvements in function but not pain after 8 weeks and in both pain and function after 26 weeks. No adverse effects were associated with acupuncture.[29]

Of all the pain related conditions, back pain is the most frequently studied using acupuncture as an intervention. In a meta-analysis of randomized controlled trials of acupuncture for low back pain, it was concluded that acupuncture is superior to the various control treatments, but insufficient evidence was available to state whether it was better than placebo needling methods.[27]

In conclusion, acupuncture appears to be a safe and potentially effective method of treating the pain and inflammation of sports-related injuries. There is sufficient evidence to suggest a physiological mechanism of action that involves neurohumoral processes that have both a central and peripheral effect. Clearly, better designed and more specific studies are needed to assess the clinical efficacy of acupuncture in various sports injuries. In addition, there is much interest in the effects that acupuncture may have on human performance, particularly as it relates to sports. Further research is needed before it can be determined what effect acupuncture may have on other aspects of athletic performance such as strength, endurance and flexibility.

Chiropractic

Box 23.3: Key Points

- Chiropractic care is utilized by a high percentage of athletes both in professional sports such as American football and baseball and in the international Olympic arena.

- Safety is generally good, although high velocity manipulation especially in the cervical region can cause serious neurological complications; anywhere from 1 in 100 000 to 1 in 1 million cases.

- The current clinical literature has focused on the use of chiropractic care for spine-related pain and suggests that it may provide short-term benefit for subacute low back pain.

- More evidence is needed to assess efficacy in athletic populations.

Chiropractic medicine is a drug-free, non-surgical branch of healthcare that considers humans as integrated beings and gives special attention to structural, spinal, musculoskeletal, neurological, vascular, nutritional, emotional and environmental relationships (Fig. 23.4). The practice and procedures of chiropractic medicine are based on academic and clinical train-

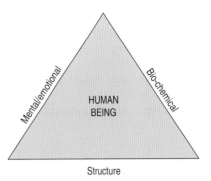

Figure 23.4 Chiropractic triangle of health.

ing received at accredited chiropractic colleges and include both diagnostic and therapeutic procedures. The mainstay of chiropractic treatments are adjustment and manipulation of the joints and associated soft tissues of the body, in particular that of the spinal column. In fact, although chiropractors may use various techniques including exercise and nutritional advice, the majority of the clinical and research literature involving chiropractic medicine has focused on spinal manipulation.

The use of spinal manipulation to treat back pain and other disorders can be traced back to writings from China in 2700 BC and Greece in 1500 BC, and the importance of spine care was written about by Hippocrates. David Daniel Palmer founded the chiropractic profession in this country in 1895 in Davenport, Iowa, thereby organizing the practice of spinal manipulation into a medical science.[30] Palmer became the founder of the Palmer School of Chiropractic, which has remained one of the most prominent chiropractic colleges in the country. During the twentieth century, chiropractic doctors gained legal recognition in all 50 states in the US, and chiropractic medicine is now practiced throughout the world.

Accordingly, chiropractic doctors are playing an increasingly active role in the treatment of athletes. They first officially participated in the care of athletes at the Olympic Games in 1980. Chiropractic medicine is now part of the sports medicine program of the US Olympic Committee. Chiropractors participate regularly in amateur sporting events, and also provide care for professional football, basketball, baseball and hockey players. Former Boston Red Sox centerfielder, Johnny Damon, was among those to popularize the use of chiropractic medicine when he stated to the press that chiropractic manipulation had eased the post-traumatic headaches he had suffered since his head-on collision with a teammate during the 2003 American League division series.

In addition, a survey of athletic trainers from 36 National Football League (NFL) teams revealed that most NFL trainers had referred players to chiropractors and that many players seek chiropractic services without official referral. A total of 31% NFL teams responding to the survey have a chiropractor on the team's medical staff.[31] Due to the widespread use of chiropractice by athletes and the involvement of chiropractors in on-field sporting events, protocols have been published to guide chiropractors in treating the most common athletic injuries that occur in each sport.[32]

Safety concerns still predominate among the medical community, especially when utilizing high velocity low amplitude (HVLA) manipulative techniques where there is an audible pop in the joint during the application of the chiropractic technique. Surveys have estimated that the incidence of vertebral artery dissection and stroke with cervical HVLA may be as low as one case in 5.8 million, based on malpractice claims, or one in 500 000 to one in 1 million, based on the report of neurologists. Data from Ontario, Canada provide estimates of serious adverse outcomes following cervical HVLA at 1.3 in 100 000. Estimates about the incidence of cauda equina syndrome following lumbar HVLA range from one case per 100 million to one in 1 million.[33]

Despite the widespread use of chiropractic in athletics, there remains a dearth of research on the use of chiropractic manipulation to treat common sports injuries. The majority of research has understandably focused on the use of spinal manipulation to treat neck or back pain. The methodological quality of these studies, however, remains low. In a study assessing the quality of reviews of spinal manipulation, 51 reviews were identified, 34 of which were positive and 17 of which were neutral. The overall methodological quality was found to be low. However, nine out of the 10 highest quality reviews were positive. Of the 34 positive reviews identified, 15 found positive conclusions only for short-term results and two made positive conclusions only for subacute back pain.[34]

A more recent randomized controlled trial compared the use of medication, acupuncture, or spinal manipulation for back or neck pain of greater than 13 weeks' duration. Subjects were excluded from this study if they had nerve root involvement, spinal anomalies other than sacralization or lumbarization of vertebrae, pathology other than mild to moderate osteoarthrosis, spondylolisthesis of L5 on S1 exceeding Grade 1 severity, a history of spinal surgery, or a leg length inequality >9 mm with postural scoliosis. The highest proportion of early recovery was found for spinal manipulation (27.3%), followed by acupuncture (9.4%) and medication (5%). In addition, manipulation achieved the best functional results with improvements of 50% on the Oswestry disability scale.[35]

Spinal manipulation is often used to treat neck pain and headache. A survey of the US population found that 6% of headache sufferers had consulted an alternative health provider, most commonly a chiropractor, within the previous year.[1] In a review of the literature on cervical manipulation and mobilization for the treatment of neck pain and headache, Hurwitz *et al.* identified 14 randomized controlled trials, two cohort studies, 14 case series, and 37 case reports. The overall methodological quality of these studies was low. The authors concluded that mobilization is likely to be of at least short-term benefit for patients with acute neck pain; manipulation is probably more effective than mobilization or physical therapy for some patients with subacute or chronic neck pain and all three treatments are likely superior to usual medical care; and, manipulation and/or mobilization may be beneficial for muscle tension type headache.[36]

MIND–BODY INTERVENTIONS

Box 23.4: Key Points

- Mind-body interventions tend to be used more for arousal regulation and performance enhancement rather than for the treatment of athletic injuries.

- There is widespread use of a variety of mind-body techniques in amateur, professional and Olympic sports including imagery, arousal regulation, meditation, biofeedback, autogenic training and hypnosis, but once again little well-designed research to support its use.

- There is some evidence in the literature to suggest that different cognitive strategies may be more effective for specific types of athletic endeavors. For example, arousal-energizing strategies may have a greater effect on performance for athletic tasks demanding high levels of strength and endurance, whereas, arousal reduction strategies may be more important to those tasks requiring greater precision and fine-motor control.

The use of psychological interventions in competitive sport for the goal of improving performance has become increasingly popular in recent years. Coaches and athletes alike readily acknowledge the importance of psychological factors in reaching high levels of athletic achievement. Sport psychologists are now commonly among the group of professionals involved in the care of sports teams and athletes. In the 1960s and 1970s, much of the focus in sport psychology was to put well-proven psychological theories to the test in laboratory settings, using motor performance as the primary outcome under study. However, in the 1980s, it became recognized that such highly controlled studies were not realistic representations of the true environment in which sporting events occurred.[37] The subsequent shift was towards more interest in applying sport psychology to real life situations. Unfortunately, research of this type is neither easy to perform nor to interpret, as the multiple variables involved make cause and effect relationships difficult to establish.

Nevertheless, an article published in the prominent New England Journal of Medicine in 1986 highlights the extensive interest in applying psychological principles to competitive sports.[38] In the article, Harvard Medical School psychiatrist, Dr Armand M. Nicholi, explains how he was hired by the New England Patriots football team in the early 1980s to provide group dynamics counseling to the coaches and team members, and to offer individual therapy sessions to certain players. Although Dr Nicholi is careful to point out that a direct causal relationship could not be determined under such uncontrolled circumstances, the team's performance improved dramatically after his interventions, and the Patriots made it to the Superbowl for the first time in 25 years.

The field of sport psychology is broad and far-reaching. Clearly, the scope of the 'mind–body' section of this chapter does not permit a review of this field, nor is that our purpose here. The goal, rather, is to discuss several of the techniques that, although they are often included within the field of sport psychology, are also considered to fall within the category of mind–body CAM interventions and to discuss their possible applications to the field of sport science. There is evidence that use of such mind–body CAM therapies is prevalent among the general population. A random telephone survey of the US population conducted in 1997, found that 18.9% of adults had used at least one mind–body therapy in the last year.[39] In addition, unlike many CAM therapies, considerable evidence exists for the efficacy of several mind–body therapies in disorders such as coronary artery disease, headaches, insomnia, incontinence, chronic low back pain, symptoms of cancer and cancer treatment, and improvement of post-surgical outcomes with moderate evidence to support their use in hypertension and arthritis.[40]

Despite their apparent prevalent use by athletes and their documented efficacy in certain medical conditions, there remain relatively few well-controlled scientific studies examining the efficacy of mind–body therapies in athletes. The mind–body CAM interventions most often used by athletes include imagery, hypnosis, meditation and biofeedback, but also may extend, in some cases, to other mental practice techniques and arousal regulation strategies. Therefore, each of these areas and their potential applications to sports and athletic performance will be briefly discussed below.

Imagery

The purposeful use of mental processes, such as imagery, for the intent of improving sports performance is perhaps one of the most popularized applications of the mind–body interaction in sports. The popular press abounds with stories from professional athletes regarding their use of imagery to enhance their performance. Retired golf professional, Jack Nicklaus, was among those to promote imagery as an important tool in sport performance. He wrote:

'I never hit a shot even in practice without having a sharp in-focus picture of it in my head. It's like a color movie. First, I 'see' the ball where I want it to finish, nice and white and sitting up high on the bright green grass. Then the scene quickly changes, and I 'see' the ball going there: its path, trajectory, and shape, even its behavior on landing. Then there's a sort of fade-out, and the next scene shows me making the kind of swing that will turn the previous images into reality. Only at the end of this short, private Hollywood spectacular do I select a club and step up to the ball'.[41]

Other competitive athletes report the frequent use of imagery strategies to enhance their performance. In a survey of athletes and coaches at a US Olympic Training Center, 90% of the athletes reported use of imagery for sport performance and 94% of coaches reported using the technique with their athletes. In this study, 97% of athletes and 100% of coaches who used imagery rated the techniques as effective.[42] A survey of elite New Zealand Olympic Class sailors found that 64% reported practicing relaxation techniques and 61% used visualization as a mental practice skill.[43] It is likely that use of imagery strategies varies based on the level of competition of the athlete with professional or elite level athletes making more frequent use of

such strategies than those participating in recreational levels of sporting activities.

The term 'imagery' may mean different phenomena to different individuals. However, the term has been defined by Richardson as follows: 'Mental imagery refers to all those quasi-sensory or quasi-perceptual experiences of which we are self consciously aware and which exist for us in the absence of those stimulus conditions that are known to produce their genuine sensory or perceptual counterparts'.[44] As further explained by Murphy, this definition touches upon several key points concerning imagery.[42] First, imagery experiences mimic sensory experiences, such as 'seeing' or 'feeling' that one is actually performing the athletic skill that is being imaged. Second, the individual is completely aware of these experiences and typically produces them purposefully, distinguishing imagery from dreaming. And, third, the imagery is experienced without the usual stimuli that produce the sensations experienced. In other words, no props should be necessary for the athlete to image performance of the skill.

Murphy has also drawn a distinction between the use of imagery to practice skills and increase learning of those skills (or mental practice) and the use of imagery to improve the performance of an already acquired skill (or psyching-up).[42] This distinction becomes more confusing when one realizes that mental practice does not necessarily require imagery, as skills can also be rehearsed verbally. In addition, 'psyching-up', which is defined as self-directed cognitive strategies used prior to skill execution with the intent of enhancing performance,[45] may be accomplished through multiple non-imaging techniques. Therefore, it is no wonder that the imagery literature is difficult to review and interpret, as even the definitions used by various researchers in the field may differ.

In addition, mental practice imagery is often distinguished from outcome imagery in which the focus of the imagery experience is not on the performance of a task but on the outcome of a task. Outcome imagery has been defined as the imagery of what happens after an action is completed and not of the action itself.[46] It has been proposed by many sport imagery theorists that mental practice imagery is likely to help in learning or improving performance of a task while outcome imagery is more likely to influence performance by affecting motivation or confidence.[47] However, in a study of 26 skilled and 25 unskilled golfers, Taylor and Shaw found that, although negative outcome imagery decreased both confidence and performance, positive outcome imagery did not increase confidence or performance in comparison to a no-imagery control group.[48] It remains unclear why negative outcome imagery would be more strongly detrimental to performance than positive imagery would be performance enhancing. In addition, the majority of studies examining outcome imagery have combined this intervention with mental practice imagery.

Although many mental practice studies have revealed a positive relationship between this type of imagery and performance, others have failed to show such a relationship. In a 1983 meta-analysis, Feltz et al. identified 98 mental practice studies with an average effect size of 0.48 standard deviations.[49] However, there are no recent comprehensive reviews of this literature available. One factor that may influence the effectiveness of imagery interventions on performance is the type of sport-related activity being studied. In particular, imagery may be more effective at enhancing performance of primarily cognitive tasks rather than those requiring gross muscular effort. A study of 120 college students of various skill levels examining the effects of imagery *versus* non-specific arousal confirmed this theory.[50] In this study, imagery interventions improved performance in free-throw shooting but not in grip-strength tasks.

Other factors that may influence the effectiveness of imagery in sport include the age, gender and skill level of the athlete, the experience of the individual with imagery use, the perspective of the imagery (internal *versus* external), and the combination of imagery with other techniques, such as relaxation.[42] It remains unclear what the benefit of combining imagery techniques with relaxation techniques may be. However, in clinical practice, relaxation techniques are often used prior to imagery practice sessions. The use of various relaxation techniques and their possible applications to sport will be discussed further in the next section.

Despite the challenges encountered by researchers in this field, imagery techniques are likely to remain popular with athletes, coaches and sport psychologists. In addition, neuroimaging studies in combination with other methods, such as studies of the effects of transcranial magnetic stimulation and studies of patients with brain injury, are beginning to elucidate the neurobiological basis of imagery. In particular, motor imagery processes appear to activate brain regions important in perception and motor control.[51] Further understanding of the underlying neural structures important in imagery processes will likely help to clarify the means by which imagery exerts its effects on performance. Clearly, however, the current state of this field remains relatively in its infancy, and further research is needed before a direct causal relationship can be established between specific imagery techniques and athletic performance.

Arousal regulation strategies

The mental and emotional state of an athlete prior to and during competitive events is often credited with affecting their performance. Therefore, within the field of sport psychology much attention has focused on interventions that may help athletes to control their arousal levels. Emotional arousal has been defined as a 'general physiological and psychological activation of the organism that varies on a continuum from deep sleep to intense excitement'.[52] In other words, arousal means how emotionally activated an athlete is before or during performance. It has been pointed out by Gould and Udry that arousal is actually a complex phenomenon that involves interacting physiological and psychological states and that, therefore, assessments of arousal should include both cognitive and somatic measures.[53] The measurement tools that are used to assess arousal become especially important in arousal regulation research.

The exact relationship between arousal and athletic performance remains to be clarified. Various theories have been proposed to try to explain this relationship. Until relatively recently, the most well accepted of these theories was the inverted-U hypothesis. The inverted-U hypothesis proposed that low arousal levels result in poor performance. Performance then improves up to a moderate level of arousal that is considered to be optimal for performance. Increases in arousal above this level, however, result in performance decrements. But, evidence for this theory has remained limited and over the last decade it has come under considerable criticism. Additional hypotheses that have emerged include the catastrophe theory, Hanin's optimal zones of functioning hypothesis, the multidimensional anxiety theory, and reversal theory.[53]

The catastrophe theory may be particularly useful to describe as it emphasizes the importance of interacting cognitive and physiologic variables. It predicts that under conditions of low cognitive anxiety the performance-arousal relationship resembles an inverted-U. However, under conditions of high cognitive anxiety, increases in physiological arousal improve performance only up to a certain point. Further increases in physiological arousal beyond this point result in a dramatic decrease in performance or catastrophe.[54] Therefore, this model emphasizes that the relationship between physiologic arousal and performance is mediated by the level of cognitive anxiety present. Once again, however, well-controlled tests of this hypothesis have not been conducted.

Theories of arousal regulation and performance suggest that there is an optimal level of arousal at which athletic performance is maximized. Athletes often do engage in pre-competition rituals in order to regulate their arousal level. The two general categories of arousal regulation strategies used by athletes include those aimed at increasing arousal, often referred to as preparatory arousal (a form of psyching-up), and those aimed at decreasing arousal or arousal reduction strategies. Therefore, depending on the level of cognitive and/or physiologic arousal experienced, the athlete may utilize strategies aimed at either increasing or decreasing arousal.

The specific athletic task being performed is likely to be another important variable in determining which arousal regulation strategy is most effective. A number of studies, for example, have found a positive relationship between preparatory arousal and strength, and there is some, although more limited, evidence for a positive relationship between preparatory arousal and muscular endurance.[45] In addition, a non-specific arousal 'psyching-up' strategy was found to improve handgrip strength, but not free-throw shooting performance, as compared to a no intervention control among college students of various skill levels.[50] Therefore, arousal-energizing strategies may have a greater effect on performance for athletic tasks demanding high levels of strength and endurance, whereas, it is conceivable that arousal reduction strategies may be more important to those tasks requiring greater precision and fine-motor control.

Relaxation techniques

Relaxation techniques have become widely used to decrease the body's physiologic response to stress and are considered an important component of what has become known as 'Mind–Body Medicine'. The Harvard Medical School cardiologist, Herbert Benson, was the first to use the now popular phrase 'the relaxation response', to describe the physiological changes of the body that are the opposite of the 'fight or flight' response.[55] Key features of the relaxation response include decreases in oxygen consumption, heart rate, respiratory rate and skeletal muscle activity. Dr Benson's initial research on relaxation techniques involved their use in treating his patients with hypertension. Since that time, these techniques have been applied successfully in a number of other conditions, including cardiac arrhythmias, headache, chronic pain, premenstrual syndrome, anxiety, mild to moderate depression and insomnia.

There are various techniques that can be used in order to invoke the relaxation response, including meditation, yoga, autogenic training, progressive relaxation, biofeedback techniques, and hypnosis with suggested deep relaxation.[55] It has been suggested that the most popular of these techniques among athletes may be biofeedback, autogenic training and progressive relaxation. As mentioned earlier in this chapter, athletes and sport psychologists may make use of a variety of techniques for arousal reduction and/or stress management.

Cognitive behavioral interventions, that combine cognitive restructuring with relaxation techniques and mental imagery, are prominently used for this purpose.[53] Cognitive behavioral interventions can be differentiated from those relaxation strategies above by their focus on altering cognitions involved in arousal regulation. A review of such techniques is beyond the scope of this chapter and the reader is referred to sport psychology textbooks for a discussion of such methods. Instead, some of the relaxation techniques, which are generally considered to be mind–body CAM therapies, and may be used by athletes for these purposes, will be discussed next.

Meditation

Meditation is a conscious mental process that induces the integrated physiologic changes known as the relaxation response. Among the physiological responses that have been noted with meditation are a marked decrease in oxygen consumption and the appearance of alpha waves (slow brain waves) on electroencephalogram.[55] Meditation may be one of the most widely used mind–body approaches for treating stress-related psychological and medical conditions, although its use by and effectiveness in athletes remains unclear. There are many different types of meditation, each with its own proponents and practitioners. A general principle of most types of meditation is maintaining a passive attitude towards one's own thoughts and the use of an alternate focus point for the mind, whether it be a word, sound, phrase, prayer, or simply the breath. Some sort of meditation has long been a part of many eastern philosophies and healing traditions. Dr Herbert Benson and Dr Jon Kabat-Zinn (at the University of Massachusetts Medical School) were among those to popularize the use of meditation for medical and psychological purposes in this country.

Transcendental meditation (or TM, as it is often called) is a form of meditation that was developed from the Yogic tradition by Maharishi Mahesh Yogi, an Indian guru and student of physics, who came to the West early in his life and trained instructors to teach this simplified technique to others.[55] In TM, a trained instructor gives the meditator a sound or phrase (mantra) that is chosen to suit the individual. The meditator then repeats this mantra over and over while sitting quietly in a comfortable position. The main purpose of repetition of the mantra is to avoid distracting thoughts. Meditators are told to assume a passive attitude and, if they notice distracting thoughts, to simply return to their mantra without judgment. In general, a regular TM practice of 20 min in the morning and 20 min in the evening is recommended.

Mindfulness meditation, a form of meditation that comes from the eastern Buddhist tradition, uses the breath rather than a mantra as its primary focus point. Again, the importance of maintaining a passive, non-judgmental attitude is emphasized and meditators are instructed that when their minds wander to simply return to paying attention to the breath. Mindfulness meditation is often practiced while sitting quietly in a comfortable position (sitting meditation) or while walking (walking meditation) with focus on the sensations experienced while moving (usually slowly), in addition to giving attention to the breath. The Stress Reduction and Relaxation Program (SR&RP) at the University of Massachusetts Medical School developed by Dr Kabat-Zinn uses a form of mindfulness meditation in participants with conditions such as cardiac disease, hypertension, asthma, headaches, chronic pain problems, seizures, sleep disorders, digestive problems, anxiety and panic, dermatologic conditions and others.[56]

Although studies of the use of meditation to treat medical problems such as these are becoming more widespread, there remains very little research on the effects of meditation in athletes. When applied in sports, meditation techniques are usually used with the intent of either hastening recovery from injury, or to enhance performance of a particular skill through arousal regulation. The possible effects of meditation on either of these outcomes, however, have not been well studied. The only study identified in the medical literature on meditation and athletic performance examined the use of a TM-like meditation technique in elite Norwegian shooters.[57] In this study, 25 elite shooters were randomized to learn meditation training once a week for 7 weeks or a control group that received no mental training. Meditators were instructed to practice the technique for 30 min daily at home during the intervention period. The competition scores of the two groups were compared for the seasons before and after the intervention. The improvement in shooting scores was significantly greater for the meditation group compared with the control group between the two seasons. No significant difference was noted between the intervention and control groups, however, for test shootings performed just before and after the intervention. Methodological weaknesses of this study include small sample size, lack of a placebo control group, and lack of standardized outcome measures.

Biofeedback

Biofeedback is a special case of operant learning that involves the use of instrumentation that provides measures of physiological functions that are not normally under voluntary control. In this way, the individual is able to modify their physiological response to stress. Many different measures can be used for biofeedback, but measures of cardiovascular function (heart rate, blood pressure); electromyogram (EMG); electrodermal response (EDR); and electroencephalogram are among the most commonly used. Within the context of sport performance, EMG and cardiovascular measures have been the most popular.[53]

The use of biofeedback as a tool to regulate arousal should not be confused with its use to improve muscle activation or contraction. Biofeedback is commonly used in the rehabilitation of sports injuries for this later purpose. When used in this manner, EMG biofeedback from a specific muscle or muscle group is monitored. This type of biofeedback is not considered a CAM therapy by most and will therefore not be discussed in this chapter. When biofeedback is used instead to decrease the overall level of arousal, the physiological functions that are measured are less specific. The effect of this type of biofeedback on sport performance is less clear.

Recently, a meta-analysis of biofeedback treatment for the treatment of essential hypertension was performed on 22 randomized controlled trials involving 905 hypertensive subjects published between 1966 and 2001. Compared with clinical or self-monitoring of blood pressure alone, biofeedback resulted in reductions in systolic and diastolic blood pressures that were greater by 7.3 mmHg and 5.8 mmHg, respectively. However, when compared with non-specific behavioral control groups the reductions that occurred with biofeedback were 3.9 mmHg for systolic and 3.5 mmHg for diastolic blood pressure. When a simple form of biofeedback was compared with relaxation-assisted biofeedback, only the relaxation-assisted form significantly decreased both systolic and diastolic blood pressures compared with non-specific behavioral controls. The authors concluded that further studies are needed to determine if biofeedback as a significant blood pressure lowering effect beyond the general relaxation response.[58]

Because biofeedback (unlike other relaxation techniques) requires costly and often cumbersome equipment, it would be important to investigate its relative effectiveness compared to other, less expensive, and easier to use techniques. However, this question has not been well investigated. It could be argued that this technique may be especially appealing to athletes because of its tangible and observable physiological responses. In one review of biofeedback interventions in sport, 42 studies were identified with 83% reporting improvement in arousal control, performance, or both.[59] The majority of these, however, had significant methodological concerns, including lack of appropriate control groups, and the findings should be interpreted with caution.[53]

Autogenic training

Autogenic training is a technique of self-hypnosis developed by Dr H.H. Sultz, a German neurologist. The technique consists of a series of six mental exercises used to elicit the bodily sensations of warmth and heaviness. This has the effect of producing the physiological changes of the relaxation response. The exercises should be practiced several times a day until the subject is able to shift voluntarily into this state of reduced stress. Autogenic training is the preferred mode of arousal regulation in many European countries.[53] Interpretation of the literature concerning autogenic training and sport is made nearly impossible by the usual combination of these techniques with imagery or other mental practice techniques.

Progressive relaxation

Progressive relaxation is a technique devised by Dr E. Jacobson, a physiologist and physician that emphasizes the relaxation of voluntary skeletal muscles. The individual systematically tenses and then relaxes muscles concentrating on the contrasting bodily sensations while at the same time maintaining a passive attitude. This technique seeks to achieve increased control over skeletal muscle until a subject is able to induce very low levels of tension in the major muscle groups, such as in the arms and legs. It has been suggested that, because progressive relaxation involves a more active approach to relaxation than other relaxation techniques, athletes find it more appealing.[53] However, the truth of this assumption and the effect of progressive relaxation on sport performance remain to be clarified.

Hypnosis

There remains little agreement among practitioners regarding the nature of hypnosis. Several different theoretical models exist. However, hypnosis is commonly viewed as an altered state of consciousness in which there is an increased receptivity to suggestion. Other characteristics of the hypnotic state include a high degree of absorption, dissociated cognitive control, a general fading of reality orientation, and an expectancy of experiencing the suggested goal. The purpose of clinical hypnosis is for the provider to produce a temporary change in perception, attention and concentration in the patient with the goal of producing a more long-standing change in behavior. With its possibility to alter functioning, it is not surprising that athletes have turned to hypnosis with the intent of impacting sport performance.

The hypnotic induction procedure usually includes suggestions of relaxation and drowsiness with the eyes closed in a comfortable position. Following the induction procedure, suggestions are made for the desired mental or physical behavior. The physiologic changes vary according to the suggested state. When deep relaxation is the suggested state, the physiologic changes of the relaxation response may be evoked.[55] Like many mind-body techniques, the primary use for hypnosis in medicine has been for pain management. The medical conditions, however, to which hypnosis has been applied as a treatment are extensive and include hypertension, asthma, peptic ulcer disease, irritable bowel syndrome, various dermatologic disorders, and diseases of immune function. The main effects reported tend to be an increased sense of well-being and of symptom reduction and behavioral changes.

The literature in sport psychology that supports the positive effects of hypnosis for improving performance is extremely limited. The few studies available have been criticized for poor control. Hypnotic states have been compared, however, to the phenomena of 'flow states' in sport. Flow states in sport are characterized by intrinsically enjoyable experiences that result in feelings of absorption, control and altered perceptions of time. It has been suggested, but it remains to be shown in scientific studies, that flow states could be accessed through hypnotic suggestion, which may result in improved athletic performance.[60]

MOVEMENT THERAPIES AND ALTERNATIVE FORMS OF EXERCISE

Box 23.5: Key Points

- Although there is use of alternative forms of exercise by athletes to optimize performance and speed recovery from injury, there is very little clinical evidence in the literature to guide care in both the general and athletic populations.

- Potential benefits of these alternative strategies include the mind–body integration during exercise and improved whole body integration in movement.

Yoga

Yoga is becoming an increasingly popular activity in the Western world. Many celebrities have promoted it for various purposes from its relaxation effects to maintaining or gaining physical fitness. For many in this country, yoga is thought of as simply an alternative form of physical exercise. Yoga classes are now available at most fitness facilities. However, yoga involves more than physical positions or 'postures', but rather is a philosophy that originated about 5000 years ago in India. The word yoga literally translates to mean 'yoke' or 'unity', meaning the union of mind, body and soul. The practice of yoga combines techniques that include not only the physical postures, or Hatha yoga, but also breathing exercises, meditation, and principles of living such as non-violence, truthfulness, purity and service that helps its practitioners to reach optimal levels of physical, mental and spiritual well-being.[61] Therefore, yoga can be thought of not only as an exercise for the physical body, but for the mind and spirit, as well, and its beneficial effects may overlap with those in the section on mind–body treatments discussed above.

There are many styles of yoga that exist and a complete review of these exceeds the scope of this chapter. There are several, however, which will be reviewed here in brief. Iyengar yoga is a form of yoga that places particular emphasis on the precision and accuracy of the poses and how to use them to achieve balance, symmetry and calm. For this reason, Iyengar yoga has been suggested by some experts to be particularly well-suited to those with back pain and other musculoskeletal problems.[61] Ashtanga yoga is a vigorous form of yoga in which a serious of postures are performed in relatively quick succession while synchronizing the breath. This form of yoga has been promoted as improving aerobic capacity as well as strength and flexibility. Viniyoga is a less well-known form as it is often taught in private session rather than large classes. In viniyoga, the concentration is on the individual's quest for self-realization, which is attained through poses, meditation, ritual and prayer. Bikram yoga is an additional form of yoga that has become extremely popular recently. Bikram is done in a heated room at approximately 100°F with the goal of warming the muscles to increase their flexibility. This form is generally not recommended for pregnant women or individuals with medical conditions aggravated by heat.

There is, unfortunately, a dearth of scientific medical literature available in western journals on the health benefits of yoga. A number of studies have been published in the Indian medical literature. However, there is evidence that interest in the healing power of yoga among western medical professionals is growing, but it is fair to say that the research on yoga and its potential uses for health and fitness is in its infancy in the west. Moreover, although yoga is being promoted as beneficial for athletes and is certainly being used by them, the specific effects that yoga practice may have on athletic performance remains to be shown in controlled studies. Among those promoting yoga for its benefits to athletic performance are Cleveland Browns' linebacker Orlando Ruff, who attributes improvements in his balance, flexibility and ability to concentrate on the game to his practice of Bikram yoga.

There is some evidence that yoga may be effective in treating certain painful medical conditions such as osteoarthritis and carpal tunnel syndrome. In a study evaluating a yoga regimen in patients with OA of the hands, patients were randomly assigned to receive either a yoga program performed once a week for 8 weeks or no treatment. The yoga group improved significantly more than the control group in pain during activity, tenderness and finger range of motion. Other trends also favored the yoga program.[62] It is unfortunate that an educational control group was not chosen for this study, as this would have controlled for attention effects and allowed more specific benefits to be attributed to yoga exercises.

In another study of 42 patients with carpal tunnel syndrome, subjects were randomized to either a yoga-based regimen of 11 upper body yoga postures and relaxation or wrist splinting. The yoga group performed their regimen twice weekly for 8 weeks. Subjects randomized to yoga had significant improvements noted in grip strength, pain intensity, and Phalen sign than subjects in the splinting group. No significant differences were noted between groups for sleep disturbance, Tinel's sign and median motor and sensory nerve conduction velocities.[63]

The Alexander Technique and the Feldenkrais Method

The Feldenkrais Method and the Alexander Technique are relatively modern methods of somatic education that focus on developing increased awareness of movements. In each case, the desired outcome is improvement in function and greater kinesthetic awareness. Both techniques were developed in educational rather than therapeutic models. Therefore, although many physical and occupational therapists may receive training in these methods and use them as part of a therapeutic regimen, neither technique was developed for the purpose of treating specific disorders. The practitioner and subject in each case are considered 'teacher' and 'student', rather than 'therapist' and 'patient'. The role of the teacher has been compared with that of a sports coach or music instructor. The greater awareness of movements that is gained allows the student to move more fluently and efficiently, which may help reduce pain, overuse injuries, muscle imbalances and performance difficulties.[64]

The Alexander Technique

The Alexander Technique was founded by Fredrick Matthias Alexander, an actor and teacher born in Australia in 1869. Alexander had developed chronic voice problems for which he sought treatment from various professionals without improvement. This led him to self-exploration and experimentation with head, neck and spine positioning.[65] Eventually, this led to the further development of these techniques in order to help others, especially those in the performing arts, and the refinement of these methods into what is now known as the Alexander Technique. There are more than 20 schools in the US certified to teach the Alexander Technique. The training involves approximately 1600 h and takes approximately 3–4 years. The American Society of the Alexander Technique is the primary governing organization for the method in the US.

Alexander believed that the positioning of the head, neck and spine was crucial to health and optimal functioning. He referred to this as the primary control. He also stressed the importance of inhibition of movement in altering habitual patterns. The technique involves both chair and table work. The focus is to lengthen and widen while maintaining proper positioning of the head, neck and spine. The student uses visual cues in addition to proprioceptive feedback. The practitioner provides hands-on guidance to reposition the student and demonstrate movements.[64]

There are very few well-designed trials examining the effectiveness of the Alexander Technique. One small study of elderly women showed small improvements in functional reach measures after group sessions of the Alexander technique once a week for 8 weeks compared with a no intervention control group.[66] Subjective improvements in balance, posture, and self-confidence were also noted. However, this study had multiple methodological issues, which makes interpretation of these findings difficult.

The Alexander technique is often used to improve breath and voice control and a small number of studies have focused on its effect on pulmonary parameters. In a study of 10 healthy volunteers who were evaluated with pulmonary function testing, significant increases were noted in peak expiratory flow and maximal inspiratory and expiratory mouth pressures after 20 weekly sessions of the Alexander Technique compared with a control group of healthy volunteers who did not undergo any treatment.[67] The Cochrane group, however, found no studies of sufficient strength evaluating the Alexander Technique and asthma management.[68]

Although there are theoretical benefits of this type of technique to athletes, there are no scientific studies on the effect of the Alexander Technique on athletic performance. Despite the lack of evidence, the technique continues to be used widely by performing artists, in particular.

The Feldenkrais Method

The Feldenkrais Method is a form of somatic movement education that integrates the body, mind and psyche through an educational model in which a trained Feldenkrais practitioner guides a client (the 'student') through movements with hands-on and verbally administered cues. The Feldenkrais Method teaches the student to integrate external feedback from the environment and internal feedback from within, while experiencing and directing movement.[69] The method incorporates both hands-on (Functional Integration) and verbally guided (Awareness through Movement) components that are based on sensorimotor developmental learning.

The Feldenkrais Method originated with Moshe Feldenkrais, born in Russia in 1904, who had training in the disciplines of mathematics, engineering, physics and martial arts. He developed this method while trying to recover from severe knee injuries, which he had incurred participating in soccer and judo. He was unsatisfied with the poor prognosis he had been given by the medical community. Using a neurodevelopmental approach, he taught himself to increase his awareness of his movements to avoid unneeded effort in his body. This was apparently successful in improving his function despite severe degeneration of his knee joints.

Since its origination, however, the Feldenkrais Method has been considered an educational, rather than a therapeutic tool. The emphasis is on teaching the student to increase awareness of their movements, which in turn helps them to function optimally. Because the focus is not aimed at treating specific impairments or diseases, there is very little scientific literature to support its use for medical purposes. A few small studies have examined its effects on patients with multiple sclerosis, chronic pain, and neck and shoulder pain syndromes.[69]

There have been no scientific studies examining the use of the Feldenkrais Method in athletes. However, the method has been used by athletes and performing artists to improve their skills and rehabilitate injuries. The Feldenkrais Method claims to improve coordination, balance, flexibility and power, and to thereby improve performance in sports, such as golf, tennis, skiing and swimming. Another aspect of the method that may be useful to athletes is its focus on the proximal muscles of the pelvis, upper thighs and hips as being important initiators of movement. In this way, it is similar to the disciplines of yoga, Pilates and martial arts, which are becoming more and more frequently practiced by athletes.

The Feldenkrais Guild of North America governs the Feldenkrais method in the US. After completing approximately 1200 h of training over the course of 3–4 years, the trainee is eligible to become a certified Feldenkrais practitioner.[64] The training consists of lectures and readings on the Feldenkrais method and on basic anatomy and biomechanics. The majority of the training is composed of hands-on experience; the trainee practices the technique, experiences it as a student, and observes the technique performed on others.

CONCLUSIONS

Despite the lack of research in the field, complementary and alternative medical therapies will continued to be used by recreational and high performance athletes to optimize performance, hasten recovery from intense training and performance sessions, and improve recovery from both acute and chronic injuries. In many cases, there is the suggestion in the literature that CAM therapies can indeed provide some benefit to athletes, however more research is needed to draw definitive conclusions. The ideal in the future would be that scientific evidence would bring CAM therapies into an integrated model of care for the athlete to fulfill the promise of providing a safe, drug free approach to maintaining high levels of performance over time.

REFERENCES

1. Eisenberg DM, Kessler RC, Foster C. Unconventional medicine in the United States: prevalence, costs, and patterns of use. N Engl J Med 1993; 328:246–252.

2. Eisenberg DM, Davis RB, Ettner SL, et al. Trends in alternative medicine use in the United States; 1990–1997: Results of a follow-up national survey. JAMA 1998; 280:1569–1575.

3. NIH. Complementary and alternative medicine use among adults: United States, 2002. Advance Data 2004; 343:1250–1270.

4. National Center for Complementary and Alternative Medicine. Online. Available: http://nccam.nih.gov/about/aboutnccam/idex.htm 16 Jan 2005.

5. Starkey C. Therapeutic modalities. Philadelphia, PA: Davis; 1993.

6. Callaghan MJ. The role of massage in the management of the athlete: a review. Br J Sp Med 1993; 27:28–32.

7. Cheung K, Hume PA, Maxwell L. Delayed onset muscle soreness: treatment strategies and performance factors. Sports Med 2003; 33:145–164.

8. Tiidus PM. Manual massage and recovery of muscle function following exercise: a literature review. J Sports Phys Ther 1997; 25:107–112.

9. Smith LL, Keating MN, Holbert D, et al. The effects of athletic massage on delayed onset muscle soreness, creatine kinase and neutrophil count: a preliminary report. J Orthop Sports Phys Ther 1994; 19:93–99.

10. Lightfoot JT, Char D, McDermott J, et al. Immediate post-exercise massage does not attenuate delayed onset muscle soreness. J Strength Cond Res 1997; 11:119–124.

11. Boone T, Cooper R, Thompson WR. A physiologic evaluation of the sports massage. Athletic Train 1991; 26:51–54.

12. Cherkin DC, Eisenberg D, Sherman KJ, et al. Randomized trial comparing traditional Chinese medical acupuncture, therapeutic massage, and self-care education for chronic low back pain. Arch Int Med 2001; 161:1081–1088.

13. Cherkin DC, Sherman KJ, Deyo RA, et al. A review of the evidence for the effectiveness, safety, and cost of acupuncture, massage therapy, and spinal manipulation for back pain. Ann Int Med 2003; 138:898–906.

14. Braddom RL, ed. Physical medicine and rehabilitation. Philadelphia, PA: WB Saunders; 2000.

15. NIH Consensus Development Panel of Acupuncture. NIH Consensus Conference. Acupuncture 1998; 280:1518–1524.

16. Pomeranz B, Chiu D. Nalozone blockade of acupuncture analgesia: endorphins implicated. Life Sci 1976; 19:1757–1762.

17. Mayer DJ, Price DD, Raffii A. Antagonism of acupuncture analgesia in man by narcotic antagonist naloxone. Brain Res 1977; 121:368–372.

18. Debreceni L. Chemical releases associated with acupuncture and electric stimulation. Crit Rev Phys Med 1993; 5:247–275.

19. Pomeranz B. Scientific basis of acupuncture. In: Stux G, Pomeranz B, eds. Basics of acupuncture. 4th edn. Berlin: Springer-Verlag; 1987:4–37.

20. Stein C, Machelska H, Binder W, et al. Peripheral opioid analgesia. Curr Opin Pharmacol 2001; 1:62–65.

21. Son YS, Park HJ, Kwon OB, et al. Antipyretic effect of acupuncture on the lipopolysaccharide-induced fever and expression of interleukin-6 and interleukin-1B mRNAs in the hypothalamus of rats. Neurosci Lett 2002; 319:45–48.

22. Yu Y, Kasahara T, Sato T, et al. Role of endogenous interferon-gamma on the enhancement of splenic NK cell activity by electroacupuncture stimulation in mice. J Neuroimmunol 1998; 90:176–186.

23. Kleinhenz J, Streitberger K, Windeler J, et al. Randomized clinical trial comparing the effects of acupuncture and a newly designed placebo needle in rotator cuff tendonitis. Pain 1999; 83:235–241.

24. Gilbertson B, Wenner K, Russell L. Acupuncture and arthroscopic acromioplasty. J Orthop Res 2003; 21:752–758.

25. Haker E, Lundeberg T. Acupuncture treatment in epicondylalgia: a comparative study of two acupuncture techniques. Clin J Pain 1990; 6:221–226.

26. Molsberger A, Hille E. The analgesic effect of acupuncture in chronic tennis elbow pain. Br J Rheumatol 1994; 33:1162–1165.

27. Audette JF, Ryan AH. The role of acupuncture in pain management. Phys Med Rehabil Clin N Am 2004; 15:749–772.

28. Ezzo J, Hadhazy V, Birch S, et al. Acupuncture for osteoarthritis of the knee: systematic review. Arthritis Rheum 2001; 44:819–825.

29. Berman BM, Lao L, Langenberg P, et al. Effectiveness of acupuncture as adjunctive therapy in osteoarthritis of the knee: a randomized, controlled trial. Ann Intern Med 2004; 141:901–910.

30. Kudlas MJ. Chiropractic. In: Leskowitz E, ed. Complementary and alternative medicine in rehabilitation. St Louis, MO: Churchill Livingstone; 2003:14–27.

31. Stump JL. The perceived utilization and role of sport chiropractors in the National Football League. J Neuromusc Syst 2001; 9:118–121.

32. Brynin R, Farrar K. Protocols for chiropractors treating athletes at athletic events. J Sports Chiropractic Rehab 2000; 14:16–20.

33. Kapral MK, Bondy SJ. Cervical manipulation and risk of stroke. CMAJ 2001; 165:907–908.

34. Assendelft WJ, Koes BW, Knipschild PG, Bouter LM. The relationship between methodological quality and conclusions in reviews of spinal manipulation. JAMA 1995; 274:1942–1948.

35. Giles LG, Muller R. Chronic spinal pain: a randomized clinical trial comparing medication, acupuncture, and spinal manipulation. Spine 2003; 28:1490–1503.

36. Hurwitz EL, Aker PD, Adams AH, et al. Manipulation and mobilization of the cervical spine: a systematic review of the literature. Spine 1996; 21:1746–1759.

37. Weinberg RS, Comar W. The effectiveness of psychological interventions in competitive sport. Sports Med 1994; 18:406–418.

38. Nicholi AM. Psychiatric consultation in professional football. NEJM 1986; 316:1095–1100.

39. Wolsko PM, Eisenberg DM, Davis RB, et al. Use of mind-body therapies. Results of a national survey. J Gen Int Med 2004; 19:43–50.

40. Astin JA, Shapiro SL, Eisenberg DM, et al. Mind-body medicine: State of the science, implications for practice. J Am Board Fam Pract 2003; 16:131–147.

41. Nicklaus J. Golf my way. New York: Simon & Schuster; 1974.

42. Murphy SM. Imagery interventions in sport. Med Sci Sport Exerc 1994; 26:486–494.

43. Legg SJ, Smith P, Slyfield D, et al. Knowledge and reported use of sport science by elite New Zealand Olympic Class sailors. J Sports Med Phys Fitness 1997; 37:213–217.

44. Richardson A. Mental imagery. New York: Springer; 1969.

45. Tod D, Iredale F, Gill N. 'Psyching-up' and muscular force production. Sports Med 2003; 33:47–58.

46. Shaw DF, Goodfellow R. Performance enhancement and deterioration following outcome imagery: testing a demand characteristics explanation. In: Cockerill I, Steinberg H, eds. Cognitive enhancement in sport and exercise psychology. Leicester: British Psychological Society; 1997:37–43.

47. Martin KA, Moritz SE, Hall CR. Imagery in sport: a literature review and applied model. Sport Psychol 1999; 13:245–268.

48. Taylor JA, Shaw DF. The effects of outcome imagery on golf-putting performance. J Sport Sci 2002; 20:607–613.

49. Feltz DL, Landers DM. The effects of mental practice on motor skill learning and performance: a meta-analysis. J Sport Psychol 1983; 5:25–57.

50. Peynircioglu ZF, Thompson JL, Tanielian TB. Improvement strategies in free-throw shooting and grip-strength tasks. J Gen Psych 2000; 127:145–156.

51. Kosslyn SM, Ganis G, Thompson WL. Neural foundations of imagery. Nat Rev Neurosci 2001; 2:635–642.

52. Gould D, Krane V. The arousal-athletic performance relationship: current status and future directions. In: Horn T, ed. Advances in sport psychology. Champaign, IL: Human Kinetics; 1992:119–141.

53. Gould D, Udry E. Psychological skills for enhancing performance: arousal regulation strategies. Med Sci Sport Exerc 1994; 26:478–485.

54. Hardy L, Parfitt G. A catastrophe model of anxiety and performance. Br J Psychol 1991; 82:163–168.

55. Benson H, Klipper MZ. The relaxation response. New York, NY: Avon Books; 2000.

56. Kabat-Zinn J. Full catastrophe living. New York, NY: Dell; 1990.

57. Solberg EE, Berglund K, Engern O, et al. The effect of meditation on shooting performance. Br J Sports Med 1996; 30:342–346.

58. Nakao M, Yano E, Nomura S, et al. Blood pressure-lowering effects of biofeedback treatment I hypertension: a meta-analysis of randomized controlled trials. Hypertens Res 2003; 26:37–46.

59. Zaichkowsky L, Fuchs C. Biofeedback applications in exercise and athletic performance. Exerc Sport Sci Rev 1988; 16:381–421.

60. Pates J, Maynard I. Effect of hypnosis on flow states and golf performance. Percept Mot Skills 2000; 91:1057–1075.

61. Fishman L, Ardman C. Relief is in the stretch: end back pain through yoga. New York: WW Norton & Company; 2005.

62. Garfinkel MS, Schumacher HR, Husain A, et al. Evaluation of a yoga based regimen for treatment of osteoarthritis of the hands. J Rheumatol 1994; 21:2341–2343.

63. Garfinkel MS, Singhal A, Katz WA, et al. Yoga-based intervention for carpal tunnel syndrome: a randomized trial. JAMA 1998; 280:1601–1603.

64. Jain S, Janssen K, DeCelle S. Alexander Technique and Feldenkrais Method: a critical overview. Phys Med Rehabil Clin N Am 2004; 15:811–825.

65 Brennan R. The Alexander Technique: a practical introduction. Shaftesbury: Element; 1998.

66 Dennis RJ. Functional reach improvement in normal older women after Alexander technique instruction. J Gerontol Med Sci 1999; 54a:M8–M11.

67 Austin JH, Ausubel P. Enhanced respiratory muscular function in normal adults after lesion in proprioceptive musculoskeletal education without exercises. Chest 1992; 102:486–490.

68 Cates DJ. Alexander technique for chronic asthma. The Cochrane Database of Systematic Reviews; 1999.

69 Cheever O, Cohen LJ. The Feldenkrais Method. In: Leskowitz E, ed. Complementary and alternative medicine in rehabilitation. St Louis, MO: Churchill Livingstone; 2003:39–50.

SECTION 3

Specific Injuries by Anatomical Location

CHAPTER 24

Athletic Head Injuries

Robert V. Cantu and Robert C. Cantu

INTRODUCTION

Sport induced head injuries have received increasing attention over the past decade. This attention is due in part to the early retirement of well-known professional athletes such as Steve Young, Troy Aikman, Pat Lafontaine, Merrill Hodge and others who have sustained multiple concussions. There is an increasing awareness of the frequency and effects of head injury in sports. This chapter will provide information to help physicians, coaches and trainers to diagnose, treat and hopefully prevent head injuries in athletes.

EPIDEMIOLOGY

Sporting activities account for an estimated 20% of the 1.54 million head injuries each year in the US.[1] High school football alone accounts for about 250,000 brain injuries each year.[1] Approximately 1 in 20 high school football players sustain a concussion in a given season.[2] Fatality due to head injury in high school football is most commonly due to a subdural hematoma (74.4%).[2] Between 1980 and 1993, 35 football players succumbed to the second impact syndrome.[2]

Although the overall number of head injuries is highest in football, many other sports pose a risk for head injury (Table 24.1). During a single season of Canadian intercollegiate ice hockey, the incidence of concussion was 1.55 per 1000 athletic exposures.[2] Concussion rates among college soccer players are estimated to be about 1 per 3000 athletic exposures.[3] Concussions occur in many other sports including wrestling, lacrosse, motor sports, cycling, diving, basketball, baseball, field hockey, gymnastics, rugby, volley ball, track and field and softball. One study sampling students from a boarding school with mandatory sports participation, reported that 97% of athletes aged 14–19 years had sustained at least one sports related concussion.[3]

Concussion is a common injury at the professional level. In the National Football League, it is estimated that 100 to 120 concussions occur per year, or about one every two to three games. In professional soccer, 52% of players have reported at least one concussion in their career.[3] The National Hockey League (NHL) has seen an increase in the number of concussions, with the rate from 1997–2002 more than triple that of the preceding decade.[4] Multiple theories have been proposed for the increase, such as bigger, faster players, new equipment, and harder boards and glass. Fortunately, the rate has reached a plateau since 1997, which was the year the NHL instituted its concussion program.

There is some evidence to suggest that younger athletes may be at higher risk for concussion. For example, the concussion rate for collegiate soccer players is estimated at 1 per 3000 athletic exposures, while the rate for high school players has been reported at 1 per 2000 exposures. Among Canadian amateur hockey players aged 15 to 20, 60% have reported sustaining a concussion during either a practice or a game. Authors have expressed concern that injury during adolescence may impair the plasticity of the developing brain.[5]

The National Athletic Trainers' Association study found gender differences in regard to concussion rates. In high school sports, females were found to be at higher risk for sustaining a concussion than males competing in the same sport. The rate in soccer was 1.14 concussions per 100 player-seasons in females and 0.92 per 100 player-seasons in males. In basketball, females had a rate of 1.04 concussions per 100 player-seasons, while males had a rate of 0.75 per 100 player-seasons, and in softball, the rate was 0.46 for females and 0.23 for males. This trend does not remain at all levels. At the collegiate level, the concussion rate for soccer and basketball players appears to be nearly identical. At the Olympic level, 89% of male and 43% of female soccer players have reported a prior history of concussion.[5]

TRAUMATIC BRAIN INJURIES

Concussion

Box 24.1: Key Points

- A concussion is a trauma-induced change in mental status that may or may not involve loss of consciousness.

- Neurochemical and structural brain changes can occur following a concussion.

- Grading of concussions helps to define severity and return to play decisions.

- Athlete should not return to competition when still symptomatic.

Definition/diagnosis

The most common head injury sustained by an athlete is a concussion. Multiple definitions of concussion exist. The word itself is derived from the Latin verb *concussus*, which means 'to shake violently'.[5] The Committee on Head Injury Nomenclature of the Congress of Neurological Surgeons defines concussion as 'a clinical syndrome characterized by immediate and transient post-traumatic impairment of neural function, such as alteration of consciousness, disturbance of vision, equilibrium, etc. due to brainstem involvement'.[3] As Kelly has stated, a concussion is a 'trauma-induced alteration in mental status that may or may not involve loss of consciousness'.[2] The American Orthopaedic Society for Sports Medicine defines concussion as 'any alteration in cerebral function caused by a direct or indirect (rotation) force transmitted to the head resulting in one or more of the following acute signs and symptoms: a brief loss of consciousness, light-headedness, vertigo, cognitive and memory dysfunction, tinnitus, blurred vision, difficulty concentrat-

ing, amnesia, headache, nausea, vomiting, photophobia, or balance disturbance. Delayed signs and symptoms may also include sleep irregularities, fatigue, personality changes, inability to perform usual daily activities, depression, or lethargy' (Table 24.2).[2]

Pathophysiology

Although some have suggested that a concussion is a physiologic disturbance without structural damage, animal and human data have shown that neurochemical and structural changes with loss of brain cells can occur. A neurochemical cascade begins within minutes following a concussion and can continue for days. It is during this period that neurons remain in a vulnerable state, susceptible to minor changes in cerebral blood flow, increase in intracranial pressure and anoxia.[6] Animal studies have shown that during this susceptible period, a decrease in cerebral blood flow that normally would have little consequence can produce extensive neuronal cell death.[4]

Following a concussion or minor traumatic brain injury, disruption of the neuronal cell membrane, stretching of axons, and opening of potassium channels lead to an efflux of potassium out of affected neurons.[3] Depolarization of neurons leads to release of glutamate, which further induces an efflux of potassium. The extracellular potassium leads to a release of excitatory amino acids and further depolarization, both serving to further increase extracellular potassium. Increased ATP is required to restore the imbalance in potassium and membrane potential. Glucose utilization increases, leading to a state of hyperglycolysis that in rat studies lasts several hours but in

Table 24.1 1989–1998 NCAA Injury Surveillance System Concussion Data

	Concussion as a percentage of all game injuries
Sports with head protection	
Ice hockey	7.5
Men's lacrosse	5.2
Football	4.5
Softball	3.6
Baseball	2.7
Sports without head protection	
Field hockey	13.0
Women's soccer	11.0
Men's soccer	9.0
Women's lacrosse	8.5
Women's basketball	8.0
Wrestling	4.3
Men's basketball	3.1

Data from the National Collegiate Athletic Association (NCAA) official website: http://www2.ncaa.org

Table 24.2 Post Concussion Signs/Symptoms

'Bell rung'
Depression
Dinged
Dizziness
Excess Sleep
Fatigue
Feeling 'in a fog'
Feeling 'slowed down'
Headache
Inappropriate emotions or personality changes
Loss of consciousness
Loss of orientation
Memory problems
Nausea
Nervousness
Numbness/tingling
Poor balance/coordination
Poor concentration, easily distracted
Ringing in the ears
Sadness
Seeing stars
Sensitivity to light
Sensitivity to noise
Sleep disturbance
Vacant stare/glassy eyed
Vomiting

humans may last significantly longer. Lactate levels increase, which can cause neuronal damage and lead to increased vulnerability to cell damage.[3]

Following a concussive injury to the brain, there is an influx of calcium into neuronal cells. Elevated intracellular calcium may activate proteases and cause cell damage or death. Oxidative phosphorylation slows, which results in decreased ATP availability and further increase in glycolysis. Cerebral blood flow has been seen to decrease 50% following concussion. This drop may further impair the neurons' ability to maintain a normal electrolyte balance.[3]

Injured cells also see a decrease in intracellular magnesium, which may not return to normal for 4 days. Decreased magnesium can cause a further influx of calcium. It is also associated with impairment of glycolysis, oxidative phosphorylation, and protein synthesis.[3]

Electrolyte imbalance usually returns to normal by 4 days post-concussion. In the hours to weeks following injury, damage may be seen in both the microtubule and neurofilament structure.[3] Structural changes may occur, such as focal axonal swelling and axonal bulbs. This swelling is also referred to as a 'retraction bulb', as the axonal ending appears severed from its distal segment, and is characteristic of diffuse axonal injury.[7]

Classification

Several attempts have been made to classify concussions based on their severity, with guidelines for return to play. The most commonly used classifications have three grades, with a type 1 described as mild, type 2 as moderate and type 3 as severe. The classification schemes vary somewhat, but are all based on clinical presentation of the athlete and duration of symptoms. Table 24.3 provides a comparison of two commonly used classifications. The Cantu classification is evidence based and requires the resolution of symptoms before final grading is made.[8]

Treatment

On the field, treatment of athletic head injuries begins with preparation, including having appropriate personnel and equipment available. For the unconscious athlete, full spine precautions should be followed, including use of a spine board and cervical collar. Maintaining an adequate airway is of primary concern. The face mask should be removed and if there is respiratory compromise, on the field intubation may be required. Continuous blood pressure monitoring is performed and cardiopulmonary resuscitative equipment should be available if needed. The shoulder pads should be loosened in the front to allow for chest compressions and defibrillation. For those patients in whom a spine injury is suspected, the Inter-Association Task Force for Appropriate Care of the Spine-Injured Athlete has outlined four instances in which the athletic helmet and chin strap should be removed (Table 24.4).[9]

The awake athlete for whom cervical spine injury has been ruled out can be helped to a sitting position. If stable in the sitting position, the athlete may be helped off the field for more detailed examination. A neurologic examination should include an assessment of level of consciousness, speech, balance, memory (antegrade and retrograde and to event), and orientation to person, place and time. Athletes should not return to play until symptoms have resolved both at rest and with exertion, such as running a sideline sprint. The primary focus is preventing a second impact that could have more severe consequences. One recent study found that some high school athletes whose symptoms were thought to have cleared quickly post concussion, scored below their baseline on neuropsychologic testing at 48 h, suggesting that perhaps no athlete with a documented concussion should return to play the same day.[10]

The use of neuropsychologic testing has received increasing attention. Given the wide variation among individuals on these tests, it is necessary to have a preseason baseline evaluation for comparison after a traumatic brain injury. A decline in neuropsychologic test results has been shown to correlate with severity of post-concussive symptoms at 1 week post-injury.[10]

Return to play decision

Because the subject does not lend itself to prospective, randomized studies, the guidelines for return to play after a concussion are based largely on retrospective analysis and judgment. A primary goal is to avoid secondary injury such as a more severe concussion or worse yet a second impact

Table 24.4   Instances When Athletic Helmet Should be Removed in the Head-Injured Patient

1	If the helmet and chin strap do not hold the head securely, such that immobilization of the helmet fails to immobilize the head
2	If the design of the helmet prevents adequate airway management even after removal of the face mask
3	If the face mask cannot be removed in a reasonable amount of time
4	If the helmet prevents immobilization for transportation in an appropriate position

Table 24.3   Classification Schemes for Concussion

	Mild: Grade 1	Moderate: Grade 2	Severe: Grade 3
Cantu	No loss of consciousness Post-traumatic amnesia <30 min Post-concussive signs/symptoms >30 min but <7 days	Loss of consciousness <1 min Post-traumatic amnesia >30 min but <24 h Post-concussive signs/symptoms >7 days	Loss of consciousness >1 min Post-traumatic amnesia >24 h
American Academy of Neurology	Transient confusion; no LOC; symptoms or abnormalities resolve in <15 min	Transient confusion; no LOC; symptoms or abnormalities last >15 min	Any LOC

syndrome. It is for this reason that athletes who remain symptomatic after even a grade 1 concussion should not return to play. Another goal is to prevent the long-term effects of multiple minor traumatic brain injuries that can lead to permanent changes such as the classic description of 'dementia pugilistica' seen in boxers. It is with these aims in mind that the guidelines in Table 24.5 were developed.

Factors other than the concussion severity must be weighed in the return to play decision. The athlete's concussion history, including total number, time between injuries, and severity of the blow causing the concussion, are important factors. When making the return to play decision, one should consider all pieces of the concussion puzzle and when in doubt, err on the side of caution; 'If in doubt, sit them out'.

A relatively recent finding is that athletes who possess the apolipoprotein E4 allele (APOE4) may be at increased risk following minor traumatic brain injuries. This allele is already known to correlate with the incidence of Alzheimer's disease. There is increasing evidence that patients who have the APOE4 allele have a worse outcome following head injury and may be predisposed to earlier onset of dementia after repetitive concussions.[11] Knowing an athlete has this allele may factor into the retirement decision after head injury.

Guidelines for return to play after concussion are developed in part to protect the injured brain from further insult as well as to try to minimize the cumulative effects that multiple concussions can cause. Boxing is perhaps most recognized for this with fighters having been described as permanently 'punch drunk' or suffering from 'dementia pugilistica'. The cumulative effects of minor traumatic head injuries are becoming better understood in many other sports as well. Athletes who have sustained prior concussions appear more prone to future head injury, often with less force required to cause impairment. In one prospective study of high school football players, those players that had sustained three prior concussions were 9.3 times more likely to demonstrate on-field signs such as loss of consciousness, anterograde amnesia, and confusion with a concussion compared to players sustaining their first concussion.[9]

Age may play a role in outcome following concussion, even between high school and college age athletes. In one prospective study, high school athletes with concussion showed prolonged memory dysfunction compared with college athletes with concussion. By 3 days post-concussion, the college athletes scored similar to age matched controls on neuropsychologic testing. At 7 days post-concussion, the high school athletes still scored below age-matched controls.[12] The exact cause for this age difference is not fully understood. Children have shown a more diffuse and prolonged cerebral swelling following traumatic brain injury compared with adults. It is hypothesized that the immature brain is more sensitive to excitotoxic brain injury and may show prolonged metabolic dysautoregulation.[13]

The grading of concussions serves as a guideline for return to play, but is clearly open to individual variation and clinical judgment. Duration of post-traumatic amnesia is one factor in the Cantu scale of concussions. In one study, the athlete's self reported memory problems at 24 h post-concussion were an indicator of the severity of the concussion. Athletes who reported memory problems on the follow-up examination, in general had longer duration of symptoms, scored worse on neurocognitive tests and had more overall symptoms.[13] All post-concussion signs and symptoms are important as is their duration, thus grading of a concussion should ideally await resolution of symptoms.

Second impact syndrome

> ### Box 24.2: Key Points
>
> - Second impact syndrome occurs in athletes still symptomatic from a prior, often minor head injury.
> - Pathophysiology believed due to a loss of vasoregulatory control in the brain resulting in massive swelling.
> - Treatment is limited and prevention is key.

Table 24.5 Guideline for Return to Play after Concussion

Grade 1	Grade 2	Grade 3
First concussion		
Athlete may return to play that day in select situations if clinical examination results are normal at rest and with exertion, otherwise return to play in 1 week	Athlete may return to play in 2 weeks if asymptomatic at rest and with exertion for 7 days	Athlete may return to play in 1 month if asymptomatic at rest and exertion for 7 days
Second concussion		
Return to play in 2 weeks if asymptomatic for 1 week	Minimum of 1 month; may return to play then if asymptomatic for 1 week; consider terminating season	Terminate season; may return to play next season if asymptomatic
Third concussion		
Terminate season; may return to play next season if asymptomatic	Terminate season; may return to play next season if asymptomatic	

Pathophysiology

A term first defined by Schneider is the second impact syndrome.[14] This syndrome occurs in an athlete who has sustained an initial head injury, most often a concussion, and returns to play while still symptomatic and sustains a second head injury. The second impact to the symptomatic brain can result in a loss of cerebral autoregulation, leading to rapid cerebral vascular congestion, increased intracranial pressure and brain herniation.[14] The condition typically occurs in adolescents aged 14–16 and is uncommon in adults. It appears to have a common pathophysiology with the 'diffuse cerebral swelling' or 'malignant brain edema' syndrome of children.

Diagnosis

Second impact syndrome typically results in a rapid decline in mental status and neurologic function. The second impact is often relatively minor, distinguishing it from other severe brain injuries such as intracranial bleeding or diffuse axonal shear. It may only be appreciated in retrospect, that the athlete was still symptomatic or suffering from post-concussive symptoms at the time of the second injury.

Treatment

Second impact syndrome requires immediate medical and sometimes surgical treatment. The main effort is to limit the severe increase in intracranial hypertension. Treatment can begin on the field with intubation and mild hyperventilation, reverse Trendelenburg positioning, and intravenous mannitol, all in an attempt to decrease intracranial pressure. On arrival at a medical facility, CT scanning should be performed to rule out other causes of rapid neurologic dysfunction, such as intracranial hemorrhage. Other medical treatments include use of barbiturates for neuroprotection and newer pharmaceutical agents such as 21-aminosteroid tirilazad mesylate. Surgical treatment is limited, but bifrontal decompressive craniectomy has been performed in refractory cases.

SEVERE TRAUMATIC BRAIN INJURY

Box 24.2: Key Points

- Approach to unconscious athlete follows the ABCs of the Advanced Trauma Life Support (ATLS) guidelines.
- Intracerebral hematoma and diffuse axonal injury result from high energy forces to the brain.
- Intracranial bleeding requires prompt diagnosis and sometimes surgical treatment.

Pathophysiology

The pathophysiology of severe traumatic brain injury can be divided into several categories: primary injury, secondary injury, inflammatory response and repair/regeneration process. The primary injury results from the initial insult to the brain during which neurons may be lost due to the physical force imparted on the cells. Secondary injury develops over minutes to hours to days and is often related to the severity of the initial impact. Expanding intracranial hematomas can also lead to secondary injury to brain cells. The inflammatory response is the first step in the body's attempt to repair the injury, but if too severe can lead to further damage. In severe traumatic brain injury, ischemia can lead to a release of oxygen free radicals. Stimulation of cyclooxygenase, monoamine oxidase, and nitric oxide synthase can result in the production of oxygen free radicals, which can cause cell membrane damage through lipid peroxidation and result in release of arachidonic acid. Production of leukotrienes and thromboxane B2 from the arachidonic acid cascade has been shown to cause neurodegeneration and result in poor outcomes in experimental models. Animal studies have used ibuprofen and indomethacin, inhibitors of cyclooxygenase, to limit the arachidonic acid cascade. These compounds have been shown to improve cerebral metabolism and reduce neurologic dysfunction in mice following brain injury.[7]

Diagnosis

Severe traumatic brain injury may take the form of a focal intracranial hematoma or a more generalized injury such as diffuse axonal injury. Both injuries typically result from high energy forces to the skull and brain, seen more commonly in sports such as auto racing or sometimes in boxing. The location of the hematoma results in the descriptive name: epidural, subdural, intracerebral.

Epidural hematomas result from bleeding above the dura, most commonly from laceration of the middle meningeal artery. Following the initial injury, the athlete may be rendered unconscious. Classically a 'lucent interval' may follow, where the person regains consciousness, followed again by rapid loss of neurologic function and consciousness as the hematoma expands resulting in increasing intracranial pressure. Diagnosis is confirmed by the characteristic appearance on CT scan (Fig. 24.1).

Subdural hematomas result from bleeding between the dura and the brain and typically arise from tearing of the venous connections between these two layers. The athlete again is usually rendered unconscious by the blow to the head, but unlike the epidural hematoma there is not commonly a lucent period. The expanding hematoma can cause rapid deterioration of neurologic status. Diagnosis is also confirmed by the appearance on CT scan (Fig. 24.1).

Intracerebral hematomas may occur in multiple areas in the brain, but most commonly in the frontal and temporal lobes.[15] Bleeding occurs from direct rupture of intracerebral vessels. Intracerebral hematomas can also occur from non-traumatic sources such as a hypertensive bleed or rupture of an aneurysm. CT scan will confirm the diagnosis (Fig. 24.1).

Diffuse axonal injury leads to 35% of all deaths after head injury and is the most common cause of the vegetative state and severe disability until death.[16] Rotational forces to the brain can result in a shearing injury to the nerve fibers at the time of injury. The amount of energy required to cause such an injury most commonly occurs in motor vehicle crashes. CT scan and MRI will show characteristic diffuse brain injury.

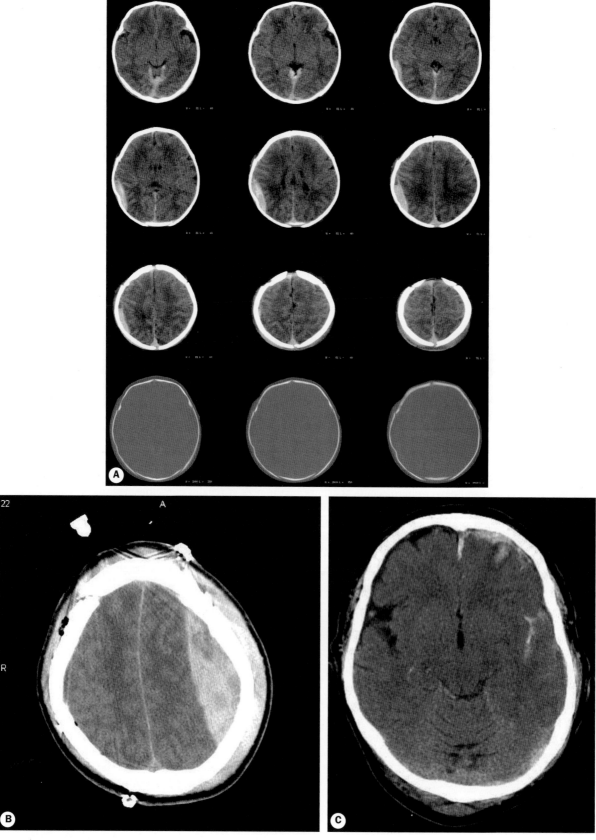

Figure 24.1 (A) CT scan appearance of epidural hematoma. (B) CT scan appearance of subdural hematoma. (C) CT scan appearance of subarachnoid hematoma.

Treatment

The initial approach to an unconscious athlete is similar to that for any traumatized patient and the ABCs of the ATLS guidelines should be followed. It is important to assume the athlete also sustained a neck injury until proven otherwise and spine precautions should be followed. The face mask on football helmets can be removed, but usually the rest of the helmet is left on and used to help stabilize the neck.

Athletes who have sustained a prolonged loss of consciousness, or exhibit neurologic deficits should be triaged to a medical center for further evaluation. Abbreviated neurologic exams such as the Glasgow Coma Scale are useful in predicting outcome after a severe head injury (Table 24.6). On arrival at a medical center a full neurologic exam should be performed including assessment of mental status, speech, memory, motor and sensory function, cranial nerve function, and reflexes (normal and abnormal). Computerized tomography scan is helpful in the evaluation of potential intracranial hemorrhage and skull fracture. An MRI study will identify more diffuse injury, such as diffuse axonal shear.

Medical/surgical treatment

The first step in medical treatment is making an accurate diagnosis. What at first may appear to be a relatively minor head injury, may actually be a developing subdural or epidural hematoma. If an athlete is suspected to have sustained such an injury, he should be triaged to the closest medical center that provides neurosurgical services. Measures to help control brain swelling such as mild hyperventilation, reverse Trendelenburg positioning, and intravenous mannitol may be used. Intracranial hematomas may require prompt craniotomy and removal, but their treatment is beyond the scope of this chapter.

Table 24.6   Glasgow Coma Scale

Sign	Evaluation	Score
Eye opening (E)	Spontaneous	4
	To speech	3
	To pain	2
	None	1
Best motor response (M)	Obeys	6
	Localizes	5
	Withdraws	4
	Decorticate	3
	Decerebrate	2
	None	1
Verbal response (V)	Oriented	5
	Confused conversation	4
	Inappropriate words	3
	Incomprehensible sounds	2
	None	1

Total EMV score by adding best response in each category. Range from 3–15.

CHRONIC BRAIN INJURY

> ### Box 24.2: Key Points
>
> - Chronic brain injury has been described primarily in boxers.
> - Advanced structural brain changes can occur over time.
> - Prevention is the best treatment.

Boxing, more than any other sport, lends itself to the study of chronic brain injury. Repetitive, relatively low-energy blows to the head over time can result in chronic injury and manifest as the 'punch drunk' condition or 'dementia pugulistica'.[17] The term 'punch drunk' was coined by Martland in 1928.[17] He described some of the symptoms as 'uncertainty in equilibrium' and 'periods of mental confusion'. As the disease advances 'slowing of muscular movements' and 'tremors of the hands' were noted, with more advanced stages leading to a parkinsonian state with encephalopathy.

Pathophysiology

Repetitive blows to the head can eventually lead to advanced structural changes in the brain. Studies on former boxers have shown the rate of traumatic encephalopathy to range from 17–50%, with number of fights and age contributing factors.[18,19] Changes found at autopsy may include such findings as a fenestrated cavum septum pellucidum, neurofibrillary tangles, amyloid angiopathy, neuritic plaques as seen in Alzheimer's disease, and degenerative changes in the substantia nigra similar to those in parkinsonism.

Diagnosis

Athletes who develop chronic brain injury typically have a history of repetitive minor head injuries. One of the earliest symptoms of traumatic encephalopathy is memory loss. Corsellis has correlated memory loss in boxers to the degree of temporal lobe neurofibrillary tangle formation.[20] Detailed neuropsychological testing can reveal early signs of brain injury, especially if a decline in scores is noted over time. In one study of 15 former and current professional fighters, the majority tested showed abnormalities on at least half of the tests in a detailed battery.[21] Other studies that may prove helpful include neuroradiographic imaging and electroencephalogram studies. As mentioned previously, boxers with the apolipoprotein E4 allele appear at higher risk for chronic brain injury.

Treatment

The mainstay of treatment for chronic brain injury is prevention. By following fighters with serial neuropsychological exams and when indicated, imaging with MRI, early signs of brain injury can be detected. Once advanced changes have occurred, there currently is little in the way of treatment that can change the course of the disease.

CONCLUSION

The ultimate goal when discussing athletic head injuries is prevention. The increased attention on head injuries in sports has made athletes, trainers, physicians and fans more aware of the potential dangers of brain injury in sports. Football was one of the first sports to focus on prevention of head and neck injury as evidenced by the rule change in 1976 prohibiting initial contact with the head (spear tackling). The number of fatalities due to head injuries in football has declined from a high of 162 during the 10 year span of 1965–1974 to a low of 32 during the 10 years of 1985–1994.

Other sports are attempting to decrease head injuries by means of rule changes, improved protective equipment, and better data collection to analyze outcomes. The National Hockey League began data collection on head injury when it instituted its concussion program in 1997.[4] Improved equipment such as the Bull Tough helmet (Bull Tough, Seguin, TX)

seems to help decrease the incidence of head injury in professional and amateur bull riders.[22] Equally important is the increasing realization by athletes that returning to competition while symptomatic from a concussion could lead to significant worsening of their symptoms and even second impact syndrome.

In conclusion, head injury is prevalent in many sports, with football resulting in the highest overall number per year in the US. What may seem to be a minor injury, such as a grade 1 concussion, can cause metabolic and potentially structural changes in the brain, making it more susceptible to further insult. Appropriate identification and on the field management of head injured athletes can limit further injury. There appears to be age and gender related differences in the rate and severity of head injury in athletics. Through increased data collection and analysis, rule changes, education and equipment development, hopefully the incidence of head injury in athletics will decline.

REFERENCES

1   McKeever CK, Schatz P. Current issues in the identification, assessment, and management of concussions in sports-related injuries. Appl Neuropsychol 2003; 10:4–11.
2   Grindel SH. Epidemiology and pathophysiology of minor traumatic brain injury. Curr Sports Med Rep 2003; 2:18–23.
3   Cooper MT, McGee KM, Anderson DG. Epidemiology of athletic head and neck injuries. Clin Sports Med 2003; 22:427–443.
4   Wennberg RA, Tator CH. National Hockey League reported concussions, 1986–1987 to 2001-2. Can J Neurol Sci 2003; 30:206–209.
5   Cantu RC. Recurrent athletic head injury: risks and when to retire. Clin Sports Med 2003; 22:593–603.
6   Echemendia RJ, Cantu RC. Return to play following sports-related mild traumatic brain injury: the role of neuropsychology. Appl Neuropsychol 2003; 10:48–55.
7   Okonkwo DO, Stone JR. Basic science of closed head injuries and spinal cord injuries. Clin Sports Med 2003; 22:467–481.
8   Cantu R. Concussion severity should not be determined until all post concussion symptoms have abated. Lancet Neurol 2004; :3437–3438.
9   Collins MW, Lovell MR, Iverson GL, et al. Cumulative effects of concussion in high school athletes. Neurosurgery 2003; 51:1175–1179.
10 Lovell MR, Collins MW, Iverson GL, et al. Grade 1 or 'Ding' concussions in high school athletes. AJSM 2003; 32:1–8.
11 Webbe FM, Barth JT. Short-term and long-term outcome of athletic closed head injuries. Clin Sports Med 2003; 22:577–592.

12 Field M, Collins MW, Lovell MR, et al. Does age play a role in recovery from sports-related concussion? A comparison of high school and collegiate athletes. J Pediatr 2003; 142:546–553.
13 Erlanger D, Kaushik T, Cantu RC, et al. Symptom-based assessment of the severity of a concussion. J Neurosurg 2003; 98:477–484.
14 Schneider RC. Head and neck injuries in football: mechanisms, treatment, and prevention. Baltimore: Williams and Wilkins; 1973.
15 Bullock R, Teasdale G. Surgical management of traumatic intracranial hematomas. In: Braackman R, ed. Handbook of clinical neurology, Vol 15: Head injury. Amsterdam: Elsevier Science; 1990:249–298.
16 McLellan DR, Adams JH, Graham DI. The structural basis of the vegetative state and prolonged coma after non-missile head injury. In: Papa I, Cohadon F, Massarotti M, eds. Le coma traumatique. Padova: Liviana Editrice; 1986:165.
17 Martland HS. Punch drunk. JAMA 1928; 91:1103–1107.
18 Roberts AH. Brain damage in boxers. London: Pitman; 1969.
19 Johnson J. Organic psychosyndrome due to boxing. Br J Psychiatry 1969; 115:45–53.
20 Corsellis JAN, Bruton CJ, Freeman-Browne D. The aftermath of boxing. Psychol Med 1973; 3:270–303.
21 Casson IR, Sham R, Campbell EA, et al. Neurological and CT evaluation of knocked-out boxers. J Neurol Neurosurg Psychiatry 1982; 45:170–174.
22 Brandenburg MA, Archer P. Survey analysis to assess the effectiveness of the bull tough helmet in preventing head injuries in bull riders: a pilot study. Clin J Sport Med 2002; 12:360–366.

CHAPTER 25

Neck Injuries

Mark R. Proctor and Robert C. Cantu

INTRODUCTION

The cervical spine brings a relatively unique set of issues to sports medicine. Unlike many other athletic injuries that predominantly affect the musculoskeletal system, neck injuries combine the challenge of a musculoskeletal injury with the potential risk of severe neurological injury. Therefore, although it may be permissible to play through the pain with an extremity injury, it is usually unsafe to return to play with neck pain until the treating medical team is absolutely certain that the vertebral column is stable and the spinal cord is not at risk. This crossover between the orthopedic and neurological implications of spine injury explains why both musculoskeletal specialties like orthopedic surgery and physiatry, as well as neurological surgeons, are often involved in the care of the spine injured patient.

The spinal cord, the most noteworthy inhabitant of the cervical spine, is (1) largely incapable of repair and regeneration and (2) serves vital functions for the individual. All neuronal transmission between the brain and extra-cranial peripheral nervous system pass through the cervical spine. The other major neck components that are susceptible to traumatic injuries in athletes are the major vascular supply to the brain, the vertebral and carotid arteries. As a result, both paralysis and stroke can occur from neck injuries. Therefore, although injuries to the cervical spine occur less frequently than other sports-related injuries, like head injury they can have a major impact on the affected individual and the sport. Sports-related injuries of the head and neck receive substantial public attention and are responsible for some of the most catastrophic athletic injuries seen, causing 70% of traumatic deaths and 20% of permanent disability related to sports.[1] In this chapter, we shall review the epidemiology of neck injuries, basic pathophysiologic mechanisms of injury, prevention, treatment and criteria for return to play of the athlete after suffering a neck injury.

EPIDEMIOLOGY

In today's society, more people are participating in athletics. As participation increases, so does the incidence of cervical injuries. Fortunately, most of the cervical injuries seen in sports are minor, and most athletes can be returned to full function.[2]

The incidence of traumatic central nervous system injury related to the spine is estimated to be 150–500 cases per 100 000 population. The percentage of these injuries related to sporting activities is thought to be 3–25%.[3] This affects both adults and children, with indications that sports-injuries may be associated with a higher injury severity in children. In a study of a large group of pediatric patients admitted for trauma, compared with non-sports injuries, sports injuries resulted in 4-fold more neck injuries.[4]

Gender differences regarding injuries of the cervical spine have not been well established but seem to follow certain patterns. It has been reported that cervical strain injuries are more prevalent in female athletes than male athletes. Male to female incidence is approximately equal in the category of herniated discs. In the category of major structural injury, studies to date have shown a significant male preponderance.[5] With increasing participation of women in contact sports that cause major structural injury, a greater incidence of these injuries may be seen in women.

Type of activity certainly has an impact on risk of neck injury. Although contact and collision sports certainly contribute to neck injuries, they can occur in a wide variety of sports. Although the injuries most visible in the public eye often occur in organized and professional sports, the majority of sports-related spine injuries appear to occur during unsupervised activities such as diving,[6] surfing and skiing.[7] These tend to be sporadic and less widely publicized, likely leading to an underestimation of the magnitude of the problem. In Japan, an extensive review of sports-related spinal cord injuries revealed a rate of 1.95 per million per annum, with the causes in order of decreasing frequency being diving, skiing, football, sky sports, judo and gymnastics. A total of 35% of patients had complete spinal injury, and 56% had related bony injury.[8]

Certain trends are prevalent with regard to sports-related injuries. It has been observed that the risk of serious spine injury in organized sports generally increases with age. Football is an excellent example of this. There is virtually no quadriplegia at the Pop Warner level (5–16 year olds), but the incidence steadily rises from junior high to high school, college and the professional level. This is because at young ages, the force of impact, a product of the individual's weight and speed, is low compared with skeletally mature participants.[9] Clearly, many of today's professional level athletes are so fast and strong that the spine could never stand the full force of a direct impact. Therefore, changes in rules and style of play are the cornerstone of protection in the current era. Protective equipment has generally not been effective at reducing cervical spine injuries.

ORGANIZED SPORTS

Box 25.1: Key Points

- Football, gymnastics, ice hockey and wrestling all have similar rates of neck injury, although in absolute numbers, football predominates in the US due to the greater number of players.

- Technique and rules changes are the most effective way to decrease the risk of spine injury. Equipment changes are less effective.

- Recreational sports like equestrian, skiing, diving and trampoline have all been associated with catastrophic neck injury.

The National Center for Catastrophic Sports Injury Research (NCCSIR) is an organization funded by the National Collegiate Athletes Association to reduce fatalities and catastrophic injuries of the head and neck in organized sports by analyzing the epidemiologic and medical data, and then recommending appropriate rules, conditioning and medical changes. Data from this organization reveals that the four sports with the highest risk of head and spine injury per 100 000 participants are football, gymnastics, ice hockey[10,11] and wrestling.[12] Although there is no statistically significant difference between the four on an incidence per 100 000 participants basis, the absolute numbers of severe head and spine injuries are highest in football because 1 800 000 youths play football annually and less than 100 000 participate in each of the other sports.

According to data from the NCCSIR, a total of 128 football players incurred permanent cervical cord injuries from 1977 through 1989. Defensive players are at greater risk for quadriplegia than offensive players, and most are injured while tackling. They recommend that to further reduce catastrophic spine injuries, players must stop using the head as a battering ram, and use the shoulder for blocking and tackling instead.[13] At high school level most cervical spine fatalities are related to football players either tackling or being tackled in a game, and almost all are fractures, dislocations or fracture-dislocations.[14] Fortunately, the trend has been improving over time. Education regarding the fundamental techniques of the game, new equipment standards, and improved medical care both on and off the playing field have led to a 270% reduction in permanent spinal cord injury from a peak of 20/year during the period 1971–1975 to 7.2 per year during the 1990s.[15] The incidence of football-related quadriplegia has decreased from a peak of 13 cases per 1 million players between 1976 and 1980,

to 3 per million from 1991 to 1993, mostly as a result of systematic research and an organized effort to eliminate high-risk behavior.[16]

Although devastating neck injuries are fortunately rare, the incidence of cervical injuries in general is relatively high. Based on a study of high school and college football players and coaches, the incidence of roentgenographic evidence of neck injuries was as high as 32% and was related to years of experience. Injury was most likely to occur to a linebacker or a defensive halfback when they tackled the ball carrier.[17] These same authors followed a single school longitudinally over 8 years and found 29% of all players in the study group sustained a head or neck injury during their college careers. The probability of a subsequent head or neck injury escalated sharply following a single incident.[18] In another study, an overall 10.8% rate of injury occurred over a 2-year study period in football, with the highest rate of injury for defensive backs and linebackers making a tackle.[19]

Ice hockey is a sport with significant risk of cervical spine injuries. In a 56-year review of Canadian hockey, 271 major spinal injuries were noted. Impact of the head with the boards is the most common mechanism of injury. Greater awareness of the problem and rules modifications have been effective in injury reduction.[11]

Other sports have a position or event at high risk of head and spine injury while the overall risks for serious injury in the sport is low. For instance, the pole vaulting event in track is high risk. Since the risks and incidence of injury are well established for most popular organized sports, such as those listed above, we will try and touch on some sports of emerging popularity, which have significant rates of injury.

Rugby, like soccer, is a sport that is prevalent worldwide and becoming increasingly popular in the US. It comes as no surprise to anyone familiar with the game that cervical spine injuries are common in this activity.[20,21] In South Africa, the region of Cape Province with a population of 10 million has seen an average of nine serious spinal cord injuries per year from rugby. It is also estimated that for every spinal cord injury there are 10 severe neck injuries from the sport.[21] The scrum seems to be the position at highest risk with a high incidence of flexion/dislocation type injuries,[22] although tacklers have a high incidence of compression fracture. In one study, 52% of the injured players were junior-level players. Conversely, in world competition, athletes sustained only 30–40% of the cervical spine injuries, indicating that experience and excellent technique are clearly protective.[23]

Gymnastics is another sport with a high incidence of cervical spine injuries (Fig. 25.1). Perhaps even more dangerous is cheerleading, which has risks similar to gymnastics but in general less structure and supervision. Whereas gymnastic events are closely monitored, cheerleaders do pyramids, jumps and flips with little guidance in technique or safety.[24]

RECREATIONAL SPORTS

Many unsupervised activities, including skiing, skating and equestrian sports, have reports of catastrophic neck injuries, but statistics on relative rate of injury are not widely studied or reviewed. Since it can never be determined how many participants there are in any given recreational sport, the rate of injury per participant can only be estimated.

Injuries to children from trampolines in the US have been defined as a national epidemic.[25] In a 6-year period from 1990–1995, there were over 249 000 trampoline-related injuries to children treated in hospital emergency rooms, with roughly 10% of injuries affecting the head and neck. Others have reported permanent paralysis as a result of trampoline related injuries.[26] Unfortunately, the rate of trampoline injuries is increasing, and they were responsible for over 6500 pediatric cervical spine injuries in 1998. This represents a 5-fold increase in just 10 years. While most have been minor, paraplegia, quadriplegia and death have all been reported.[27] Injuries resulting from child's play are common, including monkeybar and jungle gym injuries. It was estimated by the Consumer Product Safety Commission that over 200 000 injuries occurred from these and related devices from 1990–1994, of which roughly

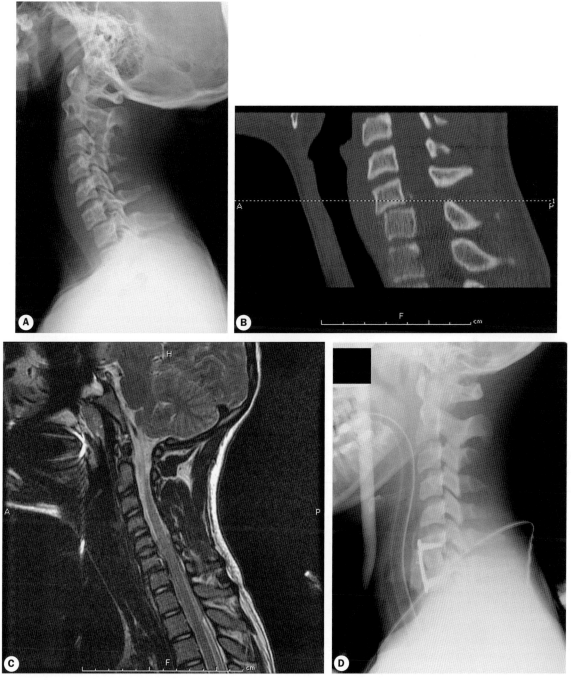

Figure 25.1 A 13-year-old gymnast who fell in the pit and felt a popping sensation. Presented with neck pain and arm numbness. Plain radiographs reveal (A) C5–6 subluxation, (B) confirmed on CT and (C) MRI. Post-surgery radiographs show reduction to normal alignment and stabilizing plate (D).

10–15% were head and neck injuries. Interestingly, the surface below the equipment did not influence the severity of injury, nor did the presence of adult supervision.[28]

Sports such as diving, although associated with significant forces to the spine, have a relatively low risk of spinal injury at the competitive level.[29] That being said, the risks at the recreational level are extremely high and unsupervised diving into shallow waters, or waters with hidden dangers such as lakes and rivers, lead to an extraordinarily high number of spine and spinal cord injuries.[6]

Equestrian accidents are also prevalent among recreational athletes. The perils of this sport were tragically brought to public attention by the catastrophic spinal cord injury of actor Christopher Reeves. In the US, more than 2300 youths are hospitalized annually due to equestrian injuries[30]; neurological injury is the leading cause of serious injury and death, with head injury occurring in 92% of patients and responsible for most deaths, while spine injury occurs in 13%.[31] With over 30 million horse riders in the US, the magnitude of the problem is potentially enormous. Likely due to the fact that more females participate in equestrian sports, more females than males are affected with cervical spine injuries, with falling from the horse being the most common mechanism.[30]

PATHOPHYSIOLOGY OF INJURY TO THE HEAD AND NECK

Box 25.2: Key Points

- Flexion injuries of the neck tend to be more common and serious than extension injuries.

- Using the head as a weapon, as in spear tackling, is the cause of many devastating spine injuries.

- Injuries can result from sudden accelerations or decelerations with no direct trauma to the head or neck.

Anatomy of the cervical spine

The cervical spine is composed of seven vertebrae joined by multiple ligaments, intervening cartilages and muscles. In the lateral view, it is curved convex forward (lordosis) (Fig. 25.2A). The ligaments consisting of elastin and collagen provide the primary stabilizing component of the cervical spine. Elastin fibers arranged in a parallel manner longitudinally allow the ligaments to stretch up to twice their length and yet return to their original length. The main ligaments are the anterior and posterior longitudinal, intertransverse and capsular, interspinal and supraspinal, and ligamentum flavum.[24]

There is significantly more muscle strength in the posterior spine than the anterior spine. This, coupled with the fact that neck movement in flexion is limited by chin contact with the sternum whereas extension is possible until the head strikes the posterior chest wall, makes extension injuries potentially more serious for an equivalent amount of force. Thus, on a purely anatomical basis, the spine is more resistant to flexion than extension. Countering this is the fact that the natural tendency of most athletes is to bend the head forward prior to or at the time of contact, so that both flexion and extension injuries are commonly seen, and in fact, flexion injuries tend to be more common and often more serious.

Causes of cervical spine injury

External forces can flex, extend, rotate, or compress the spine. With the normal head-up posture the cervical spine has a gentle lordotic curve, and forces transmitted to the head are largely dissipated in the cervical muscles. When the neck is flexed, for instance when the athlete is using his head as a weapon (spear tackling in football, which is illegal), the cervical spine becomes straight with the vertebral bodies lined up under one another (Fig. 25.2B). The forces of impact to the vertex of the head are directly transmitted from one vertebra to the next, allowing for minimal dissipation of the impact forces by the neck muscles. If the impact force exceeds the strength of the bone, it may result in fracture. At higher forces, the entire vertebra and disc may explode into the spinal canal. Analysis has shown this to be the major mechanism of cervical fracture, dislocation, and quadriplegia not only in football, but in diving and ice hockey injuries.[11,26] The fracture types seen from flexion injury include compression, anterior wedge, and chip fracture, and occasionally anterior dislocations may result when the ligaments are injured as well. With sufficient flexion one can see rupture of the posterior longitudinal, interspinal, and supraspinal ligaments as well as the ligamentum flavum. Occasionally, rupture of the posterior half of the disc is seen. Most frequently in athletes, flexion injuries result from a mobile athlete colliding with another player, an immobile structure such as the boards in hockey, or the ground. This is due to the natural tendency of the athlete to assume a flexed head position prior to contact. Flexion injury can also occur with sudden deceleration, such as when a force delivered from the front causes the athlete to stop suddenly and the head is whipped forward.

With an extension or whiplash injury, the anterior elements are disrupted and the posterior elements are compressed (Fig. 25.2). This leads to rupture of the anterior longitudinal ligament and anterior disc, with posterior bony injury to the spinous processes, facets and the neural arch. In athletics, this will often result from an unsuspecting player receiving a blow to the head or chin forcing the head back. Additionally, a sudden acceleration from a blow to the back of the body can cause the head to extend back and injure the neck. When aware of the impending contact, the athlete will usually contract the neck muscles or bend the head forward and avoid an extension injury.

Neck fractures without head trauma also may occur with sudden acceleration of the lower torso or buttocks cranially (as with a fall broken by landing on one's buttocks or by direct impact to the posterior cervical region by blunt trauma).

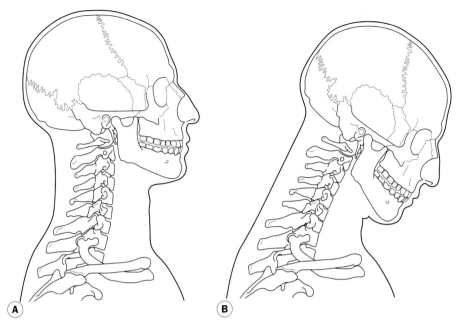

Figure 25.2   (A) In neutral posture, the cervical spine has a lordotic curvature that dissipates at the force of a blow to the cervical musculature. (B) with the neck flexed, the vertebral bodies align one above the other and directly transmits the forces of a vertex cranial blow to the vertebrae; in extension, there is distraction of the anterior elements and compression of the posterior elements.

TYPES OF SPINE INJURIES

Box 25.3: Key Points

- Injuries to the cervical spine can involve the vertebral elements, spinal cord and vascular structures, alone or in combination.

- Spinal cord injury can occur without radiographic signs of spine injury (SCIWORA).

- Brachial plexus injury, such as a stinger or burner, involves a peripheral nerve. If both upper extremities are affected, the level of pathology is the spinal cord, which is much more concerning.

- Many injuries, including disc herniations, can be treated non-operatively.

A study by Bailes *et al.* which examined a large series of athletic cervical spine injuries, gives an excellent overview of the type and severity of injury seen. Of 63 patients in their series, forty-five patients had permanent injury to the vertebral column and/or spinal cord, while 18 suffered only transient spinal cord symptoms. Football accounted for the highest number of injuries, followed by wrestling and gymnastics. Twelve patients had complete spinal cord injury, 14 patients had incomplete spinal cord injury, and 19 patients had injury to the vertebral column alone. The majority of the spinal cord lesions occurred at the C4 and C5 levels, while bony injuries of C4 through C6 predominated. A total of 25 patients required surgical stabilization, and 20 were treated with orthosis only. There was no

instance of associated systemic injuries, and hospital complications were few.[32] In this section, specific injury type will be examined.

Spinal cord injury

Traumatic lesions of the spinal cord without associated spinal column injury are relatively unusual in the older athlete, although can occur more frequently in youths (see below). Spinal cord lesions include contusion, edema and hemorrhage (Fig. 25.3). If the injury causes a complete neurological injury, recovery is generally poor.[33] As reported by the NCCSIR, all permanent spinal cord injuries have been in the cervical region, with no reports in the thoracic or lumbar region. Spinal concussion is another phenomenon that may occur, and similar to brain concussions there should be no radiographic evidence of injury despite the transient presence of neurological impairment. This will be discussed further in the section on transient neuropraxia.

Spinal cord injury without radiographic abnormality

Spinal cord injury without radiographic abnormality (SCIWORA) was an entity first identified in 1982 by Pang,[34] to describe those children with traumatic spinal cord injury with no radiographic evidence of fracture or dislocation.[35] The mechanism for this has been attributed to the elasticity of the ligamentous structures of the spine in young children, in whom substantial dislocation and spontaneous reduction is possible, with no subsequent radiographic abnormalities identified on plain films.[36] The mechanism of injury may involve

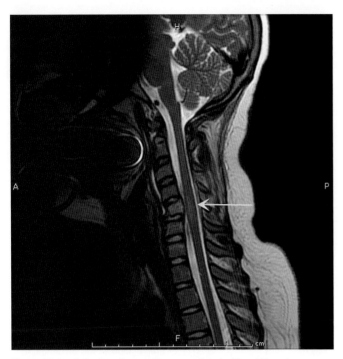

Figure 25.3 Spinal cord contusion associated with a C5 wedge compression fracture in an 8-year-old child who dived into shallow water.

either pinching of the spinal cord between[37] the vertebral body and the adjacent lamina, or a stretch of the spinal cord causing vascular injury. Because the underlying mechanism required to disrupt the spinal axis is substantial, the actual spinal cord injury tends to be quite severe and the chance of recovery is low. Most series identify a 10–20% incidence of SCIWORA, although in the current era many of these injuries are not radiographically occult. With modern MRI, most cases previously described as SCIWORA actually have demonstrable injury to the spinal cord, and even ligamentous injury can often be identified. Therefore, we can perhaps rethink SCIWORA in the current era as spinal cord injury with normal anatomic alignment after the injury, and no plain film irregularities.[38]

Stingers

Stingers or burners are colloquial terms used by athletes and trainers to describe a set of symptoms that involve pain, burning, or tingling down an arm occasionally accompanied by localized weakness.[39] The symptoms typically abate within seconds or minutes, rarely persisting for days or longer. It has been estimated that a stinger will occur at least once during the career of over 50% of athletes.[40]

There are two typical mechanisms by which stingers may occur: (1) traction on the brachial plexus or (2) nerve root impingement within the cervical neural foramen (Fig. 25.4). The majority of high-school level injuries are of the brachial

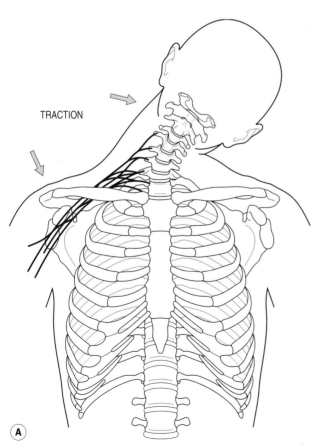

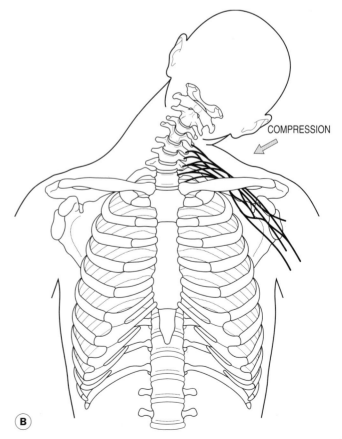

Figure 25.4 Stingers can occur either from (A) traction on the brachial plexus or (B) direct compression of exiting nerve roots.

plexus type while most at the college level and virtually all in the professional ranks result from a pinch phenomenon within the neural foramen.[24]

The brachial plexus stinger commonly involves a forceful blow to the head from the side but also can result from head extension or shoulder depression while the head and neck are fixed. Nerve root impingement usually occurs when the athlete's head is driven toward his shoulder pad. The dorsal spinal nerve root ganglion lies close to the posterior intervertebral facet joints and is pinched when the neural foramen is compressed.

With either type of stinger, the athlete experiences a shock-like sensation of pain and numbness radiating into the arm and hand. The symptoms are typically purely sensory in nature and most commonly involve the C5 and C6 dermatomes. On occasion, weakness also may be present. The most common muscles involved include the deltoid, biceps, supraspinatus and infraspinatus.

Stingers are always unilateral and never involve the lower extremities. Thus if symptoms are bilateral or involve the legs, injury to the spinal cord itself must be considered.

When stingers are not associated with any neck pain or limitation of neck movement and all motor and sensory symptoms clear within seconds to minutes, the athlete may safely return to competition. This is especially true if the athlete has previously experienced similar symptoms. If there are any residual symptoms or complaints of neck pain, return should be deferred pending further workup.

On rare occasions, a stinger may result in prolonged sensory complaints or weakness. In such a situation, an MRI of the cervical spine should be considered, to look for a herniated disc or other compressive pathology. If symptoms persist for more than 2 weeks, then electromyography should allow for an accurate assessment of the degree and extent of injury.

Some athletes seem predisposed to develop a series of recurrent stingers. It has been suggested that repeated stinger injuries over many years may lead to a proximal arm weakness and constant pain. Thus if an athlete suffers two or more stingers, particularly in rapid succession, consideration can be given to the use of high shoulder pads supplemented by a soft cervical roll which should limit lateral neck flexion and extension. Shoulder pads that elevate the point of impact off of the trapezius muscle and place the burden of impact on the scapula and clavicle can also alleviate pressure from the brachial plexus. This is more of an issue with the extremely muscular athletes seen today. Examining or changing the athlete's blocking and tackling techniques or changing the player's position also may be helpful in preventing recurrences. If the stingers repeatedly recur despite these interventions, then cessation of the causative athletic activity may be necessary.

Transient quadriplegia

Transient quadriplegia, also called spinal cord neurapraxia or concussion, is a phenomenon defined by bilateral neurological symptoms after a collision that may affect the upper extremities alone (i.e. burning hands syndrome) or both the upper and lower extremities. Unlike a stinger, the bilateral involvement implies spinal cord involvement. By definition, the symptoms do resolve, often within 15 min but occasionally lasting up to 48 h. The cause of transient quadriplegia is likely multifactorial, and may occur in athletes with or without spinal stenosis. The occurrence of cervical cord neurapraxia in pediatric patients can be attributed to the mobility of the pediatric spine rather than to congenital cervical spinal stenosis,[41] therefore being a mild form of SCIWORA. This study found no evidence of cervical spinal stenosis in children with sports-related cervical spinal cord neurapraxia.

In some athletes, spinal stenosis may be a contributing factor. Although radiographic bone measurements can suggest spinal stenosis,[42] physicians are cautioned against making the diagnosis of spinal stenosis with this technique alone. A 'Torg' ratio (ratio of spinal canal to vertebral body diameter) of less than 0.8 was initially thought to be a predictor of risk for spinal cord injury, but this has since been found to be unreliable. Although it is sensitive, in that many athletes with transient neurapraxia have a low Torg ratio, its positive predictive value is too low to be used as a screening tool in athletes.[42] This is likely because the vertebral bodies are so broad in many athletes that they may have a Torg ratio less than 0.8, despite a normal caliber spinal canal.

Instead of using absolute measurement criteria, the concept of functional stenosis is probably a more valid way of deciding when the athlete is at risk for recurrent episodes of spinal cord injury. Diagnostic technologies that view the spinal cord and other soft tissues within the vertebral canal, such as MRI or CT/myelogram, should be employed. Regardless of how the bony anatomy appears, these imaging methods can determine if the spinal cord has a normal functional reserve (defined as the space surrounding and available for the cord). These techniques alert the clinician to the presence of abnormalities such as disc protrusion, bony osteophyte, or thickening of the ligamentum not visible on plain films.

Controversy persists as to whether cervical stenosis increases the risk of spinal cord injury. Athletes who have had spinal cord symptoms from sports-related injuries and are shown to have functional spinal stenosis on MRI probably should not be allowed to return to contact sports. Though there are no hard data to back-up this recommendation, there is a body of literature in the sports medicine, neurology and radiology fields that indicates that spinal stenosis predisposes a patient to spinal cord injury.[43–45] Matsuura and his group,[45] for example, compared the spinal dimensions of 100 controls with those of 42 patients who had spinal cord injuries. They found that the control group had significantly larger sagittal spinal canal diameters than did the patients who had spinal cord injuries. Furthermore, the NCCSIR also documents several instances of permanent quadriplegia in athletes with tight spinal stenosis without fracture or demonstrated instability. Thus, following spinal cord symptoms, identification of 'functional spinal stenosis' is a contraindication to further participation in contact collision sports (Fig. 25.5). However, a single episode of transient neuropraxia in an athlete with spinal stenosis but with preserved cerebrospinal fluid-signal does not appear to increase the risk of subsequent catastrophic injury to the spinal cord.[46]

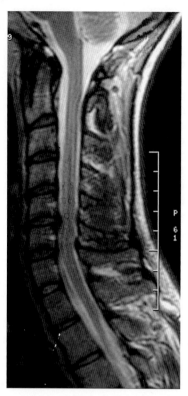

Figure 25.5 A rugby player with functional stenosis of the cervical spine due to combined effects of a congenitally narrowed spine and a C5–6 disc protrusion.

Presently, there are no good guidelines to help the physician manage an athlete with a narrow asymptomatic cervical spinal canal. When such an abnormality is encountered, management must be individualized according to the patient's symptoms, the degree of canal stenosis, and the perceived risk of permanent neurological injury.

Spinal column injury

The major concern with a cervical spinal injury is the possibility of an unstable fracture that may produce quadriplegia. In the NCCSIR registry, all cases of quadriplegia in the absence of spinal stenosis resulted from fracture dislocation of the cervical spine. At the time of injury on the athletic field, there is no way to determine the presence of an unstable fracture, and there also is no way of differentiating between a fully recoverable and a permanent case of quadriplegia. Therefore, the athlete must be transported with the head and neck immobilized to a medical facility. If the patient is fully conscious, a cervical fracture or cervical cord injury is usually accompanied by rigid cervical muscle spasm and pain that immediately alerts the athlete and physician to the presence of such an injury. It is the unconscious athlete who is susceptible to progressive cord injury if caregivers are not aware of the possibility of an unstable cervical spine fracture. With an unconscious or obviously neck-injured athlete, it is imperative that no neck manipulation be carried out on the field. Definitive treatment must await appropriate evaluation at a medical facility (see Management Section).[47]

Herniated discs

The intervertebral disc may protrude posteriorly and impact the spinal cord or nerve roots under conditions of traumatic or degenerative stress. In a series of herniated discs in athletes, 50% of the injuries were sustained in football. Sixty percent of radicular signs and symptoms were from the 4th and 5th cervical root. The roentgenographic changes were most common at the 4th and 5th intervertebral disc spaces. Most of the cases responded satisfactorily to a simple cervical collar and cervical traction. The athletes with radicular signs required on average of 5 months to return to full sports activities, and 60% of these had some residual symptoms after completion of treatment.[48] A non-operative treatment plan using a logical stepwise approach is successful in the vast majority of these patients.[49]

Vascular injury

Uncommon, but very serious neck injuries may involve the carotid and vertebral arteries (Fig. 25.6). By either extremes of lateral flexion and extension, or a forceful blow to the neck, the inner layer (intima) of the artery may be torn. This can lead to clot formation at the site of injury, resulting in emboli to the brain or, more commonly, a complete occlusion of the artery causing a major stroke. With a fracture dislocation, injury to the vertebral artery may occur, leading to a brainstem stroke. These injuries should be considered if neurological deficit exists that are not clearly from a spinal cord etiology.[24]

Diagnostic evaluation of these patients can include CT, MRI and angiography. Neuroradiologic findings of coronary artery disease can include infarction, a hyperdense artery on CT indicating thrombosis, abnormal periarterial signal on MRI, and a narrowed arterial signal column on MRA. Computed tomography alone can be an insensitive screening examination[50] and should be supplemented with CT or MR angiography.

More direct injuries to the vessels, with devastating outcomes, have been reported. One article describes three neck slash injuries in amateur ice hockey players, with one player dying of asphyxiation secondary to hemorrhage into the respiratory passage, and another exsanguinating after the neck was severed by the skate blade.[51]

MANAGEMENT OF ATHLETIC CERVICAL SPINE INJURIES

Box 25.4: Key Points

- Advanced preparation for cervical spine injuries is crucial to appropriate on-field management.

- The most important goal of management is to avoid further injury to the spinal cord by ensuring spinal stability.

- If significant neck pain or any neurological deficit exists, the cervical spine needs appropriate clinical and radiographic clearance.

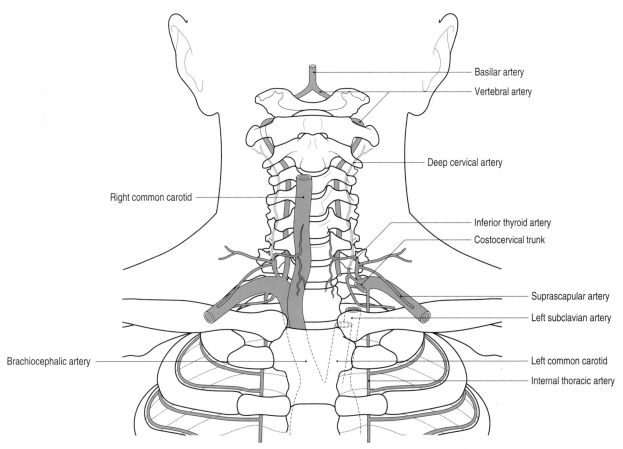

Figure 25.6 Major vascular anatomy affecting the brain, including the carotid arteries anteriorly and the vertebral arteries coming up through the foramen transversarium of the vertebral bodies.

Being prepared for neck injury is key to its on-field management. In the event of an injury, the equipment needed to evaluate and transport the injured athlete must be available. The most important goal of management of neck injury is to prevent further damage and recurrent injury.[52–54] Medical providers must use extreme caution when evaluating and treating an unconscious football player, especially when the extent of the injury remains unknown. For safety's sake, any unconscious player is presumed to have an accompanying spinal injury until proven otherwise. If the player is not breathing or the possibility of respiratory arrest exists, it is essential that certified athletic trainers and emergency medical services (EMS) providers work quickly and effectively to remove any face mask and administer care. In most situations, helmets do not need to be removed in the field. Proper management of head and neck injuries includes leaving the helmet in place whenever possible, removing only the face mask from the helmet and developing a plan to manage head- and neck-injured players using well-trained sports medicine and EMS providers. EMS agencies should work with their local high school or college athletic trainers to practice these removal techniques prior to the start of the football season.[55]

Removal of shoulder pads and helmet from a football player with suspected cervical spine injury can be particularly hazardous, and special precautions are required.[56] Stabilization of the cervical spine in an injured football player does not require routine pre-hospital removal of the helmet and shoulder pads before transport.[57] Upon arrival at a medical facility, special precautions should be employed in removing the equipment as dictated by radiographic studies. In a recent study, helmet and shoulder pads were removed under X-ray guidance with a technique consistent with that described by the National Athletic Trainers' Association (NATA). The results showed no significant change in angulation, disc height, translation and space available for the cord. Therefore, in the conscious player with no cervical injury, the protocol used by the NATA is effective in limiting cervical motion.[58]

Clearance of the cervical spine

Radiographic evaluation is only one component of clearing the cervical spine. In addition, a detailed neurological examination is carried out, and it is important to determine if the athlete has neck pain. For an athlete with no neck pain and a normal neurological exam, the cervical spine may be cleared. However, if the neurological exam is abnormal or if there is neck pain, radiographs are indicated. The first step is a lateral cervical spine radiograph. If this is normal, a complete cervical spine series of AP, odontoid, lateral, obliques and flexion-extension views may be obtained. As high as 20% of unstable cervical spine injuries are missed when the cross table lateral cervical spine radiograph is used alone.[59] Today, CT scans may often be substituted for the full X-ray evaluation, especially with the bulky size of many athletes which limits the ability to obtain high quality radiographs.

When there is spinal cord injury documented on the neurological examination, a lateral cervical spine radiograph is taken on the still neck-immobilized patient. In this instance, oblique and flexion-extension views are not taken for fear of further injuring the spinal cord. Instead, one proceeds to a CT and MRI[60] of the cervical spine to define further the extent of the trauma and presence of spinal cord compression by bone, disc or hematoma.[61]

Pediatric athletes do have some normal anatomical variants that should be considered.[62,63] The child has relative hypermobility of the upper cervical segments from C2–4. Failure to recognize this normal laxity may lead to unnecessary treatment of pseudosubluxation. The atlanto-dental space is also greater than in adults, with a distance of up to 4.5 mm being normal. In a study of almost 200 children with vertebral or spinal cord injuries, certain trends were noted. As with adults, children with complete or severe spinal injury remained with poor neurological function; however, those with moderate or mild injury regained near normal function. Most injuries were treated non-operatively, but there was a high incidence of progressive post-traumatic deformity which required eventual surgical stabilization.[64] Additional concerns arise from the expected potential for continued spine growth over time.

Because of their participation in the Special Olympics, it is important to realize that as high as 40% of children with Down's syndrome may have hypermobility of the cervical spine.[65] By far the most common abnormality is a subluxation at the atlantoaxial (C1–2) joint followed by atlanto-occipital subluxation.[66] It is often recommended that cervical spine stability be assessed in all patients with Down's syndrome who wish to participate in athletic activities, although exact guidelines do not exist for which patients require treatment and who should be excluded from play.[62]

Return to play

> ### Box 25.5: Key Points
>
> - There is no clear consensus on return to play criteria, but at a minimum, the player should have resolution of neck pain and full range of motion.
> - A player with radiographic signs of a spinal cord injury should not be allowed to return to play.
> - A broad spectrum of bony and soft tissue anomalies of the cervical spine may exist and require individualized return to play decision.
> - Prevention of injury is the key, and requires a combination of education, appropriate training, and equipment.

Despite the frequency of cervical-related injuries among athletes participating in contact and collision sports, no consensus exists within the medical field as to a standard guideline approach for return to pre-injury activity level.[67,68] In the ideal situation, it is recommended that an athlete not return to competition after a neck injury until he or she is free of neck and arm pain, has a full range of neck motion without discomfort or spasm, and neck strength in flexion, extension, and lateral bending on each side has returned to pre-injury levels. If a pre-injury profile is unknown, strength should at least be symmetrical. Also lateral neck radiographs should show return of lordotic curvature in the neutral view, and MR imaging should not reveal significant disc disease or functional spinal stenosis. Of course, not all neck injuries require a full radiographic evaluation, and the degree of evaluation should reflect the severity of initial injury.

Maroon and Bailes[32,69] have developed an alternative classification of cervical spine injuries in athletes to help with categorizing the injury and aiding in return to play criteria. They identified and then prospectively looked at three categories of injury: type I, permanent cord injury; type II, transient injury without abnormal radiographs; and type III, radiographic abnormality without neurological deficit. Their conclusions were that the type I patients were excluded from further play, type II patients were returned to play over time, and type III patients were individualized based on the abnormality.[69]

A recent study has revealed that adherence to guidelines is difficult and that little consensus exists on return to play criteria. The authors sent out 346 questionnaires to sports physicians regarding return criteria after neck injury. Only 49% of respondents reported using any type of guidelines in decision-making, and often it was not tightly adhered to. They concluded that there is no consensus on the post-injury management of many cervical spine-injured patients.[70]

Others have advocated using an anatomical basis regarding eligibility for play. Anatomical conditions included in this analysis are odontoid anomalies, spina bifida occulta, atlanto-occipital fusion, Klippel–Feil anomalies, cervical canal stenosis, spear tackler's spine and traumatic conditions of the upper, middle, and lower cervical spine, including ligamentous injuries and fractures, intervertebral disc injuries; and post-cervical spine fusion. They argue that criteria based on the anatomy be used in the decision-making process in conjunction with other such factors as the age, experience, ability of the individual, level of participation and position played, as well as the attitude and desires of the athlete and his or her parents following an informed discussion of the problem with particular regard to potential risk.[71]

Clearly, there is no consensus in this area, and different practitioners will use different criteria to formulate return to play decisions. It is highly recommended that if there is any doubt about the stability of the cervical spine, the athlete should not be allowed to return to play and further consultation or evaluation be performed.

Prevention

In best case scenarios, cervical spine injuries are problematic due to the need to assess cervical spine stability before the athlete can return to competition. At their worst, they are absolutely devastating. Due to the potential for catastrophic neurotrauma in sports, the medical team must take proper measures to prevent such injuries. Strength training of the cervical spine musculature, teaching of proper technique, and use of protective sports equipment are three primary means of attempting to prevent cervical spine injuries in sports. Improvements in equipment design have led to decreases in overall injury incidence, especially regarding significant head injury, but no available helmet can prevent catastrophic injury to the neck and cervical spine. The most effective strategy for preventing this type of injury appears to be careful instruction, training and regulations designed to eliminate head-first contact.[16] There are other avenues to assist in preventing these injuries, such as flexibility programs. The sports healthcare professional, therefore, must be knowledgeable of the needs of each individual athlete when developing prevention plans.[72]

CONCLUSION

Careful study of the pathophysiology and epidemiology of sports-related spine injuries brings to light many common features. The incidence increases as the sport becomes increasingly violent and aggressive, although most injuries are suffered in recreational sports. Poor conditioning and lack of knowledge of the proper techniques of the sport put the athlete at significant risk for neck injury. The use of the head as an offensive weapon is also a common feature of injury in organized sports. Although recognition of these features has resulted in a dramatic reduction in catastrophic neurological injury, the athlete remains at risk for neck injury. As recovery from neurological injury is often poor, and since the injuries can be so devastating, prevention remains the key to safe participation in sports at risk for neck injuries.

REFERENCES

1. Mueller FO, Cantu RC. Van Camp SP. Football. In: Mueller FO, Cantu RC, Camp SP Van, eds. Catastrophic injuries in high school and college sports. Champaign, IL: Human Kinetics; 1996:41-56.
2. Zmurko MG, Tannoury TY, Tannoury CA, et al. Cervical sprains, disc herniations, minor fractures, and other cervical injuries in the athlete. Clin Sports Med 2003; 22:513-521.
3. Kraus J. Epidemiologic features of injuries to the central nervous system. In: Anderson D, ed. Neuroepidemiology. Florida: CRC; 1991:333-357.
4. Davis JM, Kuppermann N, Fleisher G. Serious sports injuries requiring hospitalization seen in a pediatric emergency department. Am J Dis Child 1993; 147:1001-1004.
5. Kelley LA. In neck to neck competition are women more fragile? Clin Orthop Relat Res 2000; 372:123-130.
6. Albrand OW, Corkill G. Broken necks from diving accidents: a summer epidemic in young men. Am J Sports Med 1976; 4:107-110.
7. Maroon JC, Bailes JE. Athletes with cervical spine injury. Spine 1994; 21:2294-2299.
8. Katoh S, Shingu H, Ikata T, Iwatsubo E. Sports-related spinal cord injury in Japan. Spinal Cord 1996; 34:416-421.
9. Adickes MS, Stuart MJ. Youth football injuries. Sports Med 2004; 34:201-207.
10. Rampton J, Leach T, Therrien SA, et al. Head, neck, and facial injuries in ice hockey: the effect of protective equipment. Clin J Sport Med 1997; 7:162-167.
11. Tator CH, Provvidenza CF, Lapczak L, Carson J, Raymond D. Spinal Injuries in Canadian Ice Hockey: documentation of injuries sustained from 1943-1999. Can J Neurol Sci 2004; 31:460-466.
12. Wroble RR, Albright JP. Neck and low back injuries in wrestling. Clin Sports Med 1986; 5:295-325.
13. Cantu RC, Mueller FO. Catastrophic spine injuries in football (1977-1989). J Spinal Disord 1990; 3:227-231.
14. Mueller FO. Fatalities from head and cervical spine injuries occurring in tackle football: 50 years' experience. Clin Sports Med 1998; 17:169-182.
15. Cantu RC, Mueller FO. Catastrophic spine injuries in American football, 1977-2001. Neurosurgery 2003; 53:358-362.
16. Kim DH, Vaccaro AR, Berta SC. Acute sports-related spinal cord injury: contemporary management principles. Clin Sports Med 2003; 22:501-512.
17. Albright JP, Moses JM, Feldick HG, et al. Nonfatal cervical spine injuries in interscholastic football. JAMA 1976; 236:1243-1245.
18. Albright JP, McAuley E, Martin RK, et al. Head and neck injuries in college football: an eight-year analysis. Am J Sports Med 1985; 13:147-152.
19. Marzo JM, Simmons EH, Whieldon TJ. Neck injuries to high school football players in western New York State [see comment]. N Y State J Med 1991; 91:46-49.
20. Rotem TR, Lawson JS, Wilson SF, et al. Severe cervical spinal cord injuries related to rugby union and league football in New South Wales, 1984-1996. Med J Aust 1998; 168:379-381.
21. Schler A. Rugby Injuries to the cervical spine and spinal cord: a 10-year review. Clin Sports Med 1998; 17:195-206.
22. Williams P, McKibbin B. Unstable cervical spine injuries in rugby – a 20-year review. Injury 1987; 18:329-332.
23. Wetzler MJ, Akpata T, Albert T, et al. A retrospective study of cervical spine injuries in American rugby, 1970 to 1994. Am J Sports Med 1996; 24:454-458.
24. Proctor MR, Cantu RC. Head and neck injuries in young athletes. Clin Sports Med 2000; 19:693-715.
25. Smith GA. Injuries to children in the United States related to trampolines, 1990-1995: a national epidemic [see comment]. Pediatrics 1998; 101:406-412.
26. Torg JSDM. Trampoline and minitrampoline injuries to the cervical spine. Clin Sports Med 1985; 4:45-60.
27. Brown PG, Lee M. Trampoline injuries of the cervical spine. Pediatr Neurosurg 2000; 32:170-175.
28. Waltzman MLSM, Bowen AP, Bailey MC. Monkeybar injuries: complications of play. Pediatrics 1999; 103:58.
29. Badman BL, Rechtine GR. Spinal injury considerations in the competitive diver: a case report and review of the literature. Spine J: Official Journal of the North American Spine Society 2004; 4:584-590.
30. Nelson DE, Bixby-Hammett D. Equestrian injuries in children and young adults. Am J Dis Child 1992; 146
31. Hamilton MG, Tranmer BI. Nervous system injuries in horseback-riding accidents. J Trauma 1993; 34:227-232.
32. Bailes JE, Hadley MN, Quigley MR, et al. Management of athletic injuries of the cervical spine and spinal cord. Neurosurgery 1991; 29:491-497.
33. Bailes JE, Maroon JC. Management of cervical spine injuries in athletes. Clin Sports Med 1989; 8:43-58.
34. Pang D, Wilberger JE. Jr. Spinal cord injury without radiographic abnormalities in children. J Neurosurg 1982; 57:114-129.
35. Pang D, Pollack IF. Spinal cord injury without radiographic abnormality in children – the SCIWORA syndrome. J Trauma 1989; 29:654-664.
36. Kriss VM, Kriss TC. SCIWORA (spinal cord injury without radiographic abnormality) in infants and children. Clin Pediatr (Phil) 1996; 35:119-124.
37. Dickman CA, Zabramski JM, Hadley MN, et al. Pediatric spinal cord injury without radiographic abnormalities: report of 26 cases and review of the literature. J Spinal Disord 1991; 4:296-305.
38. Felsberg GJ, Tien RD, Osumi AK, et al. Utility of MR imaging in pediatric spinal cord injury. Pediatr Radiol 1995; 25:131-135.
39. Kuhlman GS. McKeag DB. The 'burner': a common nerve injury in contact sports. Am Fam Physician 1999; 60:2035-2040.
40. Feldick HG, Albright JP. Football survey reveals 'missed' neck injuries. Phys Sports Med 1976; 4:77-81.
41. Boockvar JA, Durham SR, Sun PP. Cervical spinal stenosis and sports-related cervical cord neurapraxia in children. Spine 2001; 26:2709-2713.
42. Torg JS, Naranja RJ Jr, Palov H, et al. The relationship of developmental narrowing of the cervical spinal canal to reversible and irreversible injury of the cervical spinal cord in football players. J Bone Jt Surg 1996; 78A:1308-1314.
43. Penning L. Some aspects of plain radiography of the cervical spine in chronic myelopathy. Neurology 1962; 12:513-519.
44. Eismont FJ, Clifford S, Goldberg M, Green B. Cervical sagittal spinal canal size in spine injury. Spine 1984; 9:663-666.
45. Matsuura P, Waters RL, Adkins RH, et al. Comparison of computerized tomography parameters of the cervical spine in normal control subjects and spinal cord-injured patients. J Bone Jt Surg (Am) 1989; 71:183-188.
46. Bailes JE. Experience with cervical stenosis and temporary paralysis in athletes. J Neurosurg 2005; 2:11-16.
47. Banerjee R, Palumbo MA, Fadale PD. Catastrophic cervical spine injuries in the collision sport athlete, part 2: principles of emergency care. Am J Sports Med 2004; 32:1760-1764.

48 Kumano K, Umeyama T. Cervical disk injuries in athletes. Arch Orthop Traumatic Surg 1986; 105:223–226.

49 Malanga GA. The diagnosis and treatment of cervical radiculopathy. Med Sci Sports Exerc 1997; 29:236–245.

50 Provenzale JM, Barboriak DP, Taveras JM. Exercise-related dissection of craniocervical arteries: CT, MR, and angiographic findings. J Comput Assisted Tomogr 1995; 19:268–276.

51 Vergis A, Rasanen T, Hernefalk L. Neck injuries from skate blades in ice hockey: a report of three cases. Scand J Med Sci Sports 1996; 6:352–354.

52 McAlindon RJ. On field evaluation and management of head and neck injured athletes. Clin Sports Med 2002; 21:1–14.

53 Vegso JJ, Lehman RC. Field evaluation and management of head and neck injuries. Clin Sports Med 1987; 6:1–15.

54 Warren WL Jr, Bailes JE. On the field evaluation of athletic neck injury. Clin Sports Med 1998; 17:99–110.

55 Kleiner DM, Pollak AN, McAdam C. Helmet hazards. Do's & don'ts of football helmet removal. J Emerg Med Serv 2001; 26:36–44.

56 Waninger KN. Management of the helmeted athlete with suspected cervical spine injury. Am J Sports Med 2004; 32:1331–1350.

57 Waninger KN. On-field management of potential cervical spine injury in helmeted football players: leave the helmet on![see comment]. Clin J Sport Med 1998; 8:124–129.

58 Peris MD, Donaldson WW, 3rd, Towers J, et al. Helmet and shoulder pad removal in suspected cervical spine injury: human control model. Spine 2002; 27:995–999.

59 Herzog RJ, Wiens JJ, Dillingham MF, Sontag MJ. Normal cervical spine morphometry and cervical spinal stenosis in asymptomatic professional football players: plain film radiography, multiplanar computed tomography, and magnetic resonance imaging. Spine 1991; 16:178–186.

60 Gundry CRFH. MR imaging of the spine in sports injuries. MRI Clin North Am 1999; 7:85–103.

61 Mintz DN. Magnetic resonance imaging of sports injuries to the cervical spine. Semin Musculoskeletal Radiol 2004; 8:99–110.

62 Pizzutillo P. Spinal considerations in the young athlete. Instr Course Lect 1993; 42:463–472.

63 Proctor MR. Spinal cord injury. Crit Care Med 2002; 30:489–499.

64 Osenbach RK, Menezes AH. Pediatric spinal cord and vertebral column injury. Neurosurgery 1992; 30:385–390.

65 Cope R, Olson S. Abnormalities of the cervical spine in Down's syndrome: Diagnosis, risks, and review of the literature with particular reference to the Special Olympics. South Med J 1987; 80:33–36.

66 Rosenbaum DM, Blumhagen JD, King HA. Atlantooccipital subluxation in Down's syndrome. AJR 1986; 146:1269–1272.

67 Vaccaro AR, Klein GR, Ciccoti M, et al. Return to play criteria for the athlete with cervical spine injuries resulting in stinger and transient quadriplegia/paresis. Spine J: Official Journal of the North American Spine Society 2002; 2:351–356.

68 Vaccaro AR, Watkins B, Albert TJ, et al. Cervical spine injuries in athletes: current return-to-play criteria. Orthopedics 24 2001; 24:699–703.

69 Maroon JC, Bailes JE. Athletes with cervical spine injury. Spine 1996; 21:2294–2299.

70 Morganti C, Sweeney CA, Albanese SA, et al. Return to play after cervical spine injury. Spine 2001; 26:1131–1136.

71 Torg JS, Ramsey-Emrhein JA. Management guidelines for participation in collision activities with congenital, developmental, or postinjury lesions involving the cervical spine. Clin J Sport Med 1997; 7:273–291.

72 Cross KM, Serenelli C. Training and equipment to prevent athletic head and neck injuries. Clin Sports Med 2003; 22:639–667.

CHAPTER 26

Shoulder Injuries

Jason Nielson and Peter Gerbino

INTRODUCTION

Injuries of the shoulder occur in many athletes. The overhead athlete in particular will have sport specific overuse injuries of the shoulder. The shoulder is a 4-joint entity. These joints work in synchrony to allow for smooth and powerful motions. The shoulder joint complex differs from other joints because it depends solely on its musculature for strength, synchrony, and stability for its function. Pain anywhere in this shoulder joint complex is usually due to muscle weakness. This muscle weakness leads to joint dysfunction. Evaluation and treatment of shoulder injuries is an area of active current research. Advances in diagnosis and treatment have allowed athletes to return to sports sooner and in some instances, with improved outcomes.

ACUTE TRAUMATIC SHOULDER INJURIES

Glenohumeral dislocations
Pathogenesis

Box 26.1: Key Points

- Most shoulder dislocations are anterior.
- Consider operative repair for athletes.
- Full rehabilitation after repair requires 3–4 months.

Shoulder injuries are quite common in most contact sports. Anterior shoulder dislocation occurs when the upper extremity is forced into a position of extreme external rotation and abduction. More than 90% of traumatic shoulder dislocations occur in the anterior direction. The athlete with an anteriorly dislocated shoulder will hold the extremity in external rotation and abduction. If there have been several recurrent dislocations, the shoulder can sometimes be reduced by the athlete. In most cases, muscle relaxation (often requiring medication) and pain relief are required before reduction is possible. Anterior dislocations result in tearing of the glenohumeral cap-sule (especially the inferior glenohumeral ligament) or avulsion of the anterior capsulolabral complex (Bankart lesion) or both.

Diagnosis

For posterior glenohumeral dislocations, the extremity is internally rotated and adducted. After anterior dislocations, the extremity is held in external rotation and abduction. In addition to the abnormal arm position, a posterior hollow space in the shoulder may be apparent with anterior dislocations. The axillary nerve may be injured, causing decreased sensation over the lateral shoulder as well as deltoid muscle weakness. Posterior dislocations are sometimes missed initially.

In most cases, radiographic evaluation should be obtained prior to any reduction maneuver, particularly in the skeletally immature athlete. What appears to be a shoulder dislocation may actually be a proximal humerus physeal fracture. A standard radiographic series including AP, scapular 'Y' and axillary views should be obtained. A protected 'velpeau' axillary view is usually required as the standard axillary view is not possible because of pain. Radiographs may also show glenoid or humeral head fractures that may influence treatment. All shoulder dislocations should have post-reduction radiographs to confirm reduction and to look for fractures of the humeral head (Hill–Sachs lesion) and glenoid rim that can accompany these injuries.

Treatment

An experienced physician who witnesses a shoulder dislocation may attempt to reduce the shoulder in the locker room before pain and muscle spasms prohibit relocation. More often, the shoulder is reduced at a later point by using any one of a number of techniques aided with muscle relaxants and analgesics. Recently intra-articular lidocaine injection has been shown to be as effective and less costly compared to intravenous sedation.[1]

Treatment of first time anterior glenohumeral dislocations after reduction is controversial. A majority of young competitive athletes will re-dislocate if it is not repaired surgically.[2,3] Despite this, the usual recommendation for first time dislocations remains non-operative with 4 weeks of rest in a sling and swathe in internal rotation, followed by focused therapy to restore motion and strength. One controversial report documented increased stability with decreased recurrence rates following immobilization in a position of external rotation for 3 weeks.[4] Depending on the athlete's situation, primary surgical repair may be considered, particularly if MR imaging reveals a Bankart lesion. Many authors report decreased re-dislocation rates with operative arthroscopic stabilization when compared with conventional non-operative treatment.[2,5–7] Recurrent dislocations are operatively stabilized by open or arthroscopic means.

Rehabilitation

Whether treated non-operatively or operatively, 3 to 4 months of rehabilitation are usually required to achieve pre-injury status. Initially, a 3–4 week period of immobilization is often suggested, prior to the onset of aggressive range of motion exercises. At this point range of motion as well as focusing on restoring the rotator cuff and periscapular muscle strength is performed. After strengthening the rotator cuff musculature, the larger shoulder girdle muscles are strengthened.

Following operative repair, 3–4 months is necessary to achieve adequate healing, strength, and proprioception to return to sports safely. Shoulder dislocations treated non-operatively may return to sport after pain subsides and full motion and strength are restored.

Glenohumeral subluxation

Partial dislocation (subluxation) of the glenohumeral joint can occur after single or repetitive trauma to the anterior, inferior, or posterior capsule. The glenoid labrum can be torn during dislocation or subluxation. Glenohumeral subluxations and multidirectional laxity are treated non-operatively with rotator cuff and periscapular strengthening. Only if conservative therapy fails is surgical stabilization considered. This can be performed open or arthroscopically with labrum repair and capsule plication as required.

Shoulder separations

Box 26.2: Key Points

- AC and anterior SC separations are normally treated non-operatively.
- Posterior SC dislocation is treated as a possible medical emergency.
- Long-term problems are uncommon, but can be corrected operatively.

Pathogenesis

Acute traumatic sternoclavicular dislocation may be anterior or posterior. Physical examination usually will distinguish between the two directions, but computed tomography may be necessary if swelling is prohibitive of an accurate examination. The mechanism of injury for acromioclavicular (AC) and anterior sternoclavicular (SC) separation is usually a fall directly onto the lateral shoulder with the humerus in an adducted position.

The AC joint is one of the most commonly injured in contact sports such as rugby football and hockey.

The mechanism of posterior SC injury may be the same or result from a direct blow. The ligaments around the joint are the first to tear. The posterior capsule of the SC joint is the most important restraint to anterior and posterior translation.[8] The amount of displacement determines degree of injury and possible need for reduction. This injury is a medical emergency because of the possibility of pulmonary or vascular injury. The severity of pain is related to the severity of the injury, but typically, athletes are unable to continue play. Local tenderness and deformity (in more severe degrees of injury) provide the likely diagnosis.[9]

Diagnosis

The physical examination will localize the site of dislocation and often reveal swelling, ecchymosis, deformity and tenderness. Inspection, palpation and the cross-arm test are usually adequate to assess AC or SC injuries. To visualize the severity of AC joint injury, the seated athlete is examined as distal traction is placed on both arms simultaneously. Observation of an increase in the space created between the acromion and the distal clavicle on the injured side indicated injury of the AC joint. Radiographs are obtained to help assess the degree and direction of AC separations. These include an AP view of both AC joints for comparison and an axillary view to determine anterior or posterior positioning as well as intra-articular involvement. A sternal tilt (Zanca) view may also aid in diagnosis. Sternoclavicular injuries are particularly difficult to image and may require computed tomography to see the pathology well.

In the skeletally immature athlete, physeal fracture is more likely to occur than AC or SC joint dislocation.[10] These physes may not fuse until after the age of 20. Depending on the athlete's age, the epiphysis may be difficult to visualize on X-ray, if it is still primarily cartilage.

AC separations are graded by degree of disruption and bone location. Grade I injuries are non-displaced strains to the AC ligaments. Grade II injuries have disrupted AC ligaments and intact coracoclavicular ligaments. Grade III injuries have both sets of ligaments disrupted and usually displaced more than 1 cm. Grade IV injuries are displaced posteriorly, grade V injuries are severe grade III injuries and grade VI injuries are rare and displaced inferiorly.

Treatment

Acromioclavicular separations are usually treated non-operatively.[11,12] Despite this, Mouhsine *et al.* reported only 52% of patients remained asymptomatic at an average follow-up of 6 years following conservative treatment for grade I and II AC joint separations.[13] Some grade III separations are repaired, especially in weightlifters or athletes who must wear shoulder pads. These are relative indications for surgery, and many athletes have good outcomes with conservative treatment.[14] Grades IV, V, and VI and chronic, symptomatic lesser AC separations are treated with primary repair or distal clavicle resection and stabilization.

Sternoclavicular separations are usually anterior and are treated non-operatively. Posterior SC dislocation may compromise pulmonary and neurovascular structures and are reduced operatively (Fig. 26.1).[9] Physeal fractures heal rapidly, and

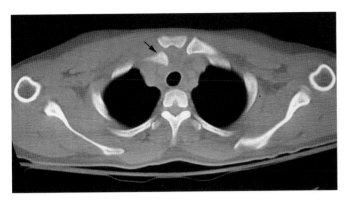

Figure 26.1 CT image of the sternoclavicular joint. Note the posterior displacement of the clavicle and its near proximity to the contents of the mediastinum.

these deformities may remodel completely with time. If field-side examination shows a posterior SC separation, emergent cardiopulmonary evaluation is required. If the injury is AC or anterior SC separation, a sling will provide comfort until full assessment is completed.

Rehabilitation

An AC separation or an anterior SC separation can be rehabilitated with general shoulder strengthening as soon as pain subsides. Operative AC and SC repairs require 4–6 weeks of healing before starting motion and strengthening. Whether treated non-surgically or surgically, 3–4 months of rehabilitation are normally required to achieve pre-injury status. Rotator cuff and periscapular muscle strength should be restored before working the larger shoulder girdle muscles.

Acromioclavicular and SC separations that are treated non-operatively can return to play as pain permits. Depending on the sport, the clavicle can be strapped or padded and the athlete returned within days or weeks. Following operative

repairs, 4 months is usually necessary to achieve adequate healing, strength, and proprioception to return to sports safely.

Fractures of the shoulder

> ### Box 26.3: Key Points
>
> - Treatment of shoulder girdle fractures depends on severity of injury and displacement.
> - Articular injuries are less forgiving and must be near anatomic.

Pathogenesis

The shoulder girdle consists of the proximal humerus, the scapula and the clavicle. Most shoulder girdle fractures occur following a lateral fall onto the shoulder or after an axial load to the humerus. They are uncommon in the athlete, but can occur secondary to high-energy trauma (Fig. 26.2). Some fractures such as a clavicle or humeral shaft fracture can be palpated readily. Others, such as some scapula fractures, may not be apparent to palpation in a muscular athlete. In the young athlete, physeal fracture of the proximal humerus is common (Fig. 26.3). Most injuries heal readily without complications.

Diagnosis

Plain radiographs consist of an anteroposterior view of the glenohumeral joint, a trans-scapular or scapular-Y lateral and an axillary view. Special views can be used to assess the anterior-inferior glenoid rim and the clavicle. If detailed osseous evaluation is needed, computed tomography is preferred.

Treatment

Management of shoulder fractures is similar in athletes and non-athletes. Since the shoulder has a large range of motion,

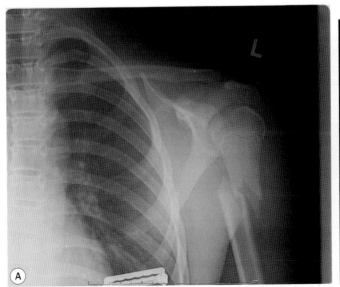
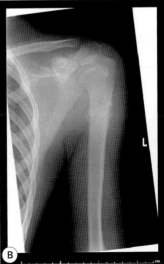

Figure 26.2 (A) AP X-ray of a displaced proximal humeral shaft fracture and (B) healing of the fracture 4 months after a ski injury.

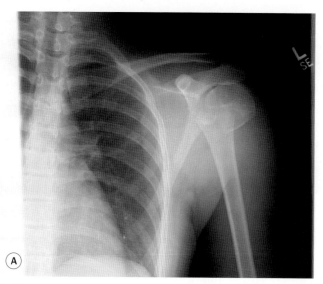

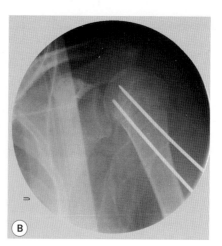

Figure 26.3 (A) AP view of a displaced proximal humeral physeal fracture. (B) Because of the degree of displacement, a percutaneous fixation was performed.

perfect anatomic reduction of proximal humerus fractures is not necessary. In adolescents or adults, the angulation should be <30° and the reduction stable. However, consideration should be given to ensuring anatomic reduction in the dominant shoulder of a throwing athlete, gymnast, or swimmer who is prone to develop overuse shoulder injury even without a fracture. Non-displaced stable fractures are treated non-surgically with immobilization and early range of motion. Displaced fractures require reduction. Displaced fractures that are unstable may require reduction and internal fixation. Children younger than 12 will remodel to a greater extent, therefore greater displacement and angulation are acceptable. Fractures of the greater tuberosity are often associated with anterior shoulder dislocations. These commonly reduce with glenohumeral relocation. Most experts accept 5 mm of displacement as the acceptable limit for indicating conservative treatment.

Clavicle fractures commonly occur in the middle third and traditionally are thought to heal acceptably with non-operative treatment using a sling or figure of 8 brace for comfort (Fig. 26.4). Recent reports have suggested that a large portion of conservatively treated patients continue to have sequela and a significant rate of non-union.[15–17] Open fractures, those in which there is interposed muscle and fractures with the skin at risk for perforation always require operative reduction and fixation.

Scapula fractures usually result from a high-energy injury and can have coexisting pulmonary injury as well as rib, clavicular and humeral fractures. Unless the glenoid is fractured and displaced more than 2 mm, scapula fractures can be treated by immobilization in a soft dressing such as a sling and swathe. Displaced articular glenoid fractures more than 2 mm should be repaired operatively.

Rehabilitation
Once the fracture has healed, strength, range-of-motion, and proprioception must be restored before play is resumed. A typical progression after bony union includes passive motion, followed by active motion and rotator cuff strengthening. Periscapular stabilization and major shoulder muscle strengthening follow in conjunction with shoulder proprioceptive training. When the bone is healed and the shoulder rehabilitated as above, the athlete may return to competition. The time-frame is variable depending on the sport.

Acute tendon rupture
Pathogenesis
Sudden severe pain in the region of a muscle following a forceful contraction (frequently as the muscle is lengthening) suggests muscle or tendon rupture. Failure occurs in hypovascular parts of the tendon or at the muscle-tendon junction. Both eccentric and concentric loads can lead to failure. Tear of the long head of the pectoralis major occurs most commonly in weight lifters and wrestlers. These tears routinely occur at the humeral insertion.[18]

Most rotator cuff tears occur at the lateral bony attachment. Patients with rotator cuff tears have night pain, weakness and have pain with impingement testing. Rupture of the long head of the biceps tendon occurs at the glenoid and causes a 'Popeye' muscle bulge at the biceps contour.

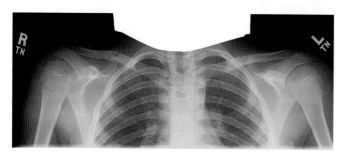

Figure 26.4 AP X-ray view of a non-displaced clavicle fracture.

Diagnosis

Muscle or tendon rupture occurs to pectoralis major, biceps long head, subscapularis and other rotator cuff muscles. Ecchymosis and asymmetric appearance of the muscular contour are common. Palpation for defects along the muscle tendon course or a prominent biceps or pectoralis major muscle bulge inconsistent with the contralateral side should raise suspicions of complete tear. Physical examination will identify most of these ruptures. Rotator cuff tears will lead to pain with impingement testing. There is pain and weakness with internal rotation (subscapularis), abduction (supraspinatus), or external rotation (infraspinatus). Magnetic resonance imaging (Fig. 26.5) or ultrasound can confirm the diagnosis.

Treatment

Except for the long head of biceps tendon, operative repair of tendon ruptures is usually necessary. Rupture of the long head of the biceps is frequently degenerative and it is difficult to achieve satisfactory repair. The resulting weakness has not been found to be significant. The biceps tendon can be left in a contracted position if the muscle bulge is cosmetically acceptable to the patient. This leads to a deficit in supination strength and some decrease in elbow flexion strength. Tenodesis to the bicipital grove in the humeral head can be done to restore normal length and appearance to the muscle-tendon complex.

After rotator cuff or pectoralis tendon repair, passive motion is begun immediately followed by active motion at 6 weeks postoperatively. Strengthening can also be started at 6 weeks. Traditionally, rotator cuff tendons have been repaired by open or mini-open means.[19] More recently, repairs are being done arthroscopically with satisfactory results and less postoperative pain.[20] Following long head of the biceps tendon rupture, the athlete may return to play as soon as pain and swelling resolve. Rehabilitation for 4–6 months is required following rotator cuff or pectoralis repair to allow adequate healing and strengthening. Outcomes of non-operative and operative treatment of pectoralis major tears have been

reported to be similar[21] but surgical repair appears to allow greater recovery of strength and improved subjective functional outcomes.[22]

OVERUSE INJURIES OF THE SHOULDER

Impingement

> **Box 26.4: Key Points**
>
> - Shoulder impingement is common and frequently secondary to another derangement.
> - Focused rotator cuff and periscapular stabilization is the main intervention.

Pathogenesis

Shoulder problems that are characterized as external impingement refer to the abnormal contact of the rotator cuff with the acromion. When the rotator cuff muscles are disproportionately weak compared with the large scapular stabilizing muscles, the humeral head translates too far anteriorly or superiorly allowing the greater tuberosity to impinge at the acromion or the coracoacromial ligament through the rotator cuff. In addition, alterations in the muscular activation sequence of the trapezius and serratus muscle have been found in young patients with impingement.[23] The resulting friction can lead to bursitis, tendonitis, tendinosis and tears. In throwing athletes, impingement is more commonly a secondary phenomenon and is usually secondary to subclinical instability with or without labral pathology. Likewise, biceps tendon injuries can cause symptoms of impingement. Reproducing the impingement confirms the diagnosis, but it is more important to discover why the muscle imbalance exists.[24]

Causes include training error (developing only the large shoulder muscles), rotator cuff tear (such as from a violent throw or fall), or repetitive motion (such as occurs in swimmers as they pull the humeral head against the coracoacromial ligament with every stroke). There are certain acromion morphologies (hooked, sloped) that may predispose to impingement, but the sport-specific repetitive use of the shoulder is a greater risk factor.[25]

Diagnosis

The history and visual inspection of the shoulder will focus the examiner on those areas requiring detailed testing. Shoulder range of motion can be simply evaluated by measuring elevation, forward flexion, adduction, external rotation in 90° of abduction, and the height along the spine that can be reached by the thumb (adduction, internal rotation). Testing internal rotation in 90° of abduction allows detection of a tight posterior capsule and tight external rotator muscles. Evaluating resisted internal rotation, external rotation, and adduction assesses rotator cuff strength. Studies have highlighted the role of scapulothoracic coordination in the development of impingement.[26] Testing serratus anterior strength and observing scapu-

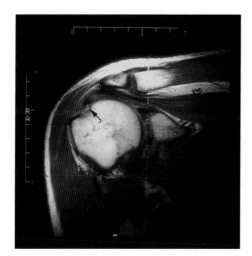

Figure 26.5 A coronal MR image of the shoulder demonstrating a tear of the supraspinatus tendon. Note the retraction of the tendon from its bony insertion of the greater tuberosity of the humerus.

lar motion as the arm moves through elevation can bring out evidence of dyskinesis. Glenohumeral joint problems are assessed with three special tests. The apprehension test leads to pain and apprehension with forced abduction and external rotation. A positive test indicates anterior glenohumeral instability. Glenohumeral translation is checked in the anterior, posterior, and inferior directions and compared to the contralateral side. Finally, loading the anterior, posterior, or superior capsule while rotating the humeral head to elicit a painful 'click' can assess the labral pathology.

MRI is the best study for evaluation of rotator cuff tears and other soft tissue injuries of the shoulder. Despite this, MRI is poor at evaluating labral tears. Use of intra-articular gadolinium with the MRI or use of CT arthrogram is better in detecting labral pathology. In many countries, ultrasound is used routinely for soft tissue evaluation of shoulder problems.[27] The technique used should be based on local availability and skill of the radiologist.

Treatment

Treatment of impingement first requires rotator cuff and periscapular strengthening and often posterior capsular stretching exercises.[28] A subacromial injection of corticosteroid may be necessary to decrease inflammation and gain sufficient pain relief to permit stretching and strengthening. If resolution does not occur or is transient, glenohumeral pathology must be considered and arthroscopic evaluation may be indicated. Further treatment may include labral repair or debridement, and capsular tightening by arthroscopic or open means. Thermal capsular shrinkage in these athletes has some distinct practical advantages, but the correction has not held-up well over time and suture plication seems to be more durable.[29]

Rehabilitation

Since shoulder impingement is in part caused by relatively weak rotator cuff muscles, strengthening the subscapularis, supraspinatus, infraspinatus, and teres minor is mandatory. The periscapular stabilizers including rhomboids, trapezius, levator scapulae and serratus anterior must be strengthened as well and may play a greater role than the cuff muscles. These periscapular muscles must be strengthened in non-operative treatment of shoulder instability as well as following operative glenohumeral repairs. The strengthening program should include the entire kinetic chain, particularly the trunk muscles.

Shoulder proprioception refers to control of the shoulder at all points of motion. Following capsular injury or surgery, proprioception must be restored prior to return to play. In general, this is accomplished by focusing on commonly used sport-specific drills. This is especially true in throwing athletes. Resumption of throwing is accomplished by slowly re-learning the muscle firing sequences as strength is restored. Restoration of muscle balance, the interplay between the cuff musculature and the scapular stabilizers, and developing stabilizer endurance are fundamental principles of rehabilitation. Any imbalance, even between the external and internal rotators can lead to excessive translation in one direction and instability or impingement. Likewise, muscle endurance needs to be balanced so that asymmetries do not develop as the athlete becomes fatigued. This concept is especially important in young athletes, throwers

and racket sport athletes who will alter their mechanics as one muscle group fatigues prematurely.

Return to play following overuse shoulder injury is governed by two factors. The first is pain within the range of motion required for the sport. The second is adequate strength and proprioception required to play the sport without increased risk of re-injury. Ideally, the shoulder (including trunk/shoulder girdle) has a full, pain-free range of motion with balanced strength and endurance and normal proprioception. If the shoulder is relatively well-balanced and pain-free and if extreme or painful motions (i.e. external rotation) can be restricted, the athlete can return to play.

Anterior impingement (swimmer's shoulder)

Box 26.5: Key Points

- Swimmer's shoulder results from an imbalance between shoulder stabilization muscles and those used for propulsion.

- Muscle balancing and technique changes can resolve symptoms.

- Both strength and endurance of that strength are important aspects of rehabilitation.

Pathogenesis

One form of external shoulder impingement is swimmer's shoulder.[30,31] Shoulder pain in the swimming athlete is common and can significantly limit activities. Most pain is caused by shoulder micro-instability[32] secondary to anterior impingement at the coracoacromial ligament. This can be precipitated secondary to the relative overdevelopment of the pectoralis major and anterior deltoid as well as changes in the recruitment patterns of the shoulder musculature.[33] A contracture of the posterior capsule causing decreased internal rotation is found. Prolonged muscle imbalances and abnormal motions of a swimmer's shoulder can lead to subclinical instability and anterior labral degeneration. Associated biceps tendonitis occurs frequently. While many swimmers have mild anterior impingement, only some become debilitated. Swimming more than 15 h per week or further than 35 km/week has been associated with more severe pathology.

Diagnosis

The athlete has pain with swimming, worsening with butterfly stroke and longer events. Diagnosis is similar to that for subacromial impingement with the exception that the impingement and pain is anterior at the coracoacromial ligament, rather than the acromion. Increased shoulder range of motion, except for decreased internal rotation, and decreased adduction strength are common.[34]

Treatment

Initially, treatment of swimmer's shoulder includes avoidance of all painful activities, use of anti-inflammatory medication to allow for physical therapy, decreasing anterior stretching and increasing stretching of the posterior capsule and external rotators. Strengthening of the rotator cuff with emphasis on external rotators is important.[34] Restoration of normal scapulo-thoracic strength and smooth motion is required. This typically includes trunk (core) strengthening as well. Surgical subacromial decompression alone, without balancing the cuff and major muscles of the shoulder, will have a low success rate.

Swimmer's shoulder is rehabilitated much the same as impingement with special emphasis on maintaining normal rotation and preventing an imbalance from developing between the strong pectoralis major and the scapular stabilizers. Like the other shoulder overuse injuries, anterior impingement that has resolved should not recur if technique and muscle balance have been optimized. If the athlete is not taught the proper training regimens, the condition will recur. Swimming is allowed when symptoms are gone.

NEUROLOGIC CONDITIONS

Neurologic injuries in athletes are uncommon. The majority are associated with contact sports. The most common injury is a stinger. A stinger is thought to be a transient neurapraxia to the brachial plexus or cervical root. Radicular symptoms, tingling, numbness and weakness are common but transient, lasting less then one minute. Diagnosis is based on physical evaluation. Further work-up is indicated with recurrent or sustained symptoms.[35] Overuse nerve injuries about the shoulder include thoracic outlet syndrome and suprascapular nerve

entrapment. Suprascapular entrapment occurs at the scapular notch and may result in severe infraspinatus atrophy. Surgical decompression at the notch is usually curative.

In the absence of abnormal anatomy, thoracic outlet syndrome is caused by poor posture, weak shoulder girdle musculature and weakness of the trapezius and levator scapula. This syndrome presents as pain, paresthesias, and/or weakness in the brachial plexus distribution. Often a diminished or thready pulse is noted with shoulder abduction. Strengthening of the supporting shoulder girdle muscles will improve the neurologic component of the syndrome.

VASCULAR CONDITIONS

Vascular injuries about the shoulder include thoracic outlet syndrome, traumatic intimal tears to the axillary or subclavian vessels, or deep vein thrombosis. Deep vein thrombosis typically presents as massive swelling of the arm, often following exercise. It is treated with anticoagulation for up to 6 months or by pharmacologic thrombolysis.[36,37] The vascular component of thoracic outlet syndrome will respond to trapezius and levator scapulae strengthening. In cases of additional cervical rib or other anatomic cause, surgical decompression may be required. The vascular surgeon treats intimal tears to shoulder girdle arteries or veins. Minor tears can be followed closely with Doppler ultrasound, MRI, or contrast angiography. Large tears must be repaired or excised.

REFERENCES

1　Miller SL, Cleeman E, Auerbach J, et al. Comparison of intra-articular lidocaine and intravenous sedation for reduction of shoulder dislocations: a randomized, prospective study. J Bone Jt Surg Am 2002; 84A:2135-2139.

2　Postacchini F, Gumina S, Cinotti G. Anterior shoulder dislocation in adolescents. J Shoulder Elbow Surg 2000; 9:470-474.

3　Arciero RA, Taylor DC. Primary anterior dislocation of the shoulder in young patients. A ten-year prospective study. J Bone Jt Surg Am 1998; 80:299-300.

4　Itoi E, Hatakeyama Y, Kido T, et al. A new method of immobilization after traumatic anterior dislocation of the shoulder: a preliminary study. J Shoulder Elbow Surg 2003; 12:413-415.

5　Romeo A, Carreira D. Outcome analysis of arthroscopic Bankart repair: Minimum two year follow-up. American Shoulder and Elbow Surgeons 16th Open Meeting, Orlando, Florida, 18 March 2000.

6　Bottoni CR, Wilckens JH, DeBerardino TM, et al. A prospective, randomized evaluation of arthroscopic stabilization versus nonoperative treatment in patients with acute, traumatic, first-time shoulder dislocations. Am J Sports Med 2002; 30:576-580.

7　Kirkley A, Griffin S, Richards C, et al. Prospective randomized clinical trial comparing the effectiveness of immediate arthroscopic stabilization versus immobilization and rehabilitation in first traumatic anterior dislocations of the shoulder. Arthroscopy 1999; 15:507-514.

8　Spencer EE, Kuhn JE, Huston LJ, et al. Ligamentous restraints to anterior and posterior translation of the sternoclavicular joint. J Shoulder Elbow Surg 2002; 11:43-47.

9　Medvecky MJ, Zuckerman JD. Sternoclavicular joint injuries and disorders. Instr Course Lect 2000; 49:397-406.

10　Kocher MS, Waters PM, Micheli LJ. Upper extremity injuries in the paediatric athlete. Sports Med 2000; 30:117-135.

11　Clarke HD, McCann PD. Acromioclavicular joint injuries. Orthop Clin North Am 2000; 31:177-187.

12　Phillips AM, Smart C, Groom AF. Acromioclavicular dislocation. Conservative or surgical therapy. Clin Orthop Relat Res 1998; 353:10-17.

13　Mouhsine E, Garofalo R, Crevoisier X, et al. Grade I and II acromioclavicular dislocations: results of conservative treatment. J Shoulder Elbow Surg 2003; 12:599-602.

14　Schlegel TF, Burks RT, Marcus RL, et al. A prospective evaluation of untreated acute grade III acromioclavicular separations. Am J Sports Med 2001; 29:699-703.

15　Nowak J, Holgersson M, Larsson S. Can we predict sequelae following fractures of the clavicle based on initial findings? A prospective study with 9-10 years follow-up. Program and Abstracts of the American Shoulder and Elbow Surgeons, 18th Open Meeting, Dallas, Texas, 16 February 2002.

16　Rokito AS, Zuckerman JD, Shaari JM, et al. A comparison of nonoperative and operative treatment of type II distal clavicle fractures. Bull Hosp Jt Dis 2002; 61:32-39.

17　Smith C, Rudd J, Crosby L. Results of operative versus non-operative treatment for 100% displaced mid-shaft clavicle fractures: A prospective randomized clinical trial. Program and Abstracts of the American Shoulder and Elbow Surgeons, 16th Open Meeting, Orlando, Florida, 18 March 2000.

18　Bak K, Cameron EA, Henderson IJ. Rupture of the pectoralis major: a meta-analysis of 112 cases. Knee Surg Sports Traumatol Arthrosc 2000; 8:113-119.

19　Warner JJ, Tetreault P, Lehtinen J, et al. Arthroscopic versus mini-open rotator cuff repair: a cohort comparison study. Arthroscopy 2005; 21:328-332.

20　Buess E, Steuber KU, Waibl B. Open versus arthroscopic rotator cuff repair: a comparative view of 96 cases. Arthroscopy 2005; 21:597-604.

21　Schepsis AA, Grafe MW, Jones HP, et al. Rupture of the pectoralis major muscle. Outcome after repair of acute and chronic injuries. Am J Sports Med 2000; 28:9-15.

22　Hanna CM, Glenny AB, Stanley SN, et al. Pectoralis major tears: comparison of surgical and conservative treatment. Br J Sports Med 2001; 35:202-206.

23　Cools AM, Witvrouw EE, Declercq GA, et al. Scapular muscle recruitment patterns: trapezius muscle latency with and without impingement symptoms. Am J Sports Med 2003; 31:542-549.

24　Mehta S, Gimbel JA, Soslowsky LJ. Etiologic and pathogenetic factors for rotator cuff tendinopathy. Clin Sports Med 2003; 22:791-812.

25　Carpenter JE, Flanagan CL, Thomopoulos S, et al. The effects of overuse combined with intrinsic or extrinsic alterations in an animal model of rotator cuff tendinosis. Am J Sports Med 1998; 26:801-807.

26　Warner JJ, Micheli LJ, Arslanian LE, et al. Scapulothoracic motion in normal shoulders and shoulders with glenohumeral instability and impingement syndrome. A study using Moire topographic analysis. Clin Orthop Relat Res 1992; 285:191-199.

27　Iannotti JP, Ciccone J, Buss DD, et al. Accuracy of office-based ultrasonography of the shoulder for the diagnosis of rotator cuff tears. J Bone Jt Surg Am 2005; 87:1305-1311.

28 Burkhart SS, Morgan CD, Kibler WB. The disabled throwing shoulder: spectrum of pathology. Part I: pathoanatomy and biomechanics. Arthroscopy 2003; 19:404–420.

29 D'Alessandro DF, Bradley JP, Fleischli JE, et al. Prospective evaluation of thermal capsulorrhaphy for shoulder instability: indications and results, two- to five-year follow-up. Am J Sports Med 2004; 32:21–33.

30 Bak K. Nontraumatic glenohumeral instability and coracoacromial impingement in swimmers. Scand J Med Sci Sports 1996; 6:132–144.

31 Rupp S, Berninger K, Hopf T. Shoulder problems in high level swimmers – impingement, anterior instability, muscular imbalance? Int J Sports Med 1995; 16:557–562.

32 Borsa PA, Scibek JS, Jacobson JA, et al. Sonographic stress measurement of glenohumeral joint laxity in collegiate swimmers and age-matched controls. Am J Sports Med 2005; 33:1077–1084.

33 Wadsworth DJ, Bullock-Saxton JE. Recruitment patterns of the scapular rotator muscles in freestyle swimmers with subacromial impingement. Int J Sports Med 1997; 18:618–624.

34 Weldon EJ, 3rd, Richardson AB. Upper extremity overuse injuries in swimming. A discussion of swimmer's shoulder. Clin Sports Med 2001; 20:423–438.

35 Koffler KM. Kelly JD 4th. Neurovascular trauma in athletes. Orthop Clin North Am 2002; 33:523–534.

36 Meyering C, Howard T. Hypercoagulability in athletes. Curr Sports Med Rep 2004; 3:77–83.

37 Thomas IH, Zierler BK. An integrative review of outcomes in patients with acute primary upper extremity deep venous thrombosis following no treatment or treatment with anticoagulation, thrombolysis, or surgical algorithms. Vasc Endovascular Surg 2005; 39:163–174.

CHAPTER 27

Hand and Wrist Injuries

Brandon E. Earp and Peter M. Waters

INTRODUCTION

Hand and wrist injuries are relatively common in sport, accounting for 3–9% of all athletic injuries.[1–3] These types of injuries are also more common in pediatric and adolescent patients than in adults.[3] They can cause significant morbidity and impairment that may substantially alter both the athletic career and future functional abilities of the patient. Prevention of injury is critical to decrease the long-term difficulties associated with many of these injuries. Protection in the form of pads and appropriately applied taping may be useful. Pre-activity stretching and adequate focus on range of motion of the entire body can also limit morbidity. Progressive resistive exercises for strengthening will improve the strength and the intrinsic protective capabilities of the body. Above all, safety in the athletic arena must be a priority for all players.

Once injury has occurred, appropriate diagnosis is important to determine the most appropriate treatment and rehabilitation program. A realistic plan for determining the timing of return to play should be explained to the athlete for planning purposes. This must take into account both the healing and rehabilitation stages that must be completed prior to safe return to sport.

Injuries may present as either acute, traumatic events, or as more subtle, chronic overuse injuries. While acute injury is often easier to diagnose (fractures, tendon injuries, dislocations), the chronic injury may ultimately lead to more long-term difficulty if left undiagnosed and untreated.

Better understanding of injury mechanisms and pathology, improvements in diagnostic methods, advances in surgical fixation for fractures, and arthroscopic techniques have significantly enhanced the ability of the physician to care for hand and wrist injuries in the athlete.[3] Specially designed splints and casts may also allow for earlier return to sport, sometimes while the injury continues to heal. Caution should be exercised; both the physician and the patient must recognize that the safety of the patient and the other players must always supersede the wishes of the player to return too quickly.

ANATOMY

Skeletal

The two bones of the forearm, the radius and ulna, articulate distally at the level of the wrist. The carpus is comprised of eight bones, of which the scaphoid and lunate articulate with the distal radius, forming the radiocarpal joint. There are two rows within the carpus – the proximal row, which includes the scaphoid, lunate, and triquetrum, and the distal row, which includes the trapezium, trapezoid, capitate, and hamate. The articulation between the rows is referred to as the midcarpal joint. The eighth carpal bone, the pisiform, sits volar to the triquetrum. There are five metacarpals that articulate with the distal row of carpal bones. Each finger has three phalanges, the proximal, middle, and distal, while the thumb has only two phalanges, the proximal and distal (Fig. 27.1).

Muscular

Motor function of the hand and wrist is controlled by muscles both extrinsic and intrinsic to the hand.

The extrinsic hand and wrist flexors originate from the medial epicondyle of the humerus and the proximal radius and ulna. The wrist flexors (flexor carpi radialis (FCR) and flexor carpi ulnaris (FCU)) insert on the distal carpus and the proximal aspect of the metacarpals. The digital flexors (flexor digitorum profundus (FDP), flexor digitorum superficialis (FDS), and flexor pollicis longus (FPL)) cross the wrist through the carpal tunnel with the median nerve. The FDP tendons insert at the proximal aspect of each digit's distal phalanx, allowing for flexion of the distal interphalangeal joints (DIP). The FDS tendons insert at the middle phalanges, providing flexion of the proximal interphalangeal joints (PIP). The FPL tendon flexes the interphalangeal joint (IP) of the thumb. At the level of the metacarpal heads, these tendons enter the flexor tendon sheath, which has multiple thickenings that are called pulleys. The pulleys maintain the tendons close to the bones, providing a mechanical advantage by preventing 'bowstringing' which would otherwise occur with flexion. The second and fourth annular pulleys, which are located along the proximal and

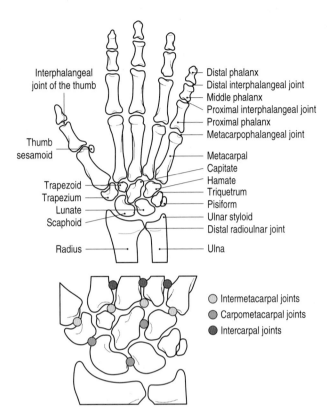

Interphalangeal
joint of the thumb

Distal phalanx
Distal interphalangeal joint
Middle phalanx
Proximal interphalangeal joint
Proximal phalanx
Metacarpophalangeal joint

Thumb
sesamoid

Metacarpal
Capitate
Hamate
Triquetrum
Pisiform
Ulnar styloid
Distal radioulnar joint

Trapezoid
Trapezium
Lunate
Scaphoid

Radius

Ulna

○ Intermetacarpal joints
○ Carpometacarpal joints
● Intercarpal joints

Figure 27.1 Bony anatomy of the hand and wrist. (From Fam AG. The wrist and hand. In: Hochberg M, Silman A, Smolen JS, eds. Rheumatology. 3rd edn. Philadelphia, PA: Mosby; 2003:641–650, with permission.)

middle phalanges respectively, are the most important for preventing tendon bowstringing during flexion.

The extrinsic hand and wrist extensors originate from the lateral epicondyle of the humerus and the proximal radius and ulna. The wrist extensors (extensor carpi radialis longus and brevis (ECRL, ECRB) and extensor carpi ulnaris (ECU)) insert at the dorsal bases of the second, third, and fifth metacarpals, respectively. The digital extensors (extensor digitorum communis (EDC), extensor indicis proprius (EIP), and extensor digiti quinti (EDQ)) allow for extension across the metacarpophalangeal joints (MCP) and through a complex extensor mechanism also coordinate with the intrinsic muscles of the hand to provide extension across the PIP and DIP joints.

The intrinsic musculature of the hand can be divided into three main divisions. The thenar muscles are located at the volar-radial aspect of the hand and allow for fine motor control of the thumb. The hypothenar muscles are located at the volar-ulnar aspect of the hand and provide abduction and opposition of the small finger. The intrinsics allow for abduction and adduction of the digits as well as extension across the PIP and DIP joints through a coordinated extensor mechanism complex with the extrinsic digital extensors (Fig. 27.2).

Neurovascular

Three major nerves cross the wrist to provide sensation in the hand. These are the radial, median, and ulnar nerves. The median and ulnar nerves innervate the hand musculature;

the median is primarily responsible for the thenar muscles, and the ulnar innervates the hypothenar and intrinsic muscles. Each of these nerves carries electrical impulses to and from the brain to allow for sensation and motion in the hand. There are two major arteries that supply oxygenated blood to the hand. After passing the level of the wrist, the ulnar artery provides the major contribution to formation of the superficial palmar arch, which is the major blood supply of the fingers. The radial artery becomes the primary contributor to the deep palmar arch of the hand, which courses more proximally than the superficial arch. There is variable continuity of the arches from each of their main supporting arteries to the other. Each digit has two volar neurovascular bundles, which contain an artery and nerve, one each on the radial and ulnar aspects. In the digit, the artery lies dorsal to the nerve; in the hand, the nerve lies dorsal (Fig. 27.3).

PHYSICAL EXAMINATION

Box 27.1: Key Points

● A thorough examination is critical to diagnosis; knowledge of anatomy is crucial.
● Observation should come before manipulation.
● Have the patient point to the problematic area with one finger.

Observation is the first step in the physical examination of the hand and wrist. The examiner should take note of the resting posture of the wrist and fingers. A normal resting posture will have the MCP joints flexed 45–70° and each of the IP joints slightly flexed up to 10°.[4] Abnormal posturing can mean fracture, ligament, or tendon injury. Any gross malalignment, edema, ecchymosis, lacerations, or skin/nail changes can indicate underlying pathology.

The patient's localization of symptoms is often most telling. It is useful to have the patient use one finger to isolate a specific region of symptoms prior to any palpation or manipulation by the examiner.

A good understanding of the surface anatomy of the hand and wrist is very important for appropriate evaluation of injuries (Fig. 27.4). This allows the examiner to focus the exam to determine which of many diagnoses are possible, and what further work-up, if any, is necessary.

A chronic examination should include the skin and nails. Skin dryness or cracking can be indicative of nerve injury. Blood supply can be assessed by palpating the radial and ulnar arterial pulses at the wrist, and by blanching the fingertips to determine capillary refill of the digits. Normal refill is <2 s. An Allen's test, performed by compressing both the radial and ulnar arteries at the wrist, which blanches the hand, and then assessing reperfusion when only one of the arteries is released, allows evaluation of the patency of the vascular arches of the hand.

Sensory function of the nerves can be evaluated in the digits by light touch and two-point discrimination using a paper clip or calipers. Normal two-point discrimination is <5 mm.[5]

Palpation of the region of interest can often localize a specific area of tenderness, crepitus, or firmness, which could indicate underlying pathology. Specific areas that should be palpated include the pisiform, hook of hamate, anatomic snuffbox, and dorsal scapholunate articulation.

Active motion by the patient is important to assess before passive manipulation. Lack of ability to flex or extend across a joint, or malalignment with motion can be assessed. As the hand is closed, fingertips should point toward the scaphoid.

The distal nail tips should be aligned when the fingers are in a partially flexed position. Wrist motion should be assessed for extension, flexion, pronation, supination, and radial and ulnar deviation. Digital motion should include flexion, extension, abduction, and adduction. The thumb's additional capability for retropulsion, and radial and palmar abduction should be examined.

Strength testing should include resisted motion across each joint. The FDS and FDP strength should be isolated by testing

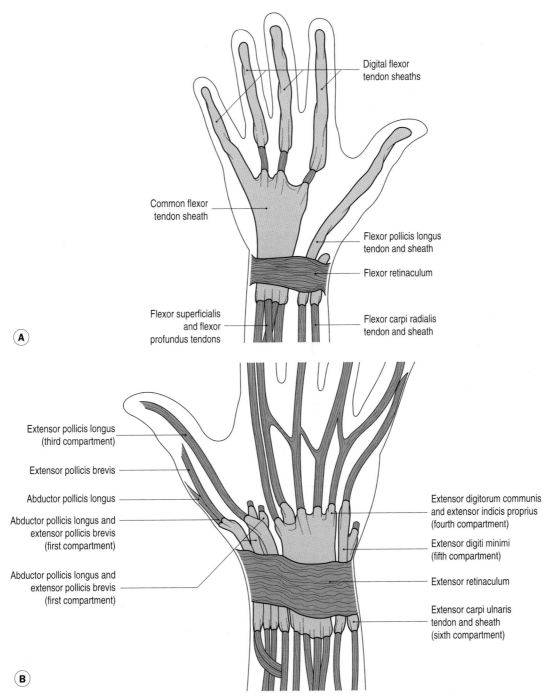

Figure 27.2 Tendons of the wrist and hand. (A) Flexor tendons. (B) Extensor tendons.

(Continued)

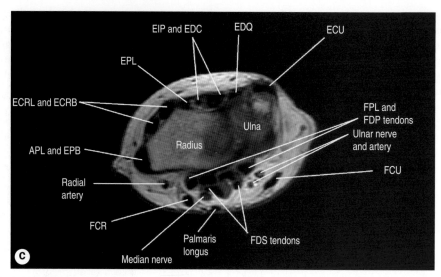

Figure 27.2 *Continued* (C) Axial MRI view of the wrist at the carpal tunnel level, showing the flexor and extensor tendons as well as major neurovascular structures as labeled. FCR, flexor carpi radialis; FPL, flexor pollicis longus; FDP, flexor digitorum profundus; FDS, flexor digitorum superficialis; FCU, flexor carpi ulnaris; APL, abductor pollicis longus; EPB, extensor pollicis brevis; ECRL and ECRB, extensor carpi radialis longus and brevis; EPL, extensor pollicis longus; EIP, extensor indicis proprius; EDC, extensor digitorum communis; EDQ, extensor digiti quinti; ECU, extensor carpi ulnaris. (Figs (A) and (B) from Fam AG. The wrist and hand. In: Hochberg M, Silman A, Smolen JS, eds. Rheumatology. 3rd edn. Philadelphia, PA: Mosby; 2003:641–650, with permission.)

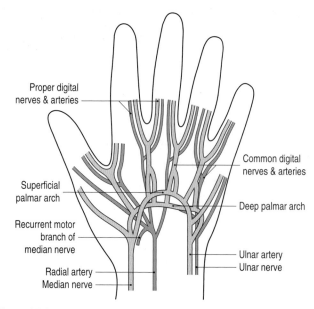

Figure 27.3 Neurovascular structures of the wrist and hand.

resisted DIP flexion for FDP strength, and by individual digit testing of resisted PIP flexion while maintaining the other digits extended. Pinch and grip strength should also be assessed.

Provocative stress testing can also elicit pain or other findings that can aid in diagnosis. These maneuvers will be discussed further in the text below.

Remember that a good examination for a hand or wrist injury should include an examination of the uninjured side.

INVESTIGATIONS

X-rays should be the first study performed and are indicated in most patients with trauma or other injury. A minimum of two views is required (a posteroanterior (PA) and lateral), but an oblique of the wrist can also be quite helpful. If a certain diagnosis is being considered, specialized views, such as a PA with clenched fist for scapholunate ligament injury, a carpal tunnel view for hook of hamate fracture, and pisotriquetral views for pathology in that area, may aid in diagnosis.

CT scans provide additional information about the bony anatomy, especially with difficult intraarticular fractures, or those involving the carpal bones, which are sometimes hard to assess with plain radiographs, given the overlapping nature of the carpus.

Bone scans can be helpful to identify regions of involvement, but do not inform the examiner of the exact process occurring. They can show stress fractures, tumors, infection, and avascular necrosis, and can be useful in the assessment of chronic wrist pain.[6]

Ultrasound can be somewhat operator dependent, but in skilled hands can localize foreign bodies, tendon injuries, soft tissue masses, and fluid collections.

MRI allows visualization of the soft tissues and can be very helpful to identify intracarpal ligament injury, triangular fibrocartilage complex (TFCC) tears and avascular necrosis. MRI scans have been used more often than bone scans for assessing both acute and chronic injuries not diagnosable by plain radiographs.

Arthrography requires an invasive process with the injection of dye into the joints, but can improve the diagnostic quality of many studies, from radiographs to MRI.[7]

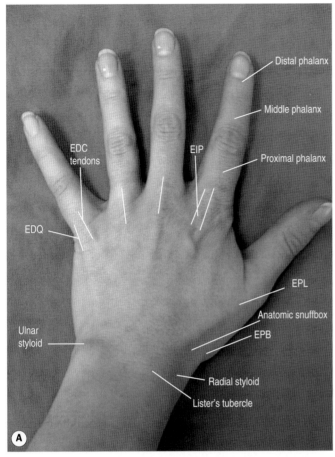
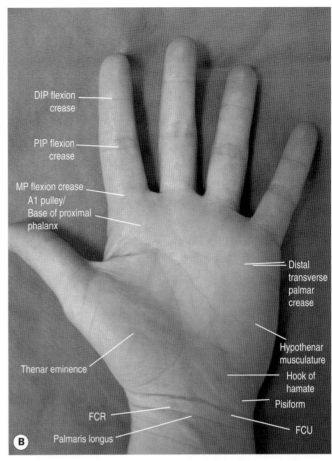

Figure 27.4 Surface anatomy of the (A) dorsal and (B) volar wrist and hand. EPB, extensor pollicis brevis; EPL, extensor pollicis longus; EIP, extensor indicis proprius; EDC, extensor digitorum communis; EDQ, extensor digiti quinti; FCR, flexor carpi radialis; FCU, flexor carpi ulnaris; DIP, distal interphalangeal; PIP, proximal interphalangeal; MP, metacarpophalangeal.

WRIST

Box 27.2: Key Points

- Always assess for other injuries when trauma has occurred.

- Examining one joint above and one below the obvious injury often leads to detection of other pathology.

- Treatment of articular fractures should attempt to restore anatomic articular alignment.

- Acute soft tissue injuries of the wrist should not be overlooked as they may lead to progressive arthrosis with time.

Acute/Traumatic Injury
Fracture

Fractures in the adult will usually unite in approximately 6 weeks; children can often heal in half of that time. Consolidation of fractures can take 12 weeks or more. Many fractures will be non-displaced or minimally displaced and will not require either reduction maneuvers or surgery. Some fractures are displaced but can be manipulated into an appropriate alignment, and with the use of splinting and/or casting can be held in place until union occurs. Still others are either unstable and cannot be held by casting alone, or may involve the articular surfaces of the bones, and if displaced will usually require surgery.

Fractures may be isolated or may involve significant injury to other organ systems. As always, injured patients must be initially assessed for airway, breathing, and circulation. During a secondary survey, bony and soft tissue injuries of the extremities are evaluated and early management is initiated.

Open fractures, where the bone has been exposed to the outside environment either from an outside-in injury, or, more commonly from an inside-out mechanism, should be detected. These skin breaks may range from complete amputations to small poke-holes and a high index of suspicion is necessary to avoid missing subtle open fractures. Once the diagnosis of an open fracture has been made, there is a surgical urgency to irrigate, débride, and stabilize the fracture. The wound should be covered with sterile saline or Betadine soaked sponges and should not be reopened for further examination until the operating room. Intravenous antibiotics, usually with a first generation cephalosporin (plus an aminoglycoside for more significant contamination, and anaerobic coverage if indicated) should be initiated. A tetanus vaccine is given if the patient has not had the vaccine in the past 5 years or if the vaccine history is not known.

Scaphoid fracture Scaphoid fractures are the most common carpal fracture, accounting for over 70% of all carpal fractures.[8] They are often sustained in a fall onto an outstretched arm. Weber and Chao have defined the biomechanics of the scaphoid fracture in the laboratory. When the wrist is positioned in more than 90° of extension and more than 10° of radial deviation, and sustains a load of over 400 kg of force, a scaphoid fracture results. When the wrist is less dorsiflexed and receives lower loads, distal radius fractures are seen (Fig. 27.5).[9]

The anatomy of the scaphoid accounts for much of the difficulty in both diagnosis and management of these fractures. The irregular shape of the scaphoid makes visualization of fractures difficult. Also, over 80% of the surface area of the scaphoid is articular, and thus there is little or no room for displacement.[10] The primary blood supply enters along the dorsal ridge of the scaphoid and flows distal to proximal through the scaphoid.[11] Fractures at or proximal to the waist of the scaphoid may sever the blood supply to the proximal fragment. Indeed, as many as one third of persons with scaphoid waist fractures will develop avascular necrosis (AVN). Due to this vascular anatomy, proximal pole fractures have an even higher rate of avascular necrosis of the proximal fragment and also have lower healing rates.

Diagnosis may be difficult and is often delayed because the fracture may not be seen on initial radiographs. Patients usually do not have any deformity of the wrist and may have very little swelling in the region. Pain is often not severe, but rather dull and aching in nature. However, any patient who presents with complaints of pain in the anatomic snuffbox region at the radial wrist should be evaluated and treated with a high degree of suspicion for this fracture. Additional radiographs such as the navicular view may aid in diagnosis. Because this fracture carries such a high rate of complications, including non-union,

malunion and avascular necrosis, a patient with pain in the area who has negative X-rays must still be treated in the short-term for a presumed scaphoid fracture. A short arm thumb spica splint helps prevent flexion, extension, supination, and pronation of the wrist temporarily. When the patient presents for re-examination in 1–2 weeks, repeat radiographs should be obtained. If the patient is no longer symptomatic and X-rays are negative, no further immobilization is necessary. If the patient continues to be symptomatic and the X-rays are negative, further work-up, most commonly including an MRI, is indicated.[12] CT scan and bone scan have also been used in this regard,[13,14] but MRI now appears to be the most definitive test for patients with acute and semi-acute wrist pain.

Once a scaphoid fracture has been diagnosed, it should be classified by location, stability, and time since injury.[15,16] This enables the treating physician to most appropriately counsel the patient on treatment recommendations.

The goal is to achieve union in an anatomic position. Studies have shown that once a scaphoid fracture displaces, carpal instability occurs.[17] The lunate assumes an extended position, and due to the intact scapholunate ligament, the proximal pole of the scaphoid also extends. The distal scaphoid flexes due to the intact attachments to the trapezium and trapezoid. A humpback deformity results. This constellation of carpal changes is also known as dorsal intercalated segment instability (DISI). Gapping at the fracture site of the scaphoid leads to a high rate of non-union and malunion. Over time, it is thought that these carpal changes will lead to progressive radiocarpal and ultimately pancarpal arthritis.[18–20]

Treatment options to achieve the goal of anatomic union can be achieved in different ways, depending on the nature, location, and age of the fracture, and on the patient's wishes. Options included cast immobilization of a variety of types *versus* internal fixation.

Non-displaced middle third fractures can be treated with a high success rate with cast immobilization. Cooney *et al.* showed a 90–100% success rate if immobilization began

Figure 27.5 Radiographs of displaced scaphoid waist fracture.

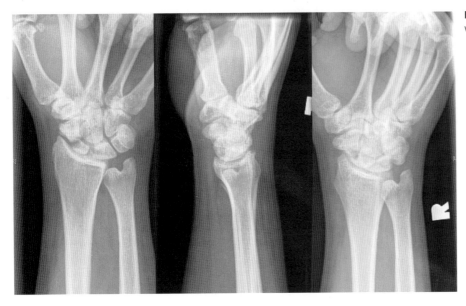

within 3 weeks of injury.[21] Many physicians prefer a long-arm cast for a period of 4–6 weeks, followed by a short arm cast once healing has begun.[22,23] Others use a short arm thumb spica throughout the immobilization period. The average time to healing for a scaphoid fracture is 8–10 weeks, and the patient should expect to be out of sport for a minimum of 3 months.

Some physicians will allow patients to play sports in their thumb spica cast, and two studies have shown over 90% healing rates with this method.[24,25] Some physicians have concerns that there may be an increased incidence of non-union that makes this practice less desirable.

Open reduction and internal fixation is usually indicated for any displaced fracture, proximal pole fractures, and for older fractures that have not had acute immobilization.[24,26,27] Fixation is usually accomplished with a headless compression screw that is buried below the level of the cartilage.

Some patients with non-displaced mid-third scaphoid fractures prefer to undergo surgery to have a compression screw placed in order to decrease the amount of time they will require cast immobilization. These fractures can often be fixed through limited incision techniques with low morbidity.[28] Time until patients return to work has been shown to be considerably less (5.8 weeks as compared with 10.2 weeks) in these patients treated surgically.[29]

Due to the difficulty in making this diagnosis, scaphoid fractures often present late, with a delayed or established non-union. Those who are symptomatic should be treated with open reduction, internal fixation and bone grafting.[30] Even in patients who are asymptomatic, surgery is recommended with internal fixation and grafting because natural history studies suggest that these patients will develop progressive arthritis.

Hook of hamate fracture

Hook of hamate fractures constitute 2–4% of all carpal fractures.[9,31–34] They are frequently diagnosed in a delayed fashion because the fracture is often not seen on standard radiographs. Patients with pain to deep palpation over the volar-ulnar hand or hypothenar region may be suspected of having this fracture. Many patients with this injury are athletes that play racquet sports, golf, bicycle riding/racing or baseball. The mechanism of injury is usually a blow to the hypothenar region of the hand, either when a bat, club, or racquet is swung and makes contact with a hard object, or if the patient falls onto the hand while holding an object across the palm.[35] If suspected, further radiographic views such as a carpal tunnel view or supinated oblique view may show the fracture. If these are not revealing, a CT scan with thin cuts through the carpus is indicated (Fig. 27.6).[36,37]

Patients with pain in this area of the hand should always be tested for ulnar nerve function, as the motor branch of the ulnar nerve curves around the hook of hamate *en route* to the more radial intrinsic musculature. Strength testing would include the first dorsal interosseous muscle (index abduction) and the adductor pollicis (thumb adductor), both of which receive innervation from this branch of the ulnar nerve.

Treatment for many hook of hamate fractures entails splinting or casting. Open reduction and fixation is appropriate for others. For patients with persistent symptoms, or even for some acute displaced or comminuted fractures, surgical exci-

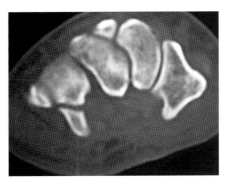

Figure 27.6 Axial CT scan of hook of hamate fracture.

sion of the small bony fragment is often indicated, as bony non-union is common.[35,38,39] Non-union is likely related to frequently delayed immobilization, but also may be due to the localization of a watershed area of vascularity at the base of the hook.[11,40,41] Return to sports in 7–10 weeks can be achieved with surgical excision.[3,35,39]

Pisiform fracture

Pisiform fractures are most often sustained in a direct blow to the region. This may occur in racquet or club sports.[42] Either fracture or other cartilage injury may lead to pisotriquetral arthrosis. Localized injection into the region can assist in diagnosis. Alternatively, a bone scan can localize abnormalities. If symptoms persist after a course of non-operative treatment, surgical excision of the pisiform can lead to symptom relief without loss in grip strength or wrist movement, and allow return to sport in 6–8 weeks.[42,43]

Triquetral fracture

Dorsal triquetral fractures were historically thought to be avulsions of the dorsal ridge. However, closer review of radiographs and cadaveric models has shown that these fractures are actually related to the abutment of either a long ulnar styloid[44] or the proximal edge of the hamate,[45] against the triquetrum, acting as a chisel to chip away a dorsal fragment from the triquetrum. This typically occurs in a position of hyperextension and ulnar deviation of the wrist. Management with a short course of immobilization has been successful in returning patients to sport in 6–8 weeks.[45]

Perilunate/lunate dislocation

Perilunate dislocation is one stage in a spectrum of wrist injury ranging from intercarpal ligament strain to lunate dislocation with complete disruption of the intercarpal ligaments. These injuries are sustained in falls onto an outstretched wrist, typically with the wrist in an extended, ulnarly deviated and supinated position.[46,47] Blunt force trauma in collision sports that mimics this type of impact can also lead to these injuries. On the initial examination, swelling and significant decreased range of motion are usually noted; however deformity may not be very pronounced. Acute carpal tunnel syndrome and median nerve contusion have both been observed with these injuries and the patient's neurovascular status should be closely documented.

Diagnosis is made on routine AP and lateral radiographs, but unfortunately can be missed if views are not acceptable or if the reviewer fails to recognize key anatomic changes associated with these injuries. On the AP view, both the proximal and distal carpal rows must be seen. They should not show disruption or overlap. The lunate should be a quadrangular shape. If it is triangular in appearance, there is a suggestion that the lunate is dislocated or that there is ligamentous disruption with extended posture of the lunate. On the lateral projection, the lunate should lie entirely within the distal radius and the capitate should rest distally within the lunate. Dorsal displacement of the capitate with respect to the lunate, and/or volar displacement of the lunate with respect to the radius indicates pathology.

As described by Mayfield,[48] the injury begins on the radial side of the wrist, frequently resulting in scapholunate ligament disruption. With higher energy injuries, the progression may continue its path ulnarly around the lunate. There may be entirely ligamentous injury, disrupting the scapholunate, midcarpal and lunotriquetral joints, or alternatively the path may be transosseous, passing through the radius, scaphoid, capitate, and triquetrum. If the lunate dislocates volarly, the injury pattern is called a lunate dislocation, and represents the most severe of the carpal disruptions. Ligamentous perilunate injuries represent disruption of the scapholunate and lunotriquetral ligaments and the capitolunate articulation. There is some variability in these injuries in that there may be a combination of ligamentous and bony disruption, for example, a trans-scaphoid perilunate dislocation (Fig. 27.7).

Treatment ranges from closed reduction and pinning to combined open volar and dorsal incisions with internal fixation and repair of ligaments.[49–52] Of primary importance is urgent closed reduction of the carpus to alleviate compression on the neurovascular structures, most importantly the median nerve. If symptoms of severe pain are unrelenting after reduction, a carpal tunnel release may be necessary acutely.

Long-term results are variable. Raab et al.[51] followed 10 patients with perilunate dislocation in the National Football League, six of whom were treated with closed reduction and pinning. Nine of these patients returned to professional football, five of them during the same season as the injury. Hildebrand et al.[52] followed 23 patients who underwent open reduction internal fixation through combined approaches. Three required wrist arthrodesis and one underwent four-corner fusion. One half of the remaining patients had radiographic arthritis and standardized, validated scoring systems, including the Disabilities of the Arm, Shoulder, and Hand (DASH) score and the Mayo wrist score showed lower scores than age matched normals, indicating functional loss. Some 73% of these patients were able to return to full duty in their former occupations.

Ligament tear

The wrist is a remarkably intricate example of the interplay between complex bony geometry and interosseous ligaments. This anatomy allows for remarkable range of motion in many planes and at the same time significant stability for functions requiring strength. When the connections between these carpal bones are changed, instability and decreased range of motion result. Changes in the mechanics can lead to increased forces across the joints and may expedite cartilage degeneration. Diagnosis and treatment of the injuries to avoid these long-term complications is critical.

Scapholunate

Scapholunate ligament injury is the most common ligamentous injury in the wrist. It often is seen following a fall onto an extended, ulnarly deviated wrist combined with a supination force, similar to the mechanism of a perilunate dislocation above. These injuries are also often seen in collision or contact sports. Indeed, a scapholunate ligament injury is the first stage of Mayfield's classification; the degree of injury is related to the energy imparted to the wrist at the time of injury.[53]

Injury to this ligament may be partial or complete. Partial tears will often have normal-appearing radiographs and further imaging with stress views, such as a clenched fist view, or even an arthrogram or MRI may be necessary for diagnosis. Both arthrogram and MRI have variable sensitivity and specificity for these ligament tears, particularly for partial tears, and ultimately, arthroscopic confirmation may be needed.[54,55] Complete tears will classically lead to an instability pattern that can be recognized on routine radiographs (Fig. 27.8). The scaphoid exerts a flexion moment on the proximal row while the triquetrum exerts an extension moment. While both bones maintain intact ligamentous attachments, the moments are balanced and allow for normal carpal motion. If the scapholunate ligament is torn, the lunate will extend due to the intact lunotriquetral ligament. The scaphoid flexes, creating what has been termed a dorsal intercalated segment instability.[56] Radiographically, this can be noted by many findings. The scaphoid ring sign is seen on an AP view. Due to the increased flexion of the scaphoid, the AP view will demonstrate the proximal pole overlapping the distal pole, appearing like a signet ring. The scapholunate interval on the AP view may be widened; a space >3 mm indicates ligamentous disruption. The lunate may have a triangular appearance rather than a quadrangular one due to its extended posture. On the lateral view, the scapholunate angle, which usually measures 30–60°, may be greater than 70°. The lunate will be volarly subluxed and extended; the normal neutral alignment of the distal radius, lunate, capitate, third metacarpal will be malaligned.[57] Note that there is significant variability among patients and so comparison views of the unaffected hand and wrist can be very helpful.

On examination, many of these patients will have significant pain and swelling acutely over the dorsal aspect of the scapholunate region. They may also have snuffbox tenderness, although this is classically associated with scaphoid fracture. Decreased range of motion is usually noted. A Watson shift test, in which pressure is placed over the volar aspect of the distal pole of the scaphoid as the wrist is brought from slight extension/ulnar deviation to radial deviation can elicit a 'shuck' as the proximal pole of the scaphoid is subluxated dorsally over the dorsal rim of the distal radius.[58] In the acute setting, many patients will not tolerate this testing due to pain. All examinations should include the contralateral wrist as a baseline.

Initial management of these patients consists of immobilization in a thumb spica splint or cast. Consultation with a hand surgeon is indicated to discuss surgical intervention, which may include ligament repair or reconstruction, or capsulodesis.[59,60] Arthroscopic evaluation may be indicated, and some partial tears may be treated with arthroscopic debridement (Fig. 27.9).[61,62]

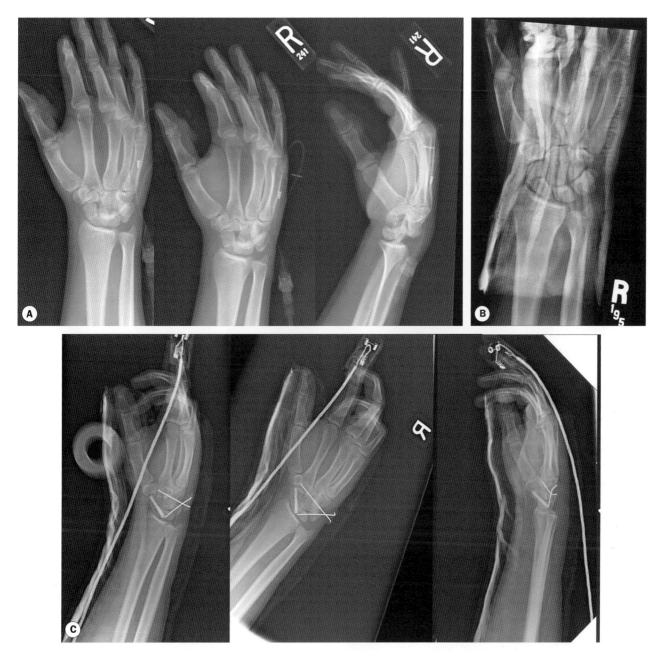

Figure 27.7 Radiographs of a trans-scaphoid fracture-dislocation. (A) Pre-reduction, (B) after closed reduction, (C) after open reduction and internal fixation.

In athletes, issues of range of motion, joint stability, pain-free activity, strength, and long-term prognosis are particularly important due to the high demands placed on these articulations. A specialized surgeon will be able to discuss options and aid the patient in making appropriate choices.

Many of these injuries go undiagnosed initially and will not present for evaluation until they have reached a chronic stage. Both motion and mechanics of the wrist are altered by scapholunate ligament tears, which may lead to abnormal loads across areas of the joint, creating inflammation and cartilage injury. With time, progression of these articular changes can lead to joint destruction, with collapse of the carpus. This condition is known as scapholunate advanced collapse (SLAC wrist). The arthrosis begins with abutment between the radial styloid and the scaphoid, progresses to involve the entire radio-scaphoid joint, and then becomes pan-carpal, usually sparing the radio-lunate joint (Fig. 27.10).[58]

Treatment for chronic diastasis is based on symptoms and the degree of arthrosis. A variety of reconstructive options including bone-retinaculum-bone autograft[63] and limited wrist fusions such as scaphocapitate or scaphotrapeziotrapezoid arthrodeses[64] have been described. For more advanced disease, proximal row carpectomy[65] or four-corner fusion[66] may be indicated for salvage.

Lunotriquetral

Lunotriquetral injuries typically arise from hyperextension of the wrist in a radially deviated, pronated wrist. They are much

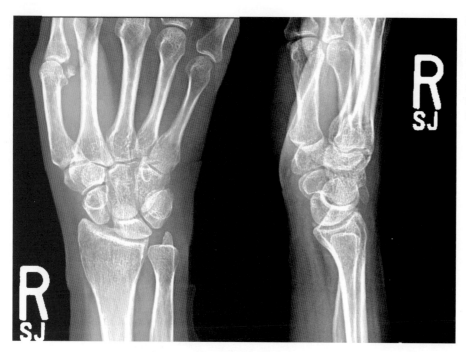

Figure 27.8 Radiographs of acute complete scapholunate ligament tear. On the posteroanterior (PA) view, there is widening of the scapholunate interval and the scaphoid has assumed a flexed position, and shows a 'ring sign'. On the lateral view, the lunate is extended from its normally neutral axis with the distal radius, capitate, and long finger metacarpal.

less frequently encountered than scapholunate tears.[67] When the lunotriquetral ligament ruptures, the intact scapholunate ligament will tend to exert a flexion force on the lunate, potentially leading to volar intercalated segment instability (VISI).[67] However, when compared with scapholunate ligament disruption, the lunotriquetral ligament is less likely to create such significant carpal instability, due to the extrinsic stabilization of the dorsal and volar ulnocarpal and volar carpal extrinsic ligaments.[67,68]

Athletes who have sustained a hyperextension injury to the wrist and who present with ulnar sided wrist pain, limited range of motion, weakness, and a 'clicking' sensation with lateral load-

ing should be examined for lunotriquetral injury.[69] They will have tenderness over the lunotriquetral region dorsally, lunotriquetral laxity and crepitus with stressed dorso-volar translation, and a snapping sensation with joint loading.[69]

Diagnosis may be delayed because plain radiographs are usually normal. Volar intercalated segment instability patterns seen on radiographs typically indicate more extensive injury, involving extrinsic ligaments as well. A wrist arthrogram may be helpful, although caution should be exercised as up to 20% of asymptomatic people may have a positive study.[70] MRI with or without enhanced indirect arthrography showed poor sensitivity but high specificity for lunotriquetral tears when compared with arthroscopy.[71]

Treatment for acute injuries should initially entail immobilization, which has been shown to be effective at achieving symptom relief in 80% of patients.[72] If symptoms persist, further diagnosis and debridement can be accomplished by arthroscopy with or without pinning.[73] Other surgical options include ligament repair or reconstruction, ulnar shortening osteotomy, and lunotriquetral arthrodesis, the latter of which has been shown to have a significant rate of non-union (40%), ulnocarpal impaction (22%), and need for revision surgery within 5 years (78%).[74] The degree of injury, duration of symptoms, and associated wrist arthrosis determine which procedure is most appropriate.

Midcarpal instability

Midcarpal instability occurs when there is disruption between the proximal and distal carpal rows, rather than within the proximal row, as seen in scapholunate and lunotriquetral disruptions. This midcarpal pattern is called 'carpal instability non-dissociative'.[66] The etiology is laxity or tearing of the volar ulnar ligaments connecting the capitate to the triquetrum, leading to loss of the normal restraints to motion between the rows.

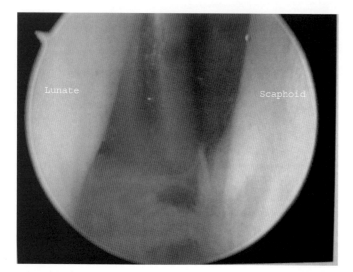

Figure 27.9 Arthroscopic view of the scapholunate interval showing a 'drive-through' sign. A probe the size of a wrist arthroscope has been passed from the midcarpal joint into the radiocarpal joint through the scapholunate disruption.

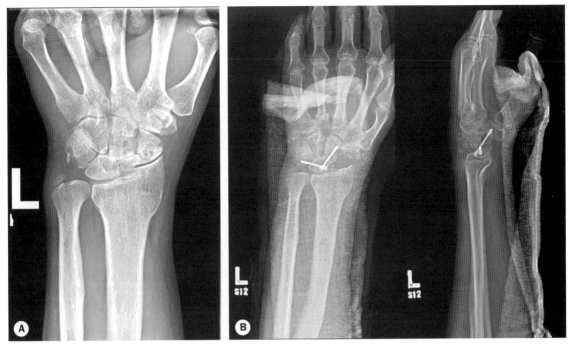

Figure 27.10 (A) Radiograph of a scapholunate advanced collapse (SLAC) wrist with pancarpal arthrosis, sparing the radiolunate joint. (B) Postoperative radiographs following a four-corner fusion, with arthrodesis of the lunate, capitate, hamate and triquetrum. The scaphoid and radial styloid have been resected.

Patients often present complaining of ulnar or diffuse wrist pain. They may demonstrate a palpable or even audible clunk when moving the wrist from radial to ulnar deviation as the proximal row fails to move smoothly from a flexed to extended position.[75] On examination, patients may show significant laxity with the ability to gently subluxate the distal row dorsally and volarly while stabilizing the proximal row. Many young athletes, particularly women, may demonstrate significant midcarpal laxity that is bilaterally symmetric and not pathologic.

Radiographic studies frequently are normal, but may show a volar intercalated segment instability pattern, as the proximal row flexes. Dynamic fluoroscopy may be most useful for diagnosis.

Treatment of this condition in athletes is frequently possible using a course of immobilization and anti-inflammatory medications. Splinting of the volar-ulnar carpus can be useful in allowing some athletes to return to play more quickly. Underlying laxity may be aided by therapy to work on strengthening of extrinsic musculature to assist in dynamic stabilization. If these modalities fail, arthroscopic debridement may achieve some symptomatic relief but does not address the underlying instability. A variety of soft-tissue procedures have been attempted with limited success.[76] Limited wrist fusion, particularly four-corner fusion has been more reliable at achieving functional return, but should be considered only as a salvage procedure in the athlete.[77]

DRUJ/TFCC injury

The triangular fibrocartilage complex (TFCC) is located between the distal ulna and the carpus, and acts to complete the arc of the distal radius, on which the proximal carpal row moves. It is comprised of a central articular disc, dorsal and volar radioulnar ligaments, meniscal homologue, ulnocarpal ligaments, and the extensor carpi ulnaris sheath. There are attachments on the ulnar border of the radius and the base of the ulnar styloid. The central portion of the TFCC is avascular; only the outer 10–15% of the periphery has a reliable vascular supply.[78]

The TFCC acts as the primary stabilizer of the distal radioulnar joint (DRUJ).[78] It also functions to support the proximal carpal row and to provide ulnocarpal stability. With axial loading, Palmer *et al.* showed that the radius supports the majority of load (82%), with the TFCC and ulna bearing a smaller load (18%). With increased ulnar variance by 2.5° mm, the load transmitted across the TFCC and ulna increases to 42%. The thickness of the TFCC has also been shown to be inversely proportional to the ulnar positive variance. Injuries to the TFCC are more common with ulnar positive variance; many procedures to address these problems focus on decreasing the ulnar positive variance.[79]

Injuries to the TFCC and DRUJ are quite common in athletes. Both direct, acute trauma and chronic, repetitive trauma can lead to tearing of the complex. Palmer *et al.* created a well-known classification of these injuries, dividing them into traumatic and degenerative groups; the traumatic group is further divided by location of the tear.[79] Traumatic tears are most commonly located centrally or peripherally and the latter may lead to DRUJ instability.

Acute trauma is usually the result of a fall onto an outstretched arm or a direct impact. Athletes competing in sports such as gymnastics, golf, and ice hockey commonly experience ulnar sided wrist pain and TFCC injury.

Patients often present with complaints of ulnar sided wrist pain. On examination, they have tenderness to palpation over the TFCC region located on the ulnar wrist between the pisiform and the ulnar styloid. They may have pain or difficulty lifting heavy objects in a supinated position. The differential diagnosis for patients with these complaints includes lunotriquetral pathology, ulnocarpal impaction, pisotriquetral arthrosis, and ECU or FCU tendonitis. DRUJ instability can be associated with TFCC injury. On examination, the piano key sign can be elicited by placing the wrists in a supported pronated position and pushing the palms into the table, which leads to dorsal subluxation of the distal ulna. The examiner can also take the radius in one hand and the ulna in the other and gently subluxate one on the other. Arthrosis of the DRUJ may lead to pain with compression of the distal radius and ulna.

Radiographic studies should be obtained to evaluate the ulnar variance of the patient. The PA view should be obtained with the shoulder abduction 90° and the elbow flexed 90° to allow for true neutral rotation at the wrist when measuring variance. Comparison views of the contralateral side are frequently helpful when trauma has occurred. Fractures or DRUJ subluxation/dislocation may be seen but most patients will have normal X-rays. A CT scan taken in three positions (neutral, full pronation, and full supination) will show DRUJ subluxation, if present.[80] TFCC tears can be assessed by arthrogram or MRI with a sensitivity of 80 and 82%, respectively, as compared with arthroscopy.[7]

Arthroscopic evaluation is indicated when patients have persistent symptoms despite a course of immobilization, activity modification, and hand therapy. This can be used for both diagnostic and therapeutic purposes, allowing for assessment of cartilage lesions, ligament pathology, TFCC tears, and dynamic instability (Fig. 27.11). Debridement of type 1A (central) TFCC tears can be performed arthroscopically, allowing for relatively rapid return to early motion and subsequently sport in 4–6 weeks.[7,81] Type 1B (peripheral) TFCC tears are in a vascularized zone, and thus are best treated with arthroscopic repair, usually requiring immobilization limiting forearm rotation for protection of the repair for 6 weeks. Return to

athletics may take 3–4 months following surgery.[82] Type 1D TFCC tears are similarly treated with repair via a trans-radial approach, allowing for healing in this avulsion-type injury.[81]

With degenerative TFCC tears, the ulnar variance should be carefully noted, and a shortening procedure presented as a surgical option for patients with ulnar positive or neutral variance. This decreases the impingement of the ulna on the ulnar-sided carpal bones, and tightens the ulnocarpal and distal radioulnar ligaments, which should improve stability.

Soft tissue injury

Wrist sprain A wrist sprain is an acute injury that causes a stretch or tearing of the ligaments of the wrist. Patients may notice swelling, tenderness to touch, pain with motion, limitations of motion, and ecchymosis. Suspected sprains with significant symptoms or with persistent symptoms past a couple of days should have X-rays taken to ensure that there is no fracture. Mild sprains can be treated with the 'RICE' principal: rest, ice, compression, and elevation. Most athletes can return to sport in 2–10 days. More significant sprains may require a short course of immobilization. Severe sprains may even require surgery (see Ligament injuries above).

Chronic/overuse injury

Box 27.3: Key Points

- Most chronic or overuse injuries are related to a relative increase in activity during a time of relative weakness.
- Non-operative modalities such as rest, activity modification, short-term immobilization, anti-inflammatory medications and therapy will lead to relief in the vast majority of cases.

Overuse injuries may be thought of as repetitive subclinical trauma that surpasses the natural ability of the body to repair and adapt. Conditions in the hand and wrist may be seen in athletes participating in a variety of sports that require repetitive force in extremes of the range of motion. Gymnastics, racquet and club sports, rowing and climbing have all been associated with these types of injuries.[83]

Athletes may notice worsened symptoms during periods of relative weakness, such as during growth spurts in adolescents, or during periods of increased strength or endurance training. Most of these injuries can be treated with rest, activity modification, anti-inflammatory medications, and perhaps a short course of immobilization. Some patients require formal therapy to address focal weakness or stiffness that may lead to difficulties around the hand and wrist. If these modalities fail, surgical intervention may be necessary.

Tendonitis

DeQuervain's syndrome DeQuervain's syndrome refers to tenosynovitis of the first dorsal compartment tendons, namely the abductor pollicis longus (APL) and the extensor pollicis brevis (EPB) (Fig. 27.2). Normally the tendon slips glide

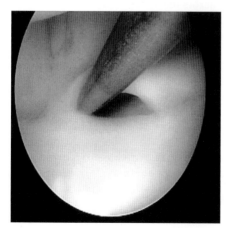

Figure 27.11 Arthroscopic view of a peripheral triangular fibrocartilage complex (TFCC) tear.

smoothly in sheaths overlying the radial styloid. Trauma or inflammation around this region can cause irritation and thickening of the sheaths surrounding the tendons. This may lead to significant radial sided wrist pain and focal tenderness to palpation just proximal to the radial styloid over these tendons. Provocative testing includes a Finklestein's test, where the patient flexes the thumb into the palm and then the wrist is gently ulnarly deviated, reproducing this localized discomfort.[84]

Treatment of patients with milder symptoms is usually with activity modification, rest and use of a long opponens splint. With more severe or persistent symptoms, steroid injection may be indicated to achieve symptomatic relief.[85] If conservative management fails to alleviate symptoms, surgical release of the first dorsal compartment may be appropriate. Care must be taken to ensure that all slips of the APL tendon and an interposed septum between the APL and EPB are identified and released (if they exist) as there is significant variability in anatomy in this region, with as many as 76% of patient having more than one slip of the APL tendon, and 60% having a dividing septum in the compartment.[86]

Intersection syndrome Intersection syndrome is a similar tenosynovitis related to inflammation at the 'intersection' between the first and second dorsal extensor compartments. The APL and EPB, otherwise known as the 'outcropper tendons' cross over the second compartment tendons (extensor carpi radialis longus and brevis – ECRL and ECRB) at this point, located typically four centimeters proximal to the wrist joint.[87] On examination, patients will have localized tenderness in that region, and may have crepitus felt or heard with wrist flexion and extension. Similar to DeQuervain's, most patients respond well to splinting, rest, anti-inflammatories, and possibly an injection, depending on severity and duration of symptoms. Surgical release can be performed in refractory cases, which entails releasing the tendon sheaths of both compartments and excising the interposed bursal tissue.[88]

Extensor carpi ulnaris (ECU) tendonitis Inflammation of the ECU tendon is not uncommon in rowing and racquet-sport athletes. It is often related to activities requiring strength in an ulnarly deviated wrist. Tenderness over the ulnar wrist, specifically over the ECU tendon can be diagnosed on examination. This condition may be related to or associated with other ulnar-sided wrist pathology, such as TFCC injury, and the patient should be examined closely for other etiologies of pain. Treatment is usually comprised of rest, activity modification, splinting, anti-inflammatory medications, and possibly steroid injection.

Some patients will also present with subluxation of the ECU tendon. This occurs when the medial wall of the tendon sheath has been torn, either due to chronic attritional tearing or an acute trauma.[89] On examination the ECU tendon can be observed to slide ulnarly over the ulnar styloid, when the patient moves the supinated wrist into ulnar deviation. There may be associated TFCC or DRUJ pathology. When the injury is noted acutely, it may respond to casting with the wrist held extended and pronated.[90] With chronic subluxation or in patients who fail

cast treatment, reconstructive procedures are indicated to allow pain-free return to sport. Any associated TFCC pathology needs to be corrected at the time of the ECU surgery.

Wrist instability

Wrist instability encompasses both acute and chronic ligamentous injury. It can range from normal laxity to complete ligamentous disruption. Chronic wrist pain may be due to subacute injury to the interosseous ligamentous structures of the wrist. Partial thickness tears may lead to dynamic instability, with impingement of flaps or fibrillation that causes synovitis and discomfort. With instability that allows for joint subluxation, chondral injury may occur, which may predispose to arthrosis. Most of the time chronic pain with laxity may be symptomatically aided by formal therapy for strengthening of the dynamic wrist stabilizers. Those with persistent symptoms may require further diagnostic workup, perhaps including arthroscopy for evaluation and treatment. More details on ligamentous injury can be found above.

Dorsal impingement syndrome/dorsal ganglion

Dorsal impingement of the wrist may be related to inflammation of the synovium and capsule of the wrist, causing pain. Mild subluxation of the carpus on the distal radius can create chondral changes, and over time may lead to osteophyte formation. Symptoms usually include pain at the extremes of wrist extension and flexion, with limitations in the flexion/extension arc. Gymnasts and other athletes who require extreme wrist extension are most prone to these problems. Conservative management will usually lead to resolution of symptoms. Sometimes surgery, either arthroscopic or open, is required to débride synovitis and osteophytes. Patients may have recurrence if they continue with similar activities postoperatively.

Another condition that may cause focal pain dorsally in the wrist is a dorsal ganglion. These may be quite large or may be occult, only seen on MRI. Most are associated with some form of scapholunate ligament injury. Doing pushups, or other activities that load the wrist in an extended position, may cause symptoms. Recurrence is over 50% following aspiration of these cysts. Following surgical excision, including eradication of the capsular stalk, recurrence is <5%.[91]

Avascular necrosis
Kienbock's disease

In Kienbock's disease, the blood supply to the lunate is interrupted, leading to avascular necrosis of the bone. Some patients may be able to recall a specific trauma to the wrist but many cannot. It is a rare condition and the etiology of the ischemic process is not well understood. Most people have two main arteries that supply the lunate, but some people only have one, which puts them at higher risk for Kienbock's. Some research has found an association of Kienbock's with ulnar negative variance of the wrist.[92]

Most patients present with a dull, aching sensation in the wrist. They may have noticed mild swelling, stiffness, and weakness. Diagnosis is made radiographically.

In Stage I, the X-rays will appear normal. MRI scan will show marrow changes consistent with AVN. Treatment should be nonoperative with immobilization and activity modification. In Stage II, the radiographs will show sclerosis, but there will not be significant collapse in the height of the lunate. In Stage IIIA, more significant lunate collapse can be seen, however, the rest of the carpus remains uninvolved. Treatment of Stages II and IIIa involves attempting to revascularize the lunate. Many different methods have been employed, include unloading the lunate by joint leveling procedures such as radial shortening osteotomies, or by trying to directly revascularize the lunate with vascularized bone grafts from the distal radius. Once the disease has progressed to Stage IIIb, the surrounding carpus has become involved, and will show signs of carpal collapse, with proximal migration of the capitate and rotatory changes noted. Limited radial sided intercarpal arthrodeses, such as the scaphotrapeziotrapezoid (STT) fusion, or proximal row carpectomy (PRC) may be indicated. In Stage IV disease, there is degenerative joint disease of the carpus, and either proximal row carpectomy, limited wrist fusion (as determined by residual joint sparing) or complete wrist fusion may be salvage procedures required to alleviate symptoms.[93]

Avascular necrosis of the scaphoid (Preiser's disease) and capitate

Non-traumatic avascular necrosis of other carpal bones including the scaphoid (Preiser's disease) and the capitate has been reported. Symptoms include dull, aching pain, with limitations in motion and functional strength. X-rays may be revealing, although in early stages, MRI may be required to visualize the marrow changes if there has not yet been cortical collapse or fragmentation. Management is similar to that of Kienbock's in early stages. For more advanced disease, management must be tailored to each patient, based on extent and location of carpal involvement.

HAND

Box 27.4: Key Points

- Rotational alignment of the digits should be assessed clinically as well as radiographically.
- Surgically-related soft tissue injury should be minimized to achieve the best results with digital fractures.

The separation of the digits of the hand allows for phenomenal independent function, but also leaves the hand and digits vulnerable to injury, due to the lack of protective surrounding structures. Rotational injury, axial loading, crushing, and falls can all create significant soft tissue and skeletal damage. Return of motion following an injury is critical in achieving maximal functional restoration. The digits become stiff quickly

when immobilized, and adherence of the soft tissue structures can affect even non-injured digits, if they are held still to allow another digit to heal.

Acute/traumatic injury
Fracture

Metacarpal fractures Metacarpal fractures in athletes most often involve a single metacarpal shaft injury that is stable.[94] These are treated with good success by casting or splinting, and return to sport can often occur with a form of immobilization while the fracture is healing.

Assessment of the rotation of the affected digit should be evaluated in flexion and extension. In extension, the digit must be straightly aligned with the other digits, and when looking end-on, the nails of all digits should have the same orientation. With wrist tenodesis-assisted digital flexion, the fingers should fall into a normal cascade without overlap, with all fingertips pointing towards the scaphoid tubercle.

The soft tissue attachments to the bony fragments may cause the fracture to displace. When the fracture is angled, shortened, or rotated into a position that is not appropriate, a reduction of the fracture, either closed or open, is required. If the manipulation can place the fracture into a stable position that may be maintained with casting or splinting, surgery is not needed. These patients need to be followed closely for the first 3 weeks to ensure that no displacement recurs. Often some type of fixation is needed to maintain the new position to allow the bone to heal with acceptable positioning; this may be either with percutaneous pins, internal plates/screws, or intramedullary devices. Surgically-related soft tissue injury should be minimized to achieve best results (Fig. 27.12).[95]

Phalangeal fractures Similar to metacarpal fractures, most phalangeal fractures in the athletes are caused by relatively low-energy mechanisms, and therefore do not have a high degree of comminution or soft tissue injury associated with them.

Distal phalangeal fractures are often of a crushing mechanism, and are frequently associated with nail bed pathology. Usually they are stable due to the multiple septae and the stabilization by the nail.

Bony mallet injuries of the distal phalanx occur when the digit is forced into a flexed position, causing an avulsion of the bony attachment of the terminal extensor tendon. Further information can be found under 'mallet finger' below.

Transverse fractures of the proximal and middle phalanges may flex or extend based on the location of the fracture. Those distal to the insertion of the FDS tendon on the middle phalanx will be extended; those proximal to the insertion will be flexed. Similarly, fractures in the proximal phalanx may have flexion of the proximal fragment by the interosseous musculature. These fractures can often be reduced into a stable, acceptable alignment, and then maintained there with buddy tape and splinting until healing has occurred. Buddy taping can allow for early active motion, which is important to decrease long-term stiffness of the digit.

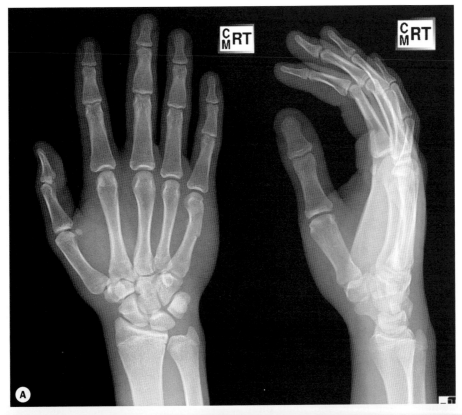

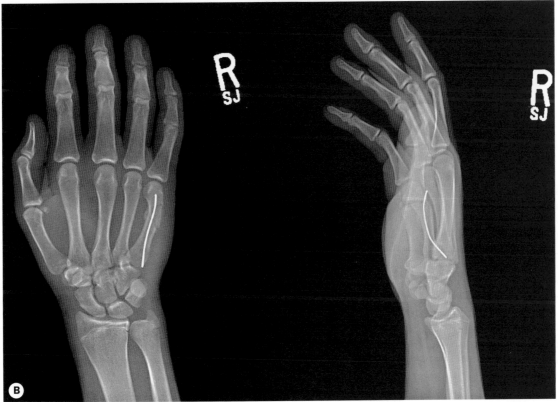

Figure 27.12 (A) Radiographs of a displaced, flexed 5th metacarpal shaft fracture. (B) Postoperative radiographs following intramedullary fixation.

Spiral or oblique fractures of the proximal and middle phalanges frequently shorten and rotate and may not be reduced and held in a stable position without operative fixation. If stable, they can be maintained with buddy taping and splinting while healing occurs. If unstable, surgery is indicated. Rotation may be assessed by the methods described under Metacarpal fractures above (Fig. 27.13).

Boxer's fracture and fight bite Fracture of the 5th metacarpal neck has been called a 'Boxer's fracture,' and is typically the result of striking a hard object with a direct blow. Most professional boxers will actually sustain a fracture of the 2nd, rather than the 5th metacarpal neck, as they are well-trained to land blows directly in the axis of the arm, providing more power to each punch. Fractures of the 5th metacarpal neck must be evaluated for displacement. They often require closed reduction and can usually be maintained in an acceptable position with immobilization. The acceptable degree of flexion of the distal fragment is debatable, with studies ranging from 20–70° as the uppermost limit of acceptable angulation.[96] Note that rotational malalignment should be addressed as this can lead to functional difficulties. Patients with some degree of flexion across their fracture should be cautioned that they will lose the cosmetic appearance of the 'knuckle' and they may feel a lump in their palm with power gripping activities.

When the blow has landed on another person, there may be lacerations or 'poke-holes' from teeth, and when these injuries are found, the injury is called a 'fight bite'. These open wounds can occur over any of the metacarpals, and when seen, there must be a presumption that the tooth penetrated the underlying joint capsule, thus exposing the metacarpal joint to oral flora. These pose a surgical urgency and should undergo irrigation and debridement to avoid the complication of a septic joint. Antibiotics should be chosen to cover oral bacteria.

Bennett's/Rolando fracture Injuries to the thumb carpometacarpal (CMC) joint are frequently associated with fracture. The most commonly seen fracture is called a Bennett's fracture, which is a two-part intraarticular fracture resulting when the thumb sustains an axial or adduction load while in a flexed position. The volar-ulnar portion of the proximal metacarpal remains attached to the volar anterior oblique, or 'beak,' ligament, leading to a fracture through the joint. The rest of the proximal metacarpal, which contains the majority of the articular surface, remains intact with the distal metacarpal, but frequently is subluxated radially and dorsally on the trapezium. This displacement is caused by the unopposed pull by the abductor pollicis longus (APL) tendon, now that the volar beak ligament is no longer attached to this portion of the metacarpal due to fracture.

Treatment usually includes closed reduction and pinning if the volar-ulnar fragment is small and a reduction with less than 1 mm step-off can be achieved. The K-wire fixation should cross the CMC joint and/or secure the first metacarpal to the second metacarpal to achieve stability while healing occurs. If the reduction cannot be achieved through closed methods, or if the fragment is sufficiently large to allow for internal fixation, an open reduction and fixation is appropriate. Internal

fixation allows for earlier range of motion exercises than pinning.[97]

Rolando's fracture similarly involves the base of the thumb metacarpal but is more extensive, in that it is a three-part fracture that entails a T- or Y-shaped intraarticular disruption. Prognosis is less favorable due to the increased injury to the articular surface. With less comminuted fractures that have larger fragments, open reduction and internal fixation is appropriate. With highly comminuted fractures, closed reduction and distraction external fixation has achieved acceptable results. These patients should be counseled that they are predisposed to degenerative joint disease in the CMC joint as a result of this injury.[98]

Joint injury

Box 27.5: Key Points

- The majority of proximal interphalangeal joint injuries can be treated with buddy taping and early mobilization.

- Operative treatment should be reserved for gross instability or irreducible dislocations, as joint stiffness can be quite problematic.

- Closed injury assessment should include testing for tendon disruption and ligament competence, as delayed diagnosis may lead to poorer outcome.

Metacarpophalangeal (MP) joint injury The MP joint is less frequently injured than the PIP joint, likely related to its position of relative protection in the hand. The border digits (index and small) are more prone to injury due to their relative exposure. Laterally directed or hyperextension forces can lead collateral ligament, volar plate injury, or dislocation.

On examination, the patient may have localized tenderness over the MP joint and may have decreased mobility of the digit. A dislocated MP joint may not be obvious on physical examination. Radiographs should be obtained to evaluate for joint dislocation, subluxation or fracture. Laxity of the collateral ligaments should be tested in extension and 30° of flexion, and compared with the uninjured side.

When attempting to reduce a subluxated or dislocated MP joint, one should not try to recreate the injury by pulling longitudinal traction or by extending the joint as this maneuver may cause the injured volar plate to become interposed between the bones, preventing reduction, and necessitating surgery. If closed reduction is achieved, further management can be obtained through splinting. If the joint is irreducible, surgical reduction is required.[99]

Gross instability of the ligaments to stress testing may require surgical repair, especially in the border digits. Other fingers can be treated closed with buddy tape and splinting (Fig. 27.14).[100,101]

Proximal interphalangeal (PIP) joint injury PIP joint injuries are very common in athletes. The joint is a hinge, which allows for flexion and extension, with significant lateral stability

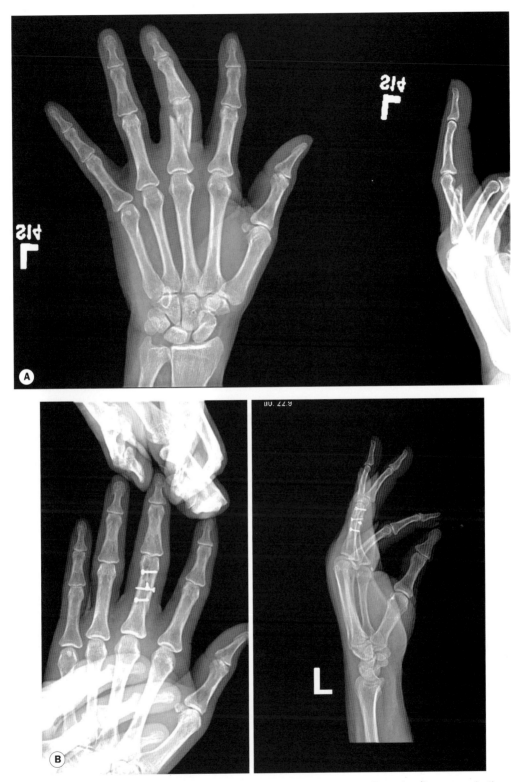

Figure 27.13   (A) Radiographs of a mal-rotated, extended phalangeal fracture. (B) Postoperative radiographs after open reduction and internal fixation.

provided by the bony architecture and the proper and accessory collateral ligaments. The volar plate provides the volar stability to prevent hyperextension. Its distal attachment is to the base of the middle phalanx; proximally the volar plate is thinner centrally and thickens laterally to form checkrein ligaments that attach to the proximal phalanx.[102]

Dislocations of the PIP joint can occur dorsally, volarly, or laterally. Dorsal dislocations occur due to hyperextension of the PIP, with volar plate disruption. This is typically from the distal attachment and may have a small avulsion fracture noted on radiograph. If the collateral ligaments are also disrupted, rotational deformity and/or lateral stress will demonstrate

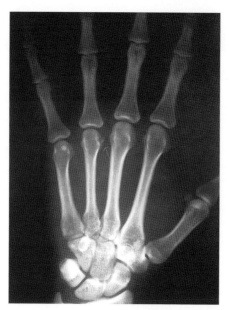

Figure 27.14 Radiographs of an avulsion fracture off of the metacarpal attachment of the radial collateral ligament of the ring finger.

instability. The most common complication of this injury is a pseudo-Boutonnière deformity with PIP flexion contracture. If there is a volar fracture and the fragment measures more than one third of the joint surface, this is an unstable injury. An examination under fluoroscopy with local anesthesia is indicated. If the joint remains concentrically reduced throughout motion, then active range of motion should be initiated. If there is instability, many treatments including extension block splinting or pinning, open reduction with internal fixation, external fixation, and volar plate arthroplasty have been described.[103]

Volar dislocations of the PIP joint are less common and require injury of the central slip mechanism, either through fracture or tendon disruption.

Most PIP joint injuries are combinations of volar plate, capsule, and collateral ligament disruptions. The majority of PIP injuries have partial soft tissue tears and can best be treated with buddy taping, short-term splinting, and early range of motion. Complete tears with gross instability (>20° of angulation compared to the uninjured side) on examination in either extension or 30° of flexion, or interposed soft tissue preventing anatomic joint reduction require operative intervention.[104]

Ligament injury
Ulnar collateral ligament (UCL) injury of the thumb metacarpophalangeal (MP) joint: 'skier's' or 'gamekeeper's' thumb

The ulnar collateral ligament of the thumb is commonly injured in sports such as skiing, football and basketball. The mechanism of injury is a radially directed force on the radially and palmarly abducted thumb, resulting in either tear of the ligament or avulsion from the attachment site on the proximal phalanx with a piece of bone.

Examination may find localized ecchymosis and tenderness over the ulnar side of the thumb MP joint. A palpable mass in this region may indicate either a fracture or a Stener lesion. A Stener lesion occurs when the adductor aponeurosis becomes interposed between the completely torn UCL and the insertion site, thus preventing it from healing to its anatomic insertion.[105]

Radiographs should be taken prior to manipulation (Fig. 27.15). If there is a displaced fragment, stress testing should not be performed, as this may cause further displacement, thus taking a possibly non-operative injury, and making it into one that requires surgery. If the fragment is non-displaced, the thought is that it has maintained position despite the stress of injury, and therefore gentle stress testing may be safely conducted without causing displacement.

Active motion should be assessed and compared with the contralateral side. Stress testing should be done in full extension of the MP and at 30° of flexion to isolate the proper and accessory collateral ligaments.[106] A local anesthetic block may be required as pain may prohibit a complete examination. More than 35° of laxity noted with valgus testing, or more than 15° of difference when compared with the non-injured side, indicates a complete tear.

Stress radiographs may also be obtained to aid in diagnosis. If these demonstrate subluxation >one third of the articular surface, repair is indicated.[107] Fragments that are displaced more than 3 mm or that involve more than 30% of the joint surface also are unlikely to heal adequately and should be treated surgically.[107]

Partial tears that maintain an endpoint within these limits detailed above can be treated non-operatively with thumb spica immobilization. If left untreated, complete tears will lead to instability and pain during attempted pinch activities, which can cause significant disability. These patients should undergo operative management.[107]

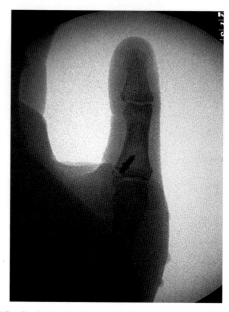

Figure 27.15 Radiograph after surgical repair of an avulsion fracture of the ulnar collateral ligament insertion associated with a 'Skier's thumb'.

Closed tendon injury
Mallet finger
A mallet finger occurs when the terminal extensor tendon either ruptures from its insertion site on the distal phalanx or there is an avulsion fracture of that insertion site. The distal interphalangeal joint assumes a flexed posture due to the unopposed pull of the intact flexor digitorum profundus.

The mechanism of injury is typically an impact resulting in forced flexion of the DIP joint.[108]

X-rays should always be obtained to see if any fracture has occurred, and to ensure that the joint is concentrically reduced (Fig. 27.16).

On examination, the patient will have no active extension across the DIP joint. There will be a flexed deformity as mentioned previously. Most acute injuries will exhibit some discomfort and swelling in the area.

If the mallet finger has no fracture, the treatment of choice is splinting in extension or slight hyperextension for 6–8 weeks. Patients may change the splint to clean and check the skin, but must maintain the position of the DIP joint in extension at all times. The splint should be worn at all times; if breaks are taken from splinting and the digit is allowed to flex, the treatment will fail. Care must be taken to not overly hyperextend the DIP joint as the dorsal skin will then blanch and could become ischemic if left this way for prolonged periods.[109] Some patients require a longitudinal K-wire across the DIP joint to maintain positioning during this time. Care should be taken to ensure that proximal interphalangeal joint motion

is encouraged to avoid long-term stiffness. After the initial treatment phase, most patients should continue to wear the splint during athletic activities and at night for another 6–8 weeks.

The bony mallet finger can be treated similarly if the fragment has less than 2 mm of displacement and there is no volar subluxation of the DIP joint on the lateral view. Serial views should be followed during this treatment to ensure that the joint remains reduced.

If there is more displacement of the bone, more than 30% of the articular surface is involved, or the joint is not concentrically reduced, some controversy exists in the literature. Most would recommend surgical treatment,[110,111] but others say that a splinting regimen is as effective.[112]

Chronic mallet fingers can attempt a course of prolonged splinting for up to 3 months, but results are usually not as good as when the splinting program is initiated within 2 weeks of injury.[113] If pain or instability becomes an issue, DIP arthrodesis is very successful in adults. In children, a dermodesis procedure is often performed.

Flexor digitorum profundus injury: 'jersey' finger
The jersey finger is so named due its occurrence when a player would get a finger, typically the ring finger, caught in another player's jersey and would sustain an avulsion of the FDP tendon. The ring finger was usually involved due to it being the longest digit when the fingers are in a flexed posture. Cadaver studies have also shown that the strength of the

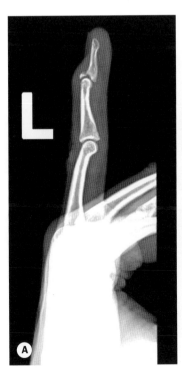
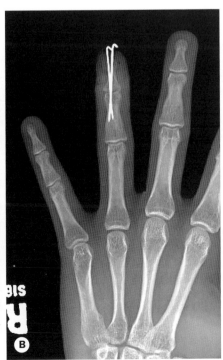
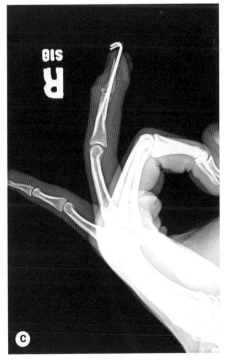

Figure 27.16 (A) Lateral radiograph of a mallet finger with subluxation of the joint. (B and C) Postoperative views following open reduction and internal fixation.

tendon insertion of the ring finger is lower than the surrounding digits.[114] The forced extension while the finger is actively flexing leads to the traumatic avulsion off of the insertion site into the volar aspect of the distal phalanx. At times, similar to a mallet finger, a piece of bone may be avulsed with the tendon.[115]

Patients with these injuries will usually have swelling, tenderness at the FDP tendon insertion site, and lack of active flexion of the DIP joint. With retraction of the tendon, the patient may also have tenderness more proximally and may notice a lump or mass in the proximal digit or the palm. Unfortunately, these FDP ruptures too often are acutely diagnosed as a finger sprain.

Radiographs should be obtained to look for avulsion fracture and displacement of the fracture, if it exists.

Leddy et al.[115,116] created a classification of these injuries to describe the degree of retraction of the tendon and also indicate the degree of vascular disruption to that tendon. Type 1 injuries retract into the palm, disrupting the blood supply from the bone, and from the long and short vinculae. These must be reattached within 7–10 days or the tendon will undergo necrosis and significant scarring. Type 2 injuries retract to the level of the PIP joint where they are held by an intact vincula longa. These should be treated within 3–6 weeks from injury. Type 3 injuries usually have an avulsed fragment attached to the tendon and therefore do not retract past the DIP joint, thus maintaining the vincula blood supply. Delayed repair can be successful. At times, an apparent type 3 injury may have both a bony avulsion and then the tendon stump may also be avulsed from the bone fragment, allowing for further retraction into the palm. This injury is classified as 3b and must be treated based on the level of tendon retraction.[115,116]

With late presentation of these injuries, occasionally delayed primary repair may be attempted. If this is not possible, most patients will choose to leave the digit without a distal flexor, as the PIP joint continues to flex normally and the deficit is usually not considerable. Patients with palm tenderness can undergo stump excision. Other patients prefer an attempt at flexor tendon grafting, which can restore active flexion to the DIP joint.[117] For patients with chronic avulsions and DIP instability, DIP arthrodesis is successful.[116]

Central slip avulsion/Boutonnière injury

Disruption of the central slip of the extensor mechanism is called a Boutonnière injury. The central slip inserts into the base of the dorsal aspect of the middle phalanx, allowing for active extension across the PIP joint. A direct blow to this region or a PIP dislocation can lead to disruption of this extensor mechanism.

Similar to the other closed tendon injuries, radiographs should be obtained to look for bony involvement and joint reduction.

On examination, the acutely injured digit may have localized swelling and discomfort over the central slip insertion site. Patients may not have deformity of the joint or loss of extension initially, if the triangular ligament is intact, allowing for appropriate positioning of the lateral bands.

Elson described a test for central slip disruption in which the PIP joint is placed into flexion. The patient then tries to

actively extend the PIP against resistance. With central slip disruption, the DIP joint will rigidly extend, while with an intact central slip, the DIP joint will remain lax.[118]

With time, the loss of the central slip will lead to overpull of the terminal tendon and hyperextension of the DIP joint. The triangular ligament will attenuate, allowing for the lateral bands to slip volarly, leading to a flexion deformity at the PIP joint.

Acute isolated central slip injuries can be treated with extension splinting for 6–8 weeks. A large or displaced fracture may require operative fixation.[119]

Chronic injuries may develop flexion contractures (Fig. 27.17), and serial casting or splint may be useful. If full passive motion can be achieved a reconstruction may be performed. If full passive motion is not possible, a staged release of the joint and tendon, followed by a reconstruction may be necessary.[120] Most patients with Boutonnière deformity achieve acceptable results without surgery.

Pulley rupture

Pulley rupture is not common but may be seen in athletes engaging in forceful cling grip with the distal phalanges, such a climbers. The annular pulleys assist in holding the flexor tendons to bone, allowing for better mechanics of the flexor system of the hand by preventing bowstringing. The A2 and A4 pulleys are most important in this regard.

Rupture of the A2 pulley usually presents acutely with pain over the volar aspect of the proximal phalanx, and more commonly affects the long and ring fingers. With complete rupture, there may be bowstringing of the tendons noted with resisted digital flexion. Most will be more subtle; ultrasound or MRI may aid in diagnosis.[121] Partial tears can be treated

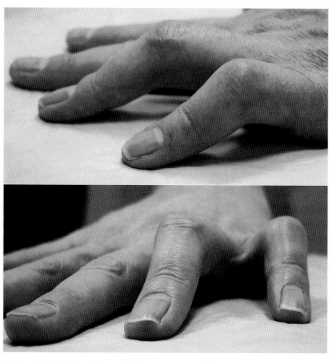

Figure 27.17 Two views of chronic Boutonnière deformity with DIP hyperextension and PIP flexion contracture.

with ring taping or ring splints to allow healing. Complete tears may require repair or reconstruction.[121]

Sagittal band rupture/MP extensor hood rupture

The extensor mechanism of the digit is quite complex. As it passes the metacarpophalangeal (MP) joint, the central tendon passes directly dorsally and the sagittal bands pass both radial and ulnarly from the tendon in a transverse fashion to maintain the central alignment and to assist in MP joint extension. These bands attach to the transverse metacarpal ligaments and the volar plate of the MP joint and act as a sling to pull the proximal phalanx into extension.

Disruption of the sagittal bands often occurs due to a direct blow, such as in boxing or other contact sports, or in a fall onto the dorsal hand. The radial side is more commonly injured. When this occurs, the extensor tendon will tend to subluxate away from the injured side, which on examination will show as the inability to extend the MP joint from a flexed position. The patient will be able to maintain the MP in an extended position against resistance because once extended the tendon will be aligned.

Acute injuries can be treated with the MP joint splinted in an extended position for 6 weeks. Chronic injuries that are symptomatic may require reconstructive procedures.[122]

Direct trauma may also lead to central disruption of the extensor hood over the MP joint. This is seen more commonly in boxers and often involves the long finger. Treatment often requires repair with immobilization postoperatively.[123]

Nail bed injuries/subungual hematoma

Nail bed injuries are usually associated with crushing injuries of the distal phalangeal region of the digit. They can also be caused by a sharp laceration. If a subungual hematoma covers more than 50% of the nail bed, research has shown that there is a 60% incidence of nail bed laceration, and many suggest that the nail plate be removed to allow for repair of the often significant nail bed injury.[124] Other studies have shown that trephination may be as effective at relieving the discomfort and providing long-term acceptable comesis, without an increase in complications.[125]

Other associated hand conditions

Box 27.6: Key Points

- Carpal tunnel syndrome in the young athlete is rare and may be associated with other medical conditions.

Trigger digit

Trigger fingers can occasionally be found in the athlete. It may be more notable in patients who participate in racquet or club sports that require tight flexion of the digits for control. A tendon nodule may develop and can be felt as a palpable lump in the palm that moves with the tendon as the digit flexes and extends. Inflammation of the tendon sheath can develop and may lead to palpable or visible 'triggering' as the nodule passes through the A1 pulley at the distal palmar crease. Note that trigger fingers are not uncommon in the general population and usually are not related to athletic participation, but can be found more frequently in patients with rheumatoid arthritis, diabetes mellitus, gout, and other disease entities that cause connective tissue disorders.[126]

Treatment with steroid injection is often curative, with success rates up to 85%.[126] If this fails, release of the A1 pulley is indicated.

Carpal tunnel syndrome

Carpal tunnel syndrome is uncommon in the younger patient, but may occasionally be seen associated with sports such as rock climbing where athletes engage in prolonged activity in a flexed wrist position.[127] These patients may develop tenosynovitis of the digital flexors, Presenting complaints usually include aching forearm and volar wrist pain, as well as paresthesias and/or numbness over the volar aspect of the radial three digits. Pain at night and difficulty sleeping are nearly universal. On examination, there may be decreased two-point discrimination and in later stages, there may be weakness of the thenar musculature. Specific testing of the abductor pollicis brevis (APB) by resisted palmar abduction is important. Provocative testing includes a Tinel's (radiating altered sensibility with percussion of the median nerve), a Phalen's test (reproduction of symptoms with the wrist held in gravity-assisted flexion with the elbows extended), and a Durkin's test (reproduction of symptoms with continuous applied pressure over the carpal tunnel). Atrophy is a late finding associated with long-standing compression.

Most patients will respond to nonoperative management with activity modification, night splints, non-steroidal anti-inflammatory drugs (NSAIDs), and possibly a steroid injection. If this fails, an electromyogram should be obtained to confirm the diagnosis. Surgical release of the carpal tunnel is rarely necessary in young athletes.[83] Other comorbidities such as mucopolysaccharidoses, dysplasias, endocrine disorders, and connective tissue abnormalities are associated with carpal tunnel syndrome in young patients and in these patients, a surgical procedure is more commonly necessary.[128] A thorough history and physical should identify these patients.

REFERENCES

1 Krahl H, Michaelis U, Pieper HG, et al. Stimulation of bone growth through sports: A radiologic investigation of the upper extremities in professional tennis players. Am J Sports Med 1994; 22:751-757.
2 Rettig AC, Ryan RO, Stone JA. Epidemiology of hand injuries in sports. In: Strickland JW, Rettig AC, eds. Hand injuries in athletes. Philadelphia, PA: WB Saunders; 1992:37-44.
3 Geissler WB. Carpal fractures in athletes. Clin Sports Med 2001; 20:167-188.
4 American Society for Surgery of the Hand. The physical examination. The hand: primary care of common problems. New York: Churchill Livingstone; 1985:3-7.
5 American Society for Surgery of the Hand. History and general examination. The hand, examination and diagnosis. 2nd edn. Edinburgh: Churchill Livingstone; 1983:3-10.
6 Akdemir UO, Atasever T, Sipahioglu S, et al. Value of bone scintigraphy in patients with carpal trauma. Ann Nucl Med 2004; 18:495-499.

7   Pederzini L, Luchetti R, Soragni O, et al. Evaluation of the triangular fibrocartilage complex tears by arthroscopy, arthrography, and magnetic resonance imaging. Arthroscopy 1992; 8:191–197.

8   Rettig AC, Patel DV. Epidemiology of elbow, forearm, and wrist injuries in the athlete. Clin Sports Med 1995; 14:289–297.

9   Weber ER, Chao EY. An experimental approach to the mechanism of scaphoid waist fractures. J Hand Surg 1978; 3A:142–148.

10 McClain EJ, Boyes JH. Missed fractures of the greater multangular. J Bone Jt Surg 1966; 48A:1625–1528.

11 Panagis JS, Gelberman RH, Taleisnik J, et al. The arterial anatomy of the human carpus. Part II: The intraosseous vascularity. J Hand Surg 1983; 8A:375–382.

12 Resnik CS. Wrist and hand injuries. Semin Musculoskel Radiol 2000; 4:193–204.

13 Ganel A, Engel J, Oster Z, et al. Bone scanning in the assessment of fractures of the scaphoid. J Hand Surg 1979; 4A:540–543.

14 Sanders WE. Evaluation of the humpback scaphoid by computed tomography in the longitudinal axial plane of the scaphoid. J Hand Surg 1986; 13A:182–187.

15 Russe O. Fracture of the carpal navicular. Diagnosis, non-operative treatment, and operative treatment. J Bone Jt Surg 1960; 42A:759–766.

16 Totterman SM, Miller RJ. MR imaging of the triangular fibrocartilage complex. Magn Reson Imaging Clin N Am 1995; 3:213–228.

17 Smith DK, Gilula LA, Amadio PC. Dorsal lunate tilt (DISI configuration): sign of scaphoid fracture displacement. Radiology 1990; 176:497–499.

18 Mack GR, Bosse MJ, Gelberman RH, et al. The natural history of scaphoid non-union. J Bone Jt Surg 1984; 66A:504–509.

19 Ruby LK, Stinson J, Belsky MR. The natural history of scaphoid non-union: A review of fifty-five cases. J Bone Jt Surg 1985; 67A:428–432.

20 Kerluke L, McCabe SJ. Nonunion of the scaphoid: A critical analysis of recent natural history studies. J Hand Surg 1993; 18A:1–3.

21 Cooney WP III, Dobyns JH, Linscheid RL. Nonunion of the scaphoid: Analysis of the results from bone grafting. J Hand Surg 1980; 5A:343–354.

22 Kuschner SH, Lane CS, Brien WW, et al. Scaphoid fractures and scaphoid nonunion. Diagnosis and treatment. Orthop Rev 1994; 23:861–871.

23 Stewart MJ. Fractures of the carpal navicular (scaphoid). A report of 436 cases. J Bone Jt Surg 1954; 36A:998–1006.

24 Rettig AC, Weidenbener EJ, Gloyeske R. Alternative management of mid-third scaphoid fractures in the athlete. Am J Sports Med 1994; 22:711–714.

25 Riester JN, Baker BE, Masher JF, et al. A review of scaphoid fracture healing in competitive athletes. Am J Sports Med 1985; 13:159–161.

26 Herbert TJ, Fisher WE, Leicester AW. The Herbert bone screw: A ten year perspective. J Hand Surg 1992; 17B:415–419.

27 Rettig AC, Kollias SC. Internal fixation of acute stable scaphoid fractures in the athlete. Am J Sports Med 1996; 24:182–186.

28 Rettig AC, Weidenbener EJ, Gloyeske R. Alternative management of mid-third scaphoid fractures in the athlete. Am J Sports Med 1994; 22:711–714.

29 Inoue G, Shionoya K. Herbert screw fixation by limited access for acute fractures of the scaphoid. J Bone Jt Surg 1997; 79B:416–421.

30 Trumble TE, Salas P, Barthel T. Robert KQ 3rd. Management of scaphoid nonunions. J Am Acad Orthop Surg 2003; 11:380–391.

31 Bishop AT, Beckenbaugh RD. Fracture of the hamate hook. J Hand Surg 1988; 13A:135–139.

32 Bowen TL. Injuries of the hamate bone. Hand 1973; 5:235–238.

33 Bryan RS, Dobyns JH. Fractures of the carpal bones other than lunate and navicular. Clin Orthop 1980; 149:107–111.

34 Murray PM, Cooney WP. Golf-induced injuries of the wrist. Clin Sports Med 1996; 15:85–109.

35 Stark HH, Jobe FW, Boyes JH, et al. Fracture of the hook of the hamate in athletes. J Bone Jt Surg 1977; 59A:575–582.

36 Greenspan A. Upper limb II–distal forearm, wrist and hand. Orthopedic radiology: a practical approach. 3rd edn. Philadelphia, PA: Lippincott Williams & Wilkins; 2000:175–176.

37 Egawa M, Asai T. Fracture of the hook of the hamate: Report of six cases and the suitability of computerized tomography. J Hand Surg 1983; 8A:393–398.

38 Morgan WJ, Slowman LS. Acute hand and wrist injuries in athletes: evaluation and management. J Am Acad Orthop Surg 2001; 9:389–400.

39 Foucher G, Schuind F, Merle M, et al. Fractures of the hook of the hamate. J Hand Surg 1985; 10B:205–210.

40 Failla JM. Hook of hamate vascularity: Vulnerability to osteonecrosis and nonunion. J Hand Surg 1993; 18A:1075–1079.

41 Vender MI, Watson HK. Acquired Madelung-like deformity in a gymnast. J Hand Surg 1988; 13A:19–21.

42 Palmieri TJ. Pisiform area pain treatment by pisiform excision. J Hand Surg 1982; 7A:477–480.

43 Lam KS, Woodbridge S, Burke FD. Wrist function after excision of the pisiform. J Hand Surg (Br) 2003; 28:69–72.

44 Levy M, Fischel RE, Stern GM, Goldberg I. Chip fractures of the os triquetrum: the mechanism of injury. J Bone Jt Surg Br 1979; 61B:355–357.

45 Hocker K, Menschik A. Chip fractures of the triquetrum. Mechanism, classification and results. J Hand Surg (Br) 1994; 19:584–588.

46 Fisk GR. Carpal instability and the fractured scaphoid. Ann R Coil Surg Engl 1970; 46:63–76.

47 Johnson RP. The acutely injured wrist and its residuals. Clin Orthop 1986; 149:33–44.

48 Mayfield JK. Mechanism of carpal injuries. Clin Orthop 1980; 149:45–54.

49 Adkison JW, Chapman MW. Treatment of acute lunate and perilunate dislocations. Clin Orthop 1982; 164:199–207.

50 Green DP. O'Brien EI': Open reduction of carpal dislocations: Indications and operative techniques. J Hand Surg 1978; 3A:250–265.

51 Raab DJ, Fischer DA, Quick DC. Lunate and perilunate dislocations in professional football players. A five-year retrospective analysis. Am J Sports Med 1994; 22:841–845.

52 Hildebrand KA, Ross DC, Patterson SD, et al. Dorsal perilunate dislocations and fracture-dislocations: questionnaire, clinical, and radiographic evaluation. J Hand Surg (Am) 2000; 25:1069–1079.

53 Mayfield JK, Johnson RP, Kilcoyne RK. Carpal dislocations: Pathomechanics and progressive perilunar instability. J Hand Surg 1980; 5A:226–241.

54 Kirschenbaum D, Sieler S, Solonick D, et al. Arthrography of the wrist: Assessment of the integrity of the ligaments in young asymptomatic adults. J Bone Jt Surg 1996; 77A:1207–1209.

55 Metz VM, Mann FA, Gilula LA. Lack of correlation between site of wrist pain and location of noncommunicating defects shown by three-compartment wrist arthrography. Am J Roentgenol 1993; 160:1239–1243.

56 Linscheid RL, Dobyns JH, Beabout JW, et al. Traumatic instability of the wrist. Diagnosis, classification, and pathomechanics. J Bone Jt Surg 1972; 54A:1612–1632.

57 Larsen CF, Mathiesen FK, Lindequist S. Measurements of carpal bone angles on lateral wrist radiographs. J Hand Surg (Am) 1991; 16:888–893.

58 Watson HK, Ballet FL. The SLAC wrist: Scapholunate advanced collapse pattern of degenerative arthritis. J Hand Surg 1984; 9A:358–365.

59 Moran SL, Cooney WP, Berger RA, et al. Capsulodesis for the treatment of chronic scapholunate instability. J Hand Surg (Am) 2005; 30:16–23.

60 Nathan R, Blatt G. Rotary subluxation of the scaphoid. Revisited Hand Clin 2000; 16:417–431.

61 Kozin SH. The role of arthroscopy in scapholunate instability. Hand Clin 1999; 15:435–444.

62 Earp BE, Waters P. Arthroscopic treatment of partial scapholunate ligament tears in pediatric and adolescent patients with chronic wrist pain. (Submitted for publication 2005).

63 Wolf JM, Weiss AP. Bone-retinaculum-bone reconstruction of scapholunate ligament injuries. Orthop Clin North Am 2001; 32:241–246.

64 Bruckner JD, Alexander AH, Lichtman DM. Acute dislocations of the distal radioulnar joint. J Bone Jt Surg 1995; 77A:958–968.

65 Inglis AE, Jones EC. Proximal-row carpectomy for diseases of the proximal row. J Bone Jt Surg 1977; 59A:460–463.

66 Watson HK, Black DM. Instabilities of the wrist. Hand Clin 1967; 3:103–111.

67 Trumble TE, Bour CJ, Smith RJ, et al. Kinematics of the ulnar carpus related to the volar intercalated segment instability pattern. J Hand Surg 1990; 15A:384–392.

68 Viegas SF, Patterson RM, Peterson PD, et al. Ulnar-sided perilunate instability: An anatomic and biomechanic study. J Hand Surg 1990; 15A:268–278.

69 Reagan DS, Linscheid RL, Dobyns JH. Lunotriquetral sprains. J Hand Surg (Am) 1984; 9:502–514.

70 Brown JA, Janzan DL, Adler BD, et al. Arthrography of the contralateral, asymptomatic wrist in patients with unilateral wrist pain. Can Assoc Radiol J 1994; 45:292–296.

71 Haims AH, Schweitzer ME, Morrison WB, et al. Internal derangement of the wrist: indirect MR arthrography versus unenhanced MR imaging. Radiology 2003; 227:701–707.

72 Cohen MS. Ligamentous injuries of the wrist in the athlete. Clin Sports Med 1998; 17:533–552.

73 Ruch DS, Poehling GG. Arthroscopic management of partial scapholunate and lunotriquetral injuries of the wrist. J Hand Surg 1996; 21A:412–417.

74 Shin AY, Weinstein LP, Berger RA, et al. Treatment of isolated injuries of the lunotriquetral ligament. A comparison of arthrodesis, ligament reconstruction and ligament repair. J Bone Jt Surg Br 2001; 83:1023–1028.

75 Brown DE, Lichtman DM. Midcarpal instability. Hand Clin 1987; 3:135–140.

76 Lichtman DM, Bruckner JD, Culp RW, Alexander CE. Palmar midcarpal instability: results of surgical reconstruction. J Hand Surg (Am) 1993; 18:307–315.

77 Goldfarb CA, Stern PJ, Kiefhaber TR. Palmar midcarpal instability: the results of treatment with 4-corner arthrodesis. J Hand Surg (Am) 2004; 29:258–263.

78 Palmer AK, Werner FW. The triangular fibrocartilage complex of the wrist – anatomy and function. J Hand Surg (Am) 1981; 6:153–162.

79 Palmer AK, Werner FW. Biomechanics of the distal radioulnar joint. Clin Orthop 1984; 187:26–35.

80 Mino DE, Palmer AK, Levinsohn EM. The role of radiography and computerized tomography in the diagnosis of subluxation and dislocation of the distal radioulnar joint. J Hand Surg (Am) 1983; 8:23–31.

81 Palmer AK. Triangular fibrocartilage disorders: Injury patterns and treatment. Arthroscopy 1990; 6:125–132.

82 Corso SJ, Savoie FH, Geissler WB, et al. Arthroscopic repair of peripheral avulsions of the triangular fibrocartilage complex of the wrist: A multicenter study. Arthroscopy 1997; 13:78–84.

83 Fulcher SM, Kiefhaber TR, Stern PJ. Upper-extremity tendinitis and overuse syndromes in the athlete. Clin Sports Med 1998; 17:433–448.

84 Finkelstein H. Stenosing tendovaginitis at the radial styloid process. J Bone Jt Surg (Am) 1930; 12:509–540.

85 Lane LB, Boretz RS, Stuchin SA. Treatment of de Quervain's disease: role of conservative management. J Hand Surg (Br) 2001; 26:258–260.

86 Bahm J, Szabo Z, Foucher G. The anatomy of de Quervain's disease. A study of operative findings. Int Orthop 1995; 19:209–211.

87 Cooney WP. Sports injuries to the upper extremity. Postgrad Med 1984; 76:45–50.

88 Grundberg AB, Reagan DS. Pathologic anatomy of the forearm: Intersection syndrome. J Hand Surg (Am) 1985; 10:299–302.

89 Rominger MB, Bernreuter WK, Kenney PJ, et al. MR imaging of anatomy and tears of wrist ligaments. Radiographics 1993; 13:1233–1246.

90 Taleisnik J. The ligaments of the wrist. In: Taleisnik J, ed. The wrist. New York: Churchill Livingstone; 1985:13–38.

91 Thornburg LE. Ganglions of the hand and wrist. J Am Acad Orthop Surg 1999; 7:231–238.

92 Gelberman RH, Salamon PB, Jurist JM, Posch JL. Ulnar variance in Kienbock's disease. J Bone Jt Surg Am 1975; 57:674–676.

93 Allan CH, Joshi A, Lichtman DM. Kienbock's disease: diagnosis and treatment. J Am Acad Orthop Surg 2001; 9:128–136.

94 Rettig AC, Ryan RO, Shelbourne KD, et al. Metacarpal fractures in the athlete. Am J Sports Med 1989; 17:567–572.

95 Kozin SH, Thoder JJ, Lieberman G. Operative treatment of metacarpal and phalangeal shaft fractures. J Am Acad Orthop Surg 2000; 8:111–121.

96 Ali A, Hamman J, Mass DP. The biomechanical effects of angulated boxer's fractures. J Hand Surg (Am) 1999; 24:835–844.

97 Kjaer-Petersen K, Langhoff O, Andersen K. Bennett's fracture. J Hand Surg (Br) 1990; 15:58–61.

98 Langhoff O, Andersen K, Kjaer-Petersen K. Rolando's fracture. J Hand Surg (Br) 1991; 16:454–459.

99 Kaplan EB. Dorsal dislocation of the metacarpophalangeal joint of the index finger. J Bone Jt Surg 1957; 39A:1081–1086.

100 Zemel NP. Metacarpophalangeal joint injuries in fingers. Hand Clin 1992; 8:745–754.

101 Ishizuki M. Injury to collateral ligament of the metacarpophalangeal joint of a finger. J Hand Surg (Am) 1988; 13:444–448.

102 Bowers WH, Wolf JW Jr, Nehil JL, Bittinger S. The proximal interphalangeal joint volar plate. I. An anatomical and biomechanical study. J Hand Surg (Am) 1980; 5:79–88.

103 Blazar PE. Steinberg DR. Fractures of the proximal interphalangeal joint. J Am Acad Orthop Surg 2000; 8:383–390.

104 McCue FC, Honner R, Johnson ME, et al. Athletic injuries of the proximal interphalangeal joint requiring surgical treatment. J Bone Jt Surg 1970; 937:52A.

105 Stener B. Displacement of the ruptured ulnar collateral ligament of the MP joint of the thumb: A clinical and anatomical study. J Bone Jt Surg 1962; 44:869–879.

106 Mack GR, Bosse MJ, Gelberman RH, et al. The natural history of scaphoid nonunion. J Bone Jt Surg (Am) 1984; 66:504–509.

107 Melone CP, Beldner S, Basuk BS. Thumb collateral ligament injuries: An anatomic basis for treatment. Hand Clin 2000; 16:345–357.

108 Abouna JM, Brown H. The treatment of mallet finger: The results in a series of 148 consecutive cases and a review of the literature. Br J Surg 1968; 55:653–667.

109 Okafor B, Mbubaegbu C, Munshi I, Williams DJ. Mallet deformity of the finger. Five-year follow-up of conservative treatment. J Bone Jt Surg Br 1997; 79:544–547.

110 Crawford GP. The molded polyethylene splint for mallet finger deformities. J Hand Surg 1984; 9A:231–237.

111 Takami H, Takahashi S, Ando M. Operative treatment of mallet finger due to intra-articular fracture of the distal phalanx. Arch Orthop Trauma Surg 2000; 120:9–13.

112 Wehbe MA, Schneider LH. Mallet fractures. J Bone Jt Surg Am 1984; 66:658–669.

113 McFarlane RM, Hampole MK. Treatment of extensor tendon injuries of the hand. Can J Surg 1973; 16:366–375.

114 Manske PR, Lesker PA. Avulsion of the ring finger flexor digitorum profundus tendon: An experimental study. Hand 1978; 10:52.

115 Leddy JP, Packer JW. Avulsion of the profundus tendon insertion in athletes. J Hand Surg 1977; 2:66.

116 Leddy JP. Avulsions of the flexor digitorum profundus. In: Strickland JW, ed. Hand clinics – flexor tendon surgery. Philadelphia, PA: WB Saunders; 1985:77–83.

117 Kotwal PP, Gupta V. Neglected tendon and nerve injuries of the hand. Clin Orthop 2005; 431:66–71.

118 Elson RA. Rupture of the central slip of the extensor hood of the finger. A test for early diagnosis. J Bone Jt Surg Br 1986; 68:229–231.

119 Leddy JP, Coyle MP. Palmar dislocation of the PIP joint. Presented at the American Society for Surgery of the Hand Conference, Seattle, September 1989.

120 Curtis RM, Reid RL, Provost JM. A staged technique for the repair of the traumatic Boutonnière deformity. J Hand Surg (Am) 1983; 8:167–171.

121 Schoffl V, Hochholzer T, Winkelmann HP, Strecker W. Pulley injuries in rock climbers. Wilderness Environ Med 2003; 14:94–100.

122 Rayan GM, Murray D. Classification and treatment of closed sagittal band injuries. J Hand Surg (Am) 1994; 19:590–594.

123 Hame SL, Melone CP Jr. Boxer's knuckle: Traumatic disruption of the extensor hood. Hand Clin 2000; 16:375–380.

124 Simon RR, Wolgin M. Subungual hematoma: association with occult laceration requiring repair. Am J Emerg Med 1987; 5:302–304.

125 Seaberg DC, Angelos WJ, Paris PM. Treatment of subungual hematomas with nail trephination: a prospective study. Am J Emerg Med 1991; 9:209–210.

126 Saldana MJ. Trigger digits: diagnosis and treatment. J Am Acad Orthop Surg 2001; 9:246–252.

127 Rooks MD. Johnston RB 3rd, Ensor CD, McIntosh B, James S. Injury patterns in recreational rock climbers. Am J Sports Med 1995; 23:683–685.

128 Meir N Van, Smet L De. Carpal tunnel syndrome in children. Acta Orthop Belg 2003; 69:387–395.

CHAPTER 28

Mid- and Low-back Injuries

Pierre A. d'Hemecourt

INTRODUCTION

Back pain is commonly seen in athletes and non-athletes. The lifetime prevalence of back pain is 60–90% of adults and up to 50% in adolescents. It is the most common cause of work disability in mid-life. Once pain has occurred, recurrence is noted in at least 30% of cases. Back pain is also a common cause of loss of playing time in sports. In professional football, 30% of players sit out for back pain[1] while 38% of tennis players lose some playing time.[2] Different sports place stress on different parts of the spine. Classic ballet and figure skating are associated with posterior element stress. Weightlifting and wrestling are often related to disc injuries. Some sports such as gymnastics with repetitive flexion and extension develop injuries to both the disc and the posterior elements. These injuries may be debilitating and require countless physician and therapy office visits. The clinician can often provide a more efficient return to activity if a standard progression of rehabilitation is followed.

The best rehabilitation is prevention. Therefore, an understanding of the injury and its predisposing factors is a starting point when pre-participation evaluations are performed. However, once an injury has occurred, an accurate diagnosis and an understanding of the phases of rehabilitation are needed. It is important look beyond the area of injury and consider the entire kinetic chain dysfunction that may have occurred subsequently or prior to the injury.

ANATOMY

The lumbar spine is unique in its position of linkage between the upper trunk and the pelvis. It is a mobile structure, bounded both inferiorly and superiorly by the more rigid structures of the thoracic spine and pelvis. It is the transition zone at each end of the lumbar spine where there is susceptibility to injury. At the inferior end, the change is more abrupt with the firm sacrum and pelvis. At this lumbosacral juncture, there is also a more acute lordotic angular change predisposing to both ante-

---

Box 28.1: Key Points

- The lumbar spine is unique in its position of flexibility between the rigid pelvis and semi rigid thoracic spine. This may predispose for injury at either end in the transition zone.
- The lumbar disc is wider than the thoracic discs.
- The adolescent disc is unique with the anular attachments to the ring apophysis and a softer growth cartilage endplate.
- The sharp lordosis at the lumbosacral juncture places increased compression forces posteriorly and shear forces at the disc.

---

rior shear and posterior compressive forces. At its upper level, the lumbar spine joins the somewhat inflexible thoracic spine. There is no sharp angular change here under normal circumstances. Instead, there is a conversion of lumbar lordosis to thoracic kyphosis. The kyphosis typically ends at T11 or T12, but may extend to L1–L2 in some individuals. The transition is also more gradual from rigidity to flexibility in a craniocaudad direction. Therefore, injuries are somewhat less common at this proximal border than the distal lumbar spine. This transitional segment spans T10 through L2.

Throughout the spine, each intervertebral level allows motion through the inherent tripod of two facet joints and the intervertebral disc. The facet joints are true diarthrodial joints with a synovial membrane. The intervertebral disc is a symphyseal joint. The facets are oriented in the sagittal plane in the mid-lumbar spine allowing more flexion. In the mid-thoracic region, they are oriented in a more frontal plane allowing some lateral bend.[3] The spine is often divided into the anterior and posterior elements. The anterior elements include everything from the anterior longitudinal ligament to the posterior longitudinal ligament, which includes the intervertebral disc and the vertebral body. The posterior elements comprise the neural arch with the pedicles, facets, pars interarticularis, lamina, transverse and spinous processes as well as the ligamentous interconnections.

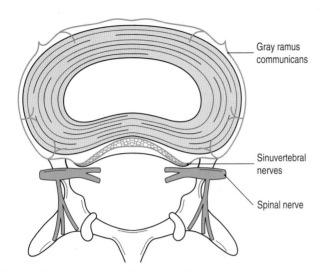

Figure 28.1   Innervation of the intervertebral disc.

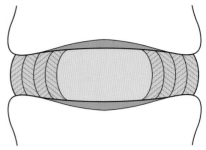

Figure 28.2   Intervertebral disc with anulus and endplate.

Anteriorly, the intervertebral discs are broadening as the transition occurs from the thoracic spine caudally. The intervertebral discs are composed of the ligamentous layers of the anulus fibrosus and the gelatinous nucleus pulposus. The anulus is comprised of 10–20 layers of concentric ligamentous lamellae with fibers obliquely oriented at 70° from the horizontal. These alternate in a crosshatched pattern that provides for torsional stablity.[4] The annular attachments are to the endplate and to Sharpey's fibers in the periphery. The endplate is hyaline cartilage that is connected to the vertebral body by the lamina cribrosa. This allows nutrient flow to the disc with hydrostatic forces. The anterior longitudinal ligament has continuous fibers with the anulus while the posterior longitudinal ligament is thinner and continuous in its length. The periphery of the annulus has dual innervation (Fig. 28.1). The sinuvertebral nerve, a branch of the spinal nerve, innervates the anulus posteriorly. The sinuvertebral nerve also innervates the posterior longitudinal ligament, the dura and the periosteum. All of these structures may contribute to back pain. The outer anterior annulus is innervated by the gray ramus communicans. At birth, there is some remnant arterial supply to the disc. However, this is non-existent by the age of 2 years.[5]

The nucleus pulposus is comprised of a few chondrocytes and fibroblast cells as well as proteoglycans and collagen. The collagen is predominantly type II. The proteoglycans are composed of a central hyaluronic acid core and attached glycosaminoglycans, predominantly chondroitin sulfate and keratin sulfate. These latter two molecules increase the osmotic gradient allowing the disc to remain hydrated. These gradually diminish in disc degeneration. Adequate hydration of the disc is dependent on the balance of the hydrostatic pressures pushing fluids from the disc and the osmotic pressures of the nucleus attracting fluid and nutrient through the lamina cribrosa of the endplate (Fig. 28.2). The nucleus comprises about 40% of the volume of the intervertebral disc.

However, in the immature spine, the attachments of the anulus are to the growth cartilage of the epiphysis and apophyseal ring. The vertebral body ends superiorly and inferiorly with the epiphyseal growth plate and overlying cartilaginous endplate and its contiguous ring apophysis (Fig. 28.3). The apophysis is attached to the outer anulus fibrosus. It has been demonstrated that this physis will separate from the subchondral bone with sheering forces. This has been shown to be the area of slippage with spondylolisthesis. Furthermore, injury to the growth zone has been demonstrated with both flexion and extension and an applied compression load.[6] The growth cartilage is the weak link in the chain in the child and adolescent spine.

In the posterior elements at the lumbosacral junction, the acute lordosis places a compressive and shear load on the facet joints and pars interarticularis. The pars may be incompletely ossified in the young spine predisposing it to injury particularly at the most lordotic part of the spine, the L5–S1 juncture. This has a demonstrated familial association. An underlying weakness here with repetitive microtrauma may result in a stress fracture referred to as a spondylolysis. Alternatively, the facet joints themselves may undergo a degenerative chondromalacia and arthrosis. The growing spine has another confounding issue with a changing sagittal alignment. From childhood to the end of adolescence, there may be an increase of about 10°

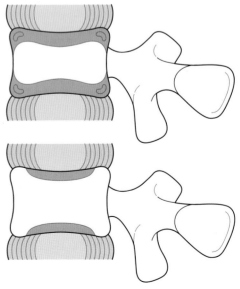

Figure 28.3   Growth cartilage in the child (above) and adult spine (below). Note the vertebral epiphysis of the child develops into the adult endplate.

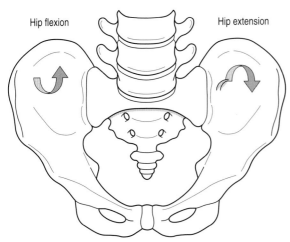

Figure 28.4 Sacroiliac joint motion.

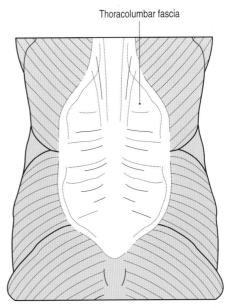

Figure 28.5 Transversus abdominus and thoracolumbar fascia.

in both lumbar lordosis and thoracic kyphosis.[7] Consequently, during the period of spinal growth, acceleration of sports participation involving spinal flexion and extension may accentuate the compressive and shear loads to the growth cartilage of the vertebral body and posterior arch.

In the posterior elements at the thoracolumbar junction, there is not an acute angular change. Nonetheless, the tight thoracolumbar fascia adds a direct compressive load. This compression may be accentuated by an excessive thoracic kyphosis.

There are other anatomic structures that must be considered in relation to mid- and low-back pain. These include the sacroiliac joint, the costovertebral junctures, the scapulothoracic articulation and the muscular stabilizers of the spine. The sacroiliac joint is where the lower spine joins the pelvic ring. Forces are transmitted across the sacroiliac joint between the trunk and lower extremities. The movement at the ileum during hip flexion is an ipsilateral posterior rotation and amplified SI compression. During hip extension, rotation of the ileum is anterior with SI distraction. The symphysis pubis is the pivot point when the lower extremities move in opposing directions (Fig. 28.4). Until puberty, the SI joint is flat. After puberty, corrugations develop into adulthood, ultimately ankylosing later in life.[8] The inferior portion is synovial, while only 25% superiorly are synovial.[9]

The upper 7 ribs have individual articulations with the sternum. The 8th, 9th and 10th ribs share a conjoined articulation. The 11th and 12th ribs are free floating. As such, the upper thoracic spine is more rigid and thus associated with less incidence of disc herniations than in the lower thoracic spine. The presence of the ribs inhibits flexion and rotation of the spine.[10] The articulation of the ribs at the costovertebral juncture is subject to subluxation that can cause inflammation, pain, and a popping sensation with rotation.

Scapula dysfunction is associated with upper-back pain, but may involve mid-back pain especially in its inferior portion. The scapula is a triangular shaped bone that is usually between the 2nd and 7th ribs. It lies 30–40° to the frontal plane. There may be bony ridges or osteophytes that rub against the ribs. There are also several bursae that assist in scapulothoracic

articulation. One is at the inferior edge and may be inflamed with repetitive pitching motion.

Finally, the muscular stabilizers of the spine must be considered. The muscular and fascia attachments of the lumbar spine and pelvis are important to the rehabilitation of back pain. Lumbar flexors consist of the psoas and the rectus abdominus. Extension is realized with the intrinsic polysegmental multifidus and the long polysegmental erector spinae group. The multifidus has the largest diameter of the group. It functions to extend the spine and control rotation due to the oblique fiber orientation.[11] The extrinsic group of extensors consists of the gluteus maximus and latissimus dorsi. They function with connections along the thoracolumbar fascia.

The thoracolumbar fascia performs several functions due to its attachments at the transverse processes, internal obliques and transversus abdominus (Fig. 28.5). Activation affords lumbar stability in forward bending and lifting. It also provides the link between the lumbar extensor and abdominal flexors with coactivation, which raises intraabdominal hydrostatic pressure to protect the spine.[12] Furthermore, there are multiple links to the pelvis and lower extremities that stabilize the spine including the gluteus medius (abduction), the adductors, as well as the small hip rotators. Injury to the lumbar spine has been shown to cause dysfunction of the lumbar stabilizers, which may prolong or cause pain themselves.[13]

BIOMECHANICS

The spine is subject to its motion and the reactive forces. These forces are known as kinematics and kinetics. Kinematics refers to the body in motion while kinetics relates a force to a mass and its motion.[14] The kinematics of spinal flexion and extension engages a shifting instantaneous axis of rotation. In spinal flexion, the axis of rotation concentrates in the nucleus pulposus with compression at the annulus and distraction at the facets. While in extension such as a gymnast in a back walk-over, there is a transfer of compressive forces to the posterior annulus and facet joints and imparts a simultaneous anterior distractive force.[15,16] As a result, injury patterns may be concurrently seen in anterior and posterior columns.[17] Flexion and extension predominantly occur at the L4–L5 and L5–S1 discs. However, this motion is part of a concerted lumbopelvic shared motion at the hip. Pelvic inflexibilities may impede sharing of this motion and apply more motion to the spine.

Spinal kinetics with sports includes intrinsic (musculotendinous inflexibility) and extrinsic (collision and ground reaction) forces affecting the spine. Spinal motion is reliant on coordinated activation of core muscles and pelvic flexibility. Excessive lumbar lordosis applies stress to the posterior arch. Intrinsic biomechanical risk factors resulting in increased lordosis include: iliopsoas inflexibility, thoracolumbar fascia tightness, abdominal weakness, genu recurvatum, and thoracic kyphosis.[18]

Axial rotation represents an intricate motion with rotation along the posterior aspect of the annulus until the facet is engaged, transferring the axis to this zygapophyseal joint. At this point, the disc is subject to shear forces along with the original torsion forces.[19] The maximal stress is at the postero-lateral disc.

PAIN GENERATION IN THE MID AND LOW BACK

There are multiple sources of mid- and low-back pain, which include the intervertebral disc, the zygapophyseal (facet) joint, nerve roots, sacroiliac joints, costovertebral joints, ligamentous and muscular tissue as well as growth cartilage (apophysis) in the young athlete. It is critical to understand that structural changes and pain do not always correlate and that there are multiple interactions in spine motion that effect pain generation in other locations of the kinetic chain.

Anteriorly, the outer one third of the anulus is innervated along with the posterior longitudinal ligament and the vertebral body. Furthermore, disc degeneration is associated with phospholipase A2 release with initiation of the inflammatory cascade particularly at the nerve root.[20] The dorsal root ganglion acts to modulate nerve transmission centrally. It is a site of production of multiple neuropeptides such as substance P and can act as a primary source of pain due to mechanical and inflammatory factors as well as vascular insufficiency.[21]

The facet joint is also recognized as a pain source.[22] This diarthrodial joint carries about 20% of the standing weight-bearing load at that segment. The median branch of the dorsal ramus from at least two levels innervates each facet.[23] Facet stimulation can produce leg and foot pain. With degeneration of the facet joint, osteophyte formation along with hypertrophy of the ligamentum flavum may produce narrowing of the intervertebral foramen. The sacroiliac joint may also produce low back and buttock pain. This will often radiate to the upper thigh. In the mid back, the costovertebral joint must also be considered.

CLINICAL EVALUATION

Box 28.2: Key Points

- The history should focus on age, gender and activity as well as a full medical history and medication review.
- The common red flags include significant pain in ages <18 or >55 years old, progressive night pain, trauma, history of cancer and immunosuppression such as systemic steroids, HIV or drug abuse.
- Cauda equina syndrome symptoms should be carefully assessed.
- Physical examination of the thoracic spine should include assessment for signs of myelopathy.

A thorough history is essential in establishing the diagnoses as well as detecting red flags. The demographics of age, gender, sport and occupational activity will often offer an initial direction. The young adult is more predisposed to discogenic disorders while the adolescent is more predisposed to spondylolytic disorders.[24] The older adult may have more osseous problems with osteophytes and stenosis or osteoporotic fractures. Gender may be significant with the male having more of a predisposition to inflammatory spondyloarthropathies and the female with more osteoporosis issues as well as fibromyalgia. Sporting activity is also quite important. Hyperextension sports such as dance, gymnastics, figure skating, as well as interior linemen are predisposed to posterior element stress fractures (spondylolysis). Flexion and torsional sports such as weight lifters, golf and racquet sports are more predisposed to disc disorders.[25] Gymnasts are also predisposed to discogenic changes at the thoracolumbar juncture from repetitive flexion and extension.[26]

The location of the pain and its relationship to activities can be quite helpful. Axial pain is pain that is in the mid to low back, with possible radiation to the buttock and upper thigh but not below the knee. Peripheral pain is below the knee and must be differentiated between referred and radicular pain. Referred pain is a non-specific pain production into the lower extremities and will not show signs of dural tension on the physical exam. Radicular pain is pain in a specific dermatome or myotome corresponding to a nerve root. This pain will be aggravated with dural tension maneuvers on the physical exam.

Pain that is flexion related such as sitting or forward bending is often due to a disc disorder, whereas a pain with extension tends to be more of a posterior element issue such as spondylolysis or facet syndrome. Pain with walking may indicate a problem with the posterior elements and/or stenosis. Peripheral pain that worsens with uphill walking is often disc related while leg pain with downhill walking is often central or lateral stenosis, referred to as neurogenic claudication. Vascular claudication will worsen with both bike and walking activities, while neurogenic claudication often is relieved in the flexed position on a bike. Pain that is worse with activities is often related to spondylolysis and sometimes an acute disc disorder. However, disc disorders are often worse after sports.

Discogenic pain is often worse in the morning after it has been hydrated in the recumbent posture. Stiffness that lasts longer than 1 h in the morning is often rheumatologic in nature. Sacroiliac pain may give some unilateral buttock pain with turning to the affected side at night. Pain at night can be due to discogenic disorders, but nocturnal pain should always raise the concern for tumors and systemic causes.

Ultimately, one must determine if there are any red flags that would indicate a more aggressive diagnostic imaging and laboratory analysis. The common red flags include significant pain in ages <18 or >55 years old, progressive night pain, trauma, history of cancer and immunosuppression such as systemic steroids, HIV or drug abuse. Also included are trauma, weight loss, systemic symptoms, crescendo pain, structural deformity, gait disturbance and inflammatory disorders suspected. Cauda equina syndrome is represented by difficulty with micturition, incontinence of bowel or bladder, loss of anal sphincter tone and saddle anesthesia.[27] This is a surgical emergency.

Previous therapy and the response are important. Previous physical therapy must be scrutinized as there is great variability in core stabilization and may simply be modality oriented with minimal stabilization. One must also determine exactly which types of injections have been done and their response. For example, even a temporary positive response to a facet injection is useful in determining the type of future injections or other therapies. Injections are often both diagnostic as well as therapeutic and may require multiple differential injections to determine the cause of pain.

The physical examination must take into account the entire kinetic chain of the spine, pelvis, upper back and lower extremities. It has been well established that incompletely rehabilitated lower extremity injuries contribute to back pain.[28] The exam should be done in a routine manner starting in the standing posture followed by a sitting exam, recumbent supine and then prone. Initially, the examiner should observe the patient in shorts noting the gait pattern, spinal curvature and the presence of a shift that may occur with a lumbar disc herniation. Thoracolumbar motion is evaluated from behind and to the side of the patient. Forward flexion tends to provoke disc symptoms while extension provokes posterior element pain. The level of forward flexion is documented by the position on the leg that the hand reaches (such as mid calf). During this motion, notation is made of any excessive kyphosis, segmental straightening, pain and scoliosis. Extension is tested again with the knees straight and noted by degrees of extension. Extension and rotation loads the facet joints while single leg hyperextension loads the unilateral facet and pars interarticularis indicating a possible spondylolysis (Fig. 28.6). Thoracolumbar rotation may produce pain and/or popping at the costovertebral juncture. Seated behind the patient, the examiner can also determine the sufficiency of sacroiliac motion with a Gillette's test. Here, the thumbs are placed on the patients two posterior superior iliac spines (PSIS) and asks the patient to march in place. As the knee moves up, the ipsilateral PSIS should move down unless there is a loss of sacroiliac motion. Finally, in the standing posture, the spinous processes are palpated. In the adolescent, tenderness here may reflect apophysitis. Toe (S1) and heel walking (L4) initiate the motor neurologic exam.

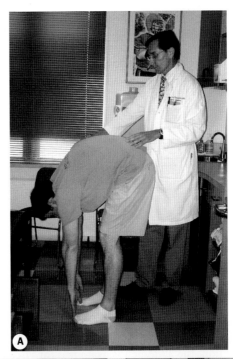

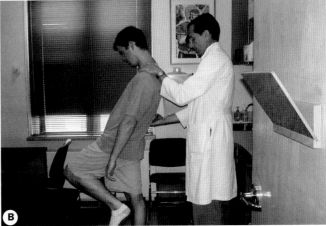

Figure 28.6   (A) Forward flexion and (B) Single leg hyperextension.

Now, the patient is asked to sit and the complete neurologic exam of the lower extremities is performed including motor, sensory and deep tendon reflexes. It is important to test for myelopathy when the thoracic region is involved. A positive test for a Babinski response and/or clonus would indicate an upper motor neuron lesion such as in the thoracic cord. While sitting, a dural tension test can be performed in the slump test. Here, the patient places his hands behind his back, rounds his shoulders forward with the head flexed and then the examiner extends the knee. A positive test will be reflected with pain into the leg.

The patient is then asked to lie recumbent. Now, pain provocation is tested in several ways. A straight leg-raising test (dural tension test) will be positive if the pain is produced into the leg at less than 70° of hip flexion. A crossed straight leg raise is more sensitive and specific. The sacroiliac joint is stressed with a FABER test. The leg is placed in the 'figure 4' posture with the knee flexed and the hip abducted and externally rotated with the heel on the contralateral thigh. The examiner has one hand on the knee and one on the contralateral anterior superior iliac spine (ASIS) and downward pressure is placed on both. Pain production in the unilateral buttock is a positive test for SI inflammation. This may be reconfirmed with a Gaenslen's test. Here, the patient is at the edge of the bed and one hip is held flexed by the examiner while the other extremity is pushed into extension over the edge of the bed. This maneuver also stresses the SI joint closest to the examiner.

While also supine, evaluation of flexibility is attained with a Thomas' test for hip flexor tightness and a popliteal angle for hamstring tightness. Having the patient hold one hip flexed with the thigh into the chest while the other leg is relaxed and passively extended performs the Thomas' test (Fig. 28.7). The examiner has a thumb on the ASIS and the point at which this moves forward as the thigh is extended is the endpoint where the angle of the thigh to the bed is measured and should be less than 30°. The popliteal angle is measured by flexing the hip to 90° and then passively extending the knee. The angle of the calf to the vertical at the point of passive resistance is the angle and should be less than 20°. Limb lengths are then measured from ASIS to the medial malleolus bilaterally. Finally, in the supine position, the abdomen is examined for visceral, pelvic and aortic abnormalities.

The patient is next in the prone position and the entire thoracolumbar spine is palpated for any point of tenderness to deep palpation. The paravertebral muscles and ribs are also

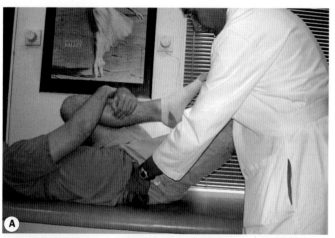

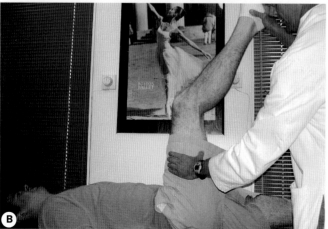

Figure 28.7 (A) Thomas' test and (B) Popliteal angle.

noted. Scapular tenderness is also noted. While supine, the upper lumbar nerve roots are tested for dural tension with a femoral stretch test. Here, the knee is first flexed and then the hip is extended. A positive test would radiate pain in a femoral nerve distribution of the anterior thigh.

Again, in a standing posture, the patient is tested for kinetic chain stability. With the hands crossed over the chest, a single leg squat is performed. Weakness of the abductors will manifest with the patient leaning to the unsupported side. Hip extensor weakness will manifest with forward bending of the torso. The patient is also asked to squat and duck walk. This will serve a screen for the ankles, knees and hips.

IMAGING STUDIES

Box 28.3: Key Points

- Plain radiographs are useful to detect developmental and congenital anomalies.
- A bone scan may also be helpful in detecting stress fractures and tumors, with the exception of multiple myeloma and purely lytic metastases.
- MRI is excellent for discogenic changes and may be very informative of posterior arch with advanced techniques to view this region.
- CT scan is the best image to define bone structural pathology.

The clinician has a number of imaging evaluation tools to assist in defining the etiology of back pain. However, it is critical to understand that all of these studies have been reported to have a high prevalence of positive findings in asymptomatic individuals.[29-31] Thus, each study should be chosen with an understanding of its positive and negative predictive values. Plain radiographs are indicated in the initial evaluation of low back pain if any of the red flags exist including the patient being under 18 or older than 55 years of age. This would include and AP and lateral view. If the pain were in the lower back, the lumbar spine would suffice. If there were involvement of the thoracic spine, a full-length thoracolumbar spine would be used. The AP view has value in looking at scoliosis, transitional vertebrae, and signs of a lytic lesion with obliteration of a pedicle. The lateral view gives excellent visualization of a spondylolisthesis, disc height, vertebral fractures and sometimes a spondylolysis. Oblique views are insensitive to picking up spondylolysis and often only add ionizing radiation.[32] However, they may be helpful in evaluation of facet arthrosis.

A technetium-99 bone scan is enhanced in its sensitivity for spinal fractures with addition of SPECT (single photon emission tomography) imaging, which offers tomographic views to the scan and increases the ability to anatomically localize a lesion.[33] Facet arthrosis may show a very similar finding to the spondylolytic lesion as they may be anatomically quite close. A bone scan may also be helpful in detecting tumors with the exception of tumors such as multiple myeloma and purely lytic metastases. A failed lumbar fusion with a pseudarthrosis may be demonstrated on bone scan.[34] A lumbar infection such as spondylodiscitis will be quite sensitive but not very specific.[35] In this setting a gallium nuclear scan would be more specific. The bone scan is used to show sacroiliac inflammation in the seronegative spondyloarthropathies. However, it is relatively in sensitive mechanical SI inflammation.[36]

Computed tomography is the gold standard for demonstrating the osseous structures. This is very useful in the traumatic situation to determine stability of the spine. The CT has also been shown to effectively classify a spondylolysis and predict its ability to heal.[37] Facet fractures and arthrosis are also well visualized. Central and lateral stenosis are well demonstrated on CT imaging. Finally, in patients with sciatic symptoms that are unable to have an MRI, myelography with CT imaging is useful to determine the extradural compression.

Magnetic resonance imaging offers excellent soft tissue and good bone resolution without any ionizing radiation. The lumbar disc herniation is well characterized as protruded (contained by the outer anulus), extruded (uncontained by the outer anulus) and sequestrated (separated from the disc). Furthermore, a high intensity zone on T2 images may indicate an anular tear.[38] Modic changes in the vertebral body adjacent to disc degeneration are also well seen. MRI images may be enhanced by gadolinium intravenous injection. This is indicated in the setting of infection, tumor, syringomyelia and delineation of recurrent disc herniation.

Initially, MRI protocols were used to analyze the disc in great detail, but the posterior elements were somewhat crudely visualized. Recently, there has been a great amount of interest in detecting a spondylolysis with the use of an MRI. By utilizing 2–3 mm MRI cuts in the sagittal and axial planes, Campbell and co-workers demonstrated equal sensitivity to a SPECT bone scan in detecting pars interarticularis stress but were somewhat equivocal in the actual delineation of the fracture.[39] This stress response is best seen with fat suppressed T2 and STIR images in the region of the pedicle and pars.

ACUTE INJURIES

Box 28.4: Key Points

- Spinal fractures should be assessed for mechanical and neurologic stability. The Denis 3 column analysis is very valuable in defining this.
- The child with spinal cord injury may present with no apparent structural injury, SCIWORA. There may be a delay in symptom onset.
- Early detection and immobilization is imperative to prevent progression of neurologic injury.

Fractures

Acute fractures of the thoracolumbar spine are infrequent in the athlete but may happen with collision sports such as ice hockey and football. These will often occur when the spine is flexed and an axial load is applied. Although these are less frequently associated with catastrophic neurologic injury than the cervical spine, they must be recognized early on the field and immobilized on a spine board to prevent further neurologic

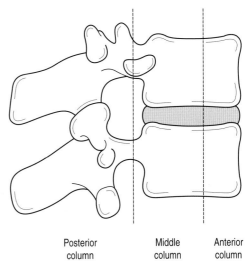

| Posterior | Middle | Anterior |
| column | column | column |

Figure 28.8 Denis three-column.

injury. The athlete should be assessed with a full advanced trauma life support protocol with assessment of airway, breathing, circulation and neurologic disability (ABCDs). It is preferable to leave the helmet on during transport along with the shoulder pads to leave the spine in alignment. However, the facemask should be removed in order to protect the airway.

Traumatic spinal injuries are often classified using the Denis' three-column theory (Fig. 28.8).[40] The anterior column contains the anterior longitudinal ligament and the anterior half of the vertebral body and anulus fibrosus. The middle column contains the posterior half of the vertebral body and anulus. The posterior column comprises the posterior arch and stabilizing ligaments. Involvement of a single column indicates stability while two-column involvement (any middle column involvement) would indicate instability. The instability may involve neurologic and/or mechanical instability with deformity progression. An initial evaluation should detail any transient weakness or paresthesia that may indicate cord involvement. Plain X-rays are obtained and an anterior compression fracture of ≤25% would indicate stability. As the fracture approaches 50% compression, a CT scan would best evaluate middle column involvement. If neurologic involvement is suspected an MRI is essential to delineate cord and soft tissue injury.

A stable thoracic compression fracture of less than 50% loss of height may be immobilized in a thoracolumbosacral orthosis (TLSO) for 6–12 weeks. Similar lumbar injuries below the level of the cord may be treated in a TLSO for 4–6 weeks. Extension exercises are started when the athlete is tolerant to these but are kept out of sports during this bracing period. Return to athletic activity is allowed when full strength and flexibility are attained along with full healing. Athletes with minimal compression fractures are allowed to return to contact sports. However, more severe compression or neurologic injury particularly in the thoracic spine may be a contraindication to contact sports. If the athlete required a single level fusion without any neurologic deficit, consideration to return to contact sports may be individualized with the full understanding by the athlete and parents of adjacent level disc degeneration. The use of instrumentation is often a contraindication to contact sports.

Pediatric patients have a unique concern of a spinal cord injury without radiographic abnormality (SCIWORA). This may be explained by the relative laxity of the spine in relation to the relatively fixed cord. Another explanation has been a transient vascular insufficiency. An MRI will often delineate an intraneural or an extraneural abnormality.[41] In the younger child, this usually involves the cervical spine with more devastating consequences. Older children have been reported to have a thoracolumbar injury. Interestingly, there is often a delay of several days before neurologic progression occurs that is often incompletely reversible. Thus, it is important to consider MRI imaging in the young child with transient neurologic complaints at the scene. Treatment usually involves 12 weeks of brace immobilization.

Acute disc herniations

Thoracic disc herniations are quite uncommon and represent about 1% of all symptomatic disc herniations.[42] The most common sites are T8–T11. However, asymptomatic thoracic disc herniations have been reported in 11–13% of individuals.[43] The coronal plane of the thoracic facets, which limit flexion and allow more lateral bending, may explain this. In the presence of a symptomatic thoracic disc herniation, a central protrusion may present with myelopathic symptoms of leg weakness and long track signs. If the herniations are lateral, radicular symptoms to the chest and abdomen may occur. However, these patients often present with axial pain located in the mid to lower thoracic spine as well as upper lumbar region.[44] An MRI is an excellent choice for imaging, as the T2 images will show a myelographic effect with the high signal of the CSF contrasted against the cord and the lower signal of the disc. However, 70% of symptomatic thoracic disc herniations will manifest disc and sometimes intrathecal calcification.[45] Calcification is better defined with CT with or without myelography.

Treatment is often conservative. Most symptomatic thoracic disc herniations do not require surgery.[46] The presence of myelopathy or progressive neurologic deficit is usually an indication for surgical intervention. However, this is less than 27% of thoracic disc herniation cases.[28] Conservative management includes extension strengthening. The athlete may return to play when they have achieved a level of full strength and are free of any symptoms. This decision in contact sports should include a full evaluation of the space around the cord similar to cervical disc disease. The athlete should be monitored as myelopathy has been noted to develop at later stages.

Lumbar disc herniations are more common, presenting in 2% of the general population.[47] These occur predominantly at the L4–L5 and L5–S1 levels and often occur with loading the spine in forward flexion and rotation such as a crew athlete. The young athlete may also have discogenic pain but with a less clear clinical presentation. They will often present with axial, non-radiating pain. Clinical findings include a loss of forward lumbar flexion, peripelvic inflexibility and possibly a sciatic shift. The pain is often worse with sitting. Dural tension signs of a straight leg raise, slump test or Lasègue test may be present. One variation of an acute disc herniation is an acute anular tear and may present with an acute popping sensation in the back. An MRI will best delineate the disc herniation and

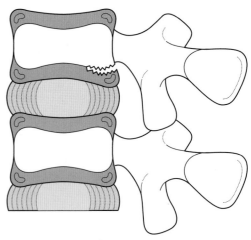

Figure 28.9 Apophyseal avulsion.

often the anular tear. This latter entity may demonstrate a high intensity zone on T2 MRI images along the posterior disc margin. The young adolescent athlete may present with an apophyseal ring avulsion as the spine goes into sudden forced flexion with an avulsion of the posterior fibrocartilage apophysis by its anular attachment (Fig. 28.9).[48] A CT scan may be needed to visualize this entity.[49]

Some 90% of disc herniations resolve within 3 months without surgical intervention. Conservative management includes a short period of rest followed by mobilization with activity modification. Flexion activities are limited. A rigid brace in 15° of lordosis may be used initially to unload the disc and allow a more rapid mobilization. The athlete is gradually advanced to a full core stabilization program with attention to kinetic chain dysfunction. Non-steroidal anti-inflammatory drugs (NSAIDS) and occasionally epidural corticosteroids are used to advance the rehabilitation process. Surgical intervention is indicated with any signs of a cauda equina syndrome, progressive neurologic deficit or refractory symptoms to conservative management. Those treated surgically may often return to sports in 6–12 weeks. Conservative management may often require 3–6 months' rehabilitation.

Muscular contusions and strains

Muscle contusions result from a direct blow to the back with a resultant hematoma. Muscular strains often occur with sudden resisted eccentric contractions. There are multiple ligaments around the spine that may be sprained with sudden stretching. Treatment of these entities involves analgesics, ice, compression, rest and gradual mobilization and stabilization. At times, the symptoms will be prolonged, which may cause kinetic chain dysfunction and require more aggressive rehabilitation.

CHRONIC INJURIES

Degenerative disc disease

Adult back pain is secondary to discogenic causes in 48% of cases.[24]

Box 28.5: Key Points

- Adult back pain is often related to the disc while the adolescent often presents with a spondylolysis.
- The adolescent performing repetitive flexion and extension may present with injury to the disc endplate at the thoracolumbar juncture (atypical Scheuermann's).
- The facet joints and sacroiliac joints are further etiologies of spinal pain.
- One must always consider inflammatory spondyloarthropathies and tumors.

The finding of a degenerative disc, the black disc, is a common finding in asymptomatic individuals and therefore should be viewed skeptically in relating it to back pain. Nonetheless, the degenerative intervertebral disc can produce phospholipase A2 which upregulates arachidonic acid and the inflammatory pathway. Irritation of the outer anulus may produce axial back pain. Disc degeneration may manifest as desiccation, anular tears, protrusion and endplate fragmentation. Furthermore, disc degeneration with adjacent endplate and cancellous edema of the vertebral body has been associated with axial back pain. This may be due to segmental instability and inflammation. This same inflammation may also cause radiculitis in the neuroforamina with secondary leg pain.

In the young athlete, repetitive flexion of the thoracolumbar spine may contribute to Scheuermann's kyphosis with resultant pain in the region of the deformity. This entity is defined as three contiguous vertebrae with at least 5° of anterior wedging, irregular endplates and a Cobb angle of at least 45°. If these same changes occur in the thoracolumbar region, the athlete may present with kyphosis of the thoracolumbar juncture and lumbar hypolordosis. This is referred to as atypical Scheuermann's or lumbar Scheuermann's.

Evaluation of these patients involves a careful exam to find their directional preference of thoracolumbar motion as well as a quantitation of the peripelvic flexibility and strength. Plain X-rays are quite helpful with Scheuermann deformities. Disc degeneration, protrusion and anular tears may be seen with MRI imaging.[50] Occasionally, discography will help delineate the symptomatic disc with an occult internal anular tear. This involves intradiscal injection of contrast to provoke typical pain as well as definition of the internal derangement with CT scanning.

Treatment of disc degeneration involves relative rest with cross-training and core stabilization that is initiated with a directional preference and graduated to a full directional stabilization as able. Most often this starts with an extension-biased program and advances to full stabilization. Short courses of NSAIDS may be quite helpful in initiating the program over the first month. Additional pain relief with tramadol may also be used. In acutely painful cases, a short term of TLSO bracing in 15° of extension may help move the patients into a more comfortable range to start stabilization. Refractory cases may respond to an epidural steroid injection particularly if radicular pain is involved. This is somewhat controversial for axial

disc pain but may also be helpful. Another alternate is intradiscal electrothermal therapy in well-selected cases with a convincing discogram provoking concordant pain and a demonstrated internal derangement. The procedure is thought to be effective through the anular shrinkage and the secondary neurolysis of the outer anulus innervation. This is effective in 53% of patients. However, this requires 4–6 months of rehabilitation.

In the adolescent athlete with Scheuermann changes, the addition of bracing is quite effective. For thoracic involvement and ongoing growth, bracing is initiated for curves greater than 45–50°. Below 50°, observation and extension exercises are indicated. Above 60–70°, surgical correction is considered. A Milwaukee brace is needed for curves above T7. Below this level, a TLSO with upper chest support may be used. Thoracolumbar and lumbar Scheuermann's respond well to TLSO bracing in 15° of extension. Extension exercises are started simultaneously.

Spondylolysis and spondylolisthesis

Spondylolysis in the athletic population represents a stress fracture from repetitive loads from the inferior articular facet at one level placing impingement on the pars interarticularis and lamina at the level below. This usually involves a fracture to the pars at L5 but may present as high as L1. This entity has been discounted as a congenital problem but has been shown to have a strong familial association.[51] The par is the weakest part of the posterior arch and is incompletely ossified in some individuals. Beutler demonstrated spondylolysis in 5% of first grade students on routine screening which showed no abnormal association with back pain on a 45-year follow-up.[52] However, the athlete usually presents with debilitating pain most often near the growth spurt. There are several reasons why the athletic spondylolysis represents a more concerning entity. During spinal development from the young spine to late adolescence, the lumbar lordosis increases with increasing posterior pressure. Repetitive extension during this period adds additional load to the posterior arch. The 6 year old with an incidental pars fracture has time to develop multiple compensatory stabilizing mechanisms from the interspinous ligaments and the anulus. Athletic spondylolysis has not had the same compensation. It is during this time that there is a small but distinct chance to develop a spondylolisthesis.

In one study, back pain in young athletes was attributed to spondylolysis in 47% of the cases. Certain high-risk sports such as gymnastics, ballet and figure skating report an incidence as high as 32% (gymnasts) and 33% (ballet). These athletes will present with activity related pain with minimal sitting or nocturnal discomfort. The examination will usually demonstrate pain on lumbar hyperextension and more specifically single leg hyperextension on the affected side. Tight hip flexors and hamstrings are often present. It is not uncommon to note a coexisting increased thoracic kyphosis. The imaging evaluation should start with an AP and lateral spine view. This will note any transitional vertebrae and may demonstrate a spondylolysis or spondylolisthesis. Since the oblique views are not sensitive and only add ionizing radiation, they are often avoided.[53,54] A bone scan with SPECT imaging is quite sensitive to detecting these lesions. MRI imaging with thin sections through the posterior elements and T2 or STIR images will demonstrate the stress response particularly at the pars region much like a SPECT bone scan.[55] Next, a CT scan isolated to the level demonstrated on MRI or SPECT scan will be accurate in assessing the state of fracture healing while minimizing radiation exposure.

Treatment options for spondylolysis are variable. Some centers report good success with sports limitation for 3–4 months along with an antilordotic physical therapy program. At Children's in Boston, an antilordotic brace is used from the start of treatment. Athletes are to refrain from sports for 4–6 weeks until they have demonstrated resolution of pain at rest and on provocative hyperextension testing. During this initial period, physical therapy addresses peripelvic flexibility and abdominal strength. If they demonstrate a normal exam at the 4–6 week visit, the athlete is advanced in the core stabilization and gradually returned to one sport providing that they remain pain free and that they continue the brace full time at 23 h per day. The brace itself will limit full participation is sports such as gymnastics, but will allow some involvement. The core stabilization at this stage adds some activation of the extensor muscles but in a neutral non hyper-extended zone such as bridges. Peripelvic and lower extremity strength are added. After 4 months of bracing, a CT may be considered to evaluate healing particularly if they are still symptomatic. In the asymptomatic athlete, the brace is weaned off over several weeks. It is critical to have an evaluation of the sport specific techniques at this stage to prevent recurrent injury. If symptoms persist at this, 4-month mark, the brace is continued. There is evidence that addition of electrical stimulation may be helpful at this point.[56] If symptoms continue to persist for 6–12 months, surgical stabilization is considered.

Minimal grade spondylolisthesis with active lesions on SPECT bone scan or MRI are treated in a similar fashion particularly in the young athlete. A mature spondylolisthesis that is symptomatic is addressed with sports limitation, antilordotic core stabilization and temporary bracing to minimize symptoms. Anti-inflammatory medication including well selected corticosteroid injections are utilized. As pain subsides, full core stabilization is attained including extension without hyperextension. Conservative management is often successful, but surgical stabilization may be needed in patients with refractory pain or radicular symptoms.[57]

Facet syndrome

Up to 40% of back pain is due to facet inflammation. This syndrome is common in athletics that involve repetitive extension. Athletes will often present with ambulatory pain that is worsened by during activities or transitional movements such as getting up from a recumbent position. Pain is often relieved with lying down. No examination technique is highly sensitive but extension with rotation may elicit some pain. The examination of spinal motion will usually elicit a flexion based directional preference. MRI imaging may demonstrate the facet irregularity along with hypertrophy of the ligamentum flavum. The facet irregularity is best seen on CT. However, all imaging is neither sensitive nor specific in predicting facet pain syn-

drome.[58] When indicated, this is most accurately diagnosed by facet joint injection of anesthetic.

Treatment is initiated with relative rest along with flexibility to address pelvic flexibility and posterior pelvic tilt. Temporary use of an anti-inflammatory may provide the ability to progress rehabilitation, which will include a flexion biased core stabilization program. Antilordotic bracing may also be helpful in the initial phases of inflammation. Fluoroscopically directed corticosteroid injections with an anesthetic may help both diagnostically and therapeutically when there is refractory pain to conservative management. This may allow the athlete to progress with therapy. However, persistence of symptoms with the above aggressive conservative therapy may indicate a radiofrequency neurotomy of the facet innervation by the medial branch primary dorsal ramus. As the pain subsides and the core stabilization is advanced, the entire kinetic chain from the lower extremities is addressed. Sports specific motion is emphasized such as the serve in tennis where extension may be gained from the knees and hips.

Costovertebral subluxation, scapular bursitis

The costovertebral joint has been demonstrated to contain nociceptors and neuropeptide substance P.[59] Sudden lateral bending with rotation may cause a sudden popping sensation in this location. This injury can become chronic with perivertebral pain and popping. No imaging study is diagnostic and often is a diagnosis of exclusion. Management involves manipulation therapy, upper back stabilization exercises and occasionally a fluoroscopically directed corticosteroid injection.

There are several bursas near the scapula at the superior border and one in the inferomedial corner, the infraserratus bursa (Fig. 28.10). These are often symptomatic in overhead sports such as pitching as well as weight training and gymnastics.[60] There will often be an associated snapping, pain and

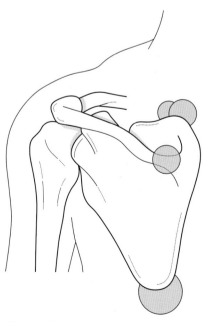

Figure 28.10 Scapular bursa.

crepitus. Evaluation should include a full review of the athlete's upper back posture as well as sport specific motion. The bursas are easily palpated with the athlete prone while adducting and internally rotating the ipsilateral arm to the contralateral scapula, the chicken wing position. Rehabilitation should address any of the scapular dyskinesia with the chest wall such as rhomboid, serratus anterior and trapezius weakness. It should also address any excessive rounding of the shoulders and kyphosis.[61] A local corticosteroid injection may be helpful with care to stay away from the chest wall. A good position for this injection is the chicken wing pose, which will retract the scapula from the chest wall.

Lordotic low back pain

During adolescent growth, the spinal growth may temporarily exceed the thoracolumbar fascia and peripelvic ability to lengthen. Consequently, with cyclic loading of the spine, there may be excessive traction and compression injuries to the spinous process and iliac crest apophyses as well as the facet joints and transitional vertebrae pseudarthrosis (Bertolotti syndrome). These athletes will often present as a spondylolysis with extension based low back pain with a reportedly normal SPECT bone scan or MRI. However, careful review may show uptake in the affected areas such as a transitional pseudarthrosis or spinous process apophysis.

Treatment centers around the antilordotic strengthening and stabilization while minimizing the injurious athletic motions such as the gymnasts back walk over. Occasionally, antilordotic bracing is needed to relieve the pressure and inflammation. With an inflamed Bertolotti pseudarthrosis, an injection of corticosteroid may be helpful.

Sacroiliac inflammation

The sacroiliac joint may become inflamed and painful as the result of a single traumatic fall onto the ischium or from repetitive asymmetrical pelvic motion. This may occur with a limb length discrepancy. The constellation of associated injury may be confusing. Primary disc involvement may present with secondary sacroiliac inflammation. Sacroiliac inflammation may also cause piriformis syndrome due to the proximity of the piriformis origin. Furthermore, the sacroiliac joint may provide the location for hematogenous seeding of infection, inflammatory disease and stress fractures. Physical findings are inconsistent and sacroiliac inflammation is most accurately diagnosed with a sacroiliac injection of an anesthetic.

Treatment revolves around correcting biomechanical issues such as a limb length discrepancy as well as addressing the asymmetric motion of certain athletic motions such as the runner remaining on the same canted surface. Core and sacroiliac stabilization are addressed with strengthening the muscles that oblique the pelvis. Predominantly, this involves rotary torso and hip rotational motion. Peripelvic strength of the hip abductors and extensors are addressed along with full lower extremity strengthening. Sacroiliac belts will provide compressive support in the initial phases of the rehabilitation. In refractory cases, a fluoroscopically directed injection to the lower

one third of the joint using anesthetic and corticosteroid may be both diagnostic and therapeutic.[62]

Inflammatory disease, spinal tumors and pseudospinal pain

The seronegative spondyloarthropathies are associated with the human leukocyte antigen (HLA) B27. These include ankylosing spondylitis (AS), Reiter's syndrome, psoriatic arthritis and enteropathic spondyloarthropathy. These often present under the age of 40 with back pain, often with sacroiliac involvement and morning stiffness lasting more than 45–60 min. AS and Reiter's syndrome are predominantly male and with an 80–90% association with HLA B27. Conversely, enteropathic and psoriatic arthritis have a 50% association with HLA B27.[63] AS may be associated with aortic insufficiency and uveitis. Ossification of the anulus will appear as marginal syndesmophytes (bamboo spine). Psoriatic arthritis may be antecedent to the skin lesions in 15% of cases. Reiter's presents with the triad of uveitis, urethritis and arthritis with implicated microbes of Shigella, Salmonella, Yersinia and Campylobacter. The enteropathic type is associated more with Crohn's than ulcerative colitis. Treatment of the spondyloarthropathies often involves anti-inflammatory medication and back extension strengthening. AS is most prone to progression with spinal deformity and spinal cord injury.[64]

Spinal tumors often present with pain. This pain is often nocturnal, progressive and constant. Primary tumors in the posterior elements are more commonly benign and in a younger population while vertebral body tumors are often malignant. Metastatic tumors are most often breast, prostate, thyroid, lung and kidney. Benign primary tumors include osteoid osteoma (<2 cm), osteoblastoma (>2 cm), osteochondroma, giant cell tumor, hemangioma, aneurysmal bone cyst and eosinophilic granuloma. With the exception of a hemangioma, these usually present under the age of 30.[65] Primary malignant tumors usually present over the age of 30. These include solitary plasmacytoma (unifocal multiple myeloma), chondrosarcoma, chordoma, lymphoma, Ewing's sarcoma and osteosarcoma. The plasmacytoma is the most common.[66] However, under the age of 30, Ewing's sarcoma and osteosarcoma are the most common. Imaging should begin with plain X-rays but may not show abnormality until there is 30–50% loss of cancellous bone.[67] A technetium-99-bone scan is sensitive but non-specific. The F-18 positron emission tomography (PET) shows improved specificity. The MRI scan especially with gadolinium demonstrates excellent definition of soft tissue and osseous changes.[48]

There are a number of abdominal, pelvic, vascular and retroperitoneal structures that may mimic spinal pain. Kidney stones are a common entity that most often presents as severe and non-positional back pain. Prostatitis may present with low back and perineal pain along with a fever. Pelvic inflammatory disease, endometriosis, and ectopic pregnancy are also considerations with back pain. Gastrointestinal contributions to back pain include pancreatitis and penetrating ulcers. Finally, in the older population, abdominal aortic aneurysms may well present with back pain.

REHABILITATION

Box 28.6: Key Points

- Rehabilitation should consider both the individual factors of diagnosis and biomechanics as well as the sport specific risk factors.
- The phases of rehabilitation include the acute, subacute, rehabilitative and sport specific phases.
- Multiple adjuncts and medications may be used to advance these phases.
- Psychologic issues sometimes impair progress and should be assessed early.

Rehabilitation in the athlete is a comprehensive task that requires a full evaluation of the patient as well as an understanding of the involved sports. There is a wide spectrum of athletic level from recreational to elite involvement. The rehabilitation will consider two aspects: individual and sport specific risk factors. Individual considerations include a precise diagnosis, age of the athlete, biomechanical and kinetic chain deficiencies. In the elite athlete or when there are concerning factors, advanced imaging may be considered to more accurately direct the spinal rehabilitation. In the younger athlete, growth and maturation are considered. In the older athlete, osteoporosis, inflexibility and strength concerns are addressed. It is critical to look beyond the diagnosis and assess the biomechanics as well as kinetic chain deficiencies that will predispose to a recurrent injury.[68] It has been well demonstrated that incompletely rehabilitated lower extremity injuries are a risk factor for back injuries.[28]

Sport-specific motions and impact are considered. Often the individual biomechanical deficiencies will accentuate the injurious motions of the activity. Technical errors of the sport specific motion may also need adjustment. Abrupt changes in sports duration, intensity, and frequency are also common errors in summer camps. Training surface for runners and dancers may also contribute to overuse injury.

The rehabilitation should be staged according to the injury. The phases include the acute phase, subacute phase, rehabilitation phase and sports specific (functional) phase. There is often overlap of these phases. However, it is important to follow through the final stages even as symptoms resolve. Incomplete rehabilitation is a common cause of recurrent injury.

Care must also be given to track the use of adjunctive care such as medication, injections, manipulation and bracing. NSAIDS are often used for short courses initially but may also assist in the progression from phase to phase. Manipulation may be quite helpful with short-term usage, particularly with sacroiliac inflammation. Corticosteroid injections are considered in refractory cases. The use of a brace is common in the adolescent athlete particularly for spondylolysis. Frequently, the brace is used through the rehabilitation and into the return to sports.

Acute and subacute phases

In the acute phase of injury, a few days of rest is helpful. Prolonged rest may be detrimental. As the pain subsides, the subacute phase is entered and the athlete is gradually mobilized. At this time, modalities such as icing, ultrasound and iontophoresis may be used. Analgesics and anti-inflammatory medication are also useful in this mobilizing process. Temporary bracing may also assist this process. This may simply be a corset brace or a more rigid brace as indicated.

In the subacute phase, the athlete may tolerate some gentle aerobic activity in the pool that may simply be treading water. Isometric muscular contraction is initiated to prevent atrophy. This would include abdominal and extensor contractions. To the extent that the athlete tolerates flexibility, these exercises may be started.

Rehabilitative phase

As the acute bleeding, swelling and/or inflammation subside, motion increases and a specific diagnosis is more attainable. The examination will elicit a directional preference so that a neutral zone of core stabilization may be initiated. Depending on the pathology, this may be more of a flexion biased or extension biased program. The neutral zone is the area of comfortable spinal motion. Gradually, this zone is expanded. Nonetheless, the entire core should be addressed as able. This includes the short and long extensors, the internal obliques, transversus abdominus, and abdominals. Any noted peripelvic, lower extremity or upper trunk weakness are also addressed (Fig. 28.11). Initially, closed chain strengthening is started. This would include floor-based exercises such as bridges and advanced to resisted machines as able. Relatively early in this phase the concept of co-activated muscular coordination is attended to with activities such as balance ball and Pilates. These activities require multiple muscle group activation as well as balance. During this period, flexibility is also stressed as indicated.

During the early rehabilitation phase, aerobic activity is also encouraged. This will often maintain the athlete's endurance and help maintain their confidence. Depending on the injury, this may be pool running, swimming, cycling, elliptical or gradually running. Certain injury patterns may be aggravated with some aerobic activities. Bicycling may aggravate disc pain with a loss of lordosis unless attention is paid to shortening the reach to the handles and lowering the seat. Rapid running will place an extension torque to the spine and aggravate facet and pars injuries. In general, the elliptical machine is well tolerated as it holds the spine in a neutral posture.

If the athlete is unable to progress during this phase, the diagnosis should be questioned and further imaging considered. It is at this time that consideration may be given to a well-selected fluoroscopic corticosteroid injection to quiet the inflammation. The decision on bracing may also be revisited if a brace was not initially chosen.

In later rehabilitation, it is important to initiate multiplanar motion that is similar to the athlete's sport. The core acts to transfer forces from the lower extremities to the arms in throwing sports. The core also acts to generate force and recoil

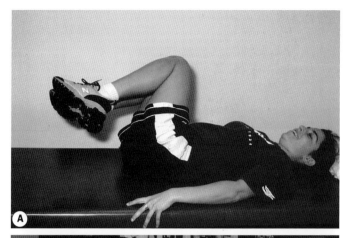

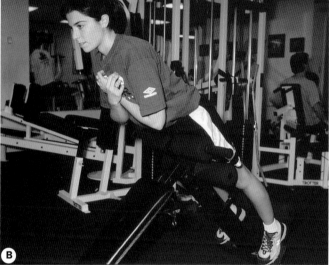

Figure 28.11 Early phase rehabilitation.

force, which requires multiple planes of motion. In preparation to return to sports, the athlete must mimic these motions in a graded fashion. This may be achieved with Therabands, resisted pulleys and free weights. Plyometrics are also gradually introduced.

Sports-specific phase

The individual's injury and biomechanics were addressed in the rehabilitative phase. During the final phase of returning to sports, the sports specific concerns should be attended to. This often involves well-trained coaches to address sports specific motion such as pitching or a golf swing. Training errors are addressed such limiting the number of gymnastic back walkovers. Training surface is reviewed particularly in dance and running. As the athlete returns to participation, the injury motions are minimized while maximizing the tolerated motions. This process is different from sport to sport.

For instance, the classic ballet dancer performs multiple extension maneuvers with arabesque and port de bras. This will naturally stress the posterior facet joints and pars interarticularis. With port de bras, the legs are maximally externally rotated during lumbar extension for aesthetics. The dancer

with femoral anteversion and poor turn out may increase the anterior pelvic tilt to release the ileofemoral ligament and achieve greater turn out. The consequence is increased lordosis. The appropriate coaching will accept the individual's natural turn out and stress abdominal strengthening.

Back pain in gymnasts is reported as high as 85%; spondylolysis is reported in up to 14%.[69] It has also been reported that gymnasts demonstrate increasing MRI changes to the disc with advancing levels of participation. In the pre-elite gymnast, 9% had disc changes while 63% at the Olympic level showed disc changes.[70] While the back walkover is often implicated in pars stress and should be minimized in the return to participation, other motions such as the back scale may increase posterior element stress if there is not good peripelvic strength for controlled motion. Furthermore, during periods of rapid growth, there is an increased risk to the gymnast for increased lordosis and injury.[71,72] Consideration to activity limitation during the growth spurt may need to be considered.

In golf and racquet sports, there are multiple combinations of rotation and lateral flexion. In these sports, there should be emphasis on keeping the shoulders and hips aligned during swinging motions. In tennis, the serve is particularly straining to the posterior elements and may be compensated for by emphasizing knee flexion to gain extension of the trunk. Furthermore, it has also been demonstrated that some increased hip extension may be trained in the tennis player.[73] The golf swing should underscore the classic swing with associated hip and shoulder motion to diminish spinal torsion. Increased club length will diminish lumbar flexion. Furthermore, the core dynamic strength must be achieved.

Bicycling is associated with back pain in up to 30% of cyclists.[74] With competitive pedaling there is progressive weakening of the abdominal muscles and decreased lordosis. This imparts pressure to the disc with a predisposition to an anular tear. This is magnified in the tucked posture. Rehabilitation should emphasize extension strengthening to maintain a normal lordotic posture on the bike. The fit of the bike is also important in the rehabilitation. The fore-aft distance (reach) and height of the handlebars are quite important. With a long reach and low handlebars, the lumbar lordosis is lost and may even be kyphotic in the lower lumbar spine. The height of the pedal is important for the sacroiliac joint. When the seat is to low, the sacrum is held fixed, there may be high repetitive forces at the SI joint from the pedaling motion of a flexed knee and hip. Essentially, the goal is to maintain a normal lumbar lordosis to decrease stress forces at the back and neck.

In football, the linemen are at risk for a back injury. This may include disc injuries from the weightlifting squat or spondylolysis. At the blocking sled, it has been demonstrated that the forces generated at L4–5 exceed tissue strength of the pars interarticularis in compression and the disc in shear forces.[75] The rehabilitation of these athletes will address a strong core with attention to speed and motion of core responsiveness. In the rehabilitation phase, the squat should be held. However, the same muscle groups may be addressed with leg press. During the early return to football, repetitive blocking sled motion should be minimized to allow tissue recovery.

These represent examples of sports that are often associated with back pain. As one is progressing with the therapy and returning to participation, there should be an emphasis that these rehabilitation conditioning programs and sport technique considerations become part of the athlete's normal training regime. In doing so, the athlete is often not only minimizing a recurrence but also often improving performance.

REFERENCES

1 Dvorak J, Junge A. Football injuries and physical symptoms: A review of the literature. Am J Sports Med 2000; 28:63-69.
2 Marks MR, Hass SS, Wiesel SW. Low back pain in the competitive tennis player. Clin Sports Med 1988; 7:277-287.
3 Bogduk N. The zygapophyseal joints. Clinical anatomy of the lumbar spine. 3rd edn. London: Churchill Livingstone; 333-341.
4 Bogduk N. The inter-body joints and intervertebral discs. Clinical anatomy of the lumbar spine. 3rd edn. London: Churchill Livingstone; 13-31.
5 Moore K. The developing human: Clinically oriented embryology. 4th edn. Philadelphia: Saunders; 1988:334-340.
6 Baranto A, Ekstrom L, Hellstrom M, et al. Fracture patterns of the adolescent porcine spine: an experimental loading study in bending-compression. Spine 2004; 30:75-82.
7 Akin C, Muharrem Y, Akin U, et al. The evolution of sagittal segmental alignment of the spine during childhood. Spine 2004; 30:93-100.
8 Bergmark A. Stability of the lumbar spine. A study in mechanical engineering. Acta Orthop Scandinav Suppl 1989; 230:20-24.
9 Dreyfuss P, Cole A, Pauza K. Sacroiliac joint injection techniques. Phys Med Rehab Clin North Am 1995; 6:112-140.
10 Oda I, Abumi K, Lü D, et al. Biomechanical role of the posterior elements, costovertebral joints, and rib cage in the stability of the thoracic spine. Spine 1996; 21:1423-1429.
11 Donisch W, Basmajian V. Electromyography of deep back muscles in man. Am J Anat 1972; 133:25-36.
12 Manning T, Plowman SA, Drake G, et al. Intra-abdominal pressure and rowing: the effect of entrainment. Med Sci Sports Exerc 1998; 30:190.
13 Richardson CA, Jull GA. Muscle control-pain control. What exercises would you prescribe? Man Ther 1995; 1:2-10.
14 Nigg BM. Biomechanics as applied to sports. In: Harries M, Williams C, Stanish WD, Micheli LJ, eds. The Oxford textbook of sports medicine. New York: Oxford Medical; 1994:94-111.
15 Letts M, Smallman T, Afanasiev R. Fracture of the pars interarticularis in adolescent athletes: a clinical biomechanical analysis. J Pediatr Orthop 1986; 6:40-46.
16 Nachemson A. The load on lumbar disks in different positions of the body. Clin Orthop Rel Res 1996; 45:107-122.
17 Itaka T, Miyake R, Katoh S, Morita T, Murasa M. Pathogenesis of sports-related spondylolisthesis in adolescents. Radiographic and magnetic resonance imaging study. Am J Sports Med 1996; 24:94-98.
18 Trepman E, Walaszek A, Micheli L. Spinal problems in the dancer. In: Solomon R, Minton S, Solomon J, eds. Preventing dance injuries: an interdisciplinary perspective. Reston: Alliance for Health, Physical Education, Recreation and Dance; 1990:103-131.
19 Farfan F, Cossette W, Robertson H, et al. The effects of torsion on the intervertebral joints: the role of torsion in the production of disc degeneration. J Bone Jt Surg 1970; 52A:468-497.
20 Kallakuri S, Cavanaugh JM, Blagoev DC. Phospholipase A2 sensitivity of the dorsal root and dorsal root ganglion. Spine 1998; 23:1297-1306.
21 Olmarker K, Storkson R, Berge O. Pathogenesis of sciatic pain: a study of spontaneous behavior in rats exposed to experimental disc herniation. Spine 2002; 27:1312-1317.
22 Eisenstein SM, Parry CR. The lumbar facet arthrosis syndrome. J Bone Jt Surg [Br] 1987; 69:3-7.
23 Bogduk N. The innervation of the lumbar spine. Spine 1983; 8:286-293.
24 Micheli L, Wood R. Back pain in young athletes. Arch Pediatr Adolesc Med 1995; 149:15-18.
25 Farfan F, Cossette W, Robertson H, et al. The effects of torsion on the intervertebral joints: the role of torsion in the production of disc degeneration. J Bone Jt Surg 1970; 52A:468-497.
26 Goldstein JD, Berger PE, Windler GE. Spine injury in gymnasts and swimmers. An epidemiologic investigation. Am J Sports Med 1991; 19:463-468.
27 Overmeer T, Linton SJ, Holmquist L, et al. Do evidence-based guidelines have an impact in primary care? A cross-sectional study of Swedish physicians and physiotherapists. Spine 2005; 30:146-151.
28 Nadler SF, Wu KD, Galski T. Low back pain in college athletes. A prospective study correlating lower extremity overuse or acquired ligamentous laxity with low back pain. Spine 1998; 23:828-843.
29 Boden SD, Davis DO, Dina TS, et al. Abnormal magnetic-resonance scans of the lumbar spine in asymptomatic subjects: a prospective investigation. J Bone Jt Surg Am 1990; 72:403-408.
30 Wiesel SW, Tsourmas N, Feffer HL, et al. A study of computer-assisted tomography: I. The incidence of positive CAT scans in an asymptomatic group of patients. Spine 1984; 9:549-551.
31 Hitselberger WE, Witten RM. Abnormal myelograms in asymptomatic patients. J Neurosurg 1968; 28:204-206.
32 Saifuddin A, White J, Tucker S, Taylor BA. Orientation of lumbar pars defects: implications for radiological and surgical management. J Bone Jt Surg (Br) 1998; 80:208-111.
33 Bellah RD, Summerville DA, Treves ST, Micheli LJ. Low back pain in adolescent athletes: Detection of stress injury to the pars intra-articularis with SPECT. Radiol 1991; 180:509-512.
34 Gates GF. SPECT bone scanning of the spine. Semin Nucl Med 1998; 28:78-94.
35 Maiuri F, Iaconetta G, Gallicchio B, Manto A, Briganti, F. Spondylodiscitis: Clinical and magnetic resonance diagnosis. Spine 1997; 22:1741-1746.
36 Slipman CW, Sterenfeld EB, Chou LH, et al. The value of radionuclide imaging in the diagnosis of sacroiliac joint syndrome. Spine 1996; 21:2251-2254.
37 Morita T, Ikata T, Katoh S, et al. Lumbar spondylolysis in children and adolescents. J Bone Jt Surg 1995; 77B:620-625.
38 Bogduk N. Point of view: Predictive signs of discogenic lumbar pain on magnetic resonance imaging with discography correlation. Spine 1998; 23:1259-1260.
39 Campbell RS, Grainger AJ, Hide IG, Papastefanou S, Greenough CG. Juvenile spondylolysis: a comparative analysis of CT, SPECT and MRI. Skeletal Radiol 2005; 34:63-73.
40 Denis F. Spinal instability so defined the three-column spine concept in spinal trauma. Clin Orthop 1984; 189:65.
41 Launay F, Leet AI, Sponseller PD. Pediatric spinal cord injury without radiographic abnormality: a meta-analysis. Clin Orthop Relat Res 2005; 433:166-170.
42 Arce CA, Dohrmann GJ. Herniated thoracic disks. Neurol Clin 1985; 3:383-392.
43 Awwad EE, Martin DS, Smith KR Jr. Asymptomatic versus symptomatic herniated thoracic discs: their frequency and characteristics as detected by computed tomography after myelography. Neurosurgery 1991; 28:180-186.
44 Garfin SR, Vaccaro AR. Thoracic disc herniations. Orthop Knowl Update 1996; 5
45 Stillerman CB, Chen TC, Couldwell WT. Experience in the surgical management of 82 symptomatic herniated thoracic discs and review of the literature. J Neurosurg 1998; 88:623-633.
46 Brown CW, Deffer PA Jr, Akmakjian J. The natural history of thoracic disc herniation. Spine 1992; 17:97-102.
47 Eismont FJ, Kitchel SH. Thoracolumbar spine. In: Stanitski CL, DeLee JC, Drez D, eds. Pediatric and adolescent sports medicine. Philadelphia: Saunders; 1994:1018-1062.
48 Itaka T, Morita T, Katoh S, Tachibani K, et al. Lesions of the posterior endplate in children and adolescents. J Bone Jt Surg 1995; 77B:951-958.
49 Peh WC, Griffith JF, Yip JK, Leong JC. Magnetic resonance imaging of the lumbar vertebral apophyseal ring fractures. Australas Radiol 1998; 42:34-37.
50 Aprill C, Bogduk N. High-intensity zone: A diagnostic sign of painful lumbar disc on magnetic resonance imaging. Br J Radiol 1992; 65: 361-369
51 Stinson J. Spondylolysis and spondylolisthesis in the athlete. Clin Sport Med 1993; 3:517-528.
52 Beutler WJ, Fredrickson BE, Murtland A, et al. The natural history of spondylolysis and spondylolisthesis: 45-year follow-up evaluation. Spine 2003; 28:1027-1035.
53 Congeni J, McCulloch J, Swanson K. Lumbar spondylolysis. A study in natural progression in athletes. Am J Sports Med 1997; 25:248-253.
54 Saifuddin A, White J, Tucker S, Taylor BA. Orientation of lumbar pars defects: implications for radiological and surgical management. J Bone Jt Surg (Br) 1998; 80:208-111.
55 Campbell RS, Grainger AJ, Hide IG, Papastefanou S, Greenough CG. Juvenile spondylolysis: a comparative analysis of CT, SPECT and MRI. Skeletal Radiol 2005; 34:63-73.
56 Friedberg R, Curtis C, Micheli L, d'Hemecourt P. Using electrical stimulation as a modality for the treatment of adolescent athletes with spondylolysis. American College of Sports Medicine Annual Meeting, Nashville TN, 2005.
57 Kwon BK, Albert TJ. Adult low-grade acquired spondylolytic spondylolisthesis: Evaluation and management. Spine 2005; 30:535-541.
58 Derby R, Bogduk N, Schwarzer A. Precision percutaneous blocking procedures for localizing pain. Part I: the posterior compartment. Pain Diag 1993; 3:89-100.

59 Erwin WM, Jackson PC, Homonko DA. Innervation of the human costovertebral joint: implications for clinical back pain syndromes. J Manipulative Physiol Ther 2000; 23:395–403.

60 Kuhn JE, Plancher KD, Hawkins RJ. Symptomatic scapulothoracic crepitus and bursitis. J Am Acad Orthop Surg 1998; 6:267–273.

61 Manske RC, Reiman MP, Stovak ML. Nonoperative and operative management of snapping scapula. Am J Sports Med 2004; 32:1554–1565.

62 Dreyfuss P, Cole A, Pauza K. Sacroiliac joint injection techniques. Phys Med Rehab Clin North Am 1995; 6:112–140.

63 Mazanec DJ. Pseudospine Pain: Conditions that mimic spine pain. In: Cole AJ, Herring SA, eds. The low back pain handbook. 2nd edn. Philadelphia: Hanley & Belfus; 2003:117–131.

64 Hayes VM, Siddiqi FN, Kondrachov D, Silbert JS. Metabolic and inflammatory diseases of the spine. In: Vaccaro A, ed. Core knowledge in orthopedics. Philadelphia: Elsevier/Mosby; 187–198.

65 Abu WA, Provenchur M. Primary bone and metastatic tumors of the cervical spine. Spine 1998; 23:2767–2777.

66 Austin LS, Grauer JN, Beiner JM, et al. Primary and metastatic spinal tumors. In: Vaccaro A, ed. Core knowledge in orthopedics. Philadelphia: Elsevier/Mosby; 226–240.

67 Shimizu K, Shikata J, Iida H, et al. Posterior decompression and stabilization for multiple metastatic tumors of the spine. Spine 1992; 17:1400–1404.

68 Standert CJ, Herring SA, Cole AJ, et al. The lumbar spine and sports. In: Cole AJ, Herring SA, eds. The low back pain handbook: A guide for the practicing clinician. 2nd edn. Philadelphia: Hanley & Belfus; 2003:385–404.

69 Hutchinson M. Low back pain in elite rhythmic gymnasts. Med Sci Sports Exerc 1999; 31:1686–1691.

70 Goldstein JD, Berger PE, Windler GE, Jackson DW. Spine injuries in gymnasts and swimmers. An epidemiologic investigation. Am J Sports Med 1991; 19:463–468.

71 Wojtys EM, Ashton-Miller JA, Huston LJ, et al. The association between athletic training time and the sagittal curvature of the immature spine. Am J Sports Med 2000; 28:490–498.

72 Caine D, Cochrane C, Caine C, et al. An epidemiologic investigation of injuries affecting young competitive female gymnasts. Am J Sports Med 1989; 17:811–820.

73 Kibler WB, Chandler TJ. Range of motion in junior tennis players participating in an injury risk modification program. J Sci Med Sport 2003; 6:51–62.

74 Schofferman J. Chronic and recurring low back pain and neck pain in bicycle riders. Spineline 2002; 3:15–19.

75 Gatt CJ, Hosea TM, Palumbo RC, et al. Impact loading of the lumbar spine during football blocking. Am J Sports Med 1997; 25:317–321.

CHAPTER 29

Hip and Pelvis Injuries

Mininder S. Kocher and Rachael Tucker

INTRODUCTION

Box 29.1: Key Points

- As significant improvements are being made in MR arthrography and hip arthroscopy, sports injuries of the hip and pelvis are increasingly being recognized.

Sports injuries of the hip and pelvis are receiving increased attention. The majority of sports injuries about the hip and pelvis are muscle sprains and soft tissue injuries that heal with non-operative supportive treatment, such as adductor strains. Repetitive overuse injuries, such as femoral neck stress fractures, and acute macro-traumatic injuries, such as avulsion fractures of the pelvis or traumatic hip dislocation, can also be seen. With the advent of hip arthroscopy and the development of more advanced imaging of the hip through MR arthrography, internal derangements of the hip such as labral tears, loose bodies and chondral injuries, are being diagnosed and treated with increased frequency. This chapter overviews the more common injuries of the hip and pelvis in athletes.

SOFT TISSUE INJURIES

Box 29.2: Key Points

- Soft tissue injuries, such as contusions and myositis ossificans, often result from direct trauma and overuse in sports.
- Contusions are related to sub-periosteal, intramuscular or subcutaneous bleeding and swelling.
  - Deep bleeding and hematoma may lead to nerve impingement.
  - Most contusions can be treated conservatively with rest, compression and ice.

- Severe contusions require more attention to flexibility and strengthening.
- Two types of myositis ossificans are myositis ossificans progressive (MOP) and myositis ossificans circumscripta (MOC).
- Early radiographic diagnosis of calcification is difficult.
- Rest and immobilization is critical to mitigate the reactive process of ossification.
- Surgical excision is available for rare refractory cases.

Contusions

Contusions around the hip and pelvis are a common injury among athletes and typically result from direct trauma over bony prominences.[1,2] They involve bleeding and swelling that can be sub-periosteal, intramuscular or subcutaneous in origin.

The most common contusion involving the hip in athletes has been coined 'hip pointer' and results from a direct blow to the iliac crest (Fig. 29.1).[1,2] On clinical examination, there is generally localized tenderness, ecchymosis and muscle spasm as a result of deep bleeding and hematoma formation around muscle insertion points. There may also be signs of nerve entrapment where large hematoma compress adjacent nerves.

Early treatment of hip contusions is conservative and aimed at minimizing complications resulting from deep bleeding and hematoma formation. This includes rest, compression and application of ice. The use of non-steroidal ant-inflammatory medications, heat therapy or massage and vigorous physiotherapy is not recommended as this may further increase bleeding. While the usefulness of hematoma aspiration is questionable, reports in the literature indicate that judicious use of corticosteroid injection may provide symptomatic relief enabling more rapid return to sports participation.[1,2]

Severe muscular contusions often require more prolonged rehabilitation, lasting 3 weeks or more and focusing on maintaining flexibility and improving strength. Return to full sports participation should not occur until full strength, range of motion and coordination has returned.[1,2] Premature return to full sports participation may result in re-injury and prolonged disability.

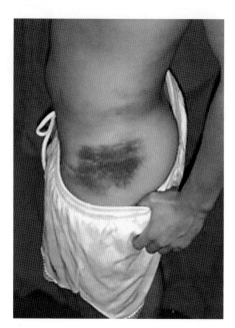

Figure 29.1 Anterolateral hip contusion.

The use of appropriate padding during sports participation may reduce the risk of contusions.[1,2]

Myositis ossificans

Myositis ossificans is a rare, benign condition characterized by heterotopic ossification of soft tissues.[2–6] There are two distinct forms of the disease, including myositis ossificans progressive (MOP) which as the name suggests leads to progressive, generalized ectopic ossifications and myositis ossificans circumscripta (MOC) in which the lesions are more localized.[6] While little is known about the etiology of this disease, it is likely that the generalized form has a genetic origin whereas the circumscribed form, which is most commonly seen following major trauma and among athletes, is likely to be a reactive complication to hematoma formation, particularly when it occurs close to the site of muscle insertion.[2,5] Irrespective of etiology, this condition can result in severe functional impairment and disability without appropriate diagnosis and treatment.[4]

Diagnosis is often delayed as radiographic evidence of calcification may not present for several weeks, however the persistence of a severe contusion or hematoma following trauma combined with a progressive loss of movement in the affected limb, should raise clinical suspicion for this condition. It is only later in the course that organized calcific deposits become evident.[2,3] This lack of definitive radiological diagnosis early in the disease can lead to misdiagnosis of malignant tumor within the bone or soft tissue and often histological examination of a biopsy specimen is the only means to accurately confirm the diagnosis.[2,3,5]

An enforced period of rest and immobilization is essential until a definitive diagnosis can be made and should continue until symptoms resolve. Subsequent rehabilitation, as recommended by Nuccion and colleagues, should involve active stretching and strengthening exercises. Both massage and active stretching should be avoided for at least 4–6 months as this will only exacerbate the reactive process resulting in increased ossification.[2]

While conservative management is usually successful for cases of localized myositis ossificans, surgical excision of the ossified mass may be required for rare refractory cases. Confirmation that the disease process is no longer active, by way of bone scan prior to surgery, may minimize the future risk of recurrence (Fig. 29.2).[2]

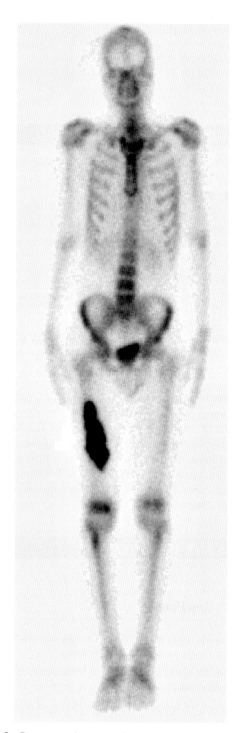

Figure 29.2 Bone scan demonstrating active right thigh myositis ossificans.

BURSITIS

Box 29.3: Key Points

- Bursitis is a painful condition that involves inflammation and enlargement of the bursa as a result of direct trauma or overuse.
  - Iliopectineal bursitis results in pain and swelling about the groin and along the femoral nerve distribution and distal edema.
  - Trochanteric bursitis presents as radiation of pain and often paresthesia along the posterior-lateral aspect of the thigh, with associated tenderness over the greater trochanter and iliotibial tract.
  - Ischial bursitis presents as pain in the buttocks and shooting pain down the back of the leg.
- Bursitis can be treated conservatively with rest, icing, and non-steroidal anti-inflammatory drugs.

A bursa is a fluid-filled, saclike structure associated with joints or bony prominence whose purpose is to act as a protective cushion. Bursitis is a painful condition that involves inflammation and enlargement of the bursa as a result of direct trauma or overuse. Athletes participating in endurance-type sports such as long distance running where the bursa is exposed to repetitive and excessive friction as well as high impact sports such as football and basketball where the risk of direct trauma are high, are at increased susceptibility for developing bursitis, especially around the hip.[2]

The iliopectineal bursa is the largest bursa surrounding the hip joint and its inflammation can result in considerable pain and disability.[7] Iliopectineal bursitis typically presents as a painful inguinal swelling with occasional radiation of pain along the femoral nerve distribution and distal edema, if compression of the femoral nerve, external iliac or common femoral vein occurs.[2,7] Flexion and external rotation of the hip provides some relief from symptoms and as a result, this is a characteristic posture assumed by patients with this condition. The etiology of iliopectineal bursitis is closely linked to the so called 'snapping hip' syndrome also known as coxa saltans and involves the snapping of the iliopsoas tendon over the iliopectineal eminence. While good results are observed with conservative management, surgical release of the iliopsoas tendon close to its insertion on the lesser trochanter is necessary for refractory cases.[2]

Trochanteric bursitis often mimics conditions affecting the hip and lower back.[8] Presentation typically involves radiation of pain and often paresthesia along the posterior-lateral aspect of the thigh, with associated tenderness over the greater trochanter and iliotibial tract.[8] As with iliopectineal bursitis, there is an etiological association with the snapping of the iliotibial band over the greater trochanter and the subsequent development of trochanteric bursitis.[9]

Ischial bursitis, also referred to as 'weaver's bottom', is an uncommon and frequently misdiagnosed cause of buttock pain.[2,10,11] While ischial bursitis typically results from direct trauma, it has also been reported among athletes participating in sports such as canoeing and horse-riding where prolonged periods of sitting are required.[10,11] Ischial bursitis typically presents with buttock pain that can be excruciating in nature and often associated with sharp, shooting pains that radiate down the back of the leg.[2,11]

Diagnosis of bursitis can typically be made on the basis of clinical signs and symptoms alone, however when imaging is warranted, ultrasound or MRI are generally considered the modalities of choice.[10,11] Although rarely performed, definitive exclusion of other more serious differentials may ultimately require needle aspiration or biopsy.[11]

First line treatment for all types of bursitis is typically conservative involving rest, ice-packs and use of oral non-steroidal anti-inflammatory drugs. If simple measures are insufficient, adjunctive injection of corticosteroids and local anesthetic directly into the bursa are often effective but only provide temporary relief of symptoms.[2]

For the rare cases that are non-responsive to conservative measures, surgical intervention may be indicated. Arthroscopic excision of the bursa is reported in the literature as a minimally invasive technique that is both safe and effective in relieving symptoms, particularly in cases of refractory trochanteric and ischial bursitis.[2,5,12] Iliopectineal bursectomies however are technically more challenging due to the close proximity to the femoral vessels and nerve and possible communication with the hip joint, increasing the inherent risk of the procedure.[2,7] In cases of iliopectineal and trochanteric bursitis attributable to coxa saltans, surgical tendon release is often successful in relieving symptoms.[2]

SNAPPING HIP SYNDROME

Box 29.4: Key Points

- Snapping hip syndrome is also known as coxa saltans and it is characterized by an audible 'snapping' sensation that can occur with normal activity. Three types are internal, external, and intra-articular. Snapping hip can be treated conservatively using activity restriction, heat therapy, stretching, and anti-inflammatory drugs. Refractory cases may require surgical intervention.

Coxa saltans is a common condition which is also referred to as 'the snapping hip'. It is characterized by an audible 'snapping' sensation that can occur during hip movement associated with exercise or normal activities of daily living. Associated hip pain is frequently but not routinely present and is localized to the anterior part of the hip or over the greater trochanter.[13,14]

This well recognized symptom-complex can be classified according to etiology into three distinct types including internal, external and intraarticular.[13,14] Traditionally, diagnosis of external and internal coxa saltans was based on clinical examination with only the intra-articular variety requiring more high-tech imaging such as MRI or CT for diagnosis. Accurate diagnosis and distinction between the three types is important for management and prognosis.

The external snapping hip is the most common form and typically affects athletes and dancers in their late teens or 20s.[14] It results from the sudden displacement of a thickened posterior border of the iliotibial band or the anterior border of the gluteus maximus muscle over the greater trochanter with hip flexion.[13,14,16] It is frequently, but not routinely, associated with hip pain and is invariably attributed to trochanteric bursitis or iliotibial tendonitis.[16] Palpation over the greater trochanter during active hip flexion is diagnostic. This diagnosis can be further corroborated by applying pressure at the level of the greater trochanter, thereby preventing the snapping sensation.[14]

Internal coxa saltans is the least common form of snapping hip and since it was first described in 1951 by Nunziata and Blumenfeld, we have gained little insight into its etiology. It results from a snapping of the iliopsoas tendon over the iliopectineal eminence (Fig. 29.3).[13,14,16] Symptoms can generally be reproduced by passive movement of the hip from an adducted and internally rotated position into flexion and external rotation.[16] Confirmation of the diagnosis is provided when application of finger pressure over the iliopsoas tendon at the level of the femoral head prevents the snapping.[14]

The intraarticular variety is distinct both in its presentation and subsequent management. Instead of the classical snapping sound, a clicking sensation is often described with hip pain being a more predominant symptom. Its etiology involves a mechanical abnormality within the joint itself, such as intra-articular loose bodies, synovial osteochondromatosis or acetabular labral tears.[14]

The diagnostic role of radiological imaging is now increasing as technology progresses. A study by Wunderbaldinger *et al.* compared the diagnostic value of various imaging techniques, including plain radiographs, ultrasound, CT and MRI, in diagnosing internal coxa saltans.[15] Among the 54 patients studied, conventional radiographs alone were able to identify the patho-etiology in 37% (20/54) compared with 46% (25/54) by ultrasound alone. When ultrasound and radiographs were used in combination, this increased to 83%. The addition of CT to the previous radiological work-up increased the rate of diagnosis to 88%. Results demonstrated that MRI was the most sensitive form of imaging with 100% diagnosis of coxa saltans. However, due to the inherent cost of this form of imaging they suggested retaining this for difficult cases only, especially where intraarticular pathology is involved.[16]

The diagnostic application of dynamic ultrasonography is likely to increase in the future. A study by Choi *et al.* demonstrated, through the use of this real-time imaging, how sudden abnormal snapping movements of the iliotibial band or gluteus maximus over the greater trochanter during joint motion or muscle contraction correlated with the painful click experienced by patients.[14,16]

While coxa saltans is a common condition, the majority of cases are infrequent and asymptomatic snapping that does not require medical intervention. For those with symptomatic snapping, conservative management is generally effective and includes avoidance of activities that produce the snapping, application of heat, stretching exercises and anti-inflammatory drugs.[14] Over a period of 6–12 months it is possible for the patient to regain full hip function with no recurrence of symptoms.

Surgical intervention is retained for the small number of patients who are refractory to conservative management or competitive athletes requiring a rapid return to sports.[13,16] Surgical correction of external coxa saltans involves excision of the greater trochanter bursa with elongation of the iliotibial band via z-plasty. The effectiveness and safety of this procedure has been documented in the literature. For those patients with refractory internal coxa saltans, surgical intervention involves lengthening of the posterolateral tendinous portion of the iliopsoas tendon. This is performed under general anesthetic as a day-stay procedure and is reported as providing effective symptomatic relief. Arthroscopy is useful where an intraarticular cause has been identified. However, where large loose bodies or synovial chondromatosis is implicated, an open approach may be warranted.[14]

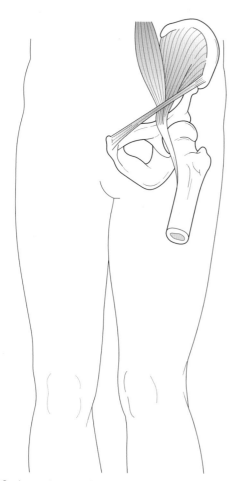

Figure 29.3 Internal coxa saltans caused by snapping of the iliopsoas tendon over the pelvic brim. (Redrawn from Dobbs MB, Gordon JE, Luhmann SJ, et al. Surgical correction of the snapping iliopsoas tendon in adolescents. J Bone Joint Surg [Am] 2002; 84:420–424).

OSTEITIS PUBIS

Box 29.5: Key Points

- Osteitis pubis is characterized by burning pain and inflammation around the pubic bones, pubic symphysis and surrounding muscular insertions, believed to be caused by periosteal trauma or repetitive micro trauma from sports related forces.

- This condition typically affects middle aged male athletes.

- Varying differential diagnoses exist, including inguinal hernias, prostatitis, and urethritis.

- Radiological imaging as a diagnostic tool in the early stages is limited, as radiographs often appear to be normal for the first few weeks of the disease.

- Most cases can be treated conservatively with rest, and anti-inflammatory drugs, and surgical intervention is rarely indicated.

Osteitis pubis is a common, self-limiting condition involving the pubic bones, pubic symphysis and surrounding muscular insertions and can result from trauma, pelvic surgery, childbirth and certain repetitive exercise.[17-19] It was first described in 1924 by the urologist Beer, in patients following suprapubic surgery and, until the 1970s, osteitis pubis was regarded as being solely infectious in origin.[17,20] The emergence of cases among athletes where there had been no history of invasive pelvic surgery highlighted the possible inflammatory origin of the disorder.[17,20]

Athletes afflicted by this condition are typically men in their 30s and 40s, who participate in sports that involve sprinting, sudden changes of direction and rapid acceleration and deceleration such as running, gymnastics, soccer, rugby, basketball and tennis.[17,21,22] While the exact cause remains controversial, periosteal trauma resulting from direct sports-related force or repetitive micro-trauma leading to subsequent inflammation and pain is thought to be the key etiological factor in osteitis pubis among athletes.[18]

Presentation is characterized by progressively worsening pain or 'burning discomfort' around the pubic region with radiation to medial aspect of the thigh, perineum and lower abdomen.[17,20]

The differential diagnosis of osteitis pubis is extensive including muscle strains and other soft tissue injuries, inguinal and femoral hernias, connective tissue disorders, prostatitis, orchitis, urolithiasis, urethritis and iatrogenic causes secondary to pelvic procedures, birth trauma, malignancy and infection.[18]

Examination typically reveals a waddling, antalgic gait, tenderness over the pubic symphysis and adductor longus insertion with a painful and reduced range of motion in one or both hips.[17,20] In addition, the patient may experience spasm of the adductor muscle with limited abduction and demonstrate a positive lateral compression test and positive cross-leg test may be seen.[17]

The diagnostic value of radiological imaging in the early stages is often limited as there is often a poor correlation between radiological findings and the site and duration of symptoms.[2] While radionuclide bone-scans (Fig. 29.4) typically show unilateral uptake around the pubic symphysis, plain radiographs are often normal for the first 2–3 weeks of the disease but occasionally demonstrate slight separation of the pubic bones with patchy sclerosis and irregular cortical margins.[17,23]

Due to the self limiting nature of the disorder, management is largely conservative, focusing on minimizing inflammation through rest, oral non-steroidal anti-inflammatory

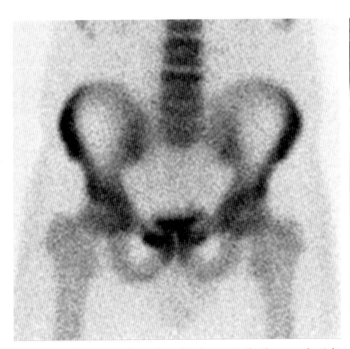
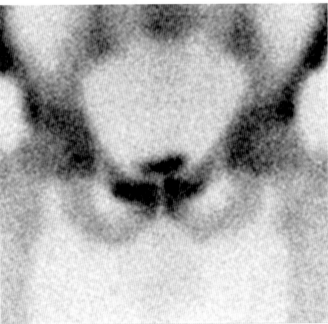

Figure 29.4 Bone scan of osteitis pubis demonstrating increased uptake at the pubic symphysis.

drugs and the occasional use of corticosteroid injections directly into the symphysis pubis.[17] Batt *et al.* reports that, on average, athletes are able to return to full sports participation within 3–6 months after a period of graduated endurance, stretching, and flexibility training with a recurrence rate of 25%.[17,21] The increasing demands and financial incentives facing professional athletes however undoubtedly influence compliance and subsequent benefit following conservative management.[18]

Surgical intervention is rarely indicated and this is reflected in the scarcity of reports in the literature. The few cases that have been reported involve primarily non-athletic women who developed osteitis pubis as a result of gynecological or obstetric causes.[18]

MUSCLE, TENDON AND LIGAMENT INJURIES

Sacroiliac sprains

Box 29.6: Key Points

- Sacroiliac sprains are characterized by pain over the sacroiliac joint, and occasionally down the lower back, groin and thigh. These sprains occur when the strength and integrity of the anterior/posterior sacroiliac, interosseous, and sacrotuberous ligaments are overcome by sudden and forceful movements such has hamstring contractions and trauma to the buttock. Symptoms can resolve effectively with conservative treatments such as bedrest, heat therapy, and oral anti-inflammatory drugs. However, corticosteroid and anesthetic injections are not recommended.

Lower back pain is a common disorder and the list of differential causes is extensive. As a result, sacroiliac sprain, due to its relative infrequency, is often overlooked.[23]

The sacroiliac joint is a complex, yet generally strong and resilient, synovial joint whose function involves the transmission of forces from the spine to the lower limbs.[23,24] Inter-individual anatomical variations are noted by Dijkstra and colleagues in terms of both sacroiliac joint surface configurations and orientation.[24] Its strength is the result of extensive ligamentous reinforcement from the anterior and posterior sacroiliac ligaments, the interosseous and sacrotuberous ligaments.[23,24]

Sacroiliac strains occur when the strength and integrity of these ligaments are overcome and this typically results from sudden and forceful movements including hamstring or abdominal muscle contraction, standing from a crouched position, or direct trauma to the buttock.[2,24] Progression of symptoms is often insidious, and according to Leblanc *et al.*, patients may have symptoms for up to seven months before seeking medical advice.[23] Thus, the link to a preceding traumatic event is often lost.[23]

Presentation typically involves pain over the sacroiliac joint with occasional referral of pain to the lower back, groin and thigh. While highly suggestive, localized tenderness over the sacroiliac joint alone is not sufficient to make the diagnosis of

sacroiliac sprain.[23] Positive findings on a few specific tests including Patrick's test, also known as Faber test, sacroiliac compression test, Gaenslen's extension test and iliac compression test provide greater diagnostic certainty.[2,23]

While radiological imaging is unhelpful in diagnosing sacroiliac sprains, it can be useful in excluding other differential causes of pain including ankylosing spondylitis, infection, fractures and malignancy.[23]

Conservative management including bedrest, application of heat, supportive bandaging, and oral anti-inflammatory medications, are generally effective in relieving acute symptoms. Typically the duration of bedrest required is brief. However, as complete healing takes 4–6 weeks, a graduated physiotherapy regime may need to replace full sports participation.[2] The use of intra-joint corticosteroid and local anesthetic injections are generally restricted to the rare cases that are refractory to conservative management.[2,23]

Adductor strains

Box 29.7: Key Points

- Adductor strains are often caused by external rotation of an abducted leg. Common clinical presentations are localized tenderness and swelling over the pubic rami, biomechanical abnormalities, and gait abnormalities. These strains should be managed with rest, ice, and compression, gradually followed by exercises to increasing range of motion and strength.

Groin pain is a common complaint in the athlete. The differential diagnosis is varied (see Table 29.1). However, adductor strains are the most common cause of groin discomfort among athletes. This is significant as groin injuries account for 2–5% of all sports injuries and up to 7% of all soccer injuries. Adductor strains typically result from forced external rotation of an abducted leg which is characteristic of the kicking motion required in soccer thereby explaining the increased prevalence of adductor strains within this sporting code.[2,25]

The diagnosis of adductor strain is largely based on clinical presentation and examination with localized tenderness and swelling over the pubic rami occurring commonly. The presence of biomechanical abnormalities such as foot and lower leg malalignment, leg length discrepancy, or gait abnormalities should also be noted as these may predispose to adductor injuries.[25]

While complete avulsion of the adductors is uncommon, strain at the musculotendinous junction is common. The gracilis muscle crosses two joints placing it at greatest susceptibility for this type of injury.[2,25] Radiological imaging by means of MRI is useful in distinguishing strains from avulsions.[25]

As with most muscle strains, initial management involves rest, ice and compression in order to minimize bleeding and swelling. This should be followed by a graduated regime

Table 29.1 Causes of Athletic Groin Pain

	Pubic	Non-pubic
Musculotendinous	Adductor tendinopathy	Iliopsoas tendinopathy
	Inguinal canal pathology	Rectus femoris tendinopathy
	Conjoint tendinopathy	Various muscle strains
	Rectus abdominus tendinopathy	
Bone	Osteitis pubis	Pelvic stress fractures
Joint	Pubic instability	Hip joint pathology
		Lumbar spine pathology
		Sacroiliac joint pathology
Nerve entrapment	Ilioinguinal nerve	
	Obturator nerve	
Genitourinary		Prostatitis
		Epididymitis
		Salpingitis

of exercises to improve range of motion and muscle strength. Recurrence is common if patients return to full sports participation before complete resolution of symptoms has occurred.[1]

NERVE ENTRAPMENT SYNDROMES

Obturator nerve entrapment

Box 29.8: Key Points

- Entrapment of the obturator nerve may cause groin pain. The extra-pelvic course within the obturator tunnel places the nerve at great risk of entrapment, especially among athletes involved in sports with repetitive kicking and twisting movements. Clinical examinations are preferred over radiographs for diagnosis. Clinical findings include medial groin pain, adductor muscle weakness and spasm. Conservative treatments are effective in acute cases, while surgical interventions may be required for chronic cases.

Chronic groin pain can be diagnostically challenging due to close proximity of a large number of anatomical structures.[26] It is only recently that entrapment of the obturator nerve has been reported in the literature as a potential cause of medial groin pain among athletes.[27]

Obturator neuropathy is caused by entrapment of the obturator nerve and this can occur at several points along its course.[2,26] The obturator nerve originates from the 2nd to 4th ventral rami of the lumbar plexus and leaves the pelvis within the obturator canal. Upon exiting the canal, it then divides into two parts with the anterior division providing motor innervation to adductor longus, adductor brevis and gracilis as well as sensory innervation to the skin of the distal two thirds of the medial thigh. The posterior division provides motor innervation to obturator externus, adductor brevis and the proximal aspect of adductor magnus.[2]

Within the pelvis, the obturator nerve is at risk of mechanical compression secondary to pelvic masses, trauma or even as a result of pregnancy.[26] While largely protected from trauma, it is the extra-pelvic course within the obturator tunnel that places the obturator nerve at greatest risk of entrapment, especially among athletes.[26,27] Cadaveric studies conducted by Harvey et al. demonstrated that localized fascial thickening at the distal end of the obturator canal is a common cause of obturator neuropathy, especially among athletes.[2,27]

Athletes participating in sports involving repetitive kicking and sideways and twisting movements appear to be at greatest susceptibility for developing this form of nerve entrapment.[26] Diagnosis is largely based on history and clinical examination due to the absence of radiological abnormalities, though needle electromyography of the adductor muscles has been shown to reliably detect entrapment in chronic cases.[2,26] Clinical presentation typically involves exercise induced medial groin pain originating at the level of adductor longus insertion, with radiation distally along the medial aspect of the thigh.[26] Bradshaw et al. likened the pain to that of 'intermittent claudication' due to the exacerbation of symptoms with exercise and resolution with periods of rest.[2,26] Reports of associated sensory changes are rare.[26] The most prominent examination findings include adductor muscle weakness, spasm.[1,28] Pain can be reproduced by passively externally rotating and abducting the affected hip While standing or internally rotating the hip against resistance.[2,26]

While conservative management involving rest, physiotherapy and use of anti-inflammatory medications can be useful in acute cases, surgical intervention is frequently required for chronic, refractory cases.[2] A case series of 32 patients by Bradshaw et al. demonstrated that surgical nerve ablation provided permanent resolution of symptoms, enabling the athletes to return to full sports competition within only a few weeks of the surgery.[2,26]

Lateral femoral cutaneous nerve entrapment (meralgia paresthetica)

Box 29.9: Key Points

- Caused by an entrapment neuropathy of the lateral femoral cutaneous nerve, meralgia paresthetica can cause pain, numbness, and paresthesia around the anterolateral thigh. This can occur at any age and spontaneously as a result of mechanical compression or iatrogenic complications from surgery. Common symptoms include numbness, pain, tingling, and decreased sensitivity to pain, touch, and temperature. Surgical interventions are more effective in less obese patients.

Meralgia paresthetica is a focal mononeuropathic symptom complex that can occur at any age and includes numbness, paresthesia and pain around the anterolateral thigh. It is caused by an entrapment neuropathy or neuroma of the lateral femoral cutaneous nerve (LFCN) and has been well documented in the literature since it was first described by Bernhardt in 1878.[2]

The LFCN is an entirely sensory nerve that supplies the skin of the anterior-lateral thigh down to the level of the knee and originates from different combinations of the first to third lumbar nerve roots.[2,29] Its superficial anatomic course through the inguinal region makes it highly susceptible to damage. Furthermore, variations in its course have been demonstrated in up to one third of individuals as shown by Keegan and Holyoke in 1962, which may explain increased susceptibility to meralgia paresthetica in some individuals.[30]

Meralgia paresthetica can occur spontaneously as a result of mechanical compression, or as an iatrogenic complication of several common orthopedic procedures including iliac crest bone grafting, pelvic osteotomy, appendicectomy and total abdominal hysterectomy.[2,29] Mechanical compression most commonly occurs at the level of the inguinal ligament as this is the most superficial part of the LFCN.[29] An anatomical study conducted by Dias Filho *et al.* demonstrated that the LFCN increased in diameter as it runs within its 'aponeurotic fascial tunnel' from the iliopubic tract to the inguinal ligament, thereby increasing the risk of entrapment.[31] Risk of compression at this point is further increased on standing and in situations or conditions where intra-abdominal pressure is increased such as pregnancy and obesity.[29] External causes such as seat belts and tight trousers which cause nerve entrapment through direct pressure can also be implicated.[29] The cause of meralgia paresthetica in athletes remains unclear, however Kho *et al.* hypothesized that the conduction block was due to local ischemia secondary to repetitive muscle stretching.[32]

Clinical presentation typically involves unilateral numbness, tingling, pain and decreased sensitivity to pain, touch and temperature in the distribution of the LFCN. Symptoms are exacerbated by palpation over the affected area, especially over the lateral inguinal ligament and on hip extension during such activities as walking or rising from a chair. Diagnosis is typically made from the characteristic history and from examination findings such as a positive Tinel sign elicited 1cm medial and inferior to the anterior superior iliac spine (ASIS).[29] In addition, electrophysiological studies or positive response to local anesthetic or steroid injection are also both diagnostic and prognostic.[33]

First-line treatment should always be conservative including minimizing periods of prolonged standing, avoiding tight clothing and use of oral analgesics.[29] While more invasive surgical procedures such as nerve decompression or ablation are viable options with largely positive results, they should be reserved for those cases where conservative management has failed.[34] Evaluation of LFCN decompression by Siu *et al.* demonstrated that 73% (33/45) and 20% (9/45) experienced complete or partial resolution of symptoms, respectively. They also demonstrated a reduced prognostic benefit in obese patients with a body mass index (BMI) >30, who were found to be 6 times more likely to have incomplete relief of symptoms following surgical decompression at long-term follow-up.[35]

Sciatic nerve entrapment

Box 29.10: Key Points

- There is no clear consensus regarding the etiology, diagnosis, and treatment in the literature. However, common clinical findings include pain around the sacroiliac joint, a greater sciatic notch, and the piriformis muscle extending down the leg. Arthroscopic release of the piriformis muscle has been shown to relieve symptoms in cases having failed conservative treatments.

The sciatic nerve is formed from the nerve roots L4–S3 of the lumbosacral plexus and along with the gluteal nerves and vessels passes through the sciatic notch with the piriformis muscle.[36] The intimate relationship between the piriformis muscle and sciatica was first described by Yeoman in 1928 but it was not until 1947 that Robinson coined the term 'piriformis syndrome' to describe this rare entrapment neuropathy and defined its cardinal features.[36,37] It is now thought that piriformis syndrome is responsible for up to 6% of all lower back pain and sciatica cases that present to general practitioners.[38,39]

The etiology of this syndrome remains unclear and at present, there is no consensus in the literature regarding diagnosis or treatment. A number of hypotheses exist to explain the cause of this rare condition, the most likely of which involves trauma to the piriformis muscle resulting in spasm, edema and contracture of the piriformis muscle causing subsequent compression of the sciatic nerve.[33,37,39]

The cardinal features as described by Robinson over 50 years ago remain valid and continue to form the basis for clinical diagnosis.[36] They include pain around the sacroiliac joint, greater sciatic notch and piriformis muscle extending down the leg, acute exacerbation of pain on hip flexion, adduction and internal rotation, a palpable, tender mass overlying the piriformis muscle, a positive Laségue sign and possible gluteal atrophy.[36,37] Also of note is the presence of 'Morton's foot' which is characterized by a prominent head of the 2nd metatarsal bone. It has been postulated that this anatomic variant may cause piriformis syndrome through promoting instability during the push-off stage of the gait cycle and a subsequent reactive contracture of the hip external rotators.[36]

Due to its infrequent presentation and lack of well-defined clinical symptoms or definitive diagnostic tests, diagnosis is often delayed or missed completely.[38] Prior to the advent of the MRI, diagnosis was largely clinical.[36,37] The role of imaging techniques such as MRI assists in diagnosis of chronic cases through the identification of atrophy and fibrous tissue replacement of the piriformis muscle but is also crucial in excluding other potential causes of sciatic pain including herniated nucleus pulposus, pelvic tumors or abscesses.[36,38]

Conservative management is generally employed initially. This includes non-steroidal anti-inflammatory drugs, injection of local anesthetic and corticosteroids combined with physiotherapy. Where non-operative management is unsuccessful, surgical release of the piriformis muscle may be necessary.[38] Dezawa *et al.* describes a new technique involving arthroscopic release of the piriformis muscle under local anesthetic. Patients were noted to gain immediate relief of symptoms and due to the minimally invasive nature of the technique were able to rapidly return to normal activity.[40]

FRACTURES

Avulsion fractures

Box 29.11: Key Points

- The incidence of avulsion fractures about the hip is increasing in children. The inherent weakness of open growth plates predisposes skeletally immature athletes to avulsion fractures resulting from sudden and unbalanced muscle contractions. Three most common sites for avulsion fractures are the anterior superior iliac spine, the anterior inferior iliac spine, and the ischial tuberosity. Clinical findings include localized pain and swelling exacerbated by passive stretching. Displaced fragments smaller than 2 cm can generally be treated conservatively.

Avulsion injuries are common among skeletally immature athletes due to the inherent weakness across the open apophysis.[1,2,41] The incidence of avulsion fractures is increasing, especially among 14–17 year olds, as a result of the growth in competitive sports participation.[2,41]

Avulsion fractures result from indirect trauma due to sudden, violent or unbalanced muscle contraction and are most commonly associated with sports such as soccer, rugby, ice hockey, gymnastics and sprinting, involving kicking, rapid acceleration and deceleration and jumping.[1,2,25] While in adults, this mechanism of injury typically causes a muscle or tendon strain, in skeletally immature athletes, the consequences are more serious due to the inherent biomechanical weakness and subsequent separation of the apophyseal region.[2] Rossi and Dragoni postulated that intensive training exposes the epiphyseal plate to repetitive tensile stress while simultaneously enhancing muscle contractility and power.[25] Clinical observations suggest that these avulsions usually occur in constitutionally 'tight' or less flexible children. This inherent weakness at the epiphyseal plate combined with the increased functional demands placed on the musculature, predisposes the subsequent avulsion injury.[25] Once the injury has occurred, the degree of bony displacement is restricted by the periosteum and surrounding fascia.[1]

While avulsion fractures can occur at any major muscle attachment, the three most common sites of avulsion injuries include the ASIS (Fig. 29.5), the anterior inferior iliac spine (AIIS) and the ischial tuberosity (Fig. 29.6) due to violent contraction of the sartorius, rectus femoris and hamstring muscles, respectively.[1,42] In addition avulsion fractures of the lesser trochanter can also occur (Fig. 29.7).

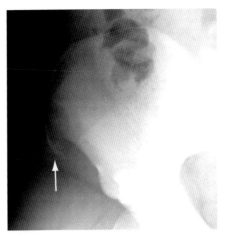

Figure 29.5 Anterior superior iliac spine (ASIS) avulsion fracture in an adolescent athlete.

Clinical presentation typically follows a traumatic incident or strenuous exercise and is characterized by acute onset of localized pain and swelling that is exacerbated on palpation and by passive stretching of the involved muscle.[1,2] Patients will characteristically assume a position that places least amount of tension on the involved muscle.[2] While clinical presentation is often diagnostic, radiological imaging is useful in determining the size of the avulsed fragment and degree of bony displacement.[1,41]

Controversy exists regarding the optimal management of avulsion fractures, particularly those involving the ischial tuberosity.[1,42] Typically, initial management will be conservative including rest, ice followed by protected weight-bearing with crutches until symptoms resolve.[1] Thereafter, progression to light isometric stretching and full weight bearing is indicated and return to full sports participation can occur once full

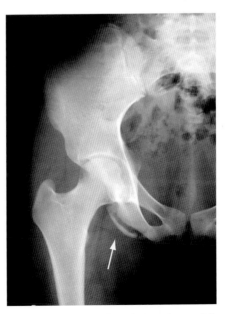

Figure 29.6 Ischial tuberosity avulsion fracture in an adolescent athlete.

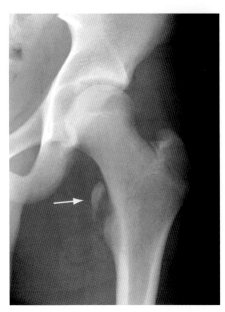

Figure 29.7 Lesser trochanteric avulsion fracture in an adolescent athlete.

strength and a pain-free range of motion is achieved.[1,41] The need for surgical intervention is rare and is based on ongoing symptoms typically and the degree of bony displacement. As a general rule, large displaced fragments greater than 2 cm are likely to require surgical fixation, however the optimal timing of surgical intervention remains unclear.[1,2,42]

Stress fractures

Box 29.12: Key Points

- Repetitive forces on bone before it can repair and remodel itself lead to stress fracture. Fatigue fractures are most common in athletes, while insufficiency fractures are common among females with hormone deficiencies.

Stress fractures involving the hip and pelvis are a well recognized but relatively rare condition affecting athletes.[43] They can be classified into two subtypes depending on the pathoetiology, fatigue and insufficiency. Fatigue fractures are the most common among athletes, particularly those participating in endurance-type sports as they are exposed to repetitive trauma which places abnormal stresses on normal bone.[43,44] Insufficiency fractures while uncommon among athletes, have been reported in females with hormonal or nutritional deficiencies, particularly long-distance runners.[43]

Repetitive loading of bone as opposed to a single traumatic event, to explain the physiological basis for stress fractures was first proposed by Detlefsen in 1937.[44] While this still remains a valid explanation, the exact etiology of stress fractures remains uncertain. The transference of excessive or abnormal forces from contracting or fatigued muscles has also been postulated.[2,44]

The reparative capacity of bone is enormous, however when exposed to repetitive forces, bone undergoes a period of temporary weakening, which manifests as a stress fracture, before its structure is reorganized and reinforced.[43,44] Knapp and Garrett explain the process of bone remodeling following periods of stress. They describe an elastic response known as the 'piezoelectric phenomenon' during periods of rest, which attempts to prevent permanent damage by the removal of surrounding lamellar bone by osteoclasts and the laying down of immature periosteal and endosteal bone by osteoblasts. Eventually, dense lamellar bone is laid down that is able to withstand the increased compressive forces it is exposed to.[45] Awareness of this process has important implications for both prevention and treatment of over-use type stress injuries.[43–45] Miller *et al.* recommend cyclical training programs as they produce the desired results without exposing single bones to excessive and repetitive stress. Moreover, rest must be a central part of every training and rehabilitation program.[43]

Pelvic stress fractures

Stress fractures involving the pubic rami represent a small 1.25% of all pelvic fractures and are most commonly seen among long-distance runners. A slightly higher incidence among females has been attributed to differences in gait.[2]

Clinical presentation typically involves pain localized to the inguinal, peroneal or adductor region which is exacerbated by exercise and relieved with rest.[2] Examination reveals an antalgic gait, exquisite tenderness to deep palpation over the pubic ramus, but a normal range of hip motion.[2,46] In addition, Noakes and his colleagues noted the presence of severe groin pain when standing unsupported on the leg corresponding to the affected side of the pelvis. The so-called 'positive standing sign' has been shown to be diagnostically useful in the absence of radiological changes.[46]

Radiological imaging by way of radionuclide bone scan can be useful in diagnosing pelvic stress fractures however, as with plain radiographs, there may be no detectable abnormalities in the first few weeks of the disease process.[43,46] The persistence of symptoms even in the absence of radiological findings always warrants further investigation and for athletes who are keen to return to competition as soon as possible, an MRI is often required to make a definitive diagnosis (Fig. 29.8). MRI can identify stress responses such as edema within the bone marrow even before a stress fracture is apparent.[43]

While the literature reports positive results from conservative management of pelvic stress fractures in the majority of cases, the optimal period of rest remains controversial. Miller *et al.* advocates use of a graduated rehabilitation program that involves three phases of gradually increasing impact and intensity taking between 3–18 weeks, whereas Nuccion and his colleagues recommend 3–5 months of complete rest from full sports participation.[2,43]

Femoral neck stress fractures

Femoral neck stress fractures are very uncommon among the adult athletic population, accounting for only 1% of all stress fractures.[47,48]

While most femoral neck stress fractures are nondisplaced at the time of presentation, the typically non-specific presenta-

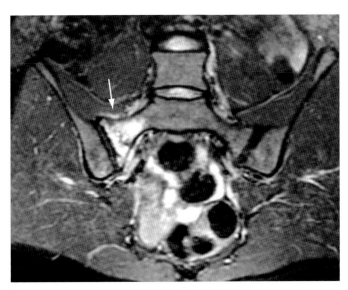

Figure 29.8 MRI identifying sacral stress fracture.

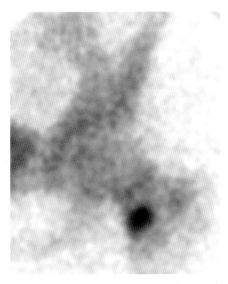

Figure 29.9 Bone scan identifying a femoral neck stress fracture.

tion and examination findings combined with an extensive list of differentials, leads to a delay in diagnosis that averages 14 weeks according to Johansson *et al.*[48,49] Progression to a displaced fracture is associated with a number of complications including avascular necrosis, non-union and varus deformity, resulting in a poor prognostic outcome.[2] Thus, a high level of clinical suspicion is required for early diagnosis, when an athlete presents with insidious groin pain, anterior thigh or knee pain that is exacerbated by exercise or weight-bearing and causes severe pain with restricted extremes of hip movement, particularly internal rotation.[2,48]

Femoral neck stress fractures that are clinically suspected but not radiologically confirmed should be treated with a period of rest and non-weight bearing for at least 7 days or until

definitive radiological changes become evident.[2] While plain radiographs are frequently normal in the first 1–2 weeks, both bone scintography and MRI (Figs 29.9, 29.10) are diagnostically very sensitive early in the course of the disease.[2]

Management is dependent on the type of fracture pattern with presence of displacement being the primary indication for surgical intervention.[2] A large number of classification systems have been reported in the literature, including Devas biomechanical classification of transverse and compression femoral neck stress fractures, which was later modified to distraction and compression fractures. Blickenstaff and Morris based their classification on the degree of displacement. Fullerton and Snowdy combined both biomechanical factors and the degree of displacement.[50–52]

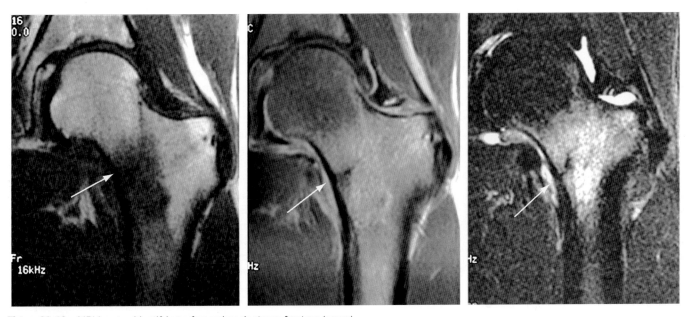

Figure 29.10 MRI images identifying a femoral neck stress fracture (arrow).

Essentially, nondisplaced fractures on the compression (medial) side are treated conservatively with rest and non-weightbearing until the patient is asymptomatic and radiographic evidence of healing is apparent. For the rare cases that don't respond to conservative management, internal fixation is warranted. In comparison, fractures on the tension side, even in the absence of displacement require urgent surgical intervention by means of internal fixation due to the high risk of subsequent displacement and poor prognosis. Fractures that have already displaced require reduction and internal fixation with a prolonged postoperative period of non- and partial weightbearing.[2]

Growth plate injuries

Box 29.13: Key Points

- SCFE is the most common hip disorder among adolescents. Many patients present with knee or thigh pain in lieu of hip pain. Stable slips allow weight-bearing while unstable hips are unable to weight bear. Delay in diagnosis can lead to further slippage. Slips are typically treated with single screw in situ fixation. Studies have shown a relationship between severity of the slip and osteonecrosis. Slippage of the contralateral hip occurs in 30-40% of the cases.

Slipped capital femoral epiphysis

Slipped capital femoral epiphysis (SCFE), as the name suggests, involves the posterior slippage of the proximal femoral epiphysis due to mechanical shearing forces, with concomitant extension and external rotation of the femoral neck and shaft (Fig. 29.11).[41] It is regarded as the most common hip disorder of adolescence, with a increased prevalence among males with peak onset around 11 years of age.[41] Increased BMI is a significant risk factor for the development of slipped capital femoral epiphysis, with both biomechanical and endocrinological factors being implicated.[53,54]

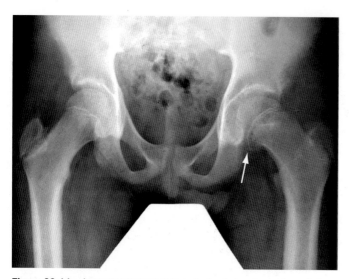

Figure 29.11 Anteroposterior pelvis radiograph demonstrating a left mild stable slipped capital femoral epiphysis.

Classification of slipped capital femoral epiphysis has traditionally been based on acuity of symptoms, and severity of the slip, however a greater emphasis is now being placed on mechanical stability due to its greater prognostic value.[41] A mechanically stable slip will allow weight-bearing whereas a patient with an unstable SCFE typically represents an acute physeal fracture, with concomitant microscopic instability resulting in pain and an inability to weight-bear.[41]

Accurate, early diagnosis of SCFE is important in preventing both short-term complications including chondrolysis and avascular necrosis of the femoral head and longer term problems such as hip dysfunction and osteoarthritis. The insidious and often ambiguous onset of symptoms, combined with the absence of radiological changes early in the condition, are common causes of delayed diagnosis.[55] Symptoms associated with a stable slip typically involve a dull ache that is exacerbated by exercise, but can be localized anywhere from the groin to the medial aspect of the knee.[41] The delayed onset of significant pain and dysfunction may allow for the progression from a stable to unstable slip, with major implications for long-term prognosis. Of interest, a retrospective study conducted by Kocher *et al.* also found that Medicaid (government-insured) patients experienced greater delays in diagnosis than those with private insurance. The same observation has been noted for a range of other conditions.[55]

Management of SCFE is fraught with challenges, especially for severe slips due to significant deformity of the femoral head and inherent risk of iatrogenic avascular necrosis and subsequent osteoarthritis.[53,56] A number of potential risks factors of avascular necrosis have been reported in the literature including the use of multiple pins, pin position and penetration, complete or partial reduction and the stability and severity of slip.[56-60] Unfortunately, at present there is a paucity in the literature regarding the optimal management of acute, unstable SCFE. A recent survey of Pediatric Orthopaedic Society of North America (POSNA) members found that 57% reported using a single threaded screw for fixation for unstable SCFE whereas 40.3% recommended three threaded screws.[61]

A retrospective study by Tokmakova *et al.* in 2003 confirmed a clear relationship between the stability and severity of the slip and subsequent post-operative risk of osteonecrosis.[56] Patients with stable lesions showed no increase in risk of osteonecrosis whereas those with unstable lesions demonstrated an increased level of risk that was proportional to the grade or severity of the slip.[56] Furthermore, Tokmakova's results indicated that *in situ* pinning without reduction using a single cannulated screw was associated with the lowest risk of iatrogenic osteonecrosis of the femoral head, irrespective of stability or severity of slip.[56]

Bilateral SCFEs have been reported to occur in 20–50% of cases, though simultaneous presentation is unusual. Despite this high incidence, the optimal management of the contralateral hip when presented with a unilateral SCFE remains controversial. The primary author advocates shared decision making which includes both the physician and patient in decision making, and takes into account outcome probabilities and patient preferences.[62]

Pathologic fractures and conditions

Box 29.14: Key Points

- Perthes disease is an idiopathic condition involving avascular necrosis of the femoral head. It affects males more often than females. Prognosis is significantly better the younger the age of child at onset. One of the most important prognostic indicators is the height of the lateral pillar. The Herring system for radiological classifications was found to be more accurate and reliable than the Catterall system. Severe forms of the disease have seen better outcome results with surgical intervention than conservative treatment.

Legg–Calvé–Perthes disease

Legg–Calvé–Perthes disease, also known as Perthes disease, is an idiopathic, self-limiting condition involving avascular necrosis of the femoral head (Fig. 29.12).[52,56] It typically presents in the 1st decade of life and for unknown reasons predominates among males aged 4–8 years, with a gender ratio of 5:1.[63] In the past 95 years, since it was first described by Legg, Calvé and Perthes, we have gained little insight into the etiology and pathophysiology of this complex condition.[41,63,64]

Pathogenesis appears complex and involves avascular necrosis, followed by resorption, collapse and subsequent repair of the capital femoral epiphysis resulting in impaired growth and development of the hip joint.[64] The natural history of the disease is variable but is largely dependent on the age of onset and the degree of femoral head involvement but is also greatly influenced by intervention.[41,63] The younger a child is at the onset of the disease, the greater the time they have for subsequent growth and remodeling.[63] Moreover, McAndrew *et al.* demonstrated that in the long term, 50% of those with childhood Perthes disease who did not receive treatment developed subsequent osteoarthritis in their 5th decade of life.[65]

Femoral head biopsies from patients with the disease have demonstrated lesions with varying degrees of necrosis and

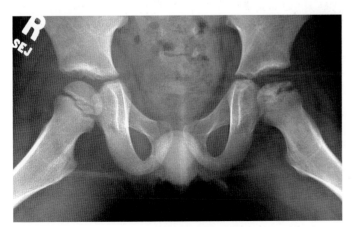

Figure 29.12 Frog pelvis radiograph demonstrating left hip Perthes disease.

repair indicating that repetitive injury to the circumflex arteries rather than a single traumatic event may be responsible for the pathological findings in Perthes disease.[64] Several hypotheses have been formulated to explain this hypovascularity. A recent study by Balasa *et al.* demonstrated that two thrombophilic risk factors: factor-V Leiden mutation and anticardiolipin antibodies which enhance intravascular clotting and increase blood viscosity are significantly associated with the disease.[64,66] Also postulated is intermittent increases in intracapsular hip pressure causing a tamponade effect and subsequent compression of the retinacular vessels as it courses through the restricted intracapsular space.[64] Unfortunately, the literature remains conflicting and there is a lack of evidence to support either of these hypotheses at present.[64]

Perthes disease is specific to the hip joint and typically presents as an insidious, unilateral painless limp.[41,63,64] If pain is present, it is usually mild, exacerbated by exercise and frequently referred to the knee. The most consistent examination findings and in fact one of the most important prognostic indicators include reduced internal rotation and abduction of the hip.[41,64] In the early stages of the disease this is attributable to muscle spasm and synovitis whereas later on in the disease, bony impingement of the femoral head on the acetabulum results in restricted hip motion.[2] The prevalence of bilateral cases reported in the literature range from 8–24% and is interestingly more common in girls.[63] A study by Guille *et al.*[1] demonstrated that the development and outcome of the disease in each hip appears to be an independent event with endocrinological etiologies such as hypoparathyroidism or skeletal dysplasias playing a role.[67]

A large number of radiological classification systems have been developed which attempt to stratify patients according to the severity of their disease, predict prognosis and provide parameters for instituting treatment.[64] The two most commonly used classification systems include the Catterall Classification which defines four groups based on the involvement of the epiphysis (25%, 50%, 75%, 100% involvement) and the Herring Classification which defines three groups according to the degree of collapse in the lateral epiphyseal pillar during the fragmentation stage.[41,64] In a comparative study by Ritterbusch *et al.*, the Herring classification system was found to be a more accurate predictor of long term outcome with greater inter-observer reliability.[68]

The treatment of Perthes disease remains highly controversial with regards to conservative versus surgical intervention.[64] The primary goals of intervention include maintenance of hip motion, pain relief and containment.[64] At present there is a lack of conclusive data in the literature regarding the indications for, and the benefits of specific treatment modalities and as a result surgical intervention largely reflects the physician's personal preference. A study conducted by Kamegaya *et al.* compared surgical versus conservative treatment and found that for patients with severe disease, surgical intervention was preferable as it improved the sphericity of the femoral head and provided greater acetabular cover.[69] The two most common surgical methods for containment include the femoral varus osteotomy and the Salter innominate osteotomy. In a comparative study by Kitakoji *et al.*, 46 patients were treated by femoral osteotomy and 30 by Salter innominate osteotomy. The clinical outcome for the two groups were similar in terms of sphericity of the femoral head, congruity of the hip and leg length discrepancy; however the acetabular coverage of the femoral head, the neck-shaft angle and the articular-trochanteric distance were closer to normal in the Salter innominate osteotomy group. The latter group were also found to have reduced scarring.[70]

Herring *et al.* who devised the Herring Lateral Pillar Classification System, conducted one of the largest studies on the topic to date and concluded that patients over the age of 8 years at the time of onset that have a Herring classification of B or B/C border have a better outcome with surgical treatment (femoral osteotomy or innominate osteotomy) than they do with non-operative treatment (brace treatment or range of motion exercises). Children that fit into group B and were <8 years old at the time of onset were shown to have favorable outcomes irrespective of treatment whereas group C children of all ages frequently had poor outcomes regardless of treatment modality.[71]

INTRAARTICULAR DERANGEMENTS

Hip dislocations

Box 29.15: Key Points

- Hip dislocations are rare due to the stability of the joint. Posterior dislocations are more common. The most common complication is avascular necrosis. The risk of this and other complications from hip dislocation can be lowered with emergent reduction. Patients can return to full activity within 3 months of reduction.

Dislocation of the hip is rare due to the inherent stability of the joint.[2,72] It is generally associated with high velocity sports such as football and rugby with the mechanism of injury involving transmission of extreme force through the long axis of the femur.[41,72]

Hip dislocations are classified according to the direction of displacement and the severity of injury. Posterior dislocations are considerably more common, accounting for up to 85% of all hip dislocations.[41,72] Clinical distinction between the two types can be largely determined by the position of the affected hip. Posterior dislocations typically present with the hip flexed, adducted and internally rotated whereas in anterior dislocations, the hip is externally rotated and abducted.[2,41]

Hip dislocations should be considered a surgical emergency due to the risk of long-term neurovascular compromise.[1,41] While early reduction has been demonstrated to significantly reduce the risk of subsequent avascular necrosis and sciatic neuropathy, pre-reduction imaging is recommended not only to define the type of dislocation but also to exclude associated injuries such as femoral neck or acetabular fractures, as it may influence management options.[1,72] In addition, a pre-reduction neurological examination is advisable to exclude sciatic nerve compromise.[1]

Nuccion describes the three basic techniques of closed reduction including the Bigelow, Allis and Stimson techniques.[2]

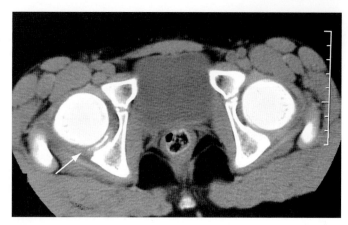

Figure 29.13 CT scan demonstrating an intraarticular loose body after right hip dislocation.

While all three methods attempt to maximize muscle relaxation around the hip joint, intravenous sedation or general anesthetic are typically required to provide sufficient relaxation for the closed reduction to be successful.[2,41] Post-reduction radiographs are recommended to ensure concentric reduction has been achieved.[41] Occasionally closed reduction is not possible and surgical intervention is indicated. Where osteochondral fragments (Fig. 29.13) or other intra-articular mechanical obstructions are preventing reduction, arthroscopic removal of the obstruction or open reduction may be necessary (Fig. 29.14).[1]

Following successful reduction, the stability of the hip should be assessed followed by 48 h of bed rest. This is followed by a 2-week period of protected weightbearing and then by a graduated strengthening program. In cases of primary dislocation where no other injuries were sustained, patients can expect to return to full activity within 3 months.[1,2,41]

The most common complication of hip dislocation is avascular necrosis of the femoral head which occurs in up to 20% of cases.[41] It is therefore recommended that a follow-up MRI is performed 3 months following the injury to exclude this.[1,41]

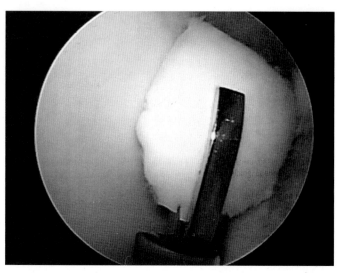

Figure 29.14 Arthroscopic removal of a loose body associated with a traumatic hip dislocation.

Acetabular labral tears

Box 29.16: Key Points

- Acetabular labral tears commonly occur anteriorly and among athletes. A clicking sensation of the hip and the internal-rotation-flexion-axial compression test are very sensitive for predicting labral tears. Most require surgical intervention. Arthroscopic debridement offers a safe and minimally invasive way to treat hip labral tears.

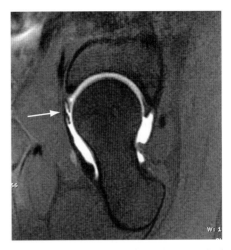

Figure 29.15 MR arthrogram demonstrating anterior labral tear.

The acetabular labrum is a thin fibrocartilaginous rim surrounding the acetabulum and acts to deepen the acetabulum and enhance articular congruency. Conflicting evidence exists regarding the biomechanical role of the acetabular labrum. While a study by Konrath et al.[73] demonstrated that the labrum does not play a fundamental role in load transmission through the hip, a more recent study by Peterson et al.[74] found that excision or removal of the labrum following trauma could adversely affect joint stability and load distribution. During the same study, Petersen also assessed the vascularity of the labrum demonstrating that only the peripheral third of the labrum receives a vascular supply from the adjacent joint capsule leaving the internal two thirds avascular. Consequently, tears occurring at watershed zones can cause destabilization of the adjacent acetabular cartilage and if left untreated have been demonstrated with the use of MRA to eventually progress to osteoarthritis.[75–77]

Acetabular labrum tears are common among athletes and typically occur anteriorly. In a review on the topic, Hickman and Peters attribute more than 60% of all labral tears to a traumatic event or acetabular dysplasias such as developmental dysplasia, Legg–Calvé–Perthes disease, neuropathic subluxation of the hip or previous episodes of septic arthritis.[77] The mechanism of injury generally involves repetitive twisting or pivoting movements resulting in hyperextension, hyperflexion or extremes of abduction.[78] Presentation classically involves acute onset unilateral hip pain or alternatively insidious hip pain that escalates over time. Associated mechanical symptoms are present in almost all cases.[2,78] A study conducted by Narvani et al. demonstrated that a clicking sensation of the hip was 100% sensitive and 85% specific for predicting labral tears.[79] Furthermore, the internal-rotation-flexion-axial compression test was 75% sensitive and 43% specific.[73] The Thomas' test was neither sensitive nor specific.[79]

Accurate diagnosis and treatment of acetabular labral tears is important not only to provide relief from pain but also in the prevention of subsequent osteoarthritis. With the advent of MR arthrography (Fig. 29.15) and the increasing popularity of hip arthroscopy (Fig. 29.16), this diagnostic and therapeutic challenge has been reduced significantly.[77]

First-line management typically involves non-operative interventions such as the use of nonsteroidal anti-inflammatory

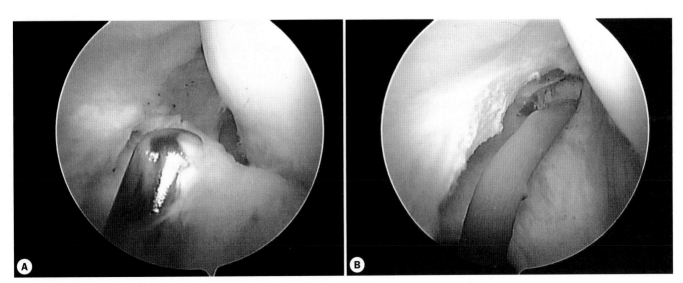

Figure 29.16 (A,B) Arthroscopic debridement of an anterior labral tear.

drugs and partial weightbearing, however surgical intervention is ultimately required in the majority of cases due to continued pain and mechanical symptoms.[77]

While the success of open arthrotomy and labral debridement is well documented in the literature, the use of arthroscopic labral debridement is increasing in popularity as it provides a relatively safe and minimally invasive treatment alternative to open arthrotomy when conservative management fails.[77] Three independent studies by Farjo et al.,[80] Hase et al.[81] and Lage et al.[82] have demonstrated that careful debridement of the torn labrum back to a stable base, while preserving the capsular labral tissue, effectively relieves pain and eliminates mechanical symptoms in those patients with no associated degenerative hip changes. Unfortunately, in patients where dysplastic or degenerative changes of the hip have been documented pre-operatively, there was no improvement in symptoms or hip function observed.[80–82] This is significant as in a study conducted by Wenger et al. of 31 patients with acetabular labral tears, 87% (27/31) had at least one structural hip abnormality on conventional radiograph and 35% had more than one abnormality. Thus, not only does pre-existing degenerative or dysplastic hip disease predispose to acetabular labral tears but it also has a major impact on treatment outcome and long-term prognosis.[83]

Hip osteoarthritis

Box 29.17: Key Points

- Although generally attributed to the elderly, premature osteoarthritis has been noted in athletes due to the repetitive and strenuous loading of the hip. Power sport athletes have been found to be predisposed to premature osteoarthritis of the hip, while endurance sport athletes were not.

Osteoarthritis is a common, degenerative disease of the weightbearing joints that primarily afflicts the elderly population and is generally attributed to a lifetime of wear and tear.[84] The development of premature osteoarthritis among a small number of athletes has highlighted the possible role of repetitive and strenuous loading of the hip joint in the early onset of the disease.[1,84,85]

It is well acknowledged that regular exercise and participation in sports improves cardiovascular health and general well-being leading to a longer lifespan.[84,85] Thus, healthy lifestyle alone may provide greater opportunity for joint wear and tear, increasing the subsequent risk of osteoarthritis.[84]

Several studies have highlighted the possible link between involvement in high level sport, particularly soccer, and an increased risk of osteoarthritis of the hip.[84,86–88] A study by Kujala et al. demonstrated a strong positive correlation between participation in mixed or power type sports and the subsequent development of premature hip osteoarthritis.[84] Interestingly however, endurance athletes such as long distance runners, while at increased risk of developing hip osteoarthritis in old age, were not predisposed to premature osteoarthritis.[84,85]

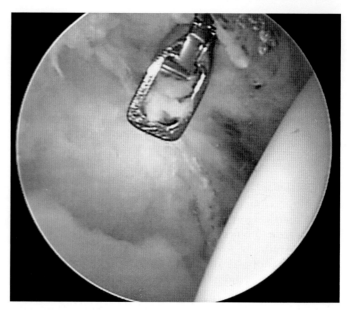

Figure 29.17 Arthroscopic debridement of an anterior acetabular chondral defect.

Hypertrophic rather than destructive osteoarthritic changes are common radiological findings among runners with osteoarthritis. These changes represent an adaptive response to trabecular microfractures that result from repetitive mechanical overload.[85]

It is not uncommon for there to be a poor correlation between radiological changes and symptoms of osteoarthritis.[85] Many of those athletes with mild osteoarthritis can be managed conservatively including oral anti-inflammatory medication and the use of supplements such as glucosamine and chondroitin sulphate.[1] The use of minimally invasive surgical technique such as arthroscopic debridement are also increasing in popularity (Fig. 29.17), leaving only those with severe debilitating symptoms to undergo hip joint replacements.[1]

HIP ARTHROSCOPY

Box 29.18: Key Points

- Hip arthroscopy is safe, minimally invasive, and enables rapid return to sports by patients.
- Hip arthroscopy can be useful and effective in treating many pediatric orthopedic conditions, such as Perthes disease, labral tears and inflammatory arthritis.
- Incidence of iatrogenic complications from hip arthroscopy, such as nerve injury and infection, is low.

The use of hip arthroscopy in the diagnosis and treatment of hip conditions was originally described by Burman in 1931.[89] Over the past 70 years, its popularity has grown and application expanded.[90–94] Today, the most recognized indication for hip arthroscopy is in the management of labral tears

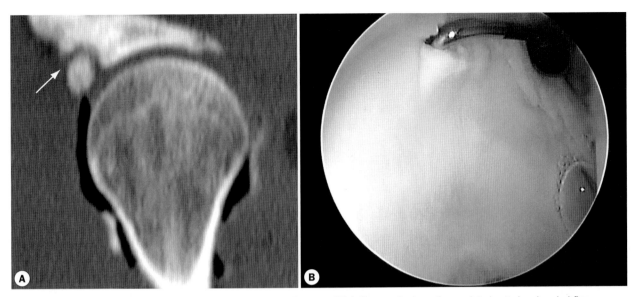

Figure 29.18   (A) CT scan demonstrating an anterior acetabular rim fracture. (B) Arthroscopic view of associated anterior chondral flap.

(Fig. 29.16) and loose bodies (Fig. 29.14). Its potential application is much broader and includes osteoarthritis (Fig. 29.17), osteonecrosis, osteochondral fractures, chondral injury (Fig. 29.18), hip dysplasia, septic arthritis, inflammatory arthritis, synovial chondromatosis, foreign bodies, ligamentum teres tears and complications following total joint arthroplasty.[95–117] While intraarticular hip conditions among athletes are relatively rare the consequences of such injuries prior to the advent of arthroscopy could be serious. Arthroscopy provides a relatively safe and less invasive alternative to traditional open arthrotomy and surgical dislocation enabling diagnosis and treatment of a wide range of intraarticular hip conditions that enables a rapid return to sporting participation.

The large majority of hip arthroscopy performed to date has involved hip disorders in adults, with the indications and outcome of hip arthroscopy in children being less well characterized.[102,107,118–123] Despite this, there exists a large array of pediatric orthopedic conditions that are amenable to and would benefit from arthroscopic intervention. Gross describes his early experience with hip arthroscopy in patients with congenital dislocation of the hip, Legg–Perthes–Calvé disease, slipped capital femoral epiphysis and neuropathic subluxation.[120] Bowen *et al.* described arthroscopic chondroplasty of unstable osteochondral lesions of the femoral head as sequelae in patients after skeletal maturity who had Legg–Perthes–Calvé disease as children.[102,121]

In a review of 24 hip arthroscopies performed in 21 patients aged 11–21 years old, Schindler *et al.* concluded that hip arthroscopy was effective for synovial biopsy and loose body removal. Schindler noted however, that as a diagnostic procedure, hip arthroscopy failed to identify the cause of symptoms in 46% of subjects.[122]

Isolated labral tears in the absence of hip dysplasia or acute traumatic dislocation is a well documented cause of hip pain and are typically anterior.[95–100] Pediatric and adolescent athletes subjected to repetitive flexion, flexion-abduction or extension-external rotation type activities such as dancers,

gymnasts and skaters appear to be at greatest risk of anterior labral tears. These patients typically present with groin pain and mechanical type symptoms with pain on hip flexion and adduction. MRI of the symptomatic hip with intra-articular contrast confirms the diagnosis.[124,125] Arthroscopic debridement has been shown to relieve symptoms and improve function.[95–100] In a study conducted by Byrd and Jones, a mean improvement in the modified Harris hip score was demonstrated among the 23 patients who underwent arthroscopic labral debridement after a minimum of 2 years follow-up.[96]

Developmental dysplasia of the hip is a common cause of intraarticular pathology in the pediatric population.[41,105] It typically presents in adolescence or young adulthood as hip pain secondary to degenerative labral tears or chondral lesions. Anterior labral tears may also result from anterior impingement from a slipped capital femoral epiphysis deformity or pistol-grip deformity.[123] Although favorable results have been reported following the arthroscopic management of intra-articular pathology resulting from developmental dysplasia of the hip, it is the view of the primary author that it is preferable to address the underlying dysplasia with a periacetabular osteotomy with or without proximal femoral osteotomy.[41,105] Following periacetabular osteotomy, patients may present with increasing hip pain and mechanical symptoms due to a degenerative labral tear. In a review conducted by the primary author of eight patients, an improvement in symptoms was demonstrated in six patients following arthroscopic debridement. The remaining two patients who had full-thickness degenerative joint disease did not improve after arthroscopic debridement leading to questions surrounding the efficacy of this approach in patients with advanced degenerative joint disease.

Loose bodies of the hip may result from traumatic injury or as a sequelae of hip disorders such as Legg–Perthes–Calvé disease, spondyloepiphyseal dysplasia, chondrocalcinosis or avascular necrosis. In patients with Legg–Perthes–Calvé disease, an unstable osteochondral fragment in the central portion of the femoral head may persist after the healing phase, particularly in patients with a flattened, aspherical head. Patients may present with pain and mechanical symptoms such as catching or locking and the loose osteochondral lesions may be visible on radiographs, CT scan or MRI. Results from the study performed by Kocher et al. indicates that arthroscopic excision provides positive results with minimal morbidity.[96,101] Patients included in this series had loose bodies associated with Legg–Perthes–Calvé disease, spondyloepiphyseal dysplasia and traumatic osteochondral fracture. Excision of these loose bodies typically resulted in a resolution of pain and mechanical symptoms during the follow-up period. The longer-term prognosis for these patients however is not as clear due to the significant asphericity of the femoral head.[46,105]

In patients with inflammatory arthritis, the literature indicates that arthroscopic synovectomy of the hip may be beneficial in terms of reducing pain and improving function.[107] Kocher et al. reported a series of three patients with inflammatory arthritis who underwent arthroscopic synovectomy for symptomatic relief due to failure of medical therapy and all three patients demonstrated improvement.[126] Arthroscopic irrigation and debridement in cases of pediatric septic arthritis of the hip have been reported.[104–106] It is the authors' preference for open arthrotomy through a limited anterior approach to the hip allowing for capsulectomy, drilling of the femoral neck to rule out associated osteomyelitis as well as thorough debridement of infected tissue and drain placement.

Reported complications of hip arthroscopy include iatrogenic injury to the articular surfaces, injury to the pudendal, lateral femoral cutaneous, femoral and sciatic nerves in addition to femoral artery injury, intra-pelvis fluid extravasation, skin pressure ulcers from traction, heterotopic ossification, instrument breakage, infection and deep venous thrombosis.[90–94] The literature indicates that the incidence of such complications is low. In the series conducted by Kocher et al. minimal complications were reported, including three cases of pudendal nerve paresthesia which resolved within three months of surgery, one broken guidewire which required arthroscopic retrieval and repeat surgery required in 7% (3/41) of labral tear procedures due to recurrent tears.

REFERENCES

1 Anderson K, Strickland S, Warren R, et al. Hip and groin injuries in athletes. Am J Sports Med 2001; 29:521-533.

2 Nuccion SL, Hunter DM, Finerman GA. Hip and pelvis: Adult. DeLee & Drez's Orthopaedic sports medicine: Principles and practice, Vol. 2. 2nd edn. Philadelphia: Saunders; 2003:1443-1462.

3 Hamida B, Hajri R, Kedadi H, et al. Myositis ossificans circumscripta of the knee improved by alendronate. Jt Bone Spine 2004; 71:114-116.

4 Okayama A, Futami M, Kyo F, et al. Usefulness of ultrasonography for early recurrent myositis ossificans. J Orthop Sci 2003; 8:239-242.

5 Sirvanci M, Ganiyusufoglu AK, Karaman K, et al. Myositis ossificans of psoas muscle: magnetic resonance imaging findings. Acta Radiol 2004; 45:523-525.

6 Ceccarelli F, Morici F, Berti L, et al. Circumscribed myositis ossificans of the iliopsoas muscle. Description of a case followed up after 1-14 years. Chir Organi Mov 2004; 89:151-159.

7 Savarese RP, Kaplan SM, Calligaro KD. Iliopectineal bursitis: an unusual cause of iliofemoral vein compression. J Vasc Surg 1991; 13:725-727.

8 Sayegh F, Potounnis M, Kapetanos G. Greater trochanter bursitis pain syndrome in females with chronic low back pain and sciatica. Acta Orthop Belg 2004; 70:423-428.

9 Zolton DJ, Clancy WG, Keene JS. A new approach to snapping hip and refractory trochanteric bursitis in athletes. Am J Sports Med 1986; :14201-14204.

10 Kim SM, Shin MJ, Ahn JM, et al. Imaging features of ischial bursitis with an emphasis on ultrasonography. Skeletal Radiol 2002; 31:631-636.

11 Cho KH, Lee SM, Lee YH, et al. Non-infectious ischiogluteal bursitis: MRI findings. Korean J Radiol 2004; 5:280-286.

12 Fox JL. The role of arthroscopic bursectomy in the treatment of trochanteric bursitis. Arthroscopy 2002; 18:E34.

13 Schaberg JE, Harper MC, Allen WC. Snapping hip syndrome. Am J Sports Med 1984; 12:361-365.

14 Allen WC, Cope R. Coxa saltans snapping hip revisited. J Am Acad Orthop Surg 1995; 3:303-308.

15 Wunderbaldinger P, Bremer C, Matuszewski L, et al. Efficient radiological assessment of the internal snapping hip syndrome. Eur Radiol 2001; 11:1743-1747.

16 Choi YS, Lee SM, Song BY, et al. Dynamic sonography of external snapping hip syndrome. J Ultrasound Med 2002; 21:753-758.

17 Andrews SK, Carek PJ. Osteitis pubis: A diagnosis for the family physician. J Am Board Fam Pract 1998; 11:291-295.

18 Williams PR, Thomas DP, Downes EM. Osteitis pubis and instability of the pubic symphysis: When operative measures fail. Am J Sports Med 2000; 28:350-355.

19 Pauli S, Willemsen P, Declerck K, et al. Osteomyelitis pubis versus osteitis pubis: a case presentation and review of the literature. Br J Sports Med 2002; 36:71-73.

20 Fricker PA, Taunton JE, Ammann W. Osteitis pubis in athletes. Infection, inflammation or injury? Sports Med 1991; 12:266-279.

21 Batt ME, McShane JM, Dillingham MF. Osteitis pubis in collegiate football players. Med Sci Sports Exerc 1995; 27:629-633.

22 Combs JA. Bacterial osteitis pubis in a weight lifter without invasive trauma. Med Sci Sports Exerc 1998; 30:1561-1563.

23 LeBlanc KE. Sacroiliac sprain. An overlooked cause of back pain. Am Fam Physician 1992; 46:1459-1463.

24 Harrison DE, Harrison DD, Troyanovich SJ. The sacroiliac joint: a review of anatomy and biomechanics with clinical implications. J Manip Physiol Ther 1997; 20:607-617.

25 Mortelli V, Smith V. Groin injuries in athletes. Am Fam Physician 2001; 64:1405-1414.

26 Bradshaw C, McCrory P, Bell S, et al. Obturator nerve entrapment. A cause of groin pain in athletes. Am J Sports Med 1997; 25:402-408.

27 Harvey G, Bell S. Obturator neuropathy. Anat Perspect Clin Orthop 1999; 363:203-211.

28 Burke G, Joe C, Levine M, et al. Tc-99 bone scan in unilateral osteitis pubis. Clin Nucl Med 1994; 19:533.

29 Grossman MG, Ducey SA, Nadler SS, et al. Meralgia paresthetica: Diagnosis and treatment. J Am Acad Orthop Surg 2001; 9:336-344.

30 Keegan JJ, Holyoke EA. Meralgia paresthetica: an anatomical and surgical study. J Neurosurg 1962; 19:341-345.

31 Dias Filho LC, Valenca MM, Guimaraes Filho FA, et al. Lateral femoral cutaneous neuralgia: an anatomical insight. Clin Anat 2003; 16:309-316.

32 Kho KH, Blijham PJ, Zwarts MJ. Meralgia paresthetica after strenuous exercise. Muscle Nerve 2005; 14

33 Silver JK. Piriformis syndrome: Assessment of current practice and literature review. Orthopedics 1998; 21:1133-1135.

34 Ivins GK. Meralgia paresthetica, the elusive diagnosis: clinical experience with 14 adult patients. Ann Surg 2000; 232:281-286.

35 Siu TL, Chandran KN. Neurolysis for meralgia paresthetica: an operative series of 45 cases. Surg Neurol 2005; 63:19-23.

36 Parziale JR, Hudgins TH, Fishman LM. Piriformis syndrome. Am J Orthop 1996; 25:819-823.

37 Barton PM. Piriformis syndrome: a rational approach to management. Pain 1991; 47:345-352.

38 Lee EY, Margherita AJ, Gierada DS, et al. MRI of piriformis syndrome. Am J Roent 2004; 183:63-64.

39 Broadhurst NA, Simmons DN, Bond MJ. Piriformis syndrome: Correlation of muscle morphology with symptoms and signs. Arch Phys Med Rehabil 2004; 85:2036-2039.

40 Dezawa A, Kusano S, Miki H. Arthroscopic release of the piriformis muscle under local anesthesia for piriformis syndrome. Arthroscopy 2003; 19:554-557.

41 Millis MB, Kocher MS. Hip and pelvic injuries in the young athlete (Section B). DeLee & Drez's Orthopaedic sports medicine: principles and practice, Vol. 2. 2nd edn. Philadelphia: Saunders; 2003:1463-1479.

42 Rossi F, Dragoni S. Acute avulsion fractures of the pelvis in adolescent competitive athletes: prevalence, location and sports distribution of 203 cases collected. Skeletal Radiol 2001; 30:127-131.

43 Miller C, Major N, Toth A. Pelvic stress injuries in the athlete: management and prevention. Sports Med 2003; 33:1003-1012.

44 Verma RB. Sherman O. Athletic stress fractures: Part 1. History, epidemiology, physiology, risk factors, radiography, diagnosis and treatment. Am J Orthop 2001; 30:798–806.

45 Knapp TP, Garrett WE Jr. Stress fractures: general concepts. Clin Sports Med 1997; 16:339–356.

46 Noakes TD, Smith JA, Lindenberg G, et al. Pelvis stress fractures in long distance runners. Am J Sports Med 1985; 13:120–123.

47 Aslam N, Gwilym S, Natarajan R. Femoral neck stress fracture in a sanitary worker. Eur J Emerg Med 2004; 11:220–222.

48 Clough TM. Femoral neck stress fracture: the importance of clinical suspicion and early review. Br J Sports Med 2002; 36:308–309.

49 Johansson C, Ekenman I, Tornkvist H, et al. Stress fractures of the femoral neck in athletes. The consequence of a delayed diagnosis. Am J Sports Med 1990; 18:524–528.

50 Devas MB. Stress fractures of the femoral neck. J Bone Jt Surg Br 1965; 47:728.

51 Blickenstaff LP, Morris JM. Fatigue fracture of the femoral neck. J Bone Jt Surg Am 1966; 48:1031.

52 Fullerton LR, Snowdy HA. Femoral neck stress fractures. Am J Sports Med 1988; 16:365.

53 Jingushi S, Suenaga E. Slipped cap femoral epiphysis: etiology and treatment. J Orthop Sci 2004; 9:214–219.

54 Poussa M, Schlenzka D, Yrjonen T. Body mass index and slipped capital femoral epiphysis. J Pediatr Orthop B 2003; 12:369–371.

55 Kocher MS, Bishop JA, Weed B, et al. Delay in diagnosis of slipped capital femoral epiphysis. Pediatrics 2004; 113:322–325.

56 Tokmakova KP, Stanton RP, Mason DE. Factors influencing the development of osteonecrosis in patients treated for slipped capital femoral epiphysis. J Bone Jt Surg 2003; 85:798–801.

57 Herman MJ, Dormans JP, Davidson RS, et al. Screw fixation of grade III slipped capital femoral epiphysis. Clin Orthop 1996; 322:77–85.

58 Blanco JS, Taylor B. Johnston CE 2nd. Comparison of single pin versus multiple pin fixation in treatment of slipped capital femoral epiphysis. J Pediatr Orthop 1992; 12:384–389.

59 Stambough JL, Davidson RS, Ellis RD, et al. Slipped capital femoral epiphysis: an analysis of 80 patients as to pin placement and number. J Pediatr Orthop 1986; 6:265–273.

60 Loder RT, Richards BS, Shapiro PS, et al. Acute slipped femoral epiphysis: the importance of physeal stability. J Bone Jt Surg Am 1993; 75:1134–1140.

61 3rd MJF, Sanders JO, Browne RH, et al. Management of unstable/acute slipped capital femoral epiphysis: results of a survey of the POSNA membership. J Pediatr Orthop 2005; 25:162–166.

62 Kocher MS, Bishop JA, Hresko MT, et al. Prophylactic pinning of the contralateral hip after unilateral slipped capital femoral epiphysis. J Bone Jt Surg 2004; 86:2658–2665.

63 Roy DR. Current concepts in Legg–Calvé–Perthes disease. Pediatr Ann 1999; 28:748–752.

64 Skaggs DL. Tolo VT. Legg–Calvé–Perthes disease. J Am Acad Orthop Surg 1996; 4:9–16.

65 McAndrew MP, Weinstein SL. A long-term follow-up of Legg–Calvé–Perthes disease. J Bone Jt Surg Am 1984; 66:860–869.

66 Balasa VV, Gruppo RA, Gluek CJ et al. Legg–Calvé–Perthes disease and thrombophilia. J Bone Jt Surg Am 2004; 86:2642–2647.

67 Guille JT, Lipton GE, Tsirikos AI, et al. Bilateral Legg–Calvé–Perthes disease: Presentation and outcome. J Pediatr Orthop 2002; 22:458–463.

68 Ritterbusch JF, Shantharam SS, Gelinas C. Comparison of lateral pillar classification and Catterall classification of Legg–Calvé–Perthes disease. Pediatr Orthop 1993; 13:200–202.

69 Kamegaya M, Saisa T, Ochiai N, et al. A paired study of Perthes disease comparing conservative management and surgical treatment. J Bone Jt Surg 2004; 86:1176–1181.

70 Kitakoji T, Hattori T, Kitoh H, et al. Which is a better method for Perthes disease: femoral varus or salter osteotomy? Clin Orthop Relat Res 2005; 430:163–170.

71 Herring JA, Kim HT, Browne R. Legg–Calvé–Perthes disease. Part 2: Prospective multicentre study of the effect of treatment on outcome. J Bone Jt Surg Am 2004; 86:2121–2134.

72 Pallia CS, Scott RE, Chao AD. Traumatic hip dislocation in athletes. Curr Sports Med Rep 2002; 1:338–345.

73 Konrath GA, Hamel AJ, Olson SA, Bay B, Sharkey NA. The role of the acetabular labrum and the transverse acetabular ligament in load transmission in the hip. J Bone Jt Surg Am 1998; 80:1781.

74 Petersen W, Petersen F, Tillmann B. Structure and vascularization of the acetabular labrum with regards to the pathogenesis and healing of labral tears. Arch Orthop Trauma Surg 2003; 123:283–288.

75 McCarthy J, Noble P, Aluisio FV, et al. Anatomy, pathologic features and treatment of acetabular labrum tears. Clin Orthop 2003; 406:38–47.

76 McCarthy JC, Noble PC, Schuck MR, et al. The Watershed labral lesion: its relationship to early arthritis of the hip. J Arthroplasty 2001; 16:81–87.

77 Hickman JM, Peters CL. Hip pain in the young adult: diagnosis and treatment of disorders of the acetabular labrum and acetabular dysplasia. Am J Orthop 2001; 30:459–467.

78 Mason JB. Acetabular labral tears in the athlete. Clin Sports Med 2001; 20: 779–790.

79 Narvani AA, Tsiridis E, Kendall S, et al. A preliminary report on prevalence of acetabular labrum tears in sports patients with groin pain. Knee Surg Sports Traumatol Arthrosc 2003; 11:403–408.

80 Farjo LA, Glick JM, Sampson TG. Hip arthroscopy for acetabular labral tears. Arthroscopy 1999; 1:132–137.

81 Hase T, Ueo T. Acetabular labral tear: arthroscopic diagnosis and treatment. Arthroscopy 1999; 15:138–141.

82 Lage LA, Patel JV, Villar RN. The acetabular labral tear: an arthroscopic classification. Arthroscopy 1999; 15:269–272.

83 Wenger DE, Kendell KR, Miner MR, et al. Acetabular labral tears rarely occur in the absence of bony abnormalities. Clin Orthop 2004; 426:145–150.

84 Kujala UM, Kaprio J, Sarna S. Osteoarthritis of weight bearing joints of lower limbs in former elite male athletes. Brit Med J 1994; 308:231–234.

85 Marti B, Knobloch M, Tschopp A, et al. Is excessive running predictive of degenerative hip disease? Controlled study of former elite athletes. Brit Med J 1989; 299:91–93.

86 Klunder KB, Rud B, Hansen J. Osteoarthritis of the hip and knee joint in retired football players. Acta Orthop Scand 1980; 51:925–927.

87 Lindberg H, Roos H, Gardsell P. Prevalence of coxarthrosis in former soccer players. Acta Orthop Scand 1993; 64:165–167.

88 Vingard E, Alfredsson L, Goldie I, et al. Sports and osteoarthritis of the hip. An epidemiological study. Am J Sports Med 1993; 21:195–200.

89 Burman MS. Arthroscopy of the direct visualization of joints. J Bone Jt Surg 1931; 13:669–695.

90 Byrd JWT. Indications and contraindications. In: Byrd JWT, ed. Operative hip arthroscopy. New York: Thieme Verlag; 1998:7–24.

91 Frich LH, Lauritzen J, Juhl M. Arthroscopy in diagnosis and treatment of hip disorders. Orthopedics 1989; 12:389–392.

92 Ide T, Akamatsu N, Nakajima I. Arthroscopic surgery of the hip joint. Arthroscopy 1991; 7:204–211.

93 McCarthy JC, Day B, Busconi B. Hip arthroscopy: applications and techniques. J Acad Orthop Surg 1995; 3:115–122.

94 Parisien S. Arthroscopy of the hip. Present status. J Dis Orthop 1985; 45:127–132.

95 Byrd JWT. Labral lesions: an elusive source of hip pain: case reports and review of the literature. Arthroscopy 1996; 12:603–612.

96 Byrd JWT, Jones KS. Prospective analysis of hip arthroscopy with 2 year follow-up. Arthroscopy 2000; 16:578–587.

97 Byrd JWT, Jones KS. Hip arthroscopy in the presence of dysplasia. Arthroscopy 2003; 19:1055–1060.

98 Dorell JH, Catterall A. The torn acetabular labrum. J Bone Jt Surg Br 1986; 68:400–403.

99 Suzuki S, Awaya G, Okada Y, et al. Arthroscopic diagnosis of ruptured acetabular labrum. Acta Orthop Scand 1986; 57:513–515.

100 Villar RN. Arthroscopic debridement of the hip. J Bone Jt Surg Br 1991; 73: 170–171.

101 Byrd JWT. Hip arthroscopy for post-traumatic loose fragments in the young active adult: three case reports. Clin Sports Med 1996; 6:129–134.

102 Bowen JR, Kumar VP, Joyce JJ, et al. Osteochondritis dissecans following Perthes disease. Arthroscopic operative treatment. Clin Orthop 1986; 209:49–56.

103 Noguchi Y, Miura H, Takasugi S, Iwamoto Y. Cartilage and labrum degeneration in the dysplastic hip generally originates in the anteriosuperior weight bearing area: An arthroscopic observation. Arthroscopy 1999; 15:496–506.

104 Blitzer CM. Arthroscopic management of septic arthritis of the hip. Arthroscopy 1993; 9:414–416.

105 Bould M, Edwards D, Villar RN. Arthroscopic diagnosis and treatment of septic arthritis of the hip joint. Arthroscopy 1993; 9:707–708.

106 Chung WK, Slater GL, Bates EH. Treatment of septic arthritis of the hip by arthroscopic lavage. J Pediatr Orthop 1993; 13:444–446.

107 Holgersson S, Brattstr MH, Morgensen B, et al. Arthroscopy of the hip in juvenile chronic arthritis. J Pediatr Orthop 1981; 1:273–278.

108 Okada Y, Awaya G, Ikeda T, et al. Arthroscopic surgery for synovial chondromatosis of the hip. J Bone Jt Surg Br 1989; 71:198–199.

109 Witwity T, Uhlmann RD, Fischer J, et al. Arthroscopic management of chondromatosis of the hip joint. Arthroscopy 1988; 4:55–56.

110 Goldman A, Minkoff J, Price A, et al. A posterior arthroscopic approach to bullet extraction from the hip. J Trauma 1987; 27:1294–1300.

111 Delcamp DD, Klaaren HE, Pompe Meerdervoort HF van. Traumatic avulsion of the ligamentum teres without dislocation of the hip. J Bone Jt Surg Am 1988; 70:933–935.

112 Gray AJR, Villar RN. The ligamentum teres of the hip: an arthroscopic classification of its pathology. Arthroscopy 1997; 13:575–578.

113 Kashiwagi N, Suzuki S, Seto Y. Arthroscopic treatment for traumatic hip dislocation with avulsion fracture of the ligamentum teres. Arthroscopy 2001; 17:67–69.

114 Mah ET, Bradley CM. Arthroscopic removal of acrylic cement from unreduced hip prosthesis. Aust NZ J Surg 1992; 62:508–510.

115 Nordt W. Giangarra CE, Levy IM, Habermann ET. Arthroscopic removal of entrapped debris following dislocation of a total hip arthroplasty. Athroscop 1987; 3:196–198.

116 Shifrin LZ, Reis ND. Arthroscopy of a dislocated hip replacement. A case report. Clin Orthop 1978; 6:213–214.

117 Vakili F, Salvati EA, Warren RF. Entrapped foreign body within the acetabular cup in total hip replacement. Clin Orthop 1980; 150:159–162.

118 Berend KR, Vail TP. Hip arthroscopy in the adolescent and pediatric athlete. Clin Sports Med 2001; 20:763–768.

119 DeAngelis NA, Busconi BD. Hip arthroscopy in the pediatric population. Clin Orthop 2003; 406:60–63.

120 Gross RH. Arthroscopy in hip disorders in children. Orthop Rev 1977; 6:43–49.

121 Lechevallier J, Bowen JR. Arthroscopic treatment of the late sequelae of Legg–Calvé–Perthes disease. J Bone Jt Surg Br 1993; 75(160)

122 Schindler A, Lechevallier JJ, Roa NS, et al. Diagnostic and therapeutic arthroscopy of the hip in children and adolescents: evaluation of results. J Pediatr Orthop 1995; 15:317–321.

123 Snow SW, Keret D, Scarangella S, et al. Anterior impingement of the femoral head: A late phenomenon of Legg–Calvé–Perthes disease. J Pediatr Orthop 1993; 13:286–289.

124 Czerny C, Hofmann S, Neuhold A, et al. Lesions of the acetabular labrum: Accuracy of MR imaging and MR arthrography in detection and staging. Radiology 1996; 200:225–230.

125 Petersilge CA, Haque MA, Petersilge WJ, et al. Acetabular labral tears: Evaluation with MR arthrography. Radiology 1996; 200:231–235.

126 Kocher MS, Kim YJ, Millis MB et al. Hip arthroscopy in children and adolescents. J Pediatr Orthop 2005; 25:680–686.

CHAPTER 30

Thigh Injuries

Gian Corrado and Pierre A. d'Hemecourt

INTRODUCTION

The upper leg or thigh contains the majority of muscle mass of the lower extremity including the hamstring, quadriceps and adductor muscle groups (Fig. 30.1). These muscles are responsible for speed and power in the running athlete, biker, skier, and in kicking sports in which powerful hip flexion is necessary including dance, soccer and karate. The need for explosive strength in activities such as football, soccer, rugby and dance leave the thigh at great risk for overuse syndromes as well as muscle and tendon tears and strains. Contact activities including hockey and football can result in sometimes disabling blunt thigh trauma. It is important for the physician in his office and at the fieldside to recognize and appropriately treat these injuries to minimize the consequences of the injury and return the athlete to play safely.

Thigh injuries are extremely common in athletes of all levels and have a wide range of severity. Blunt trauma may result in a minor contusion, which does not result in end of play and resolves without intervention. Conversely, a blunt thigh trauma may result in significant quadriceps hematoma resulting in acute compartment syndrome infrequently requiring emergent surgical intervention to prevent permanent disability from nerve, vascular and muscular damage. Muscle injury can also range from a minor strain to large tears that are slow to heal and require abstinence from play and rehabilitation for extended periods of time. Close contact with the patient, family, physical therapists, trainers and coaches is required for optimal recovery.

ADDUCTOR STRAINS

Box 30.1: Key Points

- Adductor strains are particularly prevalent in athletes participating in multiple plane sports or sports that require elevation of the leg above the waist.

- Poor conditioning, over activity and overstretching may predispose athletes to adductor strains.

- Adductor strains require prompt identification and treatment.

- An early intervention strengthening program may help prevent adductor injury in athletes involved in high risk sports.

Adductor strains are common in the general population and especially prevalent in the athlete who needs to run and skate in multiple planes such as soccer, football and hockey as well as those sports that require elevation of the leg above the waist such as karate and dance.

Anatomy

The adductors of the leg include the adductor magnus, minimus, brevis and longus, as well as the gracilis and pectinineus. The obturator nerve innervates the majority of adductors. These muscles originate from the area of the pubic ramus and insert in the proximal medial femur. The most common site of tendon injury is the musculotendinous junction.

Mechanism of injury

The athlete with an adductor strain generally has a history of gradual or sudden onset of inner thigh pain which was caused or exacerbated by quick lateral motion, lateral change in direction or forceful kicking as is often seen in the soccer player who uses the medial aspect of the foot for ball control. Poor conditioning, overuse and overstretching have all been implicated in predisposing the athlete to strains.[1]

Presentation

The patient may have tenderness along the course of the adductor muscle. More often the patient will have pain with resisted adduction and forced abduction of the hip. Occasionally in the acute injury, there may be swelling and ecchymosis over the proximal medial thigh.

Classification

Adductor strains are generally classified as degrees I–III. Degree I strains are painful without loss of function or mobility. Degree II have loss of strength and mobility without complete loss of function, whereas, a third degree will have complete loss of function.

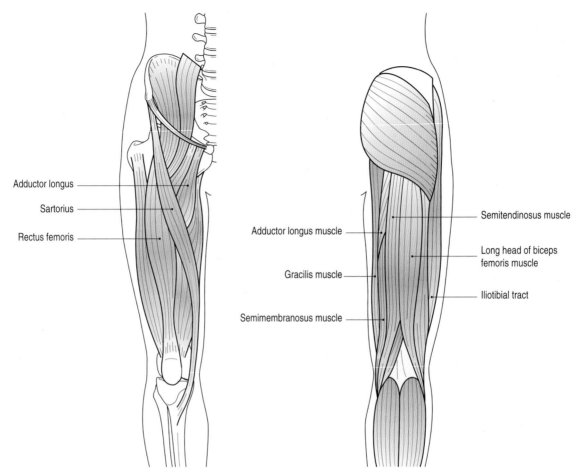

Figure 30.1   Thigh anatomy, anterior and posterior.

Imaging

Radiographs should be taken if other etiologies including osteitis pubis or avulsion fracture are being considered. An ultrasound can be used to evaluate and follow muscle or tendon injuries and rule out serious conditions including testicular torsion. MRI and CT scan can be used to further delineate the extent of a tear as well as evaluate for other possible etiologies of pain. Athletes with adductor strains require prompt identification and treatment.

Differential diagnosis

Other non-muscular causes of groin pain should be considered in the athlete with acute groin pain. Obturator nerve entrapment is an infrequent cause of groin pain which should be considered.[2] Osteitis pubis can also mimic adductor strain symptoms and may present as comorbidity.[3] Abdominal etiologies including direct and indirect inguinal hernias may produce vague pain that radiates primarily to the groin. Genitourinary causes including testicular torsion, although generally severe and sudden in onset, may have a more stuttering and less severe onset and mask as muscular groin pain. A testicular tumor or gynecologic pathology should also be considered in more indolent cases. Once the clinician is convinced that the athlete's groin pain is muscular in origin then they can begin treatment and rehabilitation.

Treatment and rehabilitation

Prevention is a crucial element of rehabilitation in previously injured and uninjured athletes involved in high risk sports. In a recent study by Tyler, professional hockey players who were identified as at risk for adductor strain were enrolled in an early intervention program attempting to minimize injury. This was a follow-up to their previous study, which found that lack of strength, not flexibility, was a risk factor for adductor strain.[4] In this study, adductor to abductor ratio of less than 80% was a positive predictor for future injury. Their strengthening program focused on concentric, eccentric and functional strengthening of adductor muscles with the clinical goal of adductor strength at 80% of abduction.[5] The program begins with warm-up, biking and adductor stretching. It then focuses on strength and uses the following exercises: sumo squats, side lunges, pelvic tilts, ball squeezes, concentric adductor strength against weight, sliding board work and finally sports specific training on the ice. The follow-up study employed this preseason strengthening program and found that all participants went without injury over the next two seasons except two players with minor first-degree strains. This concept was corroborated by a 2003 investigation by Witvrouw *et al.* in which decreased flexibility was an indicator of future risk of muscle strain for quadriceps and hamstrings but not adductor strain.[6]

The basic tenants of rehabilitation of adductor strains are the same as in all strains. These include prevention, acute management and rehabilitation and management of chronic pain and disability. In the acute phase, the principles of pneumonic rest, ice, compression and elevation (RICE) apply. Initial treatment of the athlete with a significant adductor injury should include: removal from play, compression, elevation of the involved extremity with the patient prone if possible and application of ice. Compression can be achieved with compression shorts or a hip spica wrap.

First-degree strains generally can return to play after a short period of rest but must begin a stretching and strengthening program soon after the injury. Second-degree strains can be out of play as long as 14 days depending on the severity of the injury. Post-injury, week 1 involves applying the principles of RICE, adding gentle range of motion exercises and nonsteroidal anti-inflammatory medication. When the athlete is pain free, he or she can begin a treatment regimen of progressive strengthening and stretching. Third-degree strains if not surgical are treated as severe second-degree with the addition of partial weight bearing with crutches until pain free. Good results have been reported in surgical interventions with complete rupture and refractory chronic strains.[7]

HAMSTRING INJURIES

Box 30.2: Key Points

- Hamstring injuries are most common in athletes involved in sports that require sprinting, or sports with kicking or dancing.

- The most reliable signs of hamstring injury are pain with passive hip flexion and knee extension or resisted knee flexion and hip extension.

- Multiple factors including previous injury, inadequate warm up and lack of flexibility may predispose athletes to hamstring injury.

- Acute hamstring strain should initially be treated using the RICE method before the athlete begins a progressively increasing program of strength work and stretching.

Sports that require sprinting are most prone to hamstring injuries, as this muscle group is the major power component of hip extension and knee flexion. Pain and disability for hamstring strains are a major cause of morbidity in athletes and can lead to prolonged periods of exclusion from play, as they are slow to heal.

Anatomy

The hamstring is composed of three muscles: the biceps femoris, semimembranosus, and semitendinosus. The biceps which is the most commonly injured muscle in the group originates at the proximal femur and ischial tuberosity and inserts into the proximal fibula. It is generally injured during the foot take off phase of the gait cycle. The semimembranosus and semitendinosus originate at the ischial tuberosity and insert into the proximal posterior tibia and the pes anserine, respectively. This medial muscle group is more often injured during the swing phase of the gait cycle. Most strains occur during while the hamstring is lengthening or during eccentric contraction.

Classification

Hamstring injuries are classified into three degrees of strain depending upon their severity. First-degree strains are minor injuries to the musculotendinous unit in which there is microscopic injury only. Second degree is a more severe macrotear without complete rupture of the musculotendinous unit and in third-degree strains there is rupture.

Presentation

Hamstring tears can either be acute or chronic and progressive. The athletes who suffer this injury are most often sprinters but may also be involved in sports with kicking or dancing, especially where hamstrings are stretched to their elastic limit. Proximal hamstring avulsions are also seen in water skiing. In the acute setting, injuries often begin with a tearing or popping sensation followed by pain and loss of function. With overuse injuries, the athlete may only complain initially of pain at the end of exertion, which then progresses to constant pain which precludes play. On physical examination, the posterior thigh may have tenderness at the muscle origin, musculotendinous junction, belly or insertion. There also may be a mass and ecchymosis. However, the most reliable signs are pain with passive hip flexion and knee extension or resisted knee flexion and hip extension.

Imaging

Imaging studies are rarely necessary provided the physician is confident in the diagnosis of strain and complete rupture and avulsion fracture is not in the differential diagnosis. Avulsion injuries can be easily seen on plain films. A recent small study by Brandser found that radiographs helped identify avulsion only. Computed tomography helped identify a patient with a healing ischial apophysis and that magnetic resonance imaging was useful no matter how long after the injury it was obtained.[8]

Treatment and rehabilitation

Rehabilitation and prevention of hamstring strain requires understanding of the underlying features that predispose the athlete to injury. Multiple factors have been implicated in predisposition to hamstring injury including: previous injury, inadequate warm-up, muscle fatigue, strength imbalances, lack of flexibility, poor posture, leg length discrepancy and improper technique. Hamstring muscle 'stiffness' as determined by straight leg raise was found to have a strong correlation to loss of strength, pain, muscle tenderness and creatine kinase activity suggesting traditional notions of lack flexibility as a risk factor for injury.[9] This was also the finding in Witvrouw's study in which flexibility played a major role in predicting future hamstring injuries.[6]

Multiple studies have also shown that inadequate strength also predisposes the athlete to hamstring injury.[10,11] In a large prospective cohort study of risk factors for muscle injury previous injury was by far the strongest predictor of future hamstring strain and subsequent disability.[12] Prevention of first hamstring injury through strength and flexibility training and adequate rest and rehabilitation after strain are critical to avoiding disability.

Care of the acute hamstring strain follows the classic RICE pneumonic. The athlete should be removed from play and allowed to rest for a period of days to a week. It is felt that the period of relative immobilization is required to form a granulation tissue matrix required for a strong bond with healing. Depending on the degree of injury crutches may facilitate the rest period. When the patient is pain-free gentle passive range of motion (ROM) will help facilitate scar resorption and lead to active mobilization required to avoid atrophy and regain full strength.[13] Once the patient is completely pain free throughout ROM they can begin active ROM work beginning with assisted active range of motion (AROM) or pool workouts. During this time, athletes should maintain cardiovascular fitness through swimming or cycling.

Note must be made of a relatively rare but important hamstring injury which requires surgical treatment – complete avulsion of the proximal hamstring insertion. This usually occurs as a result of dynamic eccentric overload such as can occur in water skiing. Ecchymosis occurs at the buttocks proximally, and a gap in the muscle may be palpated.

MRI can confirm the diagnosis (Fig. 30.2). If left unrepaired, the athlete is unable to run. Fortunately, late repair can also be successful, but is more hazardous, as adhesions may form on the sciatic nerve.

Following the acute treatment and early rehabilitation, the athlete may begin a progressively increasing program of strength and stretching. Early strength work can include straight-leg raises, standing hamstring curls, no-weight squats and step-ups. When these exercises become effortless, the athlete may progress to weighted exercises including curls, squats and leg-presses. Aerobic activity can be progressed from pool work to the elliptical machine or biking. Assuming the athlete is able to continue to progress with weight and strength, they may begin to attempt more sport-specific training including running, jumping and rapid deceleration. At any point, if the patient complains of pain or disability they should be encouraged to return to earlier stages of rehabilitation.

QUADRICEPS CONTUSIONS AND MYOSITIS OSSIFICANS TRAUMATICA

Box 30.3: Key Points

- Quadriceps contusion is particularly common in contact sports.
- Severe injury may be complicated by myositis ossificans.
- Removal from play and immediate initiation of treatment are vital in cases of quadriceps contusion.

Blunt trauma of the anterior thigh resulting in quadriceps contusion is a common injury, particularly in contact sports. These injuries range in severity from mild and uncomplicated with minimal loss of play and function to severe and complicated by heterotopic bone formation or myositis ossificans (MO) or by an unusual acute compartment syndrome requiring emergent surgical intervention (Fig. 30.3). The vast majority of contusions resolve without sequelae, however, MO can be challenging for the physician and athlete as many can remain symptomatic and surgical excision isn't always curative. The

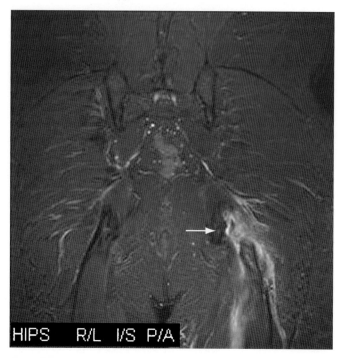

Figure 30.2   MRI of proximal hamstring strain.

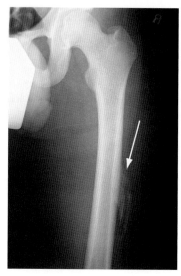

Figure 30.3   Myositis ossificans X-ray.

pathophysiology of the intramuscular bone formation has not been well delineated and therefore, the most effective mode of prevention is unclear.

Mechanism of injury

Quadriceps contusions are caused by the translation of external compressive forced which are resisted by adjacent long bone. The result is the destruction of muscle tissue and vascular tissue, which leads to muscle necrosis and bleeding. The ROM of the knee determines the severity of injury 12–24 h after injury. The contusion is considered mild when knee flexion exceeds 90°, moderate between 45 and 90° and severe when <45°.[14] Most authorities agree that mild and moderate contusions can be managed conservatively, however there is some controversy regarding severe contusions and when and if they require emergent fasciotomy. A recent review of three professional athletes with severe contusions as defined by ROM <45° had good outcomes with close observation and a conservative non-surgical approach.[15] Vascular compromise is a surgical indication.

Treatment and rehabilitation

Initial management of quadriceps contusions always requires removal from play and immediate initiation of treatment. Symptoms often do not fully evolve until 12–24 h after insult and may be aggravated by time to treatment and further contusions if the athlete is permitted to continue play. Therefore immediate rest, elevation, compression and icing are important at the fieldside when there is a significant contusion. The *West Point Update* included the much used method of resting the quadriceps in flexion in the initial treatment and focused of early flexion strength as opposed to extension maneuvers.[16] The protocol developed by Ryan *et al.* includes three phases. Phase one is control of pain, which is accomplished by rest in maximum tolerated knee, and hip flexion assisted by bandaging and tape, icing, non-steroidal anti-inflammatory drugs (NSAIDs) and avoidance of passive ROM. Occasionally, hospitalization is required for narcotic pain relief. A number of studies have shown that forceful manipulation of contused quadriceps can increase the risk of myositis ossificans. Michelsson[17] found in their rabbit model, that if they immobilized the quadriceps for the majority of the time except for 5 min of forceful manipulation that all of his subjects developed MO.

Phase two focuses on restoration of range of motion. If the patient is pain free and swelling has stabilized, they can move into this phase. Here they begin active range of motion and weight bearing as tolerated. Efforts are made to regain flexion from the quadriceps. The work done during this phase should be pain-free and if at any time the patient experiences persistent pain or signs of re-injury, they regress to the previous phase. When the athlete has regained range of motion and muscle control, it is then possible to advance to the last phase.

Phase three's goal is return to sports specific activities. Early in this phase, the athlete can begin quadriceps and overall lower extremity strengthening and this will enable a gradual process of return to sports. For instance, when a hockey player is pain-free, has regained strength and range of motion he/she may then return to the ice initially in a non-contact setting and gradually increase their ice time as long as they remain asymptomatic. Soon after this they can return to contact play with a pad to be worn at all times for up to 6 months. The development of myositis should not change management unless it becomes symptomatic.

The management of myositis ossificans, which becomes symptomatic, is difficult. It occurs in approximately 9% of quadriceps contusions and needs to be differentiated from osteosarcoma by history, physical and imaging studies if the diagnosis is in question. Early excision may lead to exacerbation of the problem and conservative management efforts need to be exhausted prior to surgical intervention. However, this may be considered in the patient with a symptomatic mature lesion in which conservative treatment has failed. The patient should repeat the above protocol after surgery.

ILIOTIBIAL BAND FRICTION SYNDROME

Iliotibial band friction syndrome (ITBFS) is a common condition in runners and cyclists, especially endurance athletes. It is caused by friction between the iliotibial band (ITB) and the lateral elements of the knee and is the most common cause of lateral knee pain in runners with an incidence over 10%.[18] This friction occurs during foot contact in the runner between the posterior edge of the ITB and the lateral epicondyle of the femur. It can be a challenging problem for athletes and caregivers, as it is often a chronic problem and its etiology is multifactorial.

Anatomy

The ITB is formed proximally by the fascial components of the gluteus maximus and medius and the tensor fascia lata. It extends distally along the lateral aspect of the thigh and inserts into the supercondylar tubercle of the lateral femoral condyle and into the anterolateral proximal tibia at Gerdy's tubercle. The ITB lies adjacent to and makes contact with the lateral femoral epicondyle and proximal insertion of lateral collateral ligament. The ITB fibers cross those of the lateral collateral ligament when the knee is in flexion enhancing lateral stability. The ITB also acts to restrict hip adduction in midstance. ITBFS occurs when a tight ITB moves from the forward position in front of the epicondyle in knee extension to the posterior position behind the epicondyle in knee flexion. It has generally been accepted that the pain was caused by an inflamed bursa below the ITB.[19] However in a radiology MRI and cadaver study there was no bursa and but small layer of fatty tissue. It also found that in knee flexion further friction was created by the fibers of the popliteus and biceps femoris.[20]

Mechanism of injury

A number of theories and studies have been done attempting to reveal the etiology of ITBFS. It has been theorized that foot biomechanics were critical in the development of this disorder, however, a recent study found no association with either pes cavus or pes planus and the overuse injury of ITBFS.[21]

An article by Orchard *et al.* proposed a biomechanical model which suggests that the degree of flexion at foot strike is a major factor in development if ITBS and that downhill runners have an increased incidence because of degree of flexion is reduced thereby increasing the contact between the ITB and epicondyle. Conversely, sprinters have a lower incidence as their degree of knee flexion at foot strike is relatively greater.[19] Messier found that runners with ITBFS were less experienced and spent a great percentage of time running on the track.[22] Fredericson *et al.* found that correction of abductor weakness alleviated symptoms in 92% of 24 runners with this syndrome.[23]

Presentation

ITBFS can usually be elicited in the history and physical. Classically a problem in runners, the patient will complain of sharp burning pain at the lateral aspect of the knee. The pain will begin during the run and generally the distanced required to elicit the pain will shorten and may eventually linger and cause pain with walking and other activities of daily living. The pain in this group can be especially symptomatic with stairs. Often the physical examination in the office is negative. The athlete may, however, have tenderness at the distal ITB where it intersects with the lateral femoral condyle. Less often the caregiver may find redness and swelling at this site. A sensitive test for eliciting pain with ITBFS can be done with the patient lying on their side facing away from the examiner with the unaffected side against the table. The affected knee is flexed and the hip slightly extended while the knee is straightened. Snapping and pain at the intersection of the ITB and lateral femoral condyle is indicative of ITBFS.

Treatment and rehabilitation

Treatment generally consists of rest, ice, non-steroidal anti-inflammatories and physical therapy. Physical therapy and treatment occur in three phases. The first phase involves rest and reduction of acute symptoms. This is followed by a stretching reduction of restriction phase. The final phase concentrates on strength and return to running. A physician may occasionally use local steroidal injections as an adjunct and in a very few number of recalcitrant cases a surgical intervention may be required.

In the first phase of rehabilitation, all efforts are aimed at the reduction of inflammation and irritation. Success is judged by objective and subjective observation with the goals of reduction of swelling, tenderness, erythema and mechanical symptoms and resolution of pain at rest. The mainstay of treatment here is avoidance of exacerbating activities particularly running. This generally includes stationary bike, elliptical and stair climbing machines. The athlete is permitted to swim while limiting their kicking, provided this activity does not elicit pain. Adjuncts to treatment include NSAIDs, ice, wraps and judicious use of local steroid injections. This phase varies in duration but may require as long as two weeks to achieve.

Once the athlete is pain free, they can begin a stretching regime meant to decrease tension of the ITB and decrease friction at its distal insertion. Three methods of achieving this are as follows:
1 Cross-legged stretch
2 Supine cross body rope stretch
3 Foam bolster (Feldenkrais roles)

After adequate stretching has been achieved, the athlete begins a strengthening program and returns to running. Exercises include squats, side-lying leg lifts, single leg squats and pelvic drops.
1 Squats
2 Single leg squats
3 Pelvic drops
4 Side-lying leg lifts

Once these have been learned in a supervised setting, the athlete can continue this training alone three to four times a week. Aerobic activity may utilize the elliptical cross-trainer if well tolerated. Once the athlete is pain free in all exercises, then there can be a gradual return to running. The athlete should be encouraged to decrease distance and intensity and return to an abbreviated course of the above treatment program. This can be tailored with physician, physical therapist, athletic trainer and coaching staff.

REFERRED PAIN AND NERVE IMPINGEMENT

There are a number of pathologies in the abdomen and pelvis that may refer pain to the groin and thigh. As mentioned above, gynecologic, testicular pathologies should be considered. In the child and adolescent, femoral head avascular necrosis and slipped capital femoral epiphysis are a concern. Osteitis pubis and sports hernias are relatively common entities. Furthermore, there are several nerve impingements that may refer pain into the thigh.

Sciatic pain

A relatively common scenario is the 'hamstring pull' that ultimately proves to be a referral from an L5–S1 disc. This may present without back pain. A straight leg raise may be positive in both. However, a slump test should only be positive with sciatic pain.

Lateral femoral cutaneous nerve (meralgia paresthetica)

For the anterior thigh, one must consider meralgia paresthetica, which is an impingement of the lateral femoral cutaneous nerve as it exits the pelvis under the lateral aspect of the inguinal ligament (Fig. 30.4). This is a pure sensory nerve derived from the L2 and L3 nerve roots. Its distribution of pain and paresthesias is the anterolateral thigh. With persistent symptoms, one must consider entrapment of the nerve along its course which would include spinal impingement in the neuroforamina, retroperitoneal and pelvic tumors, and most commonly from impingement at its exit from the pelvis.[24] Chronic trauma to the lateral inguinal ligament is common from a tight belt, obesity or pregnancy. A tight sartorius may also be an aggravating factor. Polyneuropathies from diabetes or lumbar plexopathy should also be considered.

A careful neurologic examination and pelvic exam are important. A positive Tinel at the lateral inguinal ligament just

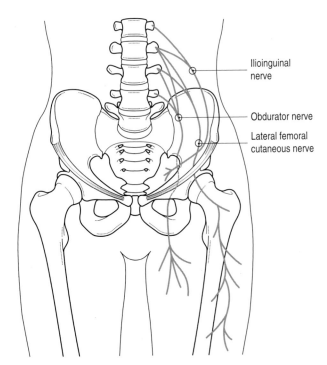

Figure 30.4 Groin and upper thigh innervation.

Labels on figure:
- Ilioinguinal nerve
- Obdurator nerve
- Lateral femoral cutaneous nerve

medial to the anterior superior iliac spine will identify an entrapment at the pelvic exit. Electrodiagnostic studies as well as lumbar and/or pelvic MRI may be helpful.

Treatment will usually focus on relieving any pressure such as a tight belt and weight management. Therapy should involve peripelvic stretches especially to the sartorius and attention to proper pelvic tilt. An adjunctive corticosteroid with anesthetic injection at the lateral inguinal ligament medial to the ASIS may be diagnostic and therapeutic. Rarely, surgical decompression is needed.[25]

Ilioinguinal nerve

The ilioinguinal nerve is derived from the nerve roots of L1 and L2. It follows the inner iliac crest and enters the inguinal canal giving innervation to the inguinal region, scrotum, labia and some of the upper medial thigh. Impingement will give pain in this distribution with weakness of the motor innervation of the internal oblique and transversus abdominus. This pain is often exertional particularly with running. Symptoms may be relieved with hip flexion and patients may walk somewhat bent over. Considerations of entrapment include the upper lumbar spine at the neuroforamina, intrapelvic pathology and inguinal canal entrapment from trauma or surgery such as a herniorrhaphy. Examination reveals tenderness of the inguinal nerve medial to the ASIS and weakness of the external ring of the inguinal canal. Imaging to the lumbar spine and/or pelvis may be indicated with an MRI. Treatment is directed to relief of the impingement along with anti-inflammatory medication and support. Local corticosteroid injections with an anesthetic are both diagnostic and often therapeutic. Refractory cases may require a surgical neurolysis.

Obturator nerve impingement

Impingement of the obturator nerve occurs in the obturator canal. This can be due to trauma, childbirth or exertional impingement in the obturator foramen. The symptoms would include pain along the medial thigh and are often accompanied by adductor weakness. There may be deep groin tenderness but typically, the adductors are non-tender. Electrodiagnostic studies may be helpful. Therapy involves message and stretching of the adductor and peripelvic region with addition of electrical stimulation. Neurolysis is indicated in refractory cases.

FEMORAL STRESS FRACTURES

Box 30.4: Key Points

- Femoral stress fractures are most common in runners and are infrequently seen in the general population.

- Athletes are more prone to stress fracture during sudden increases in duration and intensity of physical activity without appropriate rest periods.

- Women have a higher risk of stress fractures.

- For non-displaced fractures, the athlete should use crutches initially before beginning a physical therapy treatment course.

Stress fractures are most commonly seen in the tibia (50%), tarsals (25%) and metatarsals (8%).[26] They are infrequent in the general population. The incidence is higher however in runners and in the military, during basic training. Runners have been shown to bear weight up to eight times their body weight in their hips.[27] Hulkko *et al.* found the incidence to be as high as 15% in runners.[28] The incidence of femur stress fracture is relatively uncommon usually involving the femoral neck and represents only 7% of the total number of stress fractures.[26] A study by Johnson found that a greater percentage of stress fractures of the femur involve the shaft (20%) than traditionally expected.[29] Any stress fracture of the femur is considered high risk as the debilitation from delayed union, non-union and complete fracture can have significant associated morbidity.[30]

Anatomy

The femur is a long bone and is the largest and strongest in the human body. The secondary ossification centers begin at 4 months and fuse in adolescence. The femoral neck-shaft angle averages 130° and receives its blood supply from the circumflex branches of the profunda femoris. The tenuous blood supply to the head and neck make it especially prone to stress fractures.

Mechanism of injury

Stress fractures occur when bone resorption occurs more rapidly than formation during times of repetitive stress, in which the bone is deformed past its elastic limit. The athlete is more prone to this during sudden increases in duration and intensity of physical activity without proper rest periods. One theory on the development of stress fractures contends that the muscles surrounding the bone fatigue can no longer support the bone leading to microfracture, which can propagate to complete fracture at weakened sites.[31] Hormonal factors are felt to be at play as well and women have a higher risk of stress fractures.[32] Women are particularly at risk of the female triad of eating disorder, amenorrhea and osteoporosis. In this condition, their relative lack of estrogen leads to mineral deficiencies and osteoporosis, which significantly increase the risk of bone injury. The pathogenesis is multifactorial and includes extrinsic forces including training and diet and inherent features which are hormonal and genetic.

Presentation

The athlete with a femoral stress fracture will often complain of vague exertional pain that eventually will linger post exercise. Femoral neck stress fractures isolate the pain to the groin area, but may also have referred pain to the inner thigh and knee. Femoral shaft stress fracture will have mid-thigh pain and also can have referred pain to the knee. The majority of athletes will admit to an increase in duration and frequency of physical activity or will already have high endurance exercise regimens. In the absence of this historical information, the healthcare provider should have high index of suspicion for alternative diagnosis (e.g. pathologic fracture). Once the possibility of a stress fracture is recognized, the provider has a number of diagnostic studies available to confirm the diagnosis.

Imaging

If initial radiographs indicate callous formation or cortical disruption the diagnosis is generally clear and the process of injury is in the later stages. Often, however, the initial radiographs will be normal and further imaging is necessary. Computerized tomography is sensitive and may show earlier callous formation and cortical disruption. Magnetic resonance imaging and scintography are even more sensitive and may reveal an alternative diagnosis when the clinical picture is unclear. When the symptoms are vague between the hip and thigh, a bone scan will be sensitive to both areas (Fig. 30.5).

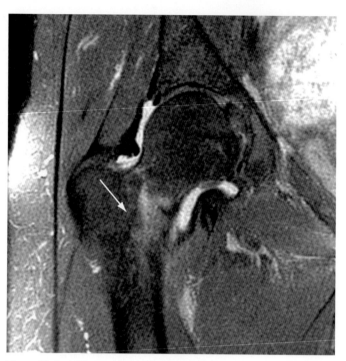

Figure 30.5 MRI of a femoral stress fracture.

Treatment and rehabilitation

For non-displaced fractures, the athlete should be placed on crutches with partial weight bearing until pain free and then can begin non-impact activities. At this point, they can begin a physical therapy treatment course with the aim of maintaining peri-pelvic, thigh and leg strength flexibility. The athlete should refrain from impact activities for at least 4–6 weeks, at which point they can slowly return to their sport provided they remain pain-free. Femoral neck stress fractures on the medial surface are compressive and most often do well. However, lateral surface neck fractures are distractive and require consideration for surgical pinning. Failure to adequately treat early stress fractures can result in displaced fractures, which are associated with a high complication rate including; osteonecrosis, non-union and recurrent fracture.[33]

REFERENCES

1 Estwanik JJ, Sloane B, Rosenberg MA. Groin strain and other possible causes of groin pain. Sports Med 1990; 18:59–65.

2 Bradshaw C, McCrory P, Bell S, Brukner P. Obturator nerve entrapment. A cause of groin pain in athletes. J Sports Med 1997; 25:402–8.

3 Batt ME, McShane JM, Dillingham MF. Osteitis pubis in collegiate football players. Med Sci Sports Exerc 1995; 27: p. 629–33.

4 Tyler TF, Nicholas SJ, Campbell RJ, McHugh MP. The association of hip strength and flexibility with the incidence of adductor muscle strains in professional ice hockey players. Am J Sports Med 2001; 29:124–128.

5 Tyler TF, Nicholas SJ, Campbell RJ, Donellan S, McHugh MP. Effectiveness of a preseason exercise program to prevent adductor muscle strains in professional ice hockey players. Am J Sports Med 2002; 30:680–683.

6 Witvrouw E, Danneels L, Asselman P, D'Have T, Cambier D. Muscle flexibility as a risk factor for developing muscle injuries in male professional soccer players: a prospective study. Am J Sports Med 2003; 31:41–46.

7 Hackney, R. The sports hernia: A cause of chronic groin pain. Br J Sports Med 1993; 27:58–62.

8 Brandser EA, el-Khoury GY, Kathol MH, Callaghan JJ, Tearse DS. Hamstring injuries: radiographic, conventional tomographic, CT, and MR imaging characteristics. Radiology 1995; 197:257–262.

9 McHugh MP, Connolly DA, Eston RG, Kremenic IJ, Nicholas SJ, Gleim GW. The role of passive muscle stiffness in symptoms of exercise-induced muscle damage. J Sports Med 1999; 27:594–599.

10 Burkett LN. Investigation into hamstring strains: The case of the hybrid muscle. J Sports Med, 1975; 3:228-231.

11 Orchard J, Marsden J, Lord S, Garlick D. Preseason hamstring muscle weakness associated with hamstring muscle injury in Australian footballers. Am J Sports Med 1997; 25: 81-85.

12 Orchard J. Intrinsic and extrinsic risk factors for muscle strains in Australian football. Am J Sports Med 2001; 29:300-3.

13 Kujala UM, Orava S, Jarvinen M. Hamstring Injuries. Current trends in treatment and prevention. Sports Med 1997; 23:397-404.

14 Jackson D, Feagin JA. Quadriceps contusions in young athletes. J Bone Joint Surg Am 1973; 55:95-105.

15 Diaz J, Fischer DA, Rettig AC, Davis TJ, Shelbourne KD. Severe quadriceps muscle contusions in athletes. A report of three cases. Am J Sports Med 2003; 31:289-93.

16 Ryan J, Wheeler JH, Hopkinson WJ, Arciero RA, Kolakowski KR. Quadriceps contusions. West Point Update. Am J Sports Med 1991; 19:299-304.

17 Michelsson J, Granroth G, Andersson LC. Myositis ossificans following forcible manipulation of the leg: a rabbit model for the study of heterotopic bone formation. J Bone Jt Surg (Am) 1980; 62:811-815.

18 Fredericson MF, Guillet M, DeBenedictis L. Quick solutions for iliotibial band syndrome. Phys Sportsmed 2000; 28:53-68.

19 Orchard JW, Fricker PA, Abud AT, Mason BR. Biomechanics of iliotibial band friction syndrome in runners. Am J Sports Med 1996; 24:375-379.

20 Muhle C, Ahn JM, Yeh L, et al. Iliotibial band friction syndrome: MR imaging findings in 16 patients and MR arthrographic study of six cadaveric knees. Radiology 1999; 212:103-110.

21 Kaufman KR, Brodine SK, Shaffer RA, Johnson CW, Cullison TR. The effect of foot structure and range of motion on musculoskeletal overuse injuries. Am J Sports Med 1999; 27:585-593.

22 Messier SP, Edwards DG, Martin DF, et al. Etiology of iliotibial band friction syndrome in distance runners. Med Sci Sports Exerc 1995; 27:951-960.

23 Fredericson M, Dowdell BC, Oestreicher N, et al. Correlation between decreased strength in hip and iliotibial band syndrome in runners. Arch Phys Med Rehabil 1997; 78:1031.

24 Ulkar B, Yildiz Y, Kunduracioglu B. Meralgia paresthetica: a long-standing performance-limiting cause of anterior thigh pain in a soccer player. Am J Sports Med 2003; 31:787-789.

25 Genitsaris M, Goulimaris I, Sikas N. Laparoscopic repair of groin pain in athletes. Am J Sports Med 2004; 32:1238-1242.

26 Matheson GO, Clement DB, McKenzie DC, Taunton JE, Lloyd-Smith DR, MacIntyre JG. Stress fractures in athletes: A study of 320 cases. Am J Sports Med 1987; 15:46-58.

27 Crowninshield RD, Johnston RC, Andrews JG, Brand RA. A biomechanical investigation of the human hip. J Biomech, 1978. 11: p. 75-85.

28 Hulkko A, Orava S. Stress fractures in athletes. J Sports Med 1987; 8:221-226.

29 Johnson AW, Weiss CB Jr, Wheeler DL. Stress fractures of the femoral shaft in athletes – more common than expected. A new clinical test. A J Sports Med 1994; 22:248-256.

30 Boden BP, Osbahr DC, Jimenez C. Low-risk stress fractures. Am J Sports Med 2001; 29:100-111.

31 McBryde AM Jr. Stress fractures in athletes. J Sports Med 1975; 3:212-217.

32 Barrow GW, Saha S. Menstrual irregularity and stress fractures in collegiate female distance runners. Am J Sports Med 1988; 16:209-216.

33 Johansson C, Ekenman I, Tornkvist H, Eriksson E. Stress fractures of the femoral neck in athletes. The consequence of a delay in diagnosis. Am J Sports Med 1990; 18:524-528.

CHAPTER 31

Knee Injuries

Peter Gerbino and Jason Nielson

INTRODUCTION

Injuries to the knee occur from single macrotrauma, repetitive microtrauma or from a relatively minor event following microtrauma. The setting in which the injury occurs and the history of the problem can accurately predict the diagnosis in most cases. Physical examination for knee injuries is injury-specific and does not always require imaging studies. Treatment and rehabilitation are constantly evolving with newer strategies employing anatomic repair, relative rest rather than absolute rest and earlier motion and return to activity.

TRAUMATIC KNEE INJURIES

Anterior cruciate ligament injury

Box 31.1: Key Points

- Reconstruction, rather than repair, is required for the symptomatic ACL tear.
- No single graft type is best for all patients.
- Young athletes need functional ACLs, but the physes must be protected.

Pathophysiology

The anterior cruciate ligament (ACL) is an internal knee ligament essential for tibio-femoral stability. After the medial collateral ligament, it is the second most commonly injured knee ligament.[1] Its primary function is to limit anterior tibial translation. It is a secondary restraint for varus and valgus stresses and internal and external rotation.

The ACL is torn during one of five circumstances: (1) sudden deceleration with strong quadriceps contraction, (2) valgus deceleration to a flexed externally rotated knee when the foot is securely fixed to the surface, (3) hyperextension of the knee, (4) hyperflexion of the knee and (5) direct valgus force to the knee.

The incidence of ACL tears is 31 in 100 000 annually.[2] Some 90% of tears occur in patients aged 15–45 years. A total of 70% of injuries are sports related[3] resulting form jumping, cutting, sudden stops or direct blows to the knee. Females playing basketball, volleyball or soccer have been found to have ACL tears at frequencies up to four times that of male counterparts.[4] Theories as to why females have more injuries include size of femoral intercondylar notch width[5,6] prior conditioning[7,8] female valgus landing pattern[9,10] hormonal influences[11] and ligament size.[4]

Diagnosis

The classic description of an ACL tear is hearing and feeling a 'pop' followed by rapid knee hemarthrosis within in 2–6 h. The athlete can rarely continue playing. A partial ACL tear will have a less dramatic presentation and an athlete with a chronic tear can have 'giving way' episodes without a 'pop' or swelling. A history of giving way or a sensation of the knee shifting is consistent with chronic ACL insufficiency.

Physical examination of the patient with acute ACL tear is both sensitive and specific.[12] The Lachman test evaluates anterior tibial translation upon the femur with the knee in 30° of flexion and the muscles relaxed. A Lachman test should always be performed on the contralateral side for comparison. Different translation of one side compared with the other side is indicative of ACL injury. More than 5 mm difference is considered to indicate complete ACL incompetence. The pivot shift test takes a fully extended knee (if the ACL is torn, the tibia subluxates anteriorly in this position) and stresses it in valgus with gradual flexion. A sudden shift, as the tibia reduces to the femur, indicates ACL and posterolateral laxity.

Imaging for ACL assessment consists of plain radiographs and MRI. Plain radiographs will show soft tissue swelling, but may show tibial spine avulsion (more common in the juvenile ACL injury) or a lateral capsular avulsion fracture (Segond fracture), that has been found to correlate with ACL tears. The MRI will show the ACL tear as well as associated bone bruises, meniscal injuries and collateral ligament tears (Fig. 31.1).

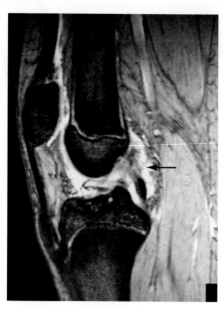

Figure 31.1 Anterior cruciate ligament (ACL) tear. Tear of the anterior cruciate ligament on sagittal T2-weighted MRI image. The normal linear structure of the ACL is not seen.

Treatment

The natural history of a torn ACL is that the ligament does not heal. Most athletic individuals will develop instability with sports and some will develop instability with activities of daily living. Further giving way episodes lead to osteoarthritis and meniscal tears.[13] Meniscal tears associated with ACL tears have a poor prognosis if repair is not accompanied by ACL reconstruction.

Initial treatment of ACL tears consists of rest, ice, compression and elevation of the knee. Immobilization with crutch walking may be needed for pain relief. Arthrocentesis is needed if hemarthrosis is particularly painful. Prolonged immobilization is discouraged and early range of motion and weight bearing help restore function.

Definitive treatment is either operative or non-operative. If there is giving way or meniscal injury requiring repair, operative reconstruction is recommended. Absent those findings, a stable knee can be evaluated for possible nonoperative care. These patients are sent to physical therapy for quadriceps and hamstring strengthening. Bracing has not been found to prevent recurrence, but is frequently preferred by patients and clinicians.

If there is a repairable meniscal tear, giving way or if the injury occurs in a high-demand athlete, reconstruction is recommended. Repair, as opposed to reconstruction, has not been successful.[14] The type of reconstruction depends upon the patient's age, activity level, associated injuries, history of other knee problems and surgeon's preference. In general, patella tendon autograft, hamstring autograft and tissue bank tendon allograft are used. All are successful and choice depends more on surgeon's experience and patient's preference, rather then improved outcome studies. Protecting the physis in the young athlete is of major concern and techniques exist to either remain completely extraphyseal or to place the graft transphyseal with only soft tissue interfacing the physis.

Posterior cruciate ligament injury

> ### Box 31.2: Key Points
>
> - PCL tears are frequently treated non-operatively.
> - PCL tears with bone avulsions should be repaired.
> - Ligament reconstruction is similar to ACL reconstruction.

Pathophysiology

PCL injuries account for 5–20% of all knee ligament injuries.[15] The PCL is an intra-articular structure and the primary stabilizer for posterior tibial translation. It is also a secondary static stabilizer for external rotation of the tibia.

The PCL is commonly injured when the knee is in flexion and a posterior force is applied to the tibia such as a dashboard injury or fall on a flexed knee. Another mode of injury is hyperextension with rotation on a planted foot. PCL injuries often occur with other injures such as meniscal and ACL tears.

The natural history of a symptomatic PCL deficient knee includes progressive pain and degeneration of the patellofemoral joint and the medial compartment. The level of patient satisfaction appears to be related to the ability of the quadriceps muscle to dynamically stabilize the knee. Parloie and Bergfield reported that the key to return to the previous activity level was dependent on the recovery of the quadriceps mechanism.[16] Current recommendations are to reconstruct PCL tears with >10 mm posterior translation.[17]

Diagnosis

The athlete often gives a history of falling on a flexed knee or sustaining a posteriorly directed force on the proximal tibia. Occasionally a pop is heard. Swelling after injury is variable secondary to concomitant tearing of the posterior capsule which dissipates the hemarthrosis. Some athletes will complain of giving way, but more often, there is no instability.

Examination may reveal an anterior tibial contusion and popliteal ecchymosis. Absence of the normal anterior tibial prominence and increased posterior tibial subluxation indicate PCL incompetence. A positive posterior drawer test is diagnostic for PCL tear. Other tests that can confirm the diagnosis are the posterior sag test, reverse pivot shift and quad active test.

A standard 4-view knee series including AP, lateral, tunnel and sunrise views should be obtained to rule out osseous pathology and avulsion injuries. MR imaging has been shown to be very specific and sensitive for PCL injury (Fig. 31.2).[18]

Treatment

Treatment of an acute PCL tear is similar to that of an ACL injury. Initially rest, ice and compression for resolution of swelling are initiated. Restoration of range of motion follows after the acute phase. Final treatment is directed toward restoration of knee motor control.

Non-operative treatment is indicated for athletes without symptomatic instability with activities. Rehabilitation in this setting includes isometric quadriceps exercises. Early hamstring strengthening is avoided to decrease subsequent

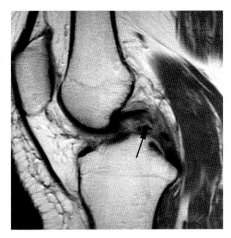

Figure 31.2 Posterior cruciate ligament tear. A sagittal MRI image of a mid-substance tear of the posterior cruciate ligament.

posterior laxity. Therapy includes early range of motion (especially extension) and quadriceps strengthening. Care is taken to avoid high loads with extension exercises to avoid high patello-femoral joint reactive forces. Closed chain exercises are used for all muscle groups, except for the hamstrings, which should be strengthened with open chain exercises. A functional PCL brace can be used for higher level activities, but this is somewhat controversial.[19]

Indications for operative treatment include bony avulsion fractures, combined ligament injuries and chronic symptomatic posterior knee instability with >10 mm posterior translation.[17,19] Surgical treatment is intended to prevent giving way and delay and or prevent long-term degenerative changes. Primary repair of avulsion injuries can result in excellent stability and function.[20]

Reconstruction typically uses auto or allograft. Special care must be taken to avoid injury to the neurovascular popliteal structures at the tibial insertion site. Techniques to avoid acute angles in the graft (tibial onlay technique) and provide better biomechanical function (double-bundle technique) continue to evolve. Knee flexion is limited in the immediate postoperative period because there is increased PCL strain with knee flexion.[21] Continuous passive motion and static quad exercises can be started early. The acute rehabilitation phase uses passive gravity assistive flexion exercises and closed chain quadriceps strengthening. During the recovery phase, avoidance of flexion past 90° until 6 weeks avoids increased strain to the graft. The functional phase of rehabilitation includes returning to full activities at 9–12 months, with full range of motion and equal strength.

Patella dislocation
Pathophysiology
Acute patella dislocation is a common injury. This occurs from a direct blow or with a valgus, external rotational force to the lower extremity. The patella dislocates in a lateral direction with osteochondral injury to the medial patellar facet, lateral femoral condyle or both in as many as 40% of

patients.[22–25] With a lateral dislocation, the medial retinaculum and patello-femoral ligaments are torn.

The true incidence of patella dislocation is difficult to determine, but has been reported to be as high as 31 of 100 000 patients. Females tend to have a higher risk in the second decade and males in the third decade of life.[26]

There appear to be two unique subsets of patients with patella dislocation. In patients with normal ligamentous stability, a truly traumatic event is needed to dislocate the patella. In this situation, the increased force required to dislocate the patella and subsequent relocation of the patella will cause greater internal derangement. The second group has constitutional ligamentous laxity. In this group, trivial trauma or activities of daily living can cause patella dislocation.

Diagnosis
The typical history of athletes with an acute patella dislocation is that of pivoting with the upper body on a planted foot. Patients report that the 'knee' is dislocated with a prominence on the lateral side. In the case where the knee remains flexed, the patella will remain laterally dislocated. Often a rapid and sizeable hemarthrosis will develop. The physician routinely sees this injury a few days after the traumatic event following spontaneous relocation and the diagnosis of patella dislocation is inferred. Patients often present with hemarthrosis, limited range of motion and tenderness to the medial patellar retinaculum. With significant internal injury, the lateral femoral condyle may also be tender.

Physical examination should include evaluation of the medial patellar restraints and patellar alignment. Thorough examination should detect focal areas of maximal tenderness and presence of a medial retinacular defect or tender area. A classic finding is apprehension when the knee is in 30° of flexion and a laterally directed force is applied to the patella. Stability of the patella should be determined by evaluating medial retinacular laxity.

Imaging for assessment in acute patellar dislocation should include the routine knee trauma series: AP, lateral, tunnel and sunrise views. Radiographic evaluation is intended to assess patellar alignment and identify osteochondral injuries. The incidence of these injuries based on radiographs ranges from 5–30%. Their incidence based on operative findings ranges from 30–70%.[23,25,27–30] Other series suggest as many as 7 of 10 patients with acute patellar dislocation will have intra-articular injuries not visualized on plain films.[31,32] MR imaging is useful in detecting soft tissue injury such as a torn medial patello-femoral ligament and detecting bone bruising, but is less reliable in detecting osteochondral fractures (Fig. 31.3).[32–34]

Treatment

Initial field treatment of the athlete consists of a thorough knee ligament evaluation. If the athlete can straighten the leg, the patella will spontaneously relocate. If this has not happened, the physician or training staff may need to assist in extending the knee to allow for relocation of the patella.

Definitive treatment of an acute patella dislocation ranges from immobilization to surgical realignment and fracture repair. Non-surgical management consists of knee immobilization for 2–3 weeks to allow healing of the medial soft tissues. Progression to range of motion exercises and strengthening follow the immobilization period. Length of immobilization and onset of therapy is a topic of debate and has not been supported in the literature by a definitive study. Many sports medicine practitioners now use a patella stabilizing brace rather than a classic immobilizer. This allows immediate physical therapy and less quadriceps atrophy.

Operative treatment is used to treat osteochondral injuries and re-establish the correct patello-femoral alignment and stability. Procedures addressing repair of osteochondral fractures range from arthroscopic debridement of cartilage flaps to internal fixation of osteochondral fracture for better congruity. Soft tissue procedures include proximal patellar realignment, reconstruction of the vastus gap, lateral release, medial plication and medial augmentation.

In patients with chronic patella dislocation and patello-femoral ligament deficiency, proximal and/or distal realignment procedures are indicated.[25,33,34] Distal realignment using an Elmslie-Trillat or Fulkerson procedure is performed when there is a large (>20°) Q-angle or with genu-valgum. Severe genu-valgum must be corrected distally to prevent patella instability.

Physical therapy plays a large role in both nonoperative and operative treatment regimens following acute patella dislocation. Structured rehabilitation should include advancing weight bearing as tolerated, regaining active and passive range of motion with closed chain exercises and bracing to medialize the patella. After regaining greater then 80% of the contra-lateral side quadriceps strength, athletes may begin progressive sport specific training. With return of full speed and cutting ability, the athlete is allowed to return to full competition. Although not proved to decrease the rate of re-dislocation,[35] McConnell taping can be used during therapy and return to sports for increased support.[26,36] Many athletes will continue to use patella controlling braces despite successful operative or non-operative treatment.

Knee dislocation

Box 31.4: Key Points

- Knee dislocation has a significant risk for vascular injury.
- A high suspicion of concomitant injuries needs to be maintained with multi-ligamentous injuries.
- Initial evaluation must assess for vascular injury.
- Acute medial collateral ligament (MCL) tears when combined with ACL/PCL injury can be treated with bracing initially.

Pathophysiology

True dislocation of the knee is a severe injury following significant force. If such an event disrupts three of the four major knee ligaments, a frank dislocation occurs and significant functional instability results.[37] The popliteal artery is tethered proximally at Hunter's canal and distally at the soleus arch making it vulnerable to injury. Vascular injury can present a risk of loss of limb. The peroneal nerve is also at risk where it wraps around the fibular head.

Classification of knee dislocation is based on the direction the tibia dislocates[38] with posterior dislocation occurring 70% of the time followed by anterior dislocation.[39] Mechanisms for posterior knee dislocation are a hyperextension injury[40] or a posteriorly directed force such as a dashboard injury.[41] Rotational dislocations are less common. A posterolateral rotational knee dislocation may be irreducible as the medial

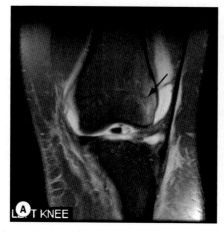
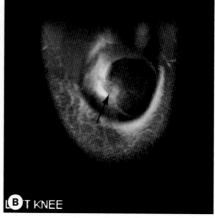

Figure 31.3 Patella dislocation. Even after spontaneous relocation of the patella, evidence can be seen consistent with patellar dislocation. (A) The lateral femoral bone bruise, and (B) the medial patellar facet bone bruise, suggest a recent dislocation. An axial MRI image shows the medial retinacular tear, a medial patellar chondral defect and lateral subluxation of the patella.

femoral condyle can buttonhole through the anterior joint capsule.[42]

The four major ligaments of the knee and the postero-medial and posterolateral corners can be injured. Sisto and Warren found that frank dislocation of the knee occurs with rupture of three of the four major knee ligaments.[37] The incidence of vascular compromise is estimated to be about 32%[43] and higher if limited to solely anterior and posterior dislocations. Peroneal or tibial nerve injuries have a reported incidence of up to 30%.[37,40,44,45] Bony lesions, including avulsion fractures of the ACL or PCL, tibial plateau fractures, or distal femoral condylar fractures have occurred with knee dislocation.

Diagnosis

The acute knee dislocation often reduces prior to presentation, but obvious deformity may be appreciated on examination. Patients with polytrauma who are sedated and intubated may not be fully diagnosed initially. The importance of early recognition of a knee dislocation is to evaluate for popliteal artery injury and observe for delayed vascular compromise.[46]

Examination should focus on vascular status of the leg alone and in comparison to the contralateral extremity. Serial vascular and neurologic examinations should be performed. Vascular compromise longer then 8 hours may require amputation,[43] so a dysvascular knee should be reduced immediately. Normal vascular status does not preclude an intimal tear that could present as dissection or occlusion later.

Imaging for a presumed knee dislocation should include a standard knee trauma series prior to manipulation to confirm direction of dislocation and to plan reduction. After knee reduction, any physical signs of ischemia indicate a vascular injury and require an immediate arteriogram. Doppler examinations and the presence of palpable pulse with capillary refill do not exclude arterial intimal damage.[47] Despite a historical tendency to obtain a screening arteriogram, it has been shown that trauma to the lower extremity with a normal vascular examination has a low incidence of vascular lesions.[48,49] For this reason, dislocations with normal vascular exams need to be followed, but not studied with an arteriogram.

Treatment

Early initial reduction of a knee dislocation is crucial. In-hospital observation is mandatory to evaluate for vascular and neurologic injuries and for compartment syndrome. Absolute acute surgical indications include clinically significant vascular injury, open or irreducible dislocation and signs of compartment syndrome.

Early definitive surgical management of the dislocated knee has been shown to have better results than late reconstruction.[37,39] Most ACL/PCL/MCL injuries are reconstructed at about 4–6 weeks, after healing of the MCL. Combined ACL/PCL/posterolateral corner injuries should be addressed surgically as early as is safely possible. This is usually at 2–3 weeks and early good result have been reported.[50]

Postoperative rehabilitation includes non-weight bearing with the knee in full extension for the first 3–6 weeks. Progressive range of motion is initiated at 6 weeks with gradual return to full weight bearing. Closed chain exercises are used for strengthening. Bracing is discontinued at 6–10 weeks when range of motion and advanced strength training are started. Return to sport occurs after adequate strength and range of motion have been achieved, usually between 6 and 10 months post reconstruction. A loss of 10–15° of terminal flexion can be expected in these severe injuries.[50]

Collateral ligament injuries

> ### Box 31.5: Key Points
>
> - Collateral ligament tears do not usually require operative repair.
> - Lateral collateral ligament (LCL) and posterolateral corner tears require direct repair or reconstruction if a varus thrust results.

Pathophysiology

The collateral ligaments, MCL and LCL, are extra-articular ligaments of the knee. They provide for valgus and varus stability. The MCL is the most commonly injured ligament of the knee.[1]

The MCL is torn during direct valgus or indirect abduction with a valgus or rotational force. Injuries are graded by degree of joint opening with stress testing. Grade I injuries cause opening of less than 5 mm, grade II injuries have an opening of 5–10 mm and grade III injuries open up >10 mm. Contact injuries cause higher-grade injuries.

The LCL is torn much less frequently and unlike the MCL, isolated injuries are uncommon. Posterolateral rotatory instability is a more common cause of lateral instability than is a pure varus deficiency. An injury to the lateral and posterolateral structures is seen frequently with injuries to the ACL. Functional results of ACL reconstruction with an undiagnosed lateral injury are poor.[51] Isolated injuries to the posterolateral corner can occur following forceful hyperflexion of the knee with external rotation.[52,53]

Diagnosis

The classic presentation of a collateral ligament injury often includes an audible 'pop' and complaints of either medial or lateral joint line pain. Often a history of instability or buckling with activities is given. Athletes have difficulty with cutting activities. A sensation of 'giving way' or feeling of instability indicates a high-grade injury. Significant lateral side injuries can have associated peroneal nerve injury.

Physical examination for injured collateral ligaments needs to include evaluation of the cruciates as well as the collateral ligaments. Findings may include tenderness over the collateral ligaments and localized swelling. Joint opening with valgus stress testing in full extension indicates laxity of the MCL and PCL. Valgus laxity at 30° of knee flexion, but not in extension, indicates isolated MCL injury. Varus laxity in full extension indicates LCL and PCL injury. Varus laxity in 30° of knee flexion indicates isolated LCL tear.

Imaging to assess collateral ligament injuries consists of routine trauma knee radiographs. These are usually normal.

Injuries such as tibial plateau fractures, PCL avulsion fractures and tibial spine avulsions can be identified. Bone avulsions from the proximal fibular head or neck may indicate lateral collateral injury. MRI has an accuracy of greater then 90% for identifying individual lateral structures (Fig. 31.4).[54] MRI can also reveal presence of bone bruises and concomitant ACL, PCL or meniscal injuries. Varus or valgus stress radiographs have been used in the immature athlete to test physeal integrity, but MRI has replaced the stress views when physeal status must be assessed.

Treatment

Initial treatment of acute collateral injuries includes rest, ice, compression and extremity elevation (RICE). Higher-grade injuries may require bracing and crutches for pain management. Range of motion of the brace should be increased as tolerated to avoid development of arthrofibrosis.

Physical therapy is the mainstay of treatment for grades I and II MCL and LCL injuries. During the acute phase, rehabilitation should be focused on regaining range of motion and minimizing quadriceps atrophy.[55] Gentle knee flexion exercises with stretching, electrical stimulation and anti-inflammatorydrugs can be helpful in edema reduction and atrophy prevention.

During the recovery phase, aerobic exercises are begun. Conditioning can be maintained through cycling, swimming with gentle leg kicks and upper body ergometric exercises. Exercise in multiple planes is begun with functional return to sport-specific activities. Both open and closed chain exercises can be utilized. Return to sports after low-grade injuries is usually 3–4 weeks, but higher-grade injuries require about 8–12 weeks.[56]

Isolated grade III MCL injures can also be treated nonoperatively due to their high rate of healing.[55,57,58] If there are concomitant injuries that are not surgically corrected, the MCL has a higher failure rate.[54,59,60] Grade III isolated LCL and posterolateral injuries do not fare as well treated nonoperatively.[54,59,60] This is especially true in patients with genu varum in whom a varus thrust may develop. Surgical repair is

needed in this setting and results are better if repair occurs within the first 2 weeks.[54]

Meniscal injury

Box 31.6: Key Points

- A locked knee with a bucket handle meniscus tear should have meniscus reduction and repair as soon as possible.
- Younger and more vascular menisci heal better than older, more complex and less vascular tears.

Pathophysiology

The meniscus was once thought to be an unimportant intra-articular structure of the knee. It is now known to play an important role in chondral protection, lubrication and stability of the knee.[61] The menisci are composed of fibrous cartilage in a semi-lunar shape. They have strong, thick peripheral attachments and are thin centrally. The medial meniscus has firm attachments to the MCL and capsule. In contrast, the lateral meniscus is more mobile, does not attach to the corresponding collateral ligament and has a posterolateral hiatus for the popliteus tendon. The greater tethering of the medial meniscus is thought to be the underlying reason for increased medial meniscal injury.[62] Lack of chondral protection caused by a resected or deformed meniscus has been shown to cause degenerative changes in the long term.[63]

The incidence of meniscal tears is up to 61 per 100 000.[64] Cadaveric studies have shown a 60% prevalence of degenerative meniscal tears.[65] Meniscal tears are classified by their overall shape, complexity, location and their plane of rupture. In addition, tears are classified either as complete or partial. Frequent mechanisms of injury include weight bearing in slight flexion while sustaining a bending or rotational force to the distal extremity. Younger patients tend to have an increased rate of vertical tears, i.e. bucket handle tears, which commonly originate at the posterior horn of the meniscus.[66,67] Older patients tend to have more degenerative meniscal tears, usually horizontal and complex in their cleavage planes.[68] With acute ACL injury, the lateral meniscus is more commonly injured and with chronic ACL deficiency, the medial meniscus is injured. This is thought to occur because of the medial meniscus' role as a secondary posterior stabilizer of the tibia.[69,70]

Diagnosis

The history should include mechanism of injury, leg position at time of injury, and immediate symptoms after injury. Some 30–40% of meniscal injuries occur in athletic competition with greater then 80% of individuals able to recall a specific mechanism of injury.[71,72] Often acute onset of sharp pain follows a twisting injury. A 'pop' or a snap may be heard. Symptoms of catching or locking suggest meniscal injury. Patients are often able to localize their symptoms to a specific area of the knee. Swelling may occur, but typically it is delayed 8–24 h after injury. Activities such as deep knee bending and twisting may be painful. Degenerative meniscal tears do not classically

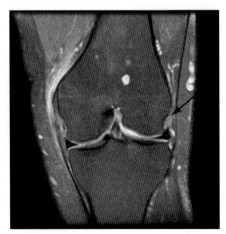

Figure 31.4 Lateral collateral ligament tear. A coronal MRI image of the lateral collateral ligament with surrounding edema at the proximal insertion of the femur.

present with a history of trauma. They cause symptoms of pain, swelling and sometimes locking with daily activities.

Physical examination for detection of meniscal injury has been reported to be about 70% accurate.[73] An antalgic gait with an altered stance phase may be noted. Mild effusions are common in the acute setting after athletic injury or with chronic meniscal injury. Quadriceps atrophy may be found within a few weeks of injury. Joint line tenderness is suggestive of meniscal injury. Lack of full extension and pain with a provocative extension 'bounce test' and provocative hyperflexion suggest displaced meniscal tear. Other provocative maneuvers include the McMurray test and the Apley compression test.

Some athletes will present with a locked knee or a 'pseudo locked' knee. A displaced bucket handle tear can cause mechanical locking of the knee, preventing full extension. A locked meniscus needs to be reduced if possible and should be repaired within the first 2 weeks of injury. After injury, the hamstrings can go into spasm and cause a 'pseudolocking' of the knee without a true mechanical extension block. As with any knee injury, the stability of the cruciates and collateral ligaments should be assessed.

Imaging for meniscal injury should include a plain radiograph. AP, lateral, tunnel and sunrise radiographs will help evaluate for degenerative changes, loose bodies, osteochondral injury and fracture. MRI has become the diagnostic test of choice, with an accuracy of 93–98% for medial tears and 90–96% for lateral tears.[74,75] When using arthroscopy as the 'gold standard', the sensitivity of MRI varies from 64% to 95% with an accuracy of 83–93% (Fig. 31.5).[76] This accuracy has been reported to be lower with younger athletes with lateral meniscal pathology.[77]

Treatment

Initial treatment of a locked knee secondary to a displaced meniscal tear should be considered urgent, requiring expedited reduction and treatment. In any other situation, the initial treatment consists of rest, ice, compression and elevation. Crutch weight bearing may be needed acutely, but patients can be allowed to weight bear as tolerated with temporary splinting for comfort. Knee flexion beyond 90° can increase pain or cause a reduced tear to displace.

The natural history of meniscal injury depends on the location and healing potential of the meniscus. Vascular supply is vital for healing of meniscal tears[78] and is determined by the location of the tear. The 'white-white' zone, located within the inner third of the meniscus, has a poor vascular supply and poor healing potential. Symptomatic tears in this zone benefit from partial meniscectomy. The 'red-white' zone has a functional blood supply at the periphery, but the inner portion is avascular. These tears have a healing potential based on the initial injury response, vascular infiltration and a fibrin scaffold evolving into fibro-cartilage.[78] 'Red-white' tears can be repaired if the meniscus is not degenerated and the tear pattern is amenable to repair. Often in the adult patient, a partial meniscectomy is performed. In young athletes, a repair is always preferred. Tears of the 'red-red' zone involve the junction of the capsule and meniscus and have a good blood supply on each side of the tear. These tears have

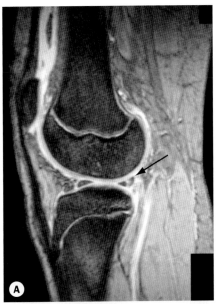

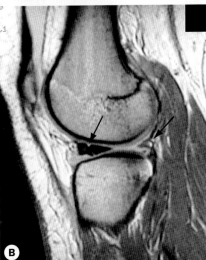

Figure 31.5 (A) This MRI image demonstrates a tear of the posterior horn of the lateral meniscus (arrow) in a patient with associated ACL tear. This meniscal tear was subsequently repaired at time of ACL reconstruction. (B) MRI image of the medial compartment of the knee. This sagittal image demonstrates a tear of the medial meniscus (arrows). This tear was clinically significant and was subsequently débrided.

the best healing potential and should routinely be repaired in all patients.

Small, stable meniscal tears are amenable to meniscal trephination and synovial abrasion to enhance the blood supply and healing potential. Larger complex and unstable tears with degeneration of the meniscus are candidates for partial meniscectomy. Optimal tears for repair include peripheral vertical tears within a few millimeters of the capsule and those secondary to acute trauma in a young, active athlete.[79,80]

Rehabilitation after meniscal injury is dependent on mode of treatment. Physical therapy following non-surgical treatment of stable meniscal tears can produce a gradual decrease in symptoms and return to activities in 6 weeks and normal function at 3 months.[81] Persistent symptomatic meniscal tears should be referred for appropriate surgical treatment.

Rehabilitation protocols after non-operative treatment and partial meniscectomy are similar. Crutches are used to unload the affected extremity and are discontinued when a pain free gait is achieved.[82] Initial treatment includes reduction of pain and swelling while increasing the range of motion and improving muscle strength.[83] Straight leg raises with adjunctive electrical stimulation can retard muscle atrophy. Aerobic exercises begin after the athlete tolerates stationary cycling or water jogging. Later modalities include closed and open chain strengthening exercises in the sagittal, coronal and transverse planes. This is done in coordination with stretching of the lower extremity. More sport specific activities follow with proprioceptive and plyometric training as the athlete returns to full activities. The ability to single leg hop, 80% return of quadriceps strength, and painless full range of motion of the knee are useful guides for readiness of an athlete to return to competition.[10] Bracing is not necessary.

Therapy protocols after meniscal repair often include a period of touch-down weight bearing, usually 4–6 weeks. In addition, hinged knee braces are used to limit the range of motion to minimize stresses on the repaired meniscus. Limitations of range of motion are often 0–40° initially with gradual increases. After this initial phase, therapy is similar to that of a partial meniscectomy.

Quadriceps tendon rupture

Box 31.7: Key Points

- Quadriceps tendon ruptures occur in older males.
- A defect and extensor lag are found.
- A strong repair and specific physical therapy yield the best outcome.

Pathophysiology

A total of 88% of quadriceps ruptures occur in patients 40 years of age or older.[84] Several pre-existing conditions increase the risk of quadriceps rupture including systemic lupus erythematosus, rheumatoid arthritis and diabetes.[85–88] The use of performance enhancing steroids has also been associated with a higher risk of quadriceps tendon rupture.[89]

The mechanism of quadriceps tendon tear is a deceleration event with the knee in partial flexion and a strong concentric quadriceps contraction against a planted lower extremity. Tears begin in the rectus femoris muscle and propagate medially and laterally. Patients often feel a sudden tear or a pop.

Diagnosis

Inability to extend the knee is typical. Athletes are usually unable to continue play. If play can be continued, a partial quadriceps tear has occurred. A rapid and large hemarthrosis is common.

There will be an effusion and a limited range of motion. A palpable defect in the quadriceps tendon is frequently found. Extensor strength is greatly decreased, but even with complete tears, some extension might be possible if the medial and lateral retinaculae remain intact. This has led to a reported rate of misdiagnosis of up to 38%.[84] Imaging of the knee should

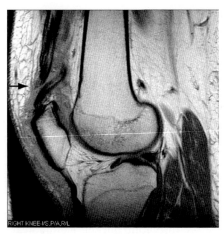

Figure 31.6 Rupture. A sagittal MRI image of the quadriceps tendon showing the discontinuity and subsequent patella infera.

include the standard trauma series and might reveal an avulsion fracture of the superior pole of the patella (Fig. 31.6). Patella infera can also be seen as there is less tension in the extensor mechanism.

Treatment

Initial treatment includes immobilization and modalities to decrease swelling such as rest, ice, compression and extremity elevation. Partial tears of the quadriceps tendon may be treated non-operatively. The knee is immobilized in extension for 4–6 weeks. Gradual progressive flexion exercises and quadriceps strengthening exercises are begun. Closed chain quadriceps exercises and straight leg lifts are the main strengthening exercises.

Treatment of complete quadriceps rupture is operative. The quadriceps mechanism has three layers and repair of the tendon should include all three. Strong non-absorbable sutures with suture anchors or patella drill holes are used. Care must be taken to repair the medial and lateral retinaculae along with the tendon to decrease postoperative extensor lag and diminution of strength. Chronic or late presenting quadriceps ruptures often require augmentation of the tendon secondary to contraction of the patellar tendon distally and contraction of the quadriceps proximally. Postoperative rehabilitation is dependent on stability of repair. Usually a short period of immobilization in extension is followed by gentle and gradual range of motion exercises. At 10–12 weeks strengthening exercises are started.

Patellar tendon rupture

Box 31.8: Key Points

- Patellar tendon ruptures occur in young athletes.
- Patellar tendinosis precedes rupture.
- Repair with heavy suture through bone tunnels in the patella.

Pathophysiology

Patellar tendon rupture is an uncommon injury and occurs in a younger population; 80% occur in patients younger then 40 years of age.[84] The distal pole of the patella is a common site of tendonitis, especially in athletes involved in jumping sports such as basketball and volleyball. Rupture often occurs at a later stage of tendinosis.[90] It has been reported that healthy tendons do not rupture.[91,92] One study found that nearly 100% of the histologic specimens of ruptured tendons had pre-existing damage.[92] The hypothesis is that repetitive jumping leads to microscopic damage. Over time, degenerative changes accumulate leaving a residual region of avascular tissue (tendinosis). Finally, the tendon fails.

Patellar tendon ruptures are usually complete (in contrast to quadriceps tendon ruptures). The mechanism of injury is similar to that of quadriceps tendon ruptures. A quadriceps contraction with eccentric loading of the lower extremity is the usual mode of failure, but concentric contraction loads can also cause rupture.

Diagnosis

Athletes usually feel a 'snap' or a 'pop'. Examination shows an effusion, lack of active extension, superior position of the patella and a palpable defect. Because of the superficial position of the patellar tendon, this injury is less frequently misdiagnosed than is a quadriceps tear. The patient is either unable to perform a straight leg raise or has a significant extensor lag.

The standard AP, lateral, tunnel and sunrise radiograph series is obtained. Patella alta is noted and avulsion fractures of the inferior pole of the patella can be appreciated, if present. MR imaging has been found to be extremely accurate in diagnosing partial or complete patellar tendon tears.[93] In the young athlete, a patella sleeve fracture can occur where the distal pole and articular surface pull free with the tendon.

Treatment

Initial treatment of patellar tendon ruptures is similar to that for quadriceps tendon ruptures and includes rest, immobilization, ice, and extremity elevation. Partial tears with no patella alta may be treated non-operatively with the knee immobilized in extension for 3–6 weeks. Gradual range of motion is then started.

Complete tears of the patellar tendon are repaired operatively. Early repairs have been found to have better results.[89] Non-absorbable sutures are used to re-approximate mid-substance tears. Avulsions off the inferior pole of the patella are repaired with heavy suture through bony tunnels in the patella. Repair of the patella retinaculum is important. Added re-enforcement, if needed, can be obtained with a heavy suture or wire, securing the patella to the tibial tubercle. It is important to take pre-operative lateral radiographs of the contralateral knee to ensure that patella alta or infera is not created with the repair.

The postoperative rehabilitation plan depends on the stability of the repair. An initial phase of immobilization is often followed by gentle range of motion exercises. Strengthening of the quadriceps mechanism begins at 10–12 weeks. Residual extensor mechanism weakness and extensor lag are the most common complications.

Acute articular cartilage injury

Box 31.9: Key Points

- Acute chondral and osteochondral injury can lead to osteoarthritis.
- Osteochondral fragments can be directly repaired, but chondral lesions are treated with microfracture, grafting or ACI.
- Restoration of articular surfaces requires joint motion with little compressive force on the repair.

Pathophysiology

Acute chondral injury occurs from direct trauma, patella dislocation, cruciate ligament tear or meniscal tear. Articular cartilage functions to provide a smooth gliding surface that minimizes friction and stress to the underlying subchondral bone. Historically, articular cartilage lesions have been classified with the Outerbridge system.[94] Grade I lesions have softening and swelling of the cartilage. Grade II lesions have fissures and fibrillation of the surface <1.25 cm in diameter. Grade III have more extensive fissuring >1.25 cm in diameter and are often referred to as having a 'crab-meat' appearance. Grade IV lesions have exposed subchondral bone.

Because of its lack of blood supply, articular cartilage healing potential is limited. Acute injury to the articular surface can be in the form of a focal chondral or osteochondral lesion. Partial thickness lesions do not heal.[95] Despite this, not all articular lesions are symptomatic. Full thickness cartilage lesions that penetrate the subchondral bone may regenerate fibrocartilage through mesenchymal cells differentiating into chondrocytes. This reparative cartilage has mechanical properties that are inferior to hyaline cartilage.

Diagnosis

Patients usually have pain with weight bearing. An effusion may be present if the subchondral bone is fractured. There may be a history of patella dislocation or other major knee injury. If there is a loose body, there may be a history of locking.

Examination of the knee includes an overall assessment for limb alignment, range of motion, the presence of an effusion and ligamentous stability. Radiographic evaluations include AP, lateral, tunnel and sunrise view. The presence of sclerosis, subchondral cysts and osteophytes are consistent with osteoarthritis. Loose bodies with a bony component can be seen radiographically. MRI images tend to underestimate the extent of cartilage lesions, but are helpful if a free cartilaginous body is present. Underlying bone bruises can also be noted, but the significance of them and their progression to further structural damage and cartilage lesions is not known.

Treatment

Operative treatment can be simple arthroscopic debridement with lavage. This is the first line option for patients with mechanical symptoms and a small lesion. This includes debridement of any loose or unstable cartilage flaps. Unstable patellae are stabilized. Any meniscal or ligament tear needs to be corrected. If the focal defect is located in a compartment that is overloaded, an osteotomy will unload that area to decrease future wear, changing the malalignment. An osteochondral fracture should be securely repaired.

Marrow stimulation techniques such as micro fracture or drilling of a defect allow reparative cartilage to form in the defect through vascular pores providing mesenchymal stem cells.[96] This does not preclude further operative treatment if necessary. For large lesions (1–2 cm), autologous transplant of osteochondral plugs[97] can be transferred from an area of decreased weight bearing to fill the lesion.[98] Autogenous chondrocyte implantation (ACI)[97] is also used in larger lesions. This is a two stage procedure and involves culturing chondrocytes from a previous biopsy and transplanting them to the defect under a periosteal patch. Fresh allograft transplants of cadaver osteochondral graft can be transplanted into the lesion and stabilized with internal fixation.[97]

Postoperative therapy protocols for micro fracture include modification of weight bearing and early range of motion, with some recommending use of continuous passive motion in the acute postoperative setting. An unloading brace for the affected compartment can decrease symptoms and lessen the forces on the healing defect. Allograft and autograft transplants also rely on early range of motion and gradual weight bearing. ACI protocols include continuous passive motion 6–8 h/day for the first 6 weeks. Strengthening of the quadriceps and hamstrings with short closed chain exercises begins at 6 weeks. Further therapy involves increasing the arc of motion and increasing resistance. Return to full sporting activities may be postponed for up to 1 year for moderate lesions and 18 months for larger lesions.

EXTENSOR MECHANISM OVERUSE INJURIES

Patello-femoral syndrome

Box 31.10: Key Points

- Patello-femoral syndrome is pain from the patella subchondral bone.
- Increased JRFs causes pain and decreasing JRFs relieves pain.
- Altering patello-femoral JRFs involves strengthening the quadriceps, and realigning the patella by nonoperative or operative means.

Pathophysiology

Patello-femoral syndrome (PFS) is a 'wastebasket' term used to describe many types of anterior knee pain. The most useful way to approach anterior knee pain is to isolate the painful structure or structures and treat each as needed. Toward that end, we define patello-femoral syndrome as anterior knee pain arising in the patellar subchondral bone.[99] The pain arises (presumably) from increased joint reactive forces (JRF) caused by

increased activity (normal patellar tracking), by excessive lateral tilt (excessive lateral pressure syndrome, ELPS) or by ELPS combined with lateral subluxation. The precise mechanism by which increased JRFs causes pain is unknown, but may simply be bone deformation.

Diagnosis

It is deceptively easy to diagnose PFS. Any patient in whom anterior-posterior patellar compression causes pain has PFS. This is called the patella compression test or patella grind test. The examiner simply pushes the patella into the trochlea to see if there is pain. Flexing the knee 30° removes the potential confounding variable of suprapatellar synovitis. Physical examination can determine if there is lateral tracking (J-sign) or a tight lateral retinaculum. If the patient becomes apprehensive when the patella is displaced laterally, this indicates possible subluxation or even prior dislocation.

Imaging studies can assist with PFS diagnosis by helping to select among the main causes of PFS. In normal tracking PFS, plain radiographs are normal or show patella alta or infera. The excessive JRF comes from excessive patello-femoral forces alone or from the patello-femoral mismatch caused by the patella alta or infera.

If ELPS has contributed to the increased JRFs and pain, 35° flexion sunrise views will show the lateral tilt. CT and MRI will also be able to show patellar tilt. If lateral subluxation has contributed to abnormal JRFs, patella overhang may be seen on CT or MRI axial views.

Treatment

Patello-femoral syndrome is treated by reducing JRFs on the patella. If the patella tracks centrally, decreasing running and jumping and strengthening the quads with short-arc or straight leg exercises is effective. If there is ELPS, medializing braces,[100] McConnell taping[101] and quad strengthening[102] are effective. Patella subluxation is treated exactly as ELPS unless surgery is required.

When non-operative interventions fail, surgical correction is useful. Patella alta and infera are very difficult to treat surgically as moving the patella proximally or distally without increasing JRFs has not been achieved predictably.

ELPS and patella subluxation can be corrected surgically. If there is tilt without subluxation, most authors recommend arthroscopic lateral retinacular release.[103] If there is subluxation, a medial reef or other medial patello-femoral ligament augmentation procedure is recommended.[104]

Sometimes, PFS is established and true chondromalacia has begun. A tibial tubercle anteriorization (Ferguson modification of the Maquet procedure) is useful. If anteriorization is combined with medialization of the tibial tubercle to correct distally based maltracking, a Fulkerson procedure is recommended.[105]

In all cases of PFS, the pre- and postoperative goals are to decrease JRFs by strengthening the quadriceps, stretching the hamstrings and optimally aligning the patella as necessary.

Patella subluxation

Pathophysiology

Patella subluxation is a common source of anterior knee pain. Subluxation occurs because of previous patella dislocation or as the result of patellar tilt and a deficient medial patello-femoral ligament. It can occur in athletes with well developed lateral quadriceps musculature and less well developed medial quadriceps. Lower limb malalignment can increase lateral patello-femoral pressure and forces that would laterally dislocate the patella. In addition, congenital trochlea dysplasia, patella alta and connective tissue laxity are risk factors for patella subluxation. The patella always subluxates laterally. Medial subluxation can occur after excessive operative medialization.

Diagnosis

Patients with patella subluxation often describe 'giving way' and a feeling of instability with pain at the anterior knee. A history of catching and noisy, painful anterior knee motion is reported. Swelling may occur, but is not typical.

Examination of the patient with patella subluxation may demonstrate abnormal alignment of the lower extremity such as an increased Q angle (angle of the quadriceps tendon to the patella tendon), genu valgum or pes planus deformity. A 'J' sign (lateral movement of the patella as the knee goes into terminal extension) may be noted. If the patient exhibits apprehension when the examiner applies a lateral force to the patella, prior subluxation episodes are probable. Retinacular tenderness should also be noted.[106] Patella alta and increased patellar mobility are common. An effusion, if present, can be from a recent patella subluxation or secondary to articular cartilage damage.

Radiographic evaluation should include standard plain films. A special 35° knee flexion sunrise view (Merchant view) has been recommended to evaluate patello-femoral congruity and assess patellar tilt. CT is useful for evaluation of femoral condyle deficiencies and to assess static patellar tilt. MR imaging is helpful to assess the articular cartilage.

Treatment

Initial non-operative physical therapy is successful for the majority of patients. Medial quadriceps strengthening to decrease lateral patello-femoral forces is the key to a good outcome. Taping[107] and bracing can be helpful in providing a medially directed force on the patella. Orthotics can be helpful with pes planus deformities to improve alignment and diminish the internal knee rotation that accompanies pronation and forces the patella laterally.

When pain is severe and physical therapy and bracing has failed, surgery is indicated. Many procedures exist including releasing the tight lateral retinaculum, plicating the medial structures, re-enforcing the medial patello-femoral ligament and bony procedures to medialize the tibial tubercle. Recently there has been more focus on the medial patello-femoral ligament. Reconstruction and augmentation of this ligament can provide good results in patients with trochlea dysplasia, collagen disorders and failed previous procedures. Lateral retinaculum release is often performed to alleviate lateral forces, but does not address the hypermobility often present in patella subluxation.[108,109] When proximal realignment procedures fail, distal realignment of the patello-femoral joint can be helpful. The Elmslie–Trillat procedure medializes the patella without increasing joint reactive forces. Patients are less prone to developing arthrosis. If arthrosis is already a concern, a Fulkerson type of osteotomy is considered. This procedure medializes and anteriorizes the patella decreasing JRF as well as correcting alignment.

Fat pad syndrome

Pathophysiology

Fat pad irritation or Hoffa's syndrome is a more and more commonly recognized cause of anterior knee pain. It is secondary to impingement and inflammation of the retro-patellar fat pad. Hypertrophy of this tissue can cause pain as it is compressed between the patella and the femoral condyle. This may lead to fat pad inflammation and/or fibrosis. Symptoms can occur after direct trauma, from chronic synovitis or subsequent to surgical intervention in the anterior knee.

Diagnosis

The pain is usually characterized by chronic infrapatellar pain which is aggravated with resisted knee extension activities. Frequently, abnormally large fat pads can be seen on either side of the patellar tendon when the knee is in extension. Examination may demonstrate tenderness with the distal patella tilted posteriorly secondary to the development of fat pad enlargement. If the fat pads are manually pushed into the patello-femoral joint during knee extension, the patient will complain of pain. Increased pain with pressure at the edges of the patellar tendon during extension of a flexed knee is a confirmatory test (Hoffa's test). Quadriceps weakness is also a common finding. Radiographic images are normal. MR images often reveal fibrotic scarring and enlargement[110] of the fat pad that is intimately connected to the anterior menisci.

Treatment

Treatment for fat pad syndrome includes gentle quadriceps stretching and strengthening exercises. Often iontophoresis and massage can help in decreasing symptoms. In cases that do not resolve with non-operative treatment, arthroscopic debridement can remove the fibrotic scar and hypertrophic synovium.[111] Pain relief is often dramatic. Other issues such as a laterally tracking patella are addressed as necessary. Rehabilitation following fat pad resection is to decrease postoperative soreness and restore strength and flexibility. Return to sports can be within 2–4 weeks.

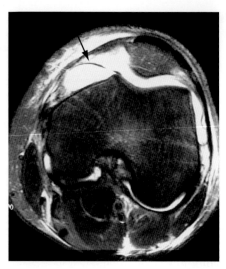

Figure 31.7   Plica syndrome. MRI image of a medial plica. A large hemarthrosis is also present.

Synovial plica syndrome

Box 31.13: Key Points

- Non-pathologic medial plicae are found in many, if not most, patients.
- Direct trauma or lateral patella tracking can cause medial plica thickening and synovitis.
- The nonarticular medial femoral condyle may be more tender than the plica that has been rubbing it.
- Excision is effective treatment.

Pathophysiology

Synovial plicae are the remnants of embryologic partitions within the knee and commonly occur in the suprapatellar, medial and infrapatellar regions of the knee. The medial plica is most common and often bilateral. The plica is attached medially at the proximal aspect of the quadriceps tendon and extends distally past the patella and over the medial femoral condyle where it inserts into the medial fat pad. The majority of knees have some form of a medial plica and most are asymptomatic. Pathologic medial plicae are felt to occur in two circumstances. A direct blow to the medial knee can cause fibrosis and enlargement of a non-pathologic plica. The enlarged plica then rubs along the medial condyle causing inflammation to both the plical synovium and nonarticular medial femoral condyle synovium. A more common occurrence is probably chronic plical rubbing of the medial condyle as a result of a lateral tracking patella. In both cases, the plica may be less tender than the nonarticular medial condyle synovium. Often there is a concomitant cartilage injury along the medial femoral condyle corresponding to chronic irritation by the plica.

Diagnosis

A painful medial plica can cause symptoms during increased patello-femoral activities, prolonged sitting or with direct trauma. Patients complain of medial knee pain and occasionally of snapping with knee flexion. Tenderness is typically found over the medial femoral condyle proximal to the joint line and can often mimic meniscal symptoms.[112,113]

Examination may reveal a snapping sensation with flexion and extension of the knee.[99] The plica can usually be palpated over the medial femoral condyle during flexion and extension of the knee. If inflamed, the plica will be tender. The non-articular medial femoral condyle will also be tender to palpation. Plain radiographs are usually normal in appearance. MR images can detect a plica and rule out other internal derangement (Fig. 31.7).

Treatment

Non-surgical management includes relative rest, ice, anti-inflammatory drugs and physical therapy. If there is a lateral tracking patella, a brace to medialize the patella can help. Iontophoresis has been helpful in improving symptoms. Therapy should include a program of progressive resistance exercises, patellar mobilization, and hamstring, iliotibial band (ITB), quadriceps and gastrocnemius stretching. Strengthening should focus on the vastus medialis oblique muscles. In cases where therapy fails to resolve symptoms, arthroscopic plica resection can be done. Results are routinely good when a careful clinical history and examination lead to the arthroscopic finding of an isolated thickened fibrotic plica.[114]

Patellar tendonitis (tendinosis)

Box 31.14: Key Points

- Most patellar 'tendonitis' is really early micro-tears and tendinosis.
- Quadriceps flexibility and progressive resistance exercises are the principle treatments.
- Excision of the degenerated tissue can relieve pain.

Pathophysiology

Patellar tendonitis occurs at the proximal insertion of the patellar tendon on the patella. It is a misnomer since the primary problem is not inflammatory. The injury is a result of recurrent micro trauma at the inferior patellar pole which has a tenuous blood supply and diminished healing potential. Pathologic specimens have revealed degeneration of the tendon without inflammatory cells (tendinosis). Decreased quadriceps and hamstring flexibility are common risk factors in the development of patellar tendonitis.[115] 'Jumper's knee', the lay term for the condition, is a more accurate name since the damage typically occurs from excessive jumping.

Diagnosis

Patients present with pain during activities requiring knee flexion, jumping or squatting. This is most common in sports requiring significant amount of jumping, such as basketball and volleyball. Pain and tenderness can be localized to the inferior patellar pole. Mild swelling and fusiform fullness can at times be appreciated. Quadriceps and hamstring tightness is a common finding. Standard radiographs are usually normal. MR images reveal areas of tendon degeneration (Fig. 31.8), but MRI has been shown to have a high rate of false positive findings in older patients.[116]

Treatment

Non-surgical treatment consists of anti-inflammatory drugs, rest, stretching and strengthening. Physical therapy should include ultrasound or iontophoresis and progressive eccentric muscle strengthening.[117] Restoration of full flexibility of the extensor mechanism is the most important factor in preventing recurrences. An elastic knee sleeve or patellar tendon strap may be helpful in decreasing symptoms. Good clinical outcomes can be achieved in patients with moderate tendinopathy. Surgical debridement with drilling of the inferior pole of the tendon is reserved for recalcitrant cases. The degenerated tissue is excised and vascular bone channels are created to promote healing at the distal pole of the patella.

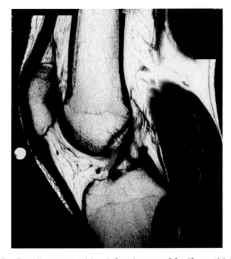

Figure 31.8 Patellar tendonitis. A focal area of fusiform thickening is noted at the proximal aspect of the patellar tendon on this sagittal MRI image. The appearance of these proximal fibers suggests tendinosis.

Iliotibial band syndrome

Box 31.15: Key Points

- ITB syndrome results from overuse of the ITB.
- Tightness, gluteus maximus overuse lead to symptoms.
- Stretching to relieve the tightness and core strengthening to relieve the gluteus maximus of its extra duties are usually curative.
- Operative release is sometimes necessary.

Pathophysiology

Iliotibial band syndrome (ITBS) is an overuse injury in the distance runner. It is the most common cause of lateral knee pain in long-distance runners.[118] ITBS is secondary to excessive friction of the iliotibial band on the lateral femoral epicondyle. The degree of knee flexion with maximum symptoms is at 30 degrees of flexion and is referred to as the 'impingement zone'.[119] Intrinsic factors such as lower extremity malalignment and leg length in equality as well as extrinsic factors such as running surface, shoe wear, training technique and downhill running can cause and worsen symptoms. Other activities requiring excessive knee flexion such as cycling, soccer and football can cause ITBS.

Diagnosis

Patients complain of activity related pain located at the lateral knee. Pain can radiate proximally or distally from the area of maximal discomfort. Symptoms are often absent with rest both before and after activities. Symptoms can be unilateral or bilateral. If unilateral, the symptoms occur on the shorter leg.

Examination of the knee reveals maximal tenderness 2 to 3 cm proximal to the lateral joint line, overlying the lateral epicondyle. A lack of joint effusion with relative maintenance of range of motion is found. Tenderness over the lateral epicondyle and ITB with range of motion of the knee is commonly found. The Ober test, which puts the ITB on stretch, increases the tenderness at the lateral epicondyle. Having the athlete hop with a flexed knee will elicit pain.[120] Evaluation lower extremity alignment is important, especially to evaluate for leg length discrepancy, genu varum and cavovarus foot with forefoot supination and compensatory foot pronation. Radiographic evaluation with plain films is usually negative. MR imaging may show edema at the area of the lateral epicondyle and possibly a thickened bursa deep to the iliotibial band at Gerdy's tubercle.

Treatment

Treatment for iliotibial band syndrome must control the inflammatory process. Use of rest, ice, anti-inflammatory drugs and iontophoresis can be helpful. Non-operative treatment is usually successful. Therapy should include stretching of the iliotibial band (Ober stretch), tensor fascia lata and the hip external rotators. Hip abductor weakness and hamstring flexibility must be addressed. Alterations in training may be very helpful, including changing running surface, direction of running if on an embankment and duration of training sessions.[119] Seat adjustment for cycling can be helpful. Foot orthotics can be useful to correct foot mechanics. Injection of corticosteroids to the bursa can be useful in difficult cases. If non-operative treatment fails, partial surgical release and decompression of the iliotibial band over the areas of maximal symptoms has been shown to be beneficial.[121,122]

Degenerative joint disease of the knee

Box 31.16: Key Points

- DJD of the knee is extremely common.
- Symptoms range from rare pain after excessive exercise to debilitating pain on a daily basis.
- Treatment is aimed at mitigating symptoms.
- Severe disease requires joint replacement.

Pathophysiology

Degenerative joint disease (DJD) or osteoarthritis is one of the most common medical problems of middle-aged and older patients. Symptomatic knee arthritis is present in about 10% of people greater the 65 years of age and has been reported to affect up to 2% of the adult population.[123] The natural history of DJD is progressive joint destruction and pain. The clinical symptoms usually progress slowly over time, with a small portion of patients remaining stable or temporarily improving. The cause of idiopathic osteoarthritis is unknown, but most studies have identified a genetic component to the condition. Osteoarthritis of a joint following trauma is felt to occur because of the primary chondral insult and/or persistent altered joint mechanics.

Diagnosis

The patient complains of chronic waxing and waning knee pain. Morning stiffness and increased pain following activity or with a decrease in barometric pressure are the classic complaints. Swelling after activity is common.

On physical examination, there is diffuse tenderness to palpation at the involved parts of the knee. An effusion may be present. Range of motion is maintained early in the process, but decreases as wear progresses. If an underlying condition such as ACL deficiency is present, signs and symptoms of that condition will be present.

Radiographic evaluation for knee DJD includes a weight bearing AP in 30° knee flexion and lateral views (Fig. 31.9). This shows how much wear has occurred and whether there are loose bodies, osteophytes, cysts or sclerosis. Long film weight bearing radiographs help to determine the mechanical axis and possible need of an osteotomy to alter this axis to unload the effected compartment. MRI is useful in DJD to access the status of degenerative meniscus tears.

Treatment

The goal in treating articular surface lesions is to decrease pain while increasing function and postpone or stop the pro-

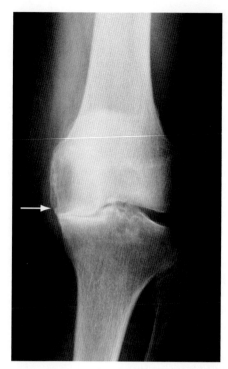

Figure 31.9 Degenerative joint disease. Plain radiographs showing significant medial compartment degenerative changes with relative maintenance of the lateral compartment.

gression of arthritis. Researchers are working to develop a biologic medium to assist the body in resurfacing the joint surface to permanently stop the progression of disease and avoid the invasive resurfacing treatments of the present.[124] Current non-operative treatment is aimed at controlling pain through the use of anti-inflammatory drugs, glucosamine sulfate, chondroitin sulfate, weight loss, increased range of motion and bracing to unload the injured compartment. Corticosteroid injections are helpful in the later progression of cartilage injury, but have limited benefit in the younger athletic population. Synthetic hyaluronic acid injections have recently been used with great success to decrease pain, increase motion and prolong cartilage wear. Physical therapy can be helpful in increasing strength and range of motion and decreasing effusions, but can do little to alter the natural progression and symptoms of cartilage injury. If malalignment is contributing to the symptoms, an unloading brace can be helpful. When the joint is beyond salvage, total joint arthroplasty is performed.

Rehabilitation following treatment is variable. To maintain joint function as the wear progresses, the therapeutic aim is to maintain strength and range of motion. If an arthroscopic procedure has been done to remove loose bodies or a symptomatic meniscal tear, restoration of function is the goal. Following total joint arthroplasty, the goals are to prevent infection and thrombosis first. Next, motion is restored. Finally, strength and function are increased.

Osgood–Schlatter syndrome

> ### Box 31.17: Key Points
>
> - Osgood–Schlatter syndrome is a stress fracture of physeal cartilage.
> - Healing occurs with adequate, pain-free rest.
> - Casting may be necessary to achieve pain-free rest.

Pathophysiology

Osgood–Schlatter syndrome (OSS) is a tibial apophysis stress fracture and is the most common traction apophysitis of the knee in younger athletes. This condition is thought to develop secondary to repetitive microtrauma to the tibial tubercle as the secondary ossification center is forming. OSS is caused by multiple submaximal avulsion fractures through the tibial apophyseal cartilage. These stress fractures are a result of repetitive concentric and eccentric quadriceps contractions and from stresses to an unbalanced, tightened extensor mechanism. Some patients will develop detached bony ossicles in the patellar tendon that can have late and chronic symptoms.[113,125]

Symptoms typically present in adolescent boys around age 13 and adolescent females at 11 or 12 years of age. This condition is activity related and is more common in athletes involved in jumping sports.[126] Symptoms are intermittent and aggravated by jumping, squatting and kneeling. Pain is localized to the inferior patellar tendon and tibial tubercle and is activity related. Pain is increased with direct blows to the anterior knee as well as acceleration and deceleration activities.

Diagnosis

Physical examination can reveal an antalgic gait with fullness of the anterior tibial tubercle. There is no joint effusion. The apophysis is tender with tenderness also at the distal patellar tendon. Tight quadriceps and hamstrings are common and often the process may occur after a rapid growth spurt. Pain is elicited with resisted extension.

Radiographic evaluation is done to rule out other osseous injuries. Plain lateral views may reveal a bony prominence of the tubercle with fragmentation of the apophysis or a free ossicle proximal to the tendon insertion.[113] Radiographic findings of >4 mm of soft tissue swelling, compared with the other unaffected knee, is suggestive of OSS.

Treatment

The symptoms of OSS are usually self-limited, with gradual resolution of pain and swelling over time. Treatment depends on the severity. Mild cases can be treated with activity modification, stretching and mild strengthening exercises. More severe symptoms warrant restriction of activities until symptoms have resolved. This can include use of a knee immobilizer or cylinder cast for 4–6 weeks. Swimming, cycling and other 'relative rest' activities can be implemented to maintain cardiovascular fitness. Therapy consists of modalities to reduce swelling and pain. Quadriceps and hamstring strengthening programs with static progressive resistance exercises should be performed.[127] In rare cases conservative treatment is not successful. Excision of the ossicle with tubercleplasty has been shown to have good results.[113,128]

Sinding–Larsen–Johansson syndrome

> ### Box 31.18: Key Points
>
> - SLJ is a stress fracture of the distal patella pole apophysis from excessive traction.
> - Treatment is exactly the same as for Osgood-Schlatter syndrome.

Pathophysiology

Sinding–Larsen–Johansson syndrome (SLJ), is an overuse traction injury of the distal pole of the patella. Avulsion fractures result from repetitive stress and micro trauma at the insertion of the patella tendon. This can be viewed as a stress fracture between the apophysis of the distal pole of the patella and the rest of the patella. The syndrome commonly affects young adolescent males, ages 9–13 years,[129,130] prior to tibial tubercle ossification. During this process, weakness of the apophysis and bone predisposes to symptoms and findings similar to Osgood–Schlatter syndrome.

Diagnosis

Symptoms include pain at the distal pole of the patella that is aggravated by jumping, running and ascending or descending stairs. Examination reveals limited range of motion with tenderness at the inferior patella pole as well as the proximal patellar tendon. There is pain with resisted extension and a weakened, tight quadriceps. Hamstring tightness is also typically found.

Plain radiographs may reveal ossifications or even a free ossicle at the distal patella pole (Fig. 31.10). The distal pole may be elongated or show fragmentation. Care must be taken to rule out a patellar sleeve fracture or a non-pathologic ossification center.[131] Radiographs can also appear normal due to the cartilaginous nature of the distal patella in this age group.

Treatment

SLJ is usually self-limited with spontaneous resolution of symptoms within 12–18 months. Treatment is similar to that of OSS and includes relative rest, activity modification, and cross training. An overall lower extremity stretching program of the quadriceps, hamstrings and Achilles is helpful utilizing eccentric quadriceps loading exercises.[117] In severe cases, a short period of immobilization can be very helpful prior to the onset of physical therapy. Return to athletic activities is allowed as symptoms decrease. Patients who fail conservative treatment with symptoms that limit function may require surgical removal of ossicles.[128,132]

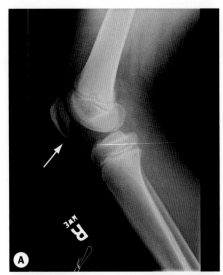

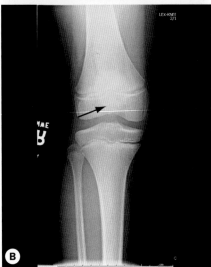

Figure 31.10 (A,B) Sinding–Larsen–Johansson syndrome.

Osteochondritis dissecans

Box 31.19: Key Points

- OCD is a subchondral stress fracture.
- Age is inversely related to healing potential.
- Stopping the insult by decreasing loads on the site decrease symptoms and will frequently allow healing.
- Some lesions must be drilled and/or stabilized before healing begins.

Pathophysiology

Osteochondritis dissecans (OCD) is a non-acute internal derangement of the subchondral bone. The changes in the underlying subchondral bone can manifest as articular softening of the overlying cartilage, articular cartilage separation, partial detachment of the lesion and osteochondral separation forming free bodies.[133] The incidence has been reported to be

4% in all knee X-rays with 29 per 100 000 in males and 18 per 100 000 in females.[134] Bilaterality is reported up 25%.[135] Some 70–80% of OCD lesions occur in the lateral aspect of the medial femoral condyle. Lateral femoral condylar lesions (20%) are usually in the posterior weight bearing region and tend to fare more poorly. The patella is involved about 10% of the time. Lesions occur in the distal half of the patella.[133,136]

The etiology of OCD is unknown. It most likely represents the accumulation of repetitive micro trauma to the subchondral bone in a vulnerable region resulting in stress fractures.[137] The natural history is dependent on multiple factors. Lesions in patients with open growth plates (juvenile OCD) have a greater healing potential[138] with more than 50% of juvenile cases demonstrating healing within 6–18 months of non-operative treatment.[133,139] The outcome in adolescent OCD is unpredictable with about 50% healing and the remainder following the course of lesions in the skeletally mature.[140] In skeletally mature patients (adult OCD), lesions have less healing potential and rarely heal without operative intervention.[133] Many develop radiographic evidence of premature degenerative joint disease.[140]

Diagnosis

Patients often complain of vague knee pain. Stiffness and swelling are common and often activity related. Mechanical symptoms of locking and catching indicate fragment instability. Physical examination may reveal tenderness of the medial femoral condyle with an effusion. Routine radiographs are diagnostic and can show a crater like defect of the subchondral bone. Radiographs should include a tunnel view, which profiles the lesion making it more apparent. Sunrise views are helpful for patellar lesions. MR imaging is sensitive and specific for early changes in OCD lesions.[136,141] MR imaging is now routinely used to stage the lesions with Stage I showing subchondral edema, Stage II showing a fluid interface, but no chondral breech, Stage III showing a 'trap door' chondral breech and Stage IV showing a loose body (Fig. 31.11).

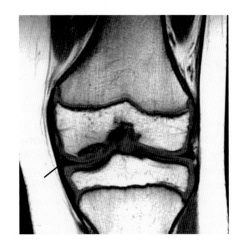

Figure 31.11 Osteochondritis dissecans. A coronal MRI image of an osteochondritis dissecans (OCD) lesion of the medial femoral condyle.

Treatment

The management of OCD is controversial, but should be based on the potential for healing. In stable juvenile lesions, non-surgical management should initially be implemented. Non-operative management will allow healing of most intact, stable OCD lesions before physeal closure. This includes relative rest to achieve a pain free state. Relative rest can mean limiting running and jumping. If this does not cause cessation of symptoms, additional interventions such as crutches or unloader braces can be used. Once pain is gone, progressive return to previous activity levels can be started. Immobilization is controversial, but casting with limited weight bearing is often used with prepubescent patients for 6–8 weeks. As symptoms dissipate, gradual return to weight bearing follows. Follow up examinations every 6–8 weeks are performed until clinical and radiographic healing. Healing is defined as the resolution of symptoms, lack of clinical findings and radiographic evidence of lesion incorporation. Physical therapy consists of non-impact activities such as cycling, swimming and strength training as well as stretching.

In skeletally mature patients or those with unstable or persistent lesions, operative management is indicated. Symptomatic, stable lesions are treated with drilling of the lesion to create vascular channels to enhance the healing process and re-vascularize the subchondral bone. Loose or unstable lesions are treated with repair. Free bodies are often found with unstable lesions. Debridement of the articular surface and excision of the fragment are often necessary in chronic fragmented lesions. After drilling or repair, a short period of immobilization (2–4 weeks) and toe-touch weight bearing is implemented. This is followed with protective weight bearing for up to 12 weeks. A hinged knee brace can be used to limit contact with the lesion by limiting range of motion. Return to full activities can occur at 12 weeks if there has been resolution of symptoms and return of strength. Using an unloader brace to shield the repair may enhance healing and allow earlier return to sports.

OTHER CAUSES OF KNEE PAIN

Most of the time, knee pain arises from acute or subacute injury. It is important to remember that knee pain can also arise from infectious, rheumatologic, neoplastic and referred causes. Detailed discussion of each of these is beyond the scope of this chapter, but each should be considered.

Infection

Septic arthritis is always a concern when there is an acutely painful knee. Even in the event of an acute traumatic event, bacterial seeding of a hemarthrosis is possible. Systemic symptoms include fever and chills. The knee is swollen and painful.

Range of motion is very painful and limited. In general, work-up includes blood cultures, complete blood count, sedimentation rate, C-reactive protein and a lyme titer in endemic regions. Further analysis includes radiographs and aspiration for cell count and cultures. Treatment of septic arthritis is thorough irrigation and debridement and appropriate antibiotic therapy.

Rheumatologic

Rheumatologic diseases are often difficult to diagnose and should be kept in the differential for knee pain that does follow traumatic injury or overuse syndrome. A family history of rheumatologic disease is important as is history of migratory pain and recurrent swelling. The diagnosis and work-up of rheumatologic disease is beyond the scope of this chapter, but in a case of knee pain that does not follow traumatic or overuse, or where several joints are involved, rheumatologic etiologies must be considered.

Neoplastic

Bone tumors usually present as pain with athletic activity. Although a straightforward presentation of PFS or Osgood–Schlatter's does not need imaging studies, any case of persistent pain requires radiographs. Continual pain without a firm diagnosis requires additional imaging and laboratory studies to rule out neoplasm.

Referred knee pain

Pain from the hip or spine can present as knee pain. In the young child, knee pain should always lead to a thorough hip examination. In the older child or adult, sciatica can present as knee pain.

CONCLUSION

There are many causes for knee pain in an athletic population. There are several traumatic injuries, overuse injuries and other sources of knee pain unrelated to sports. The context in which a given injury occurs and the history of the particular injury almost always points to the diagnosis. The physical examination is confirmatory. Imaging studies show specific pathology and help with diagnostic dilemmas.

Treatment of sports related knee injuries is also injury and patient specific. Many of the operative techniques are highly demanding. The physical therapy techniques can also be highly specific and demanding. Combining a skilled operative repair with highly refined physical therapy gets the athlete back to play sooner. Techniques for diagnosis, repair and rehabilitation continue to evolve rapidly.

REFERENCES

1 Linton RC, Indelicato PA. Medial ligament injuries. In: Delee JC, Drez D, eds. Orthopedic sports medicine principles and practice. Philadelphia: WB Saunders; 1994:1261-1274.

2 Daniel DM, Stone ML, Dobson BE, et al. Fate of the ACL-injured patient. A prospective outcome study. Am J Sports Med 1994; 22:632-644.

3 Micheo W, Frontera WR, Amy E, et al. Rehabilitation of the patient with an anterior cruciate ligament injury: a brief review. Bol Assoc Med P R 1995; 87:29-36.

4 Wilk Ke, Arrigo C, Andrews JR, et al. Rehabilitation after anterior cruciate ligament reconstruction in the female athlete. J Athletic Training 1999; 34:177-193.

5 Souryal TO, Freeman TR. Intercondylar notch size and anterior cruciate ligament injuries in athletes. A prospective study. Am J Sports Med 1993; 21:535-539.

6 LaPrade RF, Burnett QM, 2nd. Femoral intercondylar notch stenosis and correlation to anterior cruciate ligament injuries. A prospective study. Am J Sports Med 1994; 22:198-202; discussion 203.

7 Hewett TE, Stroupe AL, Nance TA, et al. Plyometric training in female athletes. Decreased impact forces and increased hamstring torques. Am J Sports Med 1996; 24:765-773.

8 Wojtys EM, Huston LJ, Lindenfeld TN, et al. Association between the menstrual cycle and anterior cruciate ligament injuries in female athletes. Am J Sports Med 1998; 26:614-619.

9 Huston LJ, Wojtys EM. Neuromuscular performance characteristics in elite female athletes. Am J Sports Med 1996; 24:427-436.

10 Urquhart MW, O'Leary JA, Giffin JR, et al. Meniscal injuries. 1. Meniscal injuries in the adult. In: DeLee JC, Drez D, Miller MD, eds. Orthopaedic sports medicine. Principles and practice, 2nd edn. Philadelphia, PA: WB Saunders; 2003:1683.

11 Liu SH, al-Shaikh R, Panossian V, et al. Primary immunolocalization of estrogen and progesterone target cells in the human anterior cruciate ligament. J Orthop Res 1996; 14:526-533.

12 O'Shea KJ, Murphy KP, Heekin RD, et al. The diagnostic accuracy of history, physical examination, and radiographs in the evaluation of traumatic knee disorders. Am J Sports Med 1996; 24:164-167.

13 Sherman MF, Warren RF, Marshall JL, et al. A clinical and radiographical analysis of 127 anterior cruciate insufficient knees. Clin Orthop 1988; 227:229-237.

14 Sherman MF, Lieber L, Bonamo JR, et al. The long-term followup of primary anterior cruciate ligament repair. Defining a rationale for augmentation. Am J Sports Med 1991; 19:243-255.

15 Kannus P, Bergfeld J, Jarvinen M, et al. Injuries to the posterior cruciate ligament of the knee. Sports Med 1991; 12:110-131.

16 Parolie JM, Bergfeld JA. Long-term results of nonoperative treatment of isolated posterior cruciate ligament injuries in the athlete. Am J Sports Med 1986; 14:35-38.

17 Wind WM Jr., Bergfeld JA, Parker RD. Evaluation and treatment of posterior cruciate ligament injuries: revisited. Am J Sports Med 2004; 32:1765-1775.

18 Gross ML, Grover JS, Bassett LW, et al. Magnetic resonance imaging of the posterior cruciate ligament. Clinical use to improve diagnostic accuracy. Am J Sports Med 1992; 20:732-737.

19 St Pierre P, Miller MD. Posterior cruciate ligament injuries. Clin Sports Med 1999; 18:199-221, vii.

20 Burks RT, Schaffer JJ. A simplified approach to the tibial attachment of the posterior cruciate ligament. Clin Orthop 1990:216-219.

21 Arms S, Johnson R, Pope M. Strain measurement of the human posterior cruciate ligament. Trans Orthop Res Soc 1984; 9:355.

22 Grogan DP, Carey TP, Leffers D, et al. Avulsion fractures of the patella. J Pediatr Orthop 1990; 10:721-730.

23 Nietosvaara Y, Aalto K, Kallio PE. Acute patellar dislocation in children: incidence and associated osteochondral fractures. J Pediatr Orthop 1994; 14:513-515.

24 Rovere GD, Adair DM. Medial synovial shelf plica syndrome. Treatment by intraplical steroid injection. Am J Sports Med 1985; 13:382-386.

25 Stanitski CL. Patellar instability in the school age athlete. Instr Course Lect 1998; 47:345-350.

26 Atkin DM, Fithian DC, Marangi KS, et al. Characteristics of patients with primary acute lateral patellar dislocation and their recovery within the first 6 months of injury. Am J Sports Med 2000; 28:472-479.

27 Casteleyn PP, Handelberg F. Arthroscopy in the diagnosis of occult dislocation of the patella. Acta Orthop Belg 1989; 55:381-383.

28 Harilainen A, Myllyen P. Operative treatment in acute patellar dislocation: Radiological predisposing factors, diagnosis and results. Am J Knee Surg 1988; 1:178.

29 Sallay PI, Poggi J, Speer KP, et al. Acute dislocation of the patella. A correlative pathoanatomic study. Am J Sports Med 1996; 24:52-60.

30 Virolainen H, Visuri T, Kuusela T. Acute dislocation of the patella: MR findings. Radiology 1993; 189:243-246.

31 Dainer RD, Barrack RL, Buckley SL, et al. Arthroscopic treatment of acute patellar dislocations. Arthroscopy 1988; 4:267-271.

32 Stanitski CL. Correlation of arthroscopic and clinical examinations with magnetic resonance imaging findings of injured knees in children and adolescents. Am J Sports Med 1998; 26:2-6.

33 Thabit G, 3rd, Micheli LJ. Patellofemoral pain in the pediatric patient. Orthop Clin North Am 1992; 23:567-585.

34 Yates CK, Grana WA. Patellofemoral pain in children. Clin Orthop 1990:36-43.

35 Cherf J, Paulos LE. Bracing for patellar instability. Clin Sports Med 1990; 9:813-821.

36 Fu FH, Stone DA. Sports injuries: Mechanisms, preventions, treatment, 2nd edn. Baltimore: Williams and Wilkins; 2001.

37 Sisto DJ, Warren RF. Complete knee dislocation. A follow-up study of operative treatment. Clin Orthop 1985:94-101.

38 Good L, Johnson RJ. The dislocated knee. J Am Acad Orthop Surg 1995; 3:284-292.

39 Frassica FJ, Sim FH, Staeheli JW, et al. Dislocation of the knee. Clin Orthop 1991:200-205.

40 Kennedy JC. Complete dislocation of the knee joint. J Bone Joint Surg Am 1963; 45:889-904.

41 Roman PD, Hopson CN, Zenni EJ, Jr. Traumatic dislocation of the knee: a report of 30 cases and literature review. Orthop Rev 1987; 16:917-924.

42 Wand JS. A physical sign denoting irreducibility of a dislocated knee. J Bone Joint Surg Br 1989; 71:862.

43 Green NE, Allen BL. Vascular injuries associated with dislocation of the knee. J Bone Joint Surg Am 1977; 59:236-239.

44 Meyers MH, Moore TM, Harvey JP, Jr. Traumatic dislocation of the knee joint. J Bone Joint Surg Am 1975; 57:430-433.

45 Welling RE, Kakkasseril J, Cranley JJ. Complete dislocations of the knee with popliteal vascular injury. J Trauma 1981; 21:450-453.

46 Wascher DC, Dvirnak PC, DeCoster TA. Knee dislocation: initial assessment and implications for treatment. J Orthop Trauma 1997; 11:525-529.

47 Cone JB. Vascular injury associated with fracture-dislocations of the lower extremity. Clin Orthop 1989:30-35.

48 Applebaum R, Yellin AE, Weaver FA, et al. Role of routine arteriography in blunt lower-extremity trauma. Am J Surg 1990; 160:221-224; discussion 224-225.

49 Trieman GS, Yellin AE, Weaver FA, et al. Evaluation of the patient with a knee dislocation: The case for selective arteriography. Arch Surg 1992; 127:1056-1063.

50 Fanelli GC, Giannotti BF, Edson CJ. Arthroscopically assisted combined anterior and posterior cruciate ligament reconstruction. Arthroscopy 1996; 12:5-14.

51 Staubli HU, Birrer S. The popliteus tendon and its fascicles at the popliteal hiatus: gross anatomy and functional arthroscopic evaluation with and without anterior cruciate ligament deficiency. Arthroscopy 1990; 6:209-220.

52 Jakob RP, Warner JP. Lateral and posterolateral rotatory instability of the knee. In: Delee JC, Drez D, eds. Orthopedic sports medicine principles and practice. Philadelphia: WB Saunders; 1994:1275-1312.

53 Hughston JC, Andrews JR, Cross MJ, et al. Classification of knee ligament instabilities. Part II. The lateral compartment. J Bone Joint Surg Am 1976; 58:173-179.

54 LaPrade R. Medial ligament complex and the posterolateral aspect of the knee. In: Arendt EA, ed. Orthopedic knowledge update. Rosemont: American Academy of Orthopedic Surgeons; 1999:327-347.

55 Reider B, Sathy MR, Talkington J, et al. Treatment of isolated medial collateral ligament injuries in athletes with early functional rehabilitation. A five-year follow-up study. Am J Sports Med 1994; 22:470-477.

56 Brukner P, Kahn K. Acute knee injuries. In: Brukner P, Kahn K, eds. Clinical sports medicine. New York: McGraw-Hill; 1997:337-371.

57 Richards DB, Kibler BW. Rehabilitation of knee injuries. In: Kibler BW, Herring SA, Press JM, eds. Functional rehabilitation of sports and musculoskeletal injuries. Gaithersburg: Aspen; 1998:244-253.

58 Reider B. Medial collateral ligament injuries in athletes. Sports Med 1996; 21:147-156.

59 Kannus P. Nonoperative treatment of grade II and III sprains of the lateral ligament compartment of the knee. Am J Sports Med 1989; 17:83-88.

60 Laprade RF, Hamilton CD, Engebretson. Treatment of acute and chronic combined anterior cruciate ligament and posterolateral knee ligament injuries. Sports Med Arthorosc Rev 1997; 5:94-99.

61 King D. The function of semilunar cartilages. J Bone Joint Surg 1936; 18:1069-1076.

62 Renstrom P, Johnson RJ. Anatomy and biomechanics of the menisci. Clin Sports Med 1990; 9:523-538.

63 Fairbank JT. Knee joint changes after meniscectomy. J Bone Joint Surg Br 1948; 30:664-670.

64 Baker BE, Peckham AC, Pupparo F, et al. Review of meniscal injury and associated sports. Am J Sports Med 1985; 13:1-4.

65 Noble J, Hamblen DL. The pathology of the degenerative meniscus lesion. J Bone Joint Surg Br 1975; 57:180-186.

66 Oberlander MA, Pryde JA. Meniscal injuries. In: Baker, CL, ed. The Hughston Clinic sports medicine book. Baltimore: Williams & Wilkins; 1995:465-472.

67 Baker BE, Peckham AC, Pupparo F. Review of meniscal injury and associated sports. Am J Sports Med 1983; 11:8-13.

68 Rodkey WG. Basic biology of the meniscus and response to injury. Sports Med Arthorosc Rev 2004, 12(1):2-7.

69 Levy IM, Torzilli PA, Warren RF. The effect of medial meniscectomy on anterior-posterior motion of the knee. J Bone Joint Surg Am 1982; 64:883-888.

70 Bellabarba C, Bush-Joseph CA, Bach BR, Jr. Patterns of meniscal injury in the anterior cruciate-deficient knee: a review of the literature. Am J Orthop 1997; 26:18-23.

71 Johnson RJ, Kettelkamp DB, Clark W, et al. Factors affecting late results after meniscectomy. J Bone Joint Surg Am 1974; 56:719-729.

72 Shakespeare DT, Rigby HS. The bucket-handle tear of the meniscus. A clinical and arthrographic study. J Bone Joint Surg Br 1983; 65:383–387.

73 Rose NE, Gold SM. A comparison of accuracy between clinical examination and magnetic resonance imaging in the diagnosis of meniscal and anterior cruciate ligament tears. Arthroscopy 1996; 12:398–405.

74 Jackson DW, Jennings LD, Maywood RM, et al. Magnetic resonance imaging of the knee. Am J Sports Med 1988; 16:29–38.

75 Polly DW, Jr., Callaghan JJ, Sikes RA, et al. The accuracy of selective magnetic resonance imaging compared with the findings of arthroscopy of the knee. J Bone Joint Surg Am 1988; 70:192–198.

76 Tuerlings L. Meniscal injuries. In: Ea IA, ed. Orthopaedic knowledge update sports medicine 2. Rosemont: AAOS; 1999.

77 Kocher MS, Zurakowski D, Micheli LJ. Diagnostic accuracy of magnetic resonance imaging of knee injuries in children and adolescents. American Orthopaedic Association 32nd Annual Meeting, Chapel Hill, NC, 1999.

78 Arnoczky SP, Warren RF. The microvasculature of the meniscus and its response to injury. An experimental study in the dog. Am J Sports Med 1983; 11:131–141.

79 Cannon WD Jr., Vittori JM. The incidence of healing in arthroscopic meniscal repairs in anterior cruciate ligament-reconstructed knees versus stable knees. Am J Sports Med 1992; 20:176–181.

80 Scott GA, Jolly BL, Henning CE. Combined posterior incision and arthroscopic intra-articular repair of the meniscus. An examination of factors affecting healing. J Bone Joint Surg Am 1986; 68:847–861.

81 Newman AP, Daniels AU, Burks RT. Principles and decision making in meniscal surgery. Arthroscopy 1993; 9:33–51.

82 DeHaven KE, Bronstein RD. Injuries to the menisci of the knee. In: Nicholas JA, Hershman EB, eds. The lower extremity and sports medicine, 2nd edn. St Louis, MO: Mosby; 1995:813–823.

83 Fontera WR, Silver JK. Essentials of physical medicine and rehabilitation. Philadelphia, PA: Hanley & Belfus; 2002.

84 Siwek CW, Rao JP. Ruptures of the extensor mechanism of the knee joint. J Bone Joint Surg Am 1981; 63:932–937.

85 Clark SC, Jones MW, Choudhury RR, et al. Bilateral patellar tendon rupture secondary to repeated local steroid injections. J Accid Emerg Med 1995; 12:300–301.

86 Karpman RR, McComb JE, Volz RG. Tendon rupture following local steroid injection: report of four cases. Postgrad Med 1980; 68:169–174.

87 Laseter JT, Russell JA. Anabolic steroid-induced tendon pathology: a review of the literature. Med Sci Sports Exerc 1991; 23:1–3.

88 McWhorter JW, Francis RS, Heckmann RA. Influence of local steroid injections on traumatized tendon properties. A biomechanical and histological study. Am J Sports Med 1991; 19:435–439.

89 Bottoni CR. LTC, Taylor DC. LTC, Arciero RA. Col (ret). 9. Knee extensor mechanism injuries in athletes. In: DeLee JC, Drez D, Miller MD, eds. Orthopaedic sports medicine. Principles and practice, 2nd edn. Philadelphia, PA: Saunders; 2003:1857–1867.

90 Jozsa L, Kannus P. Histopathological findings in spontaneous tendon ruptures. Scand J Med Sci Sports 1997; 7:113–118.

91 Davidsson L, Salo M. Pathogenesis of subcutaneous tendon ruptures. Acta Chir Scand 1969; 135:209–212.

92 Kannus P, Jozsa L. Histopathological changes preceding spontaneous rupture of a tendon. A controlled study of 891 patients. J Bone Joint Surg Am 1991; 73:1507–1525.

93 Khan KM, Visentini PJ, Kiss ZS, et al. Correlation of ultrasound and magnetic resonance imaging with clinical outcome after patellar tenotomy: prospective and retrospective studies. Victorian Institute of Sport Tendon Study Group. Clin J Sport Med 1999; 9:129–137.

94 Outerbridge RE. The etiology of chondromalacia patellae. J Bone Joint Surg Br 1961; 43-4B:752–757.

95 Campbell CJ. The healing of cartilage defects. Clin Orthop 1969; 64:45–63.

96 Frisbie DD, Trotter GW, Powers BE, et al. Arthroscopic subchondral bone plate microfracture technique augments healing of large chondral defects in the radial carpal bone and medial femoral condyle of horses. Vet Surg 1999; 28:242–255.

97 Fox JA, Kalsi RS, Cole BJ. Update on articular cartilage restoration. In: Harner CD, Vince KG, Fu FH, eds. Techniques in knee surgery. Philadelphia: Williams & Wilkins; 2003:2–17.

98 Hangody L, Fules P. Autologous osteochondral mosaicplasty for the treatment of full-thickness defects of weight-bearing joints: ten years of experimental and clinical experience. J Bone Joint Surg Am 2003; 85-88A(Suppl 2):25–32.

99 Gerbino PG, Griffin ED, d'Hemecourt PA, et al. Patellofemoral pain syndrome: Evaluation of location and intensity of pain. Clin J Pain 2006; 22:154–159.

100 D'Hondt N E, Struijs PA, Kerkhoffs GM, et al. Orthotic devices for treating patellofemoral pain syndrome. Cochrane Database Syst Rev 2002:CD002267.

101 Hinman RS, Crossley KM, McConnell J, et al. Efficacy of knee tape in the management of osteoarthritis of the knee: blinded randomised controlled trial. BMJ 2003; 327:135.

102 Crossley K, Bennell K, Green S, et al. Physical therapy for patellofemoral pain: a randomized, double-blinded, placebo-controlled trial. Am J Sports Med 2002; 30:857–865.

103 Micheli LJ, Stanitski CL. Lateral patellar retinacular release. Am J Sports Med 1981; 9:330–336.

104 Cossey AJ, Paterson R. A new technique for reconstructing the medial patellofemoral ligament. Knee 2005; 12:93–98.

105 Fulkerson JP. Operative management of patellofemoral pain. Ann Chir Gynaecol 1991; 80:224–229.

106 Fulkerson JP, Kalenak A, Rosenberg TD, et al. Patellofemoral pain. Instr Course Lect 1992; 41:57–71.

107 Pfeiffer RP, DeBeliso M, Shea KG, et al. Kinematic MRI assessment of McConnell taping before and after exercise. Am J Sports Med 2004; 32:621–628.

108 Aderinto J, Cobb AG. Lateral release for patellofemoral arthritis. Arthroscopy 2002; 18:399–403.

109 Brief LP. Lateral patellar instability: treatment with a combined open-arthroscopic approach. Arthroscopy 1993; 9:617–623.

110 Saddik D, McNally EG, Richardson M. MRI of Hoffa's fat pad. Skeletal Radiol 2004; 33:433–444.

111 Krebs VE, Parker RD. Arthroscopic resection of an extrasynovial ossifying chondroma of the infrapatellar fat pad: end-stage Hoffa's disease? Arthroscopy 1994; 10:301–304.

112 Broom MJ, Fulkerson JP. The plica syndrome: a new perspective. Orthop Clin North Am 1986; 17:279–281.

113 Mital MA, Hayden J. Pain in the knee in children: the medial plica shelf syndrome. Orthop Clin North Am 1979; 10:713–722.

114 Flanagan JP, Trakru S, Meyer M, et al. Arthroscopic excision of symptomatic medial plica. A study of 118 knees with 1–4 year follow-up. Acta Orthop Scand 1994; 65:408–411.

115 Witvrouw E, Bellemans J, Lysens R, et al. Intrinsic risk factors for the development of patellar tendinitis in an athletic population. A two-year prospective study. Am J Sports Med 2001; 29:190–195.

116 Shalaby M, Almekinders LC. Patellar tendinitis: the significance of magnetic resonance imaging findings. Am J Sports Med 1999; 27:345–349.

117 Stanish WD, Rubinovich RM, Curwin S. Eccentric exercise in chronic tendinitis. Clin Orthop 1986:65–68.

118 Orava S. Iliotibial tract friction syndrome in athletes – an uncommon exertion syndrome on the lateral side of the knee. Br J Sports Med 1978; 12:69–73.

119 Neuschwander DC. Iliotibial band syndrome. In: DeLee JC, Drez D, Miller MD, eds. Orthopaedic sports medicine. Principles and practice. Philadelphia, PA: WB Saunders; 2003:1867–1878.

120 Francdo V, Cerullo G, Gianni E. Iliotibial band friction syndrome. Operative Tech Sports Med 1997; 5:153–156.

121 Noble CA. The treatment of iliotibial band friction syndrome. Br J Sports Med 1979; 13:51–54.

122 Martens M, Libbrecht P, Burssens A. Surgical treatment of the iliotibial band friction syndrome. Am J Sports Med 1989; 17:651–654.

123 Praemer AP, Furner S, Rice DP. Musculoskeletal conditions in the United States. Rosemont: American Academy of Orthopaedic Surgeons; 1999.

124 Martinek V, Fu FH, Lee CW, et al. Treatment of osteochondral injuries. Genetic engineering. Clin Sports Med 2001; 20:403–416, viii.

125 Krause BL, Williams JP, Catterall A. Natural history of Osgood-Schlatter disease. J Pediatr Orthop 1990; 10:65–68.

126 Ferriter P, Shapiro F. Infantile tibia vara: factors affecting outcome following proximal tibial osteotomy. J Pediatr Orthop 1987; 7:1–7.

127 Micheli LJ. Special considerations in children's rehabilitation programs. In: Hunter LY, Funk FJ Jr, eds. Rehabilitation of the injured knee. St Louis, MO: Mosby; 1984.

128 Flowers MJ, Bhadreshwar DR. Tibial tuberosity excision for symptomatic Osgood-Schlatter disease. J Pediatr Orthop 1995; 15:292–297.

129 De Flaviis L, Nessi R, Scaglione P, et al. Ultrasonic diagnosis of Osgood-Schlatter and Sinding-Larsen-Johansson diseases of the knee. Skeletal Radiol 1989; 18:193–197.

130 Gardiner JS, McInerney VK, Avella DG, et al. Pediatric update No. 13. Injuries to the inferior pole of the patella in children. Orthop Rev 1990; 19:643–649.

131 Kocher MS, Micheli LJ. The pediatric knee: Evaluation and treatment. In: Insall JN, Scott WN, eds. Surgery of the knee, 3rd edn. New York: Churchill Livingstone; 2001:1356–1397.

132 Mital MA, Matza RA, Cohen J. The so-called unresolved Osgood-Schlatter lesion: a concept based on fifteen surgically treated lesions. J Bone Joint Surg Am 1980; 62:732–739.

133 Cahill BR. Osteochondritis dissecans of the knee: Treatment of juvenile and adult forms. J Am Acad Orthop Surg 1995; 3:237–247.

134 Linden B. The incidence of osteochondritis dissecans in the condyles of the femur. Acta Orthop Scand 1976; 47:664–667.

135 Bednarz PA, Paletta GA, Jr., Stanitski CL. Bilateral osteochondritis dissecans of the knee and elbow. Orthopedics 1998; 21:716–719.

136 Clanton TO, DeLee JC. Osteochondritis dissecans. History, pathophysiology and current treatment concepts. Clin Orthop 1982:50–64.

137 Cahill BR, Berg BC. 99m-Technetium phosphate compound joint scintigraphy in the management of juvenile osteochondritis dissecans of the femoral condyles. Am J Sports Med 1983; 11:329–335.

138 Kocher MS, Micheli LJ, Yaniv M, et al. Functional and radiographic outcome of juvenile osteochondritis dissecans of the knee treated with transarticular arthroscopic drilling. Am J Sports Med 2001; 29:562–566.

139 Hefti F, Beguiristain J, Krauspe R, et al. Osteochondritis dissecans: a multicenter study of the European Pediatric Orthopedic Society. J Pediatr Orthop B 1999; 8:231–245.

140 Twyman RS, Desai K, Aichroth PM. Osteochondritis dissecans of the knee. A long-term study. J Bone Joint Surg Br 1991; 73:461–464.

141 De Smet AA, Fisher DR, Graf BK, et al. Osteochondritis dissecans of the knee: value of MR imaging in determining lesion stability and the presence of articular cartilage defects. AJR Am J Roentgenol 1990; 155:549–553.

CHAPTER 32

Leg Injuries

Merrilee Zetaruk and Jeff Hyman

INTRODUCTION

'The leg' refers to the portion of the lower limb extending from the knee to the ankle. Leg pain, whether acute or overuse in nature, may result from injury to any of the structures in the region, including bone and its periosteum, muscle-tendon units, bursae, ligaments, or local neurovascular structures. Pain also may be referred from a more proximal region of the lower extremity or spine.

The tibia articulates proximally with the femur and distally with talus. The tibia and fibula articulate with each other proximally and distally via two small articular facets. The fibula also articulates with the lateral aspect of the body of the talus. Muscles, nerves and blood vessels of the leg are situated in four distinct compartments: anterior, lateral, superficial posterior and deep posterior.

Exercise-induced leg pain encompasses all leg pain which is exacerbated by activity and which usually improves with rest. The differential diagnosis includes[1,2]:
1 Medial tibial stress syndrome (MTSS)
2 Stress fractures
3 Chronic exertional compartment syndromes
4 Vascular etiologies (entrapment of arteries, endofibrosis, atherosclerosis)
5 Nerve entrapment syndromes
6 Fascial defects (muscle herniations)
7 Delayed-onset muscle soreness (DOMS)
8 Muscle strains
9 Other rarer conditions (tibiofibular instability, metabolic muscle disorders, infection, tumors)

One approach to diagnosis of exercise-induced leg pain is by anatomic location of symptoms (Table 32.1).

SHIN SPLINTS

The term 'shin splints' is non-specific and has been used over the years to describe virtually any pain in the leg resulting from overuse.[3] Shin splints most commonly refer to exertional pain along the medial border of the tibia, a frequent complaint

---

Box 32.1: Key Points

- 'Shin splints' is a non-specific term often used for exercise-related leg pain.
- Risk factors: inappropriate footwear, hard running surfaces, increased training, poor foot mechanics.

---

among runners.[3,4] Although exertional leg pain may be more precisely defined on an anatomic basis, the widespread use of the term 'shin splints' persists in our culture.

Shin splints are frequently encountered in running sports and hiking.[3–6] Contributing factors for development of exertional leg pain in runners include inappropriate footwear, hard running surfaces, and increased intensity or volume of training.[3,7] Foot mechanics play a role as well in development of symptoms.[3,4,8–10]

In order to recommend appropriate treatment for 'shin splints', the exact nature of the injury needs to be better defined in each athlete. Diagnosis should reflect a more precise, anatomic basis of pathology.[3,4] Table 32.2 summarizes the investigations that may help differentiate between common causes of exercise-related leg pain. Frequently encountered conditions to consider in evaluating the runner with exertional leg pain include medial tibial stress syndrome, tibial stress fracture, exertional compartment syndrome, and muscle-tendon unit injuries.[2,4,8,11,12]

MEDIAL TIBIAL STRESS SYNDROME

Box 32.2: Key Points

- MTSS presents with diffuse pain/tenderness over the distal third to two thirds of the medial tibia.
- Common in running and jumping sports.
- Greater risk if increased ankle pronation.
- Radiographs normal.
- Bone scan: diffuse uptake on delayed phase images.

Table 32.1   Differential Diagnosis of Exertional Leg Pain by Location of Symptoms

	Anterior	Lateral	Posterior	Medial
Chronic exertional compartment syndromes	Anterior compartment	Lateral compartment	Superficial posterior compartment	Deep posterior compartment
Stress fractures	Tibial stress fracture	Fibular stress fracture		
Nerve entrapments	Peroneal nerve (anterolateral)	Peroneal nerve (anterolateral); sural nerve (posterolateral); fibular periostitis	Sural nerve (posterolateral)	Saphenous nerve
Periostitis				Medial tibial stress syndrome
Fascial defects	Muscle hernia	Muscle hernia		
Vascular causes			Vascular: popliteal artery entrapment; external iliac artery endofibrosis	

Table 32.2   Investigations for Exertional Leg Pain

	X-rays	Bone Scan	MRI	Compartment Pressures	Other Tests
Chronic exertional compartment syndromes	Negative	Negative	Negative	Elevated (pre-exercise resting >15 mmHg and/or 1-min post exercise >30 mmHg and/or 5-min post-exercise >20 mmHg)	Nerve conduction velocities may localize compartment; often normal at rest
Stress fractures	Negative early; periosteal reaction after 2-3 weeks; fracture line (late)	Positive within 48-72 h; sensitivity near 100%	MRI positive; sensitivity similar to bone scan – greater specificity		
Nerve entrapments	Positive if bony cause of entrapment		May identify structural causes	Elevated if secondary to CECS	Nerve conduction velocities demonstrate block
Periostitis	Negative	Diffuse uptake (tibia or fibula)	MRI of limited use	Normal	
Fascial defects				Elevated if secondary to CECS	
Vascular causes			MRI may show anatomic causes of entrapment	Slightly increased in PAES	Normal or decreased ankle : brachial systolic pressure ratio post-exercise; decreased flow on Doppler ultrasound post-exertion (low sensitivity in EIAE); decreased flow with passive dorsiflexion in PAES; confirm with angiography

CECS, chronic exertional compartment syndrome; EIAE, external iliac artery endofibrosis; PAES, popliteal artery entrapment syndrome.[1,12,16,18,20,22,32,43,51,55,57,71,72,74,79,81]

Medial tibial stress syndrome is an overuse injury characterized by pain along the posteromedial aspect of the distal two thirds of the tibia. It is one of the most common causes of exercise-related leg pain and is associated with running and jumping activities.[1,2,13] Although some have suggested that the incidence of MTSS is similar in males and females,[1] a recent study noted a greater incidence of MTSS in female naval recruits compared with their male counterparts.[14]

Pathophysiology Neither the pathophysiology nor the pathological lesion in MTSS is known for certain[1]; however, the fas-

cial origin of the medial soleus has been implicated as the most probable abnormal anatomical site.[1,2,15] In a normal running gait, the foot contacts the ground in mild supination. As weight is transferred, the foot moves into pronation. Medial fibers of the soleus contract eccentrically as the foot pronates, increasing stress on the fascial origin of the medial soleus, and possibly contributing to development of MTSS.[3,13,15]

Presentation Medial tibial stress syndrome presents as dull, aching pain along the middle or distal third of the posteromedial tibia.[1,13,16] Early in the process, pain is noted near the beginning of training, improves with continued exertion, then recurs towards the end or after the workout. In these instances, pain subsides promptly with rest. With continued training, the pain becomes more severe, sharp and persistent. As it becomes more chronic, the pain may be present on ambulation or at rest.[1,13]

The pain with MTSS may be distinguished from that of a stress fracture in that it is more diffuse in MTSS and more focal in the setting of a stress fracture.[8]

The pain with MTSS is also different from chronic exertional compartment syndrome pain. In the latter, there is muscular discomfort and tightness and occasionally associated cramping and numbness of the distal extremity. It begins after running for a specified distance or duration and often resolves promptly with rest.[1]

Examination A complete musculoskeletal examination of the lower extremities, including lumbar spine, is recommended. Careful evaluation of foot and ankle mechanics should be performed, since increased pronation may be a contributing factor to the condition. The most common finding is diffuse tenderness along the posteromedial edge of the tibia, near the junction of the middle and distal thirds of the bone, and usually extends over approximately one third of the length of the tibia.[1,3,16–18] Findings on examination such as focal tenderness, leg swelling, muscle weakness, weak or absent pulses, or dysesthesias should prompt the examiner to consider other diagnoses.[1,16,18]

Investigations Plain radiographs are unremarkable in isolated MTSS.[1,16,18] Abnormalities such as periosteal reaction or cortical lucency may indicate the presence of a stress fracture rather than simple MTSS.[12,19]

Triple phase bone scans are very helpful in differentiating MTSS and tibial stress fractures (Fig. 32.1). The classical finding in MTSS is a longitudinal region of uptake along the posteromedial aspect of the tibia, seen on the delayed phase of the scan.[1] Intense uptake of isotope along the anterior and posterior cortices is referred to as the 'double stripe sign'.[16] In contrast, stress fractures appear as focal or fusiform areas of increased uptake on all three phases of bone scan.[15,17,20,21] MRI is of limited use in diagnosis of MTSS.[1,22]

Treatment The mainstay of treatment is rest of the involved extremity. All pain-inducing activities should be avoided or modified, by decreasing duration, distance, or intensity. Patients who choose activity modification need to be warned about the risks of developing a coexisting stress fracture or another overuse injury, secondary to their altered gait mechanics. Cardio-respiratory fitness can be maintained with cross-training exercises including water running, swimming, or cycling, as long as these activities are pain-free.

Ice massage three to four times daily for a few days is recommended.[1,3,23] Non-steroidal anti-inflammatories may be beneficial as well for analgesia and reduction of inflammation.[3,23] Posting of insoles or custom orthotics are indicated if there are issues related to foot or gait malalignment.

After the patient has been pain-free for a few days, walking or light running may be initiated. Patients may be advised to

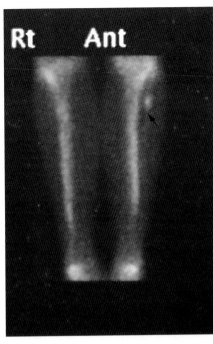

Figure 32.1 Bone scintigraphy of medial tibial stress syndrome. Diffuse radiotracer uptake along both tibiae is characteristic of this condition. Note focal area of uptake in proximal fibula which represents a concomitant stress fracture.

start at 50% of the previous intensity and distance, on soft and level surfaces. A proper warm-up and cool-down period is imperative. As long as the patient remains asymptomatic, a gradual increase in distance or duration is permitted. Athletes then may progress gradually over 3–6 weeks, as long as they remain pain-free. Once they reach their baseline distance, intensity is increased. If at any time during this progression symptoms recur, the patient should rest again, returning to an earlier stage in their progression.[3]

When these conservative measures fail, fasciotomy of the posteromedial superficial and deep fascia has been suggested.[17,24,25] Although MTSS is not a compartment syndrome, this procedure eases traction of the soleus and the deep compartment muscles on their fascial insertions.[3,15,24] At 3 months post surgery, Detmer reported 93% of subjects functioning at a level greater than their pre-operative capacity,[24] while Yates found good or excellent results in terms of pain relief in 69% of patients postoperatively.[26]

STRESS FRACTURES

Box 32.3: Key Points

- Stress fractures present with focal pain and tenderness.
- Tibia is most common site.
- Greater risk if disordered eating, menstrual irregularities or decreased bone density.

Stress fractures in bones occur when abnormal repetitive stress is applied to normal bone, resulting in bone fatigue and failure over time.[19] Stress fractures are most commonly seen in athletes and military recruits, with running being a frequently implicated activity in the genesis of this condition.[27–29] This may be due in part to the fact that ground reaction forces are two to four times body weight during running.[30] A total of 50% of stress fractures in men and 64% in women are seen in track and field athletes.[31] The tibia is the most frequent site of stress fracture (49%).[2]

Pathophysiology Stress fractures result from repetitive stress on bone either from weight bearing forces or from muscular action.[12,19] These forces may be axial, bending or torsional loads.[32] Under normal physiologic circumstances, the body's response to stress imparted to bone is a balance between resorption due to osteoclastic activity and bone formation by osteoblasts. This bone remodeling usually results in increased strength of the tissue.[19] In situations of repetitive stress to bones with inadequate recovery, particularly unaccustomed stress, the scale tips in favor of bone resorption. The resultant bone is weakened and susceptible to bone fatigue, injury and fracture.[12,19,29,33] It is theorized that when exercise is increased, the initial response by bone is to increase osteoclastic activity, with osteoblastic activity lagging behind.[29] With repeated stress, new bone formation cannot keep pace with bone resorption. The result is a thinning and weakening of cortical bone, which permits the development of microfractures. Without adequate rest to correct this imbalance, these microfractures can progress to clinical stress fractures.[33]

Risk factors Stress fractures are more likely to develop when an individual participates in unaccustomed physical activity or suddenly increases duration, intensity or frequency of training without periods of adequate rest.[12,19,29,32] Muscles which normally help to protect the bone from undue stress may permit greater transmission of force to bone when these muscles are fatigued.[12] Poor pre-participation physical condition has been cited as a predisposing factor for stress fracture.[29] This may be due to earlier muscle fatigue in these unfit individuals.[34] Athletes involved in running and jumping sports appear to be at greater risk of stress fracture than other athletes.[29,35] Training surface may affect the likelihood of stress fractures in some athletes.[19,29,33] Inappropriate footwear has also been implicated in development of stress fractures.[19,29]

Nutritional deficiencies, hormonal or menstrual dysfunction, and decreased bone density all increase the risk of stress fractures.[29,36–38] The 'female athlete triad' refers to the relationship between disordered eating, menstrual abnormalities, and osteoporosis in female athletes.[38–40] Athletes involved in sports which emphasize leanness to maximize performance, such as long-distance running, may be at increased risk of developing this triad.[38–40] Aesthetic sports such as gymnastics, figure skating, ballet and cheerleading, also emphasize a lean body type for success and are associated with higher rates of disordered eating; therefore, these athletes must be monitored closely for components of the female athlete triad.[12,38,40] Other risk factors for this triad include drive to excel at any

cost, pressure from coaches and parents, lack of nutritional knowledge, family history of eating disorders and history of abuse.

Disordered eating leads to hypothalamic dysfunction.[39] This in turn results in menstrual abnormalities such as oligomenorrhea[39,41] or amenorrhea (3–6 periods/year or >38 days/cycle). Amenorrhea may be primary (no menarche by 16 years of age) or secondary (absence of three to six consecutive menstrual cycles in those who have already reached menarche).[39,42] Such menstrual abnormalities result in decreased estrogen production. This hypoestrogenemia tilts the balance towards increased bone resorption relative to bone deposition, leading to decreased bone density.[12,39] It is in this setting that stress fractures are more likely to develop.[39]

Work-up of any female athlete with a stress fracture must include a nutritional and menstrual history. Treatment of a stress fracture in an amenorrheic athlete necessitates investigation and treatment of the menstrual abnormalities as well as the abnormal eating patterns.[38,40] A multidisciplinary approach to management of the female athlete triad involves the services not only of the physician, but also nutritionist and psychologist or psychiatrist.[38,40] Bone densitometry by dual photon radiographic absorptiometry can be used to assess bone density in these athletes.[40]

Presentation Athletes with stress fractures of the leg present with localized pain at the site of the injury, usually insidious in onset.[12,27] Symptoms may develop over days to weeks, are exacerbated by activities such as running and are initially relieved by rest.[8,12,33,43] In more severe cases, pain persists after activities or even at rest.[12,19]

Examination Focal tenderness is present over the fracture site, which may be associated with localized swelling or palpable callus in more well-established cases.[12,19,27,29] Hopping on the affected leg may precipitate symptoms.[12] Percussion of the bone may provoke pain at the site of the stress fracture.[33,44] Pain may be elicited with the use of a tuning fork over the site of the fracture.[45] Use of low-frequency ultrasound over an undiagnosed stress fracture may cause pain during treatment for an adjacent soft-tissue injury; however, the reliability of this has been called in question by some researchers.[46,47]

Tibial shaft stress fractures

Box 32.4: Key Points

- Posteromedial cortex of tibial shaft (compression side) is most common site of stress fracture.
- Anterior tibial cortex fractures (tension side) are high risk for nonunion.

Posteromedial cortex
The tibial shaft is the most common site of stress fracture.[12] Approximately half of all stress fractures in athletes are local-

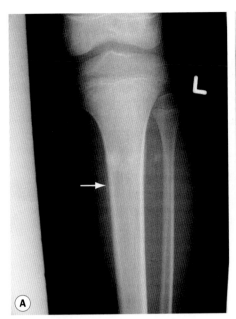 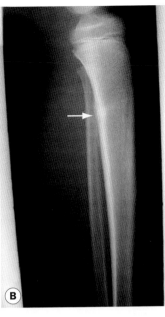

Figure 32.2 Proximal tibial stress fracture (A) anteroposterior: note sclerosis and new periosteal bone formation. (B) lateral: fracture is along posterior cortex of tibia.

ized to this region.[48] They most frequently occur at the posteromedial cortex or compression side of the tibia,[12] usually at the junction of the middle and distal thirds of the bone.[44] In young athletes, stress fractures are more commonly encountered in the proximal third of the tibia (Fig. 32.2).[44]

Anterior tibial cortex fractures

Although less frequently encountered in this area, stress fractures of the anterior tibial cortex warrant special mention. These fractures occur on the tension side of the tibia in jumping athletes.[12,23,43,44] The injury is usually localized to the middle third of the tibia where blood supply is more limited.[12] These fractures carry a significant risk of delayed or nonunion.[12,43,44] Focal tenderness is present over the mid-tibial region anteriorly. Anterior cortex tibial fractures may progress to the 'dreaded black line' fracture. This is a V-shaped, horizontally situated fracture-line (Fig. 32.3A). This appearance is due to bony resorption, and indicates non-union.[49] Bone scan may be normal at this stage.[49] This type of fracture requires prolonged healing time.[12,44] Such a fracture may progress to complete fracture if not treated aggressively (Fig. 32.3B).

Medial malleolar stress fractures

The medial malleolus is an uncommon site of stress fracture in athletes. Affected individuals will present with pain over the medial aspect of the ankle and possible ankle effusion.[12,44] As with other stress fractures of the leg, pain is aggravated by running or jumping and is alleviated by rest.[44] During running, repeated ankle dorsiflexion and tibial rotation cause stress between the medial malleolus and the tibial plafond, which may contribute to development of stress fractures of the medial malleolus.[50]

Fibular stress fractures

Stress fractures of the fibula most commonly occur in the distal third of the bone, just proximal to the inferior tibiofibular ligaments.[12,44,49] The fibula has a limited role in weight bearing; therefore, stress fractures in this region likely result from muscular contraction[12,49] and torsional forces.[49] Affected athletes present with lateral ankle pain, focal tenderness, and swelling.[44] Stress fractures also occur proximally, although this is encountered much less frequently.[44] Pain may be more diffuse over the proximal lateral aspect of the leg.[12] Tenderness is elicited over the site of the fracture.[44] The much rarer 'tibiofibular instability' should be considered as part of the differential diagnosis for proximal fibular pain and tenderness.

Investigations In contrast to radiographic imaging of acute fractures, plain X-rays are often negative for the first 23 weeks of symptoms.[12,19,43] Plain radiographs permit early detection of stress fractures in as little as 15% of cases[22]; however, periosteal reaction or cortical lucency may be seen on later images.[12,19]

Box 32.5: Key Points

- Radiographs for stress fractures are negative for first 2–3 weeks; later images may show periosteal reaction or cortical lucency.

- Bone scan is very sensitive at detecting stress fractures; positive as early as 48 h after onset of symptoms.

- MRI of stress fracture is sensitive and more specific than scintigraphy.

Bone scintigraphy (scan) is far more sensitive than plain radiography in diagnosing stress fractures,[12] with a sensitivity approaching 100%.[32] Changes on bone scan may be observed

Figure 32.3 'Dreaded black line' stress fracture: (A) Lucency represents non-union of fracture. (B) Stress fracture which progressed to complete fracture following a jump.

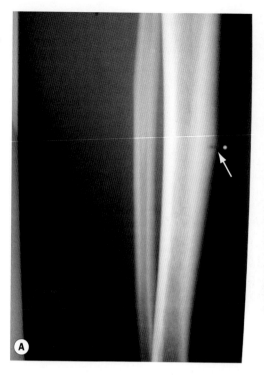
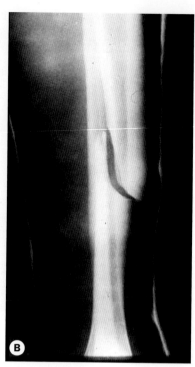

as early as 48–72 h after onset of injury[20] but may persist for up to 12–18 months. Intensity of uptake wanes over time.[12]

Magnetic resonance imaging has a similar sensitivity to bone scintigraphy in detecting stress fractures, but has a greater specificity (Fig. 32.4).[51] Other advantages of MRI over bone scintigraphy include better definition of the anatomic location and extent of the lesion, as well as lack of ionizing radiation.[12,19] MRI is less invasive than bone scintigraphy as well. Nonetheless, bone scintigraphy remains a useful tool in the diagnosis of stress fractures since access to MRI in some centres may be limited. MRI is also a more expensive test than bone scan.[20] Although CT scan is limited in its ability to detect early stress fractures, it may help differentiate between conditions which may have a similar appearance on bone scan (e.g. tumor, osteoid osteoma).[19]

Treatment For most stress fractures of the leg, avoidance of activities which provoke pain will hasten recovery and will prevent further deterioration of the injury.[12,29,44,49] Non-impact cross-training such as swimming or stationary bike permits maintenance of conditioning while facilitating healing of the stress fracture.[29,43,49] Once pain and bony tenderness settle (4–8 weeks), impact activities such as jogging may be gradually re-introduced.[12,29,43,44] As long as the athlete remains pain-free, the volume and intensity of weight-bearing activities may be increased. Most athletes are able to return to full, unrestricted training within 8–12 weeks.[49]

In severe cases, crutches or walking boot may be necessary for a brief period for pain relief and to assist ambulation.[43] Use of a pneumatic leg brace to facilitate healing and return-to-play has been proposed. It is theorized that such a brace would unload the tibia at the site of fracture, hastening healing.[12,45] In one study, athletes with tibial stress fractures were randomized

> **Box 32.6: Key Points**
>
> - Treatment of posterior cortex tibial stress fractures:
>   - pain-free activities
>   - non-impact cross-training early
>   - long pneumatic brace use shortens time to full activity.
> - Treatment of anterior cortex tibial stress fractures:
>   - 4–6 months for healing
>   - long pneumatic leg brace
>   - consider cast immobilization/non-weight bearing
>   - surgery may be necessary.

into two groups, one using a long pneumatic leg brace, the other using no casting or bracing. Both groups maintained non-impact activities such as cycling, swimming or pool running. The braced group returned to full, unrestricted activity in an average of 21 days, while the group treated without bracing required an average of 77 days to full activity.[45]

Stress fractures of the anterior tibial cortex require a more prolonged period of rest (up to 4–6 months) ranging from avoidance of provocative activities to modified activities using a pneumatic leg brace to non-weight bearing with cast immobilization.[27,49] For 'dreaded black line' fractures, a treatment regimen of long pneumatic leg brace combined with electric stimulation for 10 h/day has been proposed.[8] Athletes do not return to activity until there is evidence of cortical bridging on plain radiographs.[49] Surgery is considered if no healing has occurred after 4–6 months of conservative treatment.[12,29] Surgical options include excision and bone grafting[44] and intramedullary rod placement.[8,12,29,52] Medial malleolar stress fractures may be treated conservatively using an ankle brace

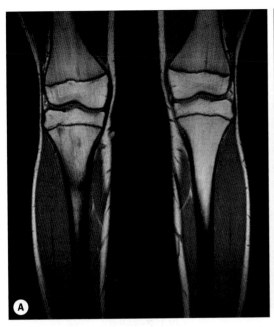
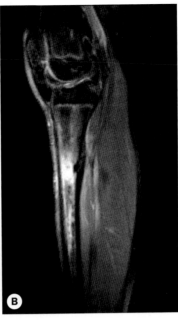

Figure 32.4 MRI appearance of tibial stress fracture. (A) coronal view, (B) sagittal view.

with a return to full activity usually by 6–8 weeks.[12,44,49] If a fracture line is seen on radiographs, immobilization for 2–3 weeks followed by a period of splinting may be necessary.[44] For athletes who desire early return to competition, internal fixation may be offered.[12,50] Bone grafting may be required for non-unions.[12]

Distal fibular stress fractures have an excellent prognosis if detected early and treated with 3–6 weeks of relative rest. If untreated, the healing time may be prolonged to 3–6 months before symptoms resolve.[12] Treatment usually entails avoidance of running and jumping for 3–4 weeks in conjunction with stretching of the calf muscles and peronei.[44] Partial weight bearing or walking boot may be necessary for pain relief early in treatment.[44,49]

CHRONIC EXERTIONAL COMPARTMENT SYNDROME

Box 32.7: Key Points

- Ache with predictable onset during activity.
- Resolves quickly with rest.
- Recurs with return to activity, even after prolonged rest.
- Anterior compartment most commonly affected.
- May have dysesthesias or foot drop.

A compartment syndrome occurs when increased interstitial pressure within an anatomically defined compartment results in compromised tissue perfusion and compression of neurovascular structures.[3,53] Compartment syndromes may be acute or chronic. Acute compartment syndrome is a surgical emergency presenting as severe pain out of proportion to the clinical history. It is seen secondary to trauma such as tibial fracture, crush injury, or circumferential burns, excessive exercise (muscle ruptures), vascular injury, externally applied pressure (a tight-fitting cast), and rarely secondary to a chronic exertional compartment syndrome (CECS). In athletes, chronic exertional compartment syndrome is more commonly encountered than the acute condition.

The prevalence of chronic exertional compartment syndrome in patients with exercise-induced leg pain may be as high as 26%.[54] It is frequently bilateral. Early studies, done mainly on military recruits, suggested that it affected men and women equally; however, more recent studies of athletic populations suggest that sportswomen may be at greater risk than men.[55,56] Anterior CECS tends to be more common than posterior and lateral CECS.[54,55] Together, anterior and deep posterior CECS make up 80% of all cases.[3,57]

Anatomy The lower leg is comprised of four compartments: anterior, lateral, superficial posterior and deep posterior.[55] A further division of the deep posterior compartment has been proposed so that a fifth compartment containing only the tibialis posterior exists.[58,59] A thorough knowledge of the compartmental anatomy of the leg, including the neurovascular components, is necessary to determine which compartment is involved in order to make the proper diagnosis.

The anterior compartment is bordered by the tibia, interosseus membrane and the fibula posteriorly. It includes the tibialis anterior, extensor digitorum longus, extensor hallucis longus and peroneus tertius. Neurovascular structures include the anterior tibial artery and vein with the deep peroneal nerve running along the interosseus membrane deep to the extensor hallucis longus. The lateral compartment is bordered anteriorly by the anterior intermuscular septum, medially by the fibula, posteriorly by the posterior intermuscular septum, and laterally by the deep fascia. It contains the peroneus longus and brevis muscles, along with the superficial peroneal nerve. The superficial peroneal nerve continues beneath the peroneus longus to emerge more distally between longus and brevis and pierce the deep fascia at the junction of the middle and lower thirds of the leg. The deep peroneal nerve leaves the lateral compartment proximally before coursing through the anterior compartment. The posterior compartments lie surrounded by the deep fascia of the leg with the deep transverse fascia separating it into two compartments. The anterior boundaries of the deep posterior compartment include the tibia, the interosseus membrane, and the fibula. Posteriorly, the border is the deep transverse fascia. The deep compartment contains the flexor digitorum longus, flexor hallucis longus, and tibialis posterior. Neurovascular structures within the deep posterior compartment include the posterior tibial artery and vein and tibial nerve. The superficial posterior compartment contains the gastrocnemius, plantaris, and soleus muscles.[58] The sural nerve lies in the fascia of the compartment[60] and courses between the heads of gastrocnemius in this compartment.[3] Some authors further subdivide the deep posterior compartment, with the tibialis posterior functioning as its own compartment. (Fig. 32.5).[3,55,59]

Muscle hernias are seen in at least 40% of patients with chronic compartment syndromes,[57] due to extremely high intracompartmental pressures. These are most often over the anterolateral compartments, at the point where the superficial peroneal nerve pierces the deep fascia.[54,57,61] This compares with the normal incidence of 5% among controls.[3]

Pathophysiology The pathophysiology of chronic exertional compartment syndrome is not definitively understood. During exercise, muscle contraction increases tissue perfusion which causes an increase in muscle size and weight by as much as 20%.[3] The fascia which borders these compartments is relatively stiff and unyielding thereby elevating the intracompartmental pressure. As exercise continues, the sustained increase in tissue pressure can lead to tissue edema with transudation of fluid into the interstitial space and disruption of the microcirculation.[3,62]

Earlier studies suggested that raised intracompartmental pressure caused relative ischemia of the involved muscles, leading to leg pain; however, some authors have questioned the existence of tissue ischemia in CECS.[63] The exact cause of pain in this condition is unclear.

Presentation Chronic exertional compartment syndrome presents as exercise-induced leg pain. It has been described as sharp, cramping, burning, aching, stabbing, or tightening; pain is referred from the underlying involved compartment.[53,55,62,64,65] Pain from the anterior or lateral compartments, innervated by the deep and superficial branches of the common peroneal nerve respectively, is usually directed over the anterolateral aspect of the shin and may radiate to the anterior ankle and the dorsum of the foot.[55] Pain from the superficial posterior compartment, innervated by the sural nerve, is referred to the upper/mid posterior calf and occasionally to the ankle.[55] Pain from the deep posterior compartment, innervated by the tibial nerve, is typically referred to the medial shin and/or distal posterior calf and may spread to the medial arch.[55] Recurrent complaints of feeling tight, tense, or achy in anatomically defined compartments are pathognomonic.[62]

Box 32.8: Key Points

- *Anterior compartment*: deep peroneal nerve (ankle dorsiflexion/sensation 1st web space).
- *Lateral compartment*: superficial peroneal nerve (ankle eversion/sensation anterolateral leg and dorsum of foot). *Note*: deep peroneal nerve may also be affected.
- *Deep posterior compartment*: tibial nerve (sensation medial arch of foot).
- *Superficial posterior compartment*: sural nerve (sensation posterolateral leg).

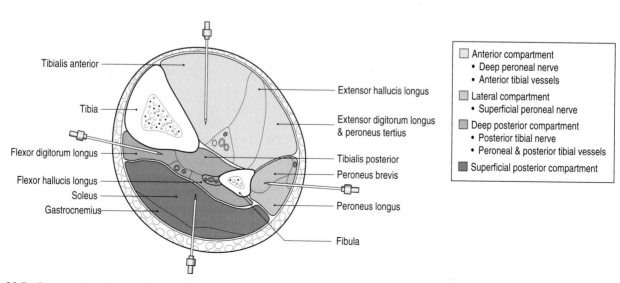

Figure 32.5 Cross-section of compartments of leg including needle position for compartment pressure monitoring.

Pain comes on at a relatively fixed point in the patient's activity. It remains constant as exercise continues, or progressively increases if exercise intensity is increased. Pain should cease or dramatically reduce within minutes of stopping but may continue overnight or until the next day in severe cases.[61,63] If the athlete continues to experience pain which prevents them from doing the same amount of exercise they did the day before, this is referred to as 'the second day phenomenon', which may occur in more severe CECS.[55] Even prolonged rest from exercise does not lead to improvement in pain on resumption of activity. In addition to exercise induced leg pain, patients with CECS rarely report neurological symptoms including dysesthesias, foot drop or loss of ankle control.[56,61]

CECS pain differs from the pain felt with isolated medial tibial stress syndrome as the latter increases upon ground contact, is felt diffusely over the medial tibial edge, and coexisting neurological symptoms are rare in MTSS. Similarly, neurological symptoms are non-existent in isolated tibial stress fractures, and the onset and disappearance of pain is more gradual. Stress fracture pain and tenderness is well localized over a focal area of the tibia.

Examination Most patients have no physical findings on initial examination at rest[55,62,65]; therefore all patients should be examined post-exercise, using the aggravating activity whenever possible. This may reveal a tense, firm compartment that is tender to deep palpation and passive stretch. All symptoms should improve within a short time after exercise cessation.

Neuromuscular examination is imperative to assess for specific nerve deficits. This assists in localizing the condition to a specific compartment. Involvement of the deep peroneal nerve in CECS of the anterior compartment may cause weakness of dorsiflexion and paresthesias of the 1st web space. CECS of the lateral compartment may have either paresthesias over the anterolateral distal shin and dorsum of the foot (superficial peroneal nerve) and/or the 1st webspace (deep peroneal nerve) associated with weakness of dorsiflexion (deep peroneal nerve) and/or eversion (superficial peroneal nerve). CECS of the deep posterior compartment may produce dysesthesias over the medial arch of the foot (tibial nerve) or cramping of the intrinsic foot muscles. Rowdon et al.[56] documented impaired vibratory sensation in subjects with CECS compared with controls, at rest and post-exercise. As previously mentioned, muscle hernias may be present,[2,17] especially over the anterolateral compartments.

Peripheral vascular examination is also important[53,55,56] to detect diminished pulses or poor capillary refill. These findings are rare, only occurring with extremely elevated compartment pressures[63]; therefore, their presence should prompt the examiner to consider other vascular causes, such as a vascular entrapment syndrome.

Investigations Radiographs, bone scintigraphy, CT, and MRI will help differentiate CECS from stress fractures, periostitis, spinal column or disc pathology, and tumors.[55,62,65] Nerve conduction studies may be indicated to confirm neurological involvement and delineate the involved compartment; however, in a small case study, Rowdon et al. found no difference in nerve conduction velocities when comparing patients with CECS and control subjects, pre- and post-exercise.[56] Arteriography, Doppler ultrasound, and ankle pressures are indicated if vascular pathology is suspected.

Box 32.9: Key Points

- Compartment pressures post-exercise are elevated in CECS; may have high resting pressure as well.
- Nerve conduction studies may detect neurological involvement.
- Treatment is surgical (fasciotomy of affected compartments).

The most useful diagnostic investigation is measurement of compartment pressures. Patients with symptoms consistent with CECS undergo pre-exercise pressure monitoring. They are then exercised to the point of reproduction of symptoms and pressures are re-evaluated at specified intervals post-exercise (Fig. 32.6). The test exercise should utilize activities as similar to the pain-producing activities as possible. Various authors have suggested different criteria for the diagnosis of CECS by compartment pressure measurements.

Most authors have observed elevated compartment pressures at rest and immediately after exercise. Two studies cited frequently in the literature are Rorabeck et al.[66] and Pedowitz et al.[57] Rorabeck's criteria include resting pre-exercise compartment pressures >10 and/or >15 mmHg at 15 min post-exercise.[66] The criteria used by Pedowitz include resting pre-exercise compartment pressure >15 and/or elevated post-exercise compartment pressure of >30 mmHg at 1 min and/or >20 mmHg at 5 min.[57]

Treatment The mainstay of treatment for CECS is surgery. Either a fasciotomy or fasciectomy is used to decrease intra-compartmental pressures and to release the compartment.[2,53,62] Conservative treatment, such as non-steroidal anti-inflammatory medications, physiotherapy, podiatry, or massage is felt to be ineffective.[3,55,62]

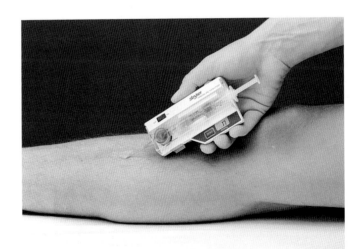

Figure 32.6 Compartment pressure monitoring. Hand-held pressure monitor used pre- and post-exercise. (Courtesy of Stryker, Kalamazoo, MI, USA.)

Postoperative recovery time is variable, with rehabilitative goals including early mobilization, and a gradual advancement through more strenuous exercise. Low impact activities such as swimming and cycling are introduced early, once ambulation is pain-free. Light running may occur between 3 and 6 weeks post-surgery and a return to full activity is anticipated within 6–12 weeks,[61,67] although return to sports participation may occur as early as 3–6 weeks postoperatively.[17]

Results for CECS surgery are very good with reports demonstrating good functional improvement or symptomatic cure in a high proportion of cases.[60] Of patients with recurrent symptoms post-surgery, some have had inadequate fasciotomy,[68] while others have been found to have a different diagnosis on further work-up.[55,69] Persistent symptoms may necessitate release of the fascia surrounding the tibialis posterior muscle as well.[70]

NEUROVASCULAR CAUSES OF LEG PAIN

Vascular causes

Leg pain due to vascular pathology in athletes is rare[71,72]; however, since it can be a cause of exercise-related leg pain and treatment differs significantly from other etiologies, it warrants discussion in this chapter. Among sedentary individuals, intermittent calf pain (claudication) may result from atherosclerotic blood vessels.[72] The athlete with vascular leg pain is more likely to have pathology referable to external iliac artery endofibrosis or popliteal artery entrapment syndrome.[72]

External iliac artery endofibrosis

External iliac artery endofibrosis is a rare narrowing of the lumen of the vessel which is the primary conduit to flow to the lower extremity.[73] It is most commonly encountered in young runners, weightlifters, rugby players and competitive cyclists.[72,73] There is a fibrotic thickening of the intima of the artery, leading to subtotal stenosis of the vessel.[72] It is thought to be due to prolonged exercise with the hip in a flexed position.[72] These lesions rarely cause significant obstruction to flow at rest or during submaximal exercise; however, during more intense exercise when muscle demand for blood flow is high, symptoms develop.[73] This condition may also affect the femoral artery.

Presentation

Affected individuals usually present with calf pain during exercise, although pain may also be present in the thigh.[72] Pain is proportional to intensity of cycling and is rapidly relieved by rest.[72] There may be concomitant numbness or a 'dead' feeling of leg.[72,73] Cyclists may also experience a loss of power during maximal efforts such as sprinting or climbing.[73]

Examination

Physical examination may reveal a bruit over the femoral artery with the hip flexed. Distal pulses may be weak or absent.[72] Examination of the patient immediately post-exercise increases the likelihood of detecting these changes.[72] Comparison of ankle to brachial systolic pressure ratios pre- and post-exercise may be helpful if the athlete develops symptoms during this exercise challenge.[72,73] Taylor and George[73]

Box 32.10: Key Points

- Calf pain ± thigh pain proportional to intensity of exercise.
- Rapidly relieved by rest.
- Most commonly seen in cyclists.
- Post-exercise ankle:brachial systolic pressure ratio <0.5.

---

found that all subjects in their study, including elite cyclists, untrained individuals and competitive cyclists who complained of exercise-induced leg pain, had resting ratios within the normal range of 1.08–1.18.[74] The study did find that in cases where exercise-induced leg pain was unilateral, the difference in ratios between legs at 1-min post-maximal exercise was significant. The authors recommended, therefore, that athletes with post-exercise ankle:brachial systolic pressure ratios <0.5 or, in the case of unilateral leg pain, a difference between sides of >0.18 at 1-min post-maximal exercise, be referred for arterial investigation for external iliac artery endofibrosis.[73]

If clinical suspicion warrants further investigation, Doppler ultrasound may be arranged to assess for impairment of flow. Unfortunately, flow normalizes rapidly with rest[72]; therefore, the likelihood of false negatives may be high. Angiography may reveal a tortuous external iliac artery with distinct stenotic lesions (Fig. 32.7).[72]

In cases of confirmed external iliac artery endofibrosis, angioplasty with possible stenting may be considered. This procedure reduces symptoms, but may not relieve pain entirely.[72]

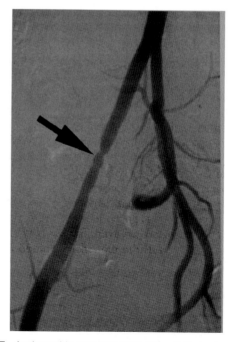

Figure 32.7 Angiographic appearance of external iliac artery endofibrosis. (From Kaufman JA. Abdominal aorta and iliac arteries. In: Kaufman JA, Lee MJ, eds. The requisites in vascular and interventional radiology. Philadelphia, PA: Mosby; 2004:277.)

Bypass surgery and open endarterectomy may be more successful in returning athletes to top-level competition.[72,75]

Popliteal artery entrapment syndrome

Box 32.11: Key Points

- Deep ache/cramp in calf or anterior leg.
- ± paresthesias in tibial nerve distribution.
- Pain disappears rapidly with rest.
- Symptoms related to intensity of exercise more than volume.
- Pain not affected by previous bouts of exercise.

Exertional leg pain in athletes may be the result of entrapment of the popliteal artery by a hypertrophic plantaris, gastrocnemius or soleus muscle.[71,72,76] This entrapment may be anatomic or functional.[76] From an anatomic standpoint, entrapment occurs as a result of an abnormal relationship between the popliteal artery and surrounding musculotendinous structures as the vessel exits the popliteal fossa.[71,72] A number of variants have been described: the accessory portion of the medial head of gastrocnemius passes behind the popliteal artery[77]; a tendinous slip arises from the medial head of the muscle; an abnormal plantaris muscle is present; multiple muscle abnormalities involving the lateral and medial heads of gastrocnemius and plantaris may exist.[72,78] In functional popliteal artery entrapment syndrome, the only anatomic anomaly noted is a hypertrophic gastrocnemius muscle.[71] In dorsiflexion, the hypertrophic gastrocnemius muscle compresses the popliteal artery, producing symptoms. In neutral, however, the popliteal artery remains widely patent with normal flow.[76]

Presentation Athletes with popliteal artery entrapment syndrome present with a deep ache in the calf or anterior leg region. Pain may have a cramp-like quality, and has been associated with coldness, blanching and paresthesias of the leg in a tibial nerve distribution.[71] The presentation may be difficult to distinguish from that of chronic exertional compartment syndrome.[72,79] Unlike exertional compartment syndrome, where symptoms in more severe cases may persist for some time after exercise is discontinued, the pain of popliteal artery entrapment syndrome disappears rapidly at rest.[13,72,79] Another distinction between these two entities is that in popliteal artery entrapment syndrome, pain is related to intensity of exercise primarily, while in exertional compartment syndrome, pain may be more closely associated with volume of exercise.[72] Unlike in exertional compartment syndrome, severity of symptoms in popliteal artery entrapment syndrome is not affected by previous bouts of exercise.[72]

Examination Physical examination may reveal bruits over the popliteal artery at rest in the setting of entrapment; however, bruits are also detected in some highly trained athletes in the absence of entrapment.[72] A more specific finding is

---

Box 32.12: Key Points

- Blood flow at rest is normal.
- Foot pulses may diminish or disappear with passive dorsiflexion and active plantarflexion.
- Doppler ultrasound and angiography should be done in neutral/active plantarflexion/active and passive dorsiflexion.

---

that of a bruit heard immediately post-exercise in athletes who exercise to the point of symptoms. Peripheral pulses may transiently decrease or disappear.[72] At rest and with the ankle in a neutral position, dorsalis pedis and posterior tibial artery pulses are generally palpable. During passive dorsiflexion and active plantarflexion of the foot, pulses may diminish or disappear.[71]

Investigations Work-up of suspected popliteal artery entrapment syndrome includes Doppler ultrasound, post-exercise ankle and brachial pressures, and angiography. Doppler ultrasound of the posterior tibial artery is performed first with the ankle in a relaxed position, then with passive dorsiflexion of the foot.[71] At rest, the blood flow is normal, but may diminish in passive dorsiflexion.[71] The diagnosis is confirmed with angiography in a neutral position, followed by active plantarflexion and active and passive dorsiflexion of the ankle during imaging.[72] Compartment pressure monitoring may be normal or slightly elevated.[79]

Treatment Initial treatment for this condition is temporary cessation of running activities and referral to a vascular surgeon.[79] Definitive treatment of popliteal artery entrapment requires release at the site of the entrapment, such as excision of muscle or division of fascial bands.[71,72] Resection of post-stenotic dilatation and vein grafting has also been proposed.[71]

Untreated, the repeated vascular compression and ensuing microtrauma to the arterial wall leads to premature localized atherosclerosis with thrombus formation.[78] These changes can result in intraluminal stenosis, poststenotic dilatation and aneurysm development.[71,76,78] There is collateral vessels formation and ultimately, serious ischemia results.[71]

With appropriate surgical intervention, athletes should be able to resume full, pain-free training within 6–8 months. In some cases, athletic performance may be improved.[71]

Atherosclerotic vessel disease

Presentation While atherosclerotic blood vessel disease is more common in older, sedentary individuals, Masters class athletes and other active older individuals with other cardiovascular risk factors may also develop this condition. Claudicant calf-pain may be the presenting symptom of this condition. As the vessel disease progresses, less and less intense exercise provokes symptoms.[72]

Examination On examination, athletes with leg pain due to atherosclerosis may have diminished or absent pulses. Bruits may be present at rest but are generally more audible after exercise.[72]

Treatment Non-surgical treatment involves angioplasty of stenotic lesions and possible vessel stenting.[72] Open endarterectomy or bypass surgery may be indicated in some individuals, depending on the extent of the disease and the availability of adequate graft vessels.[72]

Nerve compression syndromes

Peripheral nerves are vulnerable to compression or irritation at various sites in the leg, leading to exertional leg pain. Compression of the common peroneal nerve or its main branches at the fibular head is the most frequently encountered entrapment of the leg.[80] The sural and saphenous nerves may also be affected.

Common peroneal nerve entrapment

> **Box 32.13: Key Points**
>
> - Pain, numbness, dysesthesia over dorsum of foot and lateral calf.
> - Weakness of: ankle and great toe dorsiflexors; ankle evertors ('foot drop').
> - Normal deep tendon reflexes.
> - Nerve conduction studies show block at head of fibula.

The common peroneal nerve arises from the sciatic nerve above the popliteal fossa.[81] The peroneal nerve then winds around the fibular neck between the two heads of peroneus longus[81,82] and passes through the fibular tunnel between the edge of the peroneus longus muscle and the fibula.[83]

The common peroneal nerve is frequently injured by external compression at the proximal fibula, for example from bracing or casting[81,84]; however, peroneal nerve compression has also been described in athletes secondary to exercise.[85] It is postulated that compression occurs when the foot is in a plantarflexed and inverted position and the peroneal muscles are contracting, placing the taught nerve against the sharp fibrous edge of the peroneus longus muscle.[12,85] Due to the repetitive ankle motion from inversion to pronation in runners, this group of athletes may be at increased risk of common peroneal compression syndrome during exercise.[81] Runners do appear to be at increased risk of injury to this nerve.[85] Genu varum may also contribute to irritation of the common peroneal nerve.[12]

Presentation Athletes with this condition may present with pain, numbness or dysesthesia in the distribution of the common peroneal nerve.[81,86] Specifically, sensory changes over the dorsum of the foot and lateral calf are noted.[87] Pain is often vague, deep, and poorly localized.[83,86] Affected athletes may develop weakness of the ankle and great toe dorsiflexors, as well as of the ankle everters.[80,87] This presents clinically as a foot-drop or slapping gait.[80,83,87]

Examination When examined post-exercise, these athletes may demonstrate muscle weakness (ankle and great toe dorsiflexion; ankle eversion), sensory deficits on the dorsum of the

foot and lateral calf region, and a positive Tinel's sign at the fibular neck.[80,81,83,87] Deep tendon reflexes are unaffected.[83]

Investigations Unless there is a coexisting bony lesion causing compression of the nerve, investigations such as radiography, ultrasound, bone scintigraphy, and compartment pressure monitoring are normal in the setting of common peroneal nerve compression.[81] Nerve conduction studies will detect a conduction block to electrical impulses at the level of the head of the fibula.[81] Findings are increased post-exercise.[81] Electrodiagnostic studies can help differentiate foot-drop due to common peroneal nerve compression from that of L5 radiculopathy or sciatic mononeuropathy.[83] These studies can also help determine the extent of nerve injury and therefore the expected course of recovery.[83,86]

Treatment Conservative measures such as use of an ankle-foot orthosis can improve gait and prevent ankle sprains by temporarily reducing foot-drop.[80,87] Affected individuals should avoid external compression of the common peroneal nerve which occurs with leg-crossing.[83] Failing conservative treatment, surgical exploration may be warranted.[87]

Prognosis for recovery is dependent upon the severity and chronicity of symptoms. Neuropraxic injuries, the mildest form of nerve injury, affect the myelin sheath without axonal injury. These lesions may recover spontaneously within hours to days and usually within 3 months as long as compression to the nerve is relieved.[83,86] If axon loss is detected on electrodiagnostic studies, spontaneous recovery may be expected over 4–6 months.[83,86] Complete axonal disruption is the most severe form of injury and requires surgical repair and nerve reconstruction for restoration of function.[86]

Superficial peroneal nerve

The common peroneal nerve branches into the superficial and deep peroneal nerves, as it passes around the fibular neck and through the heads of peroneus longus.[81,82] The superficial peroneal nerve supplies peroneus longus and brevis, as well as sensation to the anterolateral aspect of the lower leg and dorsum of the foot.[82,83] It is rare for this nerve to be compressed at the fibular head.[80] The superficial peroneal nerve is compressed most commonly at the site where it exits the lateral compartment, approximately 8–15 cm proximal to the lateral malleolus.[12,81,88,89] Herniation through the fascia at this site may compress the nerve, leading to superficial peroneal nerve syndrome.[70,81,88] Other conditions which may produce symptoms of superficial peroneal nerve compression include direct trauma or compression of the nerve, adjacent soft-tissue mass such as lipoma, and stretch secondary to recurrent ankle sprains.[88]

Presentation Athletes with compression of this nerve present with pain, numbness or paraesthesias in the distribution of the superficial peroneal nerve (i.e. anterolateral lower leg and dorsum of foot, including second to fourth toes) during exercise and occasionally at rest (Fig. 32.8).[89,90]

Examination Clinical examination reveals decreased sensation most consistently over the dorsum of the foot after exercise.[88] Tinel's sign over the site of the compression or pain with

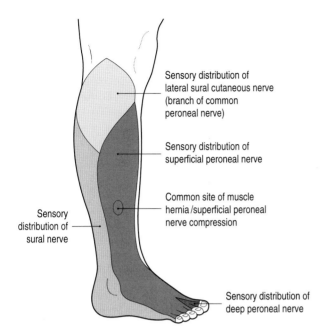

Figure 32.8 Sensory distribution of superficial peroneal nerve (SPN). Note typical location of muscle hernia/SPN compression.

passive ankle flexion/supination may be elicited.[90] Pressure over the site of entrapment while the patient actively plantarflexes and inverts the ankle may reproduce symptoms.[12] A fascial defect may be detected on palpation.

Treatment

Initial conservative treatment may include modification of aggravating activities and prevention of recurrent ankle inversions using bracing. Surgical decompression is the definitive treatment.[81]

Deep peroneal nerve

Box 32.14: Key Points

Deep peroneal nerve entrapment *versus* L5 radiculopathy

- Both may have foot drop.

- Both may have decreased sensation over dorsum of foot.

- *Ankle reflexes*: DPN entrapment, normal; L5 radiculopathy, may be depressed/absent.

- *Hip extensor strength*: DPN, normal; L5 radiculopathy, may be weak.

- *Pain in thigh*: DPN, absent; L5 radiculopathy, may be present.

- *Root stretch signs*: DPN, negative; L5 radiculopathy, positive.

The deep peroneal nerve is primarily motor, supplying the toe and ankle extensors (tibialis anterior, extensor hallucis longus and extensor digitorum longus and brevis), as well as peroneus tertius.[82,83] The sensation to the dorsal first web space is also provided by the deep peroneal nerve.[82,83] The deep branch of the peroneal nerve is more commonly affected than the super-

ficial branch, since the former is in direct contact with the fibula.[83]

Presentation/examination

Athletes with deep peroneal nerve compression may present with foot-drop and decreased sensation over the dorsal aspect of the first web space of the foot.[82,83] L5 root pathology (e.g. herniated L4–L5 disc) should be ruled out in individuals with weakness of the ankle and toe dorsiflexors, or with decreased sensation over the dorsum of the foot.[83,87] Unlike L5 radiculopathy, peroneal neuropathy is not associated with depressed or absent ankle reflexes, weakness of hip extension, or pain in the thigh region.[87,91] The presence of back pain or positive root stretch signs also suggest radiculopathy.[92]

Sural nerve

The sural nerve passes between the heads of gastrocnemius and posterior to the peroneal tendons.[12] Entrapment may occur at any site along the course of the nerve.[89] Bilateral sural nerve entrapment has been described in a hockey player. The injury resulted from compression near the top of the skate boot secondary to tight lacing at this site.[93] In a series of 18 cases, Fabre *et al.* found sural nerve compression in a fibrous arch that thickened the superficial sural aponeurosis at the site where the sural nerve passes through.[94]

Sural nerve entrapment may cause pain and paraesthesia along the postero-lateral aspect of the lower leg, extending behind the lateral malleolus and along the lateral border of the foot (Fig. 32.9).[89,93] Tenderness may be localized to a region just lateral to the musculotendinous junction of the Achilles tendon.[94] Distal neurologic examination is unremarkable.[94] Diagnosis may be confirmed with electrodiagnostic testing.[94] In Fabre's series, surgical treatment involved incision of the

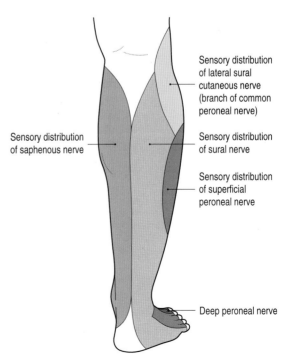

Figure 32.9 Sensory distribution of sural nerve.

thickened fibrous band at the site of sural nerve compression in the superficial sural aponeurosis.[94]

Saphenous nerve

The saphenous nerve is the longest sensory branch of the femoral nerve (L1, L2, L3 nerve roots).[81,82] It supplies sensation to the medial aspect of the leg and foot.[68,81,82,95] Although local trauma or inflammation (e.g. thrombophlebitis) may affect the nerve at the adductor canal, repeated knee flexion may also cause symptoms of claudicant pain or altered sensation in the distribution of the saphenous nerve.[81] Symptoms may be reproduced by compressing the nerve at the adductor canal[81,96] or where the nerve crosses the medial femoral condyle.[81] Tinel's sign may be present and altered sensation over the medial aspect of the leg and foot may be detected.[68,81] Conservative management includes use of analgesics and non-steroidal anti-inflammatory medications, although physiotherapeutic modalities have not been proven to reduce symptoms long-term.[97] Local injection at the exit site from the adductor canal with anesthetic or corticosteroid may be diagnostic and therapeutic.[96,97] Surgical release of the nerve may be required.[97]

STRAIN – MEDIAL HEAD OF GASTROCNEMIUS

Box 32.15: Key Points

- Feels like direct blow to medial calf.
- Focal tenderness at muscle tendon junction.
- Thompson's test negative.

The gastrocnemius muscle, overlying soleus, has two heads: medial and lateral. These heads join soleus at the tendo-Achilles, distally inserting on the calcaneus. Gastrocnemius crosses two joints, working to plantarflex the ankle and to flex the knee. Injuries to gastrocnemius tend to occur at the distal muscle–tendon junction of the medial muscle head.[13,98] Muscles that cross two joints, such as the gastrocnemius muscle, are particularly susceptible to injury.[98–100] The high proportion of fast twitch muscle fibers predisposes the gastrocnemius muscle to injury, when compared with the slow-twitch soleus muscle.[12] Eccentric loading (stretch during contraction) produces maximal tension in the muscle, setting the stage for tearing at the muscle-tendon junction.[98–100] Strains may also occur with acceleration from a dorsiflexed position.[13]

Presentation The medial head of the gastrocnemius may partially rupture during sprinting or jumping activities, particularly if an eccentric load is placed across the ankle while the knee is extended.[2,12] It has frequently been observed in tennis players, earning it the name 'Tennis Leg'.[12] Affected athletes often have a sudden, stabbing pain and may subjectively feel that they have been struck directly in the back of the calf with a ball, for example.

Examination Physical examination reveals swelling, point tenderness at the musculotendinous junction of the medial head of gastrocnemius, and possibly a palpable defect in the muscle.[2,12] Some degree of ecchymosis may be present.[17] Dorsiflexion and resisted plantarflexion are usually painful.[13] Unlike Achilles tendon ruptures, strains of the medial head of gastrocnemius are associated with a negative Thompson's test. History and physical examination are usually adequate to diagnose this injury; however, MRI can confirm the diagnosis in equivocal cases.[12]

Treatment Treatment of strains of the medial head of gastrocnemius is conservative. Rest, ice, compression and elevation (RICE) with partial weight bearing is the initial approach to the acute injury.[2,17] Use of bilateral heel wedges may be helpful.[13] Initial use of a rocker-bottom postoperative boot has also been suggested.[13] Weight bearing is increased as tolerated, and a progressive calf stretching and strengthening program is instituted when symptoms subside.[2,13,17] Full participation in sports is permitted when strength is nearly equal to the unaffected leg and symptoms have resolved.[12] In rare cases, surgery may be offered if the rupture is substantial with complete loss of muscle function[17]; however some authors feel that surgical repair of the musculotendinous junction has no more favorable outcome than non-operative care.[2] Following non-operative management, athletes can expect a full return to training in 3–12 weeks depending upon symptoms,[12,13] with most athletes resuming full training and competition within 4–6 weeks.[13]

PROXIMAL TIBIOFIBULAR JOINT DISORDERS

Box 32.16: Key Points

- *Mechanism of injury*: fall onto adducted leg with knee flexed and foot inverted/plantarflexed.
- 'Popping sensation' over lateral aspect of knee.
- May be confused with lateral meniscus tear.
- Increased anteroposterior translation of fibular head.
- Radiographs with leg internally rotated 30–90° may show widening of tibiofibular joint.

Tibiofibular ligaments stabilize the proximal tibiofibular joint.[12] This joint allows for some vertical movement of the fibula, as well as rotation in response to ankle movements. With knee flexion and extension, the fibula has slight anteroposterior movement.[12] The proximal tibiofibular joint functions to dissipate torsional loads at the ankle.[3,12]

The mechanism of injury to this joint is typically a fall onto an adducted leg with the knee flexed and foot inverted and plantarflexed.[3] The anterolateral leg muscles contract to pull the fibula anteriorly.[3] The knee is typically flexed which relaxes the fibular collateral ligament. A rotatory motion then disrupts the ligamentous restraints resulting in subluxation or dislocation in an anterolateral direction.[101]

Presentation/examination The athlete with an acute dislocation of the proximal tibiofibular joint may report a 'popping sensation' over the lateral aspect of the knee, with pain and tenderness localized to the proximal tibiofibular joint.[3,12] The fibular head may be prominent and tender.[12,101] Pain may be exacerbated by ankle flexion and extension and by ankle eversion and inversion.[3] The peroneal nerve may be injured resulting in motor dysfunction or sensory changes in the distribution of the nerve.[3,12] Chronically, patients may complain of knee instability, poorly localized lateral knee pain and loss of extension of the knee.[3] Lateral knee pain, popping and catching may be confused with lateral meniscal injury.[102] Instability of the proximal tibiofibular joint may be detected by the presence of increased anteroposterior translation of the fibular head with respect to the tibia.[3,12]

Investigations Investigations include plain radiographs with the lower leg internally rotated by various degrees (30–90°). Contralateral views may be necessary to detect widening of the tibiofibular joint.[3,12,101,103] Lateral radiographs may reveal a more anteriorly located fibular head as well.[3,103] Computed tomography helps confirm the diagnosis.[3,101]

Treatment Treatment of the acute tibiofibular joint dislocation involves closed reduction by flexing the knee to 90° and placing direct anterior or posterior pressure over the fibular head.[12] The foot is placed in dorsiflexion and eversion for this maneuver.[3] After closed reduction, some authorities advocate use of a support bandage for 6 weeks and restriction from sports for an additional 6 weeks,[101] while others suggest 2–3 weeks of immobilization in full extension or slight flexion with toe-touch weight-bearing.[3] Knee immobilizers should be removed three times daily for range-of-motion exercises.[3,12] Progressive strengthening exercises over the subsequent 3 weeks with gradual return to activities is advocated.[12]

Chronic instability may be addressed with ligament repair or reconstruction, with temporary fixation of the joint by screw or wire to permit healing. Excision of the fibular head may be necessary if pain or instability is prolonged. Fusion of the joint should be avoided, as this may lead to secondary ankle symptoms.[103]

MUSCLE HERNIATION (FASCIAL DEFECTS)

Although fascial defects with muscle herniation often occur in the setting of chronic exertional compartment syndrome, they may be observed in asymptomatic individuals as well.[2] Muscle herniation may compress the superficial peroneal nerve as it exits the fascia, resulting in tenderness at the site of the muscle herniation and symptoms in the distribution of the nerve.

Treatment is indicated in symptomatic individuals and may include fasciotomy to decompress the herniated muscle.[2] Closure of the defect, which may aggravate symptoms and precipitate an acute compartment syndrome, is contraindicated.[2,88]

DELAYED-ONSET MUSCLE SORENESS (DOMS)

Exercise that exceeds a muscle's stress tolerance can damage muscle fibres, leading to delayed-onset muscle soreness (DOMS), particularly after unaccustomed exertion.[100] Symptoms are thought to be due to reversible structural damage at the cellular level.[100] Muscles subjected to eccentric loading (e.g. running downhill) are particularly susceptible to this condition.[17,100,104] Unconditioned individuals are more likely to develop DOMS after strenuous activity. Onset of symptoms is usually within 1–2 days after exercise and peaks at 2–3 days, with resolution within 1 week of the offending activity.[100] Symptoms include muscle pain, fatigue and tenderness.[17] Treatment is symptomatic, consisting of relative rest and non-steroidal anti-inflammatories.[104]

OTHER CAUSES OF LEG PAIN

Box 32.17: Key Points

- 'Red flags' for potentially more serious causes of leg pain:
  - fever, malaise, anorexia, lethargy, night pains.
- Additional tests to consider:
  - CBC, ESR, CRP, CK, alkaline phosphatase.
  - plain radiographs/bone scintigraphy/CT/MRI.

Other more rare conditions may present with musculoskeletal pain, numbness or weakness in the leg. More serious conditions such as infection (e.g. osteomyelitis) or neoplasm, must be ruled out.[8] Systemic symptoms such as fever, anorexia, lethargy or night pains should raise the clinician's suspicion of a more concerning underlying etiology. A complete history with review of symptoms will help to identify these patients. Elevated white blood cell count, erythrocyte sedimentation rate, or C-reactive protein may assist in diagnosis;[105,106] however, values may be normal even in the setting of certain neoplasms.[106] Osteoid osteoma is a benign bone tumor which should be included in the differential diagnosis of stress fracture. Pain and tenderness is localized, much like that of a stress fracture, and bone scintigraphy demonstrates focal increased uptake. The main distinguishing features of osteoid osteoma on history are night pain and considerable pain relief with aspirin.[8] Osteochondroma of the tibia may cause compression of neurovascular structures in the leg or present with a mass (Fig. 32.10).[107] Plain radiographs, bone scintigraphy, CT and MRI each have a role in assessment of possible bone tumors.[108] Myopathic conditions are rare, but may present with exertional leg pain, progressive weakness including footdrop, or numbness.[80] Creatine kinase levels are usually elevated in these individuals, often >10 times the normal value.[80,109] More diffuse symptoms of muscle dysfunction should be sought on history, since some myopathies may affect upper and lower extremities, or both proximal and distal muscle groups.

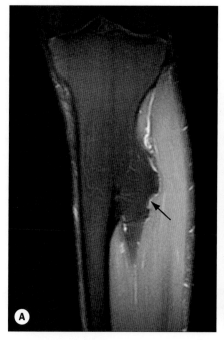
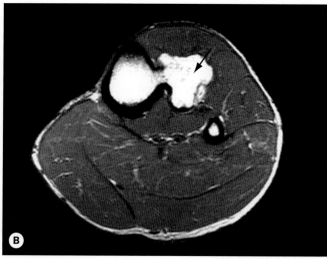

Figure 32.10   MRI of osteochondroma of proximal tibia (A) coronal view, (B) axial view.

REFERENCES

1   Kortebein PM, Kaufman KR, Basford JR, et al. Medial tibial stress syndrome. Med Sci Sports Exerc 2000; 32:27–33.
2   Touliopolous S, Hershman EB. Lower leg pain. Diagnosis and treatment of compartment syndromes and other pain syndromes of the leg. Sports Med 1999; 27:193–204.
3   Andrish JT. The leg. In: DeLee JC, Drez D, eds. DeLee & Drez's orthopaedic sports medicine: Principles and practice. 2nd edn. Philadelphia, PA: WB Saunders; 2003:2155.
4   Brukner P. Exercise-related lower leg pain: an overview. Med Sci Sports Exerc 2000; 32:1–3.
5   Hreljac A. Impact and overuse injuries in runners. Med Sci Sports Exerc 2004; 36:845–849.
6   Hreljac A, Marshall RN, Hume PA. Evaluation of lower extremity overuse injury potential in runners. Med Sci Sports Exerc 2000; 32:1635–1641.
7   Clement DB, Taunton JE, Smart GW, et al. A survey of overuse running injuries. Physician Sportsmed 1981; 9:47–58.
8   Brukner P. Exercise-related lower leg pain: bone. Med Sci Sports Exerc 2000; 32:15–26.
9   Burne SG, Khan KM, Boudville PB, et al. Risk factors associated with exertional medial tibial pain: a 12 month prospective clinical study. Br J Sports Med 2004; 38:441–445.
10 Thacker SB, Gilchrist J, Stroup DF, et al. The prevention of shin splints in sports: a systematic review of literature. Med Sci Sports Exerc 2002; 34:32–40.
11 Beck BR. Tibial stress injuries. An aetiological review for the purposes of guiding management. Sports Med 1998; 26:265–279.
12 Boden BP. The leg. In: Garrett WE, Speer KP, Kirkendall DT, eds. Principles and practice of orthopedic sports medicine. Philadelphia, PA: Lippincott; 2000:869.
13 Glazer J, Hosey RG. Soft-tissue injuries of the lower extremity. Prim Care 2004; 31:1005–1024.
14 Yates B, White S. The incidence and risk factors in the development of medial tibial stress syndrome among naval recruits. Am J Sports Med 2004; 32:772–780.
15 Michael RH, Holder LE. The soleus syndrome: a cause of medial tibial stress (shin splints). Am J Sports Med 1985; 13:87–94.
16 Bhatt R, Lauder I, Finlay DB, et al. Correlation of bone scintigraphy and histological findings in medial tibial stress syndrome. Br J Sports Med 2000; 34:49–53.
17 Clanton TO, Solcher B. Chronic leg pain in the athlete. Clin Sports Med 1994; 13:743–759.
18 Phillips GC, Armsey TD Jr. Leg injury – dance. Med Sci Sports Exerc 2003; 35:S60.
19 Spitz DJ, Newberg AH. Imaging of stress fractures in athletes. Radiol Clin North Am 2002; 40:313–331.
20 Ishibashi Y, Okamura Y, Otsuka H, et al. Comparison of scintigraphy and magnetic resonance imaging for stress injuries of bone. Clin J Sport Med 2002; 12:79–84.
21 Rupani HD, Holder LE, Espinola DA, et al. Three phase radionuclide bone imaging in sports medicine. Radiology 1985; 156:187–196.
22 Anderson MW, Ugalde V, Batt M, et al. Shin splints: MR appearance in a preliminary study. Radiology 1997; 204:177–180.
23 Fredericson M, Bergman AG, Hoffman KL, et al. Tibial stress reaction in runners - correlation of clinical symptoms and scintigraphy with a new magnetic resonance imaging grading system. Am J Sports Med 1995; 23:472–481.
24 Detmer DE. Chronic shin splints. Classification and management of medial tibial stress syndrome. Sports Med 1986; 3:436–446.
25 Holen KJ, Engebretsen L, Grøntvedt T, et al. Surgical treatment of medial tibial stress syndrome (shin splint) by fasciotomy of the superficial posterior compartment of the leg. Scand J Med Sci Sports 1995; 5:40–43.
26 Yates B, Allen MJ, Barnes MR. Outcome of surgical treatment of medial tibial stress syndrome. J Bone Joint Surg Am 2003; 85:1974–1980.
27 Batt ME, Kemp S, Kerslake R. Delayed union stress fractures of the anterior tibia: conservative management. Br J Sports Med 2001; 35:74–77.
28 Boden BP, Osbahr DC, Jimenez C. Low-risk stress fractures. Am J Sport Med 2001; 29:100–111.
29 Sanderlin BW, Raspa RF. Common stress fractures. Am Fam Physician 2003; 68:1527–1532.
30 Nigg BM, Cole GK, Bruggeman G. Impact forces during heel-toe running. J Appl Biomech 1995; 11:407–432.
31 Bennell KL, Brukner PD. Epidemiology and site specificity of stress fractures. Clin Sports Med 1997; 16:179–196.
32 Anderson MW, Greenspan A. Stress fractures. Radiology 1996; 199:1–12.
33 Maitra RS, Johnson DL. Stress fractures. Clinical history and physical examination. Clin Sports Med 1997; 16:259–274.
34 Markey KL. Stress fractures. Clin Sports Med 1987; 6:405–425.
35 Bennell K, Crossly K, Jayarajan J, et al. Ground reaction forces and bone parameters in females with tibial stress fracture. Med Sci Sports Exerc 2004; 36:397–404.
36 Boden BP, Speer KP. Femoral stress fractures. Clin Sports Med 1997; 16:307–317.
37 Nattiv A, Armsey TD. Stress injury to bone in the female athlete. Clin Sports Med 1997; 16:197–224.
38 Zetaruk MN. The young gymnast. Clin Sports Med 2000; 19:757–780.
39 Gittes EB. The female athlete triad. J Pediatr Adolesc Gynecol 2004; 17:363–365.
40 Ireland ML. Special concerns of the female athlete. Clin Sports Med 2004; 23:281–298.
41 Lebrun CM. The female athlete: exercise, osteoporosis, and birth control. In: Mellion MB, ed. Sports medicine secrets. Toronto: Mosby; 1994:38.
42 Mandelbaum BR, Nattiv A. Gymnastics. In: Reider B, ed. Sports medicine: The school age athlete, 2nd edn. Philadelphia, PA: WB Saunders; 1996:453.
43 Carr K. Musculoskeletal injuries in young athletes. Clin Fam Pr 2003; 5:385–415.

44 Puddu G, Cerullo G, Selvanetti A, et al. Stress fractures. In: Harries M, Williams C, Stanish W, Micheli LJ, eds. Textbook of sports medicine. 2nd edn. New York: Oxford University Press; 1998:649.

45 Swenson EJ Jr, DeHaven KE, Sebastianelli WJ, et al. The effects of pneumatic leg brace on return to play in athletes with tibial stress fractures. Am J Sports Med 1997; 25:322–328.

46 Boam WD, Miser WF, Yuill SC, et al. Comparison of ultrasound examination with bone scintiscan in the diagnosis of stress fractures. J Am Board Fam Pr 1996; 9:414–417.

47 Romani WA, Perrin DH, Dussault RG, et al. Identification of tibial stress fractures using therapeutic continuous ultrasound. J Orthop Sports Phys Ther 2000; 30:444–452.

48 Matheson GO, Clement DB, McKenzie C, et al. Stress fractures in athletes. A study of 320 cases. Am J Sports Med 1987; 15:46–58.

49 Wilder R, Sethi S. Overuse injuries: tendinopathies, stress fractures, compartment syndromes, and shin splints. Clin Sports Med 2004; 23:55–81.

50 Shelbourne KD, Fisher DA, Rettig AC, et al. Stress fractures of the medial malleolus. Am J Sports Med 1988; 16:60–63.

51 Deutsch AL, Coel MN, Mink JH. Imaging of stress injuries to bone: radiography, scintigraphy, and MR imaging. Clin Sports Med 1997; 16:275–290.

52 Plasschaert VF, Johansson CG, Micheli LJ. Anterior tibial stress fracture treated with intramedullary nailing: a case report. Clin J Sport Med 1995; 5:58–62.

53 Christopher NC, Congeni J. Overuse Injuries in the pediatric athlete: evaluation, initial management, and strategies for prevention. CPEM 2002; 3:118–128.

54 Styf J. Diagnosis of exercise-induced pain in the anterior aspect of the lower leg. Am J Sports Med 1988; 16:165–169.

55 Blackman PG. A review of chronic exertional compartment syndrome in the lower leg. Med Sci Sport Exerc 2000; 32:4–10.

56 Rowdon GA, Richardson JK, Hoffmann P, et al. Chronic anterior compartment syndrome and deep peroneal nerve function. Clin J Sport Med 2001; 11:229–233.

57 Pedowitz RA, Hargens AR, Mubarek SJ, et al. Modified criteria for the objective diagnosis of chronic compartment syndrome of the leg. Am J Sports Med 1990; 18:35–40.

58 Anderson JE. Grant's atlas of anatomy. 5th edn. Baltimore: Williams & Wilkins; 1983.

59 Davey J, Rorabeck C, Fowler P. The tibialis posterior muscle compartment. Am J Sports Med 1984; 12:391–397.

60 Reid DC. Exercise-induced leg pain. In: Reid DC, ed. Sports injury assessment and rehabilitation. New York: Churchill Livingstone; 1992:269.

61 Black KP, Schultz TK, Cheung NL. Compartment syndromes in athletes. Clin Sports Med 1990; 9:471–487.

62 Cetinus E, Uzel M, Bilgiç E, et al. Exercise induced compartment syndrome in a professional footballer. Br J Sports Med 2004; 38:227–229.

63 Balduini FC, Shenton DW, O'Connor KH, et al. Chronic exertional compartment syndrome: correlation of compartment pressure and muscle ischemia utilizing P-NMR spectroscopy. Clin Sports Med 1993; 12:151–165.

64 Archibold HAP, Wilson L, Barr RJ. Acute exertional compartment syndrome of the leg: consequences of a delay in diagnosis: a report of 2 cases. Clin J Sport Med 2004; 14:98–100.

65 Kruger MS. Lower extremity pain in a runner. Med Sci Sports Exerc 2003; 35:S15.

66 Rorabeck CH, Bourne RB, Fowler PJ, et al. The role of tissue pressure measurement in diagnosing chronic anterior compartment syndrome. Am J Sports Med 1988; 16:143–146.

67 Hutchison MR, Ireland ML. Common compartment syndromes in athletes: treatment and rehabilitation. Sports Med 1994; 17:200–208.

68 Pyne D, Jawad ASM, Padhiar N. Saphenous nerve injury after fasciotomy for compartment syndrome. Br J Sports Med 2003; 37:541–542.

69 Silberman MR, Shiple BJ, Collina SJ. Exercise induced leg pain – soccer. Med Sci Sports Exerc 2004; 36:S93.

70 Dunbar MJ, Stanish WD, Vincent NE. Chronic exertional compartment syndrome. In: Harries M, Williams C, Stanish W, Micheli LJ, eds. Textbook of sports medicine. 2nd edn. Oxford: Oxford University Press; 1998:669.

71 Baltopoulos P, Filippou DK, Sigala F. Popliteal artery entrapment syndrome: anatomic or functional syndrome? Clin J Sport Med 2004; 14:8–12.

72 Bradshaw C. Exercise-related lower leg pain: vascular. Med Sci Sports Exerc 2000; 32:34–36.

73 Taylor AJ, George KP. Ankle to brachial pressure index in normal subjects and trained cyclists with exercise-induced leg pain. Med Sci Sports Exerc 2001; 33:1862–1867.

74 Hirai M, Schoop W. Clinical significance of Doppler velocity and blood pressure measurements in peripheral arterial occlusive disease. Angiology 1984; 85:45–53.

75 Abraham P, Saumet JL, Chevalier JM. External iliac artery endofibrosis in athletes. Sports Med 1997; 24:221–226.

76 Turnipseed WD, Pozniac M. Popliteal entrapment as a result of neurovascular compression by the soleus and plantaris muscles. J Vasc Surg 1992; 15:285–294.

77 Bouhoutsos J, Daskalakis E. Muscular abnormalities affecting the popliteal vessels. Br J Surg 1981; 68:501–506.

78 Murray A, Halliday M, Croft RJ. Popliteal artery entrapment syndrome. Br J Surg 1991; 78:1414–1419.

79 Okragly RA, Babka BM, Briner WW. Exercise-induced leg pain. Med Sci Sports Exerc 2002; 34:S44.

80 Younger DS. Entrapment neuropathies. Prim Care 2004; 31:53–65.

81 McCrory P. Exercise-related leg pain: neurological perspective. Med Sci Sports Exerc 2000; 32:11–14.

82 Netter FH. Nerve plexuses and peripheral nerves. In: Brass A, Dingle RV, eds. The Ciba Collection of Medical Illustrations, Vol. 1 Nervous system, Part 1 Anatomy and physiology. New Jersey: Ciba Medical Education Division; 1986:113.

83 Katirji B. Peroneal neuropathy. Neurol Clin 1999; 17:567–591.

84 Ryan MM, Darras BT, Soul JS. Peroneal neuropathy from ankle-foot orthoses. Pediatr Neurol 2003; 29:72–74.

85 Leach RE, Purnell MB, Saito A. Peroneal nerve entrapment in runners. Am J Sports Med 1989; 17:287–291.

86 Hochman MG. Nerves in a pinch: imaging of nerve compression syndromes. Radiol Clin North Am 2004; 42:221–245.

87 Shapiro BE, Preston DC. Entrapment and compressive neuropathies. Med Clin North Am 2003; 87:663–696.

88 Styf J. Chronic exercise-induced pain in the anterior aspect of the lower leg. Sports Med 1989; 7:331–339.

89 Pecina M, Bojanic I, Markiewitz AD. Nerve entrapment syndromes in athletes. Clin J Sport Med 1993; 3:36–43.

90 Walker WC. Lower leg pain. In: Lillegard WA, Rucker KS, eds. Handbook of sports medicine. A symptom oriented approach. Boston: Andover Medical Publishers; 1993:150.

91 Devereaux MW. Neck pain. Prim Care 2004; 31:19–31.

92 Campbell WW. Diagnosis and management of common compression and entrapment neuropathies. Neurol Clin 1997; 15:549–567.

93 Toy BJ. Conservative treatment of bilateral sural nerve entrapment in an ice hockey player. J Athletic Train 1996; 31:68–70.

94 Fabre T, Montero C, Gaujard E, et al. Chronic calf pain in athletes due to sural nerve entrapment. Am J Sports Med 2000; 28:679–682.

95 Reid V, Cros D. Proximal sensory neuropathies of the leg. Neurol Clin 1999; 17:655–667.

96 Romanoff ME, Cory PC, Kalenak A, et al. Saphenous nerve entrapment at the adductor canal. Am J Sports Med 1989; 17:478–481.

97 Kalenak A. Saphenous nerve entrapment. Oper Tech Sports Med 1996; 4:40–45.

98 Garrett WE Jr. Muscle strain injuries. Am J Sports Med 1996; 24:2–8.

99 Anderson SJ. Lower extremity injuries in youth sports. Pediatr Clin North Am 2002; 49:627–641.

100 Boutin RD, Fritz RC, Steinbach LS. Imaging of sports-related muscle injuries. Radiol Clin North Am 2002; 40:333–362.

101 Laing AJ, Lenehan B, Ali A, et al. Isolated dislocation of the proximal tibiofibular joint in a long jumper. Br J Sports Med 2003; 37:366–367.

102 Sekiya JK, Kuhn JE. Instability of the proximal tibiofibular joint. J Am Acad Orthop Surg 2003; 11:120–128.

103 Reid DC. Internal derangement and other selected lesions of the knee. In: Reid DC, ed. Sports injury assessment and rehabilitation. New York: Churchill Livingstone; 1992:301.

104 Mellion MB. Overtraining. In: Mellion MB, ed. Sports medicine secrets. Toronto: Mosby; 1994:154.

105 Perron AD, Brady WJ, Miller MD. Orthopedic pitfalls in the ED: osteomyelitis. Am J Emerg Med 2003; 21:61–67.

106 Sherry DD, Malleson PN. The idiopathic musculoskeletal pain syndromes in childhood. Rheum Dis Clin N Am 2002; 28:669–685.

107 Resnick D. Tumors and tumor-like lesions of bone: radiographic principles. In: Resnick D, ed. Bone and Joint Imaging. 2nd edn. Toronto: WB Saunders; 1996:979.

108 Luedtke LM, Flynn JM, Ganley TJ. The orthopedists' perspective: bone tumors, scoliosis, and trauma. Radiol Clin North Am 2001; 39:803–821.

109 Fallon KE, Collins SJ, Purdam CM. Miyoshi myopathy – an unusual cause of calf pain and tightness. Clin J Sport Med 2004; 14:45–47.

CHAPTER 33

Ankle Injuries

Stephen M. Simons and Jerrad Zimmerman

Box 33.1: Key Points

- The ankle remains the single most frequent sport related joint injury.

- Common ankle sprains cause untold time lost from sport. Prompt, appropriate rehabilitation can return the athlete to the practice fields with a minimal delay.

- Injury preventive strategies, either post-injury or de novo can reduce ankle sprain frequency.

- Other ankle maladies affecting athletes include: anterior and posterior impingement syndromes, osteochondral injuries, tendonitis, peroneal tendon subluxation and a brief look at non-operatively treated ankle fractures.

INTRODUCTION

Ankle injuries remain the single most frequently injured joint in sport. This chapter reviews basic anatomy, mechanisms of injury, diagnostic strategies and clinical management recommendations for the common ankle sprain and other regional injuries.

ANATOMY

The ankle is formed by the talus, distal tibia and fibula. The distal tibial plafond, medial malleolus, and lateral malleolus comprise the ankle mortise. The talar dome fits into the ankle mortise to complete the bony components of the ankle joint. The talar dome, wider anteriorly than posteriorly, is conical shaped in the transverse plane. This increases stability of the ankle mortise when the ankle is dorsiflexed and decreases stability when the ankle is plantarflexed.[1]

The ankle has multiple stabilizing ligaments. The deltoid ligament supports the medial aspect of the ankle mortise. The deltoid ligament, aptly named because it is narrow proximally and fans out distally, extends from the distal tibia to the talus, navicular and calcaneus. The lateral ankle ligamentous structure is much less stable and is composed of three ligaments: the anterior talofibular ligament, calcaneofibular ligament, and posterior talofibular ligament. The distal tibia and fibula is stabilized by four ligaments: the interosseous membrane, anterior inferior tibiofibular ligament, posterior inferior tibiofibular ligament, and transverse tibiofibular ligament.[2] The posterior talofibular ligament runs from the posterior distal fibula to the posterior talus.

The anatomic location of the anterior talofibular ligament (ATFL) originates from the distal fibula and inserts on the lateral talus just proximal to the subtalar joint. The ATFL is a thickening of the anterior ankle capsule. The ATFL is 6–10 mm wide, 10 mm long and about 2 mm thick. The ATFL crosses the lateral ankle in the neutral position in an anterior direction making an angle of 75°. The ATFL is the most commonly injured ligament in the ankle. The ATFL functions to limit plantarflexion and internal rotation of the foot.[3]

The calcaneofibular ligament (CFL) extends distal and slightly posterior from the tip of the fibula to the lateral calcaneus. The CFL is an extracapsular ligament 2–2.5 cm in length and 6–8 mm in width. The CFL orientation forms an angle of 113–150° with the fibula when the ankle is placed in a neutral position. As the ankle is dorsiflexed, the ligament orients parallel to the long fibular axis and tightens. The CFL limits ankle mortise inversion. The CFL is the second most common injured ligament in the ankle.[3]

Ankle excursion occurs principally in the sagittal plane and to a lesser extent in the coronal and transverse planes. Sagittal plane motion is 15–20° dorsiflexion and 35–40° plantarflexion. The arc of motion while walking averages 24°, ranging from 20–36°. Coronal plane, inversion and eversion, is about 10°. Transverse plane, internal and external rotation is 15–20°.[4]

Ten tendons cross the ankle joint in four distinct compartments. The anterior compartment contains four tendons involved with dorsiflexion of the ankle. The four tendons in the anterior compartment listed from medial to lateral are tibialis anterior tendon, extensor hallucis longus tendon, extensor digitorum longus tendon, and peroneus tertius tendon. The lateral compartment holds two muscles involved in eversion of the ankle and some mild plantarflexion. The lateral compartment muscles run posterior and inferior to the lateral malleolus and insert onto the foot. They are the peroneal longus tendon and peroneal brevis tendon. The deep posterior compartment of the leg contains three muscles that cross the medial ankle joint posterior and inferior to the medial malleolus. This muscle group functions to invert the ankle and has some role in ankle plantarflexion. The tendons in the deep posterior muscle group cross the ankle posterior to the medial malleolus. The tendons lie posterior to the medial malleolus in the anterior to posterior orientation of posterior tibial tendon, flexor digitorum longus, and flexor hallucis longus. The posterior leg muscle groups combine to form the Achilles tendon that crosses the posterior ankle joint. The posterior muscle group contains the soleus, gastrocnemius, and plantaris muscles. The posterior muscle group functions as ankle plantarflexors.[1]

LATERAL ANKLE SPRAIN

Box 33.2: Key Points

- Ankle sprains are responsible for 40% of all sport related injuries.
- Early examination and identifying the specific ligaments or bone at risk is critical to proper management and return to play.
- Assessing the ankle and applying the Ottawa Ankle Rules to the 18–55-year-old athlete can guide the clinicians need to obtain radiographs.
- Ankle injury rehabilitation follows a progressive procedure returning the athlete to play on average after 14 days.
- Bracing or taping can reduce ankle re-injury rates.
- Primary ankle injury prevention by bracing or taping is possible but at some risk of performance decrement.

Ankle sprains account for about 40% of all sports related injuries. The majority of ankle sprains are on the lateral side. A total of 10% of all emergency department visits are due to ankle sprains. Ankle injuries account for 12% of missed American football practice or game time. Ankle injuries represent 53% of all basketball athletic injuries and 29% of all soccer extremity injuries.[3] The incidence of ankle injuries is 1 in 10 000 people/day.[5] The most common injury mechanism occurs when the plantarflexed foot is inverted beyond the ligamentous strain capability. The ATFL is injured first followed by the CFL. Researchers estimate rupture of the CFL requires 2–3.5 times the force needed to rupture the ATFL.[6]

The injury history focuses on sport activity, contact *versus* non-contact injury, mechanism of injury, history of previous ankle injury or instability, presence or absence of an audible pop, pain or neurologic symptoms, swelling onset, etc. The patient with a lateral ankle sprain complains of pain, swelling, and sometimes ecchymosis over the lateral ankle. The ability of the patient to bear weight on the injured ankle after a sprain helps the physician differentiate the severity of the sprain and possible need for ankle radiographs. There is generally palpable tenderness present over the injured ligaments.[3] Funder demonstrated that tenderness over the ATFL is associated with a tear of this ligament 52% of the time. Tenderness at the distal insertion of the CFL is associated with disruption to this ligament 72% of the time.[7]

Prudently evaluating ankle sprains is the subject of many studies. The Ottawa ankle rules (OAR) are perhaps the best known rules for determining the need for radiographs. These rules, developed by Stiell and colleagues in the early 1990s, potentially reduce the number of ankle radiographs performed in the emergency department by about 30%. The OAR indicating the need for ankle radiographs include tenderness with palpation of the anterior or posterior aspect of either malleolus, pain with palpation of the distal 6 cm of the distal tibia or fibula, or the inability to bear weight at the time of injury or at the time of the examination. Indications for a midfoot radiograph include tenderness along the base of the 5th metatarsal or navicular bone or inability to bear weight at the time of the examination or at the time of the injury.[8] The OAR, applied appropriately to patients aged 18–55, enjoy a nearly 100% sensitivity for detecting ankle fractures.[9] In the pediatric population when Salter I or small avulsion fractures are included in the fracture group the sensitivity of the OAR decreases to about 83%. For pediatric patients the OAR may guide your radiographic decision, but should not be your sole reasoning.[10] In questionable cases, err on the side of caution and obtain a radiograph.

Lateral ankle sprains are typically classified into three clinical grades. A grade I ankle sprain involves only stretching the ATFL with no tear and only minimal edema and pain. A grade II sprain involves tearing the ATFL with moderate pain and edema over the lateral ankle. A grade III sprain includes rupture of both the ATFL and the CFL with moderate to severe pain and swelling of the lateral ankle. A patient with a grade III ankle sprain likely will not be able to bear weight on the injured limb due to discomfort. Grade II ankle sprains may or may not cause the patient enough pain to limit weight bearing on the injured ankle.[3]

Failure to completely rehabilitate a lateral ankle sprain may result in persistent, chronic ankle pain.[11] Lateral ankle sprain rehabilitation is relatively well defined. Lateral ankle sprain rehabilitation is divided into four phases: initial phase, early rehabilitation, late rehabilitation, and functional phase. It is estimated that 10–20% of patients with lateral ankle sprains regardless of initial management will progress to lateral ankle laxity requiring more rigorous and controlled rehabilitation. The initial phase consists of rest, ice, compression and elevation (RICE). Ultrasound and electrotherapy may be of some benefit. Use of non-steroidal anti-inflammatory drugs (NSAIDs) is controversial. Theoretical detrimental effects include antiplatelet function that promotes bleeding and interferes with optimal tissue repair. However, early pain relief hastens rehabilitation progress. Common opinion endorses brief, early medication use halted within a few days of the injury.

Early gait training with or without weight bearing is essential. Early rehabilitation consists of restoring ankle range of motion with both active and passive range of motion exercise. Active range of motion therapies may include spelling the alphabet with the injured foot and ankle. Theraband resistance exercises also increase range of motion and strength. Contralateral ankle rehabilitation may hasten recovery of the injured ankle. Proprioceptive exercises performed on the contralateral, uninjured ankle, can be started immediately before such exercises could be safely done on the injured ankle. A proprioceptive crossover effect speeds the rehabilitation to the injured ankle.[12]

Late rehabilitation starts when the patient can fully bear weight. Late rehabilitation involves strength and proprioception training. Grade II or III lateral ankle injuries will cause electromyographic abnormalities, specifically, reduced peroneal nerve conduction velocity for at least 22 days.[13,14] This nerve dysfunction renders the athlete vulnerable to re-injury, especially from closed kinetic chain exercises. Early rehabilitation is ideally supervised during this vulnerable time window. Proprioception training is accomplished with multiple methods. These methods range from simple single leg standing exercises to computer monitored and controlled balance platforms. The most common form of proprioception training uses a biomechanical ankle platform system (BAPS) board. The BAPS board is available to athletic trainers, but individuals may accomplish similar goals using a simple commercially available wobble board. Proprioception training speed and difficulty should progress as the ankle improves. While completing proprioception training on the injured ankle, the athlete should also perform contralateral proprioceptive training in an effort to prevent a contralateral ankle sprain in the future.[15]

The functional phase of rehabilitation includes return to running, jumping, and sport specific activity.[16] This final phase begins when non-sporting, activities of daily living are accomplished without pain. Progression of running should start with 50% walking and 50% jogging. Once this is accomplished, the athlete may progress from running to backward running followed by patterned running. The final rehabilitation step prior to full practice is completing sport specific activities at full speed. Creative, functional tasks prepare and test the athlete's ability to return to play. A study by Crase *et al.* found that the average return to play following a lateral ankle sprain in eleven patients was 14.7 days following intensive rehabilitation.[17] Rehabilitation of chronic lateral ankle instability following a lateral ankle sprain focuses mainly on strength and proprioception training. This is accomplished in many ways but a few common rehabilitation programs make use of single leg standing training on progressively less stable surfaces and the use of a balance board.[18]

Ankle injury prevention strategies must follow adequate rehabilitation. The peroneal longus and brevis muscles intrinsically provide more than three times the resistive force to ankle inversion than tape, shoes, and braces alone or combined. Tape or an orthoses with a three-quarter top athletic shoe will increase inversion resistance by a factor of 1.77.[19] Athletic tape's propensity to loosen renders it of limited value with prolonged exercise. Ankle braces are much less prone to loosening with activity. Lace-up ankle braces are the most widely used and studied bracing technique.[20,21] Duration of ankle injury prevention strategies is not known, nonetheless, experts suggest patients should wear a protective ankle brace or tape during athletic competition for 6 months following a moderate or severe lateral ankle sprain.[22] Prophylactic bracing is more helpful for the previously injured ankle than the never before injured ankle. Mechanical stability appears less important than the proprioceptive effect of bracing.[23] Use of prophylactic

ankle devices may reduce the incidence of ankle sprain injuries in never before injured ankles.[24] The concern with using prophylactic ankle taping or bracing is their resulting decrease in function of vertical jump, shuttle run time, and sprint time of 1–5% as compared with the same athlete without ankle taping or bracing.[25]

In cases of recurrent sprains and persistent lateral instability, surgical stabilization may be necessary. The decision to proceed to surgical correction is based on history, physical findings suggesting excessive inversion instability, and stress radiographs.

Inversion AP stress radiographs must be done on both ankles. A difference in talar tilt of at least 5° and an absolute tilt of 10° on the effected side, is usually deemed evidence of frank instability of the lateral ligament complex. Surgical stabilization is done using a variety of different techniques but the common denominator of these techniques is that most are quite successful and allow the athlete to return to sports participation without instability.[26]

SYNDESMOSIS ANKLE SPRAINS

Box 33.3: Key Points

- Syndesmosis injuries are less common but require longer recovery than lateral ankle injuries.
- Oblique, mortise view radiographs are the initial test of choice. MRI can be confirmatory.
- Grade I injuries are relatively minor ligamentous injury that can be managed non-operatively.
- Grade III injuries cause, by definition, an unstable ankle and must be surgically treated.

The syndesmosis tethers the distal tibia and fibula providing a stable mortise for the talar dome within the ankle joint. Syndesmosis ankle sprains account for 1–20% of all ankle sprains.[27,28] Injury to the tibiofibular syndesmosis occurs when the ankle is subjected to extreme dorsiflexion and external rotation. A sudden widening of the ankle mortise can injure the anterior inferior tibiofibular ligament, posterior inferior tibiofibular ligament, transverse tibiofibular ligament, posterior talofibular ligament, and the interosseous membrane (Fig. 33.1).

Typically, an ankle injury happens quickly and the patient will not always give the appropriate history for a syndesmosis ankle sprain. Patients with syndesmosis ankle sprains present with symptoms similar to a lateral ankle sprain. These include pain, edema and difficulty with ambulation. In addition, syndesmosis ankle sprains will present with pain during passive dorsiflexion and external rotation of the ankle. The squeeze test was developed to help diagnose syndesmosis ankle sprains. The squeeze test involves compressing the mid-portion of the tibia and fibula. A positive test indicating a syndesmosis injury elicits pain at the ankle during compression. The external rotation stress test involves stabilizing the tibia and fibula with one

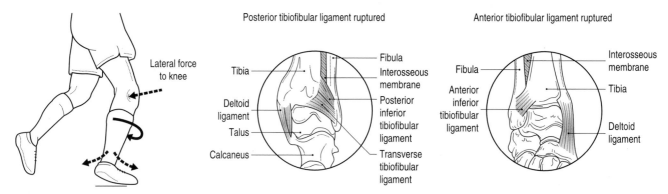

Figure 33.1 High ankle sprain. The mechanism of injury for a syndesmosis, high ankle sprain, differs from the more typical lateral ankle sprain. The foot is fixed to the ground, knee in front of the foot with ankle in dorsiflexed position. This places the wider anterior portion of the talus firmly into the ankle mortise. A forced internal or external rotation of the lower leg is accompanied by talus rotation and thus a spreading or widening force to the malleoli.

hand while the knee is flexed 90°. The other hand externally rotates the ankle. Pain with this maneuver indicates injury to the syndesmosis ligaments (Fig. 33.2).[2] The Cotton test is performed by stabilizing the distal tibia in one hand and holding the heel with the other. Then an attempt is made to displace the heel laterally. Lateral heel displacement within the ankle mortise greater than 3 mm is indicative of a syndesmosis injury. The contralateral ankle should be examined to elicit possible differences in laxity.[29]

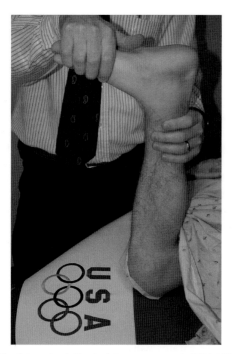

Figure 33.2 External rotation test for assessment of tibial fibular syndesmosis injury. Test can be performed in seated position or as shown in the prone position. The knee is placed at 90°. The tibia and fibula are stabilized while an external rotation force is applied to the ankle. Pain referred to the anterior ankle is a positive test. Although frequently cited to assess syndesmosis injury, test sensitivity and specificity is poor.

Syndesmosis injuries require radiograph examination to evaluate ankle mortise stability. Radiographic examination includes an AP and mortise view. The clear space 1 cm above the tibial plafond should be less than 5 mm on AP and mortise radiographs. The clear space is the distance between the distal lateral tibia and the distal medial fibula. The distal fibula and anterior tibial tubercle overlap should be >6 mm on the AP ankle view and >1 mm on the mortise view. If radiographs show widening of the clear space or decreased distal ankle bone overlap, this is suggestive of syndesmosis diastasis. Syndesmosis diastasis requires orthopedic evaluation for an unstable ankle mortise.[30] External rotation stress radiographs may show posterior tibial tubercle and distal fibula widening of greater than 5 mm on the mortise view. Delayed radiographs can reveal heterotopic ossification of the syndesmosis. Arthrography will show leakage of contrast into the distal tibiofibular syndesmosis. In recent years, the wide availability of MRI imaging has been found to give a clear and accurate assessment of both the ligaments involved and the extent of the injury.[31] Radionucleotide imaging may be helpful with diagnosing a syndesmosis injury if other imaging is not available.[32]

Syndesmosis sprains are graded based on the amount of injury to the ligaments. A grade I sprain involves syndesmosis ligament interstitial tears and tenderness during examination. A grade III sprain encompasses complete syndesmosis ligament rupture and ankle mortise instability. Grade II sprains categorize all sprains between grades I and III.[31]

Syndesmosis injury management depends on the degree of injury. Grade I injury management is non-operative. Initial management combines rest, ice, compression and elevation. The patient may or may not need crutches. External support devices may be used to support the injured ankle. The patient should begin simple rehabilitation and progress as tolerated to active rehabilitation. Grade II syndesmosis injury management is more controversial. Grade II injuries present in many ways due to the varying ligamentous injury involved. Grade II syndesmosis injury management is dependent on the physician evaluating the patient and ankle symptoms. Grade II syndesmosis injury management can be accomplished with either surgical or conservative methods. Grade III injuries require surgical management.[31] The most common procedure is placement of one or two syndesmotic screws.

Prolonged recovery following a syndesmosis injury is common. A study of National Hockey League players revealed the average return to play after a syndesmosis injury was 45 days (range 6–137) *versus* lateral ankle sprain return to play of 1.4 days (range 0–6).[33] It is important to warn the athlete and coach about this long recovery time. Their experience of quick recovery with ankle sprains needs modification when dealing with a syndesmosis sprain. The prolonged recovery time does not result in poor outcome. Following syndesmosis ankle sprains, the athlete normally regains full function. Heterotopic ossification of the damaged syndesmosis is common but usually painless. Injured syndesmoses ligaments rarely develop synostosis. Synostosis is a bony fusion between the tibia and fibula distally. Synostosis can result in pain and sometimes requires surgical excision. Starting anti-inflammatory agents, like indomethacin, two to three days after a syndesmosis injury may help prevent synostosis development. Complete syndesmosis rehabilitation reduces the incidence of recurrent ankle sprains.[31]

PERONEAL TENDON SUBLUXATION

Box 33.4: Key Points

- Peroneal subluxation can be a subtle and uncommon cause for lateral ankle pain.
- Observing the tendons translate anterior to the malleolus with provocative maneuvers suggests the diagnosis.
- Surgical fixation is usually required for chronic peroneal subluxation.

Peroneal tendon subluxation is a relatively uncommon disorder. Peroneal tendon subluxation results from peroneal longus or brevis tendon anterior translation over the lateral malleolus. The peroneal tendons normally run within the retrofibular sulcus. Injury to the superior peroneal retinaculum may permit the tendon to bowstring anteriorly and sublux over the lateral malleolus. The retinaculum usually tears from the fibula. Peroneal subluxations are often reported following skiing injuries. Acute peroneal tendon subluxation may become chronic if left untreated or treated unsuccessfully.[34]

The mechanism of action that leads to peroneal tendon subluxation is controversial. The best-described mechanism of action leading to peroneal tendon subluxation is a sudden, forceful passive dorsiflexion of the everted foot with a strong reflex contraction of the peroneal muscles and other plantarflexors. The injury may also occur with the ankle inverted. The core cause of the injury is a peroneal muscle forceful contraction tearing the superior peroneal retinaculum fibular attachment and allowing peroneal tendon anterior translation. The peroneal brevis tendon dislocates more frequently than the peroneal longus tendon.[34,35]

Eckert and Davis originally classified peroneal tendon subluxations into three grades based on operative findings. Grade I peroneal tendon subluxation is detachment of the tendon retinaculum and periosteum from the fibula. Grade II peroneal subluxation is elevation of the distal 1–2 cm of the dense fibrous lip of the retinaculum. Grade III peroneal subluxation is an avulsion of a thin fragment of bone along with the peroneal retinaculum.[36] Oden describes a second classification system. Oden's classification has the same type I and III classifications as Eckert and Davis' grade I and III. A type II injury is a retinaculum tear from its fibular attachment. An Oden's type III lesion is an anterior avulsion of the peroneal retinaculum. A type IV lesion is a posterior avulsion of the peroneal retinaculum.[37]

A peroneal tendon subluxation may be misdiagnosed as a lateral ankle sprain. The diagnosis of a peroneal tendon subluxation requires a good history and careful physical examination. An acute peroneal subluxation will usually be associated with a pop or snap and lateral ankle pain and swelling. Patients will normally not complain of ankle instability. The patient will have pain with palpation posterior to the lateral malleolus. Patients with chronic peroneal subluxation may describe snapping or popping with certain activities. Provocative testing during examination helps identify peroneal subluxation. Provocative testing consists of resisting eversion with the ankle dorsiflexed. Provocative testing will either reproduce the peroneal subluxation or cause pain. Plain radiographs may demonstrate a bony avulsion but do not usually confirm or exclude this diagnosis. MRI and ultrasound may clarify a clinically equivocal case.[34]

Acute peroneal tendon subluxation may be treated operatively or non-operatively. If the diagnosis is made acutely, which is not usual, cast immobilization in inversion may result in healing.[38] Chronic peroneal tendon subluxation requires surgical repair. Many surgical interventions are described. Surgical repair involves stabilizing the peroneal tendons within the retrofibular sulcus using bony manipulation, direct repair of the retinaculum, or reconstruction of the retinaculum using other local tissues. Chronic peroneal tendon subluxation surgical repair success rate has been reported to have good or excellent results 80–100% of the time.[39] The acute peroneal subluxation nonoperative management success rate is approximately 50%.[40] Operative reconstruction of the peroneal retinaculum in acute subluxation has a better success rate than nonoperative management. Acute peroneal subluxation operative management involves all the normal risks associated with surgery. A postoperative comparison of acute peroneal tendon operative and nonoperative management has not yet been reported.[34]

PERONEAL TENDON TEAR

Peroneal tendon tear is a very uncommon injury. It can occur in young or old patients. In young athletes, it is associated with lateral ankle sprains. Peroneal tendon tears present with posterior fibular tenderness and swelling with no appreciable subluxation. Symptoms persist for months after the original injury. MRI is usually required to confirm a tear of the peroneal longus or brevis tendon. Peroneal tendon tear is very uncommon and surgical repair of the tendon has been described as a method of treatment.[41]

ANTERIOR ANKLE IMPINGEMENT

Box 33.5: Key Points

- Anterior ankle impingement is a symptom complex of anterior ankle pain due to repetitive traction or compressive injury to the anterior aspect of the ankle.

- Lateral or oblique radiographs may reveal the typical 'kissing' osteophytes. CT or MRI may further clarify the lesion.

- Initial non-operative management includes elevating the heel and restricting dorsiflexion with tape or braces.

- Operative resection is reserved for those cases not improving with conservative care. Return to play is often within 7 weeks.

Anterior tibiotalar impingement is a symptom complex referred to the anterior ankle. The cause of anterior tibiotalar impingement is controversial. Some believe it results from repetitive anterior ankle joint capsule traction during plantarflexion. This repeated traction causes bone formation at the margin of the anterior ankle joint capsule.[29] Other researchers believe anterior tibiotalar impingement results from repetitive soft tissue injury during repetitive ankle dorsiflexion. Ballet pliés and gymnastics landings cause considerable compressive forces to the anterior ankle. The resulting repetitive compression injury causes soft tissue ossification along the anterior tibia and talus. This latter hypothesis is supported by cadaveric examination of eight ankles showing the anterior tibiotalar spurs originate distal to the anterior ankle joint capsule attachment.[42]

Anterior tibiotalar impingement presents as anterior ankle pain. The pain worsens with both terminal active and passive ankle dorsiflexion. Patients can also have pain with terminal plantarflexion. Anterior ankle edema may be present. Ankle range of motion may be limited by pain or mechanically by anterior tibial or talar osteophyte formation. A bony prominence is occasionally palpable on the anterior talus or tibia. Patients with anterior tibiotalar impingement participate in activities that require rapid acceleration and deceleration of the ankle at terminal ankle dorsi and plantarflexion.[29] Footballer's ankle and impingement exostoses are two common labels for anterior tibiotalar impingement.[43,44]

Ankle imaging helps confirm anterior tibiotalar impingement. Lateral ankle radiographs can demonstrate anterior talus or tibial osteophyte formation. Weight bearing lateral ankle radiographs during dorsiflexion may exhibit contact between the bony talus and tibia or associated osteophytes.[29] An oblique anteromedial impingement radiograph may improve sensitivity by 40% for detecting anterior talar or tibial osteophytes otherwise missed by plain ankle lateral radiographs (Fig. 33.3).[45] The tibial osteophyte is normally wider than the talar spur. The talar osteophyte peak routinely lies medial to the talar dome midline, while the tibial osteophyte peak commonly lies lateral to the talar dome midline.[46] CT imaging provides more detailed views of osteophyte formation. MRI imaging can detect soft tissue and bony edema in addition to anterior tibial and talar osteophytes. An ankle MRI may lack sensitivity and specificity in diagnosing anterior tibiotalar impingement and should be interpreted in conjunction with the findings in the physical examination.[47]

Initial management for anterior tibiotalar impingement utilizes a heel lift, appropriate rest and anti-inflammatory medications. The patient should be instructed to modify physical activity to limit ankle dorsiflexion. If initial conservative management fails then taping or bracing to limit ankle dorsiflexion may be implemented. The patient is forewarned of likely recurrent symptoms if conservative management is discontinued.

Surgical soft tissue or bony debridement can usually be performed arthroscopically, but may occasionally require arthrotomy for large osteophyte resection.[48] McDermott proposed a preoperative classification of anterior tibiotalar impingement. In a type I lesion, the lateral ankle radiograph displays an anterior tibial spur <3 mm in size. In a type II lesion, the lateral ankle radiograph shows an anterior tibial osteophyte >3 mm in size. In a type III lesion, the lateral ankle radiograph demonstrates both tibial and talar osteophytes with or without fragmentation and severe exostosis. In a type IV lesion, the lateral ankle radiograph reveals posterior, lateral, and medial destructive arthritic changes of the anterior tibiotalar joint. Anterior tibial osteophyte resection is the most common surgical intervention. Expected recovery to full athletic participation after arthroscopic debridement for type I, II and III ankles is less than 7 weeks. Type IV ankles are not candidates for arthroscopic debridement alone and usually progress to ankle arthrodesis regardless of interim management.[49]

In addition to bony impingement, certain soft tissue impingements may create similar symptoms, including pain with dorsiflexion, loss of dorsiflexion, and anterior ankle tenderness. These soft tissue inflammatory conditions include lesions of Bassett's ligament, meniscoid lesions and generalized ankle synovitis. Bassett's ligament is a distal fascicle prominence of the anterior inferior tibiofibular ligament. This prominence is felt to contact the anterior talar dome, and cause an inflammatory irritation and subsequent chondral surface damage.[50] A meniscoid lesion is a cartilaginous transformation of a torn anterior talofibular ligament. Meniscoid lesions may become compressed between the lateral malleolus and the talus. Ankle capsule synovitis may also be the cause of anterior tibiotalar impingement.[29]

Ankle rehabilitation is started 4–6 weeks after surgery. Ankle and subtalar range of motion are initially started. These range-of-motion exercises are followed by strengthening and proprioception exercises. The patient may start running and jumping 1–2 months after beginning rehabilitation.[29]

POSTERIOR ANKLE IMPINGEMENT

Posterior ankle impingement presents as posterior ankle pain occurring with ankle plantarflexion. Repetitive ankle plantarflexion compresses the tissue between the posterior tibial articular surface and os calcis. This compression results in tissue injury and inflammation. Ballet 'en pointe', soccer, and

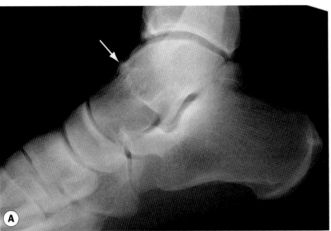 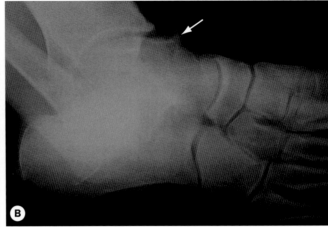

Figure 33.3 Anterior talus spur. (A) Nearly imperceptible on the lateral view. (B) An oblique view demonstrates the spur nicely. Incidental note of large, asymptomatic, os trigonum.

Box 33.6: Key Points

- Posterior ankle impingement is most common in ballet and soccer.

- Repetitive compression to posterior ankle structures include the posterior talus process or os trigonum.

- Examination findings include tenderness, swelling to the posterior ankle and pain with forced plantarflexion.

- Lateral radiographs may depict an os trigonum or large posterior talus process.

- MRI may depict the specific posterior tissues injured.

- Conservative care utilizes temporary immobilization, physical therapy modalities, stretching, proprioceptive training, and corticosteroid injections.

- Surgical intervention for those failing conservative care after 6 months enjoys excellent results.

downhill running are sporting events most commonly associated with posterior ankle impingement.[51]

Posterior ankle impingement is the result of injury to soft and bony tissue of the posterior ankle complex. Repetitive ankle plantarflexion compresses the ankle capsule, synovium, posterior tibia, os calcis, lateral process of the talus, or os trigonum. The posterior tibia and os calcis compress these tissues similar to a nut in a nutcracker during ankle plantarflexion. Posterior ankle impingement soft tissue damage leads to inflammation and hypertrophic capsulitis. These inflammatory processes cause accumulation of hypertrophic inflammatory tissue perpetuating further compression injury.[51]

The os trigonum is an accessory ossicle of the foot located posterior to the talus. Normally, a medial and lateral posterior tubercle project off the posterior talus. The posterior lateral tubercle is larger and more prominent. An os trigonum may reflect a failure of closure of the ossification center of the posterior lateral tubercle of the talus or a stress fracture through the tubercle from repetitive activity.[52] Some 7% of the adult popula-

tion exhibits an os trigonum on foot radiographs. Os trigonum occur bilaterally in 1.4% of the adult population. The ossification center between the posterior talus and lateral tubercle is usually visible in young males aged 11–13 and females aged 8–10. The ossification center normally closes 1 year after its appearance.[53] Posterior ankle impingement can be associated with a normal, edematous, or fractured os trigonum.[51]

Posterior ankle impingement can result from injury to the posterior lateral talar tubercle. Compression during forced ankle plantarflexion can fracture or bruise the posterior lateral talar tubercle.[51] Anterior ankle instability can result in posterior ankle impingement by allowing anterior translation of the talus during ankle plantarflexion. The anterior translation of the talus allows more severe impingement of the posterior ankle soft tissue and resulting posterior ankle impingement pain.[54]

Diagnosing posterior ankle impingement is dependent on history and physical examination. The patient will normally describe posterior lateral ankle pain. Tenderness results from palpation posterior to the medial or lateral malleolus. The pain can be reproduced or worsened with forced ankle plantarflexion. Swelling may or may not be present over the posterior ankle.[51]

Posterior ankle impingement imaging begins with ankle radiographs. Standard AP, lateral, and mortise views are sufficient. A standing lateral radiograph of its ankle in plantarflexion ('demipointe' in ballet) may demonstrate the impingement. Computed tomography can help visualize detailed anatomy and fractures but suffers the inability to always determine chronicity. A nuclear bone scan can demonstrate actively irritated bone by showing increased nuclear tracing uptake consistent with bone turnover. This may be helpful to distinguish acute *versus* chronic changes seen on radiographs or CT. The nuclear bone scan will not specify soft tissue injury or define the bone lesion.[51] Ankle MRI scanning can be very useful for posterior ankle impingement. Ankle MRI allows for visualization of bone contusions or fractures within the lateral talar process or os trigonum. MRI can depict pseudoarthroses of the posterolateral talus. Posterior ankle soft tissue damage seen on ankle MRI includes inflammation in the posterior synovial recess of the subtalar and tibiotalar joints and edema within the flexor hallucis longus tendon sheath (Fig. 33.4).[55]

DiStefano and Schon reported a non-operative treatment protocol for posterior ankle impingement in dancers in 2002. It is divided into acute (weeks 1 and 2), subacute (weeks 2–4), and advanced (weeks 4–6). The acute stage employs modalities, mobilization, flexibility, strengthening, proprioception training, closed chain exercises and dance technique training. The subacute stage continues with work as previously mentioned and further dance technique evaluation. The advanced stage begins further dance training with trampoline jump training. The entire treatment protocol is outlined in Table 33.1.[54] Local corticosteroid injections may also help with management of posterior ankle impingement. Cast immobilization for 3–4 weeks can be part of a conservative management plan.[51]

Operative management of posterior ankle impingement is commonly undertaken if conservative management fails. In a study by Hedrick and McBryde, 40% of ankles with posterior ankle impingement required surgical repair after failing six months of conservative therapy. Their surgical intervention employed a medial approach to resect the os trigonum or other bone fragments and debridement of any remaining inflammatory soft tissue. After resection, the patient was placed in a short leg cast for 2–3 weeks. The patient could resume normal walking with therapy at 6 weeks and regular activity at 12 weeks after surgery. In excess of 85% of the operative patients reported good to excellent results 12 months after surgery.[51] Marotta and Micheli reported a similar success rate using a lateral approach, described as theoretically safer, with less risk of neurovascular injury.[52]

Flexor hallucis longus (FHL) tendonitis is a special subset of posterior ankle impingement. Ballet imparts significant demands to the flexor tendons. Repetitive plantarflexion compression and dorsiflexion tension can cause a debilitating tendonitis along the medial side of the ankle. This is often confused with posterior tibial tendonitis. Non-operative care includes decreasing activity, ice application, physical therapy and NSAID use. Surgical debridement can be necessary if not improving.[56]

Flexor hallucis injury may co-exist with posterior impingement and os trigonum pathology. In such cases, a medial approach to the posterior ankle allows tenolysis of the FHL, and removal of the os trigonum. In cases of os trigonum impingement alone, a posterior approach is sufficient, and safer.[57]

OSTEOCHONDRAL INJURIES

Talar osteochondral injury is a common reason for chronic ankle pain. Although acute transchondral fracture can also occur it is rare compared to ankle sprain incidence and chronic osteochondral injury. Most often the talus dome is involved, but talar head lesions are also documented (Fig. 33.5).[58] Clinical suspicion is aroused as the patient complains of chronic ankle swelling, pain, instability, and catching or locking. The lesions may occur on the lateral or medial talar dome. Osteochondritis dissecans (OCD) was coined by Kappis in 1992 noting similarity to lesions in the knee. The etiology is probably injury to the subchondral bone leading to a focal osteonecrosis.

Osteochondral injuries occur on the lateral side approximately 43% of the time. Lateral defects are more commonly associated with trauma. Cadaveric studies suggest an inversion and dorsiflexion mechanism. The lateral lesion is wafer-shaped and usually located over the superior, anterior talar dome.[29]

Medial osteochondral lesions occur 57% of the time. They are more commonly located on the posteromedial talar dome and are cup shaped. They are associated with degenerative cysts and osteochondrosis.[29] Medial osteochondral lesions are less frequently associated with acute trauma as compared to lateral osteochondral lesions, and it has been suggested that repetitive stress is responsible for at least one third of the medial lesions.[48,59] Two thirds of OCD cases occur in males.

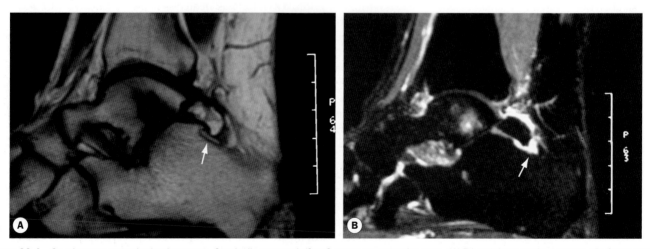

Figure 33.4 Os trigonum posterior impingement. Surgically resected after 2 years conservative care. (A) T1 weighted sagittal image. (B) Short tau inversion-recovery (STIR) image showing edema surrounding the os trigonum and infiltrating the posterior talus.

Table 33.1 Posterior Impingement Protocol

I   Acute stage (weeks 1–2)

  A   Modalities such as phonophoresis, cold whirlpool, ice and electrical stimulation

  B   Soft-tissue work/myofascial release to the gastrocnemius-soleus complex and the plantar fascia

  C   Mobilization to the talus, calcaneus, midtarsal joint, and tibiofibular joints, calcaneal and talus distractions

  D   Flexibility exercises to the gastrocnemius-soleus complex in subtalar joint neutral

  E   Strengthening exercises, using an elastic band for inversion and eversion in plantar flexion and dorsiflexion and for hip external rotators

  F   Closed chain exercises consisting of leg press, wall slides, multi-hip machine and foot intrinsic

  G   Proprioception exercises, consisting of biomechanical ankle platform system (BAPS) board in single stance with eyes open and then closed, with emphasis on proper foot placement, and balancing on a minitrampoline on the affected leg

  H   Physioball and Feldenkrais roll exercise to maintain trunk strength and stabilization

  I   Bike, swimming with no push off, and treadmill to maintain aerobic capacity

  J   Early correction of dance technique is also required. Correct turnout and use of hip external rotators, proper lower extremity alignment, and foot placement are evaluated. One-quarter *relevés* are started on two feet. Relaxation of anterior calf muscles in *demi-* and *grand-plié* are evaluated to allow proper stretch of the posterior muscles. *Tendus*, full *relevés*, and *pointe* work are not allowed at this stage.

II   Subacute stage (weeks 2–4)

  A   Continuation of modalities, soft-tissue work and mobilizations

  B   Continuation of flexibility, strengthening, stabilization, proprioception and aerobic exercises with progressions

  C   *Tendu*, *relevé*, and *pointe* technique are also evaluated and corrected. To achieve the full 180° plantarflexed position, the foot must be stretched into plantarflexion without lifting the heels up into the calf. *Tendus* and *relevés* are resumed as tolerated.

III   Advanced stage (weeks 4–6)

  A   Dance exercises are progressed to full three-quarter *relevé* and balances on *relevé* and *tendu*

  B   Jumping on the minitrampoline on two feet with progression to one foot is incorporated

  C   Dance progression to center work is instituted, and pirouettes and jumps (first with two feet, then with one) are added as tolerated

  D   Once *grande allegro* is comfortable and strong, *pointe* work may be resumed.

With permission from DiStefano and Schon 2002,[54] with permission of J Michael Ryan Publishing, Inc.

Box 33.7: Key Points

- Osteochondral injury to the talus is a common cause of chronic ankle pain, particularly in the adolescent.
- Osteochondral injury occurs nearly equally medially and laterally.
- Lateral lesions are nearly all traumatically caused, whereas one third of medial lesions may biomechanically relate.
- Classifying an OCD by CT or MRI criteria are critical to appropriate management.
- Stage I, II and medial stage III lesions may be treated non-operatively initially.
- Stage III lateral and Stage IV lesions should be treated surgically.
- Newly described Stage V lesions in adults generally do well without surgery.

Berndt and Harty first developed a staging approach for osteochondral lesions in 1959.[60] A stage I lesion is localized compression of the subchondral bone without break in the cartilage. A stage II lesion is a partially detached osteochondral fragment. The stage III lesion is a completely detached fragment remaining in place. A stage IV lesion is a displaced osteochondral fragment acting as a loose body.[61] Loomer added a stage V lesion exhibiting a stable subchondral radiolucent cyst in 1993.[62] Recently, Hepple and associates proposed a new classification system based on MRI. This also includes a stage V lesion. This classification system is better thought to guide management than Berndt and Harty's radiographic classification (Fig. 33.6).[63]

Chronic ankle pain, particularly in the adolescent, deserves a high index of suspicion for this relatively common condition. The patients may or may not have a history of ankle trauma. As previously mentioned, ankle pain, swelling, instability and catching or locking are historical clues. Careful examination may reveal tenderness directly over the talus rather than the adjacent ligaments.

Initial imaging includes standard ankle radiographs with additional plantarflexion and dorsiflexion views. Plantarflexed, oblique radiographs minimize fibular overlap and place the lesions tangential to the x-ray beam, thereby improving sensitivity for finding OCDs. MRI greatly improves evaluation of the bone and overlying chondral surface. Modern management plans rely more on these MRI findings than the X-ray changes (Fig. 33.7).[64,65]

Toll performed a meta-analysis of 32 studies encompassing the management of 582 patients with ankle osteochondral injuries.[59] Stage I, II and medial stage III lesions do well with non-operative management and are less likely to progress to arthritis. Non-weight bearing cast or bracing for 6 weeks is followed by a symptom driven gradual return to weight bearing and athletic activity. If severe symptoms persist longer than 6 months, surgical options are considered. Open or arthroscopic procedures include excision, with or without drilling, bone

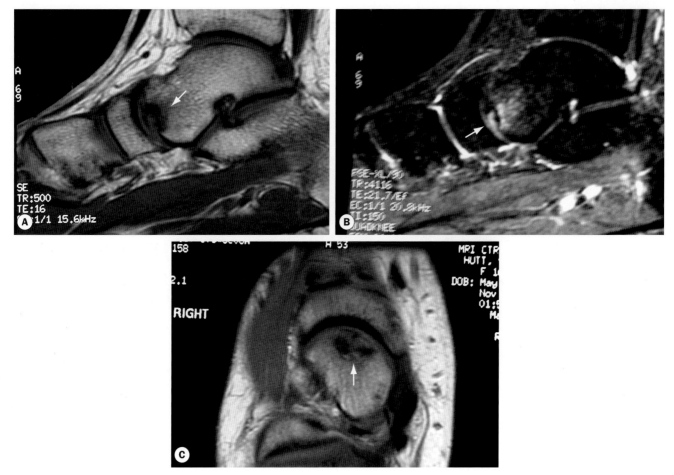

Figure 33.5 Osteochondritis dissecans (OCD) to the talus head. (A) T1 weighted sagittal MRI. (B) T2 weighted image. (C) T1 weighted transverse MRI.

grafting, internal fixation and osteochondral transplantation. Large non-displaced lesions sometimes can be secured arthroscopically with absorbable suture, buried pins, or screws. Lateral stage III and all stage IV lesions in adults are best treated surgically given their propensity to remain symptomatic, heal poorly and develop arthritis.[66] Adolescents with open physes deserved a non-operative trial period.

Shearer and colleagues reviewed 35 ankles with chronic stage V lesions, 88 months from symptom onset. Stage V lesions are usually chronic lesions and can arise from any previous osteochondral stage. Most of the patients with stage V lesions reported good to excellent overall clinical outcome following conservative care for 38 months. Lateral stage V lesions faired better than medial stage V lesions. The authors recommended non-operative management of all stage V lesions unless the symptoms were disabling or further imaging reveals an intracapsular loose body. Stage V talar osteochondral lesions are unlikely to progress to significant ankle osteoarthritis for at least 88 months after symptom onset. Patients <20 years old tend to fair worse with stage V osteochondral lesions as compared with patients over 20 years of age.[67]

Current research is being conducted on osteochondral replacement after an osteochondral injury. Research on osteo-chondral autologous transfer system (OATS), mosaicplasty and autologous chondrocyte implantation (ACI) is ongoing. OATS involves harvesting a plug of articular cartilage and bone from a donor site, usually the femoral condyle or trochlea of the patient's own knee and inserting it into the site of the osteochondral lesion. Donor site symptoms can be a complication of OATS.[68] Mosaicplasty involves harvesting multiple small fragments of articular cartilage from the femoral condyle or trochlea and arranging the multiple fragments over the osteochondral lesion. The advantage is a proposed decrease in donor site morbidity. Mosaicplasty is limited by the small fragments of transplanted tissue allowing more fibrocartilage infiltration and fragment fixation.[48] In a study by Hangody *et al.*, 36 patients with osteochondral lesions >10 mm were followed for 2–7 years after mosaicplasty. Some 94% of the patients reported good to excellent results with no donor site mortality.[69] ACI involves harvesting autologous chondrocytes and growing an articular surface *in vitro*. The *in vitro* cultured graft is then transplanted over the damaged osteochondral surface. ACI has been reported in the literature for treatment of knee osteochondral lesions with moderate success 5 years postoperatively.[48] More prospective studies need to be done to help differentiate the best osteochondral transplantation surgical technique.

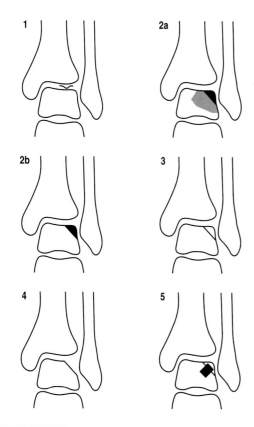

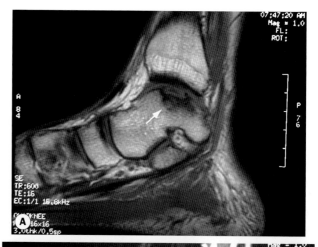

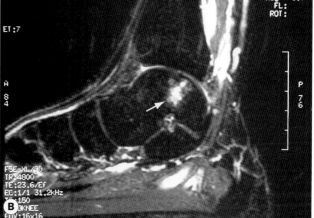

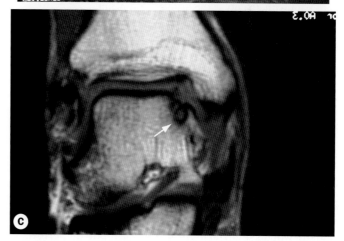

TABLE 2 Revised classification		
	Stage	Current series (*n* = 18)
Stage 1	Articular cartilage damage only	1
Stage 2a	Cartilage injury with underlying fracture and surrounding bony edema	1
Stage 2b	Stage 2a without surrounding bony edema	2
Stage 3	Detached but nondisplaced fragment	3
Stage 4	Detached and displaced fragment	2
Stage 5	Subchondral cyst formation	9

Figure 33.6   MRI based OCD classification. (From Hepple et al. 1999,[63] with permission).

POSTERIOR TIBIAL TENDINOPATHY

Box 33.8: Key Points

- Posterior tibial tendonitis presents as medial ankle pain and swelling in the absence of any specific trauma. It is associated with excessive flat foot condition.

- Relatively few acute ankle fractures are treated non-operatively. Careful attention is paid to the mortise view radiograph. Even 1–2 mm asymmetry is cause for surgical treatment.

- Medial malleolar stress fractures usually occur from overuse. The fracture is usually oriented vertical or obliquely starting at the plafond malleolus junction. Some 50% of these fractures require secondary imaging to diagnose.

Figure 33.7   Osteochondritis dissecans of dome. (A) T1 weighted image of medial stage III talus dome OCD. (B) STIR image of chronic medial stage III talus dome OCD. (C) Coronal image of medial talus dome OCD.

The posterior tibial tendon traverses the ankle posterior to the medial malleolus then inserts on the medial aspect of the navicular. In the open kinetic chain, it acts to plantarflex and invert at the ankle. During gait, it absorbs eccentric forces to stabilize the midfoot, allowing a more efficient gait. Tendinopathy occurs commonly in the general population due to a hypoperfusion zone in the area closest to the medial malleolus. Those at increased risk include women over 40, the obese and those with a pronated, planus foot. Obesity, diabetes and hypertension increase the risk of tendon rupture.[70] Among athletes, runners who inappropriately increase training and those with poor footwear are at increased risk. Dancers and ice skaters are particularly at risk for posterior tibial tendonitis. In stage I tendinopathy, the tendon is inflamed and tender, but fully intact and functional tendon. In stage II, the tendon is dysfunctional and a flexible flat foot develops. Stage III describes a fixed flat foot with a totally nonfunctional tendon and degenerative subtalar changes.

Typical symptoms include insidious onset of medial ankle pain, worse with weight bearing activity. Climbing stairs and other plantarflexion/ heel raising activities exacerbate the pain. Patients also describe an unstable feeling in the ankle while walking or running. In later stages, a change in foot structure accompanies these symptoms. Patients notice a progressively worsening flat foot or a need to use bigger shoes as the foot lengthens when the medial arch disappears. Pain or swelling posterior to the medial malleolus with a change in foot shape is highly sensitive and specific (98%) for posterior tibial tendon dysfunction in the elderly.[71]

Examination reveals tenderness along the course of the tendon, most commonly posterior and inferior to the malleolus. Patients report pain with resisted plantarflexion and inversion. Foot structure should be noted for pronation, heel valgus and medial longitudinal arch structure. With more advanced disease (Stage II or more) patients are unable to perform a single limb heel rise. Imaging serves a role in objectifying the foot deformity with plain radiographs. Subtalar and tibio-talar joint degeneration can also be evaluated. Magnetic resonance imaging can give useful anatomic information in the athlete, when medial midfoot pain with activity is the primary complaint.

Treatment starts with rest, ice non-steroidal anti-inflammatory medicines as needed and correction of biomechanical risk factors. In flat-footed runners with a short duration of symptoms, rest until pain free and orthotics may suffice as treatment. If the patient cannot perform a single leg heel rise, a short leg cast or walking boot should be used. The patient should remain in the boot until the pain ceases with this test, which may take 4–12 weeks, followed by a 1–2 week weaning from the boot. Intrinsic foot muscle strengthening and eccentric posterior tibial tendon strengthening are integral to rehabilitation.

An acutely ruptured posterior tibial tendon presents with pain radiating from the medial navicular to the medial malleolus. The acquired flat foot may not occur acutely. But the patient will have an inability invert the foot or perform a heel rise. MRI will demonstrate the rupture. This should be repaired surgically.

FRACTURES ABOUT THE ANKLE

The goal of this chapter is not to give a detailed description of the management of fractures about the ankle. Orthopedic texts handle this in great detail and with great accuracy. Suffice it to say that at the present time, fractures about the ankle can be divided into 'stable' and 'unstable' categories. Stable categories of fracture are those that do not threaten the integrity of the

mortise either medially or laterally. In such instances, fractures of the medial or lateral malleolus are felt to be potentially mechanically stable and that stability can be maintained with cast immobilization.

In the case of unstable or potentially unstable fractures, radiographs may give the impression that the integrity of the mortise has been compromised or that cast immobilization alone will be insufficient to guarantee the maintenance of the integrity of the mortise. In such cases under modern treatment management techniques, operative reduction is performed. This operative reduction generally commences with the stabilization of the lateral column of the ankle, i.e. the lateral malleolus, followed by the decision to either mechanically stabilize the medial malleolus or to even perform a surgical repair of the disrupted medial malleolar ligaments (deltoid).

Most patients treated operatively or non-operatively for malleolar fractures can return to routine sport 3 months after the injury. Return to sports requiring high-speed cutting can be as long as 6 months, even with supervised ankle physical therapy.

MEDIAL MALLEOLUS STRESS FRACTURES

Stress fractures around the ankle are quite rare. Medial malleolus stress fractures were first described by Shelbourne et al. in a series of jumping athletes.[72] Shabat reported a case in a young gymnast.[73] The authors have personally cared for two cases in runners. Relative osteopenia in the athlete may be implicated in some cases. This may be the result of the female athlete triad or relative disuse followed by rapid training escalation.

The fracture begins at the junction of the tibial plafond and the medial malleolus. The fracture is most often vertically oriented but sometimes angles obliquely medial. Repetitive rotational forces applied to the malleolus by the talus cause excessive tensile load at the plafond malleolus junction. Shelbourne suspected a biomechanical contribution by excessive forefoot pronation.

Focal ankle pain, malleolar tenderness and possible ankle swelling absent a sentinel injury should raise suspicion for this uncommon injury. The typical fracture line may be apparent on anteroposterior radiograph about 50% of the time.[72,74] If this fracture is suspected, then bone scan, MRI or subsequent radiograph can confirm.

A medial malleolar stress fracture is at risk of developing a fracture non-union or due to instability suffering a frank fracture. Treatment must consider the patients age, fracture line displacement, sport demand and return to sport urgency. The skeletally immature and adults with a non-displaced fracture can be treated conservatively with relative immobilization in a pneumatic brace or removable boot for 6 weeks followed by a gradual return to activity. Orava's five cases treated conservatively healed on average in 4 months.[74] The clinician need remain vigilant for the developing fracture non-union. Adults with complete fractures, fracture non-unions, or need for quicker return to sport, are best treated with internal fixation.

REFERENCES

1. Netter FH. Atlas of human anatomy. 3rd edn. LLC: ICON Learning Systems; 2003.
2. Taylor DC, Bassett FH. Syndesmosis ankle sprains. Phys Sportsmed 1993; 21:39-46.
3. DiGiovanni BF, Partal G, Baumhauer JF. Acute ankle injury and chronic lateral instability in the athlete. Clin Sports Med 2004; 23:1-19.
4. Simons SM, Kennedy RG. Foot and ankle. In: Roberts WO, ed. Bull's handbook of sports injuries. 2nd edn. New York: McGraw-Hill; 2004:349-369.
5. Katcherian DA. Soft-tissue injuries of the ankle. In: Dutter LD, Mizel MS, Pfeffer GB, eds. Orthopedic knowledge update: Foot and ankle. Rosemont, IL: American Academy of Orthopedic Surgeons; 1994:241-253.
6. Attarian DE, McCrackin HJ, Devito DP. Biomechanical characteristics of human ankle ligaments. Foot Ankle 1985; 6:54-58.
7. Funder V, Jorgensen JP, Andersen A, et al. Ruptures of the lateral ligaments of the ankle. Clinical diagnosis. Acta Orthop Scand 1982; 53:997-1000.
8. Stiell IG, McKnight RD, Greenberg GH, et al. Implementation of the Ottawa ankle rules. JAMA 1994; 271:827-832.
9. Nugent PJ. Ottawa Ankle Rules accurately assess injuries and reduce reliance on radiographs. J Fam Pract 2004; 53:785-788.
10. Clark KD, Tanner S. Evaluation of the Ottawa ankle rules in children. Pediatr Emerg Care 2003; 19:73-78.
11. Mizel MS, Hecht PJ, Marymont JV, Temple HT. Evaluation and treatment of chronic ankle pain. J Bone Jt Surg 2004; 86A:622-631.
12. Osborne MD, Chou LS, Laskowski ER, Smith J, Kaufman KR. The effect of ankle disk training on muscle reaction time in subjects with a history of ankle sprain. Am J Sports Med 2001; 29:627-632.
13. Nitz AJ, Dobner JJ, Kersey D. Nerve injury in grades II and III ankle sprains. Am J Sports Med 1985; 13:177-182.
14. Kleinrensink GJ, Stoeckart R, Meulstee J, et al. Lowered motor conduction velocity of the peroneal nerve after inversion trauma. Med Sci Sports Exerc 1994; 26:877-889.
15. Mattacola CJ, Dwyer MK. Rehabilitation of the ankle after acute sprain or chronic instability. J Athletic Train 2002; 37:413-429.
16. Mascaro TB, Swanson LE. Rehabilitation of the foot and ankle. Orthop Clin North Am 1994; 25:147-160.
17. Cross KM, Worrell TW, Leslie JE, Khalid RVV. The relationship between self-reported and clinical measures and the number of days to return to sport following acute lateral ankle sprains. J Orthop Sports Phys Ther 2002; 32:16-23.
18. Zöch C, Fialka-Moser V, Quittan M. Rehabilitation of ligamentous ankle injuries: a review of recent studies. Br J Sports Med 2003; 37:291-295.
19. Ashton-Miller JA, Ottaviani RA, Hutchinson Ch, et al. What best protects the inverted weightbearing ankle against further inversion. Am J Sports Med 1996; 24:800-809.
20. Gross MT, Liu HY. The role of ankle bracing for prevention of ankle sprain injuries. J Orthop Sports Phys Ther 2003; 33:572-577.
21. Gross MT, Lapp AK, Davis JM. Comparison of Swede-O-Universal ankle support and Aircast sport-stirrup orthoses and ankle tape in restricting eversion-inversion before and after exercise. J Orthop sports Phys Ther 1991; 13:11-19.
22. Osborne MD, Rizzo TD Jr. Prevention and treatment of ankle sprain in athletes. Sports Med 2003; 33:1145-1150.
23. Surve I, Schwellnus MP, Noakes T, Lombard C. A fivefold reduction in the incidence of recurrent ankle sprains in soccer players using the sport-stirrup orthosis. Am J Sports Med 1994; 22:601-606.
24. Sitler MR, Horodyski MB. Effectiveness of prophylactic ankle stabilizers for prevention of ankle injuries. Sports Med 1995; 20:53-57.
25. Burks RT, Bean BG, Marcus R, Barker HB. Analysis of athletic performance with prophylactic ankle devices. Am J sports Med 1991; 19:104-106.
26. Chrisman OD, Snook GA. Reconstruction of lateral ligament tears of the ankle. An experimental study and clinical evaluation of seven patients treated by a new modification of the Elmslie procedure. J Bone Jt Surg Am 1969; 51:904-912.
27. Boytim MJ, Fischer DA, Neuman L. Syndesmotic ankle sprains. Am J Sports Med 1991; 19:294-298.
28. Hopkinson WJ, St. Pierre P, Ryan JB, et al. Syndesmosis sprains of the ankle. Foot Ankle 1990; 10:325-330.
29. Baumhauer JF, Nawoczenski DA, DiGiovanni BF. Ankle pain and peroneal tendon pathology. Clin Sports Med 2004; 23:21-34.
30. Amendola A. Controversies in diagnosis and management of syndesmosis injuries of the ankle. Foot Ankle 1992; 13:44-50.
31. Taylor DC, Bassett FH. Syndesmosis ankle sprains. Phys Sportsmed 1993; 21:39-46.
32. Marymount JV, Lynch MA, Henning CE. Acute ligamentous diastasis of the ankle without fracture: evaluation by radionuclide imaging. Am J Sports Med 1986; 14:407-409.
33. Wright RW, Barile RJ, Surprenant DA, Matava MJ. Ankle syndesmosis sprains in national hockey league players. Am J Sports Med 2004; 32:1941-1945.
34. Safran MR, O'Malley D, Fu FH. Peroneal tendon subluxation in athletes: new exam technique, case reports, and review. Med Sci Sports Exerc 1999; 31:487-492.
35. Marti R. Dislocation of the peroneal tendons. Am J Sports Med 1977; 5:19-22.
36. Eckert WR, Davis EA. Acute rupture of the peroneal retinaculum. J Bone Jt Surg 1976; 58A:670-673.
37. Oden RR. Tendon injuries about the ankle resulting from skiing. Clin Orthop 1987; 216:63-69.
38. Arrowsmith SR, Fleming LL, Allman FL. Traumatic dislocations of the peroneal tendons. Am J Sports Med 1983; 11:142-146.
39. Escalas F, Figueras JM, Merino JA. Dislocation of the peroneal tendons. Long-term results of surgical treatment. J Bone Jt Surg Am 1980; 62:451-453.
40. Micheli LJ, Waters PM, Sanders DP. Sliding fibular graft repair for chronic dislocation of the peroneal tendons. Am J Sports Med 1989; 17:68-71.
41. Minoyama O, Uchiyama E, Iwaso H, Hiranuma K, Takeda Y. Two cases of peroneus brevis tendon tear. Br J Sports Med 2002; 36:65-66.
42. Tol JL, Dijk N van. Etiology of the anterior ankle impingement syndrome: a descriptive anatomical study. Foot Ankle Int 2004; 25:382-386.
43. McMurray TP. Footballer's ankle. J Bone Jt Surg Br 1950; 32B:68-69.
44. O'Donoghue DH. Impingement exostoses of the talus and tibia. J Bone Jt Surg Am 1957; 39A:835-852.
45. Tol JL, Verhagen RAW, Krips R, et al. The anterior ankle impingement syndrome: diagnostic value of oblique radiographs. Foot Ankle Int 2004; 25:63-68.
46. Berberian WS, Hecht PJ, Wapner KL, DiVerniero R. Morphology of tibiotalar osteophytes in anterior ankle impingement. Foot Ankle Int 2001; 22:313-317.
47. Liu SH, Nuccion SL, Finerman G. Diagnosis of anterolateral ankle impingement: a comparison between magnetic resonance imaging and clinical examination. Am J Sports Med 1997; 25:389-393.
48. Philbin TM, Lee TH, Berlet GC. Arthroscopy for athletic foot and ankle injuries. Clin Sports Med 2004; 23:35-53.
49. Scranton PE, McDermott JE. Anterior tibiotalar spurs: a comparison of open versus arthroscopic debridement. Foot Ankle 1992; 13:125-129.
50. Bassett FH, Gates HS, Billys JB, Nicolaw PK. Talar impingement by the antero-inferior tibiofibular ligament. A cause of chronic pain in the ankle after inversion sprain. J Bone Jt Surg AM 1990; 72A:55-59.
51. Hedrick MR, McBryde AM. Posterior ankle impingement. Foot Ankle 1994; 15:2-8.
52. Marotta JJ, Micheli LJ. Os trigonum impingement in dancers. Am J Sports Med 1992; 20:533-536.
53. Kelikian H, Kelikian AS. Disorders of the Ankle. Philadelphia, PA: WB Saunders; 1985.
54. DiStefano A, Schon LC. Management of posterior ankle impingement as a result of ankle instability: a case report. J Dance Med Sci 2002; 6:128-134.
55. Bureau NJ, Cardinal E, Hobden R, Aubin B. Posterior ankle impingement syndrome: MR imaging findings in seven patients. Radiology 2000; 215:497-503.
56. Omey ML, Micheli LJ. Foot and ankle problems in the young athlete. Med Sci Sports Exerc 1999; 31S:470-486.
57. Kolettis GJ, Micheli LJ, Klein JD. Release of the flexor hallucis longus tendon in ballet dancers. J Bone Jt Surg Am 1996; 78A:1386-1390.
58. Dolan AM, Mulcahy DM, Stephens MM. Osteochondritis dissecans of the head of the talus. Foot Ankle Int 1997; 18:365-368.
59. Toll JL, Struijs PAA, Bossuyt PMM, et al. Treatment strategies in osteochondral defects of the talar dome: A systematic review. Foot Ankle Int 2000; 21:119-126.
60. Berndt AL, Harty M. Transchondral fractures (osteochondritis dissecans) of the talus. J Bone Jt Surg Am 1959; 41A:988-1020.
61. Ferkel FD, Sgaglione NA. Arthroscopic treatment of osteochondral lesions of the talus: long term results. Presented at American Academy of Orthopedic Surgeons Annual Meeting, San Francisco, February 1993.
62. Loomer R, Fisher C, Lloyd-Smith R, et al. Osteochondral lesions of the talus. Am J Sports Med 1993; 21:13-19.
63. Hepple S, Winson IG, Glew D. Osteochondral lesions of the talus: A revised classification. Foot Ankle Int 1999; 20:789-793.
64. David NO. Approach alternatives for treatment of osteochondral lesions of the talus. Foot Ankle Clin 7 2002; 9(1):635-649.
65. Taranow WS, Bisignani GA, Towers JD, Conti SF. Retrograde drilling of osteochondral lesions of the medial talar dome. Foot Ankle Int 1999; 20:475-480.
66. Canale ST. Osteochondroses and related problems of the foot and ankle. DeLee and Drez's orthopaedic sports medicine. 2nd edn. Philadelphia, PA: WB Saunders; 2003.
67. Shearer C, Loomer R. Clement D. Nonoperatively managed stage 5 osteochondral talar lesions. Foot Ankle Int 2002; 23:651-654.
68. Chang E, Lenczner E. Osteochondritis dissecans of the talar dome treated with an osteochondral autograft. Can J Surg 2000; 43:217-221.
69. Hangody L, Kish G, Modis L, et al. Mosaicplasty for treatment of osteochondritis dissecans of the talus: two to seven year results in 36 patients. Foot Ankle Int 2001; 22:552-558.
70. Holmes GB, Mann RA. Possible epidemiological factors associated with rupture of the posterior tibial tendon. Foot Ankle 1992; 13:70-79.
71. Kohls-Gatzoulis J, Angel JC, Singh D, et al. Tibialis posterior dysfunction: a common and treatable cause of adult acquired flatfoot. BMJ 2004; 329:1328-1333.
72. Shelbourne KD, Fisher DA, Rettig AC, McCarroll JR. Stress fractures of the medial malleolus. Am J Sports Med 1988; 16:60-63.
73. Shabat S. Stress fractures of the medial malleolus - review of the literature and report of a 15-year-old elite gymnast. Foot Ankle Int 2002; 23:647-650.
74. Orava S, Karpakka J, Taimela S, et al. Stress fracture of the medial malleolus. J Bone Jnt Surg Am 1995; 77:362-365.

CHAPTER 34

Foot Injuries

Stephen M. Simons and Robert Kennedy

INTRODUCTION

Evolutionary adaptive changes to the human foot allowed upright, bipedal posture. The anatomic changes required for habitual bipedalism predate the expansion of the human brain. These changes, needed for single limb support, include expanding the body of the calcaneus, closing the first intermetatarsal angle, reducing first-ray mobility and dorsiflexing the toes. These modifications produce three distinct arches helpful for shock attenuation at contact followed by formation of a rigid foot that transmits muscular forces to the ground during propulsion. Mankind benefited greatly from the structural changes allowing bipedalism, but the consequential biomechanical complexities render the foot vulnerable to sports related injury.[1]

Box 34.1: Key Points

- Foot related injuries represent some of the most diverse acute and overuse injuries to detain an athlete's sports participation. As the principle interface with the playing surface, the foot is uniquely at risk of numerous types of injuries. The authors discuss the predisposing factors and mechanism of the injuries with both physical exam and important imaging studies to aid in diagnosis. Management of sport caused foot problems and common foot injuries that interfere with sport focuses on conservative therapies and indication for surgical referral. The surgeon is referred to many other authoritative texts directed at operative management.

- A detailed treatise of all sport related foot problems deserves a multi-volume text. This chapter is divided into foot locations – rearfoot, midfoot and forefoot – with additional sections on dermatologic problems and orthotics. Stress fractures, ligament sprains, tendon injuries and nerve impingements are discussed, including two stress fractures requiring special consideration – the tarsal navicular and proximal 5th metatarsal. This chapter also elucidates orthotic use for correction of biomechanical deficiency or relief from injury, including the various accommodations that can be added to the basic foot support architecture.

ANATOMY

Basic knowledge of foot anatomy is essential to understanding foot function and injuries. The bony structures of the rearfoot are the talus and calcaneus. The talus transmits forces from the foot to the leg. It articulates with the tibia and fibula superiorly. The calcaneus articulates with the talus via three facets forming the talocalcaneal joint, clinically referred to as the subtalar joint. The subtalar joint acts as a universal joint allowing the foot to adapt to terrain of various slopes. The talonavicular joint and calcaneal cuboid joint define the junction of the rearfoot and midfoot. The midfoot bones include the navicular, cuboid and three cuneiforms. The tarsometatarsal joint defines the midfoot and forefoot junction. Each of the three cuneiforms articulates with a single metatarsal while the cuboid articulates with the 4th and 5th metatarsals. It is clinically relevant to note the second metatarsal base resides in a mortise contributing to the stability of the second metatarsal. The forefoot consists of the metatarsals and phalanges. The first metatarsal, medial cuneiform and navicular is often collectively referred to as the first ray. The first metatarsal is more mobile and shorter than the lesser metatarsals. It is functionally lengthened during propulsion by the repositioning of the sesamoids from a plantar position at midstance to a distal placement on the first metatarsal head at toe-off.

REARFOOT

Plantar fasciitis

Box 34.2: Key Points

- The plantar fascia acts as a Spanish windlass to stabilize the midfoot during gait.
- Calcaneal spurs do not indicate severity or even presence of disease.
- The majority of plantar fasciitis resolves within one year with simple conservative measures.

Plantar fasciitis accounts for the majority of plantar heel pain in the athlete, and is especially common in runners. Some 10% of the general population will experience this malady at some time in their life.[2] In a majority of patients, the pain resolves spontaneously over 6–18 months, only to repeatedly recur. The plantar fascia consists of thick fibrous tissue that originates from the medial calcaneal tuberosity and inserts on the proximal phalanges of the toes. This distal attachment on the toes beyond the metatarsal-phalangeal joints (MTPs) creates a critical stabilizing role for the plantar fascia during the propulsive phase of gait. This function is likened to a Spanish windlass instead of a bowstring (Fig. 34.1). As the foot enters the terminal phase of gait, weight transfers to the plantar forefoot causing the toes to passively dorsiflex. The plantar fascia, lacking elastic qualities, exerts a tensile force pulling the calcaneus towards the toes. This action passively locks the midfoot bones into a structurally rigid foot providing a lever for propulsion. This efficient mechanism reduces the metabolic demand by the lower leg muscles.

The diagnosis is usually made on the basis of history and exam. Occasionally, differentiation from calcaneal stress fracture or other bone pathology requires imaging. Overtraining and overuse contribute to this problem in younger runners. Old and worn footwear or unsupportive footwear predisposes to plantar fascia pain. The risk of plantar fasciitis increases as the range of ankle dorsiflexion decreases, with dorsiflexion of $\leq 0°$ inferring a 23 times greater likelihood of plantar fasciitis. Individuals who spend the majority of their workday on their feet and those whose body-mass index (BMI) is $>30\,kg/m^2$ are also at increased risk for the development of the problem. These three appear to be independent risk factors for plantar fasciitis.[3]

Pain is typically worse with the first steps of the day or upon standing after prolonged sitting. Patients often report a very sharp pain in the plantar heel like stepping on glass. The pain may radiate to the plantar midfoot and forefoot or medial longitudinal arch. The discomfort often abates after a few minutes only to return later in the day when muscular fatigue fails to provide secondary support of foot function. Prolonged standing is especially problematic. Patients state that rising after sitting in the evening will exacerbate the symptoms as well. Runners often describe pain at the start of a run, resolution during the run and recurrence upon cessation of running. To compensate, sufferers will try to bear their weight on the lateral aspect of their feet or spend more time on their toes to

minimize the pressure on the heel. Calcaneal stress fractures typically will not have the improvement after painful first steps, but worsen throughout the day. Pain at night should provoke a work-up for bone tumor.

Examination of the foot reveals tenderness over the calcaneal insertion of the plantar fascia. More generally, examination of the weight bearing anatomy of the foot provides clues to the stresses applied to the plantar fascia. One should note excessive pronation/pes planus or excessive supination/pes cavus as potential biomechanical impediments. Range of motion, specifically limited weight bearing ankle dorsiflexion may predispose as mentioned above. The windlass test can be performed in both the weight bearing and non-weight bearing states. Passive dorsiflexion of the great toe while stabilizing the heel elicits pain in the plantar heel in a positive test. When done non-weight bearing, the forefoot should be loaded into dorsiflexion. This test has a low sensitivity; 32% in weight bearing and only 13.6% in non-weight bearing, but is 100% specific in both positions.[4] Examination will also help exclude other causes of heel pain. The location of tenderness will differentiate this from retrocalcaneal bursitis and Achilles enthesopathy. The absence of a bruise and heel pad atrophy eliminate those afflictions that ache in the same location as plantar fasciitis.

Imaging benefits the clinician primarily by ruling out other pathology. Plain radiographs will show a plantar calcaneal heel spur only half the time in the presence of symptoms, while 15–25% of the general asymptomatic population has heel spurs.[5] Ultrasonography can differentiate plantar fasciitis from a fascia rupture. Characteristic changes of plantar fasciitis include plantar fascia thickening, hypoechogenicity and alterations in the normal fibrous pattern.[6] Magnetic resonance imaging (MRI) will also demonstrate fascia thickening and T2 and short tau inversion-recovery (STIR) images will show increased signal in the plantar fascia indicating edema or microtears.[7]

Treatment starts with conservative measures. It must be noted that there have been no studies on treatment involving athletes only, so this information derives from the general population and expert opinion. Common strategies involve modification of the primary risk factors. Patients should avoid prolonged standing. Those involved in weight bearing athletics should try relative rest; avoiding those activities that provoke the pain and replacing with other activities.[8] In the general population, weight loss must be encouraged for the overweight and obese, though often the heel pain precludes simple exercise like walking. Patients should stretch the gastrocnemius and soleus with wall or stair stretch in both the knee flexed and extended positions. DiGiovanni and colleagues[9] found that adding a plantar fascia specific stretch provides superior pain scores, activity limitations, and patient satisfaction. Patients accomplish this by hyperextending the toes while seated with the foot on the floor. Pain also improves with cryotherapy, either by simple ice application for 20 min multiple times daily or by frozen bottle message. The frozen can or bottle technique involves rolling ones foot over a container of frozen water vigorously for 20 min.

Prefabricated and custom orthotics provides benefits as well. Prefabricated orthoses are relatively cheap and easily available. Additionally, sufferers should replace obviously worn shoes and those used for >500 miles. Night splints may pro-

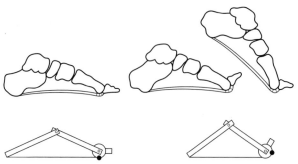

Figure 34.1 The Windlass mechanism of the plantar fascia. As the foot enters the terminal phase of stance, the toes dorsiflex as seen on the right. This action pulls the plantar fascia anteriorly, and applies a superiorly directed force to the arch of the midfoot, passively locking the midfoot bones. This provides midfoot stability during propulsion.

vide additional benefit. A Cochran review[10] cites conflicting data for this intervention. Heel cups are often prescribed for plantar heel pain. The heel cup theoretically works by providing a direct extrinsic cushion effect and an intrinsic cushion by restraining the subcalcaneal fat pad from splaying at heel contact. This cushion effect may be most helpful if the pain were due to direct local compression of plantar tissues. Since most plantar fascial heel pain is due to tensile loads applied to the plantar fascia during the propulsive phase of gait, this heel cushion is of limited value for many athletes.

Corticosteroid injection provides short-term relief. Patients report benefit up to one month, but no consistent improvement compared to placebo past that point.[10] Injection carries the risk of plantar fascia rupture (up to 10%) and fat pad atrophy. To minimize the risk of rupture, weight bearing should be limited for the 2–3 days after the procedure. Return to athletic activity should probably be delayed 3–4 weeks. The injection also causes significant discomfort to administer and patients should be warned accordingly.

In a small minority of cases, non-responsive patients require surgery for plantar fascia release. For athletes, this leads to a prolonged recovery of approximately 18 weeks until a full return.[6] Extracorporeal shock wave therapy has been used for other soft tissue afflictions. Low energy therapy does not appear to be beneficial, but high-energy treatments have shown promise. However, no definitive protocol has yet been established and the cost of the equipment prohibits wide spread use. Additionally, the procedure requires anesthetic to be tolerable. Research is ongoing and bears watching.

Plantar fascia rupture

Rupture of the plantar fascia occurs uncommonly, but may happen during athletics. Patients describe a severe tearing sensation or 'pop' in the plantar heel. Bruising, pain with passive extension of the toes and an inability to perform single leg heel raise accompany this history. Ultrasonography or magnetic resonance imaging confirm the diagnosis, but are not necessary depending on the clinical picture (Fig. 34.2).

Treatment includes a non-weight bearing period of 2–3 weeks in a short leg cast or boot then an additional 1–3 weeks weight bearing in the boot when rest pain subsides. Once pain-free with ambulation in the boot for 1 week, the boot can be discontinued. Saxena and Fullem studied this protocol in elite athletes and found an average return to athletic activity in 9±6 weeks and a return to competition in 7–40 weeks.[11]

Tarsal tunnel syndrome

Box 34.3: Key Points

- Tibial nerve compression through the tarsal tunnel occurs from trauma, biomechanical deformity and space occupying lesion.
- Tarsal tunnel syndrome may present as plantar foot paresthesias or chronic medial ankle pain.
- Surgical treatment is most successful for space occupying lesions.

Tarsal tunnel syndrome is a typical nerve entrapment syndrome often referred to as 'carpal tunnel of the foot'. The tunnel is bordered by the talus and calcaneus deep laterally while the flexor retinaculum creates the superficial 'roof'. Coursing through the tunnel is the posterior tibial tendon, flexor digitorum longus tendon, flexor hallucis tendon, posterior tibial artery and tibial nerve. The tibial nerve branches into the medial calcaneal nerve, lateral and medial plantar nerves, but the specific branching location is highly variable. The fixed nature of the posterior tibial nerve in the tunnel makes it susceptible to tension and compression. No definitive estimates of the incidence exist, but tarsal tunnel syndrome is thought to be a relatively uncommon cause of foot pain.

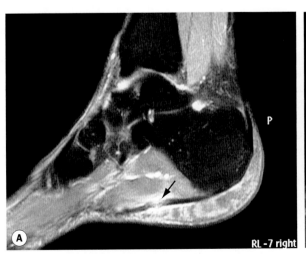
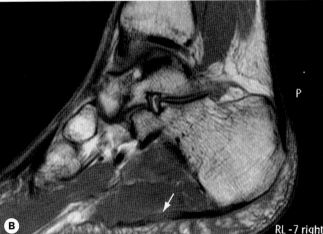

Figure 34.2 Plantar fascia rupture. (A) A short tau inversion-recovery (STIR) image showing mid-portion plantar fascia edema. (B) T1 weighted image showing mid-portion signal loss. Sudden onset mid-arch pain. Edema in the plantar fascia mid-portion and the lack of contiguous plantar fascia fibers indicates the rupture.

The etiology of tarsal tunnel syndrome is diverse and often elusive. Broadly, this includes trauma, foot deformity and space occupying lesions while a plurality of cases remain idiopathic. Trauma related nerve compression could be caused by soft tissue injury or fractures to the adjacent bones. This accounts for most cases with a clearly identifiable cause. Varicosities, bone spurs, ganglion cysts make up the most common space occupying lesions, but many different lesions have been reported.[12] Absent of a clear anatomical explanation for nerve irritation, biomechanical factors probably contribute to many cases. Both varus and valgus heel deformities have been implicated in tarsal tunnel syndrome. The valgus hind foot produces local tension on the nerve while a varus heel compresses the tunnel. An excessively pronated forefoot flattens and lengthens the foot producing a distal tension to the nerve similar to a straight leg test for radicular symptoms.

History and examination typically provide the diagnosis. The symptoms may include numbness, tingling, burning, cramping, pain or a sensation of coldness. The location varies along the plantar aspect of the foot and can be localized anywhere from the heel to the metatarsal heads and toes, or diffusely along the sole. The Valleix phenomenon describes pain that radiates proximally along the medial leg. Additionally, tarsal tunnel syndrome can be a cause of chronic medial ankle pain. Looser fitting shoes, relative rest and elevation often offer relief.

All heel and foot pain requires an assessment of foot structure and biomechanics. Additionally, attention must be paid to venous changes and swelling at the medial ankle. Percussing the tibial nerve at the flexor retinaculum that elicits paresthesias (Tinel's sign) is highly specific. However, the estimates for sensitivity vary from 50–100%.[13] The cuff test uses a blood pressure cuff to act as a tourniquet and cause venous swelling and local ischemia especially when one suspects varicosities. Finally, compressing and stretching the nerve by passive inversion and eversion may reproduce symptoms.

Imaging generally starts with plain radiographs. These may show posterior talar spurring or tarsal coalition and excludes other bony abnormality potentially causing similar symptoms. Magnetic resonance provides the best diagnostic imaging. More than 80% accuracy is demonstrated.[14] It can assess anatomic variants, edema that occurs due to venous insufficiency or tenosynovitis, and soft tissue masses that would cause localized compression of the nerve. Electrodiagnosis with electromyogram and nerve conduction studies provides additional information. The relatively high false negative rate of 9.5% precludes it from being a true gold standard.[15]

Conservative treatment focuses on correctable factors. If the patient has a flexible foot deformity, treatment includes shoe modification and orthotics. Corticosteroid injection can help reduce local inflammation. Runners may need to modify their training regimens. Return to running follows symptom control with a gradual increase in intensity. A majority of patients require surgery. Surgery includes release of the retinaculum, neurolysis of the medial and lateral plantar nerves and excision of space occupying lesions. Surgical treatment is generally successful with 80–90% of patients having objective relief of symptoms.[16,17] Patients with space occupying lesion fare better with surgery than those that have traumatic or idiopathic causes.[18] For those patients with persistent symptoms after surgery, a repeat procedure does not significantly improve outcomes.[17] Conservative measures should be thoroughly exhausted before considering operative care.

Calcaneal stress fractures

Calcaneal stress fractures must be considered in runners and marching soldiers with heel pain. Depending on the study, these place second to the metatarsals among foot stress fractures. Patients complain of plantar or diffuse heel pain worse with weight bearing activity and relieved by rest. As with other stress fractures, recent changes in training predispose to the injury. Heel striking runners may be at a higher risk. Examination may show tenderness on the plantar heel, but other causes of heel pain give the same. More specific to stress fracture, medial-lateral compression of the posterior heel gives tenderness.

Lateral view on plain radiographs may show a sclerotic line in the posterior calcaneus, perpendicular to the normal trabecular lines. Periosteal reactions appear very infrequently. Bone scintigraphy or MRI confirms the diagnosis, if necessary.

Treatment begins with rest. If the patient has pain with ambulation, the rest should be non-weight bearing until pain free. Typically, 6–8 weeks rest suffices prior to a gradual return to training. Some suggest using a rocker-bottom boot lined with cushioning to reduce and redistribute pressure as well as remind the patient to limit activity.[19] A return to full activity should take another 6–12 weeks, with correction of any biomechanical factors and appropriate shock absorption.

Posterior tibial tendinopathy

Box 34.4: Key Points

- Posterior tibial tendonitis can cause significant medial ankle pain and swelling.

- Treatment focuses on strengthening, reducing inflammation and supporting the arch.

The posterior tibial tendon traverses the ankle posterior to the medial malleolus then inserts on the medial aspect of the navicular. In the open kinetic chain, it acts to plantarflex and invert at the ankle. During gait, it absorbs eccentric forces to stabilize the midfoot, allowing a more efficient gait. Tendinopathy occurs commonly in the general population due to an area of hypoperfusion directly inferior to the medial malleolus. Those at increase risk include women over 40, the obese and those with a pronated, planus foot. Obesity, diabetes and hypertension increase the risk of tendon rupture.[20] Among athletes, runners who inappropriately increase training and those with poor footwear are at increased risk. Dancers and ice skaters are particularly at risk for posterior tibial tendonitis. Stage I tendinopathy presents as an inflamed and tender, but fully intact and functional tendon. In stage II, the tendon is dysfunctional and a flexible flat foot develops. Stage III describes a fixed flat foot with a totally nonfunctional tendon and degenerative subtalar changes.

Typical symptoms include insidious onset of medial ankle pain, worse with weight bearing activity. Climbing stairs and other plantarflexion/heel raising activities exacerbate the pain. Patients also describe an unstable feeling in the ankle while walking or running. As the tendon failure progresses, changing foot structure will accompany these symptoms. Patients report a newly acquired flat foot or a need to use bigger shoes as the foot lengthens and the medial arch disappears. Pain or swelling posterior to the medial malleolus with a change in foot shape is highly sensitive and specific (98%) for posterior tibial tendon dysfunction in the elderly.[21]

Examination reveals tenderness along the course of the tendon, most commonly posterior and inferior to the malleolus. Patients report pain with resisted plantarflexion and inversion. Foot structure should be noted for pronation, heel valgus and medial longitudinal arch structure. With more advanced disease (Stage II or more) patients are unable to perform a single limb heel rise. Imaging serves a role in objectifying the foot deformity with plain radiographs. Subtalar and tibiotalar joint degeneration can also be evaluated. The clinical diagnosis obviates the need for further imaging, but if doubt persists, a magnetic resonance imaging can give useful anatomic information.

Treatment starts with rest, ice non-steroidal anti-inflammatory medicines as needed and correction of biomechanical risk factors. Flat-footed runners with a short duration of symptoms may succeed with rest until pain-free followed by orthotic support upon return to activity. If the patient cannot perform a single leg heel rise, a short leg cast or walking boot should be used. The patient remains in the boot until the pain ceases with this test. This may take 4–12 weeks, followed by a 1–2 week weaning process from the boot. Intrinsic foot muscle strengthening and eccentric posterior tibial tendon strengthening are integral to rehabilitation. Orthotic support to the medial longitudinal arch is important for initial management and preventing symptom recurrence. A UCBL (University of California Biomechanics Laboratory) orthotic, often used in the elderly, contains walls that resist talar head and calcaneal deviation. This type of device is usually not tolerated in the running or jumping athlete.

An acutely ruptured posterior tibial tendon presents with pain radiating from the medial navicular to the medial malleolus. The acquired flat foot may not occur acutely. But the patient will have an inability invert the foot or perform a heel rise. MRI will demonstrate the rupture. This should be repaired surgically.

Lateral process of the talus fracture
Fracture of the lateral process of the talus presents similar to a severe lateral ankle sprain. A fall with inversion, extreme dorsiflexion and possibly external rotation causes this injury. The rise in popularity of snowboarding has led to a rise in the incidence of this fracture. Kirkpatrick compiles a 7-year experience from 12 Colorado ski resorts. A total of 74 lateral process fractures were seen representing 2.3% of all snowboarding injuries, 15% of all ankle injuries and 34% of all ankle frac-

tures.[22] A clinician must be highly suspicious of a snowboarder with lateral ankle pain, while this rarely occurs in sport otherwise. On examination, tenderness over the lateral process of the talus, just anterior and inferior to the lateral malleolus tip, indicates such an injury. This constitutes a possible flaw with the Ottawa ankle rules.[23] On plain radiographs, the mortise view provides the best visualization, but this view will still miss approximately 40% of these fractures. CT scan is the secondary test of choice. Additionally, multiplanar reformations are more sensitive than standard CT.

Conservative therapy is adequate treatment for minimally displaced fractures (<2 mm). Treatment starts with a non-weight bearing short leg cast for 4–6 weeks followed by protected weight bearing in a walking boot for an additional six weeks. Range of motion, strengthening and proprioception exercises are introduced at this time. Greater displacement requires surgical fixation or excision and comminuted fracture fragments should be excised. Despite appropriate therapy, a considerable number of patients continue to complain of chronic lateral ankle pain.

Sinus tarsi syndrome

Box 34.5: Key Points

- Sinus tarsi syndrome is a symptom complex of rearfoot or lateral ankle pain as well as impaired proprioception manifest as ankle instability.
- Suspected diagnosis is best evaluated by MRI.
- Treatment consists of corticosteroid injection, bracing and proprioception training.

The sinus tarsi lies anterior and inferior to the lateral malleolus in the talo-calcaneal sulcus. The sinus houses the interosseous talocalcaneal ligament and the cervical ligament as well as adipose, vessels and nerves. The syndrome consists of lateral subtalar foot pain and sometimes a feeling of instability. As with all syndromes, sinus tarsi syndrome is a constellation of symptoms following undetermined specific tissue pathology (Table 34.1). Possible injuries include interosseous ligament disruption, degenerative joint disease, nerve compression or soft tissue mass.[24] Typically, patients have excessive pronation and rear foot valgus, causing compression of this area. Palpation reveals exquisite tenderness over the sinus opening. Pain relief following an injection of local anesthetic into the sinus supports the diagnosis. Plain films show no abnormality, but MRI shows disruption of the ligaments, bone or soft tissue edema (Fig. 34.3).

Use of orthotics may reduce compression of the sinus by excess pronation. Corticosteroid injection can also be helpful, although no specific protocol has emerged. Physical therapy aids in return to play with emphasis on range of motion, strengthening, proprioception and bracing, similar to ankle sprain treatment. Cases that do not respond to these measures will do well with surgical exploration and debridement.

Table 34.1   Clinical Signs of Sinus Tarsi Syndrome

History of foot or ankle inversion sprain	Yes
Subjective instability	Yes
Tenderness	Localized to the sinus tarsi
Ankle stability	Yes/no
Anesthetic injection to the sinus tarsi	Temporary symptomatic improvement
Radiographic findings	Normal
Arthrography (subtalar)	Loss of sinus tarsi filling
Magnetic resonance imaging	Rupture of interosseous ligament or cervical ligament; bone edema, soft tissue swelling, or fibrosis at sinus tarsi
Laboratory testing (rule out systemic inflammatory process)	Negative

From Casillas MM. Ligament injuries of the foot and ankle in adult athletes. In: DeLee and Drez's orthopaedic sports medicine: Principles and practice, 2nd edn. Philadelphia, PA: WB Saunders; 2003: 2364, Table 30-E1-6, with permission.

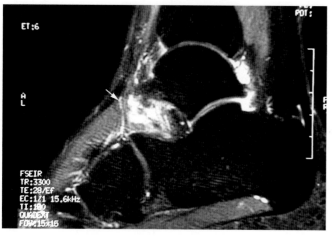

Figure 34.3   Sinus tarsi syndrome. The sinus tarsi exhibits high signal intensity on this sagittal image. MRI T2 image showing signal in the sinus tarsi. While these images show no specific ligamentous injury, the edema in the sinus is consistent with the syndrome.

MIDFOOT INJURIES

Lisfranc injuries

Box 34.6: Key Points

- High index of suspicion and early diagnosis is key to correctly managing Lisfranc sprains.

- Weight bearing radiographs, stress radiographs, or MRI are necessary diagnostic procedures for a suspected Lisfranc injury.

- Stage I Lisfranc injuries can be managed with 6 weeks, non-weight bearing immobilization, while Stage II and III sprains should be treated operatively.

Sport related tarsometatarsal joint injuries are frequently missed and underappreciated compared with the more typical high-velocity injuries from motor vehicle accidents. Early diagnosis and appropriate management are critical to the athlete's return to play and eventual foot function. The tarsometatarsal (Lisfranc) joint is formed proximally by the three cuneiforms and cuboid bone articulating distally with the five metatarsal bases. The second metatarsal base is dovetail shaped and recessed into a mortise created by the surrounding cuneiforms. This articulation is the 'keystone' to the stability of the Lisfranc joint.[25] A shallow mortise is associated with greater injury risk.[26] Strong transverse ligaments join the bases of the lesser metatarsals. The first and second metatarsal have no such intermetatarsal ligament, instead stabilization is achieved by a strong obliquely oriented ligament, the Lisfranc ligament, which links the medial cuneiform to the second metatarsal base.

The sport related incidence of Lisfranc injuries is unknown although 1 in 50 000 orthopedic trauma cases is cited.[25] Meyer *et al.* estimate a 4% incidence per year in an American college football team.[27] The mechanism of injury is attributed to direct or indirect trauma. The former occurs when a heavy object falls or rolls across the dorsum of a planted midstance foot. This mechanism occurs rarely in sport. The more common sports-related, indirect mechanism occurs as the plantarflexed foot is forcibly driven into the ground when another player lands on the heel (Fig. 34.4). A second, but similar, indirect mechanism occurs when the fully plantarflexed foot is subjected to an axial load by the athlete's own body weight. Both mechanisms injure the weaker dorsal ligaments by applying a tensile load across the dorsum of the midfoot. Khan *et al.* report a fracture/dislocation at Lisfranc's joint in a sprinter running straight down the track. Although the injury was significant, he did not suffer the usual mechanism to create this injury.[28] Historically, Lisfranc injury was an equestrian injury. The forefoot was forcefully abducted in the stirrups as the rider is thrown from the horse.

Clinical assessment begins with the history although the athlete may not accurately recall the injury. Gross deformity, seen in high velocity injuries, is usually absent in the sport injured. Midfoot swelling, inability to bear weight, possible ecchymoses and tenderness along the tarsometatarsal joints should raise suspicion for this injury. Disruption to the dorsalis pedis artery may cause hemorrhage, an increased interstitial pressure and consequent pedal compartment syndrome.[29]

Radiographic assessment

Clinical suspicion warrants a careful radiographic assessment. Initial series X-rays are negative in as many as 20–35% of cases.[25,29] The initial X-rays should include a standing anteroposterior, oblique and lateral view of the foot. Ideally, a weight bearing comparison view is obtained simultaneously. If the patient is unable to bear weight and the non-weight bearing views are inconclusive, then weight bearing views are obtained 10–14 days later or supplemental imaging is done more urgently. Several authors advocate abduction stress views, ideally performed while under anesthesia.[30,31] Nunley cites lack of standardization and inability to manually exert sufficient force, when compared with weight bearing, to reliably produce diastasis and thus assess ligamentous injury.[32] Faciszewski suggested a lateral weight bearing view to assess arch integrity. The unin-

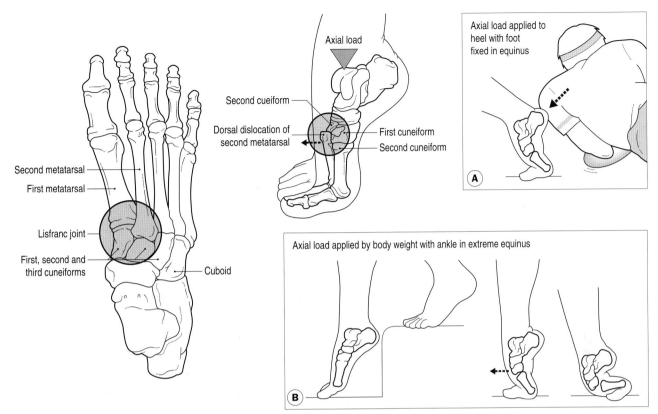

Figure 34.4 Lisfranc mechanism of injury. The most common sports related mechanism occurs when the forefoot is firmly planted on the ground and a forward directed force is applied to the heel. This occurs in (A) football when another player lands on the heel, or (B) in ballet if the dancer's weight shifts too far forward.

jured or minimally injured medial column maintains a relationship depicting the medial cuneiform superior to the proximal 5th metatarsal. The collapsed medial midfoot reverses this relationship.[33] Chiodo and Myerson believed this radiographic reversal is more useful for assessing the chronically injured foot before reconstruction.[29] Bone scintigraphy, although nonspecific is highly sensitive to osseous or periosteal injury.[34] Computed tomography may also detect anatomical disruption at the Lisfranc joint not appreciated by plain radiography.[35] Magnetic resonance imaging is especially helpful to assess ligamentous integrity in the radiographically normal foot.[36]

Several classification systems exist to help guide the clinician to the most appropriate management. Most of these classifications apply to high velocity injuries. Nunley and Vertullo proposed a classification scheme that applies to lower velocity, sport type, injury.[32] This includes the minimally injured, non-diastasis midfoot sprains. Their classification system is based on clinical findings, weightbearing radiographs, and bone scintigrams (Fig. 34.5). A Stage I sprain included inability to play due to pain in the Lisfranc region, no diastasis on weight bearing X-rays but positive bone scan results. A Stage II injury showed 1st to 2nd metatarsal bone diastasis of 1–5 mm on weight bearing AP view but no loss of medial arch on a lateral weight bearing view. Stage III had first to second metatarsal diastasis >5 mm on weight bearing AP view and loss of midfoot arch height as evidenced by reduced distance from the

proximal 5th metatarsal base to the medial cuneiform on the lateral weight bearing radiograph.

Treatment

Early recognition and appropriate management is paramount to achieve an optimum return to play and long range functional foot. Missed or misdiagnosis potentially leads to several dysfunctional untoward consequences.[37] Stage I sprains, even when delayed as long as 8 months can be successfully treated in a short leg cast or walking boot. Preferably, the patient remains non-weight bearing for 4–6 weeks.[32,38] Clinical symptoms guide the initiation and transition speed of non-weight bearing to weight bearing. Nunely used a weight bearing ankle-foot orthotic device if the patient was still symptomatic upon cast removal. Stage II and III are best operatively treated, particularly for the athlete. Good anatomical reduction is necessary for future ligamentous stability of the midfoot. Return to play varies from 6 weeks to 9 months.[31] The athlete should undergo a sport specific rehabilitation program whether treated operatively or non-operatively.

Tarsal navicular stress fractures

Tarsal navicular stress fractures previously thought quite rare are now appreciated as a very common stress fracture in track and field athletes with a propensity to afflict sprinters, hurdlers

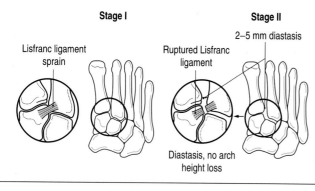

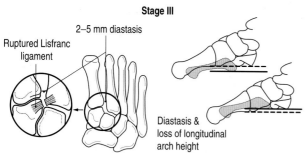

Figure 34.5 Midfoot sprain classification system. Stage I is a sprain to the Lisfranc ligament with no diastasis or arch height loss seen on radiographs but increased uptake on bone scintigrams. Stage II sprains have a first to second intermetatarsal diastasis of 1–5 mm because of failure of the Lisfranc ligament but no arch height loss. Stage III sprains display first to second intermetatarsal diastasis and loss of arch height, as represented by a decrease or inversion of the distance between the plantar aspect of the 5th metatarsal bone and the plantar aspect of the medial cuneiform bone on an erect lateral radiograph. (Redrawn from Nunley and Vertullo 2002.[32])

Box 34.7: Key Points

- Navicular stress fracture should be suspected if dorsomedial midfoot pain present.

- Conservative treatment for Type I fractures; 6 weeks non-weight bearing is necessary.

- Surgical fixation is best used for complicated Type II and all Type III fractures.

---

and middle distance runners.[39] Many other sports also suffer their fair share of these difficult stress fractures. These fractures frequently go undiagnosed for several months. The etiology of these stress fractures is speculative. Impingement or bending forces exerted by the proximal and distal tarsal bones combined with a relatively avascular middle segment are thought contributory.

History and examination

The patient presents with vague dorsal, medial midfoot pain. The pain may radiate along the medial longitudinal arch or the dorsum of the foot. One case report cited a 13-year-old female presenting with 'ankle pain'.[40] The pain begins insidiously during exertion then slowly progresses to include inactive periods and eventually forcing rest. The pain usually resolves quickly

with rest. This cyclic pattern probably contributes to the average 4 months delay to diagnosis. Examination is usually unremarkable except for tenderness directly over the apex of the navicular, a location coined the 'N' spot by Khan.[41]

Plain radiography is notoriously unreliable. Bone scan or MRI is usually required to confirm bone radiotracer uptake or edema isolated to the navicular. Saxena proposed a CT based classification system to guide clinical management.[42] Fine slice coronal CT images are evaluated for location and fracture extent and for modifiers such as avascular necrosis, cystic changes to the fracture and fracture margin sclerosis. Fractures are classified: Type 1, dorsal cortical break only; Type 2, fracture propagation into the navicular body; Type 3, fracture propagation to another cortex. Most navicular stress fractures occur in the middle third beginning at the dorsal cortex then extending in a curvilinear, plantar direction.

Treatment options depend on the fracture type, the CT identified modifiers and the athletes need to return to sport. Khan *et al*. report 89% healing with nonoperative care.[41] Quirk, writing while president of the American Orthopaedic Foot and Ankle Society, outlines the following non-operative treatment protocol.[43]

1 Six weeks on crutches with a below-the-knee non-weight bearing cast. Even those who have previously failed surgery.
2 Remove cast and examine 'N' spot. If still tender then treat with similar cast for another 2 weeks.
3 When the cast is removed permanently, design a very gradual closely supervised return to activity program.

Repeat imaging is not very helpful as CT and bone scans can remain abnormal long after the fracture is clinically ready to stress.

Saxena recommends a treatment protocol based on the CT findings.[42] Type I fractures do well with conservative care. Type II and III fractures take considerably longer to heal. Type III fractures should be treated operatively utilizing bone graft, screw fixation or both.

Type II fractures, particularly with the previously mentioned modifiers, avascular necrosis, cysts or marginal sclerosis, are also best treated surgically. In this small study the surgically treated group returned to sport on average 3.1 (±1.2) months. The conservatively treated group returned to sport on average 4.3 (±2.8) months. However, regardless of treatment chosen, the fracture type influenced the time to return to sport most. Type I fractures return to activity took 3.0 months compared with the 6.8 months for type III fractures.[42] Post-treatment rehabilitation focuses on improving ankle range of motion with gastro-Achilles stretching and addressing presumed biomechanical contributors with orthotics.

FOREFOOT INJURIES

Turf toe

Turf toe is the vernacular descriptive term used to describe injury to the capsular-ligamentous peri-articular structures of the first metatarsal-phalangeal joint (MTP).

Box 34.8: Key Points

- Grade I turf toe may return to play immediately.
- Grade II return to play averages 3–14 days and Grade III RTP in 4–6 weeks.

Anatomy

The biconvex head of the first metatarsal articulates with a shallow concavity on the proximal phalanx. Capsular thickenings form a strong plantar plate, which is firmly adherent to the proximal phalanx and loosely attached to the metatarsal neck (Fig. 34.6). Collateral ligaments consisting of a MTP ligament and a metatarsosesamoid ligament provide medial and lateral support. The abductor hallucis tendon inserts onto the medial plantar aspect of the proximal phalanx while the adductor hallucis inserts on the respective lateral side. The sesamoids are encased within two slips of the flexor hallucis brevis tendon. The first MTP range of motion varies widely from 30° plantarflexion to 80° or more dorsiflexion.[38]

Mechanisms and causes of turf toe

The most common mechanism of injury to cause turf toe is hyperextension of a great toe that is fixed to the playing surface followed by an axial load to the heel (Fig. 34.7). Less commonly, a valgus force is applied to the medial side of the toe by a directional change or an American football lineman pushing from their stance. The hyperextension mechanism leads to tensile failures of the plantar plate or collateral ligaments as well as impaction injury to the dorsal metatarsal head. Forced plantarflexion can occur in football, beach volleyball and dancers, but this 'sand toe' often behaves clinically different than turf

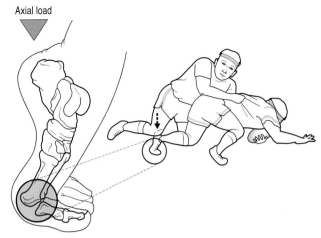

Figure 34.7   The most common mechanism of injury to cause turf toe is hyperextension of a great toe that is fixed to the playing surface followed by an axial load to the heel.

toe.[44] High frictional forces and the accompanying flexible soled shoes used when playing on artificial surfaces are thought to contribute to the higher injury rates. Aging artificial turf stiffens leading to speculation for a higher incidence of injury. However, no clinical proof is forthcoming. As artificial turf is replaced with natural surfaces or newer artificial surfaces hopefully the incidence of turf toe and other injuries will subside.[45]

Clinical and radiographic examination

Clinical assessment begins with history and/or if available, videotape review. As with many athletic injuries, immediate examination is most helpful. Inspect for deformity, swelling and ecchymoses. Palpate the joint dorsum, collateral ligaments,

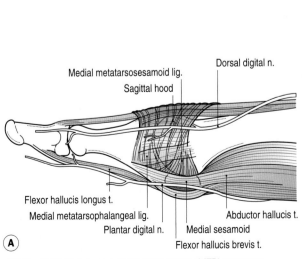

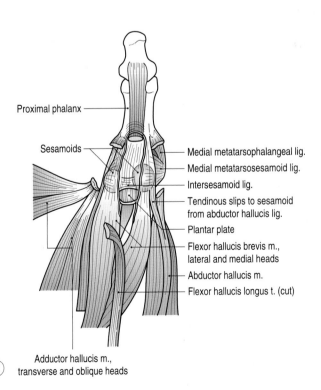

Figure 34.6   (A,B) Metatarsal-phalangeal joints (MTP) anatomy.

sesamoids and assess range of motion comparing with the unin-jured foot. Provocative tests such as varus and valgus stress test-ing; a dorsoplantar drawer test and resisted active flexion and extension are then performed within the athlete's pain tolerance.

Radiographs are necessary to assess capsular avulsions, sesamoid fractures, impaction fracture, diastasis to bipartite sesamoids, and proximal migration of the sesamoids.[44] An AP, lateral and sesamoid axial views are mandatory. The difference between the distal tip of the sesamoids and the joint should not exceed 3.0 mm tibial and 2.7 mm fibular sesamoid on the affected side *versus* unaffected side.[46] Special stress views such as a forced dorsiflexion lateral view can identify sesamoid migration, bipartite sesamoid separation and joint subluxation. Today MRI best identifies the extent of the tissue injured predicting prognosis and aiding treatment strategies.

Grading the extent of turf toe injury, proposed by Clanton and Ford, will help provide a prognosis for return to play.[47] These injuries are all quite painful initially. Therefore it may be prudent to delay grading the injury for a few days. Grade I is a minimally symptomatic stretch to the capsuloligamentous complex. There is no ecchymoses, minimal joint restriction, the athlete is able to bear weight and may athletically partici-pate with mild pain. Grade II is a partial tear to the capsulo-ligamentous complex associated with weight bearing pain, ecchymoses and joint motion restriction. Grade III is a com-plete tear of the capsuloligamentous complex, avulsion of the plantar plate from the metatarsal neck, proximal phalanx impaction into the dorsum of the metatarsal head and some-times proximal migration of the sesamoids. The athlete has severe pain, swelling, ecchymoses, motion restriction and is unable to bear weight normally.

Treatment and return to play

Initial treatment follows standard rest, ice, compression and elevation protocols. Grade I injuries may return to practice and competition without time loss. Restricting joint motion by tap-ing or inserting a stiff insole can hasten return to the field. The athlete may prefer a custom made orthotic with a Morton's extension. Grade II injuries will need more rest and usually cause a loss of playing time of 3–14 days. Grade III injuries should remain non-weight bearing for several days. Eventually the athlete slowly progresses from walking to running and cutting. Anderson believes pain free dorsiflexion of 50–60° and player position correlated with return to play.[48] This is typically 4–6 weeks for a grade III injury.

Acute surgical management is indicated for proximal migra-tion or diastasis of a bipartite sesamoid. More commonly, surgery is performed after a period of failed conservative management.

Sesamoid problems

The sesamoid bones of the first ray serve an important role in ambulation. They are encased within the flexor hallucis brevis tendon and during rest or midstance of gait reside inferior to the metatarsal head. During the late propulsive phase of gait, they act to functionally lengthen the first ray. This gives a mechanical advantage to the flexor tendons and enables a smooth lateral to medial weight transfer from the lesser metatarsals. A bipartite or multipartite sesamoid occurs in 5–33%.[49] Sesamoids can be acutely fractured with an axial load

---

Box 34.9: Key Points

- Sesamoid injury requires prompt diagnosis and withdrawal from weight bearing stress.

- Overuse sesamoid injuries are mechanically similar to patello-femoral problems.

- Radiographs are often normal. MRI or bone scan are necessary to diagnose sesamoid injury.

- Conservative care includes accomodative padding or 4-6 weeks nonweight bearing rest.

---

applied to the first metatarsal while the great toe is hyperex-tended. Most sesamoid injuries are due to overuse. They occur in runners, dancers, shot-putters, marching band and any sport that involves running. The precise tissue pathology causing the pain can be elusive. Sesamoid injuries include stress fracture (40%), sesamoiditis (30%), acute fracture (10%), osteochondri-tis (10%), osteoarthritis (5%) and bursitis (5%).[50] The medial (tibial) sesamoid is affected more commonly.[51] The sesamoids need to precisely track in their respective grooves on the metatarsal head, as they remain relatively fixed to the ground while the metatarsal head rolls into a position on top of them. The chronic problems afflicting the sesamoids are reminiscent of similar tracking pathologies at the patello-femoral joint.

With a chronic injury, patients describe a vague first metatarsal pain. They may report a pain avoidance gait by exces-sively supinating to the lateral side of the foot. Examination reveals swelling and tenderness on the plantar aspect of the first metatarsophalangeal joint. Palpation of each sesamoid individu-ally will show a localized tenderness to the bone. Passive dorsi-flexion may elicit crepitance and exacerbates the pain. Standard radiographs should include a sesamoid view. However, radi-ographs are insensitive to demonstrate chronic sesamoid injury. Bone scan or MRI can help differentiate a bipartite sesamoid from an acute or stress type fracture (Fig. 34.8).

Treating sesamoid problems begins with reducing weight bearing stress by limiting activities and avoiding high-heeled shoes. For those patients with no radiographic findings, efforts should start by taking pressure off the first metatarsopha-langeal joint utilizing a metatarsal pad, metatarsal bar or orthotic with first MTP cut out. If this is ineffective, non-weight bearing should be tried until tenderness ceases. For stress fractures, the patient is placed non-weight bearing for 6 weeks. When tenderness resolves, consider orthotics with the above-mentioned modifications to prevent future recurrence. A gradual return to full activity over 4 weeks should minimize recurrence. Surgical resection is considered after months of failed conservative care. The patient needs to understand the potential for transfer injury to the remaining sesamoid, hallux MTP or adjacent metatarsal heads. Saxena recently reported on 26 sesamoidectomies in 24 'active' individuals. The more athletic patients returned to sport on average 7.5 weeks. Active, but non-athletic patients, returned to a desired activity level at 12 weeks.[52] Complications of the surgery include scar-ring with neuroma-like symptoms, especially with fibular sesamoid resection and hallux valgus deformity with tibial sesamoid resection.

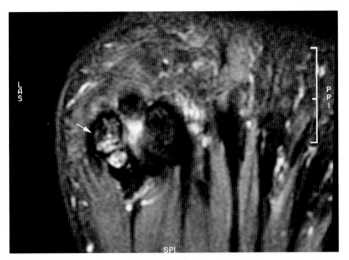

Figure 34.8 Chronic sesamoiditis. Bipartite tibial sesamoid with edema. This T2 image on MRI shows edema in a bipartite tibial sesamoid. This could have been an old sesamoid fracture, but given the 1-year time course and well corticated, smooth borders of the fragments, sesamoiditis in a bipartite sesamoid seems more likely.

Interdigital neuromas

Interdigital neuromas, although not necessarily caused by athletics, may seriously interfere with successful athletic participation. Neuroma is a common diagnostic clinical misnomer applied to a symptom complex more correctly called an interdigital neuritis. Pathologically it is caused by perineural fibrosis and demyelination to plantar interdigital or digital nerves. Repetitive irritation to the interdigital nerves occurs as they pass between the metatarsal heads and under the transverse metatarsal ligament.

Clinical presentation consists of burning type pain in the forefoot radiating into the involved toes. Pain may be aggravated with barefoot walking, but more commonly, the pain is worse with tight fitting shoes. The third interspace between the third and fourth toes is afflicted 87% of the time.[53] Branches from the medial and lateral plantar nerves merge in this interspace resulting in a larger and probably more vulnerable nerve.[54] Some, but not all patients experience an annoying or painful numbness directed to adjacent sides of the toes supplied by a single intermetatarsal nerve. Some patients will have a subtle crepitance sensation. If symptoms are present on both feet or in the hands then the practitioner needs to consider peripheral neuropathies.

Box 34.10: Key Points

- Interdigital neuromas can occur in any web space but most often affect the third and fourth toe.
- Conservative care attempts to reduce compressive and traction forces to the intermetatarsal space.
- Symptoms lasting longer than 1 year are often not successfully treated non-operatively.
- Surgical treatment provides acceptably good results in 80–85% of cases.

Direct examination includes Mulder's test performed by alternately plantarflexing one metatarsal while dorsiflexing the adjacent metatarsal. The author personally also attempts to direct the metatarsal heads towards one another with this maneuver. Unfortunately, a positive test, indicated by a painful click is present only 20% of the time.[55] Palpation and a dorsoplantar directed squeeze between the metatarsal heads usually reproduces pain. Check for decreased sensation to adjacent toes. Indirect examination clues the physician to consider other explanations for the patient's pain. Callous patterns indicate underlying pressure sources or skin lesions, equinus contracture causes increased forefoot loading and hypermobilities contribute to MTP synovitis and metatarsalgia.

Interdigital neuromas are usually diagnosed on clinical grounds. Imaging may be performed to rule out other pathologies. Radiographs may reveal stress fractures, erosive changes to the MTPs, Freiberg's infarction, etc. Gadolinium enhanced MRI is very sensitive for interdigital neuromas.

Treatment begins with nonoperative efforts to relieve direct, repetitive irritation to the nerves. Symptoms present for longer than 1 year carry a poor prognosis for non-operative success.[55] Shoe choice is the cornerstone to conservative care. The patient is well advised to seek shoes with a relatively wider and accommodating toebox, stretchable leather, and well cushioned forefoot. Elevated heels should be avoided. A well placed metatarsal pad may increase the intermetatarsal space. If fashionably acceptable, a stiff soled rocker bottom type shoe such as a hiking boot may reduce late stance phase toe dorsiflexion.

Injections with a soluble corticosteroid and local anesthetic provide diagnostic support and usually temporary therapeutic value. The injection is placed dorsally between the metatarsal heads and directed sufficiently plantar to feel a plantar fullness during injection. Extent and duration of pain relief is recorded to assist surgical decisions. Surgical resection is performed only after failing these simple treatments and the patient understands the 15–20% potential for a less than satisfactory result. Kay and Bennett[55] suggest the patient should preoperatively understand the following potentials: an incorrect diagnosis, the need to continue to wear correct shoes, the implications for true neuroma formation, the normal recovery process, numbness to the affected webspace, and further dysfunction to the forefoot.

Metatarsal stress fractures

Metatarsal stress fractures make up to 25% of stress fractures.[56] Middle metatarsal stress fractures are the originally described 'march fractures'. First metatarsal stress fractures are uncommon and 5th metatarsal stress fractures will be discussed separately. As with metatarsalgia, the forces absorbed by the second metatarsal make it most vulnerable to stress injury. Further, the proximal second metatarsal is imbedded in the cuneiforms, likely fixing its position more rigidly than the other metatarsals. The 3rd and 4th metatarsals follow in frequency of stress fracture. As with other stress fractures, a recent increase in training causes the problem. Ballet dancers uniquely suffer stress fractures at the base of the 2nd metatarsal.

Patients describe an increasing pain in the forefoot with weight bearing activity. Although biomechanics, shoewear, strength, flexibility and many other variables are implicated, rapid training change is the most likely cause. Examination

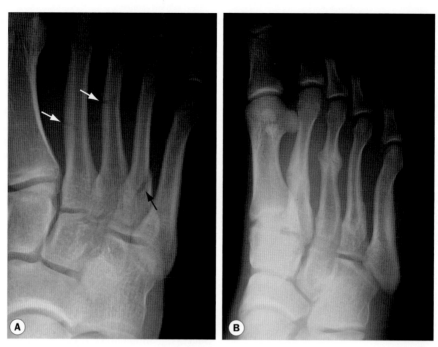

Figure 34.9 (A) A 17-year-old soccer athlete sustained an acute 4th metatarsal base fracture (black arrow). Incidental note of asymptomatic 2nd and 3rd metatarsal stress fractures (white arrows). (B) Repeat X-rays at 3 months show exuberant callous formation to 2nd and 3rd metatarsal stress fractures and solid healing to 4th metatarsal fracture.

shows focal tenderness over the affected metatarsal and sometimes dorsal forefoot swelling. Additionally, axial loading of the metatarsal will elicit pain. Patients display an inability to perform the 'hop test': hopping on the affected foot without pain. Radiographs performed within 2–3 weeks of symptom onset are often normal. A faint radiolucent fracture line, periosteal reaction, or bone callus can be seen 2–4 weeks later. Repeating X-rays or following the patient clinically with the presumption of stress fracture is most cost effective and usually diagnostically sufficient (Fig. 34.9). Bone scan or MRI can provide definitive diagnosis if the circumstances demand diagnostic accuracy and urgency.

Rest is at the forefront of treatment. Withdrawing the offending activity can treat nearly all metatarsal stress fractures. If there is still significant pain on ambulation then full or partial weight bearing restriction or using a stiff soled, postoperative shoe for the first few days or weeks is helpful. Biking and swimming substitute during this time and non-running, weight bearing exercise may be added when the patient can ambulate pain free. Running should be restricted for 4–6 weeks or until pain-free, at least 2 weeks. A gradual return to weight bearing sport is started slowly. Full training is usually successful 8 weeks after diagnosis. The clinician should perform careful biomechanical exam for structural predisposition to metatarsal stresses. This can include a hypermobile first ray, long or rigidly plantarflexed metatarsal, reversal to the transverse arch or a hallux valgus deformity. Accommodative orthotic devices can redistribute metatarsal head ground reaction forces away from the injured metatarsal.

Proximal 5th metatarsal fractures

Three main types of fracture occur at the proximal 5th metatarsal. The avulsion fracture of the tubercle accounts for

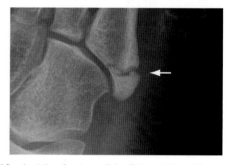

Figure 34.10 Avulsion fracture of the 5th metatarsal base.

Box 34.11: Key Points

- Metaphyseal-diaphyseal junction fractures can be treated conservatively, but intramedullary fixation is indicated for most athletes.

- Acute fracture can be differentiated from stress fracture by history, though treatment is generally the same.

- Avulsion fractures can be managed symptomatically similar to lateral ankle sprains unless displaced or involving the cubo-metatarsal joint.

most 5th metatarsal bone injuries (Fig. 34.10). The Jones' fracture describes an acute oblique fracture of the proximal diaphysis, at or just distal to the metaphyseal-diaphyseal junction (within the first 1.5 cm distal to the styloid). Finally, stress fractures of the proximal 5th metatarsal can occur at the proximal diaphysis as well (Fig. 34.11). Eponyms seem to cause confusion in this case. Various publications will refer to both of these latter two fractures as 'Jones' while others differentiate the two

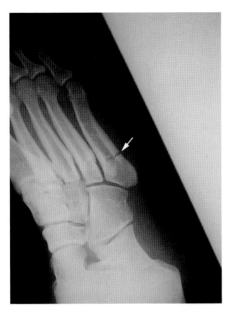

Figure 34.11   Acute Jones' fracture – metaphyseal–diaphyseal junction.

referring to only the acute fracture as a 'Jones'. The originally described fracture by Sir Robert Jones in 1902 was an acute fracture. The best way to communicate these fractures is to simply describe the radiographic findings. The Torg classification also provides some descriptive distinction. Torg Type I: No intramedullary sclerosis, fracture line with sharp margins and no widening, minimal/no cortical hypertrophy, minimal/no evidence of periosteal reaction. Type II: Fracture line involves both cortices and has periosteal reaction, widened fracture line with adjacent bone resorption, evidence of intramedullary sclerosis. Type III: Wide fracture line, periosteal new bone and radiolucency, obliteration of the medullary canal at the fracture site due to sclerosis.[57]

The avulsion fracture accompanies an ankle inversion injury during which the peroneus brevis contracts and avulses its insertion site. The Ottawa ankle rules include examination of the proximal 5th metatarsal for this reason. A lateral slip of the plantar fascia attaches to the proximal fifth and consequently is implicated to cause these avulsion fractures. Plain foot films: AP, lateral and oblique, will show the fracture, which does not displace significantly. These fractures respond well to conservative treatment, similar to that for a lateral ankle sprain. Immobilization, required only for pain control, may be discontinued with transfer to a stirrup brace for ankle support. Displaced fractures and those involving more than 30% of the cubo-metatarsal joint should be referred for surgical fixation.

The acute metaphyseal–diaphyseal fracture occurs due to an inferiorly directed force or a medial-lateral force as commonly occurs during cutting maneuvers. The lateral forefoot is fixed on the ground. When the athlete changes direction, a tensile load is applied to the lateral cortex of the proximal fifth metatarsal.[58] In this case, unlike the stress fracture, the patient reports no previous pain or tenderness to the area. Radiographs reveal a fracture line with no intramedullary sclerosis or callus formation indicating previous stress reaction (Torg type I).

Conservative treatment will suffice for most, but not for high-level athletes due to the prolonged nature of the recovery. Management starts with non-weight bearing immobilization for 6–8 weeks. After this, patients may begin weight bearing activity starting with a postoperative shoe and progressing as tolerated. Fracture union may take several additional weeks during which sport should be withheld until the union is secure by either bone or an asymptomatic fibrous union. Intramedullary screw fixation will hasten return to sport for high performance athletes. After surgery, patients are typically held non-weight bearing for 1 week followed by 2–3 weeks of weight bearing immobilization. Full return to sport can be reliably achieved by 6–10 weeks postoperatively.

A patient with pain that precedes the fracture recognition clinically differentiates a stress fracture of the proximal diaphysis from the acute fracture described above. These fractures are more commonly seen in soccer and basketball. Examination may show rear foot valgus which causes more weight to be born by the lateral column. On X-ray, medullary sclerosis and possibly callus formation will be seen. Treatment is similar to the acute fracture, however, healing is more prolonged and surgical fixation will commonly be the treatment of choice. Clapper *et al.* reported an acceptable healing rate of 72% radiographic union at average of 21 weeks following a regimen of 8 weeks non-weight bearing then weight bearing as tolerated in a cast.[59] Those who failed required surgical fixation. Bone grafting often aids healing in this chronic injury. Porter *et al.* recently reported excellent results with a 4.5 mm cannulated intramedullary screw for fixation.[60]

Metatarsalgia

Metatarsalgia refers to the pain that typically occurs near the head of the second metatarsal, but may be found at any of the metatarsal heads. Mechanical factors cause most of problems due to pressure inadequately distributed through the forefoot. Callus may form under areas of increased weight bearing, giving a clue to the pressure points of the foot. Several etiologies cause metatarsalgia. Morton's foot, with a longer second ray, and a hypermobile first ray cause increased weight through the second metatarsal head. The hypermobile first ray does not accept the normal transfer of pressure from the second metatarsal head as weight bearing courses along an arc from the lesser metatarsal heads. This forces the second metatarsal head to accept a higher burden of body weight. A fixed cavus foot, a tight Achilles' tendon and high-heeled shoes force the metatarsals to absorb more pressure. A prominent metatarsal condyle on the plantar foot additionally exposes the metatarsal head to more weight. Hammertoes also predispose to metatarsalgia as the dorsiflexed proximal phalanx will apply an inferiorly directed force to the metatarsal phalangeal joint. A tighter toe box will accentuate this complication. Synovitis of the joint, interdigital neuroma, a subluxing metatarsophalangeal joint and Freiberg's necrosis also cause pain in the metatarsal head/metatarsophalangeal joint region.

Patients will complain of pain worse with prolonged weight bearing or activities with forefoot loading. The pain begins insidiously gradually worsening with prolonged activity.

Patients will usually be able to find a point of maximal tenderness, but may describe the pain throughout the forefoot. Footwear plays an important role in all foot problems, particularly so in forefoot maladies, so inquiry into work shoe, training shoe(s) and training regimen are important.

On examination, observation of weight bearing foot structure and gait provides insight into biomechanical factors mentioned above. Calluses should also be noted for high pressure points. Palpation reveals tenderness on the plantar aspect of the metatarsal head and just distally. Axial loading does not cause as much pain, unless a joint synovitis confounds the test. This can be differentiated from a metatarsalgia because the joint disease causes pain with passive flexion and extension when the metatarsal is static and free of weight. Mobility of the first ray should be assessed with forced dorsal excursion of the distal first metatarsal. However, the accuracy of such manual testing of the first ray has been called into question when compared to reproducible machine tested mobility.[61] The MTP joint of the affected digit should be examined for subluxation with dorsal and plantar forces causing a clicking or popping sensation to both examiner and patient. The patient's shoes and inserts give clues to prominent weight bearing areas and support of the forefoot.

Imaging with plain radiographs will help exclude degenerative changes, Freiberg's necrosis of the second metatarsal head and fracture. There is little role for bone scan or MRI, unless stress fracture is indicated by history or examination. If questions about the dynamics of the foot continue, a force plate gait analysis will show the important weight bearing areas.

Adjusting footwear is key to management. Increased forefoot cushioning helps alleviate some of the problem. A stiff soled, rocker bottom shoe such as a hiking boot reduces the stress on the MTP joint. High-heeled shoes and tight toe boxes must be avoided. Metatarsal pads placed just proximal to the metatarsal heads of the lesser toes help distribute the weight proximally and reduce that born by the metatarsal heads. Cyclists should be aware that carbon fiber composite shoes produce higher forces across the plantar foot than plastic models and may contribute to metatarsalgia.[62] Horseshoe shaped padding offloads the affected area as well. Patients can create a metatarsal head cutout in the shoe inserts. These accommodations can be tried with off the shelf products and, if successful, can be incorporated into a custom orthotic. Additionally, a Morton's extension will improve first ray weight bearing in those with a hypermobile first ray. Calf stretches to increase dorsiflexion at the ankle allows a larger proportion of stance phase of gait to be spent with the heel absorbing some pressure. In some patients with prominent plantar condyles, conservative measures fail and they must consider surgery to better orient the metatarsal.

DERMATOLOGIC PROBLEMS

Corns

Corns are hyperkeratotic lesions with a central conical core. This central core of keratin distinguishes a corn from a callus. Two types of corn exist: hard corns known as heloma durum and soft corns called heloma molle. Soft corns appear between the toes and remain soft due to the moist environment. They are most commonly seen between the fourth and fifth toes due to the irritation between the 4th metatarsal head and the fifth toe. Hard corns occur most commonly on the dorsolateral fifth toe. With a hammertoe deformity, they will also be seen on the dorsal interphalangeal joint of the lesser toes. With a reducible hammertoe, a crest pad straightens the toes in weightbearing and is formed by a cotton roll placed under the interphalangeal joints of the affected toes.[63] Corn pads may reduce the direct pressure over the corn.

Calluses

Calluses are thickening of the skin in areas of pressure, friction or other irritation on the plantar foot. They may indicate prominent bones such as calluses over low riding metatarsal heads. A crescent shaped callus on the medial side of the second metatarsal head indicates inadequate weight acceptance and often a hypermobile first ray. The second metatarsal bears undue pressure. The callous is crescent shaped, apex directed toward the first ray, and usually distal to the MTP indicating terminal stance phase shear forces to the skin. Inappropriate footwear will also lead to callus formation.

Typical therapy utilizes padding around smaller calluses to relieve the pressure and pain. Doughnut shaped or 'U'-shaped padding can be cut from thin foam padding. Orthotics with cutouts for low riding metatarsal heads or Morton's extension for hypermobile first ray corrects mechanical shortcomings. Salicylic acid pads help to shrink a callus and debridement provides an immediate reduction in the callus size and pain.

Despite these treatments, the intractable plantar keratoses will persist. Prominent plantar condyles on the metatarsal head or abnormally plantar directed metatarsals predispose to this problem. Surgery may be required to elevate the distal metatarsal or remove the plantar condyles of the metatarsal heads.

Subungual hematoma

Subungual hematomas appear commonly in runners, especially on the great toe. Risk factors include a tight toebox and a short shoe or long toenail. They also occur with acute trauma.

When the hematoma causes acute pain, it requires decompression. Boring with a sterile needle, electrocautery or applying a super-heated paperclip can accomplish evacuation. Pressure relief brings near immediate pain relief. Subungual hematomas caused by a single acute event may be associated with an underlying distal phalanx fracture. Evacuation creates an open fracture environment that may require antibiotic treatment

Blisters

Friction blisters form because of sheering forces most often associated with new or poorly fitting shoes. Moisture also plays a role in this process as rubbing moist skin leads to more friction than dry. During military basic training, non-black ethnicity, use of smokeless tobacco, lack of military experience, and pes planus independently predisposed to blisters.[64]

Common places for blisters to appear include the metatarsal head area, the toes and the heel. Several preventive measures can be taken to aid athletes. Use of synthetic wicking socks reduces moisture around the foot. Knapik and colleagues found the antiperspirant aluminum chloride hexahydrate in ethyl alcohol effective for reducing blisters, but carried a high rate of skin irritation (57%).[65] Treatment of blisters depends on the size. Those <1 cm should be left intact, while larger ones should be drained under sterile conditions, leaving the overlying skin to act as a barrier to infection.[66] Protective dressings reduce continued friction, allow sport participation and assist wound healing.

Plantar warts

> ### Box 34.12: Key Points
>
> - Blisters <1 cm in diameter should be left intact, larger should be punctured leaving the skin to act as a barrier to infection.
> - Plantar warts can be differentiated from corns and calluses by the punctuate hemorrhages and disruption of skin lines seen with warts.
> - Several treatments are effective for warts, but immunotherapy has also been shown to improve warts at sites distinct from the application.

Unlike warts in other parts of the body, plantar verrucae grow inward due to the forces applied across the foot. These can cause considerable pain and may be mistaken for a corn or plantar callus. Warts can be distinguished from callouses by debriding the surface skin. Warts show a characteristic loss of normal skin lines and punctate hemorrhages (Fig. 34.12). Additionally, warts tend to be tender with squeezing while corns and callouses are tender with direct pressure. While approximately 30% of warts resolve with placebo treatments, several treatment options improve this rate.[67] Topical salicylic acid, debridement with cryotherapy and even application of duct tape are simple methods. Not all plantar warts need to be treated. Care should be taken to choose wart treatments least likely to disrupt the in-season athlete's sport participation. Immunotherapy with direct injection of candida extract may not only improve the injected wart, but has been shown to heal distant warts.[68] Warts treated with immunotherapy avoid the local tenderness caused by physical agents.

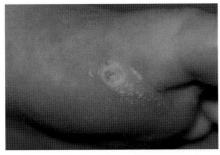

Figure 34.12 Plantar wart: central core, soft, white with pinpoint hemorrhages.

ORTHOTICS

> ### Box 34.13: Key Points
>
> - Clinical surveys suggest orthotics are helpful for managing some foot related injuries.
> - Evidence for injury prevention by orthotics is lacking.
> - Specific orthotic accommodations assist managing some injuries.

Sport use of orthotic devices, particularly by runners is a pervasive part of the culture. Rossi estimated orthotic use had grown to a US$4billion industry in 1997.[69] Orthotics are prescribed or manufactured by many different practitioners. Prescribing orthotic devices is one of the more controversial subjects in sports medicine. Areas of debate include clinical indications, benefit mechanisms, impression capture methods, orthotic materials, and relative costs. Despite these controversies, patient satisfaction surveys, acknowledging this methodology's inherent weaknesses, are quite favorable. Studies purport 33–96% partial resolution of their problem, pain relief or return to activity when treating knee pain, plantar fasciitis, shin splints, iliotibial band tendonitis and back pain.[70–75] Munderman states, 'The potential of foot orthotics for reducing pain and injuries is convincing'.[76] Contrary to patient satisfaction surveys and outcome studies favoring orthotic use, there is a substantive body of knowledge discouraging prophylactic orthotic use in an uninjured population.[77–79] Orthotic related studies encompass kinematic changes, materials, clinical outcomes, and a myriad of other variables. Methodological challenges including subject variables, testing procedures, and statistical uncertainties render it impossible to draw simplistic conclusions regarding orthotics.

For the last 30 years, rationalization for orthotics centered on balancing the foot toward some biomechanical ideal focused on the neutral subtalar position.[80] Research and clinical practice emphasized directing biomechanical movement patterns towards this ill-defined ideal. More recently, Nigg and others propose a paradigm shift to explain how orthotics and shoes might favorably influence injury reduction.[74,81–83] They suggest afferent feedback from cutaneous receptors critically determines muscle activation patterns. A positive influence by an orthotic, or the shoe, will alter the efferent muscle activation towards a favorable pattern to reduce fatigue and by inference lower injury rates. This hypothesis needs further support, but it may explain the varied clinical outcomes seen in past studies. It also proposes that the most important parameter for an orthotic is comfort. This is understandably frustrating for the clinician since predictably managing problems with orthotics is not a simple engineering task.

Injury and sport specific indications for orthotics and modifications

Turf toe and hallux rigidus Orthotic and shoe modification for turf toe is intended to reduce the need for dorsiflexion at the first MTP. A total contact orthotic (TCO) made of a firm carbon material reinforced medially can extrinsically limit the great toe dorsiflexion. This can also be effected by a steel shank, rocker sole or both placed between the layers of the shoe sole.[84] If indicated or if the athlete cannot tolerate these devices, a Morton's extension partially stiffens the medial forefoot.

Sesamoiditis A TCO incorporating a first ray cutout relieves pressure under the first MTP and allows the sesamoids to ride lower. Greater plantar pressures are directed to the second MTP. A rocker sole shoe modification may also reduce the stresses applied to the sesamoids.

Interdigital neuroma Non-operative management for an interdigital neuroma includes placing a metatarsal pad proximal to the involved web space and using a shoe with a wide toebox. These two accommodations and possibly a rocker sole may sufficiently alter the compressive and tensile forces to relieve symptoms on the neuroma.

Lesser metatarsal stress fracture The etiology of metatarsal stress fractures is multifactorial. The clinician may suspect higher stress fracture risk from a long or relatively plantarflexed metatarsal. MTP callouses, a highly mobile first or fifth ray, transverse arch reversal, or a particularly rigid pes cavus may heighten this concern. An MTP cutout can be incorporated into an orthotic to allow for a more plantarflexed position to the metatarsal head. Also, a Morton's extension can decrease weightbearing forces under the second MTP by supporting the first MTP.

Pes cavus The pes cavus foot is intrinsically rigid. Orthotic function should focus on materials that improve shock absorption. Metatarsal head and heel cushioning is used to reduce the inherently high loads focused at these locations. Excessive supination is sometimes caused by forefoot valgus deformity. A forefoot lateral wedge or valgus post may reduce this reason for heel supination.

Pes planus, posterior tibial tendonitis, plantar fasciitis As previously mentioned, orthotic prescription for prophylactic management of asymptomatic pes planus is quite controversial. Pes planus is associated with many different injuries, but certain causal relationship is lacking.[85] However, to the extent excessive pronation or pes planus is attributed to an injury such as posterior tibial tendonitis or plantar fasciitis, then orthotics designed to reduce pronation may assist the current problem and hopefully reduce the recurrence. Orthotics or full length insoles should include medial wedges applied to the rearfoot, arch, forefoot or all three. Additionally, shoes with a reinforced heel counter and denser medial mid-sole can reduce pronation.

REFERENCES

1 Bordelon RL. Foot first - evolution of man. Foot Ankle 1987; 8:125.

2 D'Maio M, Paine R, Mangine RE. Drez D. Plantar fasciitis sports. Med Rehabil Ser 1993; 16:137–142.

3 Riddle DL, Pulisic M, Pidcoe P, et al. Risk factors for plantar fasciitis: a matched case-control study. J Bone Jt Surg Am 2003; 85:872–877.

4 Garceau D De, Dean D, Requejo SM, Thordarson DB. The association between diagnosis of plantar fasciitis and Windlass test results. Foot Ankle Int 2003; 24:251–255.

5 Singh D, Angel J, Bentley G, Trevino SG. Plantar fasciitis. BMJ 1997; 315:172–175.

6 Glazer JL. Brukner P. Plantar fasciitis: Current concepts to expedite healing. Phys Sport Med 2004; 32 Online. Available: http://www.physsportsmed.com/issues/2004/1104/glazer.htm 2004

7 Buchbinder R. Plantar fasciitis. N Engl J Med 2004; 350:2159–2166.

8 Young CC, Rutherford DS, Niedfeldt MW. Treatment of plantar fasciitis. Am Fam Physician 2001; 63:467–478.

9 DiGiovanni BF, Nawoczenski DA, Lintal ME, et al. Tissue-specific plantar fascia-stretching exercise enhances outcomes in patients with chronic heel pain: a prospective randomized study. J Bone Jt Surg Am 2003; 85:1270–1277.

10 Crawford F, Thomson C. Interventions for treating plantar heel pain (Cochrane Review). The Cochrane Library (issue 4). Chichester, UK: John Wiley; 2004. Online. Available: http://www.update-software.com/abstracts/AB000416.htm 2004

11 Saxena A, Fullem B. Plantar fascia ruptures in athletes. Am J Sport Med 2004; 32:662–665.

12 Lau JT, Stavrou P. Posterior tibial nerve – primary. Foot Ankle Clin N Am 2004; 9:271–285.

13 Reade BM, Longo DC, Keller MC. Tarsal tunnel syndrome. Clin Podiatr Med Surg 2001; 18:395–408.

14 Erickson S, Quinn S, Kneeland J. MR imaging of the tarsal tunnel and related spaces: Normal and abnormal anatomical correlation. Am J Roentgenol 1990; 155:323–328.

15 Powell GD. Electrodiagnosis PG. an overview. Clin Podiatr Med Surg 1994; 11:571.

16 Gondring WH, Shields B, Wenger S. An outcome analysis of surgical treatment of tarsal tunnel syndrome. Foot Ankle Int 2003; 24:545–550.

17 Kim DH, Ryu S, Tiel RL, Kline DG. Surgical management and results of 135 tibial nerve lesions at the Louisiana State University Health Sciences Center. Neurosurgery 2003; 53:1114–1124.

18 Urguden M. Tarsal tunnel syndrome - the effect of associated features on outcome of surgery. Int Orthop 2002; 26:253–256.

19 Weber JM, Vidt LG, Gehl RS, Montgomery T. Calcaneal stress fractures. Clin Podiatr Med Surg 2005; 22:45–54.

20 Holmes GB, Mann RA. Possible epidemiological factors associated with rupture of the posterior tibial tendon. Foot Ankle 1992; 13:70–79.

21 Kohls-Gatzoulis J, Angel JC, Singh D, et al. Tibialis posterior dysfunction: a common and treatable cause of adult acquired flatfoot. BMJ 2004; 329:1328–1333.

22 Kirkpatrick DP, Hunter RE, Janes PC, et al. The snowboarder's foot and ankle. Am J Sports Med 1998; 26:271–277.

23 Chan GM, Yoshida D. Fracture of the lateral process of the talus associated with snowboarding. Ann Emerg Med 2003; 41:854–858.

24 Frey C, Feder KS, DiGiovanni C. Arthroscopic evaluation of the subtalar joint: does sinus tarsi syndrome exist? Foot Ankle Intl 1999; 20:185–191.

25 Mantas JP, Burks RT. Lisfranc injuries in the athlete. Clin Sports Med 1994; 13:719–730.

26 Peicha G, Labovitz J, Seibert FJ, et al. The anatomy of the joint as a risk factor for Lisfranc dislocation and fracture-dislocation. An anatomical and radiological case control study. J Bone Jt Surg Br 2002; 84:981–985.

27 Meyer SA, Callaghan JJ, Albright JP, Crowley ET, Powell JW. Midfoot sprains in collegiate football players. Am J Sports Med 1994; 22:392–401.

28 Khan F, Condon F, Khalid M, Dolan M. Sprinting on a running track: a rare cause of a Lisfranc dislocation. Ir Med J 2003; 96:307–308.

29 Chiodo CP, Myerson MS. Developments and advances in the diagnosis and treatment of injuries to the tarsometatarsal joint. Ortho Clin North Am 2001; 32:11–20.

30 Coss HS, Manos RE, Buoncristiani A, Mills WJ. Abduction stress and AP weightbearing radiography of purely ligamentous injury in the tarsometatarsal joint. Foot Ankle Int 1998; 19:537–541.

31 Curtis MJ, Meyerson M, Szura B. Tarsometatarsal joint injuries in the athlete. Am J Sports Med 1993; 21:497–502.

32 Nunley JA, Vertullo CJ. Classification, investigation and management of midfoot sprains. Lisfranc injuries in the athlete. Am J Sports Med 2002; 30:871–878.

33 Faciszewski T, Burks RT, Manaster BJ. Subtle injuries of the Lisfranc joint. J Bone Jt Surg AM 1990; 72:1519–1522.

34 Groshar D, Alperson M, Mendes DG, et al. Bone scintigraphy findings in Lisfranc joint injury. Foot Ankle Int 1995; 16:710–711.

35 Lu J, Ebraheim NA, Skie M, et al. Radiographic and computed tomographic evaluation of Lisfranc dislocation: A cadaver study. Foot Ankle Int 1997; 18:351–355.

36 Potter HG, Deland JT, Gusmer PB, et al. Magnetic resonance imaging of the Lisfranc ligament of the foot. Foot Ankle Int 1998; 19:438–446.

37 Philbin T, Rosenberg G, Sferra JJ. Complications of missed or untreated Lisfranc injuries. Foot Ankle Clin 2003; 8:61–71.

38 Mullen JE, O'Malley MJ. Sprains - residual instability of subtalar, Lisfranc joints, and turf toe. Clin Sports Med 2004; 23:97–121.

39 Brukner P, Bradshaw C, Khan KM. Stress fractures: A review of 180 cases. Clin J Sport Med 1996; 6:85–89.

40 Ostlie DK, Simons SM. Tarsal navicular stress fracture in a young athlete: case report with clinical, radiologic, and pathophysiologic correlations. J Am Board Fam Pr 2001; 14:381–385.

41 Khan KM, Fuller PJ, Brukner PD. Outcome of conservative and surgical management of navicular stress fracture in athletes. Am J Sport Med 1992; 20:657–666.

42 Saxena A. Results of treatment of 22 navicular stress fractures and a new proposed classification system. J Foot Ankle Surg 2000; 39:96–103.

43 Quirk R. President's guest lecture. Stress fractures of the navicular. Foot Ankle Int 1998; 19:494–496.

44 Watson TS, Anderson RB, Hodges Davis W. Periarticular injuries to the hallux metatarsophalangeal joint in athletes. Foot Ankle Clin 2000; 5:687–713.

45 Meyers MC, Barnhill BS. Incidence, causes, and severity of high school football injuries on field turf versus natural grass. A five year prospective study. Am J Sports Med 2004; 32:1626–1638.

46 Rodeo SA, Warren RF, O'Brien SJ. Diastasis of bipartite sesamoids of the first metatarsophalangeal joint. Foot Ankle 1993; 14:425–434.

47 Clanton TO, Ford JJ. Turf toe injury. Clin Sports Med 1994; 13:731–741.

48 Anderson RB. Turf toe injuries of the hallux metatarsophalangeal joint. Tech Foot Ankle Surg 2002; 1:102–111.

49 Hockenberry RT. Forefoot problems in athletes. Med Sci Sports Exerc 1999; 31:s448–s458.

50 McBryde AM, Anderson RB. Sesamoid foot problems in the athlete. Clin Sports Med 1988; 7:51–60.

51 Wilder RP, Sethi S. Overuse injuries: tendinopathies, stress fractures, compartment syndrome, and shin splints. Clin Sports Med 2004; 23:55–81.

52 Saxena A, Krisdakumtorn T. Return to activity after sesamoidectomy in athletically active individuals. Foot Ankle Int 2003; 24:415–419.

53 Giannini S, Bacchini P, Ceccarelli F, Vannini F. Interdigital neuroma: clinical examination and histopathologic results in 63 cases treated with excision. Foot Ankle Int 2004; 25:79–84.

54 Graham CE, Johnson KA, Ilstrup DM. The intermetatarsal nerve: a microscopic evaluation. Foot Ankle 1981; 2:150–152.

55 Kay D, Bennett GL. Morton's neuroma. Foot Ankle Clin N Am 2003; 8:49–59.

56 Bennell KL, Brukner PD. Epidemiology and site specificity of stress fractures. Clin Sports Med 1997; 16:179–196.

57 Strayer SM, Reece SG, Petrizzi MJ. Fractures of the proximal fifth metatarsal. Am Fam Physician 1999; 59:2516–2522.

58 Title CI, Katchis SD. Traumatic foot and ankle injuries in the athlete: acute athletic trauma. Orthop Clin N Am 2002; 33:587–598.

59 Clapper MF, O'Brien TJ, Lyons PM. Fractures of the fifth metatarsal: Analysis of a fracture registry. Clin Orthop 1995; 315:238–241.

60 Porter DA, Duncan M, Meyer SJF. Fifth metatarsal Jones fracture fixation with a 4.5 mm cannulated stainless steel screw in the competitive and recreational athlete. Am J Sports Med 2005; 33:1–8.

61 Glasoe WM. AllenMK, Saltzman CL, Ludewig PM, Sublett SH. Comparison of two methods used to assess first-ray hypermobility. Foot Ankle Int 2002; 23:248–252.

62 Jarboe NE, Quesada PM. The effects of cycling shoe stiffness on forefoot pressure. Foot Ankle Int 2003; 24:784–788.

63 Freeman DB. Corns and calluses resulting from mechanical hyperkeratosis. Am Fam Phys 2002; 11:2277–2280.

64 Knapik JJ, Reynolds K, Barson J. Risk factors for foot blisters during road marching: tobacco use, ethnicity, foot type, previous illness, and other factors. Mil Med 1999; 164:92–97.

65 Knapik JJ, Reynolds K, Barson J. Influence of an antiperspirant on foot blister incidence during cross-country hiking. J Am Acad Derm 1998; 39:202–206.

66 Freiman A, Barankin B, Elpern DJ. Sports dermatology part 1: common dermatosis. CMAJ 2004; 171:851–853.

67 Gibbs S, Harvey I, Sterling JC, Stark R. Local treatments for cutaneous warts (Cochrane Review). Cochrane Database Syst Rev 2001; 2:CD001781.

68 Johnson SM, Roberson PK, Horn TD. Intralesional injection of mumps or Candida skin test antigens: a novel immunotherapy for warts. Arch Derm 2001; 137:451–455.

69 Orthotics RWA. The miracle cure-all. Footwear News 1995; 8:22.

70 Moraros J, Hodge W. Orthotic survey. Preliminary results. J Am Podiatr Med Assoc 1993; 83:139–148.

71 Donatelli RA, Hurlbert C, Conway D. Biomechanical foot orthotics: a retrospective study. J Orthop Sports Phys Ther 1988; 10:205–212.

72 Gross ML, Davlin LB, Evanski PM. Effectiveness of orthotic shoe inserts in the long-distance runner. Am J Sports Med 1991; 19:409–412.

73 Nawoczenski DA, Cook TM, Saltzman CL. The effect of foot orthotics on three-dimensional kinematics of the leg and rearfoot during running. J Orthop Sports Phys Ther 1995; 21:317–327.

74 Nigg BM, Nurse MA, Stefanyshyn DJ. Shoe inserts and orthotics for sport and physical activities. Med Sci Sports Exerc 1999; 31:S421–S428.

75 Larsen K, Weidich F, Leboefu-Yde C. Can custom-made biomechanic shoe orthoses prevent problems in the back and lower extremities? A randomized, controlled intervention trial of 146 military conscripts. J Manipulative Physiol Ther 2002; 25:326–331.

76 Mundermann A, Nigg BM, Neil Humble R, Stefanyshyn DJ. Foot orthotics affect lower extremity kinematics and kinetics during running. Clin Biomech 2003; 18:254–262.

77 Michelson JD, Durant DM, McFarland E. The injury risk associated with pes planus in athletes. Foot Ankle Int 2002; 23:629–633.

78 Finestone A, Novack V, Farfel A, et al. A prospective study of the effect of foot orthoses composition and fabrication on comfort and the incidence of overuse injuries. Foot Ankle Int 2004; 25:462–466.

79 Ekenman I, Milgrom C, Finestone A, et al. The role of biomechanical shoe orthoses in tibial stress fracture prevention. Am J Sports Med 2002; 30:866–870.

80 Ball KA, Afheldt MJ. Evolution of foot orthotics – part 1: Coherent theory or coherent practice? 2002; 25:116–124.

81 Nawoczenski DA, Ludewig PM. Electromyographic effects of foot orthotics on selected lower extremity muscles during running. Arch Phys Med Rehabil 1999; 80:540–544.

82 Stacoff A, Reinschmidt C, Nigg BM. Effects of foot orthoses on skeletal motion during running. Clin Biomech 2000; 15:54–64.

83 Mundermann A, Stefanyshyn DJ, Nigg BM. Relationship between footwear comfort of shoe inserts and anthropometric and sensory factors. Med Sci Sports Exerc 2001; 33:1939–1945.

84 Nawoczenski DA, Janisse DJ. Foot orthosis in rehabilitation – what's new. Clin Sports Med 2004; 23:157–167.

85 Razeghi M, Batt ME. Biomechanical analysis of the effect of orthotic shoe inserts. Sports Med 2000; 29:425–438.

Index

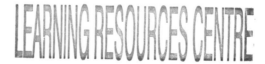